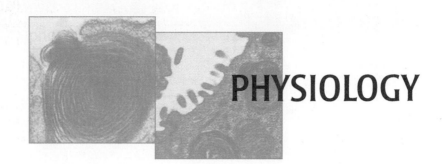

PHYSIOLOGY

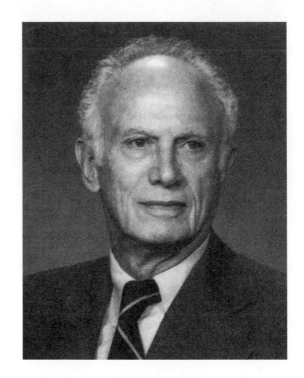

Dedication

This book is dedicated to Professor Robert M. Berne, who died October 4, 2001. Dr. Berne was a superb scientist, an acclaimed author, an excellent teacher, and a very amiable person. His devotion to the field of Physiology has inspired students and colleagues over the past half-century.

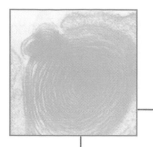

PHYSIOLOGY

Editors

ROBERT M. BERNE, MD, DSc (Hon)
PROFESSOR EMERITUS
Department of Molecular Physiology and Biological Physics
University of Virginia Health Sciences Center
Charlottesville, Virginia

MATTHEW N. LEVY, MD
PROFESSOR EMERITUS OF PHYSIOLOGY
AND BIOMEDICAL ENGINEERING
Case Western Reserve University
Cleveland, Ohio

BRUCE M. KOEPPEN, MD, PhD
PROFESSOR OF MEDICINE AND PHYSIOLOGY
Dean, Academic Affairs and Education
The Albert and Wilda Van Dusen Professor of Academic Medicine
University of Connecticut School of Medicine
Farmington, Connecticut

BRUCE A. STANTON, PhD
PROFESSOR
Department of Physiology
Dartmouth Medical School
Hanover, New Hampshire

FIFTH EDITION

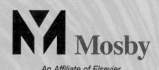
Mosby
An Affiliate of Elsevier

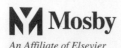

Mosby

An Affiliate of Elsevier

11830 Westline Industrial Drive
St. Louis, Missouri 63146

PHYSIOLOGY
ISBN 0-323-03390-3

NOTICE

Physiology is an ever-changing field. Standard safety precautions must be followed but as new research and clinical experience broaden our knowledge, changes in treatment and drug therapy may become necessary or appropriate. Readers are advised to check the most current product information provided by the manufacturer of each drug to be administered to verify the recommended dose, the method and duration of administration, and contraindications. It is the responsibility of the treating physician, relying on experience and knowlege of the patient, to determine dosages and the best treatment for each individual patient. Neither the Publisher nor the author assumes any liability for any injury and/or damage to persons or property arising from this publication.

The Publisher

Previous editions copyrighted 1983, 1988, 1993, 1998

Library of Congress Cataloging-in-Publication Data

Physiology/ [edited by] Robert M. Berne . . . [et al.]. — 5th ed.
    p. ; cm.
  Includes bibliographical references and index.
  ISBN 0-323-03390-3
  1. Human physiology. I. Berne, Robert M.,
  [DNLM: 1. Physiology. QT 4 P5783 2004]
  QP34.5.P496 2003
  612–dc21

2003051218

Publishing Director: William R. Schmitt
Acquisitions Editor: Jason O. Malley
Developmental Editor: Donna L. Morrissey

Printed in The United States of America

Last digit is the print number: 9 8 7 6 5 4 3 2 1

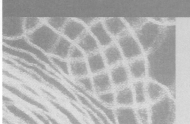

Contributors

ROBERT M. BERNE, MD, DSc (Hon)
PROFESSOR EMERITUS
Department of Molecular Physiology
  and Biological Physics
University of Virginia Health Science Center
Charlottesville, Virginia
Section IV, The Cardiovascular System

MICHELLE CLOUTIER, MD
PROFESSOR OF PEDIATRICS
University of Connecticut Health Center
Director, Asthma Center
Connecticut Children's Medical Center
Hartford, Connecticut
Section V, Respiratory System

SAUL M. GENUTH, MD
PROFESSOR OF MEDICINE
Case Western Reserve University School of Medicine
Cleveland, Ohio
Section VIII, The Endocrine System

BRUCE M. KOEPPEN, MD, PhD
PROFESSOR OF MEDICINE AND PHYSIOLOGY
Dean, Academic Affairs and Education
The Albert and Wilda Van Dusen Professor of Academic
  Medicine
University of Connecticut Health Center
Farmington, Connecticut
Section VII, The Kidney

HOWARD C. KUTCHAI, PhD
PROFESSOR, DEPARTMENT OF MOLECULAR
PHYSIOLOGY AND BIOLOGICAL PHYSICS
University of Virginia Health Sciences Center
Charlottesville, Virginia
Section I, Cellular Physiology
Section VI, The Gastrointestinal System

MATTHEW N. LEVY, MD
PROFESSOR EMERITUS OF PHYSIOLOGY
AND BIOPHYSICS AND OF BIOMEDICAL
ENGINEERING
Case Western Reserve University
Cleveland, Ohio
Section IV, The Cardiovascular System

BRUCE A. STANTON, PhD
PROFESSOR OF PHYSIOLOGY
Dartmouth Medical School
Hanover, New Hampshire
Section VII, The Kidney

ROGER S. THRALL, PhD
PROFESSOR OF MEDICINE
Director of Pulmonary Research
University of Connecticut Health Center
Farmington, Connecticut
and
Director of Clinical Research
Hospital for Special Care
New Britain, Connecticut
Section V, Respiratory System

JAMES M. WATRAS, PhD
ASSOCIATE PROFESSOR
Department of Pharmacology
University of Connecticut Health Center
Farmington, Connecticut
Section III, Muscle

WILLIAM D. WILLIS, Jr., MD, PhD
PROFESSOR AND CHAIRMAN
Department of Anatomy and Neurosciences and Director
  of Marine Biomedical Institute
The University of Texas Medical Branch
Galveston, Texas
Section II, The Nervous System

Preface

As in the previous editions of this textbook, we have attempted to emphasize broad concepts and to minimize the compilation of isolated facts. Each chapter in this edition has been altered to make the text as lucid, accurate, and current as possible. In an effort to improve comprehension, we have revised many of the illustrations, and have added many new figures. Finally, in order to emphasize broad principles, we have highlighted many of the important physiological mechanisms and critical interactions among the various organ systems.

Physiology is concerned with the function of organisms at many stages of organization, from the subcellular level to the intact organism. In the healthy human, many variables are maintained within narrow limits. The list of controlled variables includes body temperature, blood pressure, the ionic composition of the body's various fluid compartments, the blood glucose levels, and the oxygen and carbon dioxide contents of the blood. This ability to maintain the relative constancy of such critical variables, even in the face of substantial environmental changes, is known as **homeostasis.** One of the central goals of physiological research is the elucidation of homeostatic mechanisms.

In section I, **(Cellular Physiology),** of this book, and at the beginnings of several other sections, various important physiological principles are analyzed in detail. We have included considerable information about major advances in cellular and molecular biology. Such data includes the roles of membrane transport proteins and of the structure and function of ion-transporting ATPases. In order to emphasize the clinical relevance of certain advances, we have cited specific diseases in which the applicable physiological mechanism plays an important role. Scattered throughout each chapter, these clinical examples have been highlighted by enclosing them in shaded boxes.

When important principles can be represented profitably by equations, we have cited the underlying assumptions that serve as the bases of those equations. This approach provides students with a more quantitative understanding of these principles. Furthermore, because some of the readers might not favor a rigorous analytical approach, we have sequestered the more extensive mathematical analyses in shaded boxes.

Section II, **(The Nervous System),** provides a neuroanatomical framework for its presentation of contemporary cellular neurophysiology. Substantial attention has been directed toward the sensory and motor systems, because of their clinical relevance. Analysis of the fundamental principles common to the various sensory systems facilitates the comprehension of the various components of that system.

In section III, **(Muscle),** we have described the basic mechanisms of contraction in skeletal, smooth, and cardiac muscles. The characteristics of skeletal and smooth muscle are presented in detail in this section, but the description of cardiac muscle performance is divided between Sections III and IV.

In section IV, **(The Cardiovascular System),** we have dissected the system initially into its major components. One such component, namely blood composition and function, has been condensed and included as an introductory chapter in the cardiovascular section. In the subsequent chapters related to the heart and vasculature, we have first examined the functions of the individual cardiovascular components. Subsequently, we have analyzed how the various parts of the closed loop circulatory system interact under various physiological and pathological conditions.

Section V, **(The Respiratory Section)** emphasizes the physical principles that underlie the mechanics of breathing and the exchange of gas between the blood and the alveoli, and between the blood and the peripheral tissues. Furthermore, the neural and chemical processes that regulate respiration, the role of the lungs in immune defense, and certain non-respiratory functions of the lungs have been described in detail.

Section VI, **(The Gastrointestinal System),** presents first the processes of motility and secretion in the gastrointestinal tract, and then explains how these functions are integrated by neural, endocrine, and paracrine mechanisms. Furthermore, the role of ion transporters in the absorption and secretion of electrolytes in the gastrointestinal tract have been described. Subsequently, certain critical mechanisms are shown to account for the pathogenesis of various gastrointestinal disturbances.

In Section VII, **(The Kidneys),** the mechanisms by which the kidneys handle water and certain important solutes have been described in detail. The regulation of body fluid osmolality and volume, and of acid-base balance, has also been explained.

In Section VIII, **(The Endocrine System),** similarities in the functioning of the various endocrine glands are emphasized. Major new insights into the mechanisms of hormone action, the regulation of energy storage and turnover, and the processes of reproduction are presented. Discussions of the male and female gonads have been included in a common chapter to highlight the similarities between the Sertoli cell functions in spermatogenesis and the granulosa cell functions in oogenesis.

The authors of each section have presented what they believe to be the most likely mechanisms responsible for the phenomena under consideration. We have adopted this compromise to achieve brevity, clarity, and simplicity. We have not cited the specific sources for each of the assertions that appear throughout the book, but we have listed references at the end of each chapter. These references provide a current and comprehensive review of the topic.

We wish to express our appreciation to all of our colleagues and students who have provided constructive criticism during the revision of this book.

The Editors

Contents

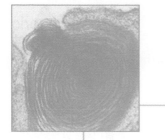

Cellular Physiology

Howard C. Kutchai

chapter one

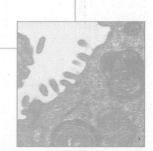

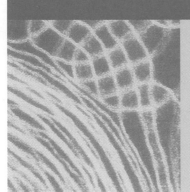

Cellular Membranes and Transmembrane Transport of Solutes and Water

CELLULAR MEMBRANES

Membranes are important components of all cells. Every cell is surrounded by a plasma membrane that separates it from the extracellular environment. The plasma membrane serves as a permeability barrier that allows the cell to maintain an interior composition far different from the composition of the extracellular fluid. The plasma membrane also contains enzymes, receptors, and antigens that play important roles in the cell's interaction with the extracellular matrix, with other cells, and with hormones and other regulatory agents in the extracellular fluid.

Membranes also enclose the various organelles of eukaryotic cells. These membranes divide the cell into discrete compartments within which particular biochemical processes take place. Many vital cellular processes actually take place in or on the membranes of the organelles. Examples of membrane-localized processes include electron transport and oxidative phosphorylation, which occur on, within, and across the mitochondrial inner membrane.

Most biological membranes have certain features in common. However, in keeping with the diversity of membrane functions, the composition and structure of the membranes differ from one cell to another and among the membranes of a single cell.

MEMBRANE STRUCTURE

The most abundant constituents of cellular membranes are proteins and phospholipids. A **phospholipid** molecule consists of a polar head group and two nonpolar, hydrophobic fatty acyl chains (Fig. 1-1, *A*). In an aqueous environment, phospholipids tend to orient with their hydrophobic fatty acyl chains away from contact with water. This orientation can be seen in the **lipid bilayer** (Fig. 1-1, *B*). Many phospholipids, when dispersed in water, spontaneously form lipid bilayers. Most of the phospholipid molecules in biological membranes have a lipid bilayer structure.

The **fluid mosaic model** of membrane structure shown in Fig. 1-2 is consistent with many of the properties of biolog-ical membranes. Note the bilayer structure of most of the membrane phospholipids. Note also that proteins are abundant in the membrane. These membrane proteins are of two major classes: (1) **integral** or **intrinsic membrane proteins** that are embedded in the phospholipid bilayer and (2) **peripheral** or **extrinsic membrane proteins** that are associated with the surface of the membrane. In general, the peripheral membrane proteins associate with the membrane by means of charge interactions with integral membrane proteins. When the ionic composition of the medium is altered, peripheral proteins are often removed from the membrane. Integral membrane proteins are embedded in the membrane by means of hydrophobic interactions with the interior of the membrane. These hydrophobic interactions can be disrupted by detergents, which make the integral proteins soluble by interacting hydrophobically with nonpolar amino acid side chains.

As the term *fluid mosaic model* suggests, cellular membranes are fluid structures. Many of the constituent molecules of cellular membranes are free to diffuse in the plane of the membrane. Most lipids and proteins move freely in the bilayer plane, but they "flip-flop" from one phospholipid monolayer to the other at much slower rates. A large, hydrophilic membrane component is unlikely to flip-flop if it must be dragged through the nonpolar interior of the lipid bilayer.

Sometimes, membrane components are not free to diffuse in the plane of the membrane. For example, acetylcholine receptors (integral membrane proteins) are sequestered at the motor end plate of skeletal muscle. Other proteins and certain lipids may be enriched in regions or domains in the membrane. Different membrane proteins are confined to the apical and basolateral plasma membranes of epithelial cells. In some cells, the cytoskeleton appears to tether certain membrane proteins. For example, the **anion exchanger,** a major protein of the human erythrocyte membrane, is bound to the spectrin network that undergirds the membrane via a protein called **ankyrin.**

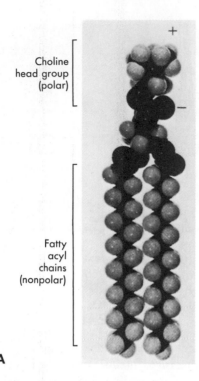

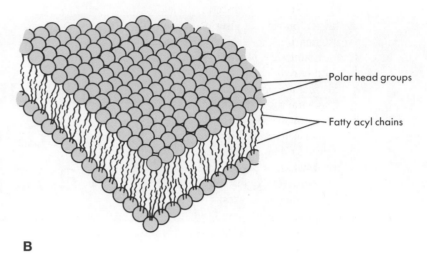

B

■ **Fig. 1-1** **A,** Structure of a membrane phospholipid molecule, in this case a phosphatidylcholine. **B,** Structure of a phospholipid bilayer. The circles represent the polar head groups of the phospholipid molecules. The wavy lines represent the fatty acyl chains of the phospholipids.

If the motor nerve that innervates a skeletal muscle is accidentally severed, the acetylcholine receptors are no longer sequestered at the motor end plate. Instead, they spread out over the entire plasma membrane of the muscle cells. The entire surface of the cell then becomes excitable by acetylcholine, a phenomenon known as **denervation supersensitivity.**

MEMBRANE COMPOSITION

Lipid Composition

Major phospholipids. In animal cell membranes, the *phospholipid bilayer is primarily responsible for the passive permeability properties of the membrane.* The most abundant phospholipids in these membranes are often the choline-containing phospholipids: the **lecithins** (phosphatidylcholines)

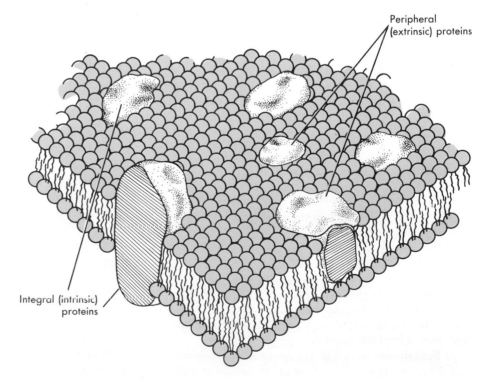

■ **Fig. 1-2** Schematic representation of the fluid mosaic model of membrane structure. The integral proteins are embedded in the lipid bilayer matrix of the membrane, and the peripheral proteins are associated with the external surfaces of integral membrane proteins.

and the **sphingomyelins.** Next in abundance are frequently the **amino phospholipids:** phosphatidylserine and phosphatidylethanolamine. Other important phospholipids that are present in smaller amounts are **phosphatidylglycerol, phosphatidylinositol,** and **cardiolipin.**

Certain phospholipids that are present in tiny amounts in the plasma membrane play vital roles in cellular signal transduction processes. **Phosphatidylinositol bisphosphate,** when cleaved by a receptor-activated phospholipase C, releases **inositol trisphosphate (IP$_3$)** and **diacylglycerol.** IP3 is released into the cytosol, where it acts on receptors in the endoplasmic reticulum to cause release of stored Ca^{2+}, which affects a wide variety of cellular processes. Diacylglycerol remains in the plasma membrane, where it participates, along with Ca^{2+}, in activating **protein kinase C,** an important signal transduction protein.

Cholesterol. Cholesterol is a major component of plasma membranes. Its steroid nucleus lies parallel to the fatty acyl chains of membrane phospholipids. Cholesterol functions as a "fluidity buffer" in the plasma membrane. It tends to keep the fluidity of the acyl chain region of the phospholipid bilayer in an intermediate range in the presence of agents, such as alcohols and general anesthetics, that would otherwise make the biological membranes more fluid.

Glycolipids. Although **glycolipids** are not abundant in plasma membranes, they have important functions. Glycolipids are found mostly in plasma membranes, where their carbohydrate moieties protrude from the external surface of the membrane. The carbohydrate parts of glycolipids frequently function as receptors or antigens.

The receptor for **cholera toxin** is the carbohydrate moiety of a particular glycolipid, ganglioside (G_{M1}). The A and B blood group antigens (Chapter 14) are the carbohydrate moieties of other gangliosides on the human erythrocyte membrane.

Membrane Proteins

The protein composition of membranes may be simple or complex. The functionally specialized membranes of the sarcoplasmic reticulum of skeletal muscle and the disks of the rod outer segment of the retina contain only a few different proteins. In contrast, plasma membranes, which perform many functions, may have more than 100 different protein constituents. Membrane proteins include enzymes, transport proteins, and receptors for hormones and neurotransmitters.

Glycoproteins. Some membrane proteins are glycoproteins with covalently bound carbohydrate side chains. As with glycolipids, the carbohydrate chains of glycoproteins are located on the external surfaces of plasma membranes. The carbohydrate moieties of membrane glycoproteins and glycolipids have important functions. The negative surface charge of cells is caused by the negatively charged sialic acid of glycolipids and glycoproteins.

Fibronectin is a large fibrous glycoprotein that helps cells attach, via cell surface glycoproteins called **integrins,** to proteins of the extracellular matrix. This linkage allows communication to take place between the extracellular matrix and the cell's cytoskeleton.

The major membrane proteins of enveloped viruses are glycoproteins. Their carbohydrate moieties appear as "spikes" that stud the outer surface of the virus. These "spikes" are necessary for the binding of the virus to a host cell.

Asymmetry of membrane proteins. The Na^+,K^+-ATPase (also called the Na^+,K^+-pump) of the plasma membrane and the Ca^{2+}-ATPase (also called the Ca^{2+}-pump) of the sarcoplasmic reticulum membrane are examples of the asymmetric distribution of membrane proteins. In both of these pumps, the cleavage of ATP occurs on the cytoplasmic face of the membrane, and some of the energy liberated is used to pump ions in specific directions across the membrane. The Na^+,K^+-ATPase pumps K^+ into the cell and Na^+ out of the cell, whereas the Ca^{2+}-ATPase actively pumps Ca^{2+} into the sarcoplasmic reticulum. In the ion-transporting ATPases, the domains that bind and hydrolyze ATP face the cytosolic side of the membrane exclusively.

MEMBRANES AS PERMEABILITY BARRIERS

Biological membranes serve as *permeability barriers.* Most of the molecules present in living systems are highly soluble in water and poorly soluble in nonpolar solvents. Such molecules are also poorly soluble in the nonpolar environment that exists within the interior of the lipid bilayer of biological membranes. As a consequence, biological membranes pose a formidable barrier to most water-soluble molecules. This barrier allows the maintenance of large differences in concentration of many substances between the cytoplasm and the extracellular fluid. However, the plasma membrane is also permeable to some substances. Thus, although it keeps out many substances, it also allows the selective passage of other substances.

The localization of various cellular processes in certain organelles depends on the barrier properties of cellular membranes. For example, the inner mitochondrial membrane is impermeable to the enzymes and substrates of the tricarboxylic acid cycle, and thus it allows the localization of this cycle in the mitochondrial matrix. Much as the walls of a house separate rooms with different functions, barriers imposed by cellular membranes organize the chemical and physical processes within the cell.

The permeability function of membranes, which allows the passage of important molecules across membranes at controlled rates, is central to the life of the cell. Examples include the uptake of nutrient molecules, the discharge of waste products, and the release of secreted molecules. As discussed in the next section, molecules may move from one side of a membrane to another without actually moving through the membrane itself. In other cases, molecules cross a particular membrane by passing through or between the molecules that make up the membrane.

TRANSPORT ACROSS, BUT NOT THROUGH, MEMBRANES

Endocytosis

Endocytosis is the process that allows material to enter the cell without passing through the plasma membrane (Fig. 1-3); it includes phagocytosis and pinocytosis. The uptake of particulate material is termed **phagocytosis** ("cell eating") (Fig. 1-3, *A*). The uptake of soluble molecules is called **pinocytosis** ("cell drinking") (Fig. 1-3, *B*).

Sometimes, special regions of the plasma membrane are involved in endocytosis. In these regions, the cytoplasmic surface of the plasma membrane is covered with bristles made primarily of a protein called **clathrin.** These clathrin-covered regions are called **coated pits,** and their endocytosis gives rise to **coated vesicles** (Fig. 1-3, *C*). The coated pits are involved in **receptor-mediated endocytosis.** In this process, specific membrane receptor proteins in the coated pits recognize and bind to the protein to be taken up. This binding often leads to aggregation of receptor-ligand complexes, and the aggregation triggers endocytosis. *Endocytosis is an active process that requires metabolic energy.* It can also occur in regions of the plasma membrane that do not contain coated pits.

Most cells cannot synthesize cholesterol, which is needed for synthesis of new membranes. Cholesterol is carried in the blood predominantly in low-density lipoproteins (LDLs). Many cells have LDL receptors in their plasma membranes. When LDL binds to these receptors, the receptor-LDL complexes migrate to coated pits, where they aggregate and are taken into the cell by receptor-mediated endocytosis. Individuals who lack LDL receptors or have defective LDL receptors have high levels of cholesterol-laden LDL in their blood. Consequently, such individuals tend to develop arterial disease (**atherosclerosis**) at an early age, which increases the risk of early heart attacks.

Exocytosis

Molecules can be ejected from cells by **exocytosis,** a process that resembles endocytosis in reverse. The release of neurotransmitters from the presynaptic nerve endings (discussed in more detail in Chapter 4) takes place by exocytosis. Exocytosis is responsible for the release of secretory proteins by many cells. A well-studied example is the release of pancreatic enzymes from the acinar cells of the pancreas. These proteins are stored in secretory vesicles in the cytoplasm of pancreatic cells. A stimulus to secrete causes the secretory vesicles to fuse with the plasma membrane and to release the vesicle contents by exocytosis.

Fusion of Membrane Vesicles

The contents of one type of organelle can be transferred to another organelle by fusion of the membranes of the organelles. In some cells, secretory products are transferred from the endoplasmic reticulum to the Golgi apparatus by fusion of vesicles. In this process, endoplasmic reticulum vesicles fuse with membranous sacs of the Golgi apparatus. Fusion of phagocytic vesicles with lysosomes allows the phagocytosed material to be digested by proteolytic enzymes in the lysosomes. The turnover of many normal cellular constituents involves their destruction in lysosomes, followed by their resynthesis. The release of secreted proteins and neurotransmitters by exocytosis requires the fusion of vesicles containing the molecules to be released with the plasma membrane of the cell.

Membrane fusion is a highly regulated process. Frequently the interaction of specific proteins in the vesicle membrane (v-SNARES) with specific proteins in the "target" membrane (t-SNARES) must precede fusion. The interaction of the SNARE proteins and the subsequent membrane fusion events are typically regulated by several different cellular proteins, including small GTPases of the Rab class.

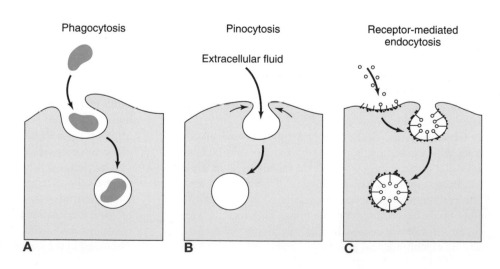

■ Fig. 1-3 Schematic depiction of endocytotic processes.
A, Phagocytosis of a solid particle.
B, Pinocytosis of extracellular fluid.
C, Receptor-mediated endocytosis by coated pits. (Redrawn from Silverstein SC et al: *Annu Rev Biochem* 46:669, 1977.)

Phagocytosis

Pinocytosis

Receptor-mediated endocytosis

Extracellular fluid

A   **B**   **C**

Influenza viruses have membrane proteins that undergo a dramatic conformational change that allows the insertion of a "fusion peptide" into the host cell plasma membrane. The fusion peptide promotes the fusion of the viral membrane with the plasma membrane of the host cell, allowing entry of the viral genome into the host cell.

TRANSPORT OF MOLECULES THROUGH MEMBRANES

The traffic of molecules through biological membranes is vital for many cellular processes. Some molecules move through biological membranes simply by diffusing among the molecules that make up the membrane. Other molecules move through membranes via specific transport proteins in the membrane.

Oxygen, for example, is a small molecule that is fairly soluble in nonpolar solvents. It crosses biological membranes by diffusing among membrane lipid molecules. Glucose, on the other hand, is a much larger molecule that is not very soluble in the membrane lipids. It enters cells via specific glucose transport proteins in the plasma membrane.

Diffusion

Diffusion occurs because of the random thermal motion, also called Brownian motion, of atoms or molecules. Diffusion eventually results in the uniform distribution of the atoms or molecules. Imagine a container divided into two compartments by a removable partition (Fig. 1-4). A much larger number of molecules of a compound is placed on side A than on side B, and then the partition is removed. Every molecule is in random thermal motion. The probability that a molecule that is located initially on side A will move to side B in a given time is equal to the probability that a molecule initially located on side B will end up on side A. Because many more molecules are present on side A, the total number of molecules moving from side A to side B will be greater than the number moving from side B to side A. Consequently, the number of molecules on side A will decrease, whereas the number of molecules on side B will increase. This process of net diffusion of molecules will continue until the concentration of molecules on side A equals that on side B. Thereafter the rate of diffusion of molecules from A to B will equal that from B to A, and no further net movement will occur; a dynamic equilibrium exists.

Range of diffusion. Diffusion is rapid when the distance over which it takes place is small. A rule of thumb is that a typical molecule takes 1 msec to diffuse 1 μm. However, the time required for diffusion increases with the square of the distance over which diffusion occurs. *Thus a 10-fold increase in the diffusion distance means that it will take 100 times longer for diffusion to reach a given degree of completion.*

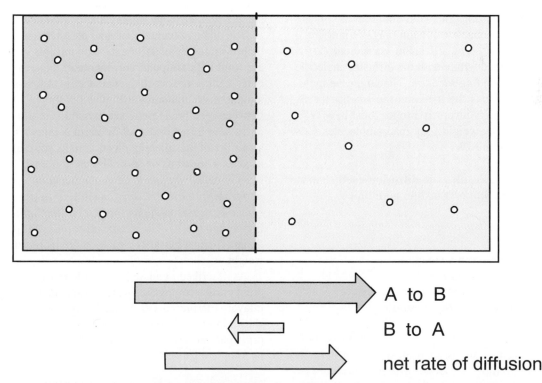

A to B

B to A

net rate of diffusion

■ Fig. 1-4   Chambers *A* and *B* are separated by a partition with holes in it. The concentration of molecules in chamber *A* is much greater than that in chamber *B*. For this reason the rate of diffusion of molecules from *A* to *B* is much greater than that from *B* to *A*. There is thus a net flux of molecules from *A* to *B*.

■ Table 1-1   The time required for diffusion to occur over various diffusion distances*

Diffusion distance (μm)	Time required for diffusion
1	0.5 msec
10	50 msec
100	5 sec
1000 (1 mm)	8.3 min
10,000 (1 cm)	14 hr

*The time required for the "average" molecule (with diffusion coefficient taken to be 1×10^{-5} cm²/sec) to diffuse the required distance was computed from the Einstein relation: $t = (\Delta X)2/2D$, where t is time and ΔX is the average diffusion distance.

Table 1-1 shows the results of calculations for a typical, small, water-soluble solute. Diffusion is extremely rapid on a microscopic scale of distance. For macroscopic distances, however, diffusion is rather slow. A cell that is 100 μm away from the nearest capillary can receive nutrients from the blood by diffusion in about 5 seconds or so. This process is sufficiently fast to satisfy the metabolic demands of many cells. However, a skeletal muscle cell that is 1 cm long cannot rely on diffusion for the intracellular transport of vital metabolites. It would take 14 hours for the diffusion of these metabolites to be completed, and this time is too great for efficient cellular metabolism. Some nerve fibers are longer than 1 m. Intracellular axonal transport systems are involved in transporting important molecules along nerve fibers. Because of the slowness of diffusion over macroscopic distances, even small multicellular organisms have evolved circulatory systems to bring the individual cells of the organisms within a reasonable diffusion range of nutrients.

Diffusion coefficient. The **diffusion coefficient** (D) is proportional to the speed with which the diffusing molecule can move in the surrounding medium. The larger the molecule and the more viscous the medium, the smaller the D. For small molecules, D is inversely proportional to $MW^{1/2}$. (MW refers to molecular weight.) For macromolecules, D is inversely proportional to $MW^{1/3}$.

For large spherical molecules the diffusion coefficient is approximated by the Stokes-Einstein equation

$$D = kT/6\pi r\eta$$

where

k = Boltzmann's constant
T = absolute temperature
r = radius of the macromolecule
η = viscosity of the medium

The numerator, kT, is directly proportional to the kinetic energy of the average diffusing molecule. The denominator is proportional to the viscous drag encountered by the molecule as it diffuses. The inverse proportionality of D to the radius of the molecule implies that D is inversely proportional to the cube root of the molecular weight. Thus, if protein A's molecular weight is 100,000

and protein B's molecular weight is 800,000, protein A will diffuse only twice as rapidly as protein B.

Diffusion across a membrane. Diffusion leads to a state in which the concentration of the diffusing species is constant in space and time. Diffusion across cellular membranes tends to equalize the concentrations on the two sides of the membrane (see Fig. 1-4). The diffusion rate across a membrane is proportional to the area of the membrane and to the difference in concentration of the diffusing substance on the two sides of the membrane. **Fick's first law of diffusion** states that

$$J = -DA \frac{\Delta C}{\Delta C} \tag{1-1}$$

where

J   = net rate of diffusion in moles or grams per unit time
D   = diffusion coefficient of the diffusing solute in the membrane
A   = area of the membrane
ΔC = concentration difference across the membrane
Δx = thickness of the membrane

Diffusive permeability of cellular membranes

Permeability to lipid-soluble molecules. The plasma membrane serves as a diffusion barrier that enables the cell to maintain cytoplasmic concentrations of many substances that differ greatly from their extracellular concentrations. As early as the turn of the twentieth century, the relative impermeability of the plasma membrane to most water-soluble substances was attributed to its "lipoid nature."

The lipoid character of the plasma membrane can be demonstrated by experiments showing that compounds that are soluble in nonpolar solvents (e.g., benzene or olive oil) enter cells more readily than water-soluble substances of similar molecular weight. Figure 1-5 shows the relationship between membrane permeability and solubility in a nonpolar solvent for a number of different solutes. The ratio of the solubility of the solute in olive oil to its solubility in water is used as a measure of solubility in nonpolar solvents. This ratio is called the *olive oil/water partition coefficient. The permeability of the plasma membrane to a particular substance increases with the "lipid solubility" of the substance.* For compounds with the same olive oil/water partition coefficient, permeability decreases with increasing molecular weight.

As described previously, the fluid mosaic model of membrane structure envisions the plasma membrane as a lipid bilayer with proteins embedded in it (see Fig. 1-2). The data shown in Fig. 1-5 support the idea that the lipid bilayer is the principal barrier to substances that permeate the membrane by simple diffusion.

Fat-soluble vitamins are absorbed by the epithelial cells of the small intestine by simply diffusing across their luminal plasma membranes. Water-soluble vitamins, by contrast, do not readily diffuse across biological mem-

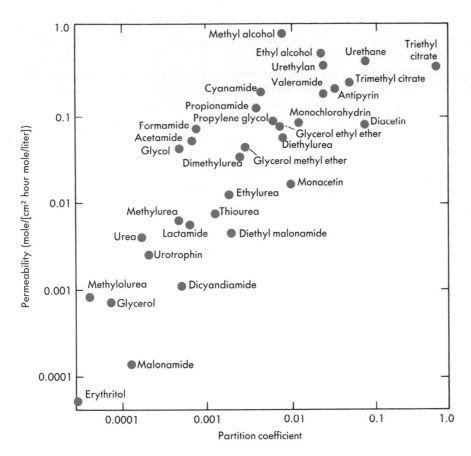

■ **Fig. 1-5** Illustration of the permeability of the plasma membrane of the alga *Chara ceratophylla* to various nonelectrolytes as a function of the lipid solubility of the solutes. Lipid solubility is represented on the abscissa by the olive oil/water partition coefficient. (Redrawn from Christensen HN: *Biological transport*, ed 2, Menlo Park, CA, 1975, WA Benjamin; data from Collander R: *Trans Faraday Soc* 33:985, 1937.)

branes, and thus special membrane transport proteins are required for absorption of water-soluble vitamins (see Chapter 33).

Permeability to water-soluble molecules. Very small, uncharged, water-soluble molecules pass through cell membranes much more rapidly than is predicted by their lipid solubility. For example, water permeates cell membranes about 100 times more rapidly than is predicted from its molecular radius and its olive oil/water partition coefficient. There are two reasons for the unusually high permeability to water. First, certain very small water-soluble molecules can pass between adjacent phospholipid molecules without actually dissolving in the region occupied by the fatty acid side chains. Second, the plasma membranes of most cells contain membrane proteins called **aquaporins** that form channels that permit a high rate of water flow. At least four isoforms of aquaporin are present in the kidney (Fig. 1-6). Mutations in aquaporins may result in defects in the ability of the kidney to produce urine that is more concentrated and more dilute than body fluids (Chapters 36 and 43).

The permeability of membranes to uncharged, water-soluble molecules decreases as the size of the molecules increases. Most plasma membranes are essentially impermeable to water-soluble molecules whose molecular weights are greater than about 200.

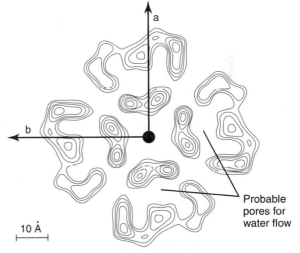

■ **Fig. 1-6** Structure of a water channel protein. Electron crystallography was used to determine the structure of aquaporin-1, a water channel protein in erythrocyte membranes and in cells of the renal proximal tubules. Section through the three-dimensional electron density map of aquaporin-1 is viewed perpendicular to the plane of the membrane. Aquaporin-1 exists in the membrane as a tetramer. Each monomer can conduct water through the membrane. (Redrawn from Cheng A et al: *Nature* 387:627, 1997.)

Because of their charge, ions are relatively insoluble in lipid solvents, and thus membranes are not very permeable to most ions. Ionic diffusion across membranes occurs mainly through protein **ion channels** that span the membrane. Some ion channels allow only specific ions to pass, whereas others allow all ions below a certain size to pass. *Some ion channels are controlled by the voltage difference across the membrane; others are controlled by neurotransmitters or other regulatory molecules* (see Chapters 3 and 4).

Although some water-soluble molecules, such as sugars and amino acids, are essential for cellular survival, they do not cross plasma membranes appreciably by simple diffusion. Plasma membranes have specific proteins that allow the transfer of vital metabolites into or out of the cell. The characteristics of membrane **protein-mediated transport** across membranes are discussed later.

Osmosis

Osmosis is defined as the flow of water across a **semipermeable** membrane from a compartment in which the solute concentration is lower to a compartment in which the solute concentration is greater. A semipermeable membrane is defined as a membrane permeable to water but impermeable to solutes. *Osmosis takes place because the presence of solute decreases the chemical potential of water.* Water tends to flow from where its chemical potential is higher to where its chemical potential is lower.

Decreasing the chemical potential of water in a solution (because of the presence of solute) also reduces vapor pressure, lowers the freezing point, and increases the boiling point of the solution as compared with pure water. Because these properties, as well as osmotic pressure, depend primarily on the concentration of the solute present rather than on its chemical nature, they are called **colligative properties.**

Osmotic pressure. In Fig. 1-7 a semipermeable membrane separates a solution from pure water. Water flows from side B to side A by osmosis because the presence of solute on side A reduces the chemical potential of water in the solution. Pushing on the piston will increase the chemical potential of the water in the solution on side A and slow the

net rate of osmotic water flow. If the force on the piston is increased gradually, a pressure is eventually reached at which net water flow stops. Application of still more pressure will cause water to flow in the opposite direction. *The pressure on side A that is just sufficient to keep pure water from entering is called the* **osmotic pressure** *of the solution on side A.*

The osmotic pressure of a solution depends on the number of particles in solution. Thus, the degree of ionization of the solute must be taken into account when osmotic pressure is calculated. A 1-M solution of glucose, a 0.5-M solution of NaCl, and a 0.333-M solution of $CaCl_2$ have approximately the same osmotic pressure. (Actually, their osmotic pressures will differ somewhat because of the deviations of real solutions from ideal behavior.) One form of **van't Hoff's law** for calculation of osmotic pressure is

$$\pi = RT(\Phi ic) \qquad (1\text{-}2)$$

where
π = osmotic pressure
R = ideal gas constant
T = absolute temperature
Φ = osmotic coefficient
i = number of ions formed by dissociation of a solute molecule
c = molar concentration of solute (moles of solute per liter of solution)

The osmotic coefficient (Φ) accounts for the deviation of the solution from the ideal. Φ depends on the particular compound, its concentration, and the temperature. Values of Φ may be greater or less than 1. Φ is less than 1 for electrolytes of physiological importance, and for all solutes Φ approaches 1 as the solution becomes more and more dilute. *The term Φic can be regarded as the osmotically effective concentration, and Φic is called the* **osmolarity** *of the solution,* with units in osmoles per liter. Sometimes a less precise estimate of osmotic pressure is computed assuming that Φ is equal to 1.

Values of Φ can be obtained from handbooks that list values of Φ for different substances as functions of concentra-

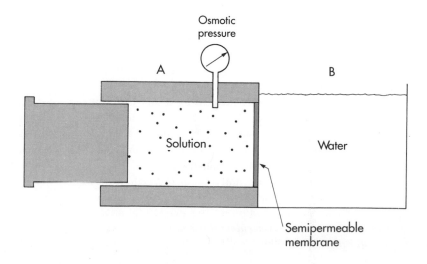

■ **Fig. 1-7** Schematic representation of the definition of osmotic pressure. When the hydrostatic pressure applied to the solution in chamber A is equal to the osmotic pressure of that solution, there will be no net water flow across the membrane.

tion. Solutions of proteins deviate greatly from ideal behavior, and different proteins may deviate to different extents. Values of the osmotic coefficient depend on the concentration of the solute and on its chemical properties. Table 1-2 lists osmotic coefficients for several solutes. These values apply, to a first approximation, to concentrations of these solutes in the extracellular fluids of mammals.

Sample calculations

1. **What is the osmotic pressure at 0° C of a 154 mM NaCl solution?**

$$\pi = RT(\Phi ic)$$

Using $\Phi = 0.93$ for NaCl from Table 1-2, we obtain

$$\pi = 22.4 \text{ L atm/mole} \times 0.93 \times 2 \times 0.154 \text{ mole/L}$$
$$= 6.42 \text{ atm}$$

2. **What is the osmolarity of this solution?**

$$\text{osmolarity} = \Phi ic$$
$$= 0.93 \times 2 \times 0.154 \text{ mole/L} = 0.286 \text{ osmolar}$$
$$= 286 \text{ milliosmolar}$$

Measurement of osmotic pressure. The osmotic pressure of a solution can be obtained by determining the pressure required to prevent water from entering the solution across a semipermeable membrane (see Fig. 1-7). It is easier, however, to estimate the osmotic pressure from another colligative property, such as depression of the freezing point. The equation that describes the osmolarity (Φic) of a solution in terms of the depression of the freezing point of water by the solute is

$$\Phi ic = \Delta T_f / 1.86 \qquad (1\text{-}3)$$

where ΔT_f is the freezing point depression in degrees centigrade. When the freezing point depression of a multicompo-

nent solution is determined, the effective osmolarity (in osmoles per liter) of the solution as a whole can be obtained.

If the total osmotic pressures of two solutions (as measured by the freezing point depression or by the osmotic pressure developed across a semipermeable membrane) are equal, the solutions are said to be **isoosmotic** (or **isosmotic**). If solution A has greater osmotic pressure than solution B, A is said to be hyperosmotic with respect to B. If solution A has less total osmotic pressure than solution B, A is said to be **hypoosmotic** with respect to B.

Osmotic swelling and shrinking of cells. The plasma membranes of most of the cells of the body are relatively impermeable to many of the solutes of the extracellular fluid but are highly permeable to water. Therefore, when the osmotic pressure of the extracellular fluid is increased, water leaves the cells by osmosis and the cells shrink. When water leaves the cell, the cellular solutes become more concentrated until the effective osmotic pressure of the cytoplasm is again equal to that of the extracellular fluid. Conversely, if the osmotic pressure of the extracellular fluid is decreased, water enters the cells. The cells will continue to swell until the intracellular and extracellular osmotic pressures are equal.

Red blood cells are often used to illustrate the osmotic properties of cells, because they are readily obtained and are easily studied. Within a certain range of external solute concentrations, the red cell behaves as an osmometer, because its volume is inversely related to the solute concentration in the extracellular medium. In Fig. 1-8 the red cell volume (the fraction of its normal volume in plasma) is plotted against the concentration of NaCl solution in which the red cells are suspended. At an NaCl concentration of 154 mM (308 mM osmotically active particles), the volume of the cells is the same as their volume in plasma; this concentration of NaCl is said to be **isotonic** to the red cell.

Isotonic NaCl solution (also known as isotonic saline) is used for intravenous rehydration or for administration of drugs to patients. Almost every patient undergoing surgery will be given an intravenous drip of isotonic saline.

A concentration of NaCl greater than 154 mM is called **hypertonic** (greater strength, causes cells to shrink); and a solution less concentrated than 154 mM is called **hypotonic** (cells swell). When red cells have swollen to about 1.4 times their original volume, some cells lyse (burst). At this volume, the properties of the red cell membrane abruptly change; hemoglobin leaks from the cell, and the membrane becomes transiently permeable to most other molecules as well.

The intracellular substances of the red blood cell that produce an osmotic pressure that just balances the osmotic pressure of the extracellular fluid include hemoglobin, K^+, organic phosphates (e.g., ATP and 2,3-diphosphoglycerate), and glycolytic intermediates. The chemical nature of the cell's contents is not important. The red cell behaves as if it

■ **Table 1-2** Osmotic coefficients (Φ) of certain solutes of physiological interest

Substance	i	Molecular weight	Φ
NaCl	2	58.5	0.93
KCl	2	74.6	0.92
HCl	2	36.6	0.95
NH_4Cl	2	53.5	0.92
$NaHCO_3$	2	84.0	0.96
$NaNO_3$	2	85.0	0.90
KSCN	2	97.2	0.91
KH_2PO_4	2	136.0	0.87
$CaCl_2$	3	111.0	0.86
$MgCl_2$	3	95.2	0.89
Na_2SO_4	3	142.0	0.74
K_2SO_4	3	174.0	0.74
$MgSO_4$	2	120.0	0.58
Glucose	1	180.0	1.01
Sucrose	1	342.0	1.02
Maltose	1	342.0	1.01
Lactose	1	342.0	1.01

From Lifson N, Visscher MB: *Osmosis in living systems*. In Glasser O, editor: *Medical physics*, vol 1, St Louis, 1944, Mosby.

■ **Fig. 1-8** The osmotic behavior of human red blood cells in NaCl solutions. At 154 mM NaCl (isotonic), the red blood cell has its normal volume. It shrinks in more concentrated (hypertonic) solutions and swells in more dilute (hypotonic) solutions. V_o and C_o are the red cell volume and intracellular solute concentration, respectively, for the red blood cell in the blood or in an isotonic solution. V and C are, respectively, the cell volume and intracellular solute concentration in a solution that is not isotonic.

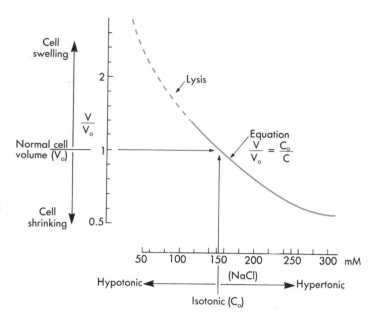

were filled with a solution of impermeant molecules with an osmotically effective concentration of 286 milliosmolar, which is the same as the osmolarity of isotonic saline:

$$\Phi_{NaCl} i_{NaCl} C_{NaCl} = 0.93 \times 2 \times 0.154 \text{ M} = \qquad (1\text{-}4)$$
$$0.286 \text{ osmolar} = 286 \text{ milliosmolar}$$

Osmotic effects of permeant solutes. In contrast to impermeant solutes, permeant solutes are solutes that are able to pass through the plasma membrane. Because of this ability, permeating solutes eventually equilibrate across the plasma membrane. For this reason, permeating solutes exert only a transient effect on cell volume.

Consider a red blood cell placed in a large volume of 0.154 M NaCl that contains 0.050 M glycerol. Initially, because the extracellular fluid contains NaCl and glycerol, the osmotic pressure of the extracellular fluid will exceed that of the cell interior, and the cell will shrink. With time, however, glycerol will equilibrate across the plasma membrane of the red cell, and the cell will swell back toward its original volume. However, *the steady-state volume of the cell is determined only by the impermeant solutes in the extracellular fluid.* In this case, the concentration of impermeant solute of the extracellular fluid (NaCl) is 154 M, which is isotonic to the red blood cells. Therefore, the final volume of the cell will be equal to the normal red cell volume. *Because the red cell ultimately returns to its normal volume, the solution (0.050 M glycerol in 0.154 M NaCl) is isotonic. Because the red cell initially shrinks when put in this solution, the solution is hyperosmotic with respect to the normal red cell.* The transient changes in cell volume depend on equilibration of glycerol across the membrane. Had we used urea (a more rapidly permeating substance), the cell would have reached steady-state volume sooner.

The following rules help predict the volume changes a cell will undergo when suspended in solutions of permeant and impermeant solutes:

1. *The steady-state volume of the cell is determined only by the concentration of impermeant solutes in the extracellular fluid.*
2. *Permeant solutes cause only transient changes in cell volume.*
3. The greater the permeability of the membrane to the permeant solute, the more rapid is the time course of the transient changes.

Magnitudes of osmotic flows caused by permeating solutes. In the preceding example, we saw that permeant solutes, such as glycerol, exert only a transient osmotic effect on cells. It is sometimes necessary to determine the rate of the osmotic flow caused by a particular permeant solute.

When a difference of hydrostatic pressure (ΔP) causes water to flow across a membrane, the rate of water flow ($\dot{V}_w$) is

$$\dot{V}_w = L \Delta P \qquad (1\text{-}5)$$

where L is a constant of proportionality, called the **hydraulic conductivity.**

Osmotic flow of water across a membrane is directly proportional to the osmotic pressure difference ($\Delta \pi$) of the solutions on the two sides of the membrane; thus,

$$\dot{V}_w = L \Delta \pi \qquad (1\text{-}6)$$

Equation 1-6 is true only for osmosis caused by *impermeant* solutes. *Permeant solutes cause less osmotic flow. The greater the permeability of a solute, the less osmotic flow it causes.* Table 1-3 shows the osmotic water flows induced across a porous membrane by solutes of different molecular size. The solutions have identical freezing points, so the

■ Table 1-3   Osmotic water flow across a porous dialysis membrane caused by various solutes*

Gradient producing the water flow	Net volume flow (μl/min)*	Solute radius (Å)	Reflection coefficient (σ)
D₂O	0.06	1.9	0.0024
Urea	0.6	2.7	0.024
Glucose	5.1	4.4	0.205
Sucrose	9.2	5.3	0.368
Raffinose	11	6.1	0.440
Inulin	19	12	0.760
Bovine serum albumin	25.5	37	1.02
Hydrostatic pressure	25		

Data from Durbin RP: *J Gen Physiol* 44:315, 1960.

*Flow is expressed as microliters per minute caused by a 1-M concentration difference of solute across the membrane. The flows are compared with the flow caused by a theoretically equivalent hydrostatic pressure.

total osmotic pressures are the same. Table 1-3 demonstrates that the larger the solute molecule, the more impermeable the membrane is to the solute, and the greater the osmotic water flow it causes.

Reflection coefficients. Equation 1-6 can be rewritten to take solute permeability into account by including σ, the **reflection coefficient.**

$$V_w = \sigma L \Delta \pi \qquad (1\text{-}7)$$

σ is a dimensionless number that ranges from 1 for completely impermeant solutes to 0 for extremely permeant solutes. σ is a property of a particular solute and a particular membrane and represents the osmotic flow induced by the solute as a fraction of the theoretical maximal osmotic flow (Table 1-3).

The mechanism by which the kidney produces urine that is more concentrated than the extracellular fluid (see Chapter 36) requires that various parts of the nephron have different reflection coefficients for important

solutes, such as NaCl and urea. The osmotic water flows induced by NaCl and urea in a particular segment of the nephron depend on the values of σ of the epithelium in that segment for these solutes.

PROTEIN-MEDIATED MEMBRANE TRANSPORT

Some substances enter or leave cells via intrinsic proteins of the plasma membrane called **transporters** (also known as **carriers**) or **channels** (Fig. 1-9). Such **protein-mediated transport** processes are able to transport substances across membranes much more rapidly than can simple diffusion.

A transporter binds the solute to be transported on one side of the membrane and then the transporter undergoes a conformational change that allows the solute to be released on the other side of the membrane (Fig. 1-9, *A*). The rate of transport is limited by the rate at which the transporter can undergo the necessary conformational changes from 10² to

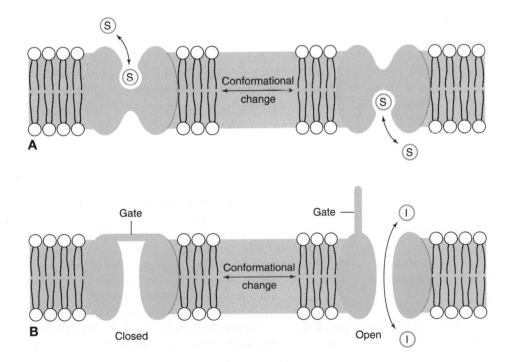

■ Fig. 1-9   Membrane transporters versus ion channels. **A,** A transporter binds the transported substance (S) from one side of the membrane and, following a conformational change, releases S at the other side of the membrane. **B,** A channel is either "open" or "closed" depending on the position of the gate. When the channel is open the conducted ion (I) can enter the channel from either side of the membrane and be conducted through the membrane.

10^4 solute molecules/sec. If the transporter has no link to metabolic energy, the transported solute will flow from the side of the membrane at which it is more concentrated to the side at which it is less concentrated. This is called **facilitated transport.** Certain transporters are linked to metabolic energy, and they can use the energy to transport the transported solute against its energy gradient from where it it less concentrated to where it is more concentrated. This is called **active transport.**

Channels are responsible for the passage of certain ions across membranes (Fig. 1-9, *B*). A channel may be either open or closed. A part of the channel protein functions as a **gate.** Random conformational changes of the conformation of the protein result in the gate alternating between open and closed positions. When the channel is open there is a direct pathway for the transported ion to flow through the channel. The rate of transport of ions through an open channel is 10^7 to 10^8 ions/sec, much greater than through a transporter. The two major classes of ion channels are **voltage-gated** ion channels and **ligand-gated** ion channels. The probability of a voltage-gated channel being open depends on the value of the transmembrane voltage difference (see Chapter 3). The probability of a ligand-gated channel being open depends on the concentration of the substance (ligand), such as acetylcholine, that regulates the channel (see Chapter 4).

In this chapter we will describe solute transport by transporters. Ion channels will be discussed later (see Chapters 3 and 4) in the context of some of the physiological phenomena that are mediated by ion channels.

Properties of Mediated Transport

1. A substance that is transported by mediated transport is transported *much more rapidly* than other molecules that are of similar molecular weight and lipid solubility and that cross the membrane by simple diffusion.
2. The transport rate shows **saturation kinetics.** As the concentration of the transported compound is increased, the rate of transport at first increases, but eventually a concentration is reached, above which the transport rate increases no further (Fig. 1-10). At this point, the transport system is said to be saturated with the transported compound. Saturation behavior of the rate (J) of mediated transport is represented by a Michaelis-Menten type of equation:

$$J = \frac{J_{max}[S]}{K_m + [S]} \qquad (1-8)$$

where J_{max} is the maximal rate of transport, [S] is the concentration of the transported substance in the compartment from which it is being removed, and K_m is the apparent Michaelis constant for the transporter. When $[S] = K_m$, $J = J_{max}/2$, so K_m can be defined as the concentration of the transported compound required for half-maximal transport.
3. The mediating protein has **chemical specificity:** only molecules with the requisite chemical structure are transported. The specificity of most transport systems is

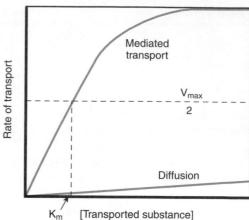

■ **Fig. 1-10**   Transport via a transport protein shows saturation kinetics. As the concentration of the transported substance increases, the rate of its transport approaches a maximal value, the V_{max} for the transporter. The concentration of the transported substance required for the transport rate to be half-maximal is termed the K_m of the transporter.

not absolute, and in general it is broader than the specificity of most enzymes. However, the lock-and-key relationship between an enzyme and its substrate can be applied to transport proteins as well.

4. Structurally related molecules may compete for transport. Typically, the presence of one transport substrate will decrease the transport rate of a second substrate by competing for the transport protein. This competition is analogous to competitive inhibition of an enzyme.
5. Transport may be inhibited by compounds that are not structurally related to transport substrates. An inhibitor may bind to the transport protein in a way that decreases the affinity of the protein for the normal transport substrate. For example, the compound **phloretin** does not resemble a sugar molecule, yet it strongly inhibits red blood cell sugar transport. Active transport systems, which require some link to metabolism, may be inhibited by metabolic inhibitors. The rate of Na^+ transport out of cells by the Na^+,K^+-ATPase is decreased by substances that interfere with ATP generation.

Facilitated Transport

Sometimes called *facilitated diffusion,* facilitated transport occurs via a transporter that does not require an input of energy. Facilitated transport has all the properties discussed previously except one: it is not generally depressed by metabolic inhibitors. Because facilitated transport processes are not linked to energy metabolism, they cannot move substances against concentration gradients. Instead, *facilitated transport systems act to equalize concentrations of the transported substances* on the two sides of the membrane.

Monosaccharides enter muscle cells by facilitated transport. Glucose, galactose, arabinose, and 3-*O*-methylglucose compete for the same carrier. The rate of transport of all

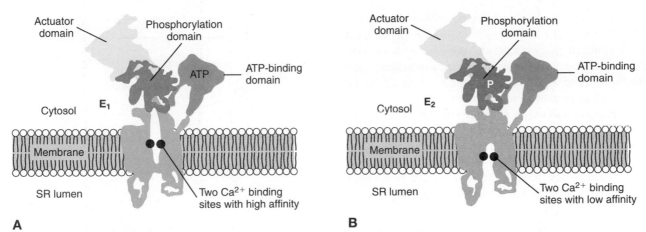

■ **Fig. 1-11**   The mechanism whereby the Ca^{2+}-ATPase of the sarcoplasmic reticulum (SR) pumps Ca^{2+} into the lumen of the SR. The intramembrane part of the protein consists mainly of 10 α-helices. Oxygen-containing amino acid residues near the center of the membrane in several of the transmembrane helices form binding sites for two Ca^{2+} ions. The Ca^{2+}-ATPase has two basic conformational states. The E_1 state (**A**) binds Ca^{2+} and ATP from the cytosol with high affinity. Movement (not illustrated) of the ATP-binding domain toward the phosphorylation domain precedes the transfer of the γ phosphate of ATP to an aspartyl residue in the phosphorylation domain. The phosphorylated intermediate can isomerize to the E_2 conformation (**B**). Conformational changes (not illustrated) in the three cytosolic domains of the protein cause movements of the intramembrane helices so that the Ca^{2+} binding sites have lower affinity and become accessible to the lumen of the SR. Ca^{2+} is then released to the lumen, which allows spontaneous release of phosphate from the protein. The dephosphorylated protein can isomerize back to the E_1 state and the transport cycle can begin again.

these substances shows saturation kinetics. The nonphysiological stereoisomer L-glucose enters the cells very slowly, and nontransported sugars, such as mannitol or sorbose, enter muscle cells very slowly, if at all. Phloretin inhibits sugar uptake, and insulin stimulates it.

Current evidence suggests that most transport proteins span the membrane and are multimeric. Figure 1-9, *A*, depicts a hypothetical dimer model that has been proposed for the monosaccharide transport protein that spans the membrane of the human red blood cell. Conformational changes of the protein, induced by monosaccharide binding, may allow a sugar molecule to enter and leave the cell.

Active Transport

Active transport processes have most of the properties of facilitated transport. In addition, *active transport systems allow the concentration of their substrates against concentration or electrochemical potential gradients. Because this process requires energy, active transport processes must be linked to energy metabolism in some way.* Active transporters may use ATP directly, or they may be linked indirectly to metabolism. If the transporter binds the transported substance with higher affinity when it faces one side of the membrane than when it faces the other side, active transport will result. For the transporter to cycle between the two affinity states requires energy. Because they depend on an input of energy, active transport processes may be inhibited by any substance that interferes with energy metabolism.

Primary active transport.   An active transport process that is linked directly to cellular metabolism, for example, by using ATP to power the transport, is called **primary active transport.**

Ion-transporting ATPases are transporters that use the energy released by ATP hydrolysis to actively transport one or more ionic species across a membrane. The Ca^{2+}-ATPase of sacoplasmic reticulum (SR) pumps two Ca^{2+} ions from the cytosol to the lumen of the SR for each ATP hydrolyzed. The Ca^{2+}-ATPase thereby lowers the Ca^{2+} concentration in the muscle cytosol to submicromolar levels and causes the muscle to relax (Chapter 12).

The mechanism of active Ca^{2+} transport by the SR Ca^{2+}-ATPase.   Structural details about the Ca^{2+}-ATPase of sarcoplasmic reticulum became available in 2000, and they have permitted increased understanding of the mechanism of ion pumping by the Ca^{2+}-ATPase (Fig. 1-11). The transporter has two basic conformations, called E_1 and E_2. In the E_1 conformation, the two Ca^{2+} binding sites have high affinity for Ca^{2+} and are accessible to the cytosol. In the E_2 conformation, the Ca^{2+} binding sites have a much lower affinity and they are accessible to the lumen of the SR. The transporter is driven around its transport cycle by first phosphorylating itself and then by being dephosphorylated (Fig. 1-11). The energy required to transverse the transport cycle is provided by ATP. Consequently, the transporter moves Ca^{2+} from the cytosol, where its concentration is low, to the lumen of the SR, where its concentration is high. This requires energy. *Because the energy is obtained directly from ATP hydrolysis this is an example of primary active transport.* A transport process that was powered by some other high-energy metabolic intermediate or that was linked directly in another way to a primary metabolic reaction would also be classified as primary active transport.

The Na$^+$,K$^+$-ATPase, a close relative of the SR Ca^{2+}-ATPase, is present in the plasma membranes of all cells. The Na$^+$,K$^+$-ATPase also cycles between E$_1$ and E$_2$ states in a cycle powered by ATP hydrolysis. In the E$_1$ conformation, the ion binding sites face the cytosol and have high affinity for Na$^+$ and low affinity for K$^+$. In the E$_2$ conformation, the ion binding sites face the extracellular fluid and have low affinity for Na$^+$ and high affinity for K$^+$. As the transporter is driven around the transport cycle from E$_1$ to E$_2$ and back to E$_1$ again, it picks up Na$^+$ from the cytosol and releases it to the extracellular fluid. It also picks up K$^+$ from the extracellular fluid and releases it into the cytosol. In each cycle of the pump one molecule of ATP is hydolyzed, three Na$^+$ ions are ejected from the cytosol, and two K$^+$ ions are taken up into the cytosol.

Due to the ion gradients created by the Na$^+$,K$^+$-ATPase, Na$^+$ tends to diffuse passively back into the cytosol and K$^+$ tends to diffuse out of the cell into the extracellular fluid. In the **steady state,** the concentrations of Na$^+$ and K$^+$ in the cytosol are constant in time because the rates of active transport of Na$^+$ and K$^+$ and the rates of their passive leakage across the plasma membrane down their electrochemical potential gradients (Chapter 2) are equal in magnitude, but opposite in direction.

Secondary active transport. The previous section emphasized that energy is required to create a concentration gradient of a transported substance. Once created, *a concentration gradient represents a store of chemical potential energy that can be harnessed to do work* (see Chapter 2). In many cell types, the concentration gradient of Na$^+$ created by the Na$^+$,K$^+$-ATPase is used to actively transport other solutes into the cell. Many cells import neutral, hydrophilic amino acids by membrane transport proteins that link the inward transport of Na$^+$ down its electrochemical potential gradient to the inward transport of amino acids against their concentration gradients (Fig. 1-12). The energy for the transport of the amino acid is not provided directly by ATP or some other high-energy metabolite, but it is provided indirectly from the gradient of Na$^+$ that is itself actively transported. Hence, the amino acid is said to be transported by **secondary active transport.** In the secondary active transport of amino acids, both the rate of amino acid transport and the extent to which the amino acid accumulates in the cell depend on the electrochemical potential gradient of Na$^+$.

In the small intestine, glucose and galactose are absorbed by Na$^+$-powered secondary active transport. The presence of Na$^+$ in the lumen enhances the absorption of glucose, and vice versa. In severe diarrheal illnesses, oral rehydration therapy is frequently employed. Patients drink a solution containing both NaCl and glucose, along with

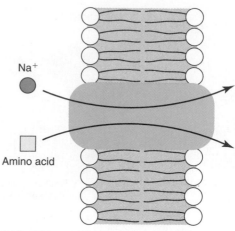

■ **Fig. 1-12** Many cells take up neutral amino acids by secondary active transport. The transport protein binds both Na$^+$ and the amino acid. Na$^+$ is transported down its electrochemical gradient, and the transport protein uses the energy released by Na$^+$ flux to transport the amino acid against a concentration gradient.

K$^+$ and HCO$_3^-$. The absorption of Na$^+$ and glucose in the small intestine helps to drive the osmotic absorption of water and thus facilitates the rehydration of the patient.

Other Membrane Transport Processes

Ion-transporting ATPases. Ion-transporting ATPases are central to the lives of all cells, from Archaebacteria to *Homo sapiens*. There are three major classes of ion-transporting ATPases: **P-type, V-type,** and **F-type ATPases.**

P-type ATPases. These ATPases are so named because their transport cycle involves a phosphorylated intermediate. The Na$^+$,K$^+$-ATPase, discussed above, is a P-type ATPase. So are the Ca^{2+}-ATPases of the sarcoplasmic reticulum, endoplasmic reticulum, and plasma membrane, and the H$^+$,K$^+$-ATPases of the gastric parietal cell, the intercalated cell of the kidney, and epithelial cells in the colon. P-type ATPases are also known as E$_1$-E$_2$ ATPases because their transport cycle involves two distinct classes of conformational states. As noted, the interconversion between the E$_1$ and E$_2$ states is driven by the phosphorylation (ATP is the phosphoryl donor) and dephosphorylation of the transporter.

V-type ATPases. The membranes of various intracellular organelles, such as lysosomes, endosomes, secretory vesicles, and storage granules, contain V-type ATPases. The V-type ATPases actively accumulate H$^+$ in the vesicle lumen. Acidification of the vesicle lumen is essential for the function of lysosomes and for the storage of neurotransmitters in synaptic vesicles.

F-type ATPases. The inner mitochondrial membrane contains an F-type ATPase, known as **ATP synthase.** Whereas P- and V-type ATPases hydrolyze ATP and use some of the energy released to actively transport ions, the ATP synthase generally uses the energy of the H$^+$ gradient that is established across the mitochondrial inner membrane by electron transport to synthesize ATP. (Because all chemical reactions

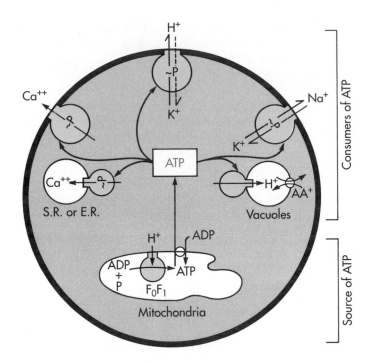

■ **Fig. 1-13**   Ion-transporting ATPases are the major sources and among the major consumers of ATP in cells. The F-type ATPase of mitochondria, ATP synthase, is the major source of ATP. P-type and V-type ATPases consume a significant fraction of the ATP utilized by cells. *SR*, Sarcoplasmic reticulum; *ER*, endoplasmic reticulum. (Modified from Pedersen PL, Carafoli E: *Trends Biochem Sci* 12:146, 1987.)

are reversible, under appropriate conditions P- and V-type ATPase can use the energy of ion gradients to produce ATP, and F-type ATPases can use ATP to actively transport H^+.) In the normal economy of animal cells, the mitochondrial ATP synthase is the major source of ATP, and the P- and V-type ATPases are major consumers of ATP (Fig. 1-13).

Calcium transport. Under most circumstances, the concentration of Ca^{2+} in the cytosol of cells is maintained at low levels, 10^{-7} M or less, whereas the concentration of Ca^{2+} in extracellular fluids is approximately 10^{-3} M. Because Ca^{2+} is an important second messenger, the cytosolic level of Ca^{2+} is subject to complex regulation. Many hormones and agonists elevate the intracellular level of Ca^{2+} by opening Ca^{2+} channels in the plasma membrane and/or in the membranes of intracellular Ca^{2+}-storage vesicles. Among the membrane transport proteins that participate in regulating the level of cytosolic Ca^{2+} are (a) the Ca^{2+}-ATPases located in plasma membranes and in the membranes of endoplasmic and sarcoplasmic reticulum, and (b) the Na^+-Ca^{2+} exchange proteins of plasma membranes.

Ca^{2+}-ATPases. Plasma membranes contain a Ca^{2+}-ATPase that helps maintain the large gradient of Ca^{2+} between the cytosol and the extracellular fluid. The plasma membrane Ca^{2+}-ATPase is a relative of the Ca^{2+}-ATPase that is responsible for sequestering Ca^{2+} in the sarcoplasmic reticulum of muscle (see Chapter 12). The plasma membrane Ca^{2+}-ATPase shares several important structural and mechanistic properties with the Ca^{2+}-ATPase of the sarcoplasmic reticulum and with the Na^+,K^+-ATPase of plasma membranes.

The plasma membrane Ca^{2+}-ATPase is regulated by **calmodulin.** In the presence of micromolar Ca^{2+}, the complex of Ca^{2+} with calmodulin binds to a specific site on the plasma membrane Ca^{2+}-ATPase. This binding causes an autoinhibitory peptide domain to dissociate from the ATP-binding site, and thus activates the Ca^{2+}-ATPase.

In addition, *most cells store Ca^{2+} in the endoplasmic reticulum or in other intracellular storage vesicles,* such as the sarcoplasmic reticulum of muscle cells. Ca^{2+} is concentrated in these vesicles by Ca^{2+}-ATPases that are members of a closely related family of Ca^{2+}-ATPases called SERCA (sarcoplasmic and endoplasmic reticulum Ca^{2+}-ATPases). The best characterized SERCA Ca^{2+}-ATPase is the Ca^{2+}-ATPase of fast skeletal muscle.

Na^+-Ca^{2+} exchange. Certain electrically excitable cells, such as those of the heart, have an additional mechanism for controlling the level of intracellular Ca^{2+}. A sodium/calcium exchange protein in their plasma membranes uses the energy in the Na^+ gradient to extrude Ca^{2+} from the cell. In heart cells, the decrease in intracellular Ca^{2+} that occurs in each diastole is caused by both the sodium/calcium exchange protein and the Ca^{2+}-ATPase of the sarcoplasmic reticulum. The Na^+-Ca^{2+} exchanger is stimulated at micromolar levels of Ca^{2+} by binding of the Ca^{2+}-calmodulin complex to a specific site of the exchanger protein.

In most cells, Ca^{2+} leaks slowly into the cell down its electrochemical potential gradient. Therefore, the energy cost of maintaining a low intracellular level of Ca^{2+} is also low. This low-energy expenditure contrasts with the cost of pumping Na^+ and K^+; *running the Na^+,K^+-pump is a major item in the energy budget of many cells.* Kidneys have an extremely high metabolic rate; most of the energy expended by the kidney is consumed by the Na^+,K^+-ATPase.

Na^+-H^+ exchange. Most cells contain a protein that mediates the one-for-one exchange of Na^+ for H^+ across the plasma membrane. This protein, the Na^+-H^+ exchanger, functions to prevent acidification of the cytosol. When the pH of the cytosol is nearly neutral, the Na^+-H^+ exchanger has a low affinity for H^+ and it is almost inactive. Acidification of the cytosol increases the affinity of the protein for H^+. Na^+ flows into the cell down its electrochemical potential gradient in exchange for the outward transport of H$^+$, and therefore the pH of the cytosol rises toward neutrality.

> Treatment of cells with certain growth factors, tumor promoters, and mitogens results in phosphorylation of the Na$^+$-H$^+$ exchanger and increases its affinity for H$^+$. Increased affinity for H$^+$ causes the exchanger to be active at neutral pH and results in persistent alkalinization of the cytosol. The activation of the Na$^+$-H$^+$ exchanger is apparently required for the stimulation of cell division by mitogens. However, the mechanism by which alkalinization contributes to an increased rate of cell division is not yet understood.

Anion exchange. Essentially all cells contain **anion exchange** proteins in their plasma membranes. Three members of the family of anion exchange proteins have been found in animal cells; the best characterized is the **band 3 protein** of human erythrocytes. These proteins mediate the exchange of an intracellular anion for an extracellular anion. Several different univalent anions are transported. Physiologically, the anions present at highest concentrations are Cl$^-$ and HCO$_3^-$. Hence, the anion-exchange protein, especially in red blood cells, is often called the **chloride-bicarbonate exchanger.**

> The chloride-bicarbonate exchanger is important in the transport of CO$_2$ from the tissues to the lungs and in the unloading of CO$_2$ from the blood in the lungs (see Chapter 28).

The anion exchanger is also involved in regulation of cell pH. Alkalization of the cytosol shifts the equilibrium of carbonic acid toward elevated bicarbonate. Consequently, elevated cell pH activates the efflux of bicarbonate in exchange for chloride and thereby shifts the cytosolic pH back toward neutrality. *Cytosolic pH is thus maintained at near-neutral*

levels by the combined actions of the anion exchanger *(which responds to alkalinization of the cytosol)* and the Na$^+$-H$^+$ exchanger *(which is activated by acidification of cytosol).*

Na$^+$,K$^+$, Cl$^-$ cotransport. Many cells, both epithelial and nonepithelial, contain a plasma membrane protein that mediates the simultaneous transport ("cotransport") of Na$^+$, K$^+$, and Cl$^-$ from the extracellular fluid to the cytosol. The stoichiometry is 1 Na$^+$: 1 K$^+$: 2 Cl$^-$, and thus the transport is electroneutral. The entry of Na$^+$ into the cell down its electrochemical potential gradient provides the energy for the active uptake of K$^+$ and Cl$^-$. In many cell types, Na$^+$, K$^+$, Cl$^-$ cotransport plays a role in fluid volume regulation. The cotransporter is activated by cell shrinking, which leads to an influx of Na$^+$, K$^+$, and Cl$^-$ and thereby generates an osmotic force to restore cell volume.

> The Na$^+$, K$^+$, Cl$^-$ cotransporter is specifically inhibited by such drugs as **furosemide** and **bumetanide,** which are known as **loop diuretics.** These diuretics inhibit the Na$^+$,K$^+$, Cl$^-$ cotransporter in the thick ascending limb of the loop of Henle, and thereby interfere with the reabsorption of Na$^+$ and Cl$^-$ from the thick ascending limb (see Chapter 35). Because the reabsorption of Na$^+$ and Cl$^-$ plays a primary role in the ability of the kidney to produce a urine of low volume and high concentration, loop diuretics are among the most powerful diuretics.

Facilitated transport of glucose. Glucose is the primary fuel for most of the cells of the body, but glucose diffuses across plasma membranes very slowly. The plasma membranes of many cell types contain transport proteins that mediate the facilitated transport of glucose and related monosaccharides. Red blood cells, hepatocytes, adipocytes, and muscle cells (skeletal, cardiac, smooth) all possess glucose transporters. Glucose uptake by these cell types does not depend on the electrochemical potential difference of Na$^+$ across the plasma membrane or in any direct way

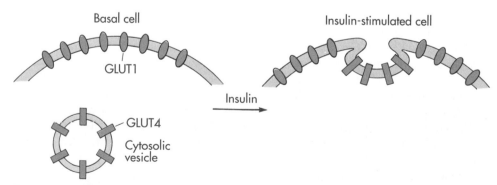

■ **Fig. 1-14** Schematic depiction of the stimulation of glucose transport in muscle or fat cells by insulin. In the basal state, glucose transporters are present in the plasma membrane (the GLUT1 isoform of the glucose transporter) and in a pool of intracellular vesicles (the GLUT4 isoform). Upon stimulation by insulin, many of the intracellular vesicles fuse with the plasma membrane, thereby increasing the total number of glucose transporters in the plasma membrane.

on cellular metabolism. Cells of adult humans contain three distinct, but highly homologous, isoforms of glucose transporters.

Stimulation of glucose transport by insulin. In adipocytes and muscle cells, the rate of transport of glucose across the plasma membrane is increased by insulin. *Insulin increases the rate of glucose transport by prompting the insertion of more glucose transport proteins into the plasma membrane.* The source of the newly inserted protein is a preformed pool of transporters in the membranes of the endoplasmic reticulum within the cell (Fig. 1-14).

In **type 1 diabetes mellitus,** also known as **insulin-dependent diabetes,** pancreatic β cells secrete very little insulin in response to elevations of blood glucose. In the absence of insulin, muscle and adipose cells must rely on the slow diffusion of glucose. Because transport of glucose into these cells is the rate-limiting step in glucose metabolism, the ability of muscle and fat cells to metabolize glucose is impaired. Consequently, in type I diabetes, these cells must turn to other fuels, such as fats, to satisfy their energy demands.

Metabolic regulation of glucose transport. The glucose uptake capacity of several different cell types is modulated in accordance with metabolic requirements. In red cells and certain neurons, glucose transport is stimulated by decreased levels of ATP and by increased levels of adenosine diphosphate (ADP) and adenosine monophosphate (AMP). Anoxia in cardiac muscle and exercise in skeletal muscle stimulate glucose transport. These responses may involve the insertion of additional glucose transporters into the plasma membrane, but most of the response is attributable to stimulation of preexisting transporters in the membrane.

The stimulation of glucose uptake in skeletal muscle by exercise does not depend on insulin. Insulin-dependent diabetics can diminish the amount of insulin required to regulate their blood glucose levels by engaging in regular exercise.

Amino acid transport. Most of the cells in the body synthesize proteins and therefore require amino acids. The synthesis of proteins is required for the turnover of cells and tissues and in such processes as wound healing. Several different amino acid transport proteins are present in plasma membranes. The amino acid transport systems include several *distinct classes of transporters:* for neutral, for basic, and for acidic amino acids. The specificities of acid transport proteins overlap significantly, and the distribution of the different transport proteins varies from one cell type to another. Some of these transport proteins are secondary active transporters powered by the concentration gradient of Na$^+$; others are facilitated transport proteins. Certain amino acid transporters in the brush border membranes of the jejunum and the renal proximal tubule are found only in epithelial cell types. Other amino acid transporters are present in almost all cell types.

ABC (*ATP-Binding Cassette*) Transporters. This class of transporters (Fig. 1-15) includes the **cystic fibrosis transmembrane regulator (CFTR),** a regulated Cl$^-$ channel that is defective in **cystic fibrosis.** Another member of the ABC transporter family is the **multiple drug resistance (MDR) transporter,** also known as P-glycoprotein. Unlike most other transporters, the MDR transporter has broad specificity; it can transport organic molecules (including many drugs used in cancer therapy), some small polypeptides, and certain lipids. By increasing the synthesis of MDR transporters many cancer cells can become resistant to the drugs used to kill them.

Transport across Epithelia

Epithelial cells are polarized with respect to their transport properties. The transport properties of the plasma membrane facing one side of the epithelial cell layer are different from those of the membrane facing the other side.

The epithelial cells of the small intestine (see Chapter 33) and the proximal tubule of the kidney (see Chapter 35) provide good examples of this polarity. The composition of membrane transport proteins in the brush border membrane that faces the lumen of the small bowel or the renal tubule differs from the transport protein composition of the basolateral plasma membrane of the cell. The **tight junctions** that join the epithelial cells side to side prevent mixing of the transport proteins of the luminal and basolateral plasma membranes. The brush border plasma membranes of these epithelia contain very few Na$^+$,K$^+$-ATPase molecules, which reside mainly in the basolateral plasma membrane. Glucose (and galactose) and neutral amino acids enter these epithelial cells at the brush border by secondary active transporters that are driven by the Na$^+$ gradient. However, these substances leave the cells at the basolateral membrane primarily by facilitated transporters (Fig. 1-16).

The tight junctions that join the cells are leaky to water and small water-soluble molecules and ions. There are thus two types of pathways for transport across the epithelia: (1)

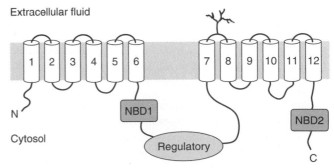

■ Fig. 1-15 An ABC transporter. ABC stands for ATP binding cassette. The cystic fibrosis transmembrane regulator and the multiple drug resistance transporter are ABC transporters. The two halves of the molecule have homologous amino acid sequences. The 12 transmembrane α-helices are shown as white cylinders and the two nucleotide binding domains, NBD1 and NBD2, are blue boxes. These proteins contain a single regulatory domain.

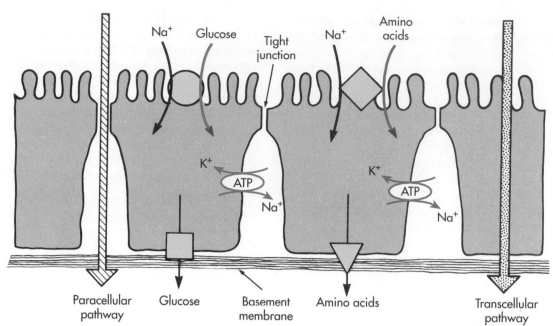

■ **Fig. 1-16** Epithelial transport processes that occur in the small intestine and renal tubules. Epithelia are polarized so that the transport processes on one side of the cell differ from those on the other side. Glucose and neutral amino acids enter the epithelial cell at the brush border via Na^+-powered secondary active transport, but they leave the cell across the basolateral membrane by facilitated transport.

transcellular pathways, through the cells, and (2) **paracellular** pathways, between the cells (Fig. 1-16).

SUMMARY

1. Biological membranes are phospholipid bilayers. Integral membrane proteins are embedded in the bilayer, and peripheral membrane proteins adhere to the surfaces of the membrane.

2. Membranes serve as permeability barriers that separate the cell from the extracellular environment and divide the cell into biochemically specialized compartments.

3. Endocytosis and exocytosis permit material to enter or leave the cell without passing through the membrane.

4. Diffusion is an effective biological transport process over microscopic distances. Only very small water-soluble molecules and lipid-soluble molecules can diffuse across biological membranes at appreciable rates.

5. Gradients of solutes across membranes power the flow of water by osmosis. The steady-state volume of cells is determined by impermeant solutes, while permeant solutes have only transient effects.

6. The osmotic water flow caused by a particular solute depends on the permeability of the membrane to that solute: the greater the permeability of the membrane to the solute, the less the osmotic water flow.

7. Biological membranes contain proteins (transporters) that transport various classes of molecules. Facilitated trans-

porters allow the transported substance to equilibrate across the membrane. Active transporters can pump the transported substances against a concentration or energy gradient. Active transport is an energy-requiring process and must be linked to metabolism.

8. Primary active transport proteins are directly linked to metabolism, frequently by consuming ATP. The Na^+,K^+-ATPase of the plasma membrane hydrolyzes ATP and uses some of the energy released to actively import K^+ and extrude Na^+.

9. Secondary active transport proteins use the gradient of another substance, frequently Na^+, to power the transport of substances such as sugars and amino acids.

10. Ion-transporting ATPases are central to the economy of the cell. The F-type ATPases of mitochondria are the primary producers of ATP. The P- and V-type ATPases of plasma and organellar membranes are major consumers of ATP.

11. Calcium ions are key second messengers. The resting cellular level of Ca^{2+} is maintained at submicromolar levels. Calcium ATPases in the plasma membrane, endoplasmic reticulum, and sarcoplasmic reticulum and sodium-calcium exchange proteins in plasma membranes play key roles in regulating the basal level of cytosolic Ca^{2+}.

12. Several types of transport proteins mediate the exchange of ions across membranes. Na^+-H^+ exchangers and anion exchangers in the plasma membranes of cells help maintain cytosolic pH near neutral. Plasma membrane Na^+, K^+, Cl^- cotransporters maintain cellular volume.

13. Facilitated transport of glucose into muscle and fat cells is rate limiting for glucose metabolism. Insulin stimulates glucose transport into these cells by promoting the insertion of additional glucose transporters into the plasma membrane.

14. Epithelial cells contain different transporters in the plasma membranes that face the opposite sides of the tissue. In most epithelia, significant transport of water and solutes occurs via the tight junctions (which are somewhat leaky) between the cells.

BIBLIOGRAPHY

Journal articles

Carruthers A: Facilitated diffusion of glucose, *Physiol Rev* 70:1135, 1990.

Christensen HN: Role of amino acid transport and counter-transport in nutrition and metabolism, *Physiol Rev* 70:43, 1990.

Fambrough DM: The sodium pump becomes a family, *Trends Neurosci* 11:325, 1988.

Finkelstein A: Water movement through membrane channels, *Curr Top Membr Transp* 21:295, 1984.

Griffith JK: Membrane transport proteins: implications of sequence comparisons, *Curr Opin Cell Biol* 4:684, 1992.

Handler JS: Overview of epithelial polarity, *Annu Rev Physiol* 51:729, 1989.

Henderson PJF: The 12-transmembrane helix transporters, *Curr Opin Cell Biol* 5:708, 1993.

Lodish HF: Anion-exchange and glucose transport proteins: structure, function, and distribution, *Harvey Lect* 82:19, 1988.

Mercer RW: Structure of the Na, K-ATPase, *Int Rev Cytol* 137C:139, 1993.

Pedersen PL, Carafoli E: Ion motive ATPases. I. Ubiquity, properties, and significance to cell function, *Trends Biochem Sci* 12:146, 1987.

Sachs G, Munson K: Mammalian phosphorylating ion-motive ATPases, *Curr Opin Cell Biol* 3:685, 1991.

Walter A, Gutknecht J: Permeability of small nonelectrolytes through lipid bilayer membranes, *J Membr Biol* 90:207, 1986.

Wright EM, Hager KM, Turk E: Sodium co-transport proteins, *Curr Opin Cell Biol* 4:696, 1992.

Books and monographs

Andreoli TE et al, editors: *Physiology of membrane disorders,* ed 2, New York, 1986, Plenum Press.

Finean JB, Michell RH, editors: *Membrane structure,* New York, 1981, Elsevier/North-Holland Biomedical Press.

Finkelstein A: *Water movement through lipid bilayers, pores, and plasma membranes: theory and reality,* New York, 1987, John Wiley.

Kaplan JH, De Weer P, editors: *The sodium pump: structure, mechanism, and regulation,* 44th Symposium of the Society of General Physiologists, New York, 1990, Rockefeller Press.

Kotyk A, Janacek K, Koryta J: *Biophysical chemistry of membrane functions,* New York, 1988, Wiley Interscience.

Läuger P: *Electrogenic ion pumps,* Sunderland, Mass, 1991, Sinauer Associates.

Martonosi AN, editor: *The enzymes of biological membranes,* ed 2, New York, 1985, Plenum Press.

Stein WH: *Channels, carriers, and pumps: an introduction to membrane transport,* San Diego, 1990, Academic Press.

chapter two

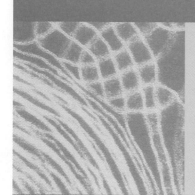

Ionic Equilibria and Resting Membrane Potentials

Most animal cells maintain an electrical potential difference (voltage) across their plasma membranes. *The cytoplasm is usually electrically negative* relative to the extracellular fluid. This electrical potential difference across the plasma membrane in a resting cell is called the resting membrane potential. The **resting membrane potential** plays a central role in the excitability of nerve and muscle cells and in certain other cellular responses. The major goal of this chapter is to explain how the resting membrane potential is generated. First, however, it is necessary to describe the principles of ionic equilibria.

IONIC EQUILIBRIA

Electrochemical Potentials of Ions

In Fig. 2-1, a membrane separates aqueous solutions in two chambers (A and B). The ion X^+ is at a higher concentration on side A than on side B. If no electrical potential difference exists between side A and side B, X^+ tends to diffuse from side A to side B, just as if it were an uncharged molecule. If, however, side A is electrically negative with respect to side B, the situation is more complex. Although X^+ still tends to diffuse from side A to side B because of the concentration difference, now X^+ also tends to move in the opposite direction (from B to A) because of the electrical potential difference across the membrane. *The direction of net X^+ movement depends on whether the effect of the concentration difference or the effect of the electrical potential difference is larger. By comparing the two tendencies—concentration and electrical—one can predict the direction of net X^+ movement.*

The quantity that allows us to compare the relative contributions of ionic concentration and electrical potential to the movement of an ion is called the **electrochemical potential** (μ) of an ion. The electrochemical potential difference of X^+ across the membrane is defined as

$$\Delta\mu(X^+) = \mu_A(X^+) - \mu_B(X^+) = RT\ln\frac{[X^+]_A}{[X^+]_B} \quad (2\text{-}1)$$
$$+ zF(E_A - E_B)$$

where

$\Delta\mu$	= electrochemical potential difference of the ion between sides A and B of the membrane
R	= ideal gas constant
T	= absolute temperature
$\ln\dfrac{[X^+]_A}{[X^+]_B}$	= natural logarithm of concentration ratio of X^+ on the two sides of the membrane
z	= charge number of the ion (+ 2 for Ca^{2+}, -1 for Cl, etc.)
F	= Faraday's number
$E_A - E_B$	= electrical potential difference across the membrane

The first term on the right-hand side of equation 2-1, $RT\ln[X^+]_A/[X^+]_B$, is the tendency of X^+ ions to move from A to B *because of the concentration difference,* and the second term, $zF(E_A - E_B)$, is the tendency of the ions to move from A to B *because of the electrical potential difference.* The first term represents the potential energy difference between a mole of X^+ ions on side A and a mole of X^+ ions on side B as a result of the concentration difference. The second term represents the potential energy difference between a mole of X^+ ions on side A and a mole of X^+ ions on side B caused by the electrical potential difference between A and B. Thus, $\Delta\mu(X^+)$ *describes the difference in potential energy that exists between a mole of X^+ ions on side A and a mole of X^+ ions on side B that results from both concentration and electrical potential differences; hence the name* **electrochemical potential difference.** The unit of electrochemical potential, and of both terms on the right-hand side of equation 2-1, is *energy/mole.*

The X^+ ions tend to move spontaneously from a higher to a lower electrochemical potential. We defined $\Delta\mu$ as the electrochemical potential of the ion on side A minus that on side B. If $\Delta\mu$ is positive, the ions tend to move from A to B; if $\Delta\mu$ is zero, there is no net tendency for the ions to move at all; if $\Delta\mu$ is negative, the ions tend to move from side B to side A.

If μ_A is greater than μ_B, ions tend to flow spontaneously *from side A to side B. To cause ions to flow from B to A, work*

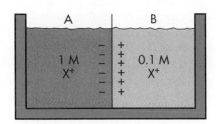

■ **Fig. 2-1** X^+ is present at 1 M in chamber A and at 0.1 M in chamber B. A concentration force for X^+ tends to cause X^+ to flow from A to B. However, chamber A is electrically negative with respect to chamber B, so an electrical force tends to cause X^+ to flow from B to A.

must be done. This work is expressed in equation 2-1: $\mu_A(X^+) - \mu_B(X^+)$. $\mu_A - \mu_B$ is the minimal amount of work that must be done to cause 1 mole of ions to flow from B to A in Fig. 2-1. Conversely, when ions flow from A to B, energy is dissipated. *This energy can be harnessed to perform work.* The maximal amount of work that can be done by 1 mole of ions flowing from A to B is μ_A to μ_B. *An electrochemical potential difference of an ion across a membrane thus represents potential energy that can be harnessed to perform work.*

What sort of work can be done by the electrochemical potential energy stored in an ion gradient? In Chapter 1, we saw that the electrochemical potential of the Na^+ gradient across the plasma membrane powers the secondary active transport of sugars and amino acids. In mitochondria, the action of the electron transport enzymes creates an electrochemical potential gradient of H^+ across the mitochondrial inner membrane. The H^+ ions flow back into the mitochondrial matrix via the ATP synthase enzyme complex in the mitochondrial inner membrane. The ATP synthase uses the energy released by the H^+ ions to drive the synthesis of ATP. Drugs, such as the poison **dinitrophenol,** that increase the permeability of the mitochondrial inner membrane to H^+ cause the H^+ gradient to collapse and prevent the synthesis of ATP.

Electrochemical Equilibrium and the Nernst Equation

In equation 2-1, $\Delta\mu$ may be thought of as the net force on the ion, whereas $RT \ln[X^+]_A/[X^+]_B$ is the force caused by the concentration difference, and $zF(E_A - E_B)$ is the force caused by the electrical potential difference. *When the latter two forces are equal and opposite,* $\Delta\mu = 0$, *and there is no net force on the ion.* When there is no net force on the ion, no net movement of the ion occurs, and the ion is said to be in **electrochemical equilibrium** across the membrane. *At equilibrium,* $\Delta\mu = 0$. From equation 2-1, therefore, at equilibrium:

$$RT\ln\frac{[X^+]_A}{[X^+]_B} + zF\,(E_A - E_B) = 0 \qquad (2\text{-}2)$$

Solving for $E_A - E_B$, we obtain

$$E_A - E_B = -\frac{RT}{zF} \ln \frac{[X^+]_A}{[X^+]_B} = \frac{RT}{zF} \ln \frac{[X^+]_B}{[X^+]_A} \qquad (2\text{-}3)$$

Equation 2-3 is called the **Nernst equation.** Because the condition of equilibrium was assumed in its derivation, *the Nernst equation is satisfied only for ions at equilibrium.* The equation is used to compute the electrical potential difference, $E_A - E_B$, *required to produce an electrical force,* $zF(E_A - E_B)$, *that is equal and opposite to the concentration force,* $RT/zF \ln[X^+]_A/[X^+]_B$.

Use of the Nernst equation. In using the Nernst equation, it is often convenient to convert the equation to a form that involves logarithm to the base 10 (log) rather than natural logarithms (ln). The formula for this conversion is ln y = 2.303 log y. Because biological electrical potentials are usually expressed in millivolts (mV), the units of R may be selected so that RT/F comes out in millivolts. At 29.2° C, the quantity 2.303 RT/F is equal to 60 mV. Because this quantity is proportional to the absolute temperature, it changes by approximately 1/273 (0.36%) for each centigrade degree. Thus, the value of 60 mV for 2.303 RT/F holds approximately for most experimental conditions in biology, and a useful form of the Nernst equation is

$$E_A - E_B = \frac{-60\text{ mV}}{z} \log \frac{[X^+]_A}{[X^+]_B} = \frac{60\text{ mV}}{z} \log \frac{[X^+]_B}{[X^+]_A} \qquad (2\text{-}4)$$

Examples of uses of the Nernst equation

Example 1   In Fig. 2-2, K^+ is 10 times more concentrated in chamber A than in chamber B. The following is a calculation of the electrical potential difference *that must exist between the chambers for K^+ to be in equilibrium across the* membrane. Because we have specified that K^+ should be in equilibrium, the Nernst equation will hold:

$$E_A - E_B = \frac{-60\text{ mV}}{+1} \log \frac{[K^+]_A}{[K^+]_B} = -(60\text{ mV}) \log \frac{0.1}{0.01}$$
$$= 60\text{ mV} \log (10) = 60\text{ mV} \qquad (2\text{-}5)$$

The Nernst equation tells us that at *equilibrium,* side A must be 60 mV negative relative to side B. We can see that this polarity is correct because the electrical force tends to drive K^+ from B to A, which counteracts the tendency for K^+ to move from A to B because of the concentration difference.

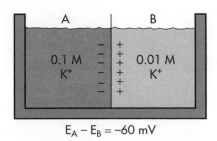

$$E_A - E_B = -60\text{ mV}$$

■ **Fig. 2-2**   A membrane separates chambers containing different K^+ concentrations. At an electrical potential difference $(E_A - E_B)$ of –60 mV, K^+ is in electrochemical equilibrium across the membrane.

This example shows that *an electrical potential difference of about 60 mV is required to balance a 10-fold concentration difference of a univalent ion.* This example thus provides a useful rule of thumb.

Example 2. When ions are not in equilibrium, the Nernst equation can be used to predict the direction in which ions will flow. For example, in Fig. 2-3 the Nernst equation can help decide whether HCO_3^- is in equilibrium. If HCO_3^- is not in equilibrium, the Nernst equation can predict the direction of net flow of HCO_3^-.

First, we must see if HCO_3^- is in equilibrium. The Nernst equation tells us the electrical potential difference, $E_A - E_B$, that will just balance the concentration difference of HCO_3^- across the membrane:

$$E_A - E_B = \frac{-60 \text{ mV}}{-1} \log \frac{[HCO_3^-]_B}{[HCO_3^-]_A}$$
$$= + (60 \text{ mV}) \log \frac{1}{0.1}$$
$$= + 60 \text{ mV} \log (10) = + 60 \text{ mV} \qquad (2\text{-}6)$$

Thus, a potential difference of +60 mV between A and B would just balance the tendency of HCO_3^- to move from A to B because of its concentration difference. However, in our example, $E_A - E_B$ is *actually* 100 mV. HCO_3^- is not in equilibrium. Now we can predict the direction in which HCO_3^- will flow. Although the electrical force is oriented in the right direction to balance the concentration force, it is 40 mV *larger* than it needs to be to just balance the concentration force. Because the electrical force on HCO_3^- is larger than the concentration force, the electrical force will determine the direction of net HCO_3^- movement. Net HCO_3^- flow will occur from B to A.

In brief, the Nernst equation can be used to predict the direction that ions tend to flow:

1. If the potential difference measured across a membrane is *equal* to the potential difference calculated from the Nernst equation for a particular ion, that ion is in *electrochemical equilibrium* across

the membrane, and no net flow of that ion will occur across the membrane.

2. If the measured electrical potential is of the same sign (positive or negative) as that calculated from the Nernst equation for a particular ion but is *larger* in magnitude than the calculated value, the electrical force is larger than the concentration force. Therefore, net movement of that particular ion tends to occur in the direction *determined by the electrical force.* Figure 2-3 meets this condition.

3. When the electrical potential difference is of the same sign but is *numerically* less than that calculated from the Nernst equation for a particular ion, the concentration force is larger than the electrical force. Therefore, net movement of that ion tends to occur in the direction *determined by the concentration difference.*

4. If the sign of the electrical potential difference measured across the membrane is opposite to that predicted by the Nernst equation for a particular ion, the electrical and concentration forces are in the same direction. Thus, that ion *cannot be in equilibrium,* and it will tend to flow in the direction determined by both electrical and concentration forces.

Gibbs-Donnan Equilibrium

The cytoplasm of a cell typically contains proteins, organic polyphosphates, nucleic acids, and other ionized substances that cannot permeate the plasma membrane. Most of these impermeant intracellular ions are *negatively charged* at physiological pH. The steady-state properties of this mixture of permeant and impermeant ions are described by the **Gibbs-Donnan equilibrium.**

Figure 2-4 *(A)* represents a model of a cell with impermeant anions. A membrane separates a solution of KCl from a solution of KY. Y^- is an anion to which the membrane is completely impermeable. The membrane is permeable to water, K^+, and Cl^-. Suppose that initially chamber A contains a 0.1 M solution of KY and that chamber B contains an equal volume of 0.1 M KCl. Because $[Cl^-]_B$ exceeds $[Cl^-]_A$, Cl^- flows from chamber B to chamber A. Negatively charged Cl^- ions flowing from side B to side A will create an electrical potential difference (side A negative) that will then cause K^+ also to flow from side B to side A. Given enough time, K^+ and Cl^- will come into equilibrium. At equilibrium, both $\Delta\mu_{K^+}$ and $\Delta\mu_{Cl^-}$ must equal zero. When both K^+ and Cl^- are at equilibrium,

$$[K^+]_A[Cl^-]_A = [K^+]_B[Cl^-]_B \qquad (2\text{-}7)$$

Equation 2-7 is called the **Donnan relation** or the **Gibbs-Donnan equation** and it holds for any univalent cation and anion pair in equilibrium between the two chambers. If other univalent ions that could attain an equilibrium distribution were present, the same reasoning and an equation similar to equation 2-7 would apply to cation-anion pairs of these ions also.

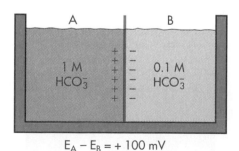

$$E_A - E_B = + 100 \text{ mV}$$

■ **Fig. 2-3**   A membrane separates chambers that contain different HCO_3^- concentrations. $E_A - E_B$ = +100 mV. HCO_3^- is not in electrochemical equilibrium. If $E_A - E_B$ were +60 mV, HCO_3^- would be in equilibrium. $E_A - E_B$ (+100 mV) is stronger than it needs to be (+60 mV) to just balance the tendency for HCO_3^- to move from A to B because of its concentration difference. Thus, net movement of HCO_3^- from B to A will occur.

The derivation of the Gibbs-Donnan equation follows from the definition of electrochemical potential. When both K^+ and Cl^- have reached equilibrium, the electrochemical potential difference of each ion across the membrane will be zero. Recalling that $z = 1$ for K^+ and $z = 1$ for Cl^-,

$$\Delta\mu_{K^+} = RT \ln \frac{[X^+]_A}{[X^+]_B} + F(E_A - E_B) = 0$$

$$\Delta\mu_{Cl^-} = RT \ln \frac{[Cl^-]_A}{[Cl^-]_B} - F(E_A - E_B) = 0$$

Adding these two equations and doing some algebra yields

$$\ln \frac{[K^+]_A}{[K^+]_B} = -\ln \frac{[Cl^-]_A}{[Cl^-]_B} = \ln \frac{[Cl^-]_B}{[Cl^-]_A}$$

which gives

$$\frac{[K^+]_A}{[K^+]_B} = \frac{[Cl^-]_B}{[Cl^-]_A}, \text{ so that } [K^+]_A[Cl^-]_A = [K^+]_B[Cl^-]_B$$

For the model situation we are considering, application of the Gibbs-Donnan equation will result in the final concentrations shown in Fig. 2-4 *(B)*.

In this Gibbs Donnan equilibrium, both K^+ and Cl^- (but not Y^-) are in electrochemical equilibrium. Because they are in electrochemical equilibrium, both K^+ and Cl^- satisfy the Nernst equation. Therefore, we can use the Nernst equation

to calculate the equilibrium transmembrane potential difference for either K^+ or Cl^-. Applying the Nernst equation to either K^+ or Cl^- results in

$$E_A - E_B = -60 \text{ mV} \log(2) = -18 \text{ mV} \tag{2-8}$$

The presence of the impermeant Y^- anions results in a negative electrical potential in the chamber that contains them. In a typical cell *the impermeant anions in the cytoplasm contribute about −10 mV to the resting membrane potential of the cytoplasm relative to the extracellular fluid.*

Note that only the permeant ions (K^+ and Cl^- in this example) attain equilibrium. The impermeant anion, Y^-, cannot reach an equilibrium distribution. It may not be evident that water also will not achieve equilibrium, unless provision is made for that to occur. The sum of the concentrations of K^+ and Cl^- ions on side A in the preceding example exceeds that on side B. *This is a general property of Gibbs-Donnan equilibria.* When the impermeant Y^- is taken into account as well, the total concentration of osmotically active ions is considerably greater on side A than on side B. Water will tend to flow by osmosis from side B to side A until the total osmotic pressure of the two solutions is equal. Then, however, ions will flow to set up a new Gibbs-Donnan equilibrium, and this requires that there be more osmotically active ions on the side with Y. All the water from side B will end up on side A unless water is restrained from moving.

Water can be restrained from moving by enclosing the solution on side A in a rigid container (Fig. 2-5). Then, as fluid flows from side B to side A, pressure will build up in chamber A. This pressure will oppose further osmotic water flow. The pressure in chamber A at equilibrium will be equal to the difference between the total osmotic pressures of the solutions in chambers A and B.

An example of a structure that restrains the movement of water is the rigid cell wall of plant cells. The cell wall allows turgor pressure to build up in the cell and partly compensates for the osmotic effects of the Gibbs-Donnan equilibrium. If

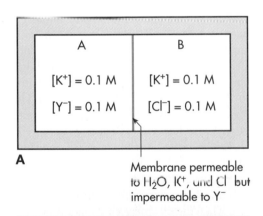

A

Membrane permeable to H_2O, K^+, and Cl^- but impermeable to Y^-

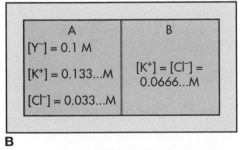

B

■ **Fig. 2-4** **A,** Before a Gibbs-Donnan equilibrium is established, a membrane separates two aqueous compartments. The membrane is permeable to water, K^+, and Cl^- but impermeable to Y^-. **B,** Ion concentrations after Gibbs-Donnan equilibrium has been attained.

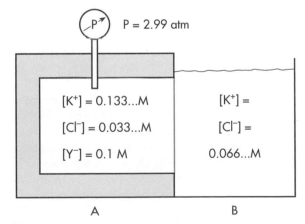

■ **Fig. 2-5** A hydrostatic pressure of 2.99 atmospheres is required to prevent water from flowing from chamber B to chamber A in the Gibbs-Donnan equilibrium in Fig. 2-4. This 2.99 atmosphere is equal to the osmotic pressure in chamber A minus that in chamber B.

a cell wall were not present, the Gibbs-Donnan equilibrium would cause osmotic pressure in the cytoplasm to build up in excess of the osmotic pressure in the extracellular fluid. This build-up of pressure would threaten the maintenance of the normal cellular volume. Animal cells, which do not have cell walls, have evolved other ways that involve ion transport processes to deal with the osmotic consequences of the Gibbs-Donnan equilibrium, which are discussed in the next section.

Regulation of Cell Volume

Both K^+ and Cl^- are nearly in equilibrium across many plasma membranes. Their distribution is influenced by the predominantly negatively charged impermeant ions, such as proteins and nucleotides, in the cytoplasm. This being the case, why does the osmotic imbalance discussed previously not cause animal cells to swell and finally burst? One reason is that *these cells actively pump Na^+ out of the cytoplasm into the extracellular fluid.* The extrusion of Na^+ decreases the osmotic pressure of the cytoplasm and increases that of the extracellular fluid. Much of the pumping of Na^+ is accomplished by the Na^+,K^+-ATPase in the plasma membrane. The Na^+,K^+-ATPase splits a molecule of ATP and uses some of the energy released to extrude three Na^+ from the cytoplasm and to pump two K^+ into the cell. Whereas K^+ is only slightly removed from an equilibrium distribution, Na^+ is pumped out against a large electrochemical potential difference.

When the ATP production of a cell is compromised (such as in the presence of metabolic inhibitors or low O_2 levels), or when the Na^+,K^+-ATPase is specifically inhibited, Na^+ enters the cell more rapidly than it can be pumped out. As a result, the cell swells.

The plasma membranes of red blood cells of patients with **hereditary spherocytosis** (HS) are about three times more permeable to Na^+ than are red cells of normal individuals. The level of Na^+,K^+-ATPase in the erythrocyte membranes of HS patients is also substantially elevated. When HS red blood cells have sufficient glucose to maintain normal ATP levels, they extrude Na^+ as rapidly as it diffuses into the cell cytosol. Hence the red blood cell volume is maintained. However, when HS erythrocytes are delayed in the venous sinuses of the spleen, where glucose and ATP are present at low levels, the intracellular ATP concentration falls. Therefore, Na^+ cannot be pumped out by the Na^+,K^+-ATPase as rapidly as it enters. The red blood cells swell owing to the osmotic effect of elevated intracellular Na^+ concentration. The spleen targets these swollen erythrocytes for destruction, and, as a consequence, HS patients become anemic.

RESTING MEMBRANE POTENTIALS

Communication between nerve cells depends on an electrical disturbance, called an **action potential,** that is propagated in the plasma membrane of the nerve cell. In striated muscle, an action potential propagates rapidly over the entire cell surface and allows the cell to contract synchronously. The action potential in nerve and muscle cells and the ionic mechanisms that account for its properties are discussed in Chapter 3.

All cells that can produce action potentials have sizable resting membrane potentials (cytoplasm negative) across their plasma membranes. Inexcitable cells also have negative resting membrane potentials, but these potentials are smaller in magnitude than those of excitable cells.

The resting membrane potential of a skeletal muscle cell is about –90 mV. By convention, we express membrane potential difference as the voltage in the cytoplasm minus that in the extracellular fluid. A negative value denotes that the cytoplasm is electrically negative relative to the extracellular fluid. The resting membrane potential is necessary for the cell to fire an action potential.

Ions that are actively transported are not in electrochemical equilibrium across the plasma membrane. As shown later in the chapter, the flow of ions across the plasma membrane, down their electrochemical potential gradients, is directly responsible for generating much of the resting membrane potential. To understand how the electrochemical potential gradient of an ion gives rise to a transmembrane difference in electrical potential, let us first consider a model system known as a **concentration cell.**

Concentration Cells

In Fig. 2-6, the membrane that separates chambers A and B is permeable to cations but not to anions. Initially, no electrical potential difference exists across the membrane. K^+ flows from A to B because of the concentration force acting on it. Cl^- has the same force on it, but it cannot flow because the membrane is impermeable to anions. The flow of K^+ from A to B will transfer net positive charge to side B and leave a very slight excess of negative charges behind on side A. *Side A will thus become electrically negative to side B* (Fig. 2-6). This electrical force is in direct opposition to the concentration force on K^+. The more K^+ that flows, the larger will be the opposing electrical force. *Net K^+ flow will stop when the electrical force just balances the concentration force,* for example when the electrical potential difference is equal to the equilibrium (Nernst) potential for K^+. That is, when

$$E_A - E_B = \frac{-60 \text{ mV}}{+1} \log \frac{[K^+]_A}{[K^+]_B}$$

$$= -(60 \text{ mV}) \log \frac{0.1}{0.01} = -60 \text{ mV} \qquad (2\text{-}9)$$

Only a very small amount of K^+ flows from A to B before equilibrium is reached. This amount of K^+ is small because the separation of positive and negative charges across the membrane requires a large amount of work. The potential difference that builds up to oppose further K^+ movement is a manifestation of that work.

The K^+ concentration difference in this example acts like a battery. The natural tendency for any ion that can flow is

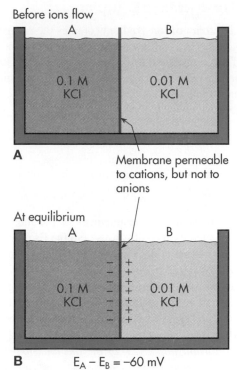

Before ions flow

At equilibrium

$E_A - E_B = -60$ mV

■ **Fig. 2-6 A,** A concentration cell. A membrane, which is permeable to cations but not to anions, separates KCl solutions of different concentrations. **B,** The concentration cell after electrochemical equilibrium has been established. The flow of an infinitesimal amount of K^+ generated an electrical potential difference across the membrane that is equal to the equilibrium potential for K^+.

to seek equilibrium; thus, K^+ tends to flow until its equilibrium potential difference is established. As explained later, when more than one type of ion can permeate a membrane, *each ion "strives" to make the transmembrane potential difference equal to its equilibrium potential. The more permeant the ion, the greater is its ability to force the electrical potential difference toward its equilibrium potential.*

Distribution of Ions Across Plasma Membranes

In most tissues, a number of ions are not in equilibrium between the extracellular fluid and the cytoplasm. Table 2-1

lists the concentrations of Na^+, K^+, and Cl^- in the extracellular fluid and in the cytoplasmic water of frog skeletal muscle. Intracellular ion concentrations for mammalian muscle are similar to those for frog muscle.

Cl^- is nearly in equilibrium across the plasma membrane of a skeletal muscle cell. We know this because the equilibrium potential of chloride, as calculated from the Nernst equation, is about equal to the measured transmembrane potential difference. K^+ has a concentration force that tends to make it flow out of the cell. The electrical force on K^+ opposes the concentration force. If the $E_{in} - E_{out}$ transmembrane potential in frog muscle were -105 mV (equal to the equilibrium potential for K^+), electrical and concentration forces on K^+ would exactly balance. However, because the actual transmembrane potential is only -90 mV, the concentration force on K^+ is greater than the electrical force. Therefore, K^+ has a net tendency to flow out of the cell.

Na^+ is the ion farthest from an equilibrium distribution. Both the concentration and the electrical forces on Na^+ tend to cause it to flow into the cell. The larger the difference between the measured membrane potential and the equilibrium potential for an ion, the larger is the net force that tends to make that ion flow. We return to this concept later in this chapter, when we discuss how these ions maintain the resting membrane potential.

Active Ion Pumping and Resting Potential

The Na^+,K^+-ATPase located in the plasma membrane uses the energy within the terminal phosphate ester bond of ATP to extrude Na^+ actively from the cell and to take K^+ actively into the cell. The Na^+,K^+-ATPase is responsible for the high intracellular K^+ concentration and the low intracellular Na^+ concentration. Because the pump moves a greater number of Na^+ ions out than K^+ ions in (three Na^+ to two K^+), *it causes a net transfer of positive charge out of the cell and thus contributes to the resting membrane potential. Because it brings about net movement of charge across the membrane, the pump is termed **electrogenic.***

The size of the pump's electrogenic contribution to the resting potential can be estimated by completely inhibiting the pump with a cardiac glycoside, such as **ouabain.** Such studies show that in some cells, the electrogenic Na^+,K^+-ATPase is responsible for a large fraction of the resting

■ **Table 2-1** Distribution of Na^+, K^+, and Cl^- across the plasma membranes of frog muscle and squid axon

	Extracellular fluid (mM)	*Cytoplasm (mM)*	*Approximate equilibrium (mV)*	*Actual resting potential*
Frog muscle				
$[Na^+]$	120	9.2	+67	
$[K^+]$	2.5	140	−105	
$[Cl^-]$	120	3 to 4	−89 to −96	−90
Squid axon				
$[Na^+]$	460	50	+158	
$[K^+]$	10	400	−96	
$[Cl^-]$	540	About 40	About −68	−70

Data from Katz B: *Nerve, muscle, and synapse,* New York, 1966, McGraw-Hill.

potential. In most vertebrate nerve and skeletal muscle cells, however, the direct contribution of the pump to the resting potential is usually small—less than 5 mV. The resting membrane potential in nerve and skeletal muscle results mainly from the diffusion of ions down their electrochemical potential gradients. The ionic gradients are maintained by active ion pumping. In other types of excitable cells, electrogenic pumping of ions may contribute more to the resting membrane potential. In certain smooth muscle cells, for example, the electrogenic effect of the Na^+,K^+-ATPase is responsible for 20 mV or more of the resting membrane potential.

> Cardiac glycosides, such as **digitalis** and related drugs, are able to increase the strength of contraction of the heart (see Chapter 16). These compounds inhibit the Na^+,K^+-ATPase. As a result of this inhibition, the intracellular level of Na^+ in cardiac cells is elevated. Each contraction of the heart is initiated by an increase in the cytosolic concentration of Ca^{2+} (see Chapter 00). For cardiac muscle to relax, Ca^{2+} must be removed from the cytosol. The removal of Ca^{2+} from the cytosol of the cardiac cells is accomplished by its being pumped into the sarcoplasmic reticulum (SR) by a Ca^{2+}-ATPase in the SR membrane and out across the plasma membrane by a plasma membrane Ca^{2+}-ATPase and by Na^+-Ca^{2+} exchangers in the plasma membrane. The Ca^{2+}-ATPase pumps Ca^{2+} into the SR; the Na^+-Ca^{2+} exchangers pump the Ca^{2+} from the SR out across the plasma membrane. (These ion transporters were described in Chapter 1.) Because cardiac glycosides increase the cytosolic Na^+ concentration, the Na^+-Ca^{2+} exchanger is not as effective in extruding Ca^{2+} from the cell. Consequently, the Ca^{2+}-ATPase can accumulate more Ca^{2+} in the SR, so that more Ca^{2+} is released from the SR to power the next cardiac contraction, which is stronger than normal because of the greater peak level of Ca^{2+} in the cytosol.

Generation of Resting Membrane Potential by Ion Gradients

The earlier discussion of concentration cells shows how an ion gradient can act as a battery. When a number of ions are distributed across a membrane, and all are removed from electrochemical equilibrium, *each ion will tend to force the transmembrane potential toward its own equilibrium potential, as calculated from the Nernst equation. The more permeable the membrane to a particular ion, the greater strength that ion will have in forcing the membrane potential toward its equilibrium potential.* In frog muscle (Table 2-1), the Na^+ concentration difference can be regarded as a battery that tries to make the transmembrane potential equal to +67 mV. The K^+ concentration difference resembles a battery that attempts to make the transmembrane potential equal to −105 mV. The Cl^- concentration difference resembles a battery trying to make the transmembrane potential equal to −90 mV.

Chord Conductance Equation

How the interplay of ion gradients creates the resting membrane potential (E_m) is illustrated by a simple mathematical model. If we consider the distribution of K^+, Na^+, and Cl^- across the plasma membrane of a cell, the following equation predicts the transmembrane potential difference across the membrane:

$$E_m = \frac{g_K}{\Sigma g} E_K + \frac{g_{Na}}{\Sigma g} E_{Na} + \frac{g_{Cl}}{\Sigma g} E_{Cl} \qquad (2\text{-}10)$$

where

$$\Sigma g = (g_K + g_{Na} + g_{Cl})$$

The gs represent the conductances of the membrane to the ions indicated by the subscripts, and the Es represent the *equilibrium potentials* of the ions denoted by their subscripts. *Conductance is the reciprocal of resistance* ($g = 1/R$). The more permeable the membrane to a particular ion, the greater is the conductance of the membrane to that ion.

Equation 2-10 is called the **chord conductance equation.** *It states that the membrane potential is a weighted average of the equilibrium potentials of all the ions to which the membrane is permeable,* in this case K^+, Na^+, and Cl^-. The weighting factor for each ion is the individual conductance of the ion in question, divided by the total ionic conductance of the membrane, Σg, or the sum of all the individual ion conductances. *Note that the sum of the weighting factors for the ions must equal 1, so that if one weighting factor becomes larger, the others must become smaller. The chord conductance equation shows that the greater the conductance of the membrane to a particular ion, the greater is the ability of that ion to bring the membrane potential toward the equilibrium potential of that ion.*

> The chord conductance equation can be derived fairly simply. As we have seen, if the transmembrane voltage is equal to the equilibrium potential for a particular ion, there will be no net flow of that ion across the membrane. However, if the membrane potential is *not* equal to the equilibrium potential for a given ion, the difference between the membrane potential and the ion's equilibrium potential can be regarded as the driving force for that ion. Because ions bear charge, ionic flow is equivalent to electrical current. Applying Ohm's law, the net current of an ion across a membrane is equal to the conductance (g) of the membrane to the ion, times the driving force on the ion ($E_m - E_{eq}$).
>
> For K^+, Na^+, and Cl^-
>
> $$\begin{aligned} I_K &= g_K (E_m - E_K) \\ I_{Na} &= g_{Na} (E_m - E_{Na}) \\ I_{Cl} &= g_{Cl} (E_m - E_{Cl}) \end{aligned} \qquad (2\text{-}11)$$
>
> where E_m is the membrane potential and I's are currents, gs are conductances, and Es are the equilibrium potentials of the ions denoted by the subscripts.
>
> In the steady state, when E_m is constant, there is no net ionic current across the membrane. If there were net cur-

rent, E_m would change. If we assume that K^+, Na^+, and Cl^- are the only important ions, the requirement that net ionic current be zero leads to

$$I_K + I_{Na} + I_{Cl} = 0 \qquad (2\text{-}12)$$

Substituting from equation 2-11 gives

$$g_K(E_m - E_K) + g_{Na}(E_m - E_{Na}) + g_{Cl}(E_m - E_{Cl}) = 0 \qquad (2\text{-}13)$$

Solving this equation for E_m gives

$$E_m = \frac{g_K}{\Sigma g}E_K + \frac{g_{Na}}{\Sigma g}E_{Na} + \frac{g_{Cl}}{\Sigma g}E_{Cl} \qquad (2\text{-}14)$$

where

$$\Sigma g = g_K + g_{Na} + g_{Cl}.$$

For the frog muscle fiber discussed earlier, the transmembrane potential = –90 mV. The membrane potential is much closer to the equilibrium potential of K^+ (–105 mV) than to Na^+ (+167 mV), because in the resting cell g_K is larger than g_{Na}. The chord conductance equation predicts that, in resting muscle, g_K is about 10 times larger than g_{Na}. This prediction has been confirmed by ion flux measurements with radioactive tracers. In other types of excitable cells, the relationship between g_K and g_{Na} may be somewhat different. Other ions also may play a role in generating the resting membrane potential. Resting membrane potentials vary from about –10 mV in human erythrocytes to around –40 mV in some types of smooth muscle and up to about –90 mV in vertebrate skeletal muscle and cardiac ventricular cells.

We have seen that K^+ has the largest resting conductance and thus has the largest influence on the resting membrane potential. For this reason, changes that occur in the concentration of K^+ in a patient's extracellular fluid will affect the resting membrane potentials of all cells. An increase in extracellular K^+ will partially depolarize cells (decrease the magnitude of the resting membrane potential), whereas a decrease in the level of extracellular K^+ will hyperpolarize cells (increase the magnitude) of the resting membrane potential. Either a depolarization or a hyperpolarization of cardiac cells (see Chapter 37) may lead to **cardiac arrhythmias,** some of which are life-threatening. **Hypokalemia** (low serum K^+) may be a result of long-term use of diuretics. **Hyperkalemia** (elevated serum K^+) occurs in acute renal failure and in a disorder called **hyperkalemic periodic paralysis,** which is characterized by episodes of muscle weakness and flaccid paralysis.

Roles of Na⁺,K⁺-ATPase in Establishing Resting Membrane Potential: Direct versus Indirect

The Na^+,K^+-ATPase establishes gradients of Na^+ and K^+ across the plasma membranes of cells. Because the amount of Na^+ pumped out is larger than the amount of K^+ pumped

in, the pump transfers net charge across the membrane and in this way *contributes directly* to the resting membrane potential. However, in vertebrate skeletal and cardiac muscle and in nerve, this *electrogenic activity of the pump is directly responsible* for only a small fraction of the resting membrane potential. The major portion of the resting membrane potential in these tissues is a result of the diffusion of Na^+ and K^+ down their electrochemical potential gradients, with each ion tending to bring the transmembrane potential toward its own equilibrium potential. This contribution to the resting membrane potential is indirectly caused by the Na^+,K^+-ATPase. The relative magnitudes of the direct and indirect contributions of the Na^+,K^+-ATPase to the resting membrane potential vary from one cell type to another.

SUMMARY

1. An ion tends to flow across a membrane if there is a concentration difference of that ion or an electrical potential difference across the membrane. The electrochemical potential difference ($\Delta\mu$) of an ion across a membrane includes the contributions of both the concentration difference and the electrical potential difference to the tendency of the ion to flow across the membrane.

2. An electrochemical potential difference of an ion across a membrane represents a difference of chemical potential energy. This potential energy difference can be harnessed to do work.

3. An ion that is distributed in equilibrium across a membrane will satisfy the Nernst equation. We can use the Nernst equation to determine whether an ion is in equilibrium or to compute what the electrical potential difference across the membrane would have to be for a particular ion to be in equilibrium.

4. Cytoplasm contains an excess of negative ions that are impermeant to the plasma membrane. A permeant univalent ion pair X^+,Z^- that can attain equilibrium across the membrane will satisfy the Gibbs-Donnan equilibrium, which is represented by the relationship: $[X]_{in}[Z]_{in} = [X]_{out}[Z]_{out}$, where "in" and "out" refer to cytoplasm and extracellular fluid, respectively.

5. All cells have a negative resting membrane potential, that is, the cytoplasm is electrically negative relative to the extracellular fluid. The diffusion of ions across the plasma membrane down their electrochemical potential gradients contributes to the resting membrane potential.

6. The flow of each ion across the plasma membrane tends to bring the resting membrane potential toward the equilibrium potential for that ion. The more conductive the membrane to a particular ion, the greater will be the ability of that ion to bring the membrane potential toward its equilibrium potential. This is described by the chord conductance equation.

7. Three processes contribute to generating the resting membrane potential: (a) ionic diffusion as just described

(major), (b) the electrogenic effect of the Na⁺,K⁺-ATPase (variable in importance), and (c) the Gibbs-Donnan equilibrium (minor in excitable cells).

BIBLIOGRAPHY

Books and monographs

Aidley DJ: *The physiology of excitable cells,* ed 4, Cambridge, 1998, Cambridge University Press.

Hille B: *Ion channels of excitable membranes,* ed 3, Sunderland, Mass, 2001, Sinauer Associates.

Junge D: *Nerve and muscle excitation,* ed 3, Sunderland, Mass, 1992, Sinauer Associates.

Kandel ER, Schwartz JH: *Principles of neural science,* ed 4, New York, 2000, Elsevier Science.

Katz B: *Nerve, muscle, and synapse,* New York, 1966, McGraw-Hill.

Keynes RD, Aidley DJ: *Nerve and muscle,* ed 2, New York, 1991, Cambridge University Press.

Läuger P: *Electrogenic ion pump,* Sunderland, Mass, 1991, Sinauer Associates.

Nicholls JG, Martin AR, Wallace BG: *From neuron to brain,* ed 4, Sunderland, Mass, 2001, Sinauer Associates.

Shepherd GM: *Neurobiology,* ed 3, New York, 1994, Oxford University Press.

chapter three

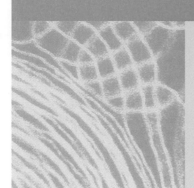

Generation and Conduction of Action Potentials

An **action potential** is a rapid change in the membrane potential followed by a return to the resting membrane potential. The size and shape of action potentials differ considerably from one excitable tissue to another (Fig. 3-1).

- An action potential is propagated with the same shape and size along the whole length of a nerve or muscle cell.
- The action potential is the basis of the signal-carrying ability of nerve cells.
- In muscle cells, an action potential allows the entire length of these long cells to contract almost simultaneously.
- Voltage-dependent ion channel proteins in the plasma membrane are responsible for action potentials.

The action potentials in the cell types shown in Fig. 3-1 differ because these cells have disparate populations of voltage-dependent ion channels.

This chapter describes how action potentials are generated and conducted in cells. Within this general discussion, the diverse action potentials of different excitable cells are also discussed and explained.

MEMBRANE POTENTIALS

Observations of Membrane Potentials

Our current knowledge about the ionic mechanisms of action potentials comes from experiments on the squid giant axon. The large diameter (up to 0.5 mm) of the squid giant axon makes it a convenient model for electrophysiological research with intracellular electrodes. The frog sartorius muscle is another useful preparation.

When a microelectrode (tip diameter <0.5 μm) is inserted through the plasma membrane of a single muscle cell of a frog sartorius muscle, a potential difference is observed between the tip of the microelectrode inside the cell and an electrode placed outside the cell. The internal electrode is approximately 90 mV negative with respect to the external electrode. This 90 mV potential difference is the **resting membrane potential** of the muscle fiber. By convention, membrane potentials are expressed as the intracellular poten-

tial minus the extracellular potential; therefore, the membrane potential of the frog sartorius muscle cell is –90 mV. In the absence of perturbing influences, the resting membrane potential remains at –90 mV. The resting potential of squid giant axons, and of many mammalian neurons, is about –70 mV.

Subthreshold Responses: The Local Response

Figure 3-2 illustrates the results of an experiment in which the membrane potential of an axon of a shore crab is perturbed by passing rectangular pulses of current across the plasma membrane. Current pulses are **depolarizing** or **hyperpolarizing,** depending on the direction of current flow. The terms *depolarizing* and *hyperpolarizing* may be confusing. A change of the membrane potential from –90 mV to –70 mV is a depolarization because it decreases the potential difference, or polarization, across the cell membrane. Conversely, a change in the membrane potential from –90 mV to –100 mV *increases* the polarization of the membrane; this change in potential is a hyperpolarization.

The larger the current that passes across the plasma membrane, the larger is the change in the membrane potential. Figure 3-2 shows that when the depolarizing current pulses reach above a certain **threshold** strength, the cell fires an action potential.

When subthreshold current pulses are passed across the plasma membrane, the size of the potential change *depends on the distance of the recording electrode from the point of current passage* (Fig. 3-3, *A*). *The closer the recording electrode to the site of current passage, the larger is the potential change.* The size of the potential change is found to *decrease exponentially with distance* from the site of current passage (Fig. 3-3, *B*). The potential change is said to be **conducted with decrement.** The distance over which the potential change decreases to 1/e (37%) of its maximal value is called the **length constant** or space constant. (*e* is the base of natural logarithms and is equal to 2.7182.) *A length constant of 1 to 3 mm is typical for mammalian nerve or muscle*

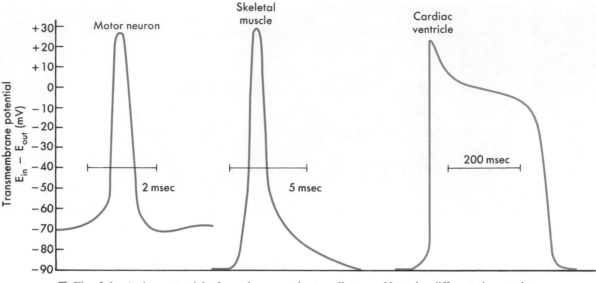

■ **Fig. 3-1**   Action potentials from three vertebrate cell types. Note the different time scales. (Redrawn from Flickinger CJ et al: *Medical cell biology,* Philadelphia, 1979, WB Saunders.)

cells. Because these potential changes are observed mainly near the site of current passage and the changes are not propagated along the length of the cell (as are action potentials), they are called **local responses.**

Action Potentials

If progressively larger depolarizing current pulses are applied to the plasma membrane, a **threshold membrane potential** can be reached at which a different sort of response, the action potential, occurs (Figs. 3-2 and 3-4). For example, the threshold value for the squid giant axon is near –55 mV. When the membrane potential reaches this value, an action potential is triggered. The action potential differs from the local response in two important ways: (1) it is a *much larger response,* in which the polarity of the membrane potential actually reverses (the cell interior becomes positive with respect to the exterior); and (2) *the action potential is propagated without decrement* down the entire length of the nerve or muscle fiber. *The size and shape of an action potential remain the same* as it travels along the fiber. Unlike a local response, its size does not decrease with distance. In addition, when a stimulus larger than the threshold stimulus is applied, the size and shape of the action potential still do not change; the size of the action potential does not increase with greater stimulus strength. A stimulus either fails to elicit an action potential (a subthreshold stimulus that leads to a local response) or it produces a full-sized action potential. For this reason, the action potential is described as an **all-or-none** response.

IONIC MECHANISMS OF ACTION POTENTIALS

Action Potentials in Squid Giant Axon

The form of an action potential of a squid giant axon is shown in Fig. 3-4. When the membrane is depolarized to the threshold, *depolarization becomes explosive.* This depolarization completely depolarizes the membrane and even **overshoots,** so that the membrane potential reverses from negative to positive. The peak of the action potential reaches about +50 mV. The membrane potential then returns toward the resting membrane potential almost as rapidly as it was depolarized. After repolarization, a transient hyperpolarization occurs that is known as the **hyperpolarizing afterpotential.** The action potential persists for about 4 msec. The following section discusses the ionic currents that cause the phases of the action potential.

Ionic Mechanism of Action Potential in the Squid Giant Axon

In Chapter 2, we saw that the resting membrane potential was the weighted sum of the equilibrium potentials for Na^+, K^+, Cl^-, and so forth. The weighting factor for each ion is the fraction that its conductance contributes to the total ionic conductance of the membrane (the chord conductance equation, equation 2-10). In the squid giant axon, the resting membrane potential (E_m) is about –70 mV. The equilibrium potential of K^+ (E_K) is about –100 mV in the squid axon. An increase in g_K would therefore hyperpolarize the membrane, while a decrease in g_K would tend to depolarize the membrane. E_{Cl} is about –70 mV, so an increase in g_{Cl} would stabilize E_m at –70 mV. An increase in g_{Na} of sufficient magnitude would cause depolarization and reversal of the membrane polarity, because E_{Na} is about +65 mV in the squid giant axon.

In a giant squid axon, the action potential is caused by successive increases in plasma membrane conductance to sodium and potassium ions. The conductance to Na^+, g_{Na}, increases very rapidly during the early part of the action potential (Fig. 3-5). Sodium conductance peaks at about the same time that the action potential peaks, and then it decreases rapidly. The potassium conductance, g_K, increases more slowly, peaks at about the middle of the repolarization phase, and then returns more slowly to resting levels.

As described in Chapter 2, the chord conductance equation shows that the membrane potential is a result of the opposing tendencies (a) of the K$^+$ gradient to bring the resting membrane potential toward the equilibrium potential for K$^+$, and (b) of the Na$^+$ gradient to bring the resting membrane potential toward the equilibrium potential for Na$^+$. *Increasing the conductance of either ion will increase its ability to pull the resting membrane potential toward its equilibrium potential.* The rapid increase in g$_{Na}$ during the early phase of the action potential causes the membrane potential to move toward the equilibrium potential for Na$^+$ (+65 mV). The peak of the action potential reaches only about +50 mV, because g$_{Na}$ quickly decreases toward resting levels, and because the increase in g$_K$, which occurs later, provides an opposing tendency to the depolarization.

The rapid return of the membrane potential toward the resting potential is caused by the rapid decrease of g$_{Na}$ and

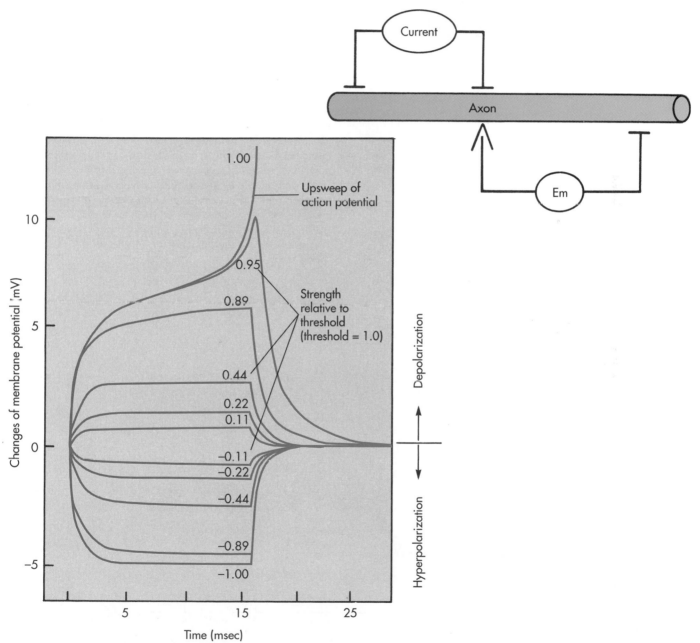

■ **Fig. 3-2** Responses of an axon of the shore crab to rectangular pulses of hyperpolarizing or depolarizing current. The change in membrane potential as recorded by an extracellular electrode is shown as a function of time. The numbers on the curves give the strength of the current relative to threshold. Note that when stimulated to threshold, the axon fires an action potential. (Redrawn from Hodgkin AL, Rushton WAH: *Proc R Soc* B133:97, 1946.)

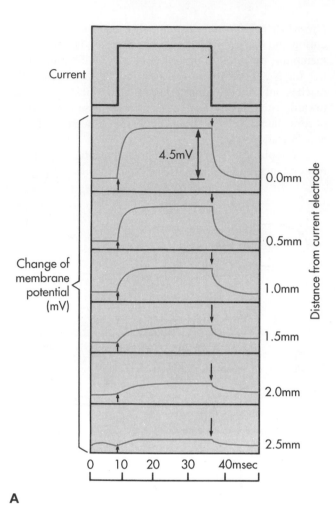

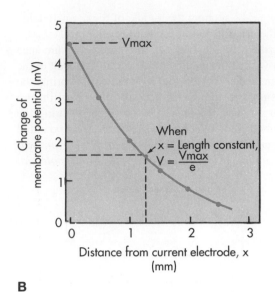

Current

4.5mV

0.0mm

0.5mm

Change of
membrane
potential
(mV)

1.0mm

1.5mm

2.0mm

2.5mm

0   10   20   30   40msec

A

Distance from current electrode

Vmax

Change of
membrane potential (mV)

When
x = Length constant,

$$V = \frac{V_{max}}{e}$$

Distance from current electrode, x
(mm)

B

■ **Fig. 3-3   A,** Responses of an axon of a shore crab to a subthreshold rectangular pulse of current recorded extracellularly by
an electrode located different distances from the current-passing
electrode. As the recording electrode is moved farther from the
point of stimulation, the response of the membrane potential is
slower and smaller. **B,** The maximal change in membrane
potential from **A** is plotted versus the distance from the point of
current passage. The distance over which the response falls to 1/e
(37%) of the maximal response is called the length constant. (**A**
Redrawn from Hodgkin AL, Rushton WAH: *Proc R Soc* B133:97,
1946.)

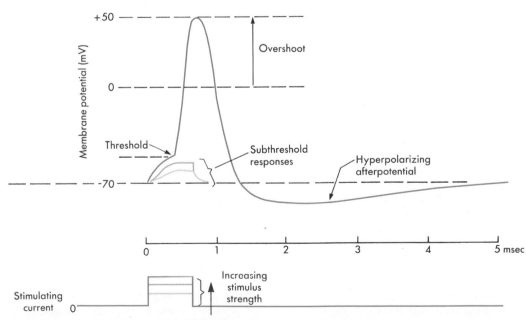

+50

Overshoot

0

Membrane potential (mV)

Threshold

Subthreshold
responses

Hyperpolarizing
afterpotential

−70

0   1   2   3   4   5 msec

Increasing
stimulus
strength

Stimulating
current   0

■ **Fig. 3-4**   Responses of the membrane potential of a squid giant axon to increasing pulses of
depolarizing current. When the cell is depolarized to threshold, it fires an action potential.

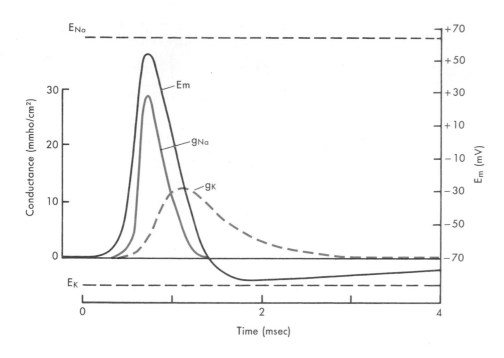

■ **Fig. 3-5** The action potential (E_m) of a squid giant axon is shown on the same time scale with the associated changes in the conductance of the axon membrane to sodium and potassium ions. (Redrawn from Hodgkin AL, Huxley AF: *J Physiol* 117:500, 1952.)

the continued increase in g_K. These conductance changes decrease the size of the Na$^+$ term in the chord conductance equation, and they increase the size of the K$^+$ term. During the hyperpolarizing afterpotential, when the membrane potential is actually more negative than the resting potential (more polarized), g_{Na} has returned to baseline levels, but g_K remains elevated above resting levels. Thus the resting membrane potential is pulled closer to the K$^+$ equilibrium potential (−100 mV) as long as g_K remains elevated.

Ion Channels and Gates

Hodgkin and Huxley proposed that the ion currents pass through separate Na$^+$ and K$^+$ channels, each with distinct characteristics, in the plasma membrane. Subsequent research supports this interpretation and has determined some of the properties of proteins that form the channels. Also the amino acid sequences of several K$^+$ and Na$^+$ channels have been determined. Research is ongoing and our knowledge of the structure of ion channels is rapidly expanding. Although the three-dimensional structure of the Na$^+$ channel remains unknown, its intramembrane domain is known to consist of several α-helices that span the mebrane and probably surround the ion channel. The Na$^+$ channel has both an **activation gate** and an **inactivation gate,** which accounts for the changes in g_{Na} during an action potential (Fig. 3-6, *A*). Groups of charged amino acid residues that form the activation and inactivation gates have been identified.

In order to enter a channel's narrowest part, known as the **selectivity filter,** an ion must shed most of the water it acquires through hydration. To strip a K$^+$ or Na$^+$ ion of its associated water molecules, negatively polarized amino acid substituents that line the pore of the channel must have a particular geometry; this precise geometry is different for K$^+$ and Na$^+$. In fact, this geometry is believed to confer specificity on an ion channel (Fig. 3-6, *B*).

The structure shown in Fig. 3-6 is characteristic of voltage-gated Na$^+$ and Ca^{2+} channels. The four repeated 6-helix motifs surround a central ion channel whose walls are partly formed by the number 6 helices and whose selectivity filter is formed by the four pore loops. Most votage-gated K$^+$ channels consist of only one of the 6-helix motifs; four such subunits are required to form a functional channel. The subunits of one class of voltage-gated K$^+$ channels contain only the number 5 and 6 helices and the intervening pore loop. The inward rectifier K$^+$ channels (Chapter 15) belong to this class of smaller K$^+$ channels, as does the K$^+$ channel from *Streptomyces lividans,* the high-resolution structure of which has recently been obtained (Fig. 3-7).

Tetrodotoxin (TTX), one of the most potent poisons known, specifically blocks the Na$^+$ channel. TTX binds to the extracellular side of the sodium channel. Tetraethylammonium (TEA$^+$), another poison, blocks the K$^+$ channel. TEA$^+$ enters the K$^+$ channel from the cytoplasmic side and blocks the channel, because TEA is unable to pass through it.

The ovaries of certain species of puffer fish, also known as blowfish, contain TTX. Raw puffer fish is a highly prized delicacy in Japan. Connoisseurs of puffer fish enjoy the tingling numbness of the lips caused by the minuscule quantities of TTX present in the flesh. Sushi chefs who are trained to remove the ovaries safely are licensed by the government to prepare puffer fish. Despite these precautions, each year several people die from eating improperly prepared puffer fish.

Saxitoxin is another blocker of Na$^+$ channels that is produced by reddish-colored dinoflagellates that are responsible for so-called **red tides.** Shellfish eat the dinoflagellates and concentrate saxitoxin in their tissues. A person who eats these shellfish may experience life-threatening paralysis within 30 minutes after the meal.

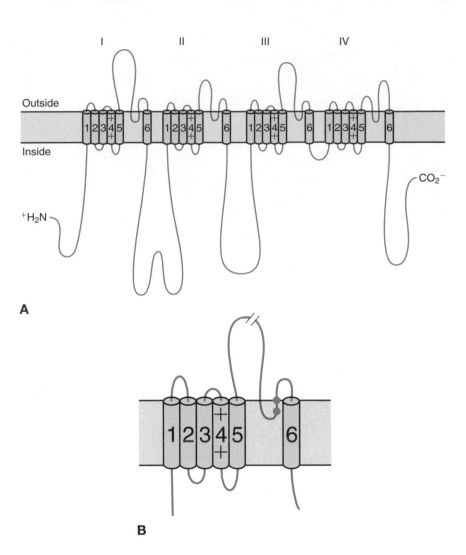

■ **Fig. 3-6**   Model of the voltage-dependent Na²⁺ channel protein. **A,** Two-dimensional model. The cylinders represent transmembrane α-helices. There are four repeats of six-cylinder domains of homologous α-helices. The S4 helices, marked with plus signs, function as voltage sensors, and movements of these helices are responsible for activation (opening) of the channel. The intracellular loop connecting domains III and IV functions as the inactivation gate: after depolarization, with a slight delay, this loop apparently swings up into the mouth of the channel to block ion conduction. **B,** Domain IV. The part of the extracellular loop that connects helices 5 and 6 and that dips into the membrane as the "pore loop" that helps form the selectivity filter of the channel. The residues indicated by solid circles are key determinants of the ionic selectivity of the channel. (**B** Redrawn from Catteral W: *J Bioenerg Biomembr* 28:219, 1996.)

Behavior of Individual Ion Channels

One way to study the behavior of individual ion channels is to incorporate either purified ion channel proteins or bits of membrane into planar lipid bilayers that separate two aqueous compartments. Electrodes placed in the aqueous compartments can then be used to monitor or impose currents and voltages across the membrane. Under some conditions only one, or only a few, ion channel(s) of a particular type may be present in the planar membrane. The ion channels spontaneously oscillate between two conductance states, an open state and a closed state (Fig. 3-8).

Another way to study individual ion channels involves the use of so-called **patch electrodes.** A fire-polished microelectrode is placed against the surface of a cell, and suction is applied to the electrode. A high-resistance seal is formed around the tip of the electrode (Fig. 3-9, *A*). The sealed patch electrode can then be used to monitor the activity of whatever channels happen to be trapped inside the seal. Sometimes, the patch trapped inside the electrode contains more than one functional ion channel of a particular type (Fig. 3-9, *B*).

Both these techniques have contributed greatly to our knowledge about the behavior of ion channels. During an action potential in a skeletal muscle cell, a rapid influx of Na⁺ ions occurs for about 1 msec. The duration of this inward Na⁺ current resembles the duration of the change in the Na⁺ conductance shown in Fig. 3-5. The overall Na⁺ current that flows into the muscle cell is caused by the opening of thousands of Na⁺ channels in response to the depolarization. However, the behavior of each individual Na⁺ channel is actually random, like the behavior of the channels shown in Figs. 3-8 and 3-9. *The probability of each channel being in the open state is increased when the membrane is depolarized to threshold.* In response to a step depolarization of a muscle cell plasma membrane (Fig. 3-10), some of the Na⁺ channels open, some do not open at all, and some open more than once. However, when the currents of a large number of channels are averaged (Fig. 3-10, *B*), it appears as if all the Na⁺ channels open in response to the depolarization and then promptly close. In other words, the "average channel" opens (activates) quickly in response to depolarization: after a short time delay, the channel then closes (inactivates), even though the applied depolarization is maintained.

Action Potentials in Cardiac and Smooth Muscle

Cardiac muscle. An action potential in a cardiac ventricular cell is shown schematically in Fig. 3-1 (see also

Chapter 15). The initial rapid depolarization and overshoot are caused by the rapid entry of Na⁺ into the cell through channels that are very similar to the Na⁺ channels of nerve and skeletal muscle. The Na⁺ channels are called **fast channels.** After the initial depolarization and overshoot, the cardiac ventricular action potential enters a plateau phase. The plateau is caused by another set of channels that is distinct from the fast Na⁺ channels. Because these channels open and close much more slowly than the fast Na⁺ channels, they are sometimes called **slow channels.** The slow channels belong to a particular class of Ca^{2+} channels, called **L-type Ca^{2+} channels.** The Ca^{2+} that enters the ventricular cell through the L-type Ca^{2+} channels during the plateau phase helps to initiate cell contraction by stimulating the release of more Ca^{2+} from the sarcoplasmic reticulum of the cell. The repolarization of the ventricular cell is brought about by the closing of the L-type Ca^{2+} channels and by a much-delayed opening of K⁺ channels. The ionic mechanisms of cardiac action potentials are discussed in more detail in Chapter 15.

Smooth muscle. Action potentials vary considerably among different types of smooth muscle (see Chapter 13). Characteristically, action potentials in smooth muscle have slower rates of depolarization and repolarization and less overshoot than do skeletal muscle action potentials. Many smooth muscle cells lack Na⁺ channels. The depolarizing phase of smooth muscle action potentials is caused primarily by Ca^{2+} channels, like those that contribute to the plateau phase in cardiac cells. Like the cardiac Ca^{2+} channels, these channels open and close slowly. The Ca^{2+} that enters via these channels is often vital for excitation-contraction coupling in smooth muscle, because some smooth muscle cells have little sarcoplasmic reticulum. Repolarization is caused by the closing of the slow Ca^{2+} channels and a simultaneous delayed opening of K⁺ channels.

PROPERTIES OF ACTION POTENTIALS
Voltage Inactivation

If a neuron or skeletal muscle cell is partially depolarized, for example, by increasing the concentration of K⁺ in the extracellular fluid, and is then stimulated to threshold, its action potential has a slower rate of rise and a smaller overshoot than does the action potential of the normally polarized cell. This is a result of two factors: (1) a smaller electrical force driving Na⁺ into the depolarized cell, and (2) voltage

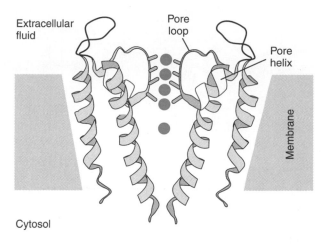

■ **Fig. 3-7** A representation of the structure of the K⁺ channel from *Streptomyces lividans,* a fungus-like bacterium. Each subunit of the channel has two transmembrane α-helices. The channel consists of four subunits; only two of the subunits are shown. The selectivity filter is formed by the pore loops of each of the four subunits. The carbonyl oxygens (green protrusions) coordinate with K⁺ (green balls) ions and thereby cause K⁺ to shed most of its waters of hydration, allowing it to pass through the pore. Shown are four positions within the selectivity filter where K⁺ may be coordinated. The bottom red ball represents a K⁺ ion in the central cavity of the ion channel. The amino acid sequence in the pore domain of this protein is nearly identical with the sequences of the homologous region of all known vertebrate voltage-gated K⁺ channels. (Redrawn from Roux B, MacKinnon R: *Science* 285:100, 1999.)

inactivation of some of the Na⁺ channels. In response to depolarization of the membrane, g_{Na} first increases and then, a short time later, decreases. The decrease in g_{Na} is caused by **voltage inactivation.** In other words, the inactivation gates of Na⁺ channels close soon after the activation gates open. Once the Na⁺ channels are inactivated, the membrane must be repolarized toward the normal resting membrane potential before the channels can be reopened. As the membrane potential is restored toward normal resting levels, more and more of the Na⁺ channels again become capable of being activated.

The explosive depolarizing phase of the action potential may be compared with a chemical explosion. Just as a chemical explosion requires a critical mass of material, *the spike of the action potential can be generated only if a critical number of Na⁺ channels are recruited.* When a cell is partly depolarized, the pool of activatable Na⁺ channels is

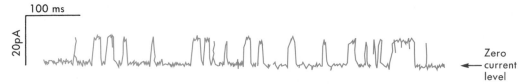

■ **Fig. 3-8** Ionic current through a single ion channel from rat muscle incorporated into a planar lipid bilayer membrane. The channel opens and closes spontaneously. The fraction of time this channel spends in the open state is a function of calcium ion concentration and membrane potential. (From Moczydlowski E, Latorre R: *J Gen Physiol* 82:511, 1983.)

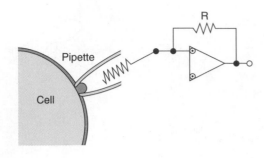

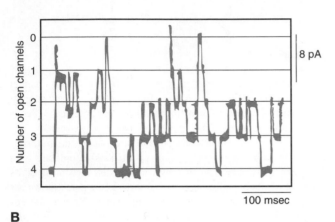

A

B

■ **Fig. 3-9** **A,** Patch electrode and circuitry required to record the ionic currents that flow through the small number of ion channels isolated in the electrode patch. **B,** Current recording from a patch electrode on the plasma membrane of a skeletal muscle cell. The five current levels show that this particular patch contains four different ion channels, each opening and closing independently of the others. (**A** Redrawn from Sigworth FJ, Neher E: *Nature* 287:447, 1980; **B** Redrawn from Hammill OP et al: *Pflügers Arch* 391:85, 1981.)

reduced; consequently, a stimulus may not be able to recruit a sufficient number of Na$^+$ channels to generate an action potential. In effect, this **voltage inactivation** of the action potential results from voltage inactivation of the Na$^+$ channels. *Voltage inactivation of Na$^+$ channels partially accounts for the important properties of excitable cells, such as refractory periods and accommodation.*

Refractory Periods

During much of the action potential, the cell is completely refractory to further stimulation. *When a cell is refractory, it is unable to fire a second action potential, no matter how strongly the cell is stimulated.* This unresponsive state is called the **absolute refractory period** (Fig. 3-11). The cell is refractory because a large fraction of its Na$^+$ channels is voltage inactivated and cannot be reopened until the membrane is repolarized. In this state the critical number of Na$^+$ channels required to produce an action potential cannot be recruited.

During the latter part of the action potential, the cell is able to fire a second action potential, *but a stronger than normal stimulus is required.* This period is called the **relative refractory period.** Early in the relative refractory period, before the membrane potential has returned to the resting potential level, some Na$^+$ channels are still voltage inactivated. Therefore, a stronger than normal stimulus is required to open the critical number of Na$^+$ channels needed to trigger an action potential. Throughout the relative refractory period, the conductance to K$^+$ is elevated, which opposes depolarization of the membrane. This increase in K$^+$ conductance also contributes to the refractoriness.

Accommodation

When a nerve or muscle cell is depolarized slowly, the normal threshold may be passed without an action potential

■ **Fig. 3-10** A patch electrode recorded the currents that flowed in small patches of rat muscle membrane in response to a 10-mV depolarization (trace *A*). Tetraethylammonium was used to block potassium channels that might have been present in the patch. The traces in curve *C* show responses to nine individual 10-mV depolarizations. The tracing in *B* is the average of 300 individual responses. Note that this average response resembles the summed response of thousands of sodium channels, as seen in measurements of whole cell Na$^+$ currents during an action potential. (Redrawn from Sigworth FJ, Neher E: *Nature* 287:447, 1980.)

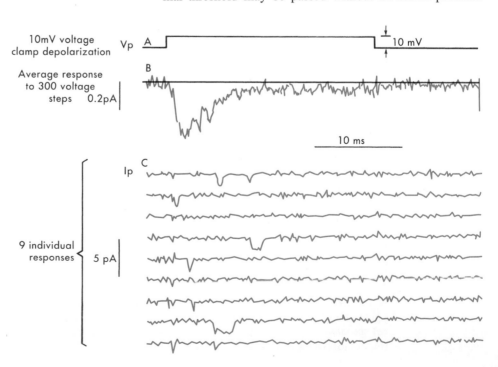

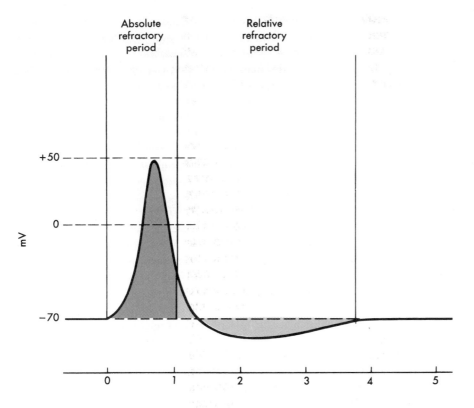

■ Fig. 3-11 The action potential of nerve and the associated absolute and relative refractory periods.

CONDUCTION OF ACTION POTENTIALS

A principal function of neurons is to transmit nerve impulses in the form of action potentials. The axons of the motor neurons of the ventral horn of the spinal cord conduct action potentials from the cell body of the neuron to a number of skeletal muscle fibers. The distance from the motor neuron to one of the muscle fibers it innervates may be longer than 1 m.

Action potentials are conducted along a nerve or muscle fiber by local current flow, just as occurs in electrotonic conduction of subthreshold potential changes. Thus, the same factors that govern the velocity of electrotonic conduction also determine the speed of action potential propagation.

The Local Response: Conduction with Decrement

Figure 3-12, *A* shows the membrane of an axon or muscle fiber that has been depolarized in a small region. In this region, the external surface of the membrane is negative relative to the adjacent membrane, and the internal face of the depolarized membrane is positively charged relative to neighboring internal areas. These potential differences cause **local currents** to flow (Fig. 3-12, *B*), which depolarize the membrane adjacent to the initial site of depolarization. These newly depolarized areas then cause current flows that depolarize other segments of the membrane still farther removed from the initial site of depolarization. This spread of depolarization is called the **local response,** and this mechanism of conduction is known as **electrotonic conduction.**

A subthreshold depolarization will be conducted electrotonically but it will diminish in strength as it moves along

being fired; this property is called **accommodation.** Na+ and K+ channels are both involved in accommodation. During slow depolarization, some of the Na+ channels that are opened by depolarization have enough time to become voltage inactivated before the threshold potential is attained. *If depolarization is slow enough, the critical number of open Na+ channels required to trigger the action potential may never be attained.* In addition, K+ channels open in response to the depolarization. The increased g_K tends to repolarize the membrane, making it still more refractory to depolarization.

In an inherited disorder, called **primary hyperkalemic paralysis,** patients have episodes of painful spontaneous muscle contractions, followed by periods of paralysis of the affected muscles. These symptoms are accompanied by elevated levels of K+ in the plasma and extracellular fluid. Some patients with this disorder have mutations of voltage-gated Na+ channels that result in a decreased rate of voltage inactivation. This results in longer-lasting action potentials in skeletal muscle cells and increased K+ efflux during each action potential. This can raise the extracellular levels of K+.

The elevation of extracellular K+ causes depolarization of skeletal muscle cells. Initially, the depolarization brings muscle cells closer to threshold, so that spontaneous action potentials and contractions are more likely. As depolarization of the cells becomes more marked, the cells accommodate because of the voltage-inactivated Na+ channels. Consequently, the cells become unable to fire action potentials and are unable to contract in response to action potentials in their motor axons.

DEPOLARIZATION

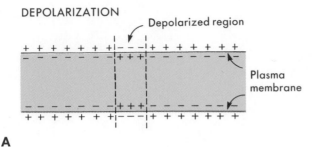

A

SPREAD OF DEPOLARIZATION

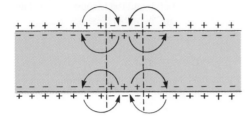

B

■ **Fig. 3-12**   Mechanism of electrotonic spread of depolarization. **A,** The reversal of membrane polarity that occurs with local depolarization. **B,** The local currents that flow to depolarize adjacent areas of the membrane and allow conduction of the depolarization.

the cell. Thus, it is **conducted with decrement.** As shown in Fig. 3-3, *B,* an electrotonically conducted signal dies away to 37% of its maximal strength over a distance of one length constant (about 1 to 2 mm) and decreases to almost nothing over about 10 mm.

How is this length constant determined? A nerve or muscle fiber has some of the properties of an electrical cable. In a perfect cable, the insulation surrounding the core conductor prevents all loss of current to the surrounding medium, so that a signal is transmitted along the cable with undiminished strength (Fig. 3-13). If we compare an unmyelinated

nerve or muscle fiber with an electrical cable, the plasma membrane will be the insulation, while the cytoplasm will be the core conductor. The membrane has a resistance (r_m) much higher than the resistance of the cytoplasm (r_{in}), but (partly because of its thinness) the plasma membrane is not a perfect insulator. *The higher the ratio of r_m to r_{in}, the less current is lost across the plasma membrane, the better the cell can function as a cable, and the longer the distance that a signal can be transmitted electrotonically without significant decrement. r_m/r_{in} determines the length constant of a cell: the length constant is equal to $\sqrt{r_m/r_{in}}$.*

Action Potential as Self-Reinforcing Signal

Many nerve and muscle fibers are much longer than their length constants (1 to 2 mm). Skeletal muscle cells can be as long as 1 to 2 cm; nerve axons can be 1 m in length. *Conduction with decrement will not work for these long cells.* For the action potential to conduct an electrical impulse with undiminished strength along the full length of these cells, the action potential reinforces itself as it is conducted along the fiber. The action potential may be said to be **propagated,** as well as conducted.

Propagation involves the generation of "new" action potentials as they spread along the length of the cell. As we saw in Fig. 3-12, the conduction of the action potential occurs via local circuit currents by the electrotonic mechanism. When the areas on either side of the depolarized region reach threshold, these areas also fire action potentials, which locally reverses the polarity of the membrane potential. The areas of the fiber adjacent to these areas are next brought to threshold by the local current flow, and these areas in turn fire action potentials. In short, propagation involves a cycle of depolarization. This cycle occurs by local current flow followed by generation of an action potential in a region of the cell membrane; this action potential is then conducted along the length of the fiber, with "new" action potentials being generated as they spread. *In this way, the*

■ **Fig. 3-13**   An axon or a muscle fiber resembles an electrical cable. Currents that flow across the membrane resistance (r_m) are lost from the cable. Currents that flow through the longitudinal resistance (r_{in}) carry the electrical signal along the cable. The larger the ratio r_m/r_{in}, the more efficient is signal transmission along the fiber and the larger is the length constant of the cell.

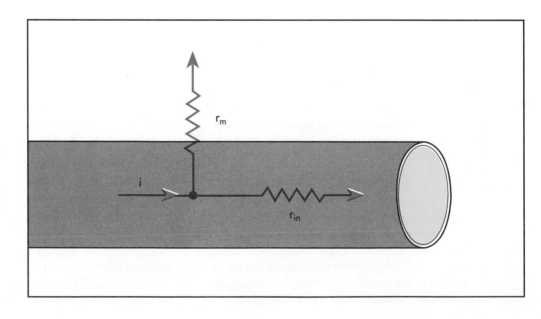

action potentials are regenerated as they spread, and the action potential propagates over long distances and keeps the same size and shape.

Because the shape and size of the action potential usually do not change, *only variations in the frequency of the action potentials can be used as the "code" for information transmission along axons.* The maximal frequency is limited by the duration of the absolute refractory period (about 2 msec) to about 500 impulses per second in large mammalian nerves.

Conduction Velocity

The speed of electrotonic conduction in a nerve or muscle fiber is determined by the electrical properties of the cytoplasm and of the plasma membrane that surrounds the fiber. The same electrical properties determine the velocity of propagation of an action potential. Therefore, although the following discussion focuses on the mechanism of electrotonic conduction, it applies equally well to the mechanism of propagation of the action potential.

Effect of fiber diameter on conduction. Fibers that are larger in diameter have a greater conduction velocity. This effect is principally caused by a decrease in resistance to conduction. As the radius (and hence the cross-sectional area) of a fiber increases, the cytoplasm along the length of the fiber becomes less resistant to conduction. Thus, action potential will be conducted faster along fibers with large diameters.

Effect of myelination on conduction. In vertebrates, certain nerve fibers are coated with **myelin;** such fibers are said to be myelinated. Myelin consists of the plasma membranes of **Schwann cells,** which wrap around and insulate the nerve fiber (Fig. 3-14). The myelin sheath consists of several to more than 100 layers of Schwann cell plasma membranes. Gaps occur in the myelin sheath every 1 to 2 mm. These gaps are known as **nodes of Ranvier,** which are about 1 μm wide. *By altering the electrical properties of the nerve fiber, myelin functions to increase the conduction velocity of the fiber.*

An unmyelinated squid giant axon with a 500-μm diameter has a conduction velocity of 25 m/sec. If conduction velocity were directly proportional to fiber radius, a human nerve fiber with a 10-μm diameter would conduct at a velocity of 0.5 m/sec. With this conduction velocity, a reflex withdrawal of the foot from a hot coal would take about 4 seconds. Although our nerve fibers are much smaller in diameter than are squid giant axons, our reflexes are much faster than 4 seconds. The myelin sheath that surrounds certain vertebrate nerve fibers is responsible for the greatly increased conduction velocity over that of unmyelinated fibers of similar diameters. A 10-μm myelinated fiber has a conduction velocity of about 50 m/sec, which is twice that of the 500-μm squid giant axon. The high conduction velocity permits reflexes that are fast enough to allow us to avoid dangerous stimuli.

How much does myelin contribute to increased conduction velocity? *A myelinated axon has a greater conduction velocity than an unmyelinated fiber that is 100 times larger*

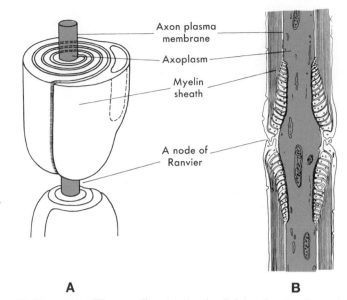

A   **B**

■ **Fig. 3-14**   The myelin sheath. **A,** Schematic drawing of Schwann cells wrapping around an axon to form a myelin sheath. **B,** Drawing of a cross section through a myelinated axon near a node of Ranvier.

in diameter (Fig. 3-15). The myelin sheath increases the velocity of action potential conduction by (1) increasing the length constant of the axon, (2) decreasing the capacitance of the axon, and (3) restricting the generation of action potentials to the nodes of Ranvier. In short, myelination greatly alters the electrical properties of the axon.

The many wrappings of membrane around the axon increase the effective membrane resistance, so that r_m/r_{in}, and thus the length constant, is much greater. Less of the conducted signal is lost through the electrical insulation of the myelin sheath, so that the amplitude of a conducted signal declines less with distance along the axon. The myelin-wrapped membrane has a much smaller electrical capacitance than does the naked axonal membrane. Hence the local currents can more rapidly depolarize the membrane as a signal is conducted. *For this reason, the conduction velocity is greatly increased by myelination.* Because of the increase in length constant and in conduction velocity, *an action potential is conducted with little decrement and at great speed from one node of Ranvier to the next.*

The resistance to the flow of ions across the many layers of Schwann cell membrane that make up the myelin sheath is so high that the ionic currents are effectively localized to the short stretches of naked plasma membrane that occur at the nodes of Ranvier. Moreover, the Na^+ and K^+ channels that participate in the action potential are highly concentrated at the nodes of Ranvier. Thus, *the action potential is regenerated only at the nodes of Ranvier* (1 to 2 mm apart), rather than being regenerated at each area along the fiber, as is the case in an unmyelinated fiber. The action potential is rapidly conducted from one node to the next (in about 20 μsec) and "pauses" to be regenerated at each node. Because the action potential appears to "jump" from one node of Ranvier to the

■ **Fig. 3-15**   Conduction velocities of myelinated and unmyelinated axons as functions of axon diameter. Myelinated axons are from cat saphenous nerve at 38° C. Unmyelinated axons are from squid and are at 20° to 22° C. Note that myelinated axons have greater conduction velocities than unmyelinated axons 100 times greater in diameter. (Based on data from Gasser HS, Grundfest H: *Am J Physiol* 127:393, 1939 [myelinated axons] and Pumphrey RJ, Young JZ: *J Exp Biol* 15:453, 1938 [unmyelinated axons].)

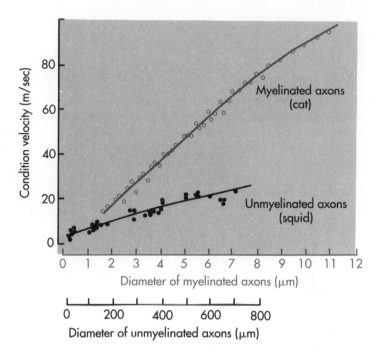

next, the process is called **saltatory** (from the Latin word *saltare,* to leap) **conduction.**

Myelinated axons are also more metabolically efficient than unmyelinated axons. The sodium-potassium pump extrudes the sodium that enters, and reaccumulates the potassium that leaves, the cell during action potentials. In myelinated axons, ionic currents are restricted to the small fraction of the membrane surface at the nodes of Ranvier. For this reason, far fewer Na^+ and K^+ ions traverse a unit area of fiber membrane, and much less ion pumping—and energy expenditure—is required to maintain Na^+ and K^+ gradients.

> In some diseases, known as **demyelinating disorders,** the myelin sheath deteriorates. In **multiple sclerosis,** scattered progressive demyelination of axons in the central nervous system results in loss of motor control. The neuropathy common in severe cases of **diabetes mellitus** is caused by demyelination of peripheral axons. When myelin is lost, the length constant, which is dramatically increased by myelination, becomes much shorter. Hence, the action potential loses amplitude as it is electrotonically conducted from one node of Ranvier to the next. If demyelination is sufficiently severe, the action potential may arrive at the next node of Ranvier with insufficient strength to fire an action potential. The axon may then fail to propagate action potentials.

SUMMARY

1. Different cell types have differently shaped action potentials because their populations of voltage-dependent ion channels differ.

2. The action potential in a squid giant axon or in a mammalian neuron is generated by the rapid opening and subsequent voltage inactivation of voltage-dependent Na^+ channels and the delayed opening and closing of voltage-dependent K^+ channels.

3. Ion channels are integral membrane proteins that have ion-selective pores. Regions of an ion channel protein act as gates that activate and inactivate the channel.

4. An ion channel typically has two states: high conductance (open) and low conductance (closed). The channel oscillates randomly between the open and closed states. For a voltage-dependent channel, the fraction of time the channel spends in the open state is a function of the transmembrane potential difference.

5. Cardiac and smooth muscle cells have L-type Ca^{2+} channels that open and close slowly and are responsible for the long duration of the action potential in these cell types.

6. The voltage inactivation of Na^+ channels is an important factor in the absolute and relative refractory periods and in the accommodation of an excitable cell to a slowly rising stimulus.

7. Local circuit currents produce electrotonic conduction. Both subthreshold signals and action potentials are conducted along the length of a cell by local circuit currents.

8. A subthreshold signal is conducted with decrement. It dies away to 37% of its maximal strength over a distance of 1 length constant. The length constant is equal to $\sqrt{r_m/r_{in}}$. A typical value for the length constant is 1 to 2 mm.

9. The action potential is propagated, rather than merely conducted; it is regenerated as it moves along the cell. In this

way, an action potential remains the same size and shape as it is conducted.

10. The velocity of conduction is determined by the electrical properties of the cell. A large-diameter cell has a faster conduction velocity.

11. Myelination dramatically increases the conduction velocity of a nerve axon. Because of myelination, an action potential is conducted very rapidly and with little decrement from one node of Ranvier to the next. Action potentials are regenerated only at the nodes of Ranvier; the internodal membrane cannot fire an action potential.

12. Because it takes much longer to generate an action potential at each node than it does for the action potential to be conducted between nodes, the action potential appears to jump from node to node; this form of conduction is called saltatory conduction.

BIBLIOGRAPHY

Journal articles

Armstrong CM, Hille B: Voltage-gated ion channels and electrical excitability, *Neuron* 20:371, 1998.

Catterall WA: From ionic currents to molecular mechanisms: the structure and function of voltage-gated sodium channels, *Neuron* 26:13, 2000.

Catterall WA: Structure and regulation of voltage-gated Ca^{2+} channels, *Annu Rev Cell Dev Biol* 16: 521, 2000.

Cooper EC, Jan LY: Ion channel genes and human neurological disease: recent progress, prospects, and challenges, *Proc Natl Acad Sci USA* 96:4759, 1999.

Neher E, Sakmann B: The patch clamp technique, *Sci Am* 266(3): 28, 1992.

Yi BA, Jan LY: Taking apart the gating of voltage-gated K^+ channels, *Neuron* 27:423, 2000.

Books and monographs

Aidley DJ: *The physiology of excitable cells,* ed 4, Cambridge, 1998, Cambridge University Press.

Aidley DJ, Stanfield P: *Ion channels: molecules in action,* Cambridge, 1996, Cambridge University Press.

Hille B: *Ionic channels of excitable membranes,* ed 3, Sunderland, Mass, 2001, Sinauer Associates.

Hodgkin AL: *The conduction of the nervous impulse,* Springfield, Ill, 1964, Charles C Thomas.

Kandel ER, Schwartz JH: *Principles of neural science,* ed 4, New York, 2000, Elsevier.

Katz B: *Nerve, muscle, and synapse,* New York, 1966, McGraw-Hill.

Levitan IB, Kaczmarek LK: *The neuron: cell and molecular biology,* ed 2, New York, 1997, Oxford University Press.

Nicholls JG, Martin AR, Wallace BG: *From neuron to brain,* ed 4, Sunderland, Mass, 2001, Sinauer Associates.

Purves D et al: *Neuroscience,* ed 2, Sunderland, Mass, 2001, Sinauer Associates.

Stevens CF: *Neurophysiology: a primer,* New York, 1966, John Wiley.

chapter four

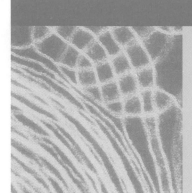

Synaptic Transmission

One electrically excitable cell may communicate with another at a **synapse,** which is a specialized structure that permits electrical communication between cells. There are two types of synapses: electrical and chemical. At an electrical synapse, the two cells are connected by a **gap junction.** (see page 48). Gap junctions permit communication between cells by the direct passage of ionic currents from one cell to the other. At a chemical synapse, the presynaptic neuron releases a **neurotransmitter substance** that binds to specific receptor proteins on the plasma membrane of the postsynaptic cell to alter its membrane potential. The neuromuscular junction, discussed in the next section, is a chemical synapse.

NEUROMUSCULAR JUNCTION

The synapses between the axons of motor neurons and skeletal muscle fibers are called **neuromuscular junctions, myoneural junctions,** or **motor end plates.** The neuromuscular junction, the first vertebrate synapse to be well characterized, serves as a model chemical synapse. An understanding of the structure and function of this junction provides the basis for understanding other, more complex synaptic interactions among neurons in the central nervous system.

Structure of the Neuromuscular Junction

As the motor nerve approaches the neuromuscular junction, it loses its myelin sheath and divides into fine terminal branches (Fig. 4-1). The terminal branches of the motor axon lie in **synaptic troughs** on the surfaces of the muscle cell. The plasma membrane of the muscle cell lining the trough is arranged into numerous **junctional folds.** The axon terminal branches contain many smooth-surfaced **synaptic vesicles** that contain **acetylcholine,** the neurotransmitter employed at this synapse. The axon terminal and the muscle cell are separated by the **junctional cleft,** which contains a carbohydrate-rich amorphous material.

Acetylcholine receptor molecules are concentrated near the mouths of the junctional folds (Fig. 4-1, *inset*). The synaptic vesicles in the nerve terminals and specialized release sites (called **active zones**) on the prejunctional membrane are situated directly opposite the mouths of the junctional folds. **Acetylcholinesterase,** the enzyme that cleaves acetylcholine into acetate and choline, is distributed on the external surface of the postjunctional membrane.

Overview of Neuromuscular Transmission

Neuromuscular transmission begins when an action potential is conducted down the motor axon to the presynaptic axon terminal. Depolarization of the plasma membrane of the axon terminal transiently opens voltage-gated calcium channels. Ca^{2+} from the interstitial fluid flows down its electrochemical potential gradient into the axon terminal. The increased concentration of Ca^{2+} in the axon terminal causes synaptic vesicles to fuse with the plasma membrane and to empty their acetylcholine into the synaptic cleft by exocytosis. Acetylcholine then diffuses across the synaptic cleft and binds to a specific acetylcholine receptor protein on the external surface of the muscle plasma membrane of the motor end plate. *The binding of acetylcholine with the receptor protein transiently increases the conductance of the postjunctional membrane to Na^+ and K^+. Ionic currents (Na^+ and K^+) result in a transient depolarization of the end plate region.* This transient depolarization is called the **end plate potential (EPP)** (Fig. 4-2). The EPP is transient because acetylcholine is quickly hydrolyzed to choline and acetate. The hydrolysis of acetylcholine is catalyzed by the enzyme **acetylcholinesterase,** which is present in high concentration on the postjunctional membrane. The steps involved in neuromuscular transmission are listed in Box 4-1.

The importance of the influx of Ca^{2+} into the axon terminal to initiate the release of transmitter is illustrated by the **Lambert-Eaton myasthenic syndrome.** Patients with this syndrome experience muscular weakness and diminished stretch reflexes. These patients produce anti-

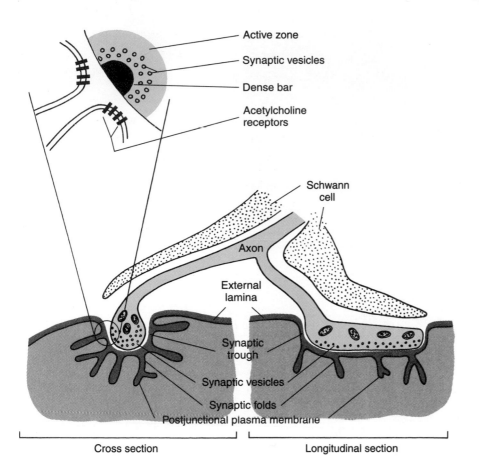

■ Fig. 4-1 The structure of the neuromuscular junction in skeletal muscle.

bodies against the Ca^{2+} channels in their motor nerve terminals. Consequently the number of Ca^{2+} channels decreases, so that less Ca^{2+} enters the nerve terminal and less neurotransmitter is released in response to each action potential.

Although it is depolarized during the course of neuromuscular transmission, *the postjunctional plasma membrane of the neuromuscular junction is not electrically excitable and does not itself fire action potentials.* After the postjunctional plasma membrane is depolarized, *regions of the muscle cell membrane immediately adjacent to the neuromuscular junction are depolarized by electrotonic conduction* (Fig. 4-2, *B*). *When these regions reach threshold, action potentials are generated.* Action potentials are propagated along the muscle fiber at high velocity and initiate the chain of events that leads to muscle contraction (see Chapter 12). Under normal circumstances, the EPP is large enough to cause an action potential in the postjunctional muscle cell.

Synthesis of Acetylcholine

Acetylcholine is produced by condensation of acetyl coenzyme A (acetyl CoA) and choline. The enzyme choline *O*-acetyltransferase, found in the motor neuron, catalyzes this reaction. Motor neurons and their axons are among the few cells able to synthesize acetylcholine; most other cells are unable to make this neurotransmitter.

Although acetyl CoA is produced by the neuron, as it is by most cells, *choline is not synthesized by the motor*

neuron. Instead, choline is obtained by active uptake from the extracellular fluid. The plasma membrane of the motor neuron has a Na^+-coupled secondary active transport system that can accumulate choline against a large electrochemical potential gradient.

■ **Box 4-1** Summary of events that occur during neuromuscular transmission

Action potential in presynaptic motor axon terminals
↓
Increase in Ca^{2+} permeability and influx of Ca^{2+} into axon terminal
↓
Release of acetylcholine from synaptic vesicles into synaptic cleft
↓
Diffusion of acetylcholine to postjunctional membrane
↓
Combination of acetylcholine with specific receptors on postjunctional membrane
↓
Increase in permeability of postjunctional membrane to Na^+ and K^+ causes EPP
↓
Depolarization of areas of muscle membrane adjacent to end plate and initiation of an action potential

EPP, End plate potential.

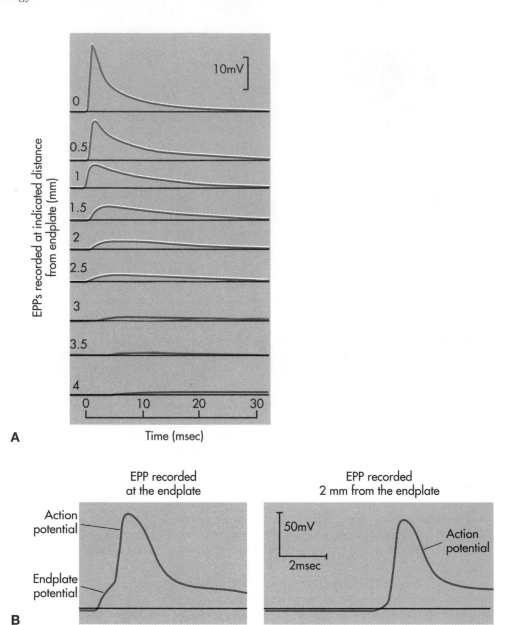

■ **Fig. 4-2** **A,** End plate potentials *(EPPs)* in a frog sartorius muscle. The preparation was treated with curare to bring the EPP just below threshold for eliciting an action potential. The EPP, recorded at increasing distances from the neuromuscular junction, decreases in amplitude and rate of rise. **B,** Intracellular recordings made at the motor end plate *(left panel)* and 2 mm away *(right panel)* in a muscle fiber of frog extensor digitorum longus. When the motor nerve was stimulated, an EPP occurred, which triggered an action potential. Both the EPP and the resultant action potential can be recorded at the end plate, but 2 mm away from the end plate only the action potential can be seen because the EPP is conducted with decrement and has substantially decayed before reaching this point on the muscle fiber. (**A** Redrawn from Fatt P, Katz B: *J Physiol* 115:320, 1951; **B** Redrawn from Fatt P, Katz B: *J Physiol* 117:109, 1952.)

Quantal Release of Transmitter

Acetylcholine is not released continuously by the prejunctional nerve ending; rather, it is released in packets, *with each packet corresponding to the release of one synaptic vesicle.* The amount of acetylcholine contained in one vesicle is called a **quantum** of acetylcholine.

The quantal release of acetylcholine is demonstrated by the small, spontaneous depolarizations known as **miniature end plate potentials (MEPPs).** MEPPs occur even if the motor neuron is not stimulated (Fig. 4-3). *An MEPP is caused by the spontaneous release of one vesicle of acetylcholine into the junctional cleft.* The frequency at which MEPPs occur is random; the average frequency is about 1 per second. The frequency of MEPPs may vary, but their amplitudes are within a relatively narrow range (Fig. 4-3).

Each MEPP depolarizes the postjunctional membrane by only about 0.4 mV on average. This depolarization is not

nearly enough to trigger an action potential in the adjacent muscle plasma membrane. Despite this major difference, MEPPs and EPPs share several similarities. The MEPP has the same time course as an EPP that is evoked by an action potential in the nerve terminal. The MEPP is also similar to the EPP in its responses to most drugs. For example, the EPP and MEPP are both increased in amplitude and prolonged by drugs that inhibit acetylcholinesterase. Also both EPPs and MEPPs are similarly depressed by compounds that compete with acetylcholine for binding to the receptor protein.

The quantal release of acetylcholine can be demonstrated in other ways as well. If the extracellular concentration of Ca^{2+} is reduced to low levels, much less Ca^{2+} enters the nerve terminal in response to an action potential, and consequently very few synaptic vesicles release their acetylcholine. Under these conditions, the size of the EPP varies in small steps, and each step is the size of an MEPP.

Miniature endplate potentials

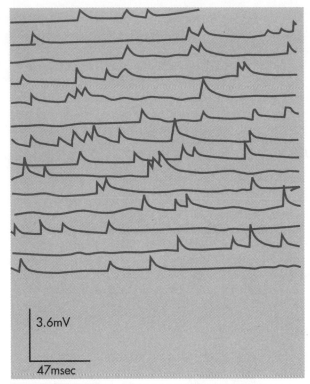

3.6mV

47msec

■ **Fig. 4-3** Spontaneous miniature end plate potentials (MEPPs) recorded at a neuromuscular junction in a fiber of frog extensor digitorum longus. (Redrawn from Fatt P, Katz B: *Nature* 166:597, 1950.)

Action of Cholinesterase and Reuptake of Choline

Acetylcholinesterase is concentrated on the external surface of the postjunctional membrane and in the external lamina. Drugs that inhibit this enzyme are called **anticholinesterases.** *In the presence of an anticholinesterase, the EPP is larger and is dramatically prolonged.*

The motor neuron cannot synthesize choline. Therefore its reuptake from the synaptic cleft provides the choline necessary for the resynthesis of acetylcholine. **Hemicholiniums** are drugs that block the choline transport system and inhibit choline uptake. Prolonged treatment with hemicholiniums depletes the store of transmitter and ultimately decreases the acetylcholine content of the quanta.

Ionic Mechanism of the End Plate Potential

The cation channels that acetylcholine opens in the postjunctional membrane differ from the voltage-gated cation channels of nerve and muscle in that they operate independently of the membrane potential. *The postjunctional channels are gated by the action of acetylcholine rather than by the transmembrane potential.* Acetylcholine receptors thus belong to the superfamily of **ligand-gated ion channels.**

Acetylcholine is the "go-between" that transmits the incoming electrical signal across the synapse. It performs this function by increasing the permeability of the postsynaptic membrane to both Na+ and K+. At the cell's resting potential, the driving force for Na+ to enter the cell is much larger than the net force that causes K+ to leave the cell. Thus a net inward ionic current will flow through the open acetylcholine receptor protein channels, which then depolarizes the postjunctional membrane (Fig. 4-2).

Acetylcholine Receptor Protein

The acetylcholine receptor protein has been extensively studied. The development of methods for isolating and purifying hydrophobic membrane proteins and the availability of snake venom neurotoxins that tightly bind to the acetylcholine receptor have been essential in these studies.

So-called α **toxins** in cobra venoms are responsible for paralyzing snakes' prey. These toxins bind to the acetylcholine binding site on the acetylcholine receptor protein and they prevent acetylcholine from binding and thereby inhibit its action. Poison arrows whose tips are dipped in **curare,** an α toxin extracted from certain plants, are used by some South American Indians to paralyze their prey.

Each motor end plate contains 10^7 to 10^8 acetylcholine receptor proteins, which are highly concentrated near the mouths of the postjunctional folds. The acetylcholine receptor protein is an integral membrane protein that spans the hydrophobic lipid matrix of the postjunctional membrane. Cholinesterase, on the other hand, is only loosely associated with the surface of the postjunctional membrane by hydrophilic interactions. The acetylcholine receptor consists of five subunits (Fig. 4-4), two of which are identical. Therefore, each receptor contains four different polypeptide chains.

Patients with a disorder called **myasthenia gravis** are unable to maintain prolonged contraction of skeletal muscle. These individuals have circulating antibodies against the acetylcholine receptor protein. Patients with this disease have a smaller number of acetylcholine receptors on the postjunctional plasma membranes and consequently the EPPs are smaller. Symptoms include muscle weakness and an inability to sustain muscle contraction. Treatment with anticholinesterases markedly improves the ability of these patients to maintain muscle contractions.

Acetylcholine receptor proteins are highly concentrated in the postjunctional membrane; very few acetylcholine receptors are located elsewhere on the muscle plasma membrane. The mechanisms responsible for localizing the acetylcholine receptors in the postjunctional membrane are not completely understood, but it is clear that the motor neuron plays a role.

If a motor axon is severed, the acetylcholine receptors in all the muscle cells it formerly innervated tend to spread out over the entire plasma membrane. The muscle cell then becomes sensitive to acetylcholine applied anywhere on its surface; this phenomenon is known as **denervation supersensitivity.**

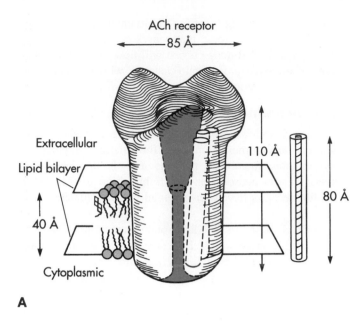

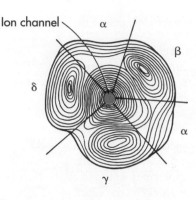

ACh receptor

85 Å

Extracellular

Lipid bilayer

110 Å

80 Å

40 Å

Cytoplasmic

A

Ion channel

α

β

δ

α

γ

B

■ **Fig. 4-4** A model of the structure of the nicotinic acetylcholine receptor protein. **A,** Viewed from the side, and **B,** viewed looking down on the acetylcholine receptor from the extracellular surface. The closed curves are electron density profiles. Five subunits surround a central ion channel. Shown are two α subunits and one each of β, γ, and δ subunits. A binding site for acetylcholine is located on each α subunit. (Redrawn from Kistler J et al: *Biophys J* 37:371, 1982.)

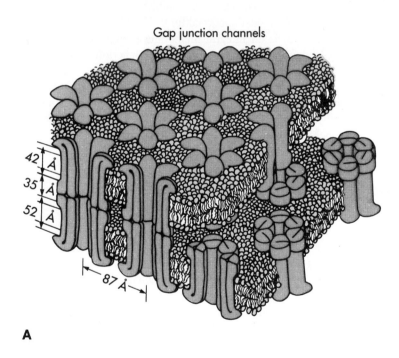

Gap junction channels

42 Å

35 Å

52 Å

87 Å

A

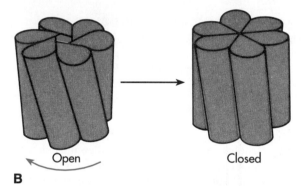

Open

Closed

B

■ **Fig. 4-5** **A,** A model for the structure of the gap junction channels. Each plasma membrane contains connexons, each of which consists of a hexagonal array of six connexin polypeptides. The connexons of the two membranes are aligned at the gap junction to form channels between the cytosolic compartments of the two cells. **B,** A model of the opening and closing of the gap junction channel. The individual connexin subunits of the connexon are proposed to twist relative to one another to open and close the central channel. (**A** Redrawn from Makowski L et al: *J Cell Biol* 74:629, 1977; **B** Redrawn from Unwin PNT, Zampighi G: *Nature* 283:45, 1980.)

ELECTRICAL SYNAPSES

Electrical synapses are present in the central nervous systems of animals, from invertebrates to mammals. **Gap junctions** (Fig. 4-5) join the two cells that participate in an electrical synapse. *A change in the membrane potential of one cell is transmitted to the other cell by the direct flow of current through the gap junction.* Because current flows directly between two cells that make an electrical synapse,

transmission takes place with essentially *no synaptic delay.* Usually, electrical synapses allow conduction in both directions. In this respect they differ from chemical synapses, which are unidirectional. Certain electrical synapses conduct more readily in one direction than in another; this property is called **rectification.**

Cells that form electrical synapses typically are joined by gap junctions. These junctions are plaquelike structures in which the plasma membranes of coupled cells are very close together (less than 3 nm). Freeze-fracture electron micrographs of gap junctions display regular arrays of intramembrane protein particles. *These intramembrane particles consist of six subunits surrounding a central channel that is accessible to water.* The hexagonal array is called a **connexon.** Each of the six subunits is a single protein (one polypeptide chain) called a **connexin** (MW about 25,000). At the gap junction, the connexons of the coupled cells are aligned to form **connexon channels** (Fig. 4-5, *A*). The channels allow the passage of water-soluble molecules up to molecular weights of 1200 to 1500 from one cell to the other. In electrical synapses, these channels are the pathways for electrical current flow between the cells.

Cells that are electrically coupled may become uncoupled by the closing of the connexon channels. The channels may close in response to an increase in intracellular concentration of Ca^{2+} or H^+ in one of the cells or in response to depolarization of one or both of the cells. A model for the mechanism that closes the channels is shown in Fig. 4-5, *B.*

Electrical synapses are widespread in the peripheral and central nervous systems of invertebrates and vertebrates. Electrical synapses are particularly useful in reflex pathways in which rapid transmission between cells (little synaptic delay) is necessary or when the synchronous response of a number of neurons is required. *Among the many nonneuronal cells that are coupled by gap junctions are hepatocytes, myocardial cells, intestinal smooth muscle cells, and the epithelial cells of the lens of the eye.*

Chemical Synapses between Neurons

When one neuron makes a chemical synapse with another, the presynaptic nerve terminal characteristically broadens to form a **terminal bouton.** At the synapse itself, the presynaptic and postsynaptic membranes are closely apposed and lie parallel to one another (Fig. 4-6). *Substantial structures stabilize the synapse.* In fact, when nervous tissue is disrupted, the relationship of the presynaptic and postsynaptic membranes at the synapse is often preserved.

Because of the structure and organization of chemical synapses, conduction is one way. The one-way conduction of chemical synapses contributes to the organization of the central nervous systems of vertebrates. The synaptic delay at chemical synapses, which is at least 0.5 msec, is mainly caused by the time required for the release of transmitter. In polysynaptic pathways, synaptic delay accounts for a significant fraction of the total conduction time.

The mode of transmission at chemical synapses is similar to that at the neuromuscular junction, in that transmission involves the release of a transmitter substance from the presynaptic cell. *At chemical synapses, the transmitter released by the presynaptic neurons alters the conductance of the postsynaptic plasma membrane to one or more ions.* A change in the conductance of the postsynaptic membrane to an ion not in equilibrium across the membrane alters the current carried by that ion. That change in ionic current alters the membrane potential of the postsynaptic cell. *In most cases, transmitters produce their effects by increasing the conductance of the postsynaptic membrane to one or more ions.*

The postsynaptic plasma membrane is specialized for chemical sensitivity rather than for electrical sensitivity. Action potentials are not produced at the synapse. The change in postsynaptic membrane potential caused by the alteration in ion currents—whether a depolarization or hyperpolarization—is conducted electrotonically over the membrane of the postsynaptic neuron. Eventually, the depolarization or hyperpolarization is conducted to the **axon hillock,** the part of the neuron where its axon originates, and then to the **initial segment,** the part of the axon very near the neuronal cell body. *In many neurons, the **axon hillock–initial segment region***

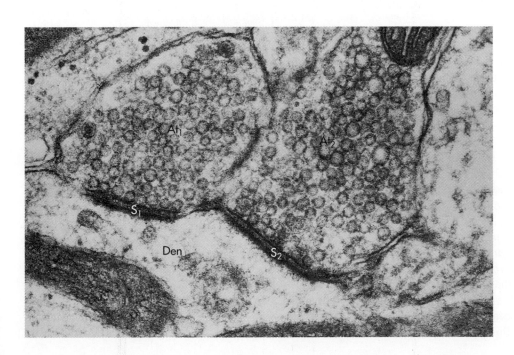

■ **Fig. 4-6** Synapses (S_1 and S_2) in the cerebral cortex. Two axon terminals (At_1 and At_2) synapse with a dendrite *(Den)* of a stellate cell. The axon terminals are packed with synaptic vesicles. (From Peters A, Palay SL, Webster H deF: *The fine structure of the nervous system,* Philadelphia, 1976, WB Saunders.)

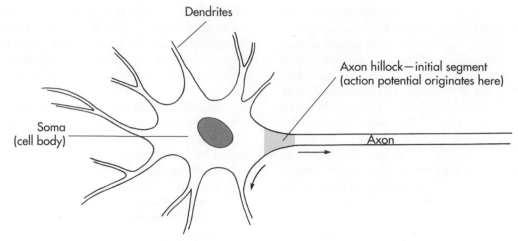

■ Fig. 4-7 A neuron. The axon hillock–initial segment region has the lowest threshold, and consequently action potentials tend to originate there.

■ Fig. 4-8 A spinal motor neuron with multiple synapses on both soma and dendrites.

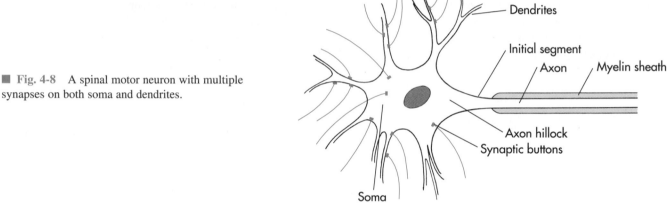

of the cell has a lower threshold than the rest of the plasma membrane of the postsynaptic cell (Fig. 4-7). An action potential will be generated at that site if the sum of all the inputs to the cell exceeds threshold. Once the action potential has been generated, it is conducted over the surface of the postsynaptic cell body and is propagated along its axon.

Input-Output Relations

The neuromuscular junction represents a simple type of synapse in which one action potential in the presynaptic cell (the input) elicits a single action potential in the postsynaptic cell (the output). In other types of synapses, the output may differ from the input. *Synapses can be classified as one-to-one, one-to-many, or many-to-one, on the basis of the relationship between input and output.*

In a **one-to-one** synapse, such as the neuromuscular junction, the input and the output are the same. A single action potential in the presynaptic cell evokes a single action potential in the postsynaptic cell. Because the output matches the input, no integration occurs at this type of synapse.

In a **one-to-many** synapse, a single action potential in the presynaptic cell elicits several action potentials in the postsynaptic cell. Axon collaterals of motor neurons make one-to-many synapses on **Renshaw cells** in the spinal cord. One action potential in the motor neuron is able to induce the Renshaw cell to fire a burst of action potentials. The burst of action potentials in the Renshaw cell inhibits the motor neuron and prevents it from being fired too frequently.

In a **many-to-one** synaptic arrangement, one action potential in a presynaptic cell is not sufficient to make the postsynaptic cell fire an action potential. *The nearly simultaneous arrival of presynaptic action potentials from several input neurons that synapse on the same postsynaptic cell is necessary to depolarize the postsynaptic cell to threshold.* The spinal motor neuron has this type of synaptic organization. Thousands of presynaptic axons synapse on each spinal motor neuron (Fig. 4-8). *Some of these axons carry excitatory inputs that depolarize the postsynaptic cell and bring it closer to its threshold. Other axons carry* *inhibitory inputs that hyperpolarize the motor neuron and take it farther away from threshold.*

Excitatory and Inhibitory Postsynaptic Potentials

A spinal motor neuron responds in one of two ways after an action potential in one of the neurons that synapses upon it. The postsynaptic response is either a transient depolarization or a transient hyperpolarization (Fig. 4-9). Because the depolarization brings the motor neuron closer to threshold, this response is called **excitatory postsynaptic potential (EPSP).** Because the hyperpolarizing response moves the motor neuron farther from its threshold, it is called an **inhibitory postsynaptic potential (IPSP).** An EPSP depolarizes the motor neuron by only about 2 mV, which is not sufficient to reach threshold. The motor neuron will reach threshold only when multiple EPSPs occur within a narrow time interval. IPSPs that occur within the same time interval as EPSPs make it less likely that the motor neuron will reach threshold. At any instant, the motor neuron is integrating its excitatory and inhibitory inputs; this process is known as **summation.**

Summation of Synaptic Inputs

Summation of inputs can occur by either spatial summation or temporal summation (Fig. 4-10). **Spatial summation** occurs when *two separate inputs* arrive almost simultaneously (Fig. 4-10, *A*). The two postsynaptic potentials are then added. If the two inputs are EPSPs, they will depolarize the postsynaptic cell about twice as much as either input alone. However, *if one input is an EPSP and the other is an IPSP, they tend to cancel one another.*

Temporal summation occurs when two or more action potentials in a single presynaptic neuron occur in rapid succession, so that the resultant postsynaptic potentials overlap in time (Fig. 4-10, *B*). A train of impulses in a *single presynaptic neuron* can change the potential of the postsynaptic cell in a stepwise manner. In this situation, each stepwise change in the postsynaptic potential is caused by one of the presynaptic impulses.

Summation of Postsynaptic Potentials

Inhibitory synapses tend to be on the cell body or **soma,** whereas excitatory synapses are more often made with **dendritic spines,** which are specialized protrusions from the shafts of dendrites. Most synapses on dendrites are made with dendritic spines. The soma is about 100 μm or less in diameter, whereas the length constant of the soma is about 1 mm. Thus, postsynaptic potentials on the soma are conducted with little decrement and are summed arithmetically. Because dendrites are much smaller in diameter than the soma, dendrites have smaller length constants than the soma. The thinner the dendrite, the smaller its length constant. Because the thinner dendrites tend to be farther from the soma, postsynaptic potentials that occur in distant dendrites are conducted to the soma with considerable decrement. In this way synaptic inputs that occur on larger dendrites that

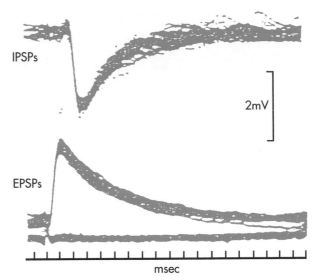

■ **Fig. 4-9** Inhibitory postsynaptic potentials *(IPSPs)* and excitatory postsynaptic potentials *(EPSPs)* recorded with a microelectrode in a cat spinal motor neuron in response to stimulation of appropriate peripheral afferent fibers. Forty traces are superimposed. (Redrawn from Curtis DR, Eccles JC: *J Physiol* 145:529, 1959.)

are closer to the soma have a greater influence on the membrane potential of the soma than do synaptic inputs that are more distant from the soma. The soma is constantly weighing and integrating the postsynaptic potentials from all of its inputs, those on the soma and those on the dendrites. The region of the motor neuron that gives rise to the axon is called the **axon hillock.** The beginning of the axon is called its **initial segment.** The axon hillock-initial segment region of the motor neuron has the lowest threshold, and thus action potentials originate there when the threshold is exceeded.

Integration at the spinal motor neuron takes place because many positive and negative inputs impinge on a single motor neuron. Integration permits fine control of the firing pattern of the spinal motor neuron.

Modulation of Synaptic Activity

The responses of a postsynaptic neuron to single action potentials in a particular presynaptic neuron are relatively constant in magnitude and time course. However, *when a presynaptic axon is stimulated repeatedly, the postsynaptic response may increase with each stimulation.* This phenomenon is called **facilitation** (Fig. 4-11, *A*). As shown in Fig. 4-11, *B,* the extent of facilitation depends on the frequency of presynaptic impulses. Facilitation dies away rapidly, within tens to hundreds of milliseconds after stimulation stops.

When a presynaptic neuron is stimulated **tetanically** (many stimuli at high frequency) for several seconds, **posttetanic potentiation** occurs. Posttetanic potentiation, like facilitation, is an enhancement of the postsynaptic response, but it lasts longer (Fig. 4-11, *C*): tens of seconds to several minutes after cessation of tetanic stimulation.

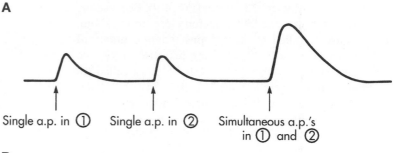

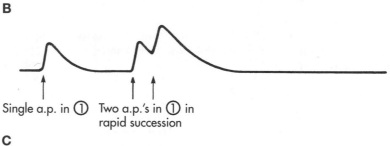

■ **Fig. 4-10** **A,** Spatial and temporal summation at a postsynaptic neuron with two synaptic inputs (*1* and *2*). **B,** Spatial summation. The postsynaptic potentials in response to single action potentials (aps) in inputs *1* and *2* occur separately and simultaneously. **C,** Temporal summation. The postsynaptic response to two impulses in rapid succession in the same input.

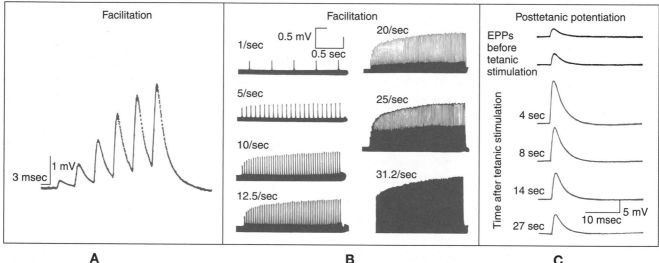

■ **Fig. 4-11** **A,** Facilitation at a neuromuscular junction. EPPs at a neuromuscular junction in toad sartorius muscle were elicited by successive action potentials in the motor axon. Neuromuscular transmission was depressed by 5 mM Mg²⁺ and 2.1 µM curare, so that action potentials did not occur. **B,** EPPs at a frog neuromuscular junction elicited by repetitively stimulating the motor axon at different frequencies. Note that facilitation failed to occur at the lowest frequency of stimulation (1/sec) and that the degree of facilitation increased with increasing frequency of stimulation in the range of frequency employed. Neuromuscular transmission was inhibited by bathing the preparation in 12 to 20 mM Mg²⁺. **C,** Posttetanic potentiation at a frog neuromuscular junction. The top two traces indicate control EPPs in response to single action potentials in the motor axon. Subsequent traces indicate EPPs in response to single action potentials after tetanic stimulation (50 impulses/sec for 20 seconds) of the motor neuron. The time interval between the end of tetanic stimulation and the single action potential is shown on each trace. The muscle was treated with tetrodotoxin to prevent generation of action potentials. (**A** Redrawn from Belnave RJ, Gage PW: *J Physiol* 266:435, 1977; **B** Redrawn from Magelby KL: *J Physiol* 234:327, 1973; **C** Redrawn from Weinrich D: *J Physiol* 212:431, 1971.)

Facilitation and posttetanic potentiation are the result of the effects of repeated stimulation on the presynaptic neuron. These phenomena do not involve a change in the sensitivity of the postsynaptic cell to transmitter. Rather, with repeated stimulation, an increased number of quanta of transmitter is released. Increased levels of intracellular calcium ions increase the transmitter release during repetitive stimulation.

Repetitive stimulation of certain synapses in the brain more persistently increases the efficacy of transmission at those synapses. This phenomenon, called **long-term potentiation,** can persist for days to weeks. Long-term potentiation is believed to be involved in the storage of memories. The increased synaptic efficacy that occurs in long-term potentiation probably involves both presynaptic (greater transmitter release) and postsynaptic (greater sensitivity to transmitter) changes.

Ca^{2+} entry into the postsynaptic region is an early required step in initiating the changes that result in long-term enhancement of the response of the postsynaptic cell to neurotransmitter. Ca^{2+} entry occurs through *N*-methyl-D-aspartate (NMDA) receptors, a class of glutamate receptors that permits Ca^{2+} influx. The entry of Ca^{2+} is believed to activate **Ca^{2+}-calmodulin kinase II,** a multifunctional protein kinase that is present in very high concentrations in postsynaptic densities. In the presence of high Ca^{2+} concentrations, this kinase can phosphorylate itself and thereby become active whether or not Ca^{2+} is present. Ca^{2+}-calmodulin kinase II is believed to phosphorylate proteins that are essential for the induction of long-term potentiation.

Long-term potentiation may also have an anatomical component. After appropriate stimulation of a presynaptic pathway, the number of dendritic spines and the number of synapses on the dendrites of the postsynaptic neurons may rapidly increase.

Changes in the presynaptic nerve terminal may also contribute to long-tem potentiation. The postsynaptic neuron may release a signal (nitric oxide [NO] has been suggested) that enhances transmitter release by the presynaptic nerve terminal.

When a synapse is repetitively stimulated for a long time, a point is reached at which each successive presynaptic stimulation elicits smaller postsynaptic responses. This phenomenon is called **synaptic fatigue** (neuromuscular depression at the neuromuscular junction). The postsynaptic cell at a fatigued synapse responds normally to transmitter applied from a micropipette; thus the defect is presynaptic. In some cases, a decrease in quantal content (the amount of transmitter per synaptic vesicle) contributes to synaptic fatigue. A fatigued synapse typically recovers within a few seconds.

Ionic Mechanisms of Postsynaptic Potentials in Spinal Motor Neurons

Much of our knowledge of synaptic mechanisms in the mammalian central nervous system is derived from studies of cat spinal motor neurons.

Excitatory postsynaptic potentials (EPSPs). The EPSP (Fig. 4-9) of the cat spinal motor neuron is caused by a *transient increase of the conductance of the postsynaptic membrane to both Na^+ and K^+* in response to the neurotransmitter. At the cell's resting potential, the driving force for Na^+ to enter the cell is much greater than the force for K^+ to leave. Hence, in response to the neurotransmitter, a net inward flow of ions occurs; inward Na^+ current depolarizes the postsynaptic cell.

Inhibitory postsynaptic potentials. The IPSP (Fig. 4-9) of cat spinal motor neurons is caused by an *increased Cl^- conductance* of the postjunctional membrane. At rest, the net tendency is for Cl^- to enter the motor neuron. The increase in Cl^- conductance that results from the release of transmitters at the inhibitory synapse allows Cl^- to enter the postsynaptic cell and hyperpolarize it.

Presynaptic inhibition. Inhibitory interactions are vital in stabilizing the central nervous system. In addition to postsynaptic inhibition, another type of inhibition called presynaptic inhibition operates at synapses. If an inhibitory input to a spinal motor neuron is stimulated tetanically and then an excitatory input to the same neuron is stimulated once, the EPSP elicited by the excitatory input may be diminished after the inhibitory volley. This type of inhibition is believed to occur by a mechanism in which axon collaterals of the inhibitory axons synapse on the excitatory nerve terminals (Fig. 4-12). Action potentials in the inhibitory nerve depolarize the excitatory nerve terminal for a long time. Although this depolarization brings the excitatory nerve terminal closer to threshold, the partial depolarization causes less Ca^{2+} to enter the cell. This change decreases the amount of transmitter released in response to an action potential. The smaller the amount of neurotransmitter released, the less is the magnitude of the excitatory postsynaptic potential.

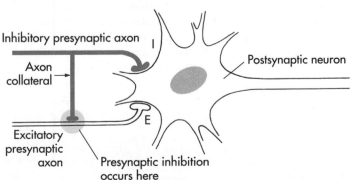

■ **Fig. 4-12** Presynaptic inhibition. Axon collaterals of the inhibitory axon *(I)* synapse on the excitatory axon terminal *(E)*. An action potential in the inhibitory axon depolarizes the excitatory axon terminal. The depolarized excitatory axon terminal will release less transmitter in response to an action potential in the excitatory neuron *(E)*.

NEUROTRANSMITTERS AND NEUROMODULATORS

Identification of Transmitter Substances

Certain compounds that may function as neurotransmitters are called **candidate** or **putative neurotransmitters.** These putative neurotransmitters are usually concentrated in specific neurons or in specific neuronal pathways.

It is often difficult to prove that a substance is the transmitter at a particular synapse. *A putative transmitter (X) must satisfy the following criteria before it is accepted as a proven transmitter at a particular synapse:*

1. The presynaptic neurons must contain X and must be able to synthesize it.
2. X must be released by the presynaptic neurons in response to appropriate stimulation.
3. Microapplication of X to the postsynaptic membrane must mimic the effects of stimulation of the presynaptic neuron.
4. The effects of presynaptic stimulation and of microapplication of X should be altered in the same way by drugs.

Identifying a putative neurotransmitter may involve determining whether (a) the presynaptic cell contains the enzymes involved in biosynthesis of the transmitter or the transporters for transmitter reuptake, or (b) whether the postsynaptic cell contains receptors for the putative transmitter.

Some transmitters have rapid and transient effects on the postsynaptic cell. Other transmitters have effects that are much slower in onset and that last for minutes or even hours. Most known neurotransmitters fall into three major chemical classes: amines, amino acids, and oligopeptides.

Neurotransmitters

Acetylcholine. As discussed previously, acetylcholine is the transmitter used by all motor axons that arise from the spinal cord. Acetylcholine also plays a central role in the autonomic nervous system; it is the transmitter for all autonomic preganglionic neurons as well as for postganglionic parasympathetic fibers. The Betz cells of the motor cortex use acetylcholine as their transmitter. The basal ganglia, which are involved in the control of movement, contain high levels of acetylcholine. Thus acetylcholine is probably an important neurotransmitter in the basal ganglia. In addition, acetylcholine may be the transmitter in many other central neural pathways.

Deficits in pathways involving acetylcholine (**cholinergic pathways**) in the brain have been implicated in some forms of **senile dementia** (e.g., **Alzheimer's disease**). Treatment with long-lasting anticholinergic drugs that penetrate the blood-brain barrier may improve cognitive function in some individuals suffering from dementia.

Biogenic amine transmitters. Among the amines that may serve as neurotransmitters are **norepinephrine, epinephrine, dopamine, serotonin,** and **histamine.**

Dopamine, norepinephrine, and epinephrine are **catecholamines,** and they share a common biosynthetic pathway that starts with the amino acid, tyrosine. Tyrosine is converted to L-dopa by the enzyme tyrosine hydroxylase. L-Dopa is converted to dopamine by a specific decarboxylase. In dopaminergic neurons, the pathway stops here. In noradrenergic neurons, another enzyme, dopamine β-hydroxylase, converts dopamine to norepinephrine. Norepinephrine is the primary transmitter for postganglionic sympathetic neurons. Chromaffin cells in the adrenal medulla add a methyl group to norepinephrine to produce the hormone, epinephrine.

Neurons that contain high levels of dopamine are prominent in the midbrain regions known as the **substantia nigra** and the **ventral tegmentum.** Some of the axons of these neurons terminate in the corpus striatum, where they participate in controlling complex movements. The degeneration of dopaminergic synapses in the corpus striatum occurs in **Parkinson's disease,** and this degeneration may be a major cause of the muscular tremors and rigidity that characterize this disease. Treatment of some Parkinson's patients with L-**dopa,** a precursor of dopamine, improves motor control.

In contrast, the hyperactivity of dopaminergic synapses may be involved in some forms of **psychosis.** **Chlorpromazine** and related antipsychotic drugs inhibit the dopamine receptors on postsynaptic membranes and thus diminish the effects of dopamine released from presynaptic nerve terminals.

Serotonin (5-hydroxytryptamine)-containing neurons are present in high concentration in certain nuclei located in the brainstem. Serotonergic neurons may be involved in temperature regulation, sensory perception, onset of sleep, and control of mood and have been implicated in the aggressive behavior of certain animal species.

Histamine is present in certain neurons in the hypothalamus. The functions of these presumably histaminergic neurons are not yet known.

Amino acid transmitters. **Glycine,** the simplest amino acid, is an inhibitory neurotransmitter released by certain spinal interneurons.

γ-Aminobutyric acid (GABA) is not incorporated into proteins, nor is it present in all cells (as are the other naturally occurring amino acids). *GABA is produced from glutamate by a specific decarboxylase present only in certain neurons in the central nervous system.* Among the cells that contain GABA are some neurons in the basal ganglia, cerebellar Purkinje cells, and certain spinal interneurons. *In all known cases, GABA functions as an inhibitory transmitter. It is the most common transmitter in the brain.* GABA may be the neurotransmitter at as many as one third of the synapses in the brain.

The postsynaptic receptors for glycine and GABA are both ligand-gated Cl⁻ channels that allow the influx of Cl⁻ to hyperpolarize the postsynaptic neuron.

General **anesthetics** prolong the open time of GABA receptor chloride channels and thus prolong the inhibition of the postsynaptic neurons at GABA-ergic synapses. GABA receptors may be a principal target of general anesthetics.

Glutamate and **aspartate,** which are dicarboxylic amino acids, strongly excite many neurons in the brain. Glutamate is the most common excitatory neurotransmitter in the brain. Five classes of **excitatory amino acid (EAA) receptors** have been identified (see below).

Nitric oxide (NO). NO is a transmitter at synapses between inhibitory motor neurons of the enteric nervous system and gastrointestinal smooth muscle cells (see Chapter 31). NO also functions as a neurotransmitter in the central nervous system. It is an unusual neurotransmitter because it is neither packaged into synaptic vesicles nor released by exocytosis. It is highly permeant and simply diffuses from its site of production to neighboring cells. The enzyme **NO synthase** catalyzes the production of NO as a product of the oxidation of arginine to citrulline. This enzyme is stimulated by an increase in cytosolic Ca^{2+}.

In addition to serving as a neurotransmitter, NO functions as a cellular signal transduction molecule both in neurons and in nonneuronal cells (such as vascular smooth muscle, see Chapter 20). One way NO functions as a signal transduction molecule is by regulating guanylyl cyclase, the enzyme that produces cyclic guanosine monophosphate (GMP) from guanosine triphosphate (GTP). NO binds to a heme group in soluble guanylyl cyclase and potently stimulates the enzyme. The stimulation of this enzyme leads to an elevation of cyclic GMP in the target cell. The cyclic GMP can then influence multiple cellular processes.

Neuroactive Peptides

Certain cells release peptides that act at very low concentrations to excite or inhibit neurons. To date, more than 25 of these so-called **neuroactive peptides** or **neuropeptides,** ranging from 2 to about 40 amino acids long, have been identified. Some of these neuropeptides are listed in Box 4-2. Neuropeptides typically affect their target neurons at lower concentrations than the "classic" neurotransmitters discussed previously, and the actions of neuropeptides usually last longer than those of neurotransmitters.

Neuropeptides may act as hormones, as neurotransmitters, or as neuromodulators. In fact, a number of neuropeptides are more familiar as hormones, which are substances that are released into the blood and that reach their target cells via the circulation. A number of neuropeptides act as true transmitters at particular synapses and as neuromodulators at other synapses. Both neurotransmitters and neuromodulators are typically released near the surface of a target cell and they diffuse to the target cell. A neurotransmitter, as discussed earlier, acts to change the conductance of the target cell to one or more ions, thereby changing the membrane potential of the target cell. A neuromodulator, on the other hand, modulates synaptic transmission. A neuromodulator

■ **Box 4-2**   Some neuroactive peptides

Gut-brain peptides

Vasoactive intestinal polypeptide (VIP)
Cholecystokinin octapeptide (CCK-8)
Substance P
Neurotensin
Methionine enkephalin
Leucine enkephalin
Motilin
Insulin
Glucagon

Hypothalamic-releasing hormones

Thyrotropin-releasing hormone (TRH)
Luteinizing hormone–releasing hormone (LHRH)
Somatostatin (growth hormone releasing-inhibiting factor, or SRIF)

Pituitary peptides

Adrenocorticotropin (ACTH)
β-Endorphin
α-Melanocyte-stimulating hormone (α-MSH)

Others

Dynorphin
Angiotensin II
Bradykinin
Vasopressin
Oxytocin
Carnosine
Bombesin

From Snyder SH: *Science* 209:976, 1980.

may act presynaptically to change the amount of transmitter released in response to an action potential, or it may act on the postsynaptic cell to modify its response to the neurotransmitter. Box 4-3 lists differences between nonpeptide neurotransmitters and peptide neurotransmitters.

In many instances, neuropeptides coexist in the same nerve terminals with classic transmitters (Table 4-1). In some of these cases, the neuropeptide is released along with the transmitter in response to nerve stimulation.

The neurotransmitter-containing vesicles are released from vesicles docked at active sites as previously described at the neuromuscular junction (Fig. 4-1). Neuropeptide is released at sites on the soma more distant from the synaptic cleft; these release sites do not involve active zones or other specialized structures. Because the voltage-gated Ca^{2+} channels are located near the active zones, low-frequency stimulation of the postsynaptic cell raises the level of Ca^{2+} locally near the active zones, and it promotes the release of neurotransmitter without concomitant release of neuropeptide. Higher-frequency stimulation of the presynaptic neuron produces increased Ca^{2+} everywhere in the nerve terminal, and it leads to release of neuropeptide as well as of neurotransmitter.

Synthesis of neuropeptides. Nonpeptide neurotransmitters are synthesized in nerve terminals by pathways that involve soluble enzymes and simple precursors. Neuropeptides are synthesized in the neuronal cell body. They are encoded

■ Box 4-3   Distinctions between classical nonpeptide neurotransmitters and peptide neurotransmitters

Nonpeptide transmitters	Peptide transmitters
Synthesized and packaged in nerve terminal	Synthesized and packaged in cell body; transported to nerve terminal by fast axonal transport
Synthesized in active form	Active peptide formed when it is cleaved from a much larger polypeptide that contains several neuropeptides
Usually present in small, clear vesicles	Usually present in large, electron-dense vesicles
Released into a synaptic cleft	May be released some distance from the postsynaptic cell
	There may be no well-defined synaptic structure
Action of many terminated because of uptake b presynaptic terminal by Na^+-powered active transport	Action terminated by proteolysis or by the peptide diffusing away
Typically, action has short latency and short duration (msec)	Action may have long latency and may persist for many seconds

■ Table 4-1   Examples of the coexistence within the same nerve terminal of a classical transmitter and a neuropeptide*

Transmitter	Peptide
Acetylcholine	Vasoactive intestinal peptide (VIP)
Norepinephrine	Somatostatin
	Enkephalin
	Neurotensin
Dopamine	Cholecystokinin (CCK)
	Enkephalin
Epinephrine	Enkephalin
Serotonin	Substance P
	Thyrotropin-releasing hormone (TRH)

From Schwartz JH: In Kandel ER, Schwartz JH, editors: *Principles of neural science,* New York, 1981, Elsevier Science.
*Evidence for the coexistence of a classic transmitter substance with a neuroactive peptide has been reported for these combinations. With the information thus far available, it is not yet possible to determine the specificity of the pairs and their physiological significance.

in the cell's DNA and transcribed into messenger RNA (mRNA); synthesis of the neuropeptide takes place on polyribosomes bound to the endoplasmic reticulum where the mRNA is translated. Secretory vesicles containing the neuropeptide are released from the mature face of the Golgi complex. The secretory vesicles are moved by **fast axonal transport** (Fig. 4-13) to the axon terminal, where they function as synaptic vesicles.

Some neuropeptides are synthesized as preprohormones (see also Chapter 43). Cleavage of a signal sequence converts a preprohormone to a prohormone. Proteolytic cleavage of the prohormone may then release one or more active peptides. In some cases, one prohormone may contain several active peptide sequences. For example, the prohormone of the opioid peptide, β-endorphin, is a 31,000-dalton polypeptide that contains several active sequences. One cleavage of the prohormone releases adrenocorticotropic hormone (ACTH) and β-lipotropin. Cleavage of ACTH releases yet another hormone, melanocyte-stimulating hormone (α-MSH), and cleavage of β-lipotropin releases α-MSH and a number of active β-endorphins.

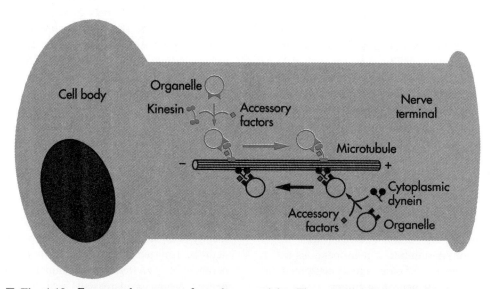

■ Fig. 4-13   Fast axonal transport of membrane vesicles. The network of microtubules that runs the length of the axon serves as the pathway for fast axonal transport of vesicles from the cell body to the nerve terminal and in the reverse direction. Most of the microtubules are oriented with their plus (rapidly growing) ends toward the nerve terminal. Kinesin and dynein are microtubule-associated motor proteins that function to transport the vesicles toward the nerve terminal and the cell body, respectively. Other proteins, called accessory factors, are required for transport of vesicles. (Modified from Sheetz MP, Steuer ER, Schroer TA: *Trends Neurosci* 12:474, 1990.)

Opioid peptides. **Opiates** are drugs derived from the juice of the opium poppy.

> Opiates are useful therapeutically as powerful **analgesics** (pain relievers). They exert their analgesic effect by binding to specific opiate receptors. The binding of opiates to their receptors is stereospecifically inhibited by a morphine derivative called **naloxone.**

Compounds that are not derived from the opium poppy, but that exert direct effects by binding to opiate receptors, are called **opioids.** *Operationally, opioids are defined as direct-acting compounds whose effects are stereospecifically antagonized by naloxone.*

The three major classes of endogenous opioid peptides in mammals are **enkephalins, endorphins,** and **dynorphins.** Enkephalins are the simplest opioids; they are pentapeptides. Dynorphin and the endorphins are somewhat longer peptides that contain one or the other of the enkephalin sequences at their N-terminal ends.

Opioid peptides are widely distributed in neurons of the central nervous system and intrinsic neurons of the gastrointestinal tract. Within these neurons, opioid peptides are found in vesicles that resemble synaptic vesicles. The endorphins are discretely localized in particular structures of the central nervous system, whereas the enkephalins and dynorphins are more widely distributed. Opioids inhibit neurons in the brain involved in the perception of pain. Opioid peptides are among the most potent analgesic (pain-relieving) compounds known.

Nonopioid neuropeptides. Most of the known neuropeptides are not opioids. **Substance P,** a peptide of 11 amino acids, is present in specific neurons in the brain, in primary sensory neurons, and in plexus neurons in the wall of the gastrointestinal tract. Substance P was the first so-called **gut-brain peptide** to be discovered. The wall of the gastrointestinal tract is richly innervated with neurons that form networks or plexuses (see also Chapter 31). The intrinsic plexuses of the gastrointestinal tract exert primary control over its motor and secretory activities. These enteric neurons contain many of the neuropeptides, including substance P, that are found in the brain and spinal column. Substance P is involved in pain transmission and has a powerful effect on smooth muscle.

Substance P is probably the transmitter employed at synapses made by primary sensory neurons (their cell bodies are in the dorsal root ganglia) with spinal interneurons in the dorsal horn of the spinal column. Enkephalins act to decrease the release of substance P at these synapses and thereby inhibit the pathway for pain sensation at the first synapse in the pathway.

Vasoactive intestinal polypeptide (VIP) is a member of a family of neuropeptides related to the hormone **secretin.** VIP was first discovered as a gastrointestinal hormone, but it is now known to be a neuropeptide also.

VIP is widely distributed in the central nervous system and in the intrinsic neurons of the gastrointestinal tract. In neurons in the brain, VIP has been localized in synaptic vesicles. VIP may function as an inhibitory transmitter of vascular and nonvascular smooth muscle and as an excitatory transmitter to glandular epithelial cells.

Secretin, glucagon, and **gastric inhibitory polypeptide (GIP),** whose functions as gastrointestinal hormones have been well characterized, have sequence homology with VIP. Although these peptides have also been found in particular neurons in the central nervous system, their functions in these neurons remain undetermined.

Cholecystokinin (CCK) is a member of a group of neuropeptides that includes **gastrin** and **cerulein,** which have similar C-terminal sequences. CCK is a well-known gastrointestinal hormone that elicits contraction of the gallbladder (see Chapter 32). One form of CCK is present in particular neurons of the central nervous system.

Neurotensin is present in enteric neurons and in the brain. When neurotensin is injected into cerebrospinal fluid at low concentrations, it lowers body temperature. Thus, neurotensin may function in temperature regulation.

Other Neuromodulators

Some important neuromodulators are not peptides. Purines and purine nucleotides (adenosine triphosphate [ATP]) and nucleosides (adenosine) function as neuromodulators in the central, autonomic, and peripheral nervous systems. Substances that serve as neurotransmitters may also act as neuromodulators. In some cases, a transmitter binds to receptors on the presynaptic neuron that released it, thereby regulating its own release.

NEUROTRANSMITTER RECEPTORS
Two Classes of Neurotransmitter Receptors

Many neurotransmitter receptors, such as the acetylcholine recptor, are ligand-gated ion channels. Such neurotransmitters are also called **ionotropic receptors.** The binding of the neurotransmitter alters (usually increases) the probability of the ion channel being in the open state. Certain other neurotransmitter receptors are not ligand-gated ion channels, but rather are participants in the first step in a signal transduction cascade that alters the function of an ion channel in the postsynaptic membrane. Such neurotransmitter receptors are called **metabotropic receptors.** Metabotropic receptors discussed below include $GABA_B$ receptors and so-called metabotropic glutamate receptors. Binding of transmitter to an ionotropic receptor typically results in postsynaptic events that are rapid in both onset and decay, lasting several milliseconds. By contrast, metabotropic receptors mediate postsynaptic phenomena that may persist from many milliseconds to minutes.

Inhibitory Receptors: GABA and Glycine Receptors

The most common inhibitory synapses in the central nervous system use either glycine or GABA as their transmitter. Glycine-mediated inhibitory synapses predominate in the spinal cord, whereas GABA-ergic synapses are the most numerous synapses in the brain.

GABA and glycine receptors, and most other neurotransmitter receptors, belong to a superfamily of **ligand-gated ion channels.** The probability of these channels opening and the average time a channel stays open are controlled by the concentration of the neurotransmitter for which the receptor is specific. The nicotinic acetylcholine receptor (Fig. 4-4) is the best studied member of the ligand-gated ion channel superfamily.

Despite their different ion specificities, important similarities exist between GABA and glycine receptors and the nicotinic acetylcholine receptor. All these channels are composed of five subunits that surround a central ion channel. The protein subunits share similarities in amino acid sequence and in tertiary structure. Although these channels contain five distinct subunits, only one or two subunit isoforms are typically required to form a functional ion channel. Different cell types in the central nervous system may have different receptor subtypes that consist of different combinations of subunit isoforms. Evolution appears to have created a variety of subunit isoforms from which a particular cell type can pick and choose in constructing its own multimeric ligand-gated receptor subtype.

GABA and glycine receptors are ligand-gated Cl^- channels that mediate Cl^- influx into neurons. The Cl^- current hyperpolarizes and thus inhibits the neurons. Two major types of GABA receptors have been identified—$GABA_A$ and $GABA_B$. The $GABA_A$ receptor is a GABA-mediated Cl^- channel. Five distinct protein subunits can form $GABA_A$ receptors, and different $GABA_A$ receptor subtypes are composed of different combinations of the subunits. The $GABA_B$ receptor is metabotropic. Binding of GABA to this receptor activates a heterotrimeric GTP-binding protein (G-protein, Chapter 5), which leads to activation of K^+ channels, and hence hyperpolarization of the postsynaptic cell, and to inhibition of Ca^+ channels.

> $GABA_A$ receptors are the targets of two major classes of drugs: **benzodiazepines** and **barbiturates.** Benzodiazepines (e.g., diazepam) are widely used antianxiety and relaxant drugs. Barbiturates are used as sedatives and anticonvulsants. Both classes of drugs bind to distinct sites on $GABA_A$ receptors and enhance the opening of the receptors' Cl^- channels in response to GABA.

Excitatory Amino Acid Receptors

Glutamate is the major neurotransmitter that mediates synaptic excitation in the central nervous system. Glutamate receptors are also known as **excitatory amino acid (EAA) receptors.** At present, five subtypes of EAA receptors have been recognized (Table 4-2), classified principally by the synthetic amino acid analogs to which they bind tightly and specifically. Four of the subtypes are ligand-gated ion channels; the fifth subtype is a receptor (called the

■ **Table 4-2**   Different classes of excitatory amino acid receptors

Receptor class	Properties
AMPA	Widely distributed in CNS; channel-selective for Na^+ and K^+; formerly known as quisqualate receptor
NMDA	Widely distributed in CNS; channel-selective Ca^{2+}, Na^+, and K^+; blocked by Mg^{2+}; block relieved by depolarization
Kainate	Present in specific areas of CNS
L-AP4	Not widely distributed; may function as a presynaptic glutamate receptor that inhibits glutamate release
Metabotropic	Not an ion channel; mobilizes IP3 and increases intracellular Ca^{2+}

CNS, Central nervous systems.

metabotropic EAA receptor) that is indirectly linked to an ion channel.

Two EAA receptors, the **AMPA** and **NMDA** receptors, are widely distributed in the central nervous system. Stimulation of AMPA receptors by glutamate or another agonist elicits an EPSP caused by flow of Na^+ and K^+. Stimulated NMDA receptors permit flow of Ca^{2+} as well as Na^+ and K^+. NMDA receptors are blocked by extracellular Mg^{2+} at physiological levels. The Mg^{2+} block is relieved when the cell is depolarized. Thus, physiologically, the first response to glutamate is depolarization of the postsynaptic cell by glutamate acting on AMPA receptors. This depolarization relieves the Mg^{2+} block of NMDA receptors, which then respond by permitting Ca^{2+} influx and further depolarization of the postsynaptic cell. NMDA receptors are also regulated by glycine, which binds to the receptor to enhance current flow in response to glutamate.

Cellular and Molecular Mechanisms of Neurotransmitter Release

The lipid and protein components of synaptic vesicles are synthesized in the neuronal soma and they travel to the nerve ending via fast axonal transport (Fig. 4-13). Neuropeptides are synthesized in the soma and packaged there into large electron-dense core vesicles, which are transported down the axon to the nerve ending. The smaller synaptic vesicles that contain classic small molecule neurotransmitters are filled with transmitter in the nerve ending. Catecholamine-containing vesicles are small and have an electron-dense core. Vesicles containing other small molecule transmitters are small and appear clear in electron micrographs. Small synaptic vesicles are formed by budding off from early endosomes (Fig. 4-14). The classic neurotransmitter is synthesized in the nerve terminal and accumulated in the synaptic vesicles by secondary active transporters that catalyze the exchange of neurotransmitters for H^+ ions. The H^+ ion gradient is generated by a V-type ATPase (see Chapter 1) in the vesicle membrane.

The large vesicles that release neuropeptides may fuse with the presynaptic membrane at multiple locations to release

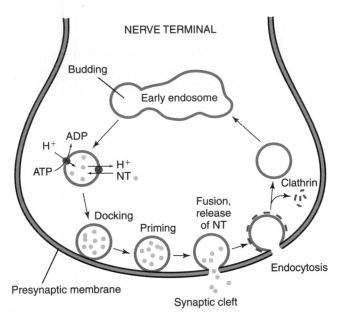

NERVE TERMINAL

Budding

Early endosome

ADP
H⁺
ATP
H⁺
NT

Clathrin

Docking

Priming

Fusion, release of NT

Endocytosis

Presynaptic membrane

Synaptic cleft

■ **Fig. 4-14**   The synaptic vesicle cycle. A synaptic vesicle is budded from a late endosome and is filled with neurotransmitter *(NT).* The filled vesicle docks at an active site and then, after a time delay, undergoes priming. Upon an increase in the local [Ca²⁺] the synaptic vesicle fuses with the plasma membrane and releases NT into the synaptic cleft. The empty vesicle is coated with clathrin and endocytosed. In the cytosol, the endocytosed vesicle loses its clathrin coat and fuses with the late endosome.

their contents. The small vesicles that contain nonpeptide neurotransmitters can fuse with the presynaptic membrane only at specific sites, called **active zones.** To become competent to fuse with the presynaptic membrane at an active zone, a small vesicle must first **dock** at the active zone. Then it must undergo a **priming** process before the vesicle can fuse and release its transmitter into the synaptic cleft in response to an increase in the local cytoplasmic concentration of Ca²⁺. Due to the entry of Ca²⁺ into the nerve terminal through voltage-gated ion channels, the local concentration of Ca²⁺ in the nerve terminal rises and triggers the fusion of a small fraction of the docked vesicles. The fused vesicles release transmitter into the synaptic cleft. The empty vesicles are coated with clathrin, are rapidly internalized and subsequently fuse with early endosomes, the compartment from which new synaptic vesicles form by budding. Thus the protein and lipid components of the synaptic vesicles rapidly cycle within the nerve terminal. On the order of 25 proteins may play roles in docking, priming, and fusion. Some of these proteins are cytosolic, and others are proteins of the vesicle membrane or of the presynaptic membrane. Although functions of most of these proteins are incompletely understood, knowledge of the molecular details of transmitter release, which will not be discussed in detail here, has increased dramatically in recent years.

As with other exocytotic processes (Chapter 1) neurotransmitter release involves SNARE proteins: v-SNARES in the vesicle membrane and t-SNARES on the (target) presynaptic plasma membrane. Zipper-like interactions between **synaptobrevin** (a v-SNARE) and **syntaxin** and **SNAP-25** (two t-SNARES) bring the vesicle membrane and the presynaptic plasma membrane close together prior to fusion.

Toxins produced by *Clostridium botulinum* cause a disease known as **botulism.** This organism produces several toxins that are proteases that specifically cleave SNARE proteins involved in neurotransmitter release. Botulinum toxins types B, D, F, and G cleave the v-SNARE synaptobrevin. The t-SNARE syntaxin is cleaved by botulinum toxin type C, whereas SNAP-25, also a t-SNARE, is cleaved by botulinum toxins types A and E.

SUMMARY

1. The neuromuscular junction is the best characterized chemical synapse in vertebrates. Acetylcholine released by the prejunctional nerve terminal binds to acetylcholine receptors in the postjunctional membrane to open ion channels conductive to Na⁺ and K⁺. The resultant ion flow across the postjunctional membrane causes a depolarization, called an end plate potential.

2. The end plate potential is terminated by the hydrolysis of acetylcholine by the enzyme acetylcholinesterase.

3. When acetylcholine is hydrolyzed, the choline liberated in the synaptic cleft is actively transported back into the nerve terminal.

4. The release of acetylcholine is quantal. A quantum corresponds to the amount of acetylcholine in a single presynaptic vesicle.

5. Direct electrical transmission between neighboring cells is mediated by gap junctions.

6. An action potential in an excitatory input to a spinal motor neuron causes an excitatory postsynaptic potential that depolarizes the motor neuron and brings it closer to threshold.

7. An action potential in an inhibitory input causes an inhibitory postsynaptic potential that hyperpolarizes the motor neuron.

8. The efficacy of synaptic transmission depends on the timing and frequency of action potentials in the presynaptic neuron. Facilitation, posttetanic potentiation, and long-term potentiation are examples of increased efficacy of synaptic transmission in response to previous multiple stimulations of a synapse.

9. Acetylcholine, biogenic amines, glutamate, glycine, and γ-aminobutyric acid (GABA) are important neurotransmitters in the central nervous system.

10. Glycine and γ-aminobutyric acid are the major transmitters at inhibitory synapses in the central nervous system.

11. Glutamate is the major excitatory neurotransmitter in the central nervous system. There are five classes of excitatory amino acid (EAA) receptors.

12. Many neuroactive peptides function as neuromodulators or neurotransmitters in the central nervous system.

BIBLIOGRAPHY

Journal articles

Amara SC, Sonders MS: Neurotransmitter transporters as molecular targets for addictive drugs, *Drug Alcohol Depend* 51:87, 1998.

Bennett MK: Ca^{2+} and the regulation of neurotransmitter secretion, *Curr Opin Neurobiol* 7:316, 1997.

Hokfelt T et al: Neuropeptides: an overview, *Neuropharmacology* 39:1337, 2000.

Jahn R, Sudhof TC: Membrane fusion and exocytosis, *Annu Rev Biochem* 68:863, 1999.

Kandel ER: The molecular biology of memory storage: a dialogue between genes and synapses, *Science* 294(5544):1030, 2001.

Karlin A: Emerging structure of the nicotinic acetylcholine receptors, *Nature Rev Neurosci* 3:102, 2002.

Kennedy MB: On beyond LTP: long-term potentiation, *Learn Memory* 6:417, 1999.

Luscher C et al: Synaptic plasticity and dynamic modulation of the postsynaptic membrane, *Nature Neurosci* 3:545, 2000.

Sudhof TC: The synaptic vesicle cycle revisited, *Neuron* 28:317, 2000.

Books and monographs

Aidley DJ: *The physiology of excitable cells,* ed 4, Cambridge, 1998, Cambridge University Press.

Eccles JC: *The physiology of synapses,* Berlin, 1964, Springer-Verlag.

Hall Z: *An introduction to molecular neurobiology,* Sunderland, Mass, 1992, Sinauer Associates.

Kandel ER, Schwartz JH: *Principles of neural science,* ed 4, New York, 2000 McGraw-Hill.

Katz, B: *Nerve, muscle, and synapse,* New York, 1966, McGraw-Hill.

Levitan IB, Kaczmarek LK: *The neuron: cell and molecular biology,* ed 3, New York, 2002, Oxford University Press.

Nicholls JG et al: *From neuron to brain,* ed 4, Sunderland, Mass, 2001, Sinauer Associates.

Purves G et al: *Neuroscience,* ed 2, Sunderland, Mass, 2001, Sinauer Associates.

chapter five

Membrane Receptors, Second Messengers, and Signal Transduction Pathways

Basic cellular processes are regulated by a host of substances. Some regulatory substances, such as steroid hormones (Chapter 39), enter the cell and influence the transcription of certain genes. Other regulatory substances, such as most neurotransmitters and peptide hormones, exert their influences from outside the cell. This chapter discusses regulatory substances and the ways in which they influence cellular processes.

OVERVIEW

The first step in the action of an extracellular regulatory substance is to bind to specific protein receptors on the extracellular surface of the plasma membrane of the target cells. For example, the neurotransmitters discussed in Chapter 4 bind to a receptor in order to bring about a response. The receptor is a ligand-gated ion channel, and the response of the cell is a ligand-induced ionic current. In this example, the ligand-gated ion channel protein is both the receptor and the **effector** for the action of the neurotransmitter. For most regulatory molecules, however, a more complex series of events takes place between the binding of a regulatory substance to its specific membrane receptor and its final effects on cellular function. Extracellular regulatory molecules exert their effects on cells via **signal transduction pathways.**

Signal Transduction Pathways

In most signal transduction pathways, the binding of a regulatory substance to its plasma membrane receptors alters the activities of particular cellular proteins and thereby causes a cellular response. Although many regulatory substances exist, there are relatively few signal transduction pathways. Our knowledge of these pathways is increasing at such a rapid rate that a comprehensive discussion of this subject is beyond the scope of this book. Therefore, only certain well-understood signal transduction pathways are emphasized, especially those that are relevant to topics discussed in subsequent chapters.

Extracellular Regulatory Substances

The regulatory compounds we consider in this chapter are often classified as endocrine, neurocrine, or paracrine substances. **Endocrine** regulatory substances (hormones) are released by endocrine cells. Hormones reach their target cells, which may be far from the endocrine cells, via the bloodstream. **Neurocrine** regulators are released by neurons in the immediate vicinity of the target cells. Neurotransmitters are neurocrine substances, as are most of the neuromodulators discussed in Chapter 4. **Paracrine** substances are released by cells that are not immediately adjacent to the target cells, but they are sufficiently close for the paracrine substance to reach the target cells by diffusion. For example, histamine is a paracrine agonist of gastric HCl secretion (see Chapter 32). Histamine is released by enterochromaffin-like (ECL) cells in the gastric mucosa, and it reaches the acid-secreting parietal cells by diffusion. Paracrine regulators are secreted by one cell type, and they act upon cells of a different type. However, some cells release regulators that act on that cell itself or on its neighbors of the same cell type. This type of regulation is called **autocrine** regulation. For example, certain nerve terminals release autocrine substances that act on receptors on the nerve terminal to influence the subsequent release of neurotransmitter.

TYPES OF SIGNAL TRANSDUCTION PATHWAYS

This section provides a brief overview of some of the major signal transduction pathways that have been characterized. After this section, the discussion turns to a more detailed description of certain of these pathways.

Protein Kinases and Phosphatases in Signal Transduction Pathways

Frequently, the final step in a signal transduction pathway is the phosphorylation of particular proteins that play central roles in eliciting cellular responses. When these effector proteins are phosphorylated, their activities may be enhanced or inhibited. **Protein kinases** in the cell are responsible for phosphorylating particular proteins, whereas **protein phosphatases** catalyze the removal of phosphates from proteins. The state of phosphorylation of an effector protein depends on the balance of the activities of the kinase that phosphorylates it and the phosphatase that dephosphorylates it. Protein phosphatases are discussed later in this chapter.

Often, a signal transduction pathway alters the activity of a protein kinase in response to the binding of the regulatory molecule, often called an **agonist,** to its membrane receptor. The major classes of agonist-activated protein kinases are shown in Fig. 5-1.

Frequently, binding of an agonist to its membrane receptors brings about a change in the cytosolic concentration of a compound called a **second messenger,** which then increases the activity of a protein kinase. Second messengers include **cAMP, cGMP, Ca^{2+}, inositol-1,4,5-trisphosphate (IP$_3$),** and **diacylglycerols.** Cells contain protein kinases that are modulated by each of these second messengers. In the following paragraphs, we discuss some of these second messengers and the protein kinases they modulate.

Cells contain protein kinases whose activities are enhanced by the second messengers, cyclic AMP and cyclic GMP. These kinases are called **cyclic AMP-dependent protein kinases** and **cyclic GMP-dependent protein kinases,** respectively.

The activities of **calmodulin-dependent protein kinases** are enhanced when they bind to a complex consisting of Ca^{2+} and a protein called calmodulin. Calmodulin is a protein (MW 16,700) that is present in all cells; in some cells calmodulin accounts for 1% of the total cellular protein. Calmodulin binds four Ca^{2+} ions; the Ca^{2+}-calmodulin complex then regulates a host of other intracellular proteins, many of which are not kinases.

Protein kinases of the **protein kinase C** family are activated by Ca^{2+}, diglycerides, certain membrane phospholipids, and certain breakdown products of membrane phospholipids.

Insulin and some **growth factors** bind to membrane receptors that are themselves protein kinases. These receptors, called protein tyrosine kinase receptors, are discussed later in this chapter and in Chapter 41.

G Protein–Mediated Signal Transduction Pathways

Many hormones, neuromodulators, and other regulatory compounds that alter cellular processes do so by signal transduction pathways that involve **heterotrimeric GTP-binding**

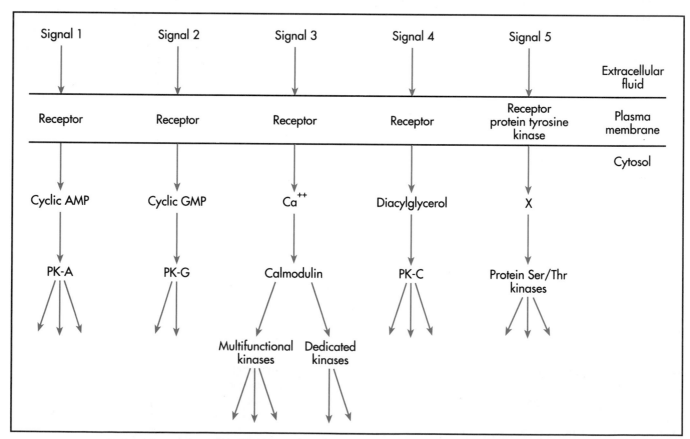

■ **Fig. 5-1**   Frequently the final step in a signal transduction pathway is the phosphorylation of an effector protein by a protein kinase. Five major signal transduction pathways of mammalian cells that involve protein kinases are depicted in this diagram. *PK-A,* Cyclic AMP-dependent protein kinase; *PK-G,* cyclic GMP-dependent protein kinase; *PK-C,* protein kinase C; *X,* signaling pathways described later. (Adapted from Cohen P: *Trends Biochem Sci* 17:408, 1992.)

proteins, also called **G proteins.** (Another class of GTP-binding proteins, monomeric GTP-binding proteins, is discussed later.) A G protein is a molecular switch (Fig. 5-2) that can exist in two states. In its activated ("on") state, a G protein has a higher affinity for GTP. In the inactivated ("off") state, G protein preferentially binds GDP. When agonist molecules bind to them, some membrane receptors interact with a G protein to promote conversion of the G protein to its activated state by binding GTP. The activated G protein can then interact with many **effector proteins,** most notably enzymes or ion channels, to alter their activities. The activated G protein has GTPase activity, so that the bound GTP is eventually hydrolyzed to GDP, and the G protein reverts to its inactive state (Fig. 5-2).

Among the most important targets of activated G proteins are molecules that change the cellular concentrations of the second messengers cAMP, cGMP, Ca^{2+}, IP_3, and diacylglycerol (Fig. 5-3). G protein-mediated mechanisms are powerful modulators of adenylyl cyclase and cGMP phosphodiesterase, the enzymes responsible for the synthesis of cAMP and the breakdown of cGMP, respectively. Ca^{2+} channels may be modulated directly by G proteins or indirectly by second messenger–dependent protein kinases. Other effectors that are modulated by G proteins include certain K^+ channels and phospholipases C, A_2, and D.

In brief, a G protein-protein kinase-mediated signal transduction pathway involves the following events (Fig. 5-3):

1. A hormone or other regulatory molecule binds to its plasma membrane receptor.
2. The ligand-bearing receptor interacts with a G protein and activates it, and the activated G protein binds GTP.
3. The activated G protein interacts with one or more of the following: adenylyl cyclase; cGMP phosphodiesterase; Ca^{2+} or K^+ channels; or phospholipases C, A_2, or D to activate or inhibit them.
4. The cellular level of one or more of the following second messengers increases or decreases: cAMP, cGMP, Ca^{2+}, IP_3, or diacylglycerol.

5. The increase or decrease of the concentration of a second messenger changes the activity of one or more second messenger–dependent protein kinases, such as cyclic AMP–dependent protein kinase, cGMP–dependent protein kinase, calmodulin-dependent protein kinase, or protein kinase C; or the change in second messenger concentration activates an ion channel.
6. The level of phosphorylation of an enzyme or an ion channel is altered, or an ion channel activity changes and brings about the final cellular response.

Membrane Phospholipids and Signal Transduction Pathways

Another class of extracellular agonists binds to receptors that activate, via a G protein called G_q, the β isoform of **phospholipase C.** This isoform cleaves phosphatidylinositol-4,5-bisphosphate (a phospholipid present in minute quantities in the plasma membrane) into **inositol-1,4,5-trisphosphate** **(IP_3)** and **diacylglycerol** (Fig. 5-4). Both IP_3 and diacylglycerol are second messengers. IP_3 binds to specific ligand-gated Ca^{2+} channels in the endoplasmic reticulum and releases Ca^{2+}, thus increasing its cytosolic concentration. The Ca^{2+} channel of the endoplasmic reticulum has a structure similar to that of the Ca^{2+} channel of the sarcoplasmic reticulum, which is involved in excitation-contraction coupling in skeletal and cardiac muscle (see Chapters 12 and 16). Diacylglycerol, together with Ca^{2+}, activates another important class of protein kinases, called **protein kinase C.** Among the substrates of protein kinase C are proteins involved in the control of cellular growth and proliferation.

The enzymes **phospholipase A_2 (PLA_2)** and **phospholipase D** are also activated by some agonists via G protein-dependent pathways. These enzymes act on membrane phospholipids, and products of these reactions also activate protein kinase C (discussed later). PLA_2 cleaves the number 2 fatty acid from membrane phospholipids. Because some of the phospholipids contain arachidonic acid, PLA_2-mediated cleavage of these phospholipids releases significant amounts of **arachidonic acid.** Arachidonic acid is an effector mole-

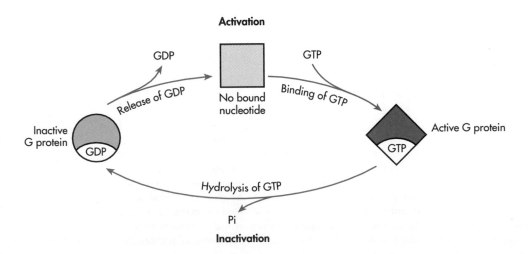

Activation

GDP — Release of GDP → No bound nucleotide — Binding of GTP → GTP

Inactive G protein (GDP) — Active G protein (GTP)

Hydrolysis of GTP → Pi

Inactivation

■ **Fig. 5-2** The activity cycle of a GTP-binding protein (G protein). The inactive form of the G protein *(circle)* binds GDP. Interaction of the G protein with a ligand-bearing membrane receptor promotes a conformational change leading to the release of GDP and the binding of GTP. The GTP bound form of the G protein *(diamond)* is the active form that interacts with proteins such as adenylyl cyclase and ion channels to alter their activities. The G protein has an intrinsic GTPase activity; hydrolysis of GTP converts the G protein back to its inactive state.

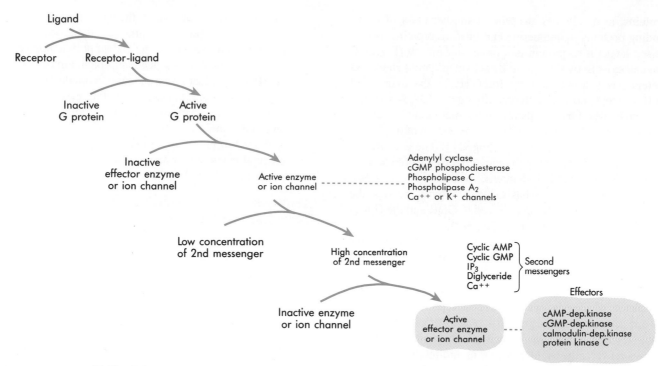

■ **Fig. 5-3**   A schematic depiction of the signal transduction cascade by which an extracellular ligand such as a peptide hormone can bind to its receptor so as to activate a G protein and, via the cascade, lead to the activation or inactivation of an ion channel, a protein kinase, or a phospholipase. At each level of the cascade, amplification can occur. For the sake of simplicity, the figure indicates that occupation of receptor by ligand leads to an *increase* in a second messenger, which causes an *activation* of an enzyme or ion channel. In reality, there are numerous cases in which receptor occupation leads to a *decreased* concentration of second messenger and cases in which increased second messenger results in *inactivation* of an enzyme or ion channel.

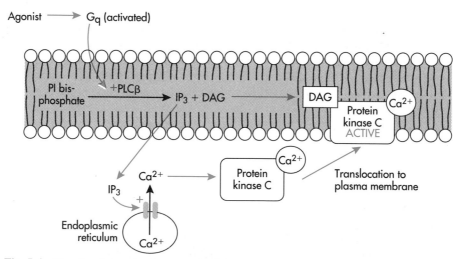

■ **Fig. 5-4**   The signal transduction pathway activated by the hydrolysis of inositol phospholipids of the plasma membrane. Some agonists bind to receptors that activate the G_q class of heterotrimeric G proteins. Activated G_q stimulates the activity of phospholipase Cβ to hydrolyze the minor membrane phospholipid phosphatidylinositol-4,5-bisphosphate. This cleavage releases IP_3 and diacylglycerol (DAG), both of which are second messengers. IP_3 binds to a specific Ca^{2+} channel in the endoplasmic reticulum membrane, causing Ca^{2+} to be released. Ca^{2+} binds to cytosolic protein kinase C, causing protein kinase C to bind to the cytoplasmic surface of the plasma membrane. Diacylglycerol, together with Ca^{2+}, activates protein kinase C to phosphorylate important cellular effector proteins.

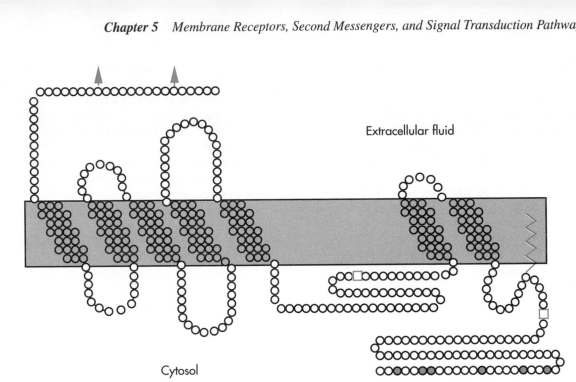

Extracellular fluid

Cytosol

■ **Fig. 5-5** Proposed structure of the human β_2-adrenergic receptor. Sites for *N*-linked glycosylation of the extracellular domain are indicated by arrows. Phosphorylation of the receptor promotes its desensitization (bound agonist elicits diminished response). *Colored circles* indicate serine and threonine residues near the C terminus that are phosphorylated by β-adrenergic receptor kinase. *Colored squares* indicate amino acids that are phosphorylated by cyclic AMP–dependent protein kinase. Phosphorylation of the receptor is involved in its regulation. The colored zigzag line represents covalently bound palmitic acid. (Modified from Dohlman HG et al: *Annu Rev Biochem* 60:653, 1991.)

cule in its own right, as well as the precursor for the cellular synthesis of **prostaglandins, prostacyclins, thromboxanes, and leukotrienes,** which are important classes of potent regulatory molecules. Arachidonic acid can also be produced from the breakdown of diacylglycerols.

Prostaglandins, prostacyclins, and thromboxanes are synthesized from arachidonic acid via the **cyclooxygenase-dependent pathway.** Leukotrienes are derived from arachidonic acid via the **lipoxygenase-dependent pathway.** One of the antiinflammatory actions of corticosteroids (see Fig. 45-20) is to inhibit the phospholipase A_2 that releases arachidonic acid from phospholipids. Aspirin and other non-steroidal antiinflammatory agents inhibit the oxidation of arachidonic acid by cyclooxygenase.

Protein Tyrosine Kinases

Proteins with intrinsic **protein tyrosine kinase** activity represent a family of membrane receptors that is not linked to G proteins. When an agonist (such as a growth factor) binds to these receptors, their tyrosine kinase activity is stimulated, and they phosphorylate specific effector proteins on particular tyrosine residues. The other protein kinases that have previously been discussed only phosphorylate proteins on serine and threonine residues. The receptor for the hormone insulin and receptors for many growth factors are tyrosine kinases. Most growth factor receptors dimerize when a growth factor binds to them. Dimerization activates the tyrosine kinase activity. Often, the activated receptors phosphorylate themselves, a process called **autophosphorylation.**

G Protein–Linked Membrane Receptors

Membrane receptors that mediate agonist-dependent activation of G proteins make up a protein family with more than 1000 members. This family includes α and β-adrenergic receptors, muscarinic acetylcholine receptors, serotonin receptors, adenosine receptors, olfactory receptors, rhodopsin, and receptors for most peptide hormones. The members of the G protein–coupled receptor family (Fig. 5-5) have seven transmembrane α helices, each consisting of 22 to 28 predominantly hydrophobic amino acids. Many subtypes of G protein–linked receptors exist for certain ligands, such as acetylcholine, epinephrine, norepinephrine, and serotonin. The subtypes are distinguished by differing affinities for competing agonists and antagonists.

The remainder of this chapter focuses in more detail on the mechanisms of these signal transduction pathways.

HETEROTRIMERIC G PROTEINS

As we have seen, GTP-binding proteins, also known as G proteins, bind and hydrolyze GTP. They serve as molecular switches that regulate a host of intracellular processes. The active form of a G protein has a high affinity for GTP (Fig. 5-2). The intrinsic GTPase activity of the G protein hydrolyzes GTP, which causes the G protein to revert to its inactive GDP-bound form. Active G proteins modulate many vital cellular activities by binding to and modifying the activity of certain important enzymes and ion channels. Two classes of G proteins are known: **heterotrimeric G proteins** and

monomeric proteins (also called **low-molecular-weight** or **small G proteins**).

A heterotrimeric G protein has three subunits: an α subunit (40,000 to 45,000 daltons), a β subunit (about 37,000 daltons), and a γ subunit (8000 to 10,000 daltons). Currently, we know of 22 different genes that encode subunits, at least 5 genes that encode β subunits, and about 12 genes that encode β subunits in mammals. In most G proteins, the β and γ subunits are tightly associated with one another. Some heterotrimeric G proteins and the signal transduction pathways they mediate are listed in Table 5-1.

Heterotrimeric G proteins function as intermediaries between the plasma membrane receptors for over 100 different extracellular regulatory substances (e.g., hormones, neuromodulators) and the intracellular processes they control. Simply put, binding of the regulatory substance to its receptor activates the G protein; the activated G protein then either stimulates or inhibits an enzyme or an ion channel.

Inactive G proteins exist primarily as αβγ heterotrimers, with GDP in their nucleotide-binding sites. The interaction of a heterotrimeric G protein with a ligand-bearing receptor causes its α subunit to change to the active form, which has a higher affinity for GTP and a lower affinity for the βγ pair. Therefore, the activated α subunit releases GDP, binds GTP, and then dissociates from βγ. In most G proteins, the dissociated α subunit then interacts with the next protein in the signal transduction pathway. *In some G proteins, however, the βγ dimer is responsible for all or some of the receptor-mediated response.*

Regulation of adenylyl cyclase. Cyclic AMP was the first of the second messengers to be discovered, and the regulation of adenylyl cyclase, which is the enzyme that produces cAMP, is the prototype for G protein–mediated signal transduction pathways.

Adenylyl cyclase is subject to both positive and negative control by G protein–mediated pathways (Fig. 5-6). In

---

■ Table 5-1 Selected mammalian heterotrimeric GTP-binding proteins classified on the basis of their α subunits*

G protein	Activated by receptors for	Effectors	Signaling pathways
G_s	Epinephrine, norepinephrine, histamine, glucagon, ACTH, luteinizing hormone, follicle-stimulating hormone, thyroid-stimulating hormone, and others	Adenylyl cyclase Ca²⁺ channels	↑cAMP ↑Ca²⁺ influx
G_{olf}	Odorants	Adenylyl cyclase	↑cAMP (olfaction)
G_{t1} (rods)	Photons	cGMP phosphodiesterase	↓cGMP (vision)
G_{t2} (cones)	Photons	cGMP phosphodiesterase	↓cGMP (color vision)
G_{i1}, G_{i2}, G_{i3}	Norepinephrine, prostaglandins, opiates, angiotensin, many peptides	Adenylyl cyclase Phospholipase C Phospholipase A₂ K⁺ channels	↓cAMP ↑Inositol trisphosphate, diacylglycerol, Ca²⁺ Arachidonate release
G_q	Acetylcholine, epinephrine	Phospholipase Cβ	Membrane polarization ↑Inositol trisphosphate, diacylglycerol, Ca²⁺

Modified from Bourne HR, Sanders DA, McCormick F: *Nature* 348:125, 1990.
ACTH, Adrenocorticotropic hormone; *cAMP*, cyclic AMP; *cGMP*, cyclic GMP.
*There is more than one isoform of each class of α subunit; more than 20 distinct α subunits have been identified.

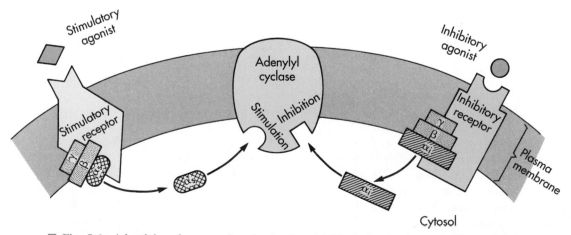

■ Fig. 5-6 Adenylyl cyclase may be stimulated or inhibited via signal transduction pathways. Receptors for agonists that stimulate adenylyl cyclase activate G_s, whose $α_s$ subunit dissociates from βγ and then interacts with adenylyl cyclase to stimulate it. Receptors for agonists that inhibit adenylyl cyclase activate G_i, whose $α_i$ subunit inhibits adenylyl cyclase.

positive control, the binding of a stimulatory ligand, such as epinephrine acting through β-adrenergic receptors, activates heterotrimeric G proteins with α subunits of the type called α_s (*s* for stimulatory). Activation of the G_s-type G protein by the ligand-bearing receptor causes its α_s subunit to bind GTP and then to dissociate from βγ. α_s then interacts with adenylyl cyclase to activate it.

Other regulatory substances, such as epinephrine acting at α_2 receptors and adenosine acting on α_1 receptors, participate in negative or inhibitory control of adenylyl cyclase. These regulatory substances activate G_i-type G proteins that have α subunits of a type called α_i (*i* for inhibitory). Binding of the inhibitory ligand to its receptor activates the G_i-type G protein and causes its α_i subunit to dissociate from the βγ dimers. The activated α_i binds to and inhibits adenylyl cyclase.

> **Cholera** causes a watery diarrhea that can rapidly lead to dehydration and death if not promptly treated. The diarrhea is caused by a toxin produced by the bacterium *Vibrio cholerae*. A component of the cholera toxin enters the cells and catalyzes the covalent addition of ADP-ribose to the $G_s\alpha$ subunit. This reaction permanently activates G_s, which results in persistent activation of adenylyl cyclase. As a consequence, cyclic AMP is permanently elevated. The brush border membrane that faces the lumen of the small intestine contains an electrogenic chloride channel that opens when cyclic AMP levels are elevated (see Chapter 33). The persistent activation of this Cl⁻ channel causes Cl⁻, Na⁺, and water to pour into the lumen of the small intestine. The result of this secretion is persistent watery diarrhea of as much as 20 L per day.

Direct modulation of ion channels by G proteins. In Chapter 4, several ligand-gated ion channels that are modulated directly by an extracellular agonist, such as acetylcholine or γ-aminobutyric acid, were discussed. Other ion channels are regulated by second messenger-mediated mechanisms that involve G proteins. The regulation of these ion channels takes place after G proteins are activated in the second step of the signal transduction cascade.

Some ion channels, however, are *directly modulated by G proteins and do not involve a second messenger.* The binding of acetylcholine to M_2 muscarinic receptors in the heart and in certain neurons, for instance, leads to the activation of a specific class of K⁺ channels. Acetylcholine binding to the muscarinic receptor activates a G protein of the G_i subclass. The activated α_i subunit then dissociates from the βγ dimer. *The βγ dimer directly interacts with a particular class of K⁺ channels* to increase their probability of opening. The action of acetylcholine on muscarinic receptors to increase K⁺ conductance of the pacemaker cells in the sinoatrial node of the heart is one of the major mechanisms whereby para-sympathetic nerves cause slowing of the heart rate (see Chapter 15).

Monomeric GTP-Binding Proteins

Cells contain another family of GTP-binding proteins called **monomeric GTP-binding proteins;** they are also known as low-molecular-weight G proteins or small G proteins (MW 20,000 to 35,000 daltons). Table 5-2 lists the major subfamilies of monomeric GTP-binding proteins and some of their properties. The Ras-like and Rho-like monomeric GTP-binding proteins are involved in signal transduction pathways that link growth factor receptor tyrosine kinases to their intracellular effects. Among the processes that are regulated by pathways that involve monomeric GTP-binding proteins are polypeptide chain elongation in protein synthesis, proliferation and differentiation of cells, neoplastic transformation of cells, control of the actin cytoskeleton and linkages between the cytoskeleton and the extracellular matrix, transport of vesicles among different organelles, and exocytotic secretion.

Monomeric GTP-binding proteins, like their heterotrimeric cousins, are molecular switches that alternate between an "on" (activated) state and an "off" (inactivated) state (Fig. 5-2). However, the activation and inactivation of the monomolecular GTP-binding proteins involve additional regulatory proteins that do not operate on the heterotrimeric G proteins (Fig. 5-7). Monomeric GTP-binding proteins are activated by **guanine nucleotide exchange factors (GEFs)** and inactivated by **GTPase-activating proteins (GAPs).** Therefore, activation and inactivation of monomeric GTP-binding proteins are probably controlled by signals that influence the activity of GEFs or GAPs, rather than by direct effects on the monomeric G protein.

Second Messenger-Dependent Ion Channels

Most cellular responses mediated by G protein-coupled pathways involve second messenger-dependent protein kinases. However, in some responses, the second messenger acts directly on an ion channel to produce a response. Some cells have a class of K⁺ channels that is directly activated by the level of Ca^{2+} in the cytosol. When intracellular Ca^{2+} rises, **Ca^{2+}-activated K⁺ channels** are activated, which leads to repolarization or hyperpolarization of the cell. Both vision and olfaction involve ion channels that are gated by second messengers.

Visual transduction (see Chapter 8) depends on cGMP–gated ion channels. When a person is in a dark room, the level of cGMP in rod photoreceptors is high. Consequently, the **cGMP-activated Na⁺ channels** in the rod plasma mem-

■ Table 5-2   Subfamilies of monomeric GTP-binding proteins and some of the intracellular processes they regulate

Subfamily	Cellular effects
Ras-like proteins	Control growth and differentiation
Rho-like proteins (including Rac)	Control polymerization of actin filaments and their assembly into particular structures such as focal adhesions
Rab-like proteins	Control vesicle trafficking by helping target vesicles to particular membranes
ARF-like proteins	Regulate the assembly and disassembly of vesicle coat proteins and thereby control vesicle traffic

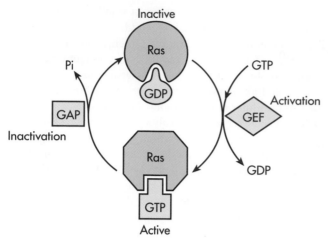

■ Fig. 5-7   The activity cycle of Ras, a monomeric GTP-binding protein. Other monomeric GTP-binding proteins have a similar activity cycle. The activation of Ras is stimulated by a GEF (guanine nucleotide–exchange factor), which promotes the binding of GTP and the release of GDP, thereby activating the small G protein. The inactivation of Ras is promoted by a GAP (GTPase-activating protein), which stimulates the hydrolysis of the bound GTP, thus inactivating Ras.

brane are open, and the entry of Na^+ into the rod cell maintains its depolarized state. **Rhodopsin** is a member of the family of G protein-coupled receptors, and it is activated by light. When activated, it interacts with and activates a heterotrimeric G protein called **transducin (G_t).** Activated transducin interacts with cGMP phosphodiesterase to greatly increase its activity, and thereby to rapidly decrease the intracellular cGMP concentration. Consequently, the cGMP–activated Na^+ channels close and the rod cell is hyperpolarized. Hyperpolarization of rod cells is necessary for visual signals to be conducted to the brain.

Olfaction (see Chapter 8) involves cAMP–gated ion channels. Humans and other vertebrates are able to distin-

guish a large number of different **odorants.** Many of these odorants interact with G protein-coupled receptors in the plasma membrane of olfactory receptor cells. The odorant-bearing receptor activates G_{olf}, a heterotrimeric G protein. Activated **G_{olf},** in turn, stimulates adenylyl cyclase to produce cyclic AMP. Elevated cyclic AMP levels activate **cyclic AMP–gated Na^+ channels** in the plasma membrane of the olfactory receptor cell. Na^+ inflow leads to depolarization of the receptor, which may trigger an action potential in the axon of the olfactory receptor cell.

SECOND MESSENGER-DEPENDENT PROTEIN KINASES

Cyclic AMP was first identified as a second messenger during investigations of the mechanisms involved in the hormonal control of glycogen synthesis and breakdown (see Chapters 40 and 41). Researchers found that the hormonal regulation of glycogen metabolism involves the phosphorylation of rate-determining enzymes that participate in these metabolic pathways by cAMP–dependent protein kinases.

Cyclic AMP-Dependent Protein Kinase

In the absence of cAMP, cAMP-dependent protein kinase is composed of four subunits: two regulatory subunits and two catalytic subunits. The presence of the regulatory subunits greatly inhibits the enzymatic activity of the complex. Therefore, activation of the enzymatic activity of cAMP-dependent protein kinase must involve the dissociation of the regulatory subunits from the complex.

Activation takes place when micromolar levels of cAMP are present. Each regulatory subunit binds two molecules of cAMP. The binding of cAMP induces a conformational change in the regulatory subunits and diminishes their affinity for binding the catalytic subunits. Hence, the regulatory subunits dissociate from the catalytic subunits, and the catalytic subunits become activated (Fig. 5-8). The active

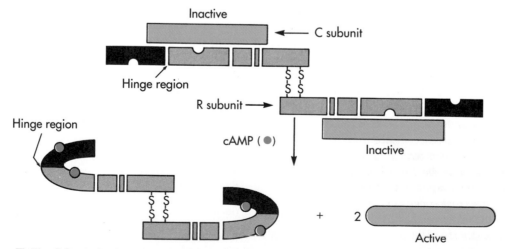

■ Fig. 5-8   Activation of cyclic AMP–dependent protein kinase. The two regulatory subunits (R subunit) of the R_2C_2 complex are held together by two disulfide bonds. Binding of two molecules of cyclic AMP to each R subunit causes flexion in a hinge region of each R subunit and the release of the two active catalytic subunits (C subunits). (Adapted from Taylor S: *J Biol Chem* 264:8443, 1989.)

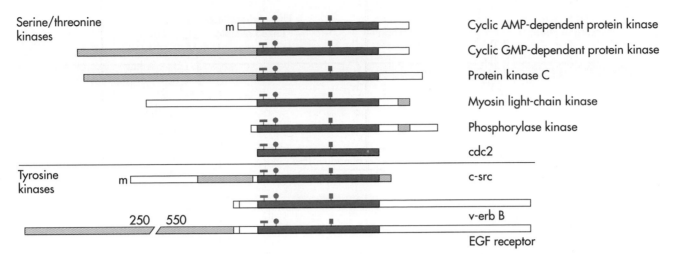

■ **Fig. 5-9** The protein kinase family. All known protein kinases share a common catalytic core *(solid color)* that contains ATP- and peptide-binding domains and the active site where phosphoryl transfer occurs. Conserved residues are aligned with lysine 72 *(colored circle)*, aspartate 184 *(colored square)*, and the glycine-rich loop *(small colored rectangle)* of the catalytic subunit of cyclic AMP–dependent protein kinase. Regions important for regulation are cross-hatched. Sites of covalent attachment of myristic acid are indicated by *m*. This fatty acid helps to anchor the protein kinase to the plasma membrane. (Adapted from Taylor S et al: *Annu Rev Cell Biol* 8:429, 1992.)

catalytic subunit phosphorylates target proteins on particular serine and threonine residues.

Comparison of the amino acid sequence of cAMP–dependent protein kinase with representatives of the other classes of protein kinases shows that despite vast differences in their regulatory properties, the different classes of protein kinases share a common catalytic core with high amino acid homology (Fig. 5-9). The core structure includes the ATP-binding domain and the enzyme's active center, where the transfer of phosphate from ATP to the acceptor protein occurs. Regions of the kinases outside the catalytic core are involved in regulation of the kinase activities.

The catalytic core that is conserved among all known protein kinases consists of two lobes. The smaller of the two lobes contains an unusual ATP-binding site, whereas the larger lobe contains the peptide-binding site. Many protein kinases also contain a regulatory region known as a **pseudosubstrate domain.** The amino acid sequence of this site resembles the phosphorylation sites of substrate proteins. The pseudosubstrate region binds to the active site of the protein kinase and inhibits the phosphorylation of true substrates of the protein kinase. Activation of the kinase may involve phosphorylation or a noncovalent allosteric modification of the protein kinase to remove the inhibition of the pseudosubstrate domain. Tissue specificity is attained in pathways that use cAMP as the second messenger in three ways. First, the distribution of receptors for agonists is different in different tissues. Second, the proteins that are phosphorylated by cAMP–dependent protein kinase (protein kinase A) are different in different tissues. Third, some cells have proteins that anchor protein kinase A near its target proteins. These anchoring proteins are called **A kinase-associated proteins (AKAPs).**

Calmodulin-Dependent Protein Kinases

A host of vital cellular processes, including release of neurotransmitters, secretion of hormones, and muscle contraction, are regulated by the cytosolic level of Ca^{2+}. One way that Ca^{2+} exerts control over these processes is by binding to the protein calmodulin. The Ca^{2+}-calmodulin complex can then influence the activity of many different proteins, among them a group of protein kinases known as **calmodulin-dependent protein kinases** (Fig. 5-10). Some calmodulin-dependent protein kinases, such as myosin light chain kinase and phosphorylase kinase, have only one cellular substrate. Others are multifunctional and phosphorylate more than one substrate protein.

Myosin light chain kinase plays a central role in the regulation of contraction of smooth muscle (see Chapter 13). Elevation of the cytosolic Ca^{2+} concentration in a smooth muscle cell stimulates the activity of myosin light chain kinase; the resultant phosphorylation of the regulatory light chains of myosin allows contraction of smooth muscle cells to proceed.

Calmodulin-dependent protein kinase II is among the most abundant proteins in the nervous system; it accounts for as much as 2% of total protein in certain regions of the brain. This kinase participates in the mechanism by which an increase in Ca^{2+} concentration in a nerve terminal causes exocytotic release of neurotransmitter. Its preferred substrate is a protein called **synapsin,** which is present in nerve terminals and binds to the external surface of synaptic vesicles. When synapsin I is bound to vesicles, it apparently prevents exocytosis; phosphorylation of synapsin I causes it to dissociate from the vesicles, and it allows the vesicle to release neurotransmitter by exocytosis.

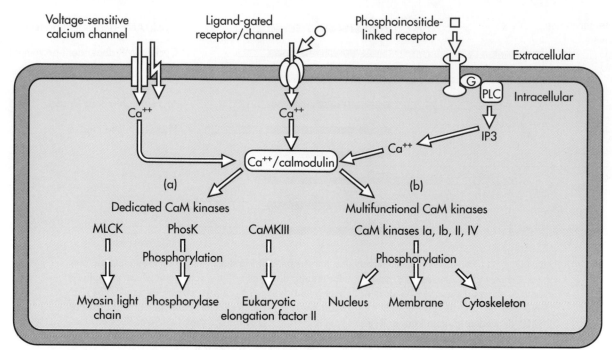

Fig. 5-10 Calmodulin-dependent protein kinases are the final steps in many signal transduction pathways that are elicited by an increase in cytosolic Ca^{2+} levels. Cytosolic Ca^{2+} may rise because of Ca^{2+} influx via a voltage- or ligand-gated ion channel or by the release of Ca^{2+} from internal stores by IP_3. The complex of Ca^{2+} with calmodulin activates calmodulin-dependent protein kinases. Dedicated calmodulin (CaM)-dependent protein kinases phosphorylate specific effector proteins such as the regulatory light chain of myosin, phosphorylase, and elongation factor II. Multifunctional calmodulin-dependent protein kinases phosphorylate multiple proteins of the nucleus or cytoskeleton or membrane proteins. *PLC,* Phospholipase C; *MLCK,* myosin light chain kinase; *PhosK,* phosphorylase kinase; *CaMKIII,* calmodulin-dependent kinase III. (Adapted from Schulman H: *Curr Opin Cell Biol* 5:247, 1993.)

Protein Kinase C

Protein kinase C plays a vital role in the control of certain cellular processes. The primary action of certain lipophilic tumor-promoting substances, most notably the **phorbol esters,** is to activate protein kinase C directly. Activation of protein kinase C powerfully stimulates cell division in many cell types. It also converts normal cells with controlled growth properties into transformed cells that grow uncontrollably.

The best known pathway of activation of protein kinase C is as follows. In an unstimulated cell, much of the protein kinase C is present in the cytosol and is inactive. When cytosolic levels of Ca^{2+} rise, Ca^{2+} binds to protein kinase C. The binding of Ca^{2+} causes protein kinase C to bind to the inner surface of the plasma membrane, where it can be activated by the diacylglycerol that is produced by the hydrolysis of phosphatidylinositol bisphosphate. Membrane phosphatidylserine is also a potent activator of certain isoforms of protein kinase C, once the enzyme has bound to the membrane.

About 10 different isoforms of protein kinase C have been discovered (Table 5-3). Although particular subtypes are present in many or most mammalian cells, the γ and ε subtypes are found predominantly in certain cells of the central nervous system. In addition to being differentially distributed among the cells and tissues of the body, the subtypes of protein kinase C also appear to be differentially regulated (Table 5-3). Some of the subtypes may be bound to the plasma membrane in unstimulated cells and thus do not require elevated Ca^{2+} for activation. Some of the isoforms of protein kinase C are activated by arachidonic acid, by other unsaturated fatty acids, or by lysophospholipids.

An initial, short-lived activation of protein kinase C may be caused by diacylglycerol, which is released when phospholipase Cβ is activated, and by Ca^{2+}, which is released from internal stores by IP_3 (Fig. 5-11). A longer-lasting activation of protein kinase C may be caused by receptor-activated phospholipases A_2 and D. These enzymes act primarily on phosphatidylcholine, a major membrane phospholipid. Phospholipase A_2 cleaves the number 2 fatty acid from phosphatidylcholine to liberate a fatty acid (mostly unsaturated fatty acids) and a lysophosphatidylcholine. Both of these products activate certain protein kinase C isoforms (Table 5-3). Receptor-activated phospholipase D cleaves phosphatidylcholine to produce phosphatidic acid and choline. The phosphatidic acid is further broken down to diacylglycerol, which participates in long-term stimulation of protein kinase C.

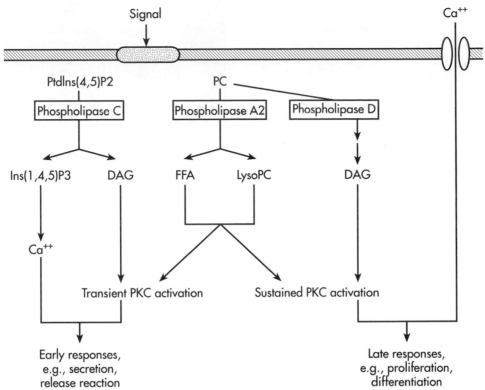

■ Fig. 5-11 Activation of protein kinase C *(PKC)* by degradation of membrane phospholipids. Rapid and transient activation of PKC is effected by IP_3 *[Ins(1,4,5)P_3]* and diacylglycerol *(DAG)* formed by the degradation of phosphatidylinositol bisphosphate *[PtdIns(4,5)P_2]* by a specific receptor-activated phospholipase C. Slower and more sustained activation of PKC is caused by degradation of phosphatidylcholine *(PC)* by receptor-activated phospholipases A_2 and D. Free fatty acids *(FFA)*, lysolecithin *(lysoPC)*, and diacylglycerol *(DAG)* released by these enzymes acting on PC stimulate PKC. (Adapted from Asaoka Y et al: *Trends Biochem Sci* 17:414, 1992.)

■ Table 5-3 Properties of mammalian isozymes of protein kinase C

Group	Subspecies	Apprent molecular mass (Da)	Activators	Tissue expression
cPKC	α	76,799	Ca^{2+}, DAG, PS, FFA, LysoPC	Universal
	βI	76,790	Ca^{2+}, DAG, PS, FFA, LysoPC	Some tissues
	βII	76,933	Ca^{2+}, DAG, PS, FFA, LysoPC	Many tissues
	γ	78,366	Ca^{2+}, DAG, PS, FFA, LysoPC	Brain only
nPKC	δ	77,517	DAG, PS	Universal
	ε	83,474	DAG, PS, FFA	Brain and others
	η (L)	77,972	?	Lung, skin, heart
	θ	81,571	?	Skeletal muscle (mainly)
aPKC	ζ	67,740	PS, FFA	Universal
	λ	67,200	?	Ovary, testis, and others

From Asaoka Y et al: *Trends Biochem Sci* 17:414, 1992.
DAG, Diacylglycerol; *PS,* phosphatidylserine; *FFA, cis*-unsaturated fatty acids; *LysoPC,* lysophosphatidylcholine.

TYROSINE KINASES

Receptor Tyrosine Kinases

The receptors for certain peptide hormones and growth factors are proteins with a glycosylated extracellular domain, a single transmembrane sequence, and an intracellular domain with protein tyrosine kinase activity. Members of this superfamily (Fig. 5-12) of peptide receptors include the receptors for insulin and related growth factors, epidermal growth factor (EGF), nerve growth factor (NGF), platelet-derived growth factor (PDGF), colony-stimulating factor (CSF), fibroblast growth factor (FGF), and hepatocyte growth factor (HGF). The binding of hormone or growth factor to its receptor triggers multiple cellular responses, including Ca^{2+} influx, increased Na^+-H^+

exchange, stimulation of the uptake of sugars and amino acids, and stimulation of phospholipase Cβ and hydrolysis of phosphatidylinositol bisphosphate.

The known protein–tyrosine kinase receptors fall into eight subfamilies, four of which are shown in Fig. 5-12. In general, the mechanism by which these receptors trigger cellular responses begins with the binding of ligand (the hormone or growth factor) to the receptor, which results in dimerization of the receptor-ligand complexes. The dimerization enhances binding affinity and activates the protein–tyrosine kinase activity of the receptor. Each monomer in a dimer phosphorylates the other monomer on multiple tyrosine residues. The tyrosines that are phosphorylated reside in the kinase insert regions of subfamilies III and IV, or in the carboxyl terminal tail of the receptor. (In contrast to receptor tyrosine kinases, phosphorylation of the receptor protein on serines or threonines by other kinases, such as protein kinase C, may diminish the tyrosine kinase activity of the receptor.) In subclass II receptors, the insulin receptor family, the unliganded receptor exists as a disulfide-linked dimer, and binding of insulin results in a conformational change of both "monomers." This conformational change enhances insulin binding and activates the receptor's tyrosine kinase activity, which leads to enhanced autophosphorylation of the receptor.

Protein tyrosine kinases that are "out of control" play a central role in cell transformation and cancer. In some cell types, growth factor receptor mutation causes the receptor to actively phosphorylate tyrosines, regardless of the presence or absence of the growth factor. Other tumor cells secrete a growth factor and overexpress its receptor. This situation leads to abnormally high rates of protein–tyrosine kinase activity.

Monomeric GTP-binding proteins of the Ras family (Table 5-2) are involved in coupling the binding of mitogenic ligands and their tyrosine–protein kinase receptors to the intracellular effects on cell proliferation that result. When Ras is inactive, cells cannot respond to the growth factors that operate via receptor tyrosine kinases.

Mutations in Ras may produce overactive forms of Ras that constitutively activate the effectors that ultimately lead to cell division. These effectors are normally active only in the presence of growth factors. As a result of the continued activation of these effectors, cell growth may be uncontrolled. Approximately 30% of human cancers involve mutated Ras proteins.

Activation of Ras by an activated receptor tyrosine kinase in turn activates a signal transduction pathway that ultimately

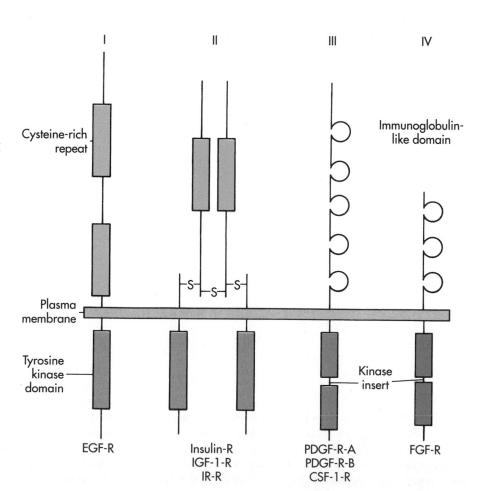

■ **Fig. 5-12** The structures of four subfamilies of receptor protein–tyrosine kinases are depicted; eight subfamilies have been identified. Subfamilies I and II have extracellular domains with cysteine-rich repeat sequence domains *(light color)*, whereas the extracellular domains of subclasses III and IV have immunoglobulin-like regions *(loops)*. The protein–tyrosine kinase domains *(solid color)* are the most conserved sequences. A short intracellular region, the kinase insert region (quite variable in length), and the carboxyl terminal tail are sites of regulation of protein kinase activity. *EGF,* Epidermal growth factor; *IGF-1,* insulin-like growth factor-1; *IR,* insulin-related protein; *PDGF,* platelet-derived growth factor; *CSF-1,* colony-stimulating factor-1; *FGF,* fibroblast growth factor. (Adapted from Ullrich A, Schlessinger J: *Cell* 61:203, 1990.)

turns on the transcription of certain key genes that promote cell growth. The **MAP (mitogen-activated protein) kinase cascade** (Fig. 5-13) is involved in the responses to activated Ras. Protein kinase C also activates the MAP kinase cascade. Thus, the MAP kinase cascade is an important point of convergence for multiple effectors that promote cellular proliferation. Moreover, there is significant cross talk between the protein kinase C and the tyrosine kinase pathways near their starting points. For example, the γ isoform of phospholipase C is activated by binding to activated Ras; this activation turns on protein kinase C via activation of phospholipid hydrolysis.

Receptor-Associated Tyrosine Kinases

The receptors for **growth hormone, prolactin,** and **erythropoietin** (as well as receptors for interferon and many cytokines) are not themselves protein kinases. However, upon activation, these receptors form signaling complexes with intracellular tyrosine kinases that bring about their intracellular effects (Fig. 5-14). Because they are not true receptor tyrosine kinases, but rather bind to them, these receptors are called **receptor-associated tyrosine kinases.** The mechanism by which these receptors induce intracellular effects begins when a hormone binds to the receptor, which induces dimerization of the hormone receptor. The receptor dimer binds one or more members of the **Janus family of tyrosine kinases (JAK).** The JAKs then cross-phosphorylate one another and also phosphorylate the receptor. Members of the **signal transducers and activators of transcription (STAT)** family bind to phosphotyrosine domains on the complex of receptor and JAK proteins. The STAT proteins are phosphorylated by the JAKs and then dissociate from the signaling complex. Finally, the phosphorylated STAT proteins form dimers that move into the nucleus to activate the transcription of certain genes.

Specificity of the receptor for each hormone derives partly from the particular members of the JAK and STAT family that are recruited to the signaling complex. In some instances, the signaling complex also activates the MAP kinase cascade via the same adapter proteins used by the receptor tyrosine kinases. Some of the responses to receptor tyrosine kinase ligands also involve the JAK-STAT pathway.

PROTEIN PHOSPHATASES AND THEIR MODULATION

Phosphorylation of proteins is one of the most important means by which protein activities are regulated. The extent of phosphorylation of a regulated protein results from the activities of the protein kinase that phosphorylates that protein and of the protein phosphatase that dephosphorylates it. In addition to the different types of protein kinases that we have discussed, all cells also contain **protein phosphatases** that reverse the effects of protein phosphorylation. In keeping with the classification of protein kinases, protein phosphatases are classified as **serine-threonine protein phosphatases** or **tyrosine protein phosphatases.**

Serine-Threonine Protein Phosphatases

The serine-threonine protein phosphatases are a large family of structurally related molecules. Currently, they are classified as type 1 (**PP-1**) or type 2 (**PP-2**). The type is based on the subunit of phosphorylase kinase they prefer to dephosphorylate. PP-1s prefer the β subunit, whereas PP-2s prefer the α subunit of phosphorylase kinase (Table 5-4). The PP-2s are subclassifed into PP-2A, PP-2B, and PP-2C, based on their regulation by divalent cations. PP-2A does not require divalent cations for activity. PP-2B has an absolute requirement for the Ca^{2+}-calmodulin complex. PP-2C absolutely requires Mg^{2+}. PP-2B is also called **calcineurin,** and it is especially abundant in certain regions of the brain. PP-1 and the PP-2s can also be distinguished by their inhibition by **okadaic acid** (Table 5-4), a complex fatty acid produced by marine dinoflagellates. Okadaic acid is as potent a tumor promoter as the phorbol esters, presumably because both okadaic acid and phorbol esters enhance the phosphorylation of certain substrates of protein kinase C.

PP-1s and PP-2s contain a catalytic core with a significantly homologous amino acid sequence. The PP-2s appear to be mainly cytosolic enzymes. In contrast, PP-1 in the liver is bound to glycogen particles; in muscle, PP-1 is bound to glycogen, to the sarcoplasmic reticulum, and to the myofibrils (the contractile proteins). Cytosolic PP-1 is relatively inactive. Protein subunits of PP-1 are responsible for the binding of PP-1 to specific cellular structures, and this binding appears to direct the activity of PP-1 toward particular physiological substrates.

The activity of PP-1 is also regulated by two classes of **endogenous inhibitor proteins: I-1** and **I-2.** I-1 is an effective inhibitor only when it is phosphorylated by protein kinase A. Phosphorylated I-1 has a high affinity for PP-1. By binding PP-1 and removing it from the subunit that attaches it to glycogen or to other cellular structures, it inactivates PP-1. The complex regulation of PP-1 suggests that it plays a key role in cellular regulation.

Protein Tyrosine Phosphatases

Protein tyrosine phosphatases (PTPases) are not structurally homologous to serine-threonine protein phosphatases. In contrast, all the protein kinases apparently derive from a common ancestor protein kinase. Figure 5-15 schematically depicts four of the approximately 65 PTPases currently known. Note that although two of the PTPases are small cytosolic proteins, two other PTPases are larger transmembrane proteins. On the basis of their structures, the transmembrane PTPases are probably receptors whose PTPase activity is modulated by extracellular ligands.

Both of the transmembrane PTPases shown in Fig. 5-15 are important molecules. **CD45** is the leukocyte common antigen that is crucial in cell-mediated immune responses. **LAR** (leukocyte common antigen-related protein) has extracellular sequences that are highly homologous to the neural cell adhesion molecule (N-CAM), which is important in the development of the nervous system.

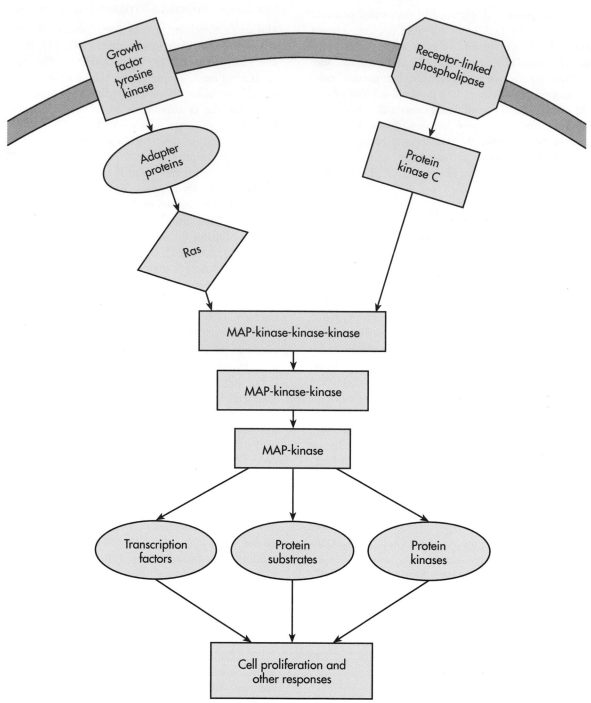

■ **Fig. 5-13** The MAP (mitogen-activated protein) kinase cascade is involved in the cell proliferative responses elicited by agonists that stimulate protein kinase C and by growth factors that act on membrane protein tyrosine kinase receptors. Protein kinase C phosphorylates MAP-kinase-kinase-kinase to activate it. Activated Ras activates MAP-kinase-kinase-kinase by binding to it. The cascade results in phosphorylation and activation of MAP kinase, which in turn phosphorylates transcription factors, protein substrates, and other protein kinases that are important in eliciting proliferation and other cellular responses. Activation of Ras depends on "adapter proteins" that bind to phosphotyrosine domains on the activated growth factor receptors. The adapter proteins bind to and activate a GEF (guanine nucleotide-exchange factor) that in turn activates Ras.

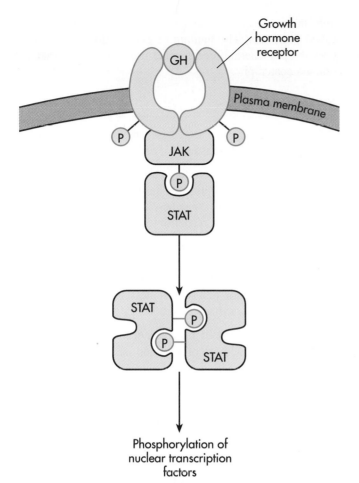

■ **Fig. 5-14** Receptors for growth hormone *(GH)*, prolactin, and certain other ligands have no intrinsic tyrosine kinase activity. The growth hormone receptor dimerizes in response to GH binding. The dimeric receptor binds one or more JAK tyrosine kinases, which phosphorylate themselves and the receptor. STAT tyrosine kinases bind to the complex and are phosphorylated. The phosphorylated STATs dissociate as dimers that are translocated into the nucleus, where they phosphorylate key transcription factors. *JAK,* Janus family of tyrosine kinases; *STAT,* signal transducers and activators of transcription.

ATRIAL NATRIURETIC PEPTIDE RECEPTOR–GUANYLYL CYCLASES

Atrial natriuretic peptide (ANP) is released by cells of the atrium of the heart in response to an elevation of atrial pressure

(see Chapters 36, 43, and 45). This hormone then acts to increase the excretion of NaCl and water by the kidney (see Chapter 36) and to diminish the constriction of certain blood vessels. Membrane receptors for ANP are notable because *the receptors themselves* possess guanylyl cyclase activity. This activity is stimulated when ANP is bound to the receptor. ANP receptors have an extracellular ANP-binding domain, a single transmembrane helix, and an intracellular guanylyl cyclase domain. The binding of ANP to the receptor stimulates the guanylyl cyclase activity and elevates intracellular levels of the second messenger, cGMP, without the intermediation of a G protein or any other signal transducing protein.

The elevated cGMP concentration that occurs when ANP binds to its receptor stimulates cGMP–dependent protein kinase. In contrast to the cAMP–dependent protein kinase, which has regulatory and catalytic subunits, the regulatory and catalytic domains of cGMP–dependent protein kinase reside on a single polypeptide chain. cGMP–Dependent kinase then phosphorylates intracellular proteins to evoke various cellular responses.

NITRIC OXIDE

Nitric oxide (NO) is a paracrine mediator that is released by endothelial cells and by certain neurons. Because NO is rapidly oxidized, its biological lifetime is only several seconds. For this reason, NO affects only cells in the immediate vicinity of the cell that produces it. NO stimulates a soluble guanylyl cyclase in the target cell and thereby elevates the intracellular concentration of cGMP in the target cell, thus stimulating cGMP–dependent protein kinase.

The production of NO is catalyzed by **NO synthase,** a Ca^{2+}-calmodulin–dependent enzyme that accelerates the conversion of arginine to citrulline plus NO. An increase in cytosolic Ca^{2+} levels is often the stimulus for enhanced formation and release of NO. This substance is released by nerve terminals of cerebellar granule cells and acts on postsynaptic cerebellar Purkinje cells. NO is also released by endothelial cells in response to agonists such as acetylcholine, which acts on muscarinic receptors to increase intracellular Ca^{2+}. NO released by these endothelial cells dilates nearby vascular smooth muscle cells (see Chapter 20). In addition, NO is one of the neurotransmitters released by neurons of the enteric nervous system. Acting on gastrointestinal smooth muscle cells, NO inhibits their contractile activity (see Chapter 20).

■ **Table 5-4** Properties of subtypes of serine-threonine protein phosphatases

Subtype	PP-1	PP-2A	PP-2B	PP-2C
Preference for the α or β subunit of phosphorylase kinase	β subunit	α subunit	α subunit	α subunit
Inhibition by I-1 and I-2	Yes	No	No	No
Absolute requirement for divalent cations	No	No	Yes (Ca^{2+})	Yes (Mg^{2+})
Stimulation by calmodulin	No	No	Yes	No
Inhibition by okadaic acid (Ki)	Yes (20 nM)	Yes (0.2 nM)	Yes (5 μM)	No
Phosphorylase phosphatase activity	High	High	Very low	Very low

From Cohen P: *Annu Rev Biochem* 58:453, 1989.

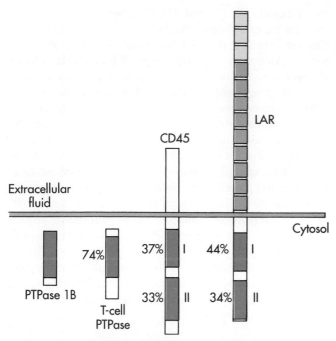

Extracellular
fluid

Cytosol

74%

37% | I

44% | I

33% | II

34% | II

PTPase 1B

T-cell
PTPase

CD45

LAR

■ **Fig. 5-15** Protein tyrosine phosphatases (PTPases) schematically depicted. About 65 different PTPases have been identified. Shown are two small cytosolic PTPases: PTPase 1B from human placenta and T-cell PTPase from human T lymphocytes. Also shown are two transmembrane PTPases: CD45 (the leukocyte common antigen) and LAR (leukocyte common antigen-related protein). The solid-colored cytosolic segments of each protein are the PTPase catalytic domains. The homology among catalytic domains is indicated by percent identities to the catalytic domain of PTPase 1B. The extracellular domains of LAR are homologous to N-CAM (neural cell adhesion molecule). The lighter-colored domains are homologous to the IgG-like domains; the intermediate-colored domains are homologous to the non–IgG-like domains of N-CAM. (Adapted from Tonks NK, Charbonneau H: *Trends Biochem Sci* 14:497, 1989.)

DOWN-REGULATION AND DESENSITIZATION OF RECEPTORS

Prolonged exposure of a cell to a particular agonist often causes the cell to become less responsive to that agonist. This comes about in two ways: **down-regulation,** which refers to a decrease in the number of the receptors, and **desensitization,** which means a decreased responsiveness to the agonist. Down-regulation occurs by receptor-mediated endocytosis of receptors via coated pits (Chapter 1) and their subsequent degradation in lysosomes. Prolonged exposure of cells to epidermal growth factor (EGF) and to many other agonists for protein tyrosine kinase receptors elicits down-regulation via endocytosis and degradation. G-protein coupled receptors may be phosphorylated when cAMP is elevated in the cytosol. Phosphorylation of the receptor desensitizes the receptor; that is to say phosphorylation decreases the receptor's ability to influence its effector protein, for example, adenylyl cyclase. Phosphorylation of the β-adrenergic receptor by a specific protein kinase per-

mits the receptor to associate with a regulatory protein, called β-arrestin. The binding of **β-arrestin** both desensitizes the β-adenergic receptor and promotes its internalization via coated pits.

SUMMARY

1. Many regulatory substances exert their effects on cellular processes via signal transduction pathways.

2. Heterotrimeric GTP-binding proteins serve as intermediaries between (a) a receptor that has been activated by binding an agonist and (b) enzymes and ion channels whose activity is modulated in response to agonist binding.

3. A GTP-binding protein is activated by interacting with an agonist-bearing receptor. It then changes the activity of an enzyme or an ion channel, and thereby alters the intracellular concentration of a second messenger, such as cAMP, cGMP, Ca^{2+}, IP3, or diacylglycerol.

4. An increased level of one or more second messengers may increase the activity of a second messenger-dependent protein kinase: cAMP–dependent protein kinase, cGMP–dependent protein kinase, calmodulin-dependent protein kinase, or protein kinase C.

5. Many cellular processes are regulated via the phosphorylation of enzymes and ion channels.

6. Certain membrane receptors for hormones and growth factors are protein tyrosine kinases or are associated with tyrosine kinases that are activated by binding of the agonist.

7. Monomeric GTP-binding proteins are intermediaries between (a) the binding of growth factors to their protein–tyrosine kinase receptors and (b) the downstream effects on cellular proliferation. The small G proteins also regulate the function of the actin cytoskeleton and intracellular vesicular trafficking.

8. Protein phosphatases, which are themselves subject to complex regulation by agonists and second messengers, reverse the effects of protein phosphorylation.

BIBLIOGRAPHY

Journal articles

Berridge MJ: Inositol trisphosphates and calcium signalling, *Nature* 361:315, 1993.

Berridge MJ: Elementary and global aspects of calcium signaling, *J Exp Biol* 200:315, 1997.

Birnbaumer L: Receptor-to-effector signaling: roles for beta gamma dimers as well as alpha subunits, *Cell* 71:1069, 1992.

Bourne HR: How receptors talk to trimeric G proteins. *Curr Opin Cell Biol* 9:134, 1997.

Bourne HR, Sanders DA, McCormick F: The GTPase superfamily: conserved structure and molecular mechanism, *Nature* 349:117, 1991.

Charbonneau H, Tonks NK: 1002 protein phosphatases?, *Annu Rev Cell Biol* 8:463, 1992.

Cohen P: Signal integration at the level of protein kinases, protein phosphatases and their substrates, *Trends Biochem Sci* 17:408, 1992.

Fantl WJ, Johnson DE, Williams LT: Signalling by receptor tyrosine kinases, *Annu Rev Biochem* 62:453, 1993.

Ferris CD, Snyder SH: Inositol 1,4,5-trisphosphate-activated calcium channels, *Annu Rev Physiol* 54:469, 1992.

Gudermann T, Kalkbrenner, Schultz G: Diversity and selectivity of receptor-G protein interactions, *Annu Rev Pharmacol Toxicol* 36:429, 1996.

Hall A: Ras-related proteins, *Curr Opin Cell Biol* 5:265, 1993.

Hamm HE, Gilchrist A: Heterotrimeric G proteins, *Curr Opin Cell Biol* 8:189, 1996.

Harden TK: G-protein regulated phospholipase C: identification of component proteins, *Adv Sec Messenger Phosphoprot Res* 26:11, 1992.

Hille B: G-protein-coupled mechanisms and nervous signaling, *Neuron* 9:187, 1992.

Hobbs AJ: Soluble guanylate cyclase: the forgotten sibiling, *Trends Pharmacol Sci* 18:484, 1997.

Iniguez-Lluhi J, Kleuss C, Gilman AG: The importance of G protein beta-gamma subunits, *Trends Cell Biol* 3:230, 1993.

Jaken S: Protein kinase C isozymes and substrates, *Curr Opin Cell Biol* 8:168, 1996.

Khokhlatchev AV et al: Phosphorylation of the MAP kinase ERK2 promotes its homodimerization and nuclear translocation, *Cell* 93:605, 1998.

Krupnick JG, Benkovic JL: The role of receptor kinases and arrestins in G protein-coupled receptor regulation, *Annu Rev Pharmacol Toxicol* 38:289, 1998.

Lamb TD, Pugh EN Jr: G protein cascades: gain and kinetics, *Trends Neurosci* 15:291, 1992.

Linder ME, Gilman AG: G proteins, *Sci Am* 267:36, 1992.

Lowy DR, Willumsen BM: Function and regulation of Ras, *Annu Rev Biochem* 62:851, 1993.

Meldolesi J: Multifarious IP3 receptors, *Curr Biol* 2:393, 1992.

Michell RH: Inositol lipids in cellular signalling mechanisms, *Trends Biochem Sci* 17:274, 1992.

Nishida E, Gotoh Y: The MAP kinase cascade is essential for diverse signal transduction pathways, *Trends Biochem Sci* 18:128, 1993.

Nishizuka Y: Intracellular signaling by hydrolysis of phospholipids and activation of protein kinase C, *Science* 258:607, 1992.

Nishizuka Y: Signal transduction: crosstalk, *Trends Biochem Sci* 17:367, 1992.

Posada J, Cooper JA: Molecular signal integration. Interplay between serine, threonine, and tyrosine phosphorylation, *Mol Biol Cell* 3:583, 1992.

Ruderman JV: MAP kinase and the activation of quiescent cells, *Curr Opin Cell Biol* 5:207, 1993.

Schindler C, Darnell JE Jr: Transcriptional responses to polypeptide ligands: the JAK-STAT pathway, *Annu Rev Biochem* 64:621, 1995.

Schlessinger J, Ullrich A: Growth factor signaling by receptor tyrosine kinases, *Neuron* 9:383, 1992.

Schulman H: The multifunctional Ca^{2+}/calmodulin-dependent protein kinases, *Curr Opin Cell Biol* 5:247, 1993.

Singer WD, Brown HA, Sternweis PC: Regulation of eukaryotic phosphatidylinositol-specific phospholipase D, *Annu Rev Biochem* 66:475, 1997.

Tang W-J, Gilman AG: Adenylyl cyclases, *Cell* 70:869, 1992.

Taylor CW, Marshall ICB: Calcium and inositol 1,4,5-trisphosphate receptors: a complex relationship, *Trends Biochem Sci* 17:403, 1992.

Vieira AV, Lamaze C, Schmid SL: Control of EGF receptor signalling by clathrin-mediated endocytosis, *Science* 274:2086, 1996.

Walton KM, Dixon JE: Protein tyrosine phosphatase, *Annu Rev Biochem* 62:101, 1993.

Wedel BJ, Garbers DL: New insights on the functions of the guanyl cyclase receptors, *FEBS Lett* 410:29, 1997.

Whitmarsh AJ, Davis RJ: Structural organization of MAP-kinase signaling modules by scaffold proteins in yeast and mammals, *Trends Biochem Sci* 32:481, 1998.

Books and monographs

Alberts B et al: *Molecular biology of the cell,* ed 4, New York, 2002, Garland.

Barritt GJ: *Communication within animal cells,* Oxford, 1992, Oxford Science Publications.

Houslay MD, Milligan G, editors: *G-proteins as mediators of cellular signalling processes,* New York, 1990, John Wiley.

Lodish H et al: *Molecular cell biology,* ed 4, New York, 2000, Scientific American Books.

Peroutka SJ, editor: *G-protein-coupled receptors,* Boca Raton, Fla, 1994, CRC Press.

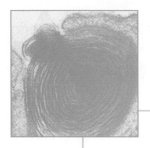

section two

The Nervous System

William D. Willis, Jr.

chapter six

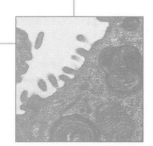

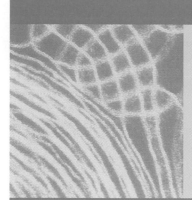

The Nervous System: Its Peripheral and Central Components

The nervous system is a communications network that allows an organism to interact in appropriate ways with its environment. In the sense used here, the environment includes both the external environment (the world outside the body) and the internal environment (the contents of the body). The nervous system includes sensory components that detect environmental events, integrative components that process and store sensory and other data, and motor components that generate movements and glandular secretions. The nervous system can be divided into peripheral and central parts, each with further subdivisions.

CELLULAR ORGANIZATION OF THE NERVOUS SYSTEM

The nervous system consists of a highly complex aggregation of cells, part of which forms a communications network and part of which forms a supportive matrix. The communications network is composed of numerous neural circuits.

Neurons

For its communicative activities, the functional unit of the nervous system is the **neuron** (Fig. 6-1). The typical neuron has a receptive surface that consists of a **cell body,** or **soma,** and several branchlike **dendrites** that receive **synapses** or neuron-to-neuron connections. Another neurite that extends from the soma is the **axon.** An axon makes synaptic connections with other neurons or with effector cells.

The nervous system forms a communications network through **neural circuits** made up of such synaptically interconnected neurons. Neural activity is generally coded by sequences of **action potentials** propagated along the axons in the neural circuits (see Chapter 3). The coded information is passed from one neuron to the next by **synaptic transmission** (see Chapter 4). In synaptic transmission, the action potentials that reach a **presynaptic ending** usually release a **neurotransmitter** substance. The *neurotransmitter* either

excites the **postsynaptic cell,** possibly to discharge one or more action potentials, or it **inhibits** the activity of the postsynaptic cell. Axons not only transmit information in neural circuits, but also convey chemical substances toward or away from the synaptic terminals by **axonal transport** (see page 84).

The **soma** of a neuron contains the **nucleus** and **nucleolus.** It also possesses a well-developed biosynthetic apparatus for manufacturing membrane constituents, synthetic enzymes, and other chemical substances needed for the specialized functions of nerve cells. The neuronal biosynthetic apparatus includes **Nissl bodies,** which are stacks of rough endoplasmic reticulum, and a prominent **Golgi apparatus.** The soma also contains numerous **mitochondria** and cytoskeletal elements, including **neurofilaments** and **microtubules.**

Dendrites are extensions of the neuronal cell body. In some neurons the dendrites are more than 1 mm long, and they account for more than 90% of the surface area. The proximal dendrites (near the cell body) contain Nissl bodies and parts of the Golgi apparatus. However, the main cytoplasmic organelles in dendrites are microtubules and neurofilaments. Traditionally dendrites have not been regarded as electrically excitable. However, we now know that the dendrites of many neurons have voltage-dependent conductances. These often depend on calcium channels that, when activated, produce calcium spikes.

The **axon** of a neuron arises from the soma (or sometimes from a dendrite) in a specialized region called the **axon hillock.** The length of axons varies with the neuronal type. Some axons do not extend much beyond the length of the dendrites, whereas others may be a meter or more long. The axon contains smooth endoplasmic reticulum and a prominent cytoskeleton. The axon hillock and axon differ from the soma and proximal dendrites in that they lack rough endoplasmic reticulum, free ribosomes, and Golgi apparatus. For this reason, axons degenerate when disconnected from the cell body (see page 85).

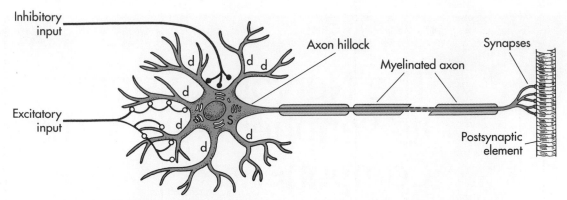

■ **Fig. 6-1** Schematic diagram of an idealized neuron and its major components. Most afferent input from axons of other cells terminates in synapses on the dendrites *(d)*, although some may terminate on the soma *(S)*. Excitatory terminals tend to terminate more distally on dendrites than do inhibitory ones, which often terminate on the soma. (Redrawn from Williams PL, Warwick R: *Functional neuroanatomy of man,* Edinburgh, 1975, Churchill Livingstone.)

Neuroglia

The other cellular elements of the nervous system are the **neuroglia** ("nerve glue"; Fig. 6-2), or supportive cells. Neuroglial cells in the human CNS outnumber neurons by an order of magnitude: there are about 10^{13} neuroglia and 10^{12} neurons.

Neuroglia do not participate directly in the short-term communication of information through the nervous system, but they do assist in that function. For example, some types of neuroglial cells provide many axons with **myelin sheaths** that speed up the conduction of action potentials along axons (see Chapter 3). This increase in conduction velocity allows some axons to communicate rapidly with other cells over relatively long distances. Other axons have a metabolic function, including biodegradation of neurotransmitter molecules.

Neuroglial cells in the peripheral nervous system (PNS) that support the activity of neurons include **Schwann cells** and **satellite cells,** and in the central nervous system (CNS) **they include astrocytes** and **oligodendroglia** (Fig. 6-2). **Microglia** and **ependymal cells** are also considered to be central neuroglial cells.

Astrocytes (named for their star shape) help regulate the microenvironment of neurons in the CNS, although they contact only a part of the surfaces of central neurons. However, their processes surround groups of synaptic endings and isolate these from adjacent synapses. Astrocytes also have **foot processes** that contact the capillaries and the connective tissue at the surface of the CNS, the **pia mater** (see Fig. 6-2). These foot processes may help limit the free diffusion of substances into the CNS. Astrocytes can actively take up K+ ions and neurotransmitter substances, which they can metabolize. Thus the astrocytes serve to buffer the extracellular environment of neurons with respect to both ions and neurotransmitters. The cytoplasm of astrocytes contains glial filaments, which provide mechanical support for CNS tissue. After injury, the astrocytic processes that contain these glial filaments hypertrophy and form a glial "scar."

Axons may be ensheathed or bare. Many axons are surrounded by a **myelin sheath,** which is a spiral multilayered wrapping of glial cell membrane (Figs. 6-1 and 6-3, *B*). **Unmyelinated axons** lack a myelin sheath, but in the PNS

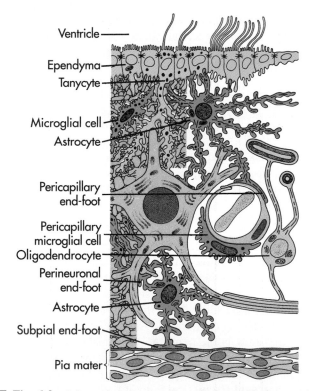

■ **Fig. 6-2** Schematic representation of nonneural elements in the central nervous system. Two astrocytes *(darker color)* are shown ending on a neuron's soma and dendrites. They also contact the pial surface and/or capillaries. An oligodendrocyte *(lighter color)* provides the myelin sheaths for axons. Also shown are microglia *(darker color)* and ependymal cells *(lighter color).* (Redrawn from Williams PL, Warwick R: *Functional neuroanatomy of man,* Edinburgh, 1975, Churchill Livingstone.)

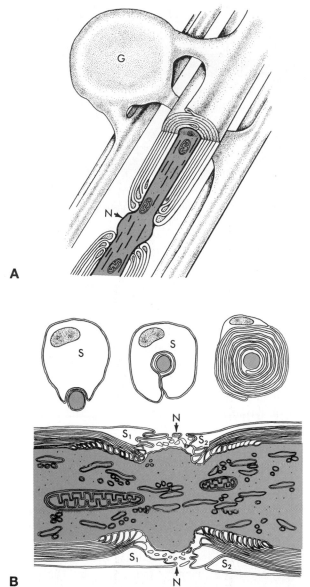

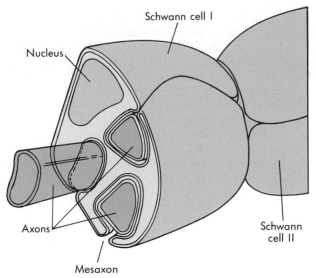

■ **Fig. 6-4** Three-dimensional impression of the appearance of a bundle of unmyelinated axons enwrapped by Schwann cells. The cut face of the bundle is seen to the left. One of the three unmyelinated axons is represented as protruding from the bundle. A mesaxon is indicated, as is the nucleus of the Schwann cell. To the right, the junction with adjacent Schwann cells is depicted.

A

B

■ **Fig. 6-3** Myelin sheaths of axons. **A,** Myelinated axons in the central nervous system. A single oligodendrocyte *(G)* emits several processes, each of which winds in a spiral fashion around an axon to form the myelin sheath. The axon *(color)* is shown in cutaway. The myelin from a single oligodendrocyte ends before the next wrapping from another oligodendrocyte. The bare axon between sheaths is the node of Ranvier *(N)*. Conduction of action potentials is saltatory down the axon, skipping from node to node. **B,** Myelinated axon in the peripheral nervous system. A Schwann cell forms a myelinated sheath for peripheral axons in much the same fashion as oligodendrocytes do for central ones, except that each Schwann cell myelinates a single axon. The top shows a cross-sectional view of progressive stages in myelin sheath formation by a Schwann cell *(S)* around an axon *(color)*. The bottom shows a longitudinal view of a myelinated axon *(color)*. The node of Ranvier *(N)* is shown between adjacent sheaths formed by two Schwann cells *(S₁ and S₂)*. (Redrawn from Patton HD et al: *Introduction to basic neurology,* Philadelphia, 1976, WB Saunders.)

they are surrounded by Schwann cells (Fig. 6-4). In the CNS myelinated axons are ensheathed by the membranes of **oligodendroglia** (Fig. 6-3, *A*), and unmyelinated axons are bare.

Myelin increases the speed of action potential conduction, in part by limiting the flow of ionic current during action potentials to the **nodes of Ranvier** (the unmyelinated portions of the axon at the junctions between adjacent sheath cells). This action results in **saltatory conduction,** which is the skipping of nerve impulses from node to node (see Chapter 3).

Satellite cells encapsulate dorsal root and cranial nerve ganglion cells and regulate their microenvironment in a fashion similar to that employed by astrocytes.

Microglia are latent phagocytes. When the CNS is damaged, the microglia help remove the cellular products of the damage. They are assisted by neuroglia and by other phagocytes that invade the CNS from the circulation.

Ependymal cells form the epithelium that separates the CNS from cerebrospinal fluid (CSF) in the ventricles. Many substances diffuse readily across the ependyma, which lie between the extracellular space of the brain and the CSF. The CSF is secreted in large part by specialized ependymal cells of the choroid plexuses, located in the ventricular system.

Most neurons in the adult nervous system are postmitotic cells (although there may also remain some precursor neurons or **stem cells**). Many glial precursor cells are present in the adult brain, and they can still divide and differentiate. Therefore, the cellular elements that give rise to most intrinsic **brain tumors** in the adult brain are the glial cells. For example, brain tumors can be derived from astrocytes (which vary in malignancy from the

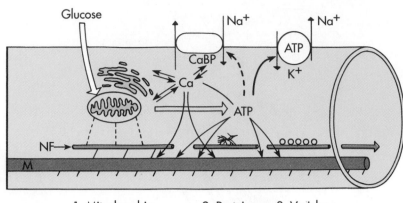

Fig. 6-5 Axonal transport has been proposed to depend on the movement of transport filaments. Energy is required and is supplied by glucose. Mitochondria control the level of cations in the axoplasm by supplying adenosine triphosphate *(ATP)* to the ion pumps. An important cation for axonal transport is calcium. Transport filaments *(red bars at bottom of drawing)* move along the cytoskeleton (microtubules, *M,* or neurofilament, *NF)* by means of cross-bridges. Transported components attach to the transport filaments.

slowly growing **astrocytoma** to the rapidly fatal **glioblastoma multiforme**), from oligodendroglia **(oligodendroglioma),** or from ependymal cells **(ependymoma).** Meningeal cells can also give rise to slowly growing tumors **(meningiomas)** that compress brain tissue, as do Schwann cells (e.g., **"acoustic neurinomas,"** which are tumors formed by Schwann cells of the eighth cranial nerve). In the brain of infants, neurons that are still dividing can sometimes give rise to **neuroblastomas** (e.g., of the roof of the fourth ventricle) or **retinoblastomas** (in the eye).

Axonal Transport

Most axons are too long to allow efficient movement of substances from the soma to the synaptic endings simply by diffusion. Membrane and cytoplasmic components that originate in the biosynthetic apparatus of the soma and of the proximal dendrites must be distributed along the axon (especially to the presynaptic elements of synapses) to replenish secreted or inactivated materials. A special transport mechanism, called **axonal transport,** accomplishes this distribution (Fig. 6-5).

Several types of axonal transport exist. Membrane-bound organelles and mitochondria are transported relatively rapidly by **fast axonal transport.** Substances, such as proteins, that are dissolved in cytoplasm are moved by **slow axonal transport.** In mammals fast axonal transport proceeds as rapidly as 400 mm/day, whereas slow axonal transport occurs at about 1 mm/day. Synaptic vesicles, which travel by fast axonal transport, can travel from the soma of a motor neuron in the spinal cord to a neuromuscular junction in a person's foot in about $2^1/_2$ days. In comparison, the movement of many soluble proteins over the same distance can take nearly 3 years.

Axonal transport requires metabolic energy and involves calcium ions. Microtubules provide a system of guidewires along which membrane-bound organelles move (Fig. 6-5). Organelles attach to microtubules through a linkage similar to that between the thick and thin filaments of skeletal muscle fibers. Calcium triggers the movement of the

organelles along the microtubules. Special microtubule-associated motor proteins, called **kinesin** and **dynein,** are required for axonal transport.

Axonal transport occurs in both directions. Transport from the soma toward the axonal terminals is called **anterograde axonal transport.** This process involves kinesin, and it allows the replenishment of synaptic vesicles and of enzymes that are responsible for neurotransmitter synthesis in synaptic terminals. Transport in the opposite direction, which is driven by dynein, is called **retrograde axonal transport.** This process returns synaptic vesicle membrane to the soma for lysosomal degradation.

Certain viruses and toxins can be conveyed by axonal transport along peripheral nerves. For example, **herpes zoster,** the virus of chicken pox, invades dorsal root ganglion cells. The virus may be harbored by these neurons for many years. However, eventually the virus may become active, because of a change in immune status. The virus may then be transported along the sensory axons to the skin. A new outbreak of skin lesions may then occur and produce **"shingles,"** a painful rash in the dermatomal distribution of one or more spinal nerves. Another example is the axonal transport of **tetanus toxin.** *Clostridium tetani* bacteria may grow in a dirty wound, and if the person had not been vaccinated against tetanus toxin, the toxin can be transported retrogradely in the axons of motor neurons. The toxin can escape into the extracellular space of the spinal cord ventral horn and block the synaptic receptors for inhibitory amino acids. This process can result in tetanic convulsions.

NERVOUS TISSUE REACTIONS TO INJURY

Injury to nervous tissue elicits responses by neurons and neuroglia. Severe injury causes cell death. Once a neuron is lost, it cannot be replaced, because neurons are postmitotic cells.

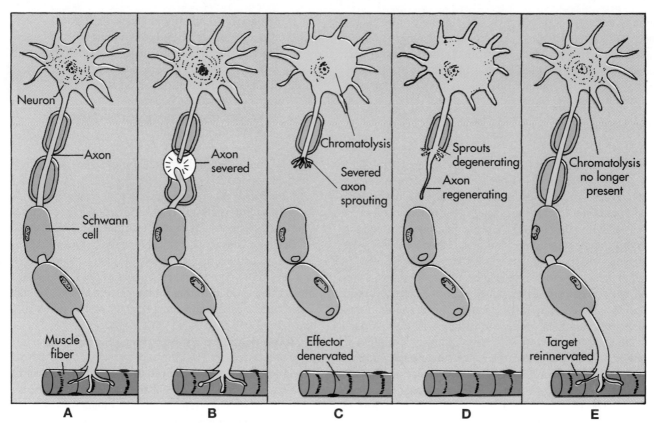

■ Fig. 6-6 **A,** Normal motor neuron innervating a skeletal muscle fiber. **B,** Motor axon has been severed, and the motor neuron is undergoing chromatolysis. **C,** This is associated in time with sprouting and, in **D,** with regeneration of the axon. The excess sprouts degenerate. **E,** When the target cell is reinnervated, chromatolysis is no longer present.

Degeneration

When an axon is transected, the soma of the neuron may show an "axonal reaction" or chromatolysis. Normally, Nissl bodies stain well with basic aniline dyes that attach to the ribonucleic acid of the ribosomes (Fig. 6-6, *A*). After injury to the axon (Fig. 6-6, *B*), the neuron attempts to repair the axon by making new structural proteins. During the axonal reaction, the cisterns of the rough endoplasmic reticulum become distended with the products of protein synthesis. The ribosomes appear to be disorganized, and the Nissl bodies are stained weakly by basic aniline dyes. This process, called **chromatolysis,** alters the staining (Fig. 6-6, *C*). In addition, the soma may swell and become rounded, and the nucleus may assume an eccentric position. These morphological changes reflect the cytological processes that accompany increased protein synthesis.

Because the axon cannot synthesize new protein, the axon distal to the transection dies (Fig. 6-6, *C*). Within a few days, the axon and all of the associated synaptic endings disintegrate. If the axon had been myelinated, the myelin sheath fragments, and it is eventually phagocytozed and removed. However, in the PNS the Schwann cells that had formed the myelin sheath remain viable, and in fact they undergo cell division. This sequence of events was originally described by Waller and is called **wallerian degeneration.**

If the axons that provide the sole or predominant synaptic input to a neuron or to an effector cell are interrupted, the postsynaptic cell may undergo **transneuronal degeneration** and even death. The best known example of this is the atrophy of skeletal muscle fibers after their innervation by motor neurons has been interrupted.

Regeneration

After an axon is lost through injury, many neurons can regenerate a new axon. The proximal stump of the damaged axon develops **sprouts** (see Fig. 6-6, *C*). In the PNS, these sprouts elongate, and they grow along the path of the original nerve if this route is available (Fig. 6-6, *D*). The Schwann cells in the distal stump of the nerve not only survive the wallerian degeneration, but they also proliferate and form rows along the course previously taken by the axons. **Growth cones** of the sprouting axons find their way along the rows of Schwann cells, and they may eventually reinnervate the original peripheral target structures (Fig. 6-6, *E*). The Schwann cells then remyelinate the axons. The rate of regeneration is limited by the rate of slow axonal transport to about 1 mm/day.

In the CNS, transected axons also sprout. However, proper guidance for the sprouts is lacking, because the oligodendroglia do not form a path along which the sprouts can grow. This limitation may be a consequence of the fact that a single oligodendroglial cell myelinates many central axons, whereas a single Schwann cell provides myelin for only a single axon in the periphery. Alternatively, different chemical signals may affect peripheral and central attempts at regeneration differently. Another obstacle is the formation of a glial scar by astrocytes.

Trophic Factors

A number of proteins are now known to affect the growth of axons and the maintenance of synaptic connections. The best studied of these substances is **nerve growth factor (NGF)**. NGF was initially thought to enhance the growth and maintain the integrity of many neurons of neural crest origin, including the small dorsal root ganglion cells and the autonomic postganglionic neurons. However, we now believe that NGF also affects some neurons in the CNS.

Other growth factors have also been described, including **brain-derived growth factor, neurotrophin 3, neurotrophin 4, neurotrophin 5,** and **ciliary neurotrophic factor.** Some of these factors affect the growth of large dorsal root ganglion cells or motor neurons. Probably, a large assortment of growth factors plays a role in the growth and maintenance of neurons in the peripheral and central nervous systems.

NGF is secreted by target cells and it binds to special receptors that are located on neurons that synapse with the target cells. The bound NGF and receptor are internalized, and the NGF is transported retrogradely to the soma. NGF may act directly on the nucleus and affect the production of enzymes responsible for neurotransmitter synthesis and axonal growth. NGF receptors include both a low-affinity form and the higher-affinity tyrosine kinase receptor, known as TRK_A. Other neurotrophic factors bind to the same low-affinity receptor and also to one of the other high-affinity tyrosine kinase receptors, known as TRK_B or TRK_C.

GENERAL FUNCTIONS OF THE NERVOUS SYSTEM

The general functions of the nervous system include **sensory detection, information processing,** and **behavior.** *Learning and memory are special forms of information processing that permit behavior to change appropriately in response to previous environmental challenges.* Other systems, such as the endocrine and immune systems, share these functions, but the nervous system is specialized for them.

Excitability is a cellular property of neurons. This property involves electrical signals that enable the neurons to receive and transmit information. Excitability is manifested by electrical events such as **action potentials, receptor potentials,** and **synaptic potentials** (see Section I). Chemical events often accompany these electrical events.

Sensory detection is the process whereby neurons **transduce** environmental energy into neural signals. Sensory detection is accomplished by special neurons called **sensory receptors.** Various forms of energy can be sensed, including mechanical forces, light, sound, chemicals, temperature, and, in some animals, electrical fields.

Information processing includes the following:
1. The transmission of information in neural networks
2. The transformation of signals by combining them with other signals (**neural integration**)
3. Storage of information in and retrieval of information from memory
4. Use of sensory information for **perception**
5. Thought processes
6. Learning
7. Planning and implementation of motor commands
8. Emotions

Information processing, including learning and memory, depends on **intercellular communication** in neural circuits. The mechanisms involve both electrical and chemical events.

Behavior consists of the totality of the organism's responses to its environment. Behavior may be covert, as in **cognition,** but it is often readily observable as a motor act, such as a **movement** or an **autonomic response.** In humans, **language** constitutes a particularly important set of behaviors.

THE PERIPHERAL NERVOUS SYSTEM

The **peripheral nervous system (PNS)** provides an interface between the environment and the CNS. It includes sensory (or primary afferent) neurons, somatic motor neurons, and autonomic motor neurons. Autonomic motor neurons are discussed in Chapter 11.

Primary Afferent Neurons

Primary afferent neurons are connected peripherally to **sensory receptors,** which are specialized structures that transduce changes in environmental energy. Sensory receptors provide information to the organism about its external and internal environment. In general, that information is then transmitted to the CNS by trains of nerve impulses in primary afferent neurons. The cell bodies of primary afferent neurons are located in dorsal root and cranial nerve ganglia. Each primary afferent neuron has two types of processes: (1) a peripheral process that extends distally within a peripheral nerve to reach the appropriate sensory receptors, and (2) a central process that enters the CNS through a dorsal root or a cranial nerve (Fig. 6-7).

Types of Sensory Receptors. Sensory receptors can be classified according to whether they provide information about the external environment (**exteroceptors**), the internal environment (**interoceptors**), or the position of the body in space (**proprioceptors**). Another more detailed classification is given in Table 6-1.

Functions of Sensory Receptors

Transduction. Sensory systems are designed to respond to the environment. *Stimulation is the action of environmental energy on the body through activation of one or more sensory receptors.* A **stimulus** is the environmental event that excites sensory receptors, which then provide information about the stimulus to the CNS. The **response** to the stimulus is the effect that the stimulus has on the organism.

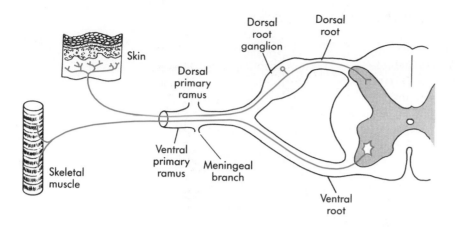

■ **Fig. 6-7** A diagram of the spinal cord, spinal roots, and spinal nerve. A primary afferent neuron is shown with its cell body in the dorsal root ganglion and its central and peripheral processes distributing, respectively, to the spinal cord gray matter and to a sensory receptor in the skin. An α-motor neuron is shown to have its cell body in the spinal cord gray matter and to project its axon out the ventral root to innervate a skeletal muscle fiber.

■ **Table 6-1** Classification of sensory receptors

Special	Vision, audition, taste, olfaction, balance
Superficial	Touch, pressure, flutter, vibration, tickle, warmth, cold, pain, itch
Deep	Position, kinesthesia, deep pressure, deep pain
Visceral	Hunger, nausea, distention, visceral pain

From Willis WD, Grossman RG: *Medical neurobiology,* ed 3, St. Louis, 1981, Mosby.

Responses can be recognized at several levels; these include (1) receptor potentials in sensory receptors, (2) transmission of action potentials along axons in sensory pathways, (3) synaptic events in sensory neural networks, (4) motor activity triggered by sensory stimulation, and ultimately (5) behavioral events. The process that enables a sensory receptor to respond usefully to a stimulus is called **sensory transduction.**

Environmental events that involve sensory transduction can be mechanical, thermal, chemical, or other forms of energy; the type of transduction depends on the sensory apparatus that serves as a transducer. Although humans cannot sense electrical or magnetic fields, other animals can respond to such stimuli. For example, many fish have electroreceptors, and various fish and birds use the earth's magnetic field to orient themselves during migration.

Figure 6-8 shows how different types of stimuli can alter the membrane properties of sensory receptor neurons that transduce such stimuli. Figure 6-8, *A* illustrates how a **chemoreceptor** responds when a chemical stimulant reacts with **receptor molecules** on the plasma membrane of the sensory receptor. (Note the distinction between a sensory receptor, which includes one or more cells, and a receptor molecule, which is a protein inserted into the membrane of a cell.) The reaction between the chemical stimulant and the receptor molecules opens ion channels, which enables the influx of ionic current that depolarizes the sensory receptor. In Fig. 6-8, *B,* the ion channel of a **mechanoreceptor** opens in response to the application of a mechanical force along the membrane; this stimulus opens the ion channel and allows an influx of current to depolarize the sensory receptor. In Fig. 6-8, *C,* the ion channel of a cell, called a **pho-**

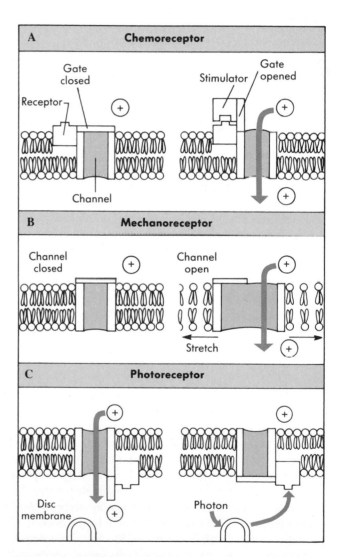

■ **Fig. 6-8** Conceptual models of transducer mechanisms in three types of receptors. **A,** Chemoreceptor; **B,** mechanoreceptor; **C,** vertebrate photoreceptor. (See text.)

toreceptor (because it responds to light), is open in the dark and closed when a photon is absorbed by pigment on the disc membrane. In this case, an influx of current (called a **dark current**) occurs in the dark; the current ceases when light is applied. When the current stops, the photoreceptor hyperpolarizes.

As illustrated in Fig. 6-9, sensory transduction generally produces a **receptor potential** in the peripheral terminals of the axon of a primary afferent neuron. The **receptor potential** is usually a depolarizing event that results from inward current flow, which brings the membrane potential of the sensory receptor toward the threshold needed to trigger an action potential. For example, in Fig. 6-9 a mechanical stimulus distorts the ending of a mechanoreceptor. This distortion causes inward current flow at the end of the axon, and longitudinal and outward current flow along the axon. The outward current produces a depolarization (the receptor potential), which might exceed threshold for an action potential. In this case the action potential is generated in a trigger zone at the first node of Ranvier of the afferent fiber. In photoreceptors, however, the receptor potential is hyperpolarizing, as mentioned above. Information transmission in the retina is discussed in Chapter 8.

In some sensory receptors, the primary afferent fiber terminates on a separate, peripherally located sensory cell. For example, in the **cochlea,** primary afferent fibers end on **hair cells.** Sensory transduction in such sense organs is made more complex by this arrangement. In the cochlea, a receptor potential arises in the hair cells in response to sound (see Chapter 8). The receptor potential is oscillatory. In each oscillatory cycle, however, when the membrane of the hair cell is depolarized, the hair cell releases an excitatory neurotransmitter onto the primary afferent terminal. The result is a **generator potential,** which in turn depolarizes the primary afferent fiber. The generator potential brings the membrane potential of the primary afferent fiber toward the threshold potential that fires nerve impulses.

Adaptation is a characteristic property of sensory receptors; it makes them better suited to signal particular kinds of sensory information. In **slowly adapting receptors,** a prolonged stimulus produces a repetitive discharge in the primary afferent neurons that supply the sensory receptors. However, in **rapidly adapting receptors,** the same stimulus produces a brief response (only a few discharges). These different rates of adaptation may reflect either a maintained or a transient receptor potential in the sensory receptor. The functional implication of the adaptation rate is that different temporal features of a stimulus can be analyzed by receptors with different adaptation rates. For example, during an indentation of the skin, a slowly adapting receptor may respond repetitively at a rate proportional to the amount of indentation (Fig. 6-10, *A*). Conversely, rapidly adapting receptors in the skin respond best to transient mechanical stimuli. The information signaled may reflect stimulus velocity (Fig. 6-10, *B*) or acceleration (Fig. 6-10, *C*), rather than the amount of skin indentation.

Receptive Fields. The relationship between the location of a stimulus and the activation of particular sensory neurons is a major theme in sensory physiology. The **receptive field** of a sensory neuron is the region that, when stimulated, affects the discharge of the neuron. For example, a sensory

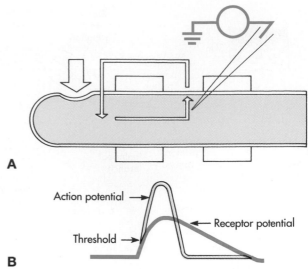

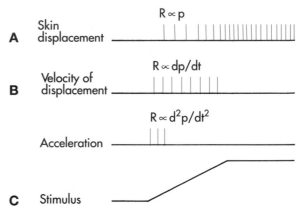

A, The current flow produced by stimulation of a mechanoreceptor at the site indicated by the arrow and an intracellular recording from a node of Ranvier. **B,** The receptor potential produced by the current and an action potential that may be superimposed on the receptor potential if the latter exceeds threshold.

■ **Fig. 6-9** A, The current flow produced by stimulation of a mechanoreceptor at the site indicated by the arrow and an intracellular recording from a node of Ranvier. **B,** The receptor potential produced by the current and an action potential that may be superimposed on the receptor potential if the latter exceeds threshold.

■ **Fig. 6-10** Responses of slowly and rapidly adapting mechanoreceptors to displacement of the skin. The discharges of the primary afferent fibers supplying the receptors during a ramp and hold stimulus (shown at the *bottom*) are termed the response *(R)*. **A,** R is proportional to skin position *(p)*. The receptor is slowly adapting and signals skin displacement. **B,** R is a function of the velocity of displacement *(dp/dt)*. **C,** R is a function of the acceleration *(d²p/dt²)*. These receptors are rapidly adapting, but signal different, dynamic features of the stimulus.

receptor might be activated by indentation of only a small area of skin. That area is the **excitatory receptive field** of the sensory receptor. A neuron in the CNS might be excited by stimulation of a receptive field several times as large as that of a sensory receptor (Fig. 6-11). The reason that CNS sensory neurons often have larger receptive fields than do sensory receptors is that CNS sensory neurons may receive information from many sensory receptors, each with a slightly different receptive field. The receptive field of the

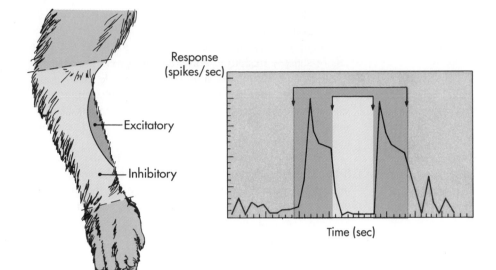

■ **Fig. 6-11** Excitatory and inhibitory receptive fields of a central somatosensory neuron located in the SI (primary) somatosensory cerebral cortex. The excitatory receptive field is on the forearm and is surrounded by an inhibitory receptive field. The graph shows the response to an excitatory stimulus and the inhibition of that response by a stimulus applied in the inhibitory field.

CNS neuron is the sum of the receptive fields of the sensory receptors that influence the CNS neuron. The location of the receptive field is determined by the location of the sensory transduction apparatus responsible for signaling information about the stimulus to the sensory neuron.

Generally, the receptive fields of sensory receptors are excitatory. However, a central sensory neuron can have either an excitatory or an **inhibitory receptive field.** For example, the somatosensory neuron illustrated in Fig. 6-11 had both excitatory and inhibitory receptive fields. This cell was located in the primary somatosensory cerebral cortex (SI cortex; see Chapter 7). Inhibition results from data processing in sensory neural circuits and is mediated by inhibitory interneurons.

Sensory Coding. Sensory neurons encode stimuli. In the process of sensory transduction, one or more aspects of the stimulus must be encoded in a way that can be interpreted by the CNS. The encoded information is an abstraction based on (1) which sensory receptors are activated, (2) the responses of sensory receptors to the stimulus, and (3) information processing in the sensory pathway. Some of the aspects of stimuli that may be encoded include the **sensory modality, spatial location, threshold, intensity, frequency,** and **duration.** Other aspects of stimuli that are encoded are presented in relation to particular sensory systems in later chapters.

A **sensory modality** is a readily identified class of sensation. For example, maintained mechanical stimuli applied to the skin result in sensations of **touch** or **pressure,** and transient mechanical stimuli may evoke sensations of **flutter** or **vibration.** Other cutaneous modalities include cold, warmth, and pain. Vision, audition, position, taste, and smell are examples of noncutaneous sensory modalities. The encoding of sensory modality is done by labeled-line sensory channels in most sensory systems. A **labeled-line sensory channel** consists of a set of neurons that is devoted to a particular sensory modality. For example, the visual pathway includes neurons in the retina, the lateral geniculate nucleus of the thalamus, and the visual areas of the cerebral cortex (see Chapter 8). The normal means for activating the visual system is by

light that strikes the retina. Neurons of the retina process the information and then transmit signals along the visual pathway. However, mechanical or electrical stimulation of neurons in the visual pathway (e.g., by indentation of the eye, which will activate retinal neurons mechanically) also produces a visual sensation, although a distorted one. Thus neurons of the visual system can be regarded as a labeled line, which, when activated by whatever means, causes a visual sensation.

The **spatial location** of a stimulus is signaled by the activation of the particular population of sensory neurons whose receptive fields are affected by the stimulus. The information may be encoded in the CNS by a neural map. For example, a **somatotopic map** is formed by arrays of neurons in the somatosensory cortex that receive information from corresponding locations on the body surface (see Chapter 7). In the visual system, points on the retina are represented by neuronal arrays that form **retinotopic maps** (see Chapter 8). In the auditory system the frequency of sounds is represented in **tonotopic maps** (see Chapter 8). In some cases an inhibitory receptive field or a contrasting border between an excitatory and an inhibitory receptive field can have localizing value. Resolution of two different adjacent stimuli may depend on excitation of partially separate populations of neurons and on inhibitory interactions.

A **threshold stimulus** is the weakest stimulus that can be reliably detected. For detection, a stimulus must produce receptor potentials that are large enough to activate one or more primary afferent fibers. Weaker intensities of stimulation can produce subthreshold receptor potentials; however, such stimuli would not excite central sensory neurons, and so could not be perceived. Furthermore, the number of primary afferent neurons that need to be excited for sensory detection depends on the requirements for **spatial** and **temporal summation** in the sensory pathway (see Chapter 4). In some sensory systems a stimulus at the threshold for detection must be much greater than the threshold for activation of the most responsive primary afferent neurons.

Thus a stimulus that excites some primary afferent neurons may not be perceived. On the other hand, if a stimulus is perceived, at least one primary afferent neuron has to be excited beyond threshold.

An example of a difference in the thresholds of sensory receptors and for perception is in the peripheral encoding of pain. Painful stimuli activate the sensory receptors, which are called nociceptors. Recordings have been made from nociceptors in human nerves. A technique, called microneurography, has been used, in which a microelectrode is inserted into a peripheral nerve in a conscious subject. Recordings from the axon of an individual nociceptor have demonstrated that minimal activation of the axon under observation might not cause pain. This can be explained if more than one nociceptive afferent axon at a time needs to be activated to produce pain, because central nociceptive processing requires spatial summation. Alternatively, a nociceptor may need to be activated more than once because temporal summation might be needed. In fact, it appears that a single cutaneous nociceptor needs to discharge at a rate of 3 Hz or more before pain is perceived, and pain is more intense when more than one nociceptor is activated.

Stimulus **intensity** may be encoded by the mean frequency of discharge of sensory neurons. The relationship between stimulus intensity and response can be plotted as a stimulus-response function. For many sensory neurons, the stimulus-response function approximates an exponential curve. The general equation for such a curve is

$$\text{Response} = \text{Constant} \times (\text{stimulus} - \text{threshold stimulus})^n$$

The exponent, n, can be less than, equal to, or greater than 1. Stimulus-response functions with fractional exponents are found for many mechanoreceptors. **Thermoreceptors,** which detect changes in *temperature,* have linear stimulus-response curves (exponent of 1). **Nociceptors,** which detect *painful* stimuli, may have linear or positively accelerating stimulus-response functions (i.e., the exponent for these curves is 1 or more).

The processing of pain in the nociceptive pathways of the CNS is characterized by positively accelerating curves. The positively accelerating stimulus-response functions of nociceptors help explain the urgency that is experienced as the pain sensation increases.

Another way in which stimulus **intensity** is encoded is by the number of sensory receptors that are activated. A stimulus at the threshold for perception may activate just one or just a few primary afferent neurons of an appropriate class, whereas a strong stimulus of the same type may excite many similar receptors. Central sensory neurons that receive input from this particular class of sensory receptor would be more powerfully activated as more primary afferent neurons dis-

charge. Greater activity in central sensory neurons is perceived as a stronger stimulus.

Stimuli of diferent intensities may also activate different sets of sensory receptors. For example, a weak mechanical stimulus applied to the skin might activate only mechanoreceptors, whereas a strong mechanical stimulus might activate both mechanoreceptors and nociceptors. In this case the sensation evoked by the stronger stimulus would be more intense, and the quality would be different.

Stimulus **frequency** can be encoded by the intervals between the discharges of sensory neurons. Sometimes the interspike intervals correspond exactly to the intervals between stimuli (Fig. 6-12). In other cases, a given neuron may discharge at intervals that are multiples of the interstimulus interval.

A third method for encoding information is by the **patterns of nerve impulses,** which are sequences of nerve impulses that result in synaptic transmission of information to a new set of neurons. The communicated information is coded in terms of the structure of the nerve impulse trains. Several different types of nerve impulse codes have been proposed. A commonly used code depends on the **mean discharge frequency.** For example, in many sensory systems, increases in the intensity of a stimulus cause a greater frequency of discharge of the sensory neurons. Other candidate codes depend on the **time of firing,** the **temporal pattern,** and the **duration of bursts.**

Stimulus **duration** may be encoded in slowly adapting sensory neurons by the duration of enhanced firing. The beginning and end of a stimulus may be signaled by transient discharges of rapidly adapting sensory receptors.

Conduction Velocities of the Axons of Primary Afferent Neurons. The peripheral processes of primary afferent neurons that supply different types of sensory receptors have characteristic ranges of conduction velocity. For example, some sensory receptors in muscle are supplied by the largest myelinated axons in the peripheral nervous system, the

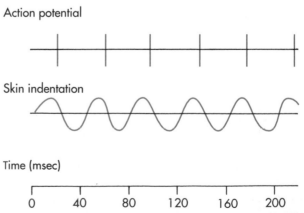

■ **Fig. 6-12** Coding for the frequency of stimulation. Discharge of a rapidly adapting cutaneous mechanoreceptor in phase with a sinusoidal stimulus. The action potentials are shown at the top and the stimulus in the middle trace.

■ Table 6-2   Types of sensory receptors

Type	Group	Subgroup	Diameter (μm)	Conduction velocity (m/sec)	Tissue supplied	Function
Afferent						
A	I	Ia	12-20	72-120	Muscle	Afferents from muscle spindle primary endings
		Ib			Muscle	Afferents from Gogli tendon organs
	II		6-12	36-72	Muscle	Afferents from muscle spindle secondary endings
	Beta				Skin	Afferents from pacinian corpuscles, touch receptors
	III		1-6	6-36	Muscle	Afferents from pressure-pain endings
	Delta				Skin	Afferents from touch, temperature, and pain receptors
C	IV		<1	0.5-2	Muscle	Afferents from pain receptors
	Dorsal root				Skin	Afferents from touch, pain, and temperature receptors

From Willis WD, Grossman RG: *Medical neurobiology,* ed 3, St. Louis, 1981, Mosby.

group I afferent fibers. Other sensory receptors in muscle are innervated by medium-sized (**group II**) or small (**group III**) myelinated axons or by unmyelinated (**group IV**) axons. The largest myelinated axons that supply cutaneous sensory receptors are comparable in size to the medium-sized muscle afferent fibers. They are sometimes also called group II fibers, but more commonly they are referred to as **Aβ** afferent fibers. Small myelinated and unmyelinated cutaneous afferent fibers are classed as **Aδ** fibers and **C** fibers, respectively.

Table 6-2 lists some of the types of sensory receptors that are associated with different sized axons of primary afferent neurons that supply muscle or skin. The terminology used for different sized axons that supply joints is the same as that for muscle, and that for viscera is the same as that for skin.

SOMATIC MOTOR NEURONS

Contractions of skeletal muscle fibers are responsible for movements of the body. Skeletal muscle fibers are innervated by large neurons, called **α-motor neurons,** in the ventral horn of the spinal cord or in cranial nerve nuclei. These neurons are large, multipolar neurons that range in size up to 70 μm in diameter. Their axons leave the spinal cord through the ventral roots (Fig. 6-7). The motor axons distribute to the appropriate skeletal muscles through peripheral nerves, and they terminate with synapses, called **neuromuscular junctions** or **end plates,** on skeletal muscle fibers.

A given skeletal muscle is supplied by a group of α-motor neurons located in a **motor nucleus.** In the ventral horn, a motor nucleus is typically a sausage-shaped array of motor neurons that extends over several spinal cord segments. Motor nuclei that supply different muscles are arranged somatotopically in the ventral horn. In the cervical and lumbosacral enlargements, the motor nuclei that supply the axial muscles of the body are in the medial part of the ventral horn, whereas the motor nuclei that innervate the limb muscles are in the lateral part of the ventral horn.

*A **motor unit** is an α-motor neuron, its motor axon, and all of the skeletal muscle fibers that it supplies.* Each skeletal muscle fiber in mammals is supplied by just one α-motor neuron. However, a given α-motor neuron may innervate a variable number of skeletal muscle fibers; the number depends on how fine a control of the muscle is required. For highly regulated muscles, such as the eye muscles, an α-motor neuron may supply only a few skeletal muscle fibers. However, in a proximal limb muscle, such as the quadriceps femoris, a single α-motor neuron may innervate thousands of skeletal muscle fibers.

The motor unit can be regarded as the basic unit of movement. When an α-motor neuron discharges under normal circumstances, all of the muscle fibers of the motor unit contract. A given α-motor neuron may participate in a variety of reflexes and in voluntary movements. Because decisions about whether or not the synaptic input from various sources will cause particular muscle fibers to contract is made at the level of the α-motor neuron (in mammals), these motor neurons have been termed **the final common pathway.**

Another type of motor neuron is called the **γ-motor neuron.** γ-Motor neurons are smaller than α-motor neurons; they have a soma diameter of about 35 μm. The γ-motor neurons that project to a particular muscle are located in the same motor nucleus as the α-motor neurons that supply that muscle. γ-Motor neurons do not supply ordinary skeletal muscle fibers. Instead, they synapse on specialized striated muscle fibers, the **intrafusal muscle fibers,** that are found within muscle spindles (see Chapter 9). Table 6-3 shows the sizes of the axons of somatic motor neurons and their conduction velocities.

*The skeletal muscle fibers that belong to a given motor unit are called a **muscle unit.*** All of the muscle fibers in a muscle unit are of the same histochemical type (i.e., they are either all type I, type IIB, or IIA). The motor units that twitch

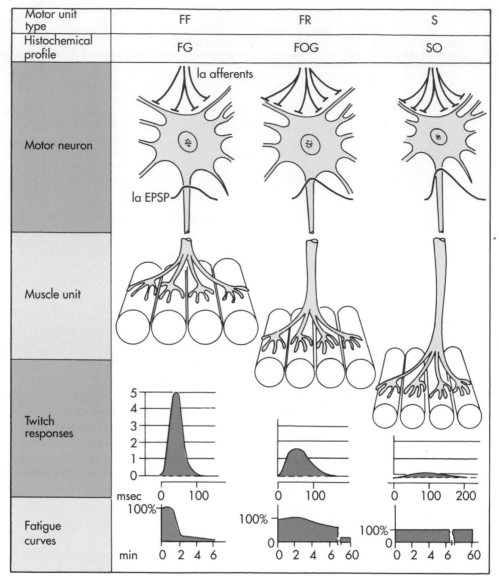

Motor unit type	FF	FR	S
Histochemical profile	FG	FOG	SO

■ **Fig. 6-13**   Summary of features of motor units in a mixed muscle (medial gastrocnemius of cat). Relative sizes are shown for motor neurons, muscle fibers, monosynaptic excitatory postsynaptic potentials evoked by volleys in group Ia afferent fibers, and twitch responses. *EPSP,* Excitatory post-synaptic potential; *FG,* fast glycolytic; *FOG,* fast oxidative-glycolytic; *SO,* slow oxidative; *FF,* fast fatigable; *FR,* fast fatigue resistant; *S,* slow.

■ Table 6-3   Characteristics of axons of somatic motor neurons

Type	Group	Subgroup	Diameter (μm)	Conduction velocity (m/sec)	Tissue supplied	Function
A	α		12-20	72-120	Muscle	Motor supply of extrafusal skeletal muscle fibers
	γ		2-8	12-48	Muscle	Motor supply of intrafusal muscle fibers

From Willis WD, Grossman RG: *Medical neurobiology,* ed 3, St. Louis, 1981, Mosby.

slowly and resist fatigue are classified as **S** (slow), and they have type I fibers. S motor units depend on oxidative metabolism for their energy supply and their contractions are weak (Fig. 6-13). The muscle units with fast twitches are **FF** (fast, fatigable) and **FR** (fast, fatigue resistant). FF muscle units have type IIB fibers, they use glycolytic metabolism, and they have strong contractions, but they fatigue easily. FR muscle units have type IIA fibers and rely on oxidative metabolism; their contractions are of intermediate force, and these muscle units resist fatigue.

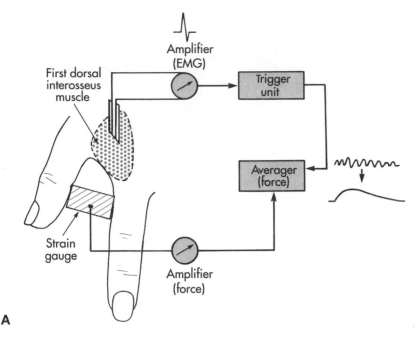

A

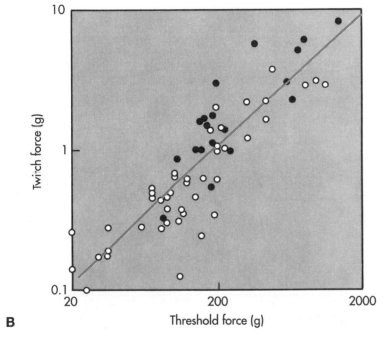

B

■ **Fig. 6-14**   Relationship between the threshold for recruitment and the force developed by a motor unit as studied during voluntary contraction of the first dorsal interosseus muscle of the human. **A,** Experimental arrangement for detecting the force developed by a single motor unit during voluntary contraction. The action potential of the motor unit is used to trigger an averager, which then samples the muscle force. **B,** Weaker motor units are recruited before stronger ones. (From Milner-Brown HS, Stein RB, Yemm R: *J Physiol [Lond]* 230:359, 1973.)

A clinically useful way to monitor the activity of motor units is **electromyography.** An electrode is placed within a skeletal muscle to record the summed action potentials of the skeletal muscle fibers of a muscle unit (Fig. 6-14). If no spontaneous activity is noted, the patient is asked to contract the muscle voluntarily to increase the activity of motor units in the muscle. As the force of voluntary contraction increases, more motor units are **recruited.** In addition to the recruitment of more motor neurons, contractile strength is affected by the rate of discharge of the active α-motor neurons.

Electromyography is employed for various purposes. For example, the conduction velocity of motor axons can be estimated by measuring the difference in latency of motor unit potentials when a peripheral nerve is stimulated at two sites that are separated by a known distance. Another use is to observe fibrillation potentials that occur when muscle fibers are denervated. Fibrillation potentials are spontaneously occurring action potentials in single muscle fibers. These spontaneous potentials contrast with motor unit potentials, which are larger and have a longer duration, because they represent the action potentials in a set of muscle fibers that belongs to a motor unit.

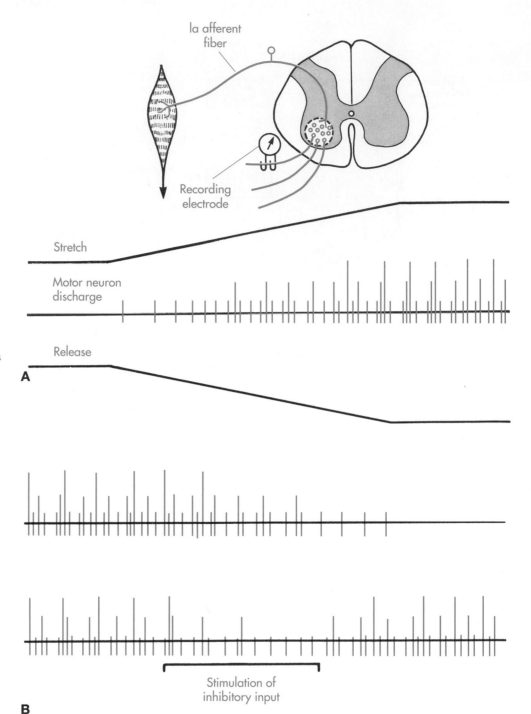

■ **Fig. 6-15** The size principle in the recruitment of motor neurons. The schematic at the top shows a Ia afferent fiber from a muscle spindle and recording electrodes on a dissected ventral root filament arising from homonymous motor neurons. **A,** Excitation. As a muscle is stretched, the increased activity of the Ia afferent fibers first recruits the smaller motor neurons. As the stretch increases, successively larger motor neurons are recruited. On release from stretch, the larger motor neurons stop discharging first and the smaller motor neurons last. **B,** Inhibition. Activating an inhibitory input to the motor neuron pool first silences the larger motor neurons and then successively smaller motor neurons. (From Eyzaguirre C, Fidone SJ: *Physiology of the nervous system: an introductory text,* ed 2, St. Louis 1975, Mosby.)

The first motor units to be activated, either by voluntary effort or during reflex action (see Chapter 9), are those with the smallest motor axons (Fig. 6-15); these motor units generate the smallest contractile forces and allow the initial contraction to be finely graded (cf. Fig. 6-14). As more motor units are recruited, the motor neurons with progressively larger axons become involved, and they generate progressively larger amounts of tension. This orderly recruitment of motor units is called the **size principle,** because the motor units are recruited in order of motor axon size. The size principle depends on the fact that small γ-motor neurons are

activated by excitatory postsynaptic potentials that exceed those in large α-motor neurons (Fig. 6-13).

Autonomic motor neurons are discussed in Chapter 11.

THE CENTRAL NERVOUS SYSTEM

The central nervous system (CNS), among other functions, gathers information about the environment from the PNS; processes this information and perceives part of it; organizes reflex and other behavioral responses; is responsible for cognition, learning, and memory; and plans and executes

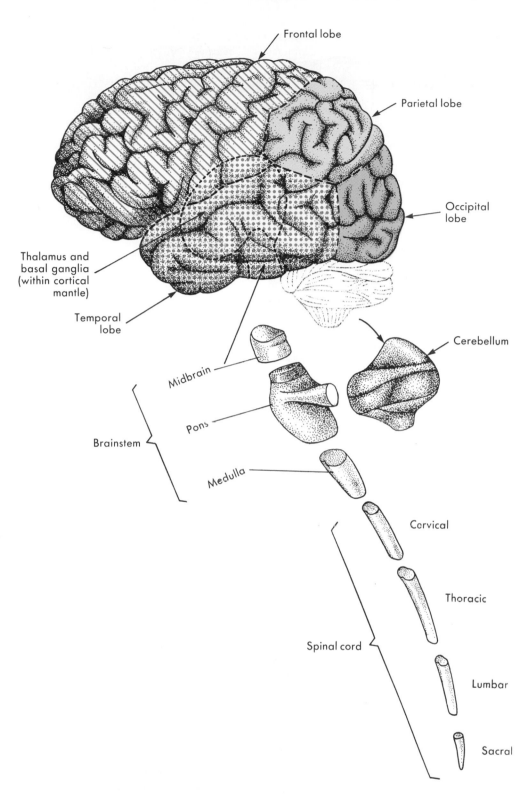

Frontal lobe

Parietal lobe

Occipital lobe

Thalamus and basal ganglia (within cortical mantle)

Temporal lobe

Cerebellum

Midbrain

Pons

Brainstem

Medulla

Cervical

Thoracic

Spinal cord

Lumbar

Sacral

■ **Fig. 6-16**   Exploded view showing the major components of the central nervous system. Also shown are the four major divisions of the cerebral cortex: the occipital lobe *(darker color)*, parietal lobe *(lighter color)*, frontal lobe *(hatching),* and temporal lobe *(stippling).* (Redrawn from Kandel ER, Schwartz JH: *Principles of neuroscience,* New York, 1981, Elsevier North-Holland.)

voluntary movements. The CNS includes the **spinal cord** and the **brain** (Fig. 6-16).

The spinal cord (lower part of Fig. 6-16) can be subdivided into a series of regions, each composed of a number of segments (in humans, 8 cervical, 12 thoracic, 5 lumbar, 5 sacral, and 1 coccygeal). Based on embryological development, the brain can be subdivided into five regions: the

myelencephalon, the **metencephalon,** the **mesencephalon,** the **diencephalon,** and the **telencephalon** (Fig. 6-16). In the adult brain the myelencephalon includes the **medulla oblongata** (or medulla); the metencephalon includes the **pons** and **cerebellum;** the mesencephalon is the **midbrain;** the diencephalon includes the **thalamus** and **hypothalamus;** and the telencephalon includes the **basal ganglia** and the **cerebral**

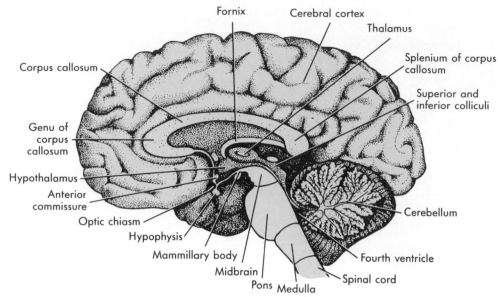

■ **Fig. 6-17**   Midsagittal section of the brain. Note the relationships among the cerebral cortex, cerebellum, thalamus, and brainstem plus the location of various commissures. (Redrawn from Kandel ER, Schwartz JH: *Principles of neuroscience,* New York, 1981, Elsevier North-Holland.)

■ **Table 6-4**   Parts and functions of the central nervous system

Region	Subdivision	Functions
Spinal cord		Sensory input; reflex organization; somatic and autonomic motor output
Myelencephalon	Medulla	Cardiovascular control; respiratory control; brainstem reflexes
Metencephalon	Pons	Respiratory and urinary bladder control; vestibular control of eye movements
	Cerebellum	Motor control; motor learning
Mesencephalon	Midbrain	Acoustic relay; control of eye movements; motor control
Diencephalon	Thalamus	Sensory and motor relay to cerebral cortex
	Hypothalamus	Autonomic and endocrine control
Telencephalon	Basal ganglia	Motor control
	Cerebral cortex	Sensory perception; cognition; learning and memory; motor planning and voluntary movement

cortex. The cerebral cortex is further divided into various lobes; they are named after the overlying bones of the skull: the **frontal, parietal, temporal,** and **occipital** lobes. The right and left **cerebral hemispheres** are connected across the midline by a massive bundle of axons, the **corpus callosum** (Fig. 6-17).

The major functions of the different parts of the CNS are listed in Table 6-4.

ENVIRONMENT OF THE CNS NEURON

The local environment of most CNS neurons is controlled, such that neurons are normally protected from extreme variations in the composition of the extracellular fluid that bathes them. This control is provided by regulation of the CNS circulation, the presence of a blood-brain barrier, the buffering function of neuroglia, and the exchange of substances between the **cerebrospinal fluid (CSF)** and the extracellular fluid of the CNS.

The cranial cavity contains the brain, blood, and CSF (Fig. 6-18). The human brain weighs about 1350 g; approximately 15%, or 200 ml, is extracellular fluid. The intracranial blood volume is about 100 ml as is the cranial volume of CSF. Thus the extracellular fluid space in the cranial cavity totals approximately 400 ml.

The Blood-Brain Barrier

The movement of large molecules and highly charged ions from the blood into the brain and spinal cord is severely restricted (see Fig. 6-18). The restriction is at least partly caused by the barrier action of tight junctions between the capillary endothelial cells of the CNS. Neuroglia, called astrocytes, may also help limit the movement of certain substances. For example, astrocytes can take up potassium ions and thus regulate the K^+ concentration in the extracellular space. Some pharmaceutical agents, such as penicillin, are removed from the CNS by transport mechanisms.

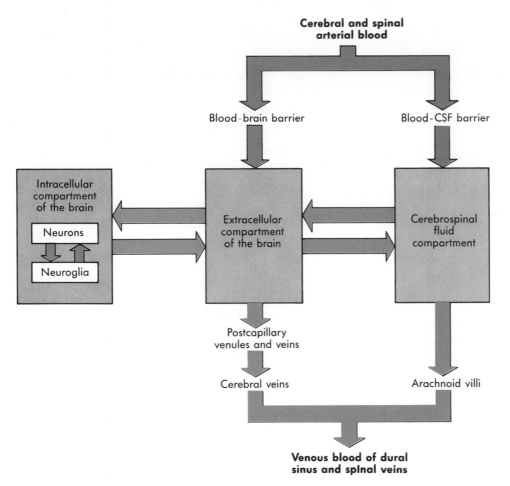

■ **Fig. 6-18**   The structural and functional relationships involved in the blood-brain and blood-CSF barriers. Substances entering the neurons and glial cells (i.e., intracellular compartment) must pass through the cell membrane. Arrows indicate direction of fluid flow under normal conditions.

The blood-brain barrier can be disrupted by pathology of the brain. For example, **brain tumors** may allow substances that are otherwise excluded to enter the brain from the circulation. This fact can be exploited radiologically by introducing into the circulation a substance that normally cannot penetrate the blood-brain barrier. If the substance can be imaged, its leakage into the region occupied by the brain tumor can be used to demonstrate the distribution of the tumor.

Cerebrospinal Fluid

Within the substance of the brain is the **ventricular system,** a series of spaces filled with CSF. CSF cushions the brain and regulates the extracellular environment of neurons. The CSF is formed largely by the **choroid plexuses,** which are covered by specialized ependymal cells. The choroid plexuses are located in the lateral, third, and fourth ventricles. The **lateral ventricles** are located within the two cerebral hemispheres. These connect with the **third ventricle** through the **interventricular foramena** (of Monro). The third ventricle lies in the midline between the diencephalon on the two sides. The **cerebral aqueduct** (of Sylvius) traverses the midbrain and connects the third ventricle with the **fourth ventricle.** The fourth ventricle is interposed between the

pons and medulla below and the cerebellum above. The **central canal** of the spinal cord continues caudally from the fourth ventricle, although in adult humans, the canal is generally not patent.

The CSF escapes from the ventricular system into the **subarachnoid space** through three apertures (the **medial aperture** of Magendie and the two **lateral apertures** of Luschka) that are located in the roof of the fourth ventricle. After it leaves the ventricular system, the CSF circulates through the subarachnoid space that surrounds the brain and spinal cord. Regions where these spaces are distended are called **subarachnoid cisterns.** An example is the **lumbar cistern,** which surrounds the lumbar and sacral spinal roots below the level of termination of the spinal cord. *The lumbar cistern is the target for lumbar puncture,* a procedure used clinically to sample the CSF. A large part of the CSF is removed by bulk flow through the valvular **arachnoid villi** into the dural venous sinuses in the cranium.

The volume of the CSF within the cerebral ventricles is approximately 35 ml, and that in the subarachnoid spaces is about 100 ml. About 0.35 ml of CSF is produced each minute. This rate allows the CSF to be turned over approximately four times daily.

The pressure in the CSF column is about 120 to 180 mm H_2O when a person is recumbent. The rate at which CSF

■ Table 6-5   Constituents of CSF and blood

Constituent	Lumbar CSF	Blood
Na$^+$ (mEq/L)	148	136-145
K$^+$ (mEq/L)	2.9	3.5-5
Cl$^-$ (mEq/L)	120-130	100-106
Glucose (mg/dl)	50-75	70-100
Protein (md/dl)	15-45	6.8×10^3
pH	7.3	7.4

From Willis WD, Grossman RG: *Medical neurobiology*, ed 3, St. Louis, 1981, Mosby.

is formed is relatively independent of the pressure in the ventricles and subarachnoid space, as well as of the systemic blood pressure. However, the absorption rate of CSF is a direct function of the CSF pressure.

The extracellular fluid within the CNS communicates directly with the CSF. Thus, the composition of the CSF indicates the composition of the extracellular environment of neurons in the brain and spinal cord. The main constituents of CSF in the lumbar cistern are listed in Table 6-5. For comparison, the concentrations of the same constituents in the blood are also given. The CSF has a lower concentration of K$^+$, glucose, and protein, but a greater concentration of Na$^+$ and Cl$^-$ than does blood. Furthermore, the CSF contains practically no blood cells. The increased concentration of Na$^+$ and Cl$^-$ enables the CSF to be isotonic to blood, despite the much lower concentration of protein in the CSF.

Obstruction of the circulation of CSF leads to increased CSF pressure and **hydrocephalus,** an abnormal accumulation of fluid in the cranium. In hydrocephalus the ventricles become distended, and if the pressure increase is sustained, brain substance is lost. When the obstruction is within the ventricular system or in the roof of the fourth ventricle, the condition is called a **noncommunicating hydrocephalus.** If the obstruction is in the subarachnoid space or the arachnoid villi, it is known as a **communicating hydrocephalus.**

SUMMARY

1. Sensory, integrative, and motor components of the nervous system permit the body to interact with the environment.

2. The neuron is the functional unit of the nervous system. Neurons contain a nucleus and nucleolus, Nissl bodies (rough endoplasmic reticulum), Golgi apparatus, mitochondria, neurofilaments, and microtubules.

3. Information is conveyed through neural circuits by action potentials in the axons of neurons and by synaptic transmission between axons and the dendrites and somas of other neurons or between axons and effector cells.

4. Neuroglial cells include astrocytes (regulate the CNS microenvironment), oligodendroglia (form CNS myelin), Schwann cells (form PNS myelin), ependymal cells (line the

ventricles), and microglia (CNS macrophages). Neuroglial cells that provide myelin sheaths speed up the conduction velocities of axons.

5. Chemical substances are distributed along the axons by fast or by slow axonal transport; the direction of axonal transport may be anterograde or retrograde.

6. Damage to the axon of a neuron causes an axonal reaction (chromatolysis) in the cell body and wallerian degeneration of the axon distal to the injury. Regeneration of PNS axons is more likely than of CNS axons.

7. The growth and maintenance of axons are affected by trophic factors, such as nerve growth factor.

8. General functions of the nervous system include excitability, sensory detection, information processing, and behavior. Different types of neurons are specialized for different functions.

9. The peripheral nervous system (PNS) includes primary afferent neurons and the sensory receptors that they innervate, somatic motor neurons, and autonomic neurons.

10. The cell bodies of primary afferent neurons are in dorsal root or cranial nerve ganglia.

11. Sensory receptors include exteroceptors, interoceptors, and proprioceptors. Stimuli are environmental events that excite sensory receptors; responses are the effects of stimuli; sensory transduction is the process by which stimuli are detected.

12. Sensory transduction is accomplished in different ways by different sensory receptors, but in general it involves the production of a receptor potential.

13. Sensory receptors may be slowly or rapidly adapting.

14. A receptive field is the region that, when stimulated, causes a response in sensory neurons.

15. Sensory receptors encode modality, spatial location, threshold, intensity, frequency, and duration of stimuli.

16. Neurons encode information by labeled lines, neural maps, and patterns of nerve impulses.

17. Primary afferent fibers can be subdivided according to the different receptor types that they supply and by their size.

18. α-Motor neurons innervate skeletal muscle fibers; a motor unit includes an α-motor neuron, its axon, and a set of skeletal muscle fibers. γ-Motor neurons are smaller than α-motor neurons and supply intrafusal muscle fibers in muscle spindles.

19. Muscle fibers in a motor unit form a muscle unit; all of the muscle fibers of a muscle unit are of the same histochemical type (slow; fast, fatigable; or fast, fatigue resistant).

20. The activity of motor units can be monitored by electromyography.

21. Motor units are recruited in an orderly fashion during voluntary or reflex activity; the first units to be recruited are those with the smallest motor axons and contractile force (size principle).

22. The central nervous system (CNS) includes the spinal cord and brain. The brain includes the medulla, pons, cerebellum, midbrain, thalamus, hypothalamus, basal ganglia, and cerebral cortex.

23. CNS extracellular fluid composition is regulated by the cerebrospinal fluid (CSF), the blood-brain barrier, and the astrocytes.

24. Choroid plexuses form CSF. CSF leaves the ventricles through the roof of the fourth ventricle, traverses the subarachnoid space, and returns to the circulation through arachnoid villi.

25. CSF differs from blood in having a lower concentration of K^+, glucose, and protein and a higher concentration of Na^+ and Cl^-; CSF normally lacks blood cells.

BIBLIOGRAPHY

Journal articles

Bray GM, Rasminsky M, Aguayo AJ: Interactions between axons and their sheath cells, *Annu Rev Neurosci* 4:127, 1981.

Burke RE: Motor unit properties and selective involvement in movement, *Exercise Sports Sci Rev* 3:31, 1975.

Deadwyler SA, Hampson RE: The significance of neural ensemble codes during behavior and cognition, *Annu Rev Neurosci* 20:217, 1997.

García Añoveros J, Corey DP: The molecules of mechanosensation, *Annu Rev Neurosci* 20:567, 1997.

González-Scarano F, Baltuch G: Microglia as mediators of inflammatory and degenerative diseases, *Annu Rev Neurosci* 22:219, 1999.

Huang EJ, Reichardt LF: Neurotrophins: roles in neuronal development and function, *Annu Rev Neurosci* 24:677, 2001.

Ip NY, Yancopoulos GD: The neurotrophins and CNTF: two families of collaborative neurotrophic factors, *Annu Rev Neurosci* 19:491, 1996.

Johnston D et al: Active properties of neuronal dendrites, *Annu Rev Neurosci* 19:165, 1996.

Landis DMD: The early reactions of non-neuronal cells to brain injury, *Annu Rev Neurosci* 17:133, 1994.

Lewin GR, Barde YA: Physiology of the neurotrophins, *Annu Rev Neurosci* 19:289, 1996.

Liu Y, Edwards RH: The role of vesicular transport proteins in synaptic transmission and neural degeneration, *Annu Rev Neurosci* 20:125, 1997.

Matthews G: Neurotransmitter release, *Annu Rev Neurosci* 19:219, 1996.

Parker AJ, Newsome WT: Sense and the single neuron: probing the physiology of perception, *Annu Rev Neurosci* 21:227, 1998.

Rekling JC et al: Synaptic control of motoneuronal excitability, *Physiol Rev* 80:767, 2000.

Reyes A: Influence of dendritic conductances on the input-output properties of neurons, *Annu Rev Neurosci* 24:653, 2001.

Rubin LL, Staddon JM: The cell biology of the blood-brain barrier, *Annu Rev Neurosci* 22:11, 1999.

Sofroniew MV, Howe CL, Mobley WC: Nerve growth factor signaling, neuroprotection, and neural repair, *Annu Rev Neurosci* 24:1217, 2001.

Steward O, Schumann EM: Protein synthesis at synaptic sites on dendrites, *Annu Rev Neurosci* 24:299, 2001.

Udin SB, Fawcett JW: Formation of topographic maps, *Annu Rev Neurosci* 11:289, 1988.

Vallee RB, Bloom GS: Mechanisms of fast and slow axonal transport, *Annu Rev Neurosci* 14:59, 1991.

Verkhratsky A, Orkand RK, Kettenmann H: Glial calcium: homeostasis and signaling function, *Physiol Rev* 78:99, 1998.

Wechsler-Reya R, Scott MP: The developmental biology of brain tumors, *Annu Rev Neurosci* 24:385, 2001.

Westbury DR: A comparison of the structures of alpha- and gamma-spinal motoneurones of the cat, *J Physiol* 325:79, 1982.

Books and monographs

Akoev GN, Andrianov GN: Synaptic transmission in the mechano- and electroreceptors of the acousticolateral system. In Ottoson D, editor: *Progress in sensory physiology 9,* Berlin, 1989, Springer-Verlag.

Basmajian JV: *Muscles alive: their functions revelaed by electromyography,* Baltimore, 1967, Williams & Wilkins.

Binder MD, Mendell LM, editors: *The segmental motor system,* New York, 1990, Oxford University Press.

Burgess PR, Perl ER: Cutaneous mechanoreceptors and nociceptors. In Iggo A, editor: *Handbook of sensory physiology,* vol II, *Somatosensory system,* Berlin, 1973, Springer-Verlag.

Burke RE: Motor units: anatomy, physiology and functional organization. In Brookhart JM, Mountcastle VB, editors: *Handbook of physiology: the nervous system,* vol II, Bethesda, Md, 1981, American Physiological Society.

Cajal SR: *Degerneration and regernation of the nervous system,* New York, 1959, Hafner Publishing.

Cajal SR: *The neuron and the glial cell,* Springfield, Ill, 1984, Charles C Thomas.

Henneman E, Mendell LM: Functional organization of motoneuron pool and its inputs. In Brookhart JM, Mountcastle VB, editors: *Handbook of physiology: the nervous system,* vol II, Bethesda, Md., 1981, American Physiological Society.

Kandel ER, Schwartz JH, Jessell TM: *Principles of neural science,* ed 4, New York, 2000, Elsevier.

Millen JW, Woollam DHM: *The anatomy of the cerebrospinal fluid,* New York, 1962, Oxford University Press.

Mountcastle VB: Central nervous system mechanisms in mechanoreceptive sensibility. In Brookahrt JM, Mountcastle VB, editors: *Handbook of physiology: the nervous system,* vol. III, Bethesda, Md, 1984, American Physiological Society.

Nicholls JG, Martin AR, Wallace BG: *From neuron to brain,* ed 3, Sunderland, Mass, 1992, Sinauer Associates.

Paxinos G, editor: *The human nervous system,* San Diego, 1990, Academic Press.

Shepherd GM: *Neurobiology,* ed 3, New York, 1994, Oxford University Press.

Whitfield IC: *Nerocommunications: an introduction,* New York, 1984, John Wiley & Sons.

Willis WD, Coggeshall RE: *Sensory mechanisms of the spinal cord,* ed 2, New York, 1991, Plenum Press.

Willis WD, Grossman RG: *Medical neurobiology,* ed 3, St. Louis, 1981, Mosby.

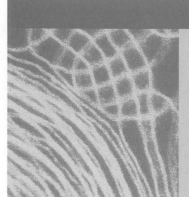

chapter seven

The Somatosensory System

SENSORY PATHWAYS

A sensory pathway is simply a set of sensory neurons arranged in series (Fig. 7-1). First-, second-, third-, and higher-order neurons are sequential elements in a given sensory pathway. In addition, several parallel sensory pathways are often involved in transmitting similar sensory information. We describe the neural elements that form the somatosensory system below. Most of the other sensory systems have a comparable arrangement, as will be discussed in Chapter 8.

SOMATOSENSORY SYSTEM

The somatosensory system (or somatovisceral sensory system) transmits information from sensory receptor organs in the skin, muscles, joints, and viscera to the cerebral cortex. Information arising from these sensory receptors first reaches the spinal cord or brainstem by way of **first-order neurons,** which are primary afferent neurons. The cell bodies of the primary afferent neurons are located in dorsal root (Fig. 7-1) or cranial nerve ganglia. Each ganglion cell gives off an axon that branches into a peripheral process and a central process. The **peripheral processes** terminate peripherally as sensory receptors (or on accessory cells). The **central processes** enter either the spinal cord through a dorsal root or the brainstem through a cranial nerve. A central process typically gives rise to numerous collateral branches that end synaptically on several **second-order neurons.**

The analysis of somatosensory information involves the contralateral thalamus and cerebral cortex. Somatosensory information reaches the thalamus by means of the axons of second-order neurons, which cross to the other side of the central nervous system (CNS) either in the spinal cord or in the brainstem. These crossed axons then travel rostrally to the thalamus, where they synapse on **third-order neurons** of the somatosensory system (Fig. 7-1).

The third-order somatosensory neurons in turn project to the somatosensory regions of the cerebral cortex, where they synapse on **fourth-order neurons** (Fig. 7-1). Fourth and **higher-order neurons** in the same and other cerebral corti-

cal areas, as well as in subcortical structures that receive cortical connections, process the information further. At some undetermined site the sensory information results in **perception,** which is a conscious awareness of the stimulus.

The most important ascending somatosensory pathways that carry information from the body are the **dorsal column–medial lemniscus path** and the **spinothalamic tract.** The projection that carries somatosensory information from the face is the **trigeminothalamic tract.** We will emphasize these pathways. There are also several ancillary somatosensory pathways that will mentioned only briefly.

The sensory modalities that are mediated by the somatosensory system include touch-pressure, flutter-vibration, proprioception (position sense and joint movement), thermal sense (warmth and cold), pain, and visceral distension. The sensory receptors that are responsible for signaling these sensory modalities will now be discussed.

SOMATOVISCERAL SENSORY RECEPTORS
Cutaneous Receptors

Cutaneous receptors can be subdivided according to the type of stimulus to which they respond. The major types of cutaneous receptors include **mechanoreceptors, thermoreceptors,** and **nociceptors.**

Mechanoreceptors. Mechanoreceptors respond to mechanical stimuli, such as stroking or indenting the skin, and they can adapt rapidly or slowly. A rapidly adapting receptor is one that discharges at the onset (and often at the offset) of a stimulus. A slowly adapting receptor continues to discharge so long as the stimulus is maintained.

Rapidly adapting cutaneous mechanoreceptors include **hair follicle receptors** in hairy skin, **Meissner's corpuscles** in glabrous (nonhairy) skin, and **Pacinian corpuscles** in subcutaneous tissue (Fig. 7-2, *A*). Hair follicle receptors and Meissner's corpuscles respond best to stimuli that are repeated at rates of about 30 to 40 Hz, whereas Pacinian corpuscles respond best to stimuli that are repeated at about 250 Hz.

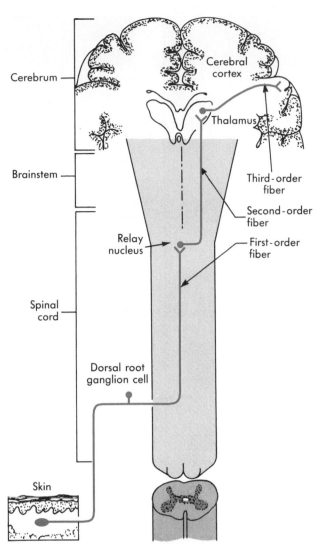

Fig. 7-1 General arrangement of sensory pathways. First-, second-, and third-order neurons are shown. Note that the axon of the second-order neuron crosses the midline, so that sensory information from one side of the body is transmitted to the opposite side of the brain.

Labels in figure: Cerebrum; Cerebral cortex; Thalamus; Brainstem; Third-order fiber; Second-order fiber; Relay nucleus; First-order fiber; Spinal cord; Dorsal root ganglion cell; Skin

Slowly adapting cutaneous mechanoreceptors include **Merkel cell endings** and **Ruffini endings** (Fig. 7-2, *B*) and **C-mechanoreceptors.** Merkel cell receptors have punctate receptive fields, whereas stretching the skin, even at some distance away from the receptor terminals, activates Ruffini endings.

The axons of all of these receptor types are myelinated. Most of the axons are Aβ fibers, although one class of hair follicle receptor, the down-hair receptor, is supplied by Aδ fibers. C-mechanoreceptors are innervated by unmyelinated axons and they respond best to slowly moving stimuli, such as stroking. C-mechanoreceptors have only recently been found in humans, although they are common in other mammals, such as cats.

Thermoreceptors. Thermoreceptors are sensitive to the temperature of the skin. The two types of thermoreceptors in the skin are **cold** and **warm receptors.** Both types are slowly

adapting, although they also discharge phasically when skin temperature changes rapidly (Fig. 7-3, *A*). Thermoreceptors are among the few receptor types that discharge spontaneously under normal circumstances. The receptors are active over a broad range of temperatures (Fig. 7-3, *B*). At a moderate skin temperature, such as 35°C, both types of receptor may be active. However, as the skin is warmed, the cold receptors become inactive; conversely, as the skin is cooled, the warm receptors become inactive. Warm receptors also stop discharging as the temperature reaches the **noxious** (damaging) range (above 45°C). Therefore these receptors cannot signal heat pain.

The stimulus-response curve for cold receptors in Fig. 7-3, *B* shows that the mean discharge frequencies of these fibers would not allow the CNS to discriminate between temperatures at points above and below the peak of the curve. However, over a certain range of temperature, cold receptors discharge in bursts (Fig. 7-3, *A*). These bursts may provide information that allows the CNS to distinguish between the activity of cold receptors exposed to higher versus lower temperatures. In addition, another class of cold receptors is activated only when the temperature of the skin is lowered below a certain point. Most cold fibers are supplied by Aδ fibers, and most warm receptors by C fibers.

Nociceptors. Nociceptors respond to stimuli that threaten or damage the organism. The two major classes of cutaneous nociceptors are the **Aδ mechanical nociceptors** and the **C-polymodal nociceptors,** although several other types exist. As their names suggest, the Aδ mechanical nociceptors are supplied by finely myelinated afferent fibers, and the C-polymodal nociceptors by unmyelinated fibers. The Aδ mechanical nociceptors respond to strong mechanical stimuli, such as pricking the skin with a needle or crushing the skin with forceps. They typically do not respond to noxious thermal or chemical stimuli, unless they have previously been sensitized (see below). C-polymodal nociceptors, on the other hand, respond to several types of noxious stimuli, including mechanical, thermal (Fig. 7-4), and chemical stimuli. Many C-nociceptors (and some Aδ nociceptors) contain vanilloid receptors (VR1 receptors) in their surface membranes, which are activated by heat, low pH, and the vanilloid substance, capsaicin.

Nociceptors may undergo **peripheral sensitization** after they are exposed to a strong noxious stimulus. Sensitized nociceptors respond more vigorously to a noxious stimulus, because their threshold for activation is lowered (Fig. 7-4). This more vigorous response can lead to **hyperalgesia,** which is characterized by an increase in the pain produced by stimulation at a given intensity, and by a decrease in the pain threshold (see below in the section on **Pain**). The nociceptors may also develop a background discharge, which may produce spontaneous pain.

Sensitization of primary afferent nociceptors occurs when chemical products, such as K+, bradykinin, serotonin, histamine, and eicosanoids (prostaglandins and leukotrienes), are released near nociceptor terminals in

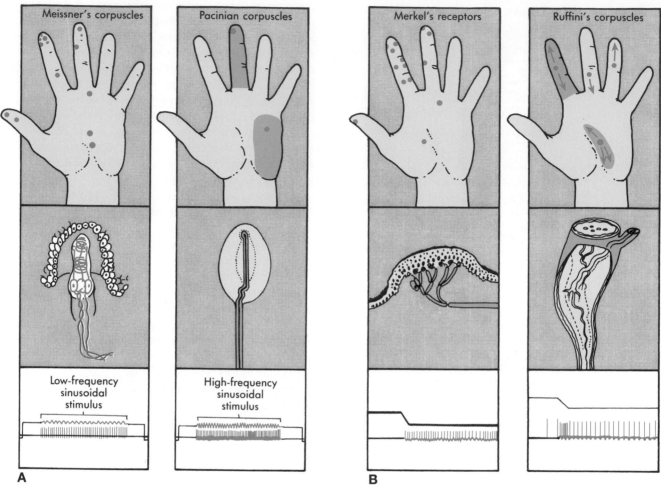

■ **Fig. 7-2**   The receptive fields of several types of cutaneous mechanoreceptors are shown in the top row of drawings. **A,** Rapidly adapting mechanoreceptors: Meissner corpuscles and Pacinian corpuscles. **B,** Slowly adapting mechanoreceptors: Merkel receptors and Ruffini corpuscles. The second row of drawings shows the morphology of the receptors; the third row shows the responses to sinusoidal stimuli (**A**) or to step indentations of the skin (**B**).

response to tissue damage or to inflammation. For example, a noxious stimulus applied to the skin may destroy cells near a nociceptor (Fig. 7-5, *A*). The dying cells release K$^+$, which depolarizes the nociceptor. Dying cells also release proteolytic enzymes that react with circulating globulins to form bradykinin. Bradykinin then binds to a receptor on the membrane of the nociceptor and activates a second messenger system, which in turn sensitizes the ending. Other chemical agents, such as serotonin released from platelets, histamine from mast cells, and eicosanoids from various cellular elements, also contribute to sensitization, either by opening ion channels or by activating second messenger systems. Many of these substances also act on blood vessels, immune cells, platelets, and other effectors that participate in inflammation.

Nociceptors are often responsible for the initiation of inflammation. The type of inflammation for which

nociceptors are responsible is called **neurogenic inflammation.**

Activation of a nociceptor terminal releases various chemicals, such as the peptides, substance P (SP), and calcitonin gene-related peptide (CGRP). These agents may be released not only from the same terminal that is stimulated, but also from other terminals of the same nociceptor through an **axon reflex** (Fig. 7-5, *B*). A nerve impulse established in one branch of a nociceptor conducts centrally through the parent axon to elicit a sensory response. However, it also spreads antidromically into other branches of the axon in the skin. As the nerve impulse invades these peripheral branches of the nociceptor, SP and CGRP are released into the skin (Fig. 7-5, *B*). SP and CGRP cause several effects, including vasodilation and increased capillary permeability. The effects of SP and CGRP augment the effects of other agents released from damaged cells, and from platelets,

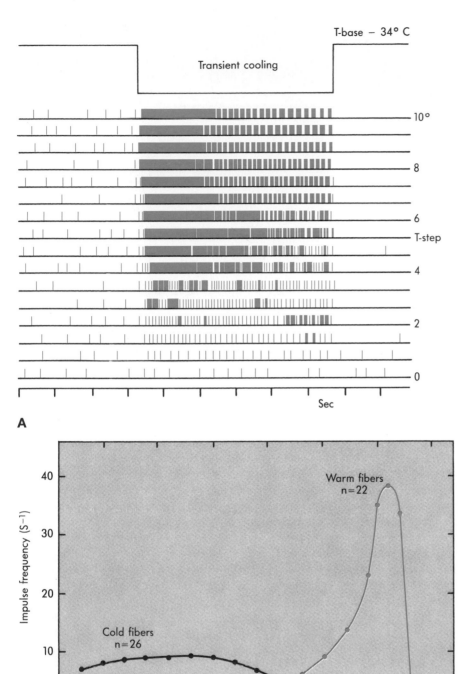

Fig. 7-3 **A,** Responses recorded from the afferent supplying a cold receptor to graded cooling pulses. **B,** Average static discharge rates for populations of cold and warm receptors. (**A,** from Darian-Smith I, Johnson KD, Dykes R: *J Neurophysiol* 36:325, 1973; **B,** from Hensel H, Kenshalo DR: *J Physiol* 204:99, 1969.)

mast cells, and invading leukocytes. The resultant inflammation leads to a typical series of cutaneous changes, such as reddening and warming caused by the increased blood flow, swelling caused by **neurogenic edema,** and pain and tenderness due to the sensitization of nociceptors. These responses constitute the classic signs and symptoms of inflammation, namely **rubor** (redness), **calor** (heat), **tumor** (swelling), and **dolor** (pain).

Muscle, Joint, and Visceral Receptors

Skeletal muscle also contains several types of sensory receptors. These are chiefly mechanoreceptors and nociceptors, although some muscle receptors may possess thermosensitivity or chemosensitivity. The best-studied muscle receptors are the **stretch receptors,** which include muscle spindles and Golgi tendon organs. Although these are important in sensing movement and position (proprioception), they may be even more important in motor control. Their structure and

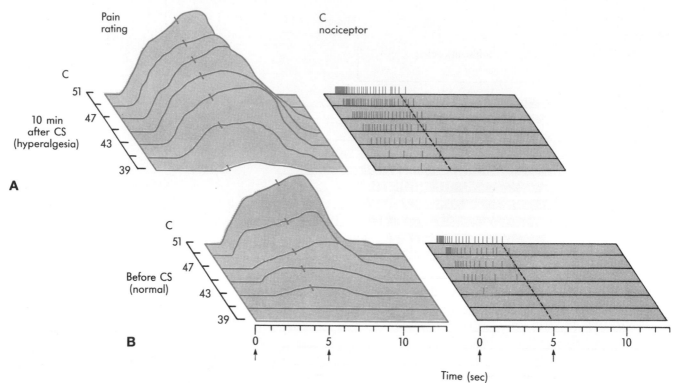

■ Fig. 7-4 A, Curves show magnitude ratings of pain in a human in response to heat pulses applied to the hairy skin before and after a mild burn. Arrows indicate the beginning and end of the stimuli. **B,** The responses of a C-polymodal nociceptor innervating the hairy skin in a monkey in response to the same heat pulses before and after the mild burn. (From LaMotte RH, Thalhammer JG, Robinson CJ: *J Neurophysiol* 50:1, 1983.)

function are discussed in Chapter 9. **Nociceptors** in muscle respond to pressure applied to the muscle and to release of metabolites, especially during ischemia. Muscle nociceptors are supplied by medium-sized and small myelinated axons (groups II and III) or by unmyelinated afferent fibers (group IV). Other muscle receptors with fine afferent fibers are regarded as **ergoreceptors,** which signal the work of muscles.

Joints are associated with several types of sensory receptors, such as rapidly and slowly adapting **articular mechanoreceptors** and **articular nociceptors.** The rapidly adapting mechanoreceptors include Pacinian corpuscles, which respond to transient mechanical stimuli, such as vibration. The slowly adapting receptors are Ruffini endings, which respond best to extreme movements of a joint. These endings signal pressure or torque applied to the joint. Joint mechanoreceptors are innervated by medium-sized (group II) afferent fibers. Joint nociceptors are activated by hyperextension or hyperflexion, although many articular nociceptors fail to respond to normal joint movements. If sensitized by inflammation, however, the nociceptors respond to movements or to weak pressure stimuli, which normally do not activate these receptors. Joint nociceptors are innervated by finely myelinated (group III) or unmyelinated (group IV) primary afferent fibers.

The viscera are sparsely supplied with sensory receptors. These visceral receptors are usually involved in reflexes and have little to do with sensory experience. However, some visceral **mechanoreceptors** are responsible for the sensation of distension, and **visceral nociceptors** signal visceral pain. Pacinian corpuscles are present in the mesentery and in the capsules of visceral organs, such as the pancreas. These presumably signal transient mechanical stimuli. Whether some forms of visceral pain result from overactivity of mechanoreceptor afferent fibers that supply viscera is still controversial. Many viscera, however, do have specific nociceptors. Visceral nociceptors may be inactive under normal circumstances, but they become active after they are sensitized by injury or inflammation.

Microneurography

The sensory functions of various cutaneous sensory receptors have been studied in human subjects using a technique known as microneurography, in which a fine metal microelectrode is inserted into a nerve trunk in the arm or leg. When a recording can be made from a single sensory axon, the receptive field of the fiber is mapped. Most of the various types of sensory receptors that have been studied in experimental animals have also been found in humans.

In some humans it has been possible, after the receptive field of a sensory axon has been characterized, to stimulate the same sensory axon through the microneurography electrode. In these experiments, the subject is asked to locate the perceived receptive field of the sensory axon, which turns out to be identical to the mapped receptive field. Repetitive

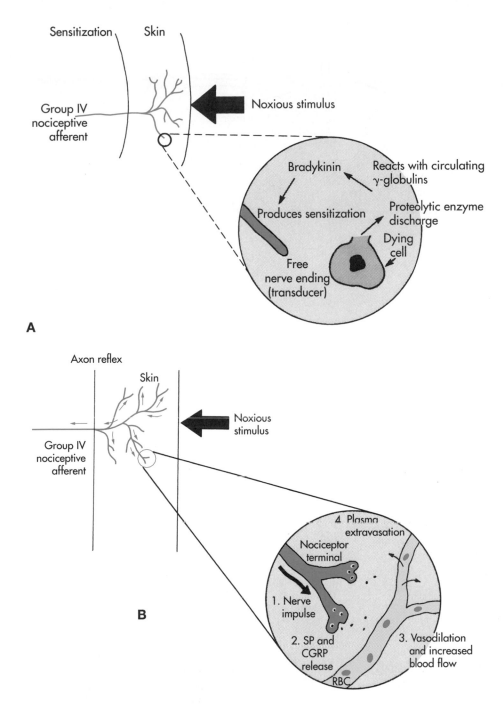

A

B

■ **Fig. 7-5** **A,** sensitization of the terminals of a nociceptor. A noxious stimulus that causes damage to cells results in the local release of proteolytic enzymes that react with circulating proteins to produce bradykinin. Bradykinin then binds to a receptor on the membrane of the nociceptive afferent fiber and sensitizes it (after activation of a second messenger system). The nociceptor is now more responsive to further stimulation. Other agents that would have similar effects include prostaglandins, serotonin, histamine, leukotrienes, and K^+ ions, although these have different actions at the membrane level (e.g., serotonin would act on a receptor that opens an ion channel). **B,** Release of substance P (SP) and calcitonin gene–related peptide (CGRP) from a nociceptor after an axon reflex causes changes in the local environment. One action is vasodilation, resulting in reddening of the skin and warming. Another is increased capillary permeability, resulting in plasma extravasation. *RBC,* Red blood cell.

stimulation is usually required to evoke a sensation, but the sensations produced by individual nerve fibers are perceived as pure sensations that match the properties of the receptors. The quality of the sensations remains the same, regardless of the frequency of stimulation. For example, stimulation of the afferent fiber of a Meissner corpuscle causes a sensation of flutter, of a Pacinian corpuscle, a sensation of vibration, and of a Merkel receptor, a sensation of maintained touch. If the frequency of stimulation of Meissner or Pacinian corpuscles is increased, the perceived frequency of flutter or of vibration increases. However, an increase in the frequency of stimulation of Merkel endings augments the intensity of

the sensation of touch or pressure. Higher-frequency stimulation does not cause the quality of the sensation to change, for example, to pain.

The axons of most Ruffini endings so far tested do not produce a sensation when they are stimulated, but stimulation of these endings has recently been shown to cause sensations of either touch or of joint position. Central summation is probably required for most Ruffini endings to produce a sensation, and the sensation can be either touch-pressure or position sense.

Activation of individual Aδ nociceptors causes a pricking pain. Stimulation of C-polymodal nociceptors produces either

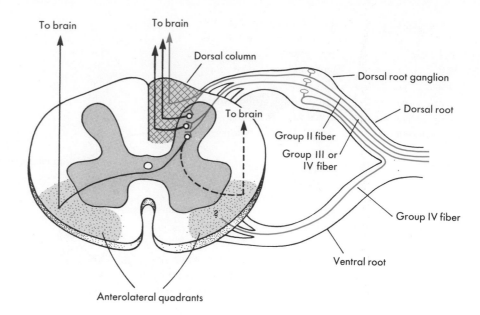

■ **Fig. 7-6** Entry of large and small primary afferent fibers into the spinal cord. Primary afferent fibers have their cell bodies in the dorsal root ganglion. The central processes of the large fibers enter the spinal cord through the medial part of the dorsal root and join the dorsal funiculus. Collaterals synapse in the spinal cord gray matter. The central processes of small afferent fibers enter the cord through the lateral part of the dorsal root (or in some cases through the ventral root). Collaterals from primary afferent axons in the dorsolateral fasciculus synapse in the dorsal horn. Some of the second-order neurons project to the brain, either through the contralateral ventrolateral funiculus or through ipsilateral pathways in the dorsal or lateral funiculus.

a burning pain or, in some cases, an itch. In the case of C fibers, the microneurography electrode usually activates more than one afferent fiber.

SPINAL ROOTS AND DERMATOMES

As shown in Fig. 7-6, axons of the peripheral nervous system (PNS) enter or leave the CNS through the spinal roots (or through cranial nerves). The **dorsal root** on one side of a given spinal segment is composed entirely of the central processes of dorsal root ganglion cells. The **ventral root** consists chiefly of motor axons, including α-motor axons, γ-motor axons (see Chapter 9), and, at certain segmental levels, autonomic preganglionic axons (see Chapter 11). Ventral roots also contain many primary afferent fibers; the role of these fibers is still unclear.

Primary afferent fibers in the adult are distributed both peripherally and centrally. The pattern of innervation is determined during embryological development. In the adult, a given dorsal root ganglion supplies a specific cutaneous region, which is called a **dermatome.** Many dermatomes become distorted during development, chiefly because of the rotation of the upper and lower extremities as they are formed, and also because humans maintain an upright posture. However, the sequence of dermatomes can readily be understood if depicted on the body of a person in a quadrupedal position (Fig. 7-7).

> Although a dermatome receives its densest innervation from the corresponding spinal cord segment, collateral branches of primary afferent fiberss of several adjacent spinal segments also supply the dermatome. Thus, transection of a single dorsal root causes little sensory loss in the corresponding dermatome. Anesthesia of any given dermatome requires interruption of several successive dorsal roots.

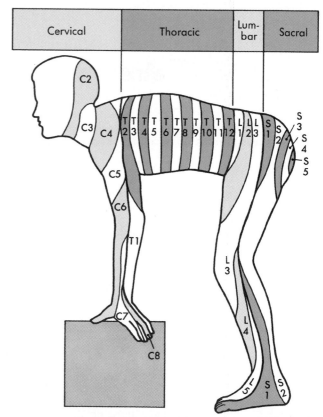

■ **Fig. 7-7** Dermatomes represented on a drawing of a person assuming a quadrupedal position.

Just before they penetrate the spinal cord, the large myelinated primary afferent fibers assume a medial position in the dorsal root, whereas the fine myelinated and unmyelinated fibers shift to a lateral position. The large, medially placed afferent fibers enter the dorsal column, where they bifurcate to send one branch rostrally and another branch caudally. These branches travel through several segments, and some ascend to the medulla as part of the dorsal column–medial lemniscus pathway (see page 101). The axons in the dorsal funiculus give off collaterals that pass ventrally into the gray matter of the spinal cord. These transmit sensory information to neurons in the dorsal horn and also provide the afferent limb of reflex pathways.

INNERVATION OF THE FACE BY THE TRIGEMINAL NERVE

The arrangement of primary afferent fibers that supply the face is comparable to that of fibers that supply the body. Peripheral processes of neurons in the trigeminal ganglion pass through the ophthalmic, maxillary, and mandibular divisions of the trigeminal nerve to innervate dermatome-like regions of the face. The trigeminal nerve also innervates the teeth, oral and nasal cavities, and cranial dura mater.

Elderly people are sometimes susceptible to a condition of chronic pain known as **trigeminal neuralgia.** People with this condition experience spontaneous episodes of severe, often lancinating pain in the distribution of one or more branches of the trigeminal nerve. Often, the pain is triggered by weak mechanical stimulation in the same region. A major contributing factor to this painful state appears to be mechanical damage to the trigeminal ganglion by an artery that impinges on the ganglion. Surgical displacement of the artery can often resolve the condition.

SOMATOSENSORY PATHWAYS OF THE DORSAL SPINAL CORD

Dorsal Column–Medial Lemniscus Pathway

The ascending branches of many large myelinated primary afferent nerve fibers travel rostrally in the dorsal funiculus of the spinal cord (Fig. 7-6) all the way to the caudal medulla. These axons are the first-order neurons of the dorsal column–medial lemniscus pathway. Second-order neurons that receive synaptic input from the ascending branches of primary afferent fibers in the dorsal funiculus are located in the dorsal column nuclei of the caudal medulla.

Neurons in the dorsal column nuclei respond similarly to the primary afferent fibers that synapse on them. The main differences between the responses of dorsal column neurons and of primary afferent neurons are (1) dorsal column neurons have larger receptive fields, because multiple primary afferent fibers synapse on a given dorsal column neuron; (2) dorsal column neurons sometimes respond to more than one class of sensory receptor, owing to convergence of several different types of primary afferent fibers on the second-order neurons; and (3) dorsal column neurons often have inhibitory receptive fields that are mediated through interneuronal circuits in the dorsal column nuclei.

Neurons in the dorsal column nuclei project their axons across the midline and through the medial lemniscus to the contralateral thalamus. The third-order neurons are located in the ventral posterior lateral (VPL) nucleus. The third-order neurons in the thalamus then project to the somatosensory areas of the cerebral cortex.

The pathway in the trigeminal system that is equivalent to the dorsal column–medial lemniscus path involves a relay from primary afferent fibers that supply the face in the main sensory nucleus of the trigeminal nerve. Second-order neurons in this nucleus send their axons across the midline and through the trigeminothalamic tract to the ventral posterior medial (VPM) nucleus of the contralateral thalamus. Third-order neurons of the VPM nucleus project to the somatosensory cerebral cortex.

At all levels of the dorsal column–medial lemniscus pathway, there is a precise somatotopic arrangement of the neurons and their axons. This arrangement is clearly demonstrated at the cerebral cortical level, where a **sensory homunculus** can be used to represent the somatotopic map (Fig. 7-8). The leg is represented on the medial aspect of the somatosensory cortex, and the arm is represented on the lateral aspect. The input to these areas is transmitted via the VPL thalamic nucleus. The face representation is just dorsal to the lateral fissure, and its input is from the VPM nucleus. The homunculus appears distorted, because regions of the body and face that are more densely innervated make use of more of the cortical circuitry than do regions that are less densely innervated.

Ancillary Somatosensory Pathways of the Dorsal Spinal Cord

Other pathways that carry somatosensory information and that ascend in the dorsal part of the spinal cord on the same side as the afferent input include (1) the spinocervical tract, (2) the postsynaptic dorsal column pathway, and (3) collaterals of the dorsal spinocerebellar tract that end in a medullary nucleus, just rostral to the dorsal column nuclei. All of these pathways relay in the upper cervical spinal cord or medulla via neurons that project to the contralateral VPL nucleus. The latter, in turn, relays information to the somatosensory cortex. The sensory functions of these ancillary somatosensory pathways include tactile sense and nociception (the spinocervical tract and the postsynaptic dorsal column pathway) and position sense (the collateral branches of the dorsal spinocerebellar tract),

Sensory Functions of the Dorsal Spinal Cord Pathways

Somatosensory pathways that ascend in the dorsal part of the spinal cord are at least partially responsible for the following sensory modalities: flutter-vibration, touch-pressure, proprioception, visceral distension, and visceral pain.

Flutter-vibration. **Flutter** refers to the recognition of transient, low-frequency mechanical stimuli. In clinical testing, this often involves sensory responses to brief applications of a wisp of cotton or brief taps on the skin. The

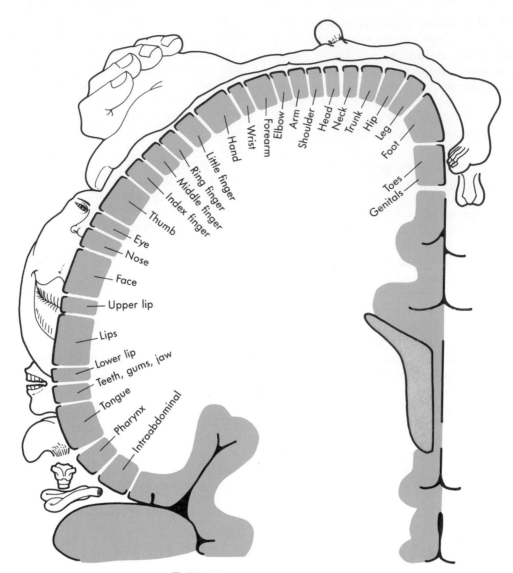

■ Fig. 7-8   Sensory homunculus.

sensory receptors that detect flutter include hair follicles and Meissner corpuscles. Several parallel ascending sensory tracts convey information that is used for flutter sensation. These tracts include the dorsal column–medial lemniscus pathway, the spinocervical tract, and the postsynaptic dorsal column path. In addition, the spinothalamic tract in the ventral part of the cord is partly responsible for flutter sensation, as discussed later in this chapter. **Vibratory sense** involves recognition of transient, high-frequency stimuli. A common clinical test of vibratory sense is discrimination of whether a tuning fork placed against a bony prominence is vibrating. Pacinian corpuscles detect high-frequency vibration. The information is transmitted through the dorsal column–medial lemniscus pathway.

Touch-pressure. Maintained skin indentation is recognized in touch-pressure. The receptors include Merkel cell and Ruffini endings. The ascending pathways that convey information from these receptors include the dorsal column–medial lemniscus and the postsynaptic dorsal column paths.

Proprioception. The senses of **joint movement** and **joint position** are included in proprioception. The sensory information arises from receptors in muscle, joints, and skin. For proximal joints, such as the knee, the most important information is derived from the activity of muscle spindles in the muscles that move the joint. In distal joints, such as those of the fingers, Ruffini endings in skin and joint receptors also contribute. All of the information required for proprioception in the upper extremity ascends in the dorsal column–medial lemniscus pathway. However, a major part of the information needed for proprioception in the lower extremity depends on collaterals of the dorsal spinocerebellar tract that relay in the medulla.

Visceral sensations. The feeling of fullness of certain viscera, such as the urinary bladder, is one example of a visceral sensation. Information about visceral distension arises from stretch receptors in the wall of the viscus and is transmitted by way of the dorsal column–medial lemniscus pathway. Recently, the dorsal column–medial lemniscus pathway has been found to be largely responsible for mediating visceral pain.

> **Effects of interruption of dorsal cord pathways.** A lesion that interrupts pathways that ascend in the dorsal part of the spinal cord will result in deficits in tactile discrimination, vibratory sense, position sense, and visceral sensation. Particularly affected is the ability to recognize figures drawn on the skin (**graphesthesia**) and tactile recognition of objects placed in the hand (**stereognosis**). Some tactile function remains, and it allows localization of a tactile stimulus and a flutter sensation. Cutaneous pain and temperature sensations are unaffected, but visceral pain is substantially diminished.

SOMATOSENSORY PATHWAYS OF THE VENTRAL SPINAL CORD

Spinothalamic Tract

The spinothalamic tract is the most important sensory pathway for somatic pain and thermal sensations. It also contributes to tactile sensation. The first-order neurons are primary afferent fibers from nociceptors, thermoreceptors, and mechanoreceptors. The second-order neurons are in the spinal cord (rather than in the caudal medulla, as in the dorsal column–medial lemniscus pathway). The axons of spinothalamic tract cells cross to the opposite side within the spinal cord. They then ascend to the brain in the ventral part of the lateral funiculus, where they terminate on third-order neurons in the thalamus. However, the spinothalamic tract ends not only in the VPL nucleus, but also in several other thalamic nuclei, including those in the intralaminar complex. Nociceptive signals are then forwarded to several cortical areas, including not only the somatosensory cortex, but also cortical areas that are involved in affective responses, such as the cingulate gyrus and the insula, which have limbic system functions.

The cells of origin of the spinothalamic tract are found chiefly in the spinal cord dorsal horn. Most spinothalamic tract cells receive an excitatory input from nociceptors in the skin, but many can also be excited by noxious stimulation of muscle, joints, or viscera. Effective cutaneous stimuli include noxious mechanical, thermal, and chemical stimuli. Some spinothalamic tract cells are excited by activity in cold or warm thermoreceptors or in sensitive mechanoreceptors. Thus, different spinothalamic tract cells respond in a manner appropriate for signaling noxious, thermal, or mechanical events.

Some nociceptive spinothalamic tract cells receive a convergent excitatory input from several different classes of cutaneous sensory receptors. For example, a given spinothalamic neuron may be activated weakly by tactile stimuli, but more powerfully by noxious stimuli (Fig. 7-9, *A*). Such neurons are called **wide-dynamic range cells,** because they are activated by stimuli with a wide range of intensities. Wide-dynamic range neurons mainly signal noxious events; the

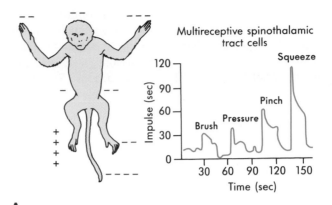

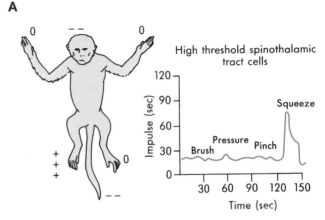

■ **Fig. 7-9 A,** Responses of a wide-dynamic-range or multireceptive spinothalamic tract cell. **B,** Responses of a high-threshold spinothalamic tract cell. The figures indicate the excitatory *(plus signs)* and inhibitory *(minus signs)* receptive fields. The graphs show the responses to graded intensities of mechanical stimulation. *Brush* is with a camel's hair brush repeatedly stroked across the receptive field. *Pressure* is applied by attachment of an arterial clip to the skin. This is a marginally painful stimulus to a human. *Pinch* is by attachment of a stiff arterial clip to the skin and is distinctly painful. *Squeeze* is by compressing a fold of skin with forceps and is damaging to the skin.

weak responses to tactile stimuli appear to be ignored by higher centers. However, in certain pathological conditions, these neurons may be sufficiently activated by tactile stimuli to evoke a sensation of pain. This would explain some pain states in which the activation of mechanoreceptors causes pain (**mechanical allodynia**). Other spinothalamic tract cells are activated only by noxious stimuli. Such neurons are often called **high-threshold** or **nociceptive-specific cells** (see Fig. 7-9, *B*).

The neurotransmitters released by nociceptors that activate spinothalamic tract cells include the excitatory amino acid, glutamate, and any of several peptides, such as SP, CGRP, and vasoactive intestinal polypeptide (VIP). Glutamate appears to act as a fast transmitter by its action on non–*N*-methyl-D-aspartic acid (non-NMDA) excitatory amino acid receptors. However, with repetitive stimulation, glutamate can also increase the activity, or **wind-up,** through an action mediated by NMDA receptors. Peptides appear to act as neuromodulators. For example, through a combined action with an excitatory amino acid, such as glutamate, SP can produce a long-lasting increase in the responses of spinothalamic tract cells; this enhanced responsiveness is called **central sensitization.** CGRP seems to increase SP release and to prolong the action of SP by inhibiting its enzymatic degradation.

Spinothalamic tract cells often have inhibitory receptive fields. Inhibition may result from weak mechanical stimuli, but usually the most effective inhibitory stimuli are noxious ones. The nociceptive inhibitory receptive fields may be very large and may include most of the body and face (see Fig. 7-9, *A*). Such receptive fields may account for the ability of various physical manipulations, including transcutaneous electrical nerve stimulation and acupuncture, to suppress pain (see discussion below in the section on **Pain**). Neurotransmitters that can inhibit spinothalamic tract cells include the inhibitory amino acids, γ-aminobutyric acid (GABA) and glycine, as well as monoamines and the endogenous opioid peptides (see page 114).

Ancillary Somatosensory Pathways of the Ventral Spinal Cord

Other pathways that transmit somatosensory information and ascend in the ventrolateral part of the spinal cord include the spinoreticular tract and the spinomesencephalic tract.

Spinoreticular tract neurons often have large, sometimes bilateral, receptive fields, and the effective stimuli include noxious ones. The reticular formation, which projects to the intralaminar complex of the thalamus and then to wide areas of the cerebral cortex, is involved in attentional mechanisms and arousal (see Chapter 7). Reticulospinal projections also contribute to the descending systems that control pain transmission.

Many cells of the **spinomesencephalic tract** respond to noxious stimuli, and the receptive fields may be small or large. The terminations of this tract are in several midbrain nuclei, including the **periaqueductal gray,** which is an important component of the endogenous analgesia system. Motivational responses may also result from activation of the periaqueductal gray. For example, stimulation in the periaqueductal gray can cause vocalization and aversive behavior. Information from the midbrain is relayed not only to the thalamus, but also to the amygdala, a part of the limbic system. This provides one of several pathways by which noxious stimuli can trigger emotional responses.

Sensory Functions of the Ventral Spinal Cord Pathways

The most important sensations mediated by ventral spinal cord pathways are pain and termperature. However, they also contribute to flutter sensation. The spinothalamic tract alone is insufficient for the recognition of the direction of a tactile stimulus, and discrimination is much more accurate when the dorsal column–medial lemniscus path is intact. This can be tested clinically by drawing numbers on the fingertip (graphesthesia). Graphesthesia is lost when the dorsal column–medial lemniscus pathway is interrupted, but not when the spinothalamic tract is interrupted. Thermal sense, which includes the two submodalities of cold and warm, appears to depend on input from cold and warm receptors to spinothalamic tract cells in the dorsal horn.

Effects of interruption of ventral spinal cord pathways, including the spinothalamic tract. Both the sensory-discriminative and the motivational-affective components of pain are lost on the contralateral side of the body when the spinothalamic tract and accompanying ventral spinal cord pathways are interrupted. This motivated the development of the surgical procedure known as **anterolateral cordotomy.** This procedure was formerly used to treat pain in many individuals, especially those suffering from cancer. This operation is now used infrequently, because of improvements in drug therapy and because pain often returns months to years after an initially successful cordotomy. The return of pain may reflect either an extension of the disease or the development of a central pain state (see later discussion). In addition to the loss of pain sensation, anterolateral cordotomy produces a loss of sensation of cold and warmth on the contralateral side of the body. Careful testing may reveal a minimal tactile deficit as well, but the intact sensory pathways of the dorsal part of the spinal cord provide sufficient tactile information that any loss caused by interruption of the spinothalamic tract is insignificant.

SENSATION FROM THE FACE

Trigeminal Tactile and Proprioceptive Pathways

Primary afferent fibers that supply the face, teeth, oral and nasal cavities, and cranial meninges synapse in several brainstem nuclei, including the main sensory nucleus and the spinal nucleus of the trigeminal nerve. The mesencephalic nucleus of the trigeminal nerve is comparable to a portion of the trigeminal ganglion. The other trigeminal nucleus is the motor nucleus of the trigeminal nerve, whose motor neurons project to skeletal muscles of the head through the trigeminal nerve.

The pathway through the main sensory nucleus resembles the dorsal column–medial lemniscus pathway. This sensory nucleus relays tactile information to the contralateral VPM thalamic nucleus by way of the trigeminothalamic tract. Third-order neurons in the VPM nucleus project to the face area of the somatosensory cortex.

The mesencephalic nucleus of the trigeminal nerve is unusual, in that the neurons in this nucleus are actually the cell bodies of primary afferent proprioceptive neurons. These neurons, in turn, innervate stretch receptors in the muscles of mastication and in other muscles of the head. The central processes of these neurons project to the trigeminal motor nucleus and to other brainstem nuclei.

Trigeminal Nociceptive and Thermoreceptive System

Nociceptive and thermoreceptive information that originates from regions of the head is processed in a fashion similar to that for the trunk and limbs. Pain in the trigeminal distribution is particularly important, because it includes both tooth and headache pain.

The primary afferent fibers of nociceptors and thermoreceptors in the head enter the brainstem through the trigeminal nerve (some also enter through the facial, glossopharyngeal, and vagus nerves). These fibers then descend through the brainstem to the upper cervical spinal cord through the spinal tract of the trigeminal nerve. Some mechanoreceptive afferent fibers also join the spinal tract. Axons in the spinal tract synapse on second-order neurons in the spinal nucleus. These neurons transmit information concerning sensations of pain and temperature to the contralateral VPM nucleus through the trigeminothalamic tract. The spinal nucleus also projects to the intralaminar complex and other thalamic nuclei, in a fashion similar to the spinothalamic tract. These thalamic nuclei in turn project to the somatosensory cerebral cortex for sensory discrimination of pain and temperature, and to other cortical regions that are responsible for motivational-affective responses.

PAIN

Nociceptive sensory information that leads to pain is particularly important because of the medical implications of pain. Several aspects of pain mechanisms will be discussed in more detail.

Pain is a complex phenomenon and includes both sensory-discriminative and motivational-affective components. That is, pain is a sensory experience that is accompanied by emotional responses and by somatic and autonomic motor adjustments. Presumably the sensory-discriminative component of pain depends on the spinothalamic and trigeminothalamic projections to the VPL and VPM nuclei. This nociceptive information is then transmitted to the SI and SII regions of the cerebral cortex (see page 113). Sensory processing at these and higher levels of the cortex results in (1) the perception of the quality of pain (e.g., pricking, burning, or aching), (2) the location of the painful stimulus, (3) the intensity of the pain, and (4) the duration of the pain.

The motivational-affective responses to painful stimuli include attention and arousal, somatic and autonomic reflexes, endocrine responses, and emotional changes. These account collectively for the unpleasant nature of painful stimuli. The motivational-affective responses depend on activity transmitted in several ascending pathways, including not only the spinothalamic and trigeminothalamic, but also the spinoreticular and the spinomesencephalic tracts. Cortical areas that are involved in these responses include the cingulate gyrus and the insula. In addition, several recently discovered pathways connect the spinal cord directly with the limbic areas, including the amygdala, but without a thalamic relay.

Types of pain

Nociceptive pain. Pain that is associated with the discharges of nociceptors is called **nociceptive pain.** However, several additional pain states can develop because of changes in the sensitivity of primary afferent nociceptors or of central nociceptive neurons, such as spinothalamic tract cells.

Hyperalgesia and allodynia. As previously mentioned, primary afferent nociceptors may become sensitized after the skin or other tissue is injured. A painful stimulus may therefore become even more painful, because the nociceptive afferents are more readily activated and they discharge at higher rates in response to a given stimulus. This state is known as **primary hyperalgesia.**

In addition, a surrounding area of skin may also become tender, because nociceptive neurons in the spinal cord, including the spinothalamic tract cells, become sensitized. If a noxious stimulus evokes more pain than it does in normal skin, the condition is called **secondary hyperalgesia.** If a normally innocuous tactile or thermal stimulus evokes pain, the condition is called **allodynia.** Central sensitization of nociceptive neurons may be due in part to the activation of second messenger systems in the dorsal horn neurons.

Referred pain. Referred pain is defined as pain that is perceived as coming from an area that is remote from its actual origin. For example, in angina pectoris, the pain is caused by ischemia of the heart. However, the ischemic heart pain may be referred to the inner aspect of the left arm. Referred pain originates from deep structures, including muscle and viscera, and it is poorly localized. In contrast, pain that originates from the skin is generally well localized, presumably because spinothalamic tract cells have relatively discrete cutaneous receptive fields. Also, the ascending system through which they signal is organized somatotopically. In angina pectoris, the area of pain referral is in the T1 dermatome, which corresponds to the spinal cord level that provides the main sensory innervation of the heart.

One explanation of referred pain is that many spinothalamic neurons receive excitatory input not only from the skin, but also from muscle and viscera. The spinal cord segments that innervate the dermatomes that contain the cutaneous receptive field of the cell correspond to the segments that innervate the muscle or viscus. The activity in a population of spinothalamic tract cells may be interpreted by subjects as originating in specific somatic structures, based on their learning this association during childhood. Subsequently, activation of these neurons by pathological input from visceral nociceptors is misinterpreted as resulting from stimulation of superficial parts of the body.

Neuropathic pain. Pain sometimes occurs in the absence of nociceptor stimulation. This type of pain is most likely to occur after damage to peripheral nerves or to parts of the CNS that are involved in transmitting nociceptive information. Pain caused by damage to neural structures is called **neuropathic pain.** Neuropathic pain states include **peripheral neuropathic pain,** which may follow damage to a peripheral nerve, and **central neuropathic pain,** which sometimes occurs after damage to CNS structures.

Examples of pain secondary to damage to a peripheral nerve are **causalgia** and **phantom limb pain.** Causalgia may develop after traumatic damage to a peripheral nerve. Even though evoked pain is reduced, the area innervated by the damaged nerve may develop severe pain. Such pain may be very difficult to treat, even with strong analgesic drugs. The pain is caused in part by spontaneous activity that develops in dorsal root ganglion cells; such activity may be attributed to an upregulation of sodium channels. In some cases, the pain seems to be maintained by sympathetic neural activity, because sympathetic nerve block may alleviate the pain. Sympathetic involvement may relate to the sprouting of damaged sympathic postganglionic axons into the dorsal root ganglia, and it may be accompanied by an upregulation of adrenoreceptors in primary afferent neurons. Phantom limb pain follows traumatic amputation in some individuals. Such phantom pain is clearly not caused by activation of nociceptors, because these receptors are no longer present in the area in which pain is felt.

Lesions of the thalamus or at other levels of the spinothalamocortical pathway may cause **central pain,** which is a severe, spontaneous pain. However, interruption of the nociceptive pathway by the same lesion may simultaneously prevent or reduce the pain evoked by peripheral stimulation. The mechanism of such trauma-induced pain caused by neural damage is poorly understood. The pain appears to depend on changes in the activity and response properties of more distant neurons in the nociceptive system.

Inhibition of Pain

As previously mentioned, because spinothalamic tract neurons have inhibitory receptive fields activation of inhibitory mechanisms might be useful for relieving pain.

The **gate control theory of pain** explains how innocuous stimuli may inhibit the responses of dorsal horn neurons that transmit information about painful stimuli to the brain. This theory asserts that pain transmission may be prevented by innocuous inputs mediated by large myelinated afferent fibers, whereas pain transmission may be enhanced by inputs that are carried over fine afferent fibers. The inhibitory interneurons in the superficial dorsal horn may serve as the gating mechanism. A commonly experienced example of the application of this mechanism is rubbing a painful area to reduce pain. A medical therapy designed to activate the gate control mechanism is transcutaneous electrical nerve stimulation **(TENS).** In this procedure, application of electric shocks to the skin in the painful area reduces pain.

Noxious stimuli applied to any location within a large area of the body can also inhibit indirectly the discharges of nociceptive dorsal horn neurons. The noxious stimuli activate pathways that ascend to the brainstem. Neural activity in these ascending pathways excite axons that descend from the brainstem to inhibit nociceptive neurons in the spinal cord (see the description of the endogenous analgesia system described below). This inhibitory system is referred to as **diffuse noxious inhibitory controls.** Acupuncture may be a way to activate this system, as it resembles TENS.

HIGHER PROCESSING OF SOMATOSENSORY INFORMATION

Thalamus

The medial lemniscus and the spinothalamic tract synapse in the VPL nucleus of the thalamus. Several other parallel sensory tracts also terminate in the VPL nucleus. The trigeminothalamic tracts from the main sensory and spinal nuclei of the trigeminal nerve synapse in the VPM nucleus of the thalamus.

The responses of many neurons in the VPL and VPM nuclei resemble those of first- and second-order neurons in the ascending tracts. The responses may be dominated by a particular type of sensory receptor. The receptive field may be small, but is probably larger than that of a primary afferent fiber. The receptive fields are contralateral to the thalamic neuron, and the location of the thalamic neuron is systematically related to that of the receptive field. In other words, the VPL and VPM nuclei are somatotopically organized. The lower extremity is represented by neurons in the lateral part of the VPL nucleus, the upper extremity by neurons in the medial part of the VPL nucleus, and the face by neurons in the VPM nucleus.

Thalamic neurons often have inhibitory, as well as excitatory, receptive fields. The inhibition may actually take place in the dorsal column nuclei or in the dorsal horn of the spinal cord. However, inhibitory circuits are also located within the thalamus. The VPL and VPM nuclei contain inhibitory interneurons (in primates, but not in rodents), and some of the inhibitory interneurons in the reticular nucleus of the thalamus project into the VPL and VPM nuclei. The inhibitory neurons intrinsic to the VPL and VPM nuclei and in the reticular nucleus use GABA as their inhibitory neurotransmitter.

One difference between neurons in the VPL and VPM nuclei and sensory neurons at lower levels of the somatosensory system is that thalamic neuron excitability depends on the stage of the sleep–wake cycle and on the presence or absence of anesthesia. During a state of drowsiness or during barbiturate anesthesia, thalamic neurons tend to undergo an alternating sequence of excitatory and inhibitory postsynaptic potentials. The alternating bursts of discharges in turn intermittently excite neurons in the cerebral cortex. Such excitation and inhibition result in an alpha rhythm or in spindling in the electroencephalogram (see Chapter 10). This alternation of excitatory and inhibitory postsynaptic potentials during these two states may reflect the level of excitation of thalamic neurons by excitatory amino acids that act at non-NMDA and NMDA receptors. It may also reflect the inhibition of the thalamic neurons by recurrent pathways through the reticular nucleus.

The spinothalamic tract and the part of the trigeminothalamic tract that originates in the spinal nucleus of the trigeminal nerve also project to the central lateral nucleus of the intralaminar complex of the thalamus, as well as to other nuclei of the medial thalamus. The intralaminar nuclei are not somatotopically organized, and they project diffusely to the cerebral cortex, as well as to the basal ganglia. The projection of the central lateral nucleus to the SI cortex may be involved in arousal of this part of the cortex and in selective attention.

Destruction of the VPL or VPM nuclei diminishes sensation on the contralateral side of the body or face. The sensory qualities that are lost reflect those that are transmitted mainly by the dorsal column–medial lemniscus pathway and its trigeminal equivalent. The sensory-discriminative component of pain sensation is also lost. However, the motivational-affective component of pain is still present if the medial thalamus is intact. Presumably, pain persists because of the spinothalamic and spino-reticulothalamic projections to this part of the thalamus. In some individuals, a lesion of the somatosensory thalamus results in a central pain state, known as **thalamic pain,** which is a form of **central pain.** However, pain that is indistinguishable from thalamic pain can also be produced by lesions in the brainstem or cortex.

Somatosensory Cortex

Third-order sensory neurons in the VPL and VPM nuclei of the thalamus project to the somatosensory cortex. The main somatosensory receiving areas of the cortex are called the SI and SII areas. The SI cortex (or primary somatosensory cortex) occupies much of the postcentral gyrus, and the SII cortex (secondary somatosensory cortex) is in the superior bank of the lateral fissure.

As previously discussed (see page 111), the **SI cortex,** like the somatosensory thalamus, has a somatotopic organization (Fig. 7-8). The **SII cortex** also contains a somatosensory map, as do several other less understood areas of the cortex. In the SI cortex, the face is represented in the lateral part of the postcentral gyrus, above the lateral fissure. The hand and the rest of the upper extremity are represented in the dorsolateral part of the postcentral gyrus and the lower extremity on the medial surface of the hemisphere. The map of the surface of the body and face of a human on the postcentral gyrus is called a **sensory homunculus.** The map is distorted, because the greatest volume of neural tissue is devoted mostly to the densely innervated regions, such as the perioral area and the thumb and other digits.

The sensory homunculus is an expression of place coding of somatosensory information. A locus in the SI cortex encodes the location of a somatosensory stimulus on the surface of the body or face. For example, the brain knows that a certain part of the body has been stimulated because certain neurons in the postcentral gyrus are activated.

The SI cortex has several morphological and functional subdivisions, and each subdivision has a somatotopic map like that shown in Fig. 7-8. These subdivisions were originally described by Brodmann, and they were based on the arrangements of neurons in the various layers of the cortex, as seen in Nissl-stained preparations. The subdivisions are therefore known as Brodmann areas 3a, 3b, 1, and 2. Cutaneous

input dominates in areas 3b and 1, whereas muscle and joint input dominates in areas 3a and 2. Thus separate cortical zones are specialized for the processing of tactile and proprioceptive information. The inputs to these cortical areas are from distinct parts of the VPL and VPM nuclei.

Within any particular area of the SI cortex, all of the neurons along a line perpendicular to the cortical surface have similar response properties and receptive fields. The SI cortex is thus said to have a **columnar organization.** A comparable columnar organization has also been demonstrated for other primary sensory receiving areas, including the primary visual and auditory cortices (see Chapter 8). Nearby cortical columns in the SI cortex may process information for different sensory modalities. For example, the cutaneous information that reaches one cortical column in area 3b may come from rapidly adapting mechanoreceptors, whereas the information that reaches a neighboring column might be from slowly adapting mechanoreceptors.

Besides being responsible for the initial processing of somatosensory information, the SI cortex also begins higher-order processing, such as feature extraction. For example, certain neurons in area 1 respond preferentially to a stimulus that moves in one direction across the receptive field, but not in the opposite direction (Fig. 7-10). Such neurons presumably contribute to the perceptual ability to recognize the direction of an applied stimulus.

Effects of lesions of the somatosensory cortex. A lesion of the SI cortex in humans causes sensory changes similar to those produced by a lesion of the somatosensory thalamus. However, usually only a part of the cortex is involved, and so the sensory loss may be confined, for example, to the face or to the leg, depending on the location of the lesion with respect to the sensory homunculus. The sensory modalities most affected are discriminative touch and position sense. Graphesthesia and stereognosis are particularly disturbed. Pain and thermal sensation may be relatively unaffected, although a loss of pain may follow cortical lesions. Conversely, cortical lesions can result in a central pain state that resembles thalamic pain.

Association Cortex

The SI cortex is connected with many other cortical areas, such as the SII cortex, the motor cortex, supplementary sensory and motor cortices, and the parietal association cortex. The parietal association cortex also receives input from other sensory systems, notably from the visual system. A major function of the parietal association cortex is the relationship of the body to extrapersonal space. For example, this part of the cortex on one side helps to coordinate hand and eye movements on the contralateral side. In humans the posterior parietal cortex of the nondominant hemisphere is particularly involved in spatial relations, whereas that in the dominant hemisphere is concerned with language (see Chapter 10).

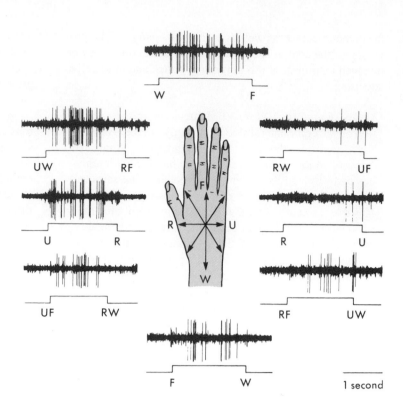

■ **Fig. 7-10**   Feature extraction by cortical neurons. The responses were recorded from a neuron in the somatosensory cortex of a monkey. The direction of a stimulus was varied, as shown by the arrows in the drawing. Note that the responses were greatest when the stimulus moved in the direction from *UW* to *RF* and least from *RW* to *UF. R,* Radial side; *U,* ulnar side; *F,* fingers; *W,* wrist. (From Costanzo RM, Gardner EP: *J Neurophysiol* 43:1319, 1980.)

Effects of a lesion in the parietal association cortex. A lesion of the parietal association cortex on the non-dominant side with respect to language causes deficits in the ability to relate to extrapersonal space. When an affected person is asked to copy geometric figures, the figures are distorted. For example, the numbers of a clock face may all be drawn on the side of the clock that corresponds to the normal side of the person with the lesion (**constructional apraxia**). The person may deny the existence of the contralateral side of the body (**neglect syndrome**) and have difficulty in dressing on that side. The individual with a lesion may also have difficulty reading maps, driving, or performing other activities that require spatial orientation.

Centrifugal Control of Somatosensation

Sensory experience is not just the passive detection of environmental events. Instead, it more often depends on exploration of the environment. Tactile cues are sought by moving the hand over a surface. Visual cues result from scanning visual targets with the eyes. Thus, sensory information is often received as the result of activity in the motor system. Furthermore, transmission in pathways to the sensory centers of the brain is regulated by descending control systems. These systems allow the brain to control its input by filtering the incoming sensory messages. Important information can be attended to and unimportant information can be ignored.

The tactile and proprioceptive somatosensory pathways are regulated by descending pathways that originate in the SI and motor regions of the cerebral cortex. For example, corticobulbar projections to the dorsal column nuclei help control sensory input that is transmitted by the dorsal column–medial lemniscus pathway.

Of particular interest is the descending control system that regulates the transmission of nociceptive information. This system presumably suppresses excessive pain under certain circumstances. For example, it is well known that soldiers on the battlefield, accident victims, and athletes in competition often feel little or no pain at the time a wound occurs or a bone is broken. At a later time, pain may develop and become severe. Although the descending regulatory system that controls pain is part of a more general centrifugal control system that modulates all forms of sensation, the pain control system is so important medically that it is distinguished as a special system called the **endogenous analgesia system.**

Several centers in the brainstem and descending pathways from these contribute to the endogenous analgesia system. For example, stimulation in the periaqueductal gray, the locus coeruleus, or the medullary raphe nuclei inhibits nociceptive neurons at spinal cord and brainstem levels, including spinothalamic tract and trigeminothalamic tract cells (Fig. 7-11, *A*). Other inhibitory pathways originate in the sensorimotor cortex, the hypothalamus, and the reticular formation.

The endogenous analgesia system can be subdivided into two components: one component uses one of the endogenous **opioid peptides** as neurotransmitters or modulators and the other does not. The endogenous opioids are neuropeptides that activate one of several types of opiate receptors. Some

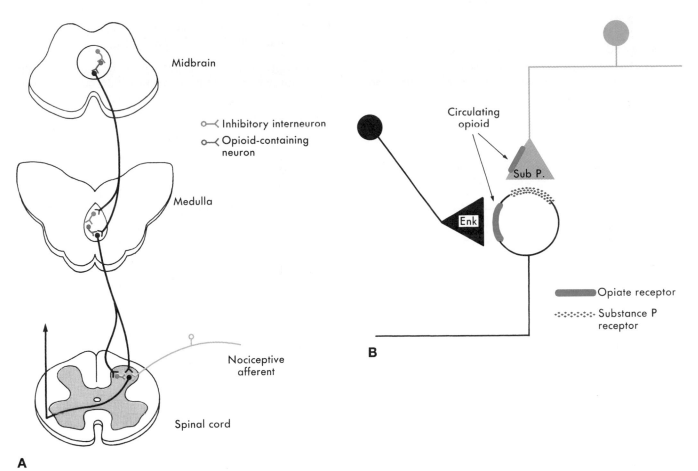

Fig. 7-11   A, Some of the neurons thought to play a role in the endogenous analgesia system. Neurons in the midbrain periaqueductal gray activate the raphe-spinal tract, which in turn inhibits nociceptive spinal neurons, such as those of the spinothalamic tract. Interneurons containing opioid substances are involved in the system at each level. **B,** Possible presynaptic and postsynaptic sites of action of enkephalin *(Enk)*. The presynaptic action might prevent the release of substance P *(SubP)* from nociceptors. (Redrawn from Henry JL: In Porter R, O'Connor M, editors: *Ciba Foundation Symposium 91,* London, 1982, Pitman.)

of the endogenous opioids include enkephalin, dynorphin, and β-endorphin. Opiate analgesia can generally be prevented or reversed by the narcotic antagonist naloxone. Therefore, naloxone is often used to determine whether analgesia is mediated by an opioid mechanism.

The opioid-mediated endogenous analgesia system can be activated by exogenous administration of morphine or other opiate drugs. Thus one of the oldest medical treatments for pain depends on the triggering of a sensory control system. Opiates typically inhibit neural activity in nociceptive pathways. Two sites of action have been proposed for opiate inhibition, presynaptic and postsynaptic (Fig. 7-11, *B*). The presynaptic action of opiates on nociceptive afferent terminals is thought to prevent the release of excitatory transmitters, such as substance P. The postsynaptic action produces an inhibitory postsynaptic potential. How can an inhibitory neurotransmitter activate descending pathways? One hypothesis is that the descending analgesia system is under tonic inhibitory control by inhibitory interneurons in both the midbrain and the medulla. The action of opiates would inhibit

the inhibitory interneurons and thereby disinhibit the descending analgesia pathways.

Some endogenous analgesia pathways operate by neurotransmitters other than opioids and thus are unaffected by naloxone. One way of engaging a nonopioid analgesia pathway is through certain forms of stress. The analgesia so produced is a form of **stress-induced analgesia.**

Many neurons in the raphe nuclei use serotonin as a neurotransmitter. Serotonin can inhibit nociceptive neurons and presumably plays an important role in the endogenous analgesia system. Other brainstem neurons release catecholamines, such as norepinephrine and epinephrine, in the spinal cord. These catecholamines also inhibit nociceptive neurons; therefore catecholaminergic neurons may contribute to the endogenous analgesia system. Furthermore, these monoamine neurotransmitters interact with endogenous opioids. Undoubtedly, many other substances are involved in the analgesia system. In addition, there is evidence for the existence of endogenous opiate antagonists that can prevent opiate analgesia.

SUMMARY

1. Sensory neurons have cell bodies in sensory nerve ganglia. They connect peripherally to a sensory receptor and centrally to second-order neurons. Higher-order neurons are in the contralateral thalamus and cortex.

2. Skin contains mechanoreceptors, thermoreceptors, and nociceptors. Mechanoreceptors may be rapidly or slowly adapting. Thermoreceptors include cold and warm receptors. Aδ and C nociceptors may be sensitized by release of chemical substances from damaged cells.

3. Peripheral release of substances, such as peptides, from nociceptors may contribute to inflammation. Muscle, joints, and viscera have mechanoreceptors and nociceptors.

4. Large primary afferent fibers enter the dorsal funiculus through the medial dorsal root; collaterals synapse in the deep dorsal horn, intermediate zone, and ventral horn. Small primary afferent fibers enter the dorsolateral fasciculus through the lateral dorsal root; collaterals synapse in the dorsal horn.

5. Trigeminal primary afferent fibers supply the face, oral and nasal cavities, and dura. The cell bodies are in the trigeminal ganglion or, if proprioceptive, the mesencephalic nucleus.

6. Ascending branches of large primary afferent fibers synapse on second-order neurons in the dorsal column nuclei, which project in the medial lemniscus to the contralateral thalamus and synapse on third-order neurons of the ventral posterior lateral (VPL) nucleus.

7. The equivalent trigeminal pathway relays in the main sensory nucleus and contralateral ventral posterior medial (VPM) nucleus.

8. The spinocervical tract, the postsynaptic dorsal column path, and the part of the dorsal spinocerebellar tract that relays in the nucleus act in parallel with the dorsal column–medial lemniscus path.

9. The dorsal spinal cord pathways signal the sensations of flutter-vibration, touch-pressure, and proprioception. They also contribute to visceral sensation, including visceral pain.

10. The spinothalamic tract includes nociceptive, thermoreceptive, and tactile neurons; its cells of origin are mostly in the dorsal horn, and the axons cross, ascend in the ventrolateral funiculus, and synapse in the VPL and intralaminar nuclei of the thalamus.

11. The equivalent trigeminal pathway relays in the spinal nucleus and projects to the contralateral VPM and intralaminar nuclei.

12. The spinothalamic relay in the VPL nucleus helps account for the sensory-discriminative aspects of pain. Parallel nociceptive pathways in the ventrolateral funiculus are the spinoreticular and spinomesencephalic tracts; these and the spinothalamic projection to the medial thalamus contribute to the motivational-affective aspects of pain.

13. Referred pain is explained by convergent input to spinothalamic tract cells from the body wall and from viscera.

14. Damage to a peripheral nerve or to the central nociceptive pathway may result in neuropathic pain, such as causalgia, phantom limb pain, or thalamic pain.

15. The VPL and VPM nuclei are somatotopically organized and contain inhibitory circuits. The somatosensory cortex includes the SI and SII regions; these are also somatotopically organized.

16. The SI cortex contains columns of neurons with similar receptive fields and response properties. Some SI neurons are involved in feature extraction. The association cortex of the parietal lobe is concerned with extrapersonal space.

17. Transmission in somatosensory pathways is regulated by descending control systems. The endogenous analgesia system regulates nociceptive transmission, and it uses transmitters such as the endogenous opioid peptides, norepinephrine, and serotonin.

BIBLIOGRAPHY

Journal articles

Besson JM, Chaouch A: Peripheral and spinal mechanisms of nociception, *Physiol Rev* 67:67, 1987.

Boivie J, Leijon G, Johansson I: Central post-stroke pain: a study of the mechanisms through analysis of the sensory abnormalities, *Pain* 37:173, 1989.

Caterina MJ, Julius D: The vanilloid receptor: a molecular gateway to the pain pathway, *Annu Rev Neurosci* 24:487, 2001.

Colby CL, Goldberg ME: Space and attention in parietal cortex, *Annu Rev Neurosci* 22:319,1999.

Constanzo RM, Gardner, EP: A quantitative analysis of responses of direction-sensitive neurons in somatosensory cortex of awake monkeys, *J Neurophysiol* 43:1319, 1980.

Darian-Smith I, Johnson KO, Dykes R: "Cold" fiber population innervating palmar and digital skin of the monkey: response to cooling pulses, *J Neurophysiol* 36:325, 1973.

Fields HL, Heinricher MM, Mason P: Neurotransmtters in nociceptive modulatory circuits, *Annu Rev Neurosci* 14:219, 1991.

Hensel H, Kenshalo DR: Warm receptors in the nasal region of cats, *J Physiol* 204:99, 1969.

Johnson KPO, Hsiao SS: Neural mechanisms of tactual form and texture perception, *Annu Rev Neurosci* 15:227, 1992.

LaMotte RH, Thalhammer JG, Robinson CJ: Peripheral neural correlates of magnitude of cutaneous pain and hyperalgesia: a comparison of neural events in monkey with sensory judgements in human, *J Neurophysiol* 50:1, 1983.

Romo R, Salinas E: Touch and go: decision-making mechanisms in somatosensation, *Annu Rev Neurosci* 24:107, 2001.

Schaible HG, Schmidt RF: Effects of an experimental arthritis on the sensory properties of fine articular afferent units, *J Neurophysiol* 54:1109, 1985.

Torebjork HE, Vallbo AB, Ochoa J: Intraneural microstimulation in man: its relation to specificity of tactile sensations, *Brain* 110:1509, 1987.

Books and monographs

Akil H, Lewis JW: *Neurotransmitters and pain control,* Basel, 1987, Karger.

Belmonte C, Cervero F, editors: *Neurobiology of nociceptors,* Oxford, Oxford University Press, 1996.

Bonica JJ: *The management of pain,* Philadelphia, 1990, Lea & Febiger.

Carli G, Zimmermann M, cditors: *Towards the neurobiology of chronic pain,* Elsevier, Amsterdam, 1996.

Creutzfeldt OD: *Cortex cerebri,* Oxford, 1995, Oxford University Press.

Geppetti P, Holzer P, editors: *Neurogenic inflammation,* Boca Raton, Fla, 1996, CRC Press.

Light AR: *The initial processing of pain and its descending control: spinal and trigeminal systems,* Basel, 1992, Karger.

Jones EG: *The thalamus,* New York, 1985, Plenum Press.

Mountcastle VB: *Perceptual neuroscience: the cerebral cortex,* Cambridge, Mass, 1998, Harvard University Press.

Penfield W, Jasper H: *Epilepsy and the functional anatomy of the human brain,* Boston, 1954, Little, Brown & Co.

Wall PD, Melzack R: *Textbook of pain,* ed 3, Edinburgh, 1994, Churchill Livingstone.

Willis WD: *The pain system,* Basel, 1985, Karger.

Willis WD, Coggeshall RE: *Sensory mechanisms of the spinal cord,* ed 2, New York, 1991, Plenum Press.

Willis WD, editor: *Hyperalgesia and allodynia,* New York, 1992, Raven Press.

chapter eight

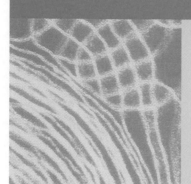

The Special Senses

Encephalization is an evolutionary trend in which special sensory organs develop in the heads of animals, along with corresponding neural systems in the brain. These special sensory systems, which include the visual, auditory, vestibular, olfactory, and gustatory systems, allow the animal to detect and analyze light, sound, and chemical signals in the environment, as well as to signal the position of the head.

THE VISUAL SYSTEM

Vision is one of the most important special senses in humans. We depend on vision and audition for most human communication. The visual system detects and interprets photic stimuli. In vertebrates, effective photic stimuli are electromagnetic waves between 400 and 750 nm long; such wavelengths constitute **visible light.**

The eye can distinguish two aspects of light, its **brightness** (or luminance) and its **wavelength** (or color). Light enters the eye and impinges on **photoreceptors** of a specialized sensory epithelium, the **retina.** The photoreceptors include rods and cones. **Rods** have low thresholds for detecting light and operate best under conditions of reduced lighting **(scotopic vision).** However, rods neither provide well-defined visual images nor contribute to color vision. **Cones,** by contrast, are not as sensitive as rods to light, and so operate best under daylight conditions **(photopic vision).** Cones are responsible for high visual acuity and color vision.

Information processing within the retina is performed by **retinal interneurons,** and the output signals are carried to the brain by the axons of **retinal ganglion cells.** The axons travel in the **optic nerves;** some cross to the opposite side of the brain in the **optic chiasm,** and others continue on the same side. Posterior to the optic chiasm, the axons of retinal ganglion cells pass through the **optic tracts** and synapse in nuclei of the brain. The main visual pathway in humans is through the **lateral geniculate nucleus** (LGN) of the thalamus. This nucleus projects through the **optic radiation** to the **visual cortex** (see page 127). Other extrageniculate visual pathways relay in the **superior colliculus, pretec-**

tum, and **hypothalamus.** These participate in orientation of the eyes, control of pupil size, and circadian rhythms, respectively.

Structure of the Eye

The wall of the eye is formed of three concentric layers (Fig. 8-1). The outer layer, or the fibrous coat, includes the transparent **cornea,** with its epithelium (the **conjunctiva**), and the opaque **sclera.** The middle layer, or vascular coat, includes the iris and the choroid. The **iris** contains both radially and circularly oriented smooth muscle fibers, which make up the pupillary dilator and sphincter muscles. The **choroid** is rich in blood vessels that supply the outer layers of the retina, and it also contains pigment. The inner coat of the eye is the neural layer or retina. The functional part of the retina covers the entire posterior eye except for the "blind spot," which is the **optic nerve head** or **optic disc** (see Fig. 8-1). Visual acuity is highest in the central part of the retina, in an area called the **macula lutea.** The **fovea** is a pitlike depression in the middle of the macula, where visual targets are focused. Tributaries of the central artery and vein of the retina nourish the inner retinal layers. These vessels course with the optic nerve, diverge from the optic nerve head, and spread over the inner surface of the retina. However, the vessels avoid the macula.

Besides the retina, the eye contains a lens, to focus light on the retina, and fluids called the **aqueous** and **vitreous humor.** These fluids are located in the **anterior** and **posterior chambers** and in the space behind the lens, and they help maintain the shape of the eye. The aqueous humor is secreted by the epithelium of the **ciliary body** into the posterior chamber of the eye. The aqueous humor then circulates through the pupil and into the anterior chamber, where it is drained by the **canal of Schlemm** into the venous system. The aqueous humor pressure, which is normally less than 22 mm Hg, determines the pressure within the eye. The vitreous humor is a gel composed of extracellular fluid that contains collagen and hyaluronic acid; unlike the aqueous humor, however, it turns over very slowly.

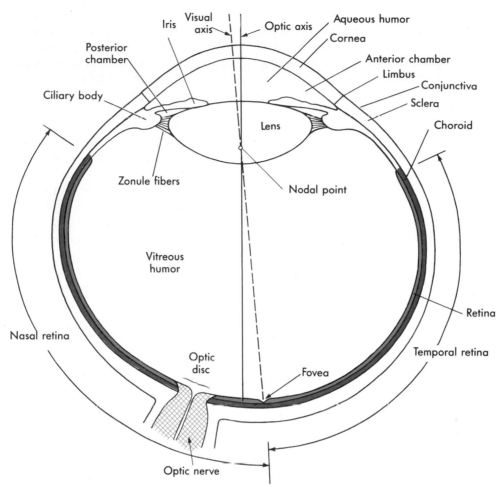

■ Fig. 8-1   View of a horizontal section of the right eye. (Redrawn from Wall GL: *The vertebrate eye and its adaptive radiation,* Bloomfield Hills, Mich., 1942, Cranbrook Institute of Science.)

If aqueous humor is not absorbed adequately, the **intraocular pressure** increases, a condition known as **glaucoma.** An increase in intraocular pressure can cause blindness by impeding blood flow to the retina.

A number of functions of the eyes are under muscular control. Externally attached extraocular muscles aim the eyes toward an appropriate visual target (see Chapter 9). These are innervated by the **oculomotor, trochlear,** and **abducens** nerves. Several muscles are also found within the eye (intraocular muscles). The **pupillary dilator** and **sphincter muscles** allow the iris to act as a diaphragm to control pupil size; this action is similar to that of the diaphragm of a camera, and it controls the amount of entering light. The dilator is activated by the sympathetic nervous system and the sphincter by the parasympathetic nervous system (through the oculomotor nerve).

The shape of the lens is also affected by muscular action. **Suspensory ligaments** (or **zonule fibers**), which attach to the wall of the eye at the ciliary body (see Fig. 8-1), hold the lens in place behind the iris. Because they surround the lens and its suspensory ligaments, the **ciliary muscles** act as a

sphincter. When the ciliary muscles are relaxed, the tension exerted by the suspensory ligaments flattens the lens. When the ciliary muscles contract, they reduce the tension on the suspensory ligaments; this process allows the somewhat elastic lens to assume a more spherical shape. The ciliary muscles are activated by the parasympathetic nervous system (via the oculomotor nerve).

Physiology of light absorption by the eye. Light enters the eye through the cornea and passes through a series of transparent fluids and structures, which are collectively called the **dioptric media.** These fluids and structures consist of the cornea, aqueous humor, lens, and vitreous humor. Normally, light from a visual target is focused sharply on the retina by the cornea and the lens, which bend or refract the light. The cornea has a refractive power of 43 diopters[*] (D) and is the major refractive element of the eye. However, because the lens can change shape, the refractive power of the lens can vary between 13 and 26 D. In this way, the lens allows the eye to accommodate either to near or to distant objects.

---

[*]The diopter describes the refractile power of a lens and equals the reciprocal of the focal length of the lens, in meters.

For instance, when light from a distant visual target enters the normal eye (one with a relaxed ciliary muscle), the target is in focus on the retina. However, if the eye is directed at a nearby visual target, the light is initially focused behind the retina (i.e., the image at the retina is blurred) until accommodation occurs. The ciliary muscle contracts and the zonule fibers relax; the image is sharpened when the convexity of the lens increases as a result of these muscular changes.

Although the optic axis of the human eye passes through the nodal point of the lens and reaches the retina at a point between the fovea and the optic disc (see Fig. 8-1), the eye is directed by the oculomotor system at a point, called the **fixation point,** on the visual target. Light from the fixation point passes through the nodal point and is focused on the fovea; the light courses along the visual axis. Light from the remainder of the visual target is focused on the retina surrounding the fovea.

Proper focus of light on the retina depends not only on the lens, but also on the iris. The iris acts like the diaphragm in a camera, not only in regulating the amount of light entering the eye, but more importantly in controlling the depth of field of the image and the amount of spherical aberration produced by the lens. When the pupil is constricted, the depth of field is increased, and the light is directed through the central part of the lens, where spherical aberration is minimal. Pupillary constriction occurs reflexly when the eye accommodates for near vision. Thus, when a person reads or does other fine visual work, the quality of the image is improved by the optical system of the eye.

Another factor that affects the quality of the image is light scatter. Light scatter is minimized in the eye by restric-

tion of the light path and by absorption of stray light by pigment in the choroid and by the retinal pigment epithelium (Fig. 8-2). Again, the eye is similar to a camera in these respects. In a camera, light scatter is also prevented by limiting the light path and by covering the interior of the camera with black paint.

Defects in focusing are caused by a discrepancy between the size of the eye and the refractive power of the dioptric media. For example, in **myopia** (near-sightedness), the images of distant objects are focused in front of the retina. Concave lenses correct this problem. Conversely, in **hypermetropia** (far-sightedness), the images of distant objects are focused behind the retina; this problem can be corrected with convex lenses. However, temporary focusing is also possible by accommodation, which may fatigue the ciliary muscles and cause eyestrain. In **astigmatism,** an asymmetry exists in the radii of curvature of different meridians of the cornea or lens (or sometimes of the retina). Astigmatism can often be corrected with lenses that possess appropriately matched radii of curvature.

As an individual ages, the elasticity of the lens gradually declines. As a result, accommodation of the lens for near vision becomes progressively less effective, a condition called **presbyopia.** A young person can change the power of the lens by as much as 14 D. However, by the time a person reaches 40 years of age, the amount of accommodation halves, and after 50 years it decreases to 2 D or less. Presbyopia can be corrected by convex lenses.

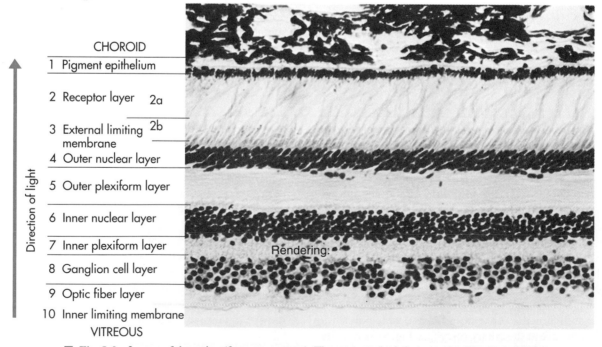

CHOROID
1 Pigment epithelium
2 Receptor layer 2a
3 External limiting 2b
  membrane
4 Outer nuclear layer
5 Outer plexiform layer
6 Inner nuclear layer
7 Inner plexiform layer
8 Ganglion cell layer
9 Optic fiber layer
10 Inner limiting membrane
VITREOUS

Direction of light

Rendering:

■ **Fig. 8-2** Layers of the retina (from a macaque). The arrow at the left shows the direction of light impinging on the retina. Nissl stain. (Courtesy of RE Weller.)

Retina

Layers of the retina. The 10 layers of the retina are shown in Fig. 8-2. The retina begins with the **pigment epithelium** (layer 1), which is just inside the choroid. As previously mentioned, the pigment epithelium absorbs stray light, and thereby reduces light scatter. The pigment cells have tentacle-like processes that extend into the photoreceptor layer and surround the outer segments of the rods and cones. These processes prevent transverse scatter of light between photoreceptors. In addition, they probably serve a mechanical function in maintaining the contact between layers 1 and 2. Other important functions of pigment cells include (1) phagocytosis of the ends of the outer segments of the rods, which are continuously shed, and (2) reconversion of metabolized photopigment into a form that can be reused after it is transported back to the photoreceptors.

The **outer** and **inner** segments of the photoreceptors form the **receptor layer** (layer 2) of the retina (see Fig. 8-2). The structure of the photoreceptors is shown in Fig. 8-3.

The junction between layers 1 and 2 of the retina in adults represents the surface of fusion between the anterior and posterior walls of the embryonic optic cup. Because this junction is structurally weak, it can separate, and thus result in **retinal detachment.** Retinal detachment causes loss of vision, due to the displacement of the retina from the focal plane of the eye. It can also lead to death of the photoreceptor cells, which are maintained by the blood supply of the choroid (the photoreceptor layer itself is avascular).

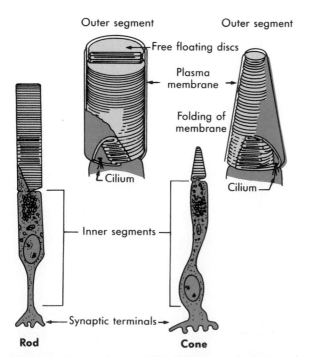

Fig. 8-3 Rods and cones. The drawings at the bottom show the general features of a rod and a cone. The insets show the outer segments.

The photoreceptors form an organized surface that light strikes. Light rays that originate from different parts of the visual target correspond point-to-point to particular photoreceptors. Therefore, the geometry of the retina, and in particular that of the photoreceptors, must be maintained for normal vision to take place. Retinal glial cells, known as **Müller cells,** play an important role in maintaining the geometry of the retina. Müller cells are oriented radially, parallel to the light path through the retina. The outer ends of the Müller cells form tight junctions with the inner segments of the photoreceptors. The numerous connections made between Müller cells and inner segments give the appearance of a continuous layer in the light microscope (see Fig. 8-2). This layer is called the **external limiting membrane** (layer 3 of the retina).

Inside the external limiting membrane is a layer of nuclei (see Fig. 8-2) called the **outer nuclear layer** (layer 4 of the retina). This layer contains the nuclei of the rods and cones.

The next layer of the retina (layer 5) is called the **outer plexiform layer** (Fig. 8-2). This layer contains presynaptic and postsynaptic elements of synapses that lie between the photoreceptors and retinal interneurons, including bipolar cells and horizontal cells.

The next layer of the retina is the **inner nuclear layer** (layer 6 of the retina). This layer contains the cell bodies and nuclei of various cell types, including the retinal interneurons (bipolar cells, horizontal cells, amacrine cells, and interplexiform cells) and the Müller cells.

The next layer is the **inner plexiform layer** (layer 7 of the retina). This layer contains the presynaptic and postsynaptic elements of the synapses between retinal interneurons, including the bipolar and amacrine cells, and the ganglion cells.

Layer 8 of the retina is the **ganglion cell layer.** As previously mentioned, the ganglion cells are the output cells of the retina. They transmit visual information to the brain.

The axons of the retinal ganglion cells form the **optic fiber layer** (layer 9 of the retina). The axons pass across the vitreous surface of the retina, and thereby avoid the macula, and then they enter the optic disc. They leave the eye in the optic nerve. The portions of the ganglion cell axons that are in the optic fiber layer remain unmyelinated, but the axons become myelinated after they reach the optic disc and nerve. The lack of myelin where the axons cross the retina is a specialization that helps permit light to pass through the inner retina with minimal distortion.

The innermost layer of the retina is the **inner limiting membrane** (layer 10 of the retina). This layer is formed by projections of the Müller cells.

Structure of photoreceptors: rods and cones. The photoreceptors include the rods and the cones. Each photoreceptor cell is composed of a cell body, an inner and an outer segment that extends into layer 2, and a synaptic terminal (Fig. 8-3). The outer segments of rods are longer than those of cones, and they contain stacks of freely floating membrane discs that are rich in rhodopsin molecules. The outer segments of cones also contain membranous discs that are associated with photopigment. However, the outer segments of cones are not as long as those of rods, and the disc membranes consist of infoldings of the surface membrane. *Rods contain much more photopigment than do cones. The greater photopigment content of rods accounts in part for their greater sensitivity to light.* A single photon can elicit a rod response, whereas several hundred photons are required for a cone response.

The inner segments of the photoreceptors are connected to the outer segments by a modified cilium that contains nine pairs of microtubules, but that lacks the two central pairs of microtubules that are found in most cilia. The inner segments

contain a number of organelles, including numerous mitochondria.

The photopigment is synthesized in the inner segment and incorporated into the membranes of the outer segment. In rods, the pigment is inserted into new membranous discs that are then displaced distally, until they are eventually shed at the apex of the outer segment. There, they are phagocytized by the pigment cell epithelium. This process determines the rodlike shape of the outer segments of rods. In cones, the photopigment is inserted randomly into the membranous folds of the outer segment, and shedding, comparable to that seen in rods, does not take place.

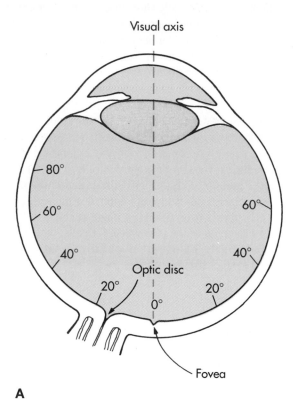

■ **Fig. 8-4** The drawing on the right shows the location of the fovea (0 degrees) and different parts of the retina at varying degrees of eccentricity from the fovea. The graph below plots the density of cones and rods as a function of retinal eccentricity from the fovea. Note that cone density peaks at the fovea, rod density peaks at an eccentricity of about 20 degrees, and no photoreceptors occur in the optic disc. (Redrawn from Cornsweet TN: *Visual perception,* New York, 1970, Academic Press.)

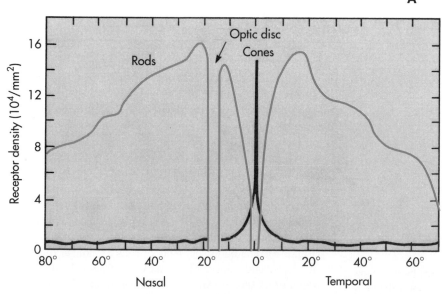

Regional variations in the retina

Fovea. The fovea, which is a depression in the macula lutea, is the region of the retina that has the highest visual resolution. Correspondingly, the image from the fixation point is focused on the fovea. The retinal layers in the foveal region are unusual because several of them appear to be pushed aside. This arrangement allows light to reach the photoreceptors without having to pass through the inner layers of the retina, and thereby reduces distortion of the image. The fovea has cones with unusually long and thin outer segments. This cone shape permits a high packing density. In fact, cone density is maximal in the fovea (see Fig. 8-4). The cones provide high visual resolution, which matches the high quality of the image provided to the fovea.

Optic disc. The *optic disc* lacks photoreceptors, and therefore lacks photosensitivity. Thus, the optic disc is a "blind spot" in the visual surface of the retina. A person normally ignores the blind spot, both because the corresponding part of the visual field can be seen by the contralateral eye, and because of the psychological process in which incomplete visual images tend to be completed perceptually. However, the blind spot can be mapped, as demonstrated by Fig. 8-5.

As mentioned, the axons of the retinal ganglion cells cross the retina in the optic fiber layer (layer 9) and enter the optic nerve at the optic disk. The axons in the optic fiber layer pass around the macula and avoid the fovea, as do the blood vessels that supply the inner layers of the retina. The optic diṣk can be visualized on physical examination by use of an **ophthalmoscope.** The normal optic disk has a slight depression in its center. Changes in the appearance of the optic disk are important clinically. For example, the depression may be exaggerated by loss of ganglion cell axons **(optic atrophy)** or the optic disk may protrude into the vitreous space, because of edema **(papilledema)** caused by an increased intracranial pressure.

Visual pigments. Light must be absorbed in order for it to be detected by the retina. Light absorption is accomplished by the visual pigments, which are located in the outer segments of the rods and cones. The pigment found in the outer segments of rods is **rhodopsin,** or visual purple (so named because it has a purple appearance after green and blue light have been absorbed). Three variants of visual pigment are found in different cone types. Rhodopsin absorbs light best at a wavelength of 500 nm, whereas the cone pigments absorb best at 420 nm (blue), 531 nm (green), or 558 nm (red). However, the absorption spectra of these visual pigments overlap considerably (Fig. 8-6).

Rhodopsin contains a chromophore, called **retinal,** which is the aldehyde of **retinol,** or vitamin A. Retinol is derived from carotenoids, such as β-carotene, the orange pigment found in carrots. Like other vitamins, retinol cannot be synthesized by humans; instead it is derived from food sources. Individuals with a severe vitamin A deficiency suffer from **"night blindness,"** a condition in which vision is defective in poor illumination.

Rhodopsin is formed when a retinal isomer, known as 11-*cis*-retinal, is combined with a glycoprotein, known as opsin. When rhodopsin absorbs light, it is "boosted" to a higher energy level. This boost causes a series of chemical

■ **Fig. 8-5** If one eye is closed and the page is held about 30 cm from the open eye, when one of the symbols is fixated, the other will disappear as the page is moved back and forth. For the right eye, the fixation point should be the circle and for the left eye the cross.

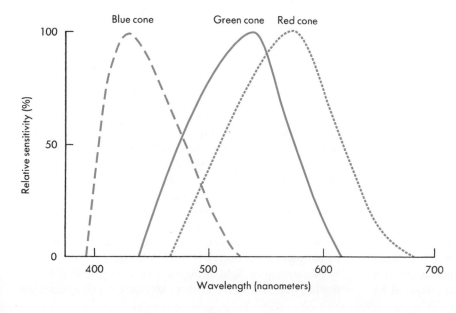

■ **Fig. 8-6** The spectral sensitivity of the three types of cones in the human retina is shown. Note that the curves overlap.

changes that lead to isomerization of 11-*cis*-retinal to all-*trans*-retinal, release of the bond with opsin, and conversion of the retinal to retinol. The separation of all-*trans*-retinal from opsin causes bleaching of the visual pigment, that is, the pigment loses its purple color.

Visual adaptation. **Light adaptation** is associated with *a reduction in the amount of rhodopsin, which in turn reduces visual sensitivity.* Light adaptation, which occurs rapidly, within seconds, favors cone vision because the rhodopsin in rods bleaches more readily than do the cone pigments.

Bleached rhodopsin must be regenerated. As all-*trans*-retinal is formed during light adaptation, it is transported to the retinal pigment cell layer, where it is reduced, isomerized, and esterified. As all-*trans*-retinal is converted back to 11-*cis*-retinal, it is transported back to the photoreceptor layer, taken up by outer segments, and recombined with opsin to regenerate the bleached rhodopsin. *The regeneration of photopigment is one mechanism involved in **dark adaptation,** a process that results in an increase in visual sensitivity.* Cones adapt more rapidly to darkness than do rods, but their adapted threshold is relatively high. Thus, cones do not function when the ambient light level is low. By contrast, rods adapt to darkness slowly, but their sensitivity increases. Within 10 minutes in a dark room, rod vision is more sensitive than cone vision.

Dark adaptation is very familiar to moviegoers, who must wait several minutes after entering the darkened theater before they can see an empty seat. Although the theater is dark and rod vision is operative, visual acuity is low and colors are not distinguished (this is called **scotopic vision**). When the movie is projected, light adaptation allows cone function to resume (this is called photopic vision) and visual acuity and color vision are restored.

Color vision. The three visual pigments in cone outer segments have opsins that differ from the opsin found in rhodopsin. As a result of these differences, the three types of cone pigments absorb light best in the blue, green, or red parts of the visible light spectrum (Fig. 8-6). According to the **trichromacy theory,** the differences in absorption are presumed to account for color vision.

The basis of the trichromacy theory is that a suitable mixture of three other colors can produce any color. Because three types of cone pigments exist, it has been proposed that these pigments in some way provide for a neural analysis of color mixing. However, a neural system must also exist for the analysis of color brightness, because absorption of light by a visual pigment depends in part on the wavelength and in part on the intensity of the light (Fig. 8-6). A given wavelength of light at a particular intensity may be absorbed by two or three of the visual pigments found in cones. However, absorption by one of the pigments will be greater than absorption by the others. If the intensity, but not the wavelength, of the light is changed, the ratio of absorption will remain constant. By comparing the effectiveness of aborption of light of different wavelengths by the different types of cones, the visual system can distinguish different colors. At least two different kinds of cones are required for color vision. The presence of three kinds decreases the ambiguity in distinguishing colors when all three absorb light, and it ensures that at least two types of cones will absorb most wavelengths of visible light.

Observations on color blindness are consistent with the trichromacy theory. In **color blindness,** a genetic defect (sex-linked recessive), one or more cone mechanisms are lost. Normal people are **trichromats,** because they have three cone mechanisms. Individuals who have lost one of the cone mechanisms are called **dichromats.** When the long wavelength cone mechanism is lost, the resulting condition is called **protanopia;** loss of the medium wavelength system causes **deuteranopia;** and loss of the short wavelength system causes **tritanopia. Monochromats** have lost all three cone mechanisms (or in some cases, two of these).

Other theories of color vision have also been proposed. The **opponent-process** theory is based on the observation that certain pairs of colors are perceived as if these colored lights activate opposing neural processes. Green and red are opposed, as are yellow and blue, and black and white. For example, if a gray area is surrounded by a green ring, the gray area appears to acquire a reddish color. Furthermore, a greenish-red or a bluish-yellow color does not exist. These observations have led to the proposal that neurons activated by green are inhibited by red. Similarly, neurons excited by blue are inhibited by yellow. Neurons with these characteristics are found both in the retina and at higher levels of the visual pathway.

A recent theory, the retinex theory, attributes color vision to the combined action of neural activity at several levels, including the retina and cerebral cortex, of the visual system. All of these theories of color vision may be applicable.

Visual transduction. The transduction of visual signals involves the hyperpolarization of the rods and cones. Transmission of visual signals thus differs from the usual manner of signal transduction, in which the sensory receptors are depolarized.

When light is absorbed by rhodopsin, the signal is amplified in the rods by a special transduction mechanism. This amplification mechanism, along with the large amount of photopigment in the outer segments of the rods, accounts for the extraordinary sensitivity of rods, which can detect a single photon after full dark adaptation. In the dark, rods have open sodium channels (Fig. 8-7). A net influx of Na^+ results in a continuous current, called the dark current. The dark current causes the rods to be maintained in a constant state of depolarization (the "resting potential" is about -40 mV). As a consequence of this constant depolarization, neurotransmitter (considered to be glutamate) is tonically released at the rod synapses on bipolar and horizontal cells. The intracellular Na^+ concentration is kept at a steady-state level by the pumping action of Na^+,K^+-ATPase.

Absorption of light activates a G-protein, called **transducin.** This G-protein, in turn, activates **cyclic guanosine**

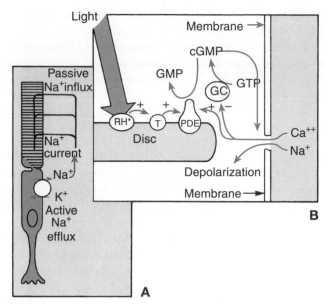

Fig. 8-7 **A,** A drawing of a rod. The flow of dark current is indicated, as well as the Na pump. **B,** The sequence of second messenger events that follow absorption of light is shown. *Rh,* Rhodopsin; *T,* transducin; *PDE,* phosphodiesterase; *GC,* guanylate cyclase; *cGMP,* cyclic guanosine monophosphate; *GTP,* guanosine triphosphate.

monophosphate (cGMP) phosphodiesterase, which is associated with the rhodopsin-containing discs, hydrolyzes cGMP to 5^1-GMP, and lowers the cGMP concentration in the rod cytoplasm (Fig. 8-7). cGMP normally keeps the sodium channels open. A reduction in cGMP concentration therefore causes the channels to close and the membrane to hyperpolarize. Amplification is the result of the ability of a single rhodopsin molecule to activate hundreds of transducin molecules; in addition, each phosphodiesterase molecule hydrolyzes thousands of cGMP molecules per second.

Similar events occur in cones, but the membrane hyperpolarization occurs more quickly than in rods, perhaps because the intracellular distances are shorter in cones.

Retinal circuitry. A diagram of the basic circuitry of the retina is shown in Fig. 8-8. Photoreceptors *(R)* synapse on the dendrites of bipolar cells *(B)* and horizontal cells *(H)* in the outer plexiform layer. The horizontal cells make transverse connections with bipolar cells, and they receive input from interplexiform cells *(I)*. Bipolar cells synapse on the dendrites of ganglion cells *(G)* and on the processes of amacrine cells *(A)* in the inner plexiform layer. Amacrine cells connect with ganglion cells, other amacrine cells, and interplexiform cells.

Several features of this circuitry are noteworthy. The input to the retina is provided by light striking the photoreceptors. The output is carried by the axons of retinal ganglion cells to the brain. Information is processed within the retina by the interneurons. The most direct pathway through

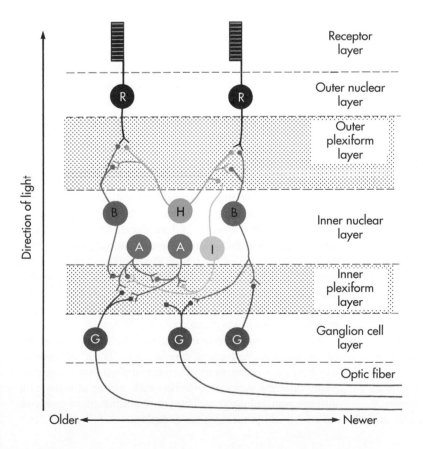

Fig. 8-8 Basic retinal circuitry. The arrow at the left indicates the direction of light through the retina. *R,* Photoreceptors; *B,* bipolar cells; *H,* horizontal cells; *A,* amacrine cells; *I,* interplexiform cells; *G,* ganglion cells.

the retina is from the photoreceptors to the bipolar cells, and then to the ganglion cells. A more indirect pathway involves the photoreceptors, bipolar cells, amacrine cells, and ganglion cells. Horizontal cells provide lateral interactions between adjacent pathways. Interplexiform cells allow interactions to occur from the inner to the outer retina.

Contrasts in rod and cone pathway functions. Rod and cone pathways have several important functional differences, based partly on the differences in their phototransduction mechanisms and partly on retinal circuitry. As we have previously described, rods have more photopigment and a better signal amplification system than do cones, and there are many more rods than cones. Thus, rods function better in dim light (scotopic vision). However, they contain a single photopigment, and so they cannot signal color differences. Furthermore, many rods converge on single bipolar cells. Therefore, rods cannot provide high-resolution vision, because the effective receptive field for the rod pathway is large. In bright light, rhodopsin is bleached. Hence, rods no longer function under photopic conditions, because of light adaptation. *Loss of rod function results in night blindness.*

Cones have a higher threshold to light and so they are not activated in dim light after dark adaptation. However, they operate very well in daylight. They provide high-resolution vision, because only a few cones converge on bipolar cells in the cone pathways, and no convergence occurs in the fovea; here the cones make one-to-one connections to bipolar cells. As a result of the smaller convergence, cone pathways have very small receptive fields. Therefore, the cone pathways can resolve stimuli that originate from sources very close to each other. Cones also respond to sequential stimuli with good temporal resolution. Finally, cones have three different cone photopigments. Thus, they can discriminate among wavelengths and can participate in color vision. Loss of cone function results in functional blindness; rod vision is not sufficient for normal visual requirements.

Synaptic interactions. The distances between retinal components are short. Hence, receptor and synaptic potentials are sufficient for most of the activity in retinal circuits, and action potentials are not required in most of the interneurons. Only the ganglion cells and some amacrine cells generate action potentials. It is unclear why amacrine cells have action potentials, but ganglion cells must generate them to transmit information over the relatively long distance from the retina to the brain.

Although receptor potentials in photoreceptors are hyperpolarizing, synaptic potentials in the retina can be either hyperpolarizing or depolarizing. Hyperpolarizing events reduce neurotransmitter release from the synaptic terminals of a retinal interneuron, whereas depolarizing events increase neurotransmitter release.

Receptive field organization. The activation of the receptive fields of retinal ganglion cells constitutes an important step in visual information processing, because these fields reflect the characteristics of visual signals that are conveyed to the brain. The receptive fields of photoreceptors and retinal interneurons determine the receptive fields of the retinal ganglion cells.

The receptive field of an individual photoreceptor is small and circular. Light in the receptive field will hyperpolarize the photoreceptor cell. The photoreceptor cell will therefore release less neurotransmitter.

A bipolar cell that receives input from a photoreceptor can have either of two types of receptive fields. Both are described as having a center-surround organization, in which the light that strikes the central region of the receptive field either excites or inhibits the bipolar cell. Also, the light that strikes the annular region of the receptive field that surrounds the central region has the converse effect. One type of receptive field has a centrally located excitatory region, surrounded by an inhibitory annulus. This type of receptive field is called an **on-center, off-surround** receptive field. The other type of receptive field has an **off-center, on-surround** arrangement.

The receptive fields of bipolar cells depend on input from photoreceptors and from horizontal cells. The response to stimulation of the center of the receptive field reflects direct connections from only a few photoreceptors. If the neurotransmitter tonically released by the photoreceptor hyperpolarizes the bipolar cell, light that strikes the photoreceptor and that hyperpolarizes it will reduce the release of the neurotransmitter, and hence the bipolar cell will be depolarized (disinhibited) and thus excited. On the other hand, if the neurotransmitter tonically released by the photoreceptor is depolarizing, the bipolar cell will be hyperpolarized (disfacilitated). The surround response results when light impinges on adjacent photoreceptors and changes the activity of horizontal cells. The pathway through the horizontal cells results in a response that is opposite in sign to that produced more directly by the photoreceptors that mediate the center response.

The neurotransmitter used in the retinal pathway from photoreceptor cells to bipolar cells and to horizontal cells is an excitatory amino acid, probably glutamate. Excitatory amino acids depolarize off-center bipolar cells, as well as horizontal cells, through activation of ionotropic glutamate receptors. They hyperpolarize on-center bipolar cells through an action on metabotropic glutamate receptors.

If light strikes both the photoreceptors that cause the surround response and those responsible for the center response, the bipolar cell may not respond at all, because of the opposing actions from the center and surround. Thus, many bipolar cells do not signal changes in the intensity of light that strikes a large area of the retina. On the other hand, a small beam of light moving across the receptive field may sequentially alter dramatically the activity of the bipolar cell, as the light crosses the receptive field from surround to center and then back again to surround.

Amacrine cells receive input from different combinations of on-center and off-center bipolar cells. Thus, their receptive fields are mixtures of on-center and off-center regions. Many different types of amacrine cells utilize at least eight different neurotransmitters. Thus, the contributions of amacrine cells to visual processing are complex.

Ganglion cells may receive a dominant input from amacrine cells, a mixed input from amacrine and bipolar cells, or a dominant input from bipolar cells. When the amacrine cell input dominates, the receptive fields of ganglion cells tend to be diffuse, and they are either excitatory or inhibitory. On the other hand, when bipolar cells dominate the input, the ganglion cells have a center-surround organization, similar to that of bipolar cells.

P, M, and W cells. Experiments have shown that in primates, retinal ganglion cells can be subdivided into three general types, called **P cells, M cells,** and **W cells.** P and M cells are fairly homogeneous groups, whereas W cells are heterogeneous. P cells are so named because they project to the parvocellular layers of the lateral geniculate nucleus (LGN); M cells project to the magnocellular layers of the LGN. P and M cells have center-surround receptive fields; hence, they are presumably controlled by bipolar cells. Some W cells also have center-surround receptive fields, but many have diffuse receptive fields. Thus, they are probably influenced chiefly through amacrine cell pathways.

Several of the physiological differences among these cell types correspond to morphological differences (Table 8-1). For example, P cells have smaller receptive fields (which correspond to smaller dendritic trees) and more slowly conducting axons than do M cells. In addition, P cells have tonic responses to visual stimuli, show more linear summation of responses than do M cells, and respond better to small stimuli than to large stimuli. M cells have phasic, nonlinear responses to complex stimuli; such responses cannot be predicted from the responses to simple stimuli. P cells respond differently to different wavelengths of light, whereas M cells

■ Table 8-1   Properties of retinal ganglion cells

Properties	P cells	M cells	W cells
Cell body and axon	Medium-sized	Large	Small
Dendritic tree	Restricted	Extensive	Extensive
Receptive field			
Size	Small	Medium	Large
Organization	Center-surround	Center-surround	Diffuse Poorly responsive
Adaptation	Tonic	Phasic	
Linearity	Linear	Nonlinear	
Wavelength	Sensitive	Insensitive	Insensitive
Luminance	Insensitive	Sensitive	Sensitive

are not sensitive to differences in wavelength. On the other hand, M cells are more sensitive to luminance than are P cells. W cells have large, diffuse receptive fields (which correspond to extensive dendritic fields), and slowly conducting axons, and they respond poorly to visual stimuli.

The Visual Pathway

Retinal ganglion cells transmit information to the brain by way of the optic nerve, optic chiasm, and optic tract. Figure 8-9 shows the relationships between a visual target *(arrow)*, the retinal images of the target in the two eyes, and the projections of retinal ganglion cells to the two hemispheres of the brain. The eyes and the optic nerves, chiasm, and tract are viewed from above.

The visual target, an arrow, is in the visual fields of both eyes (see Fig. 8-9). The visual target in this case is so long

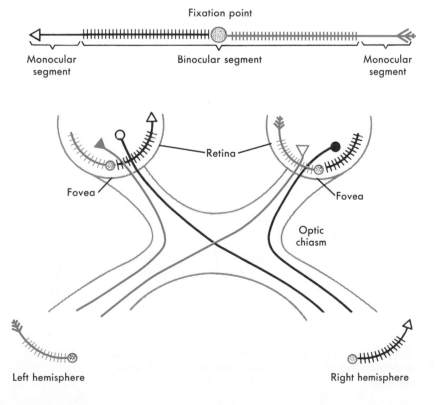

■ **Fig. 8-9**   Relationships between a visual target, images on the retinas of the two eyes, and the projections of the ganglion cells carrying visual information about these images. The image is so large that it extends into the monocular segments of the eyes where the image is seen in only one eye.

that it extends into the monocular segments of each retina (i.e., one end of the target can be seen only by one eye, and the other end only by the other eye). The shaded circle at the center of the target shows the fixation point. The image of the target is reversed on the retinas by the lens system. The left half of the visual target is imaged on the nasal retina of the left eye and the temporal retina of the right eye. Thus, the left visual field is seen by the left nasal retina and the right temporal retina. Similarly, the right half of the visual target is imaged on and seen by the left temporal retina and the right nasal retina.

The projections of retinal ganglion cells may be uncrossed or crossed, depending on the location of the ganglion cell (Fig. 8-10). For example, a given axon from the left retina may pass through the left optic nerve, the left side of the optic chiasm, and the left optic tract to terminate in the brain on the left side. Alternatively, an axon in the left retina may pass through the left optic nerve, cross to the opposite side in the optic chiasm, and then pass through the right optic tract to end in the right side of the brain. *Axons that remain uncrossed arise from ganglion cells in the temporal retina, whereas axons that do cross arise from ganglion cells in the nasal retina.* This arrangement results in the representation of the left field of vision in the right side of the brain and of the right field of vision in the left side of the brain (see Fig. 8-10).

The axons of retinal ganglion cells can synapse in any of several nuclei of the brain. The main pathway for vision relays in the LGN, which is one of the sensory nuclei of the thalamus. The LGN in turn projects to the **primary visual cortex** or **striate cortex** by way of the **optic radiation** (Fig. 8-10). As the optic radiation passes caudally, it fans out, and some of the fibers loop forward in the temporal lobe as **Meyer's loop.** The axons in Meyer's loop carry information derived from the lower half of the appropriate hemiretinas. Thus the axons in Meyer's loop represent the contralateral upper visual field. Axons that pass caudally through the parietal lobe in the optic radiation represent the contralateral lower visual field.

The optic radiation ends in the striate cortex, which is located dorsal and ventral to the calcarine fissure in the occipital lobe. The gyrus dorsal to the calcarine fissure is the **cuneus,** and the gyrus ventral to that fissure is the **lingual gyrus.** The cuneus receives information from the upper part

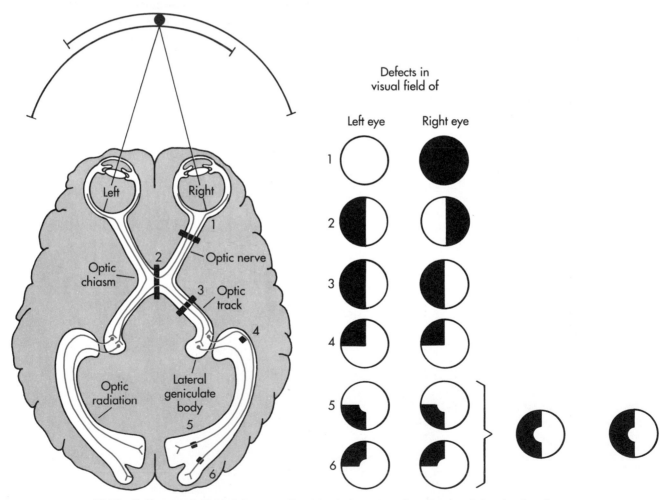

■ **Fig. 8-10**   Visual field defects produced by lesions at various levels of the visual pathway. *1,* Right optic nerve; *2,* optic chiasm; *3,* optic tract; *4,* Meyer's loop; *5,* cuneus; *6,* lingual gyrus; *bracket,* occipital lobe (with macular sparing).

of the appropriate hemiretinas, and the lingual gyrus receives information from the lower hemiretinas. Thus the cuneus represents the contralateral lower visual field, and the lingual gyrus the upper visual field.

Visual field defects

Interruption of the visual pathway at any level will cause a defect in the appropriate part of the visual field (Fig. 8-10). For example, a lesion of the retina, or interruption of the optic nerve on one side, produces either **blindness** or a **scotoma** in that eye. Damage to the optic nerve fibers as they cross in the optic chiasm results in loss of vision in both temporal fields of vision; this condition is known as **bitemporal hemianopsia.** This condition occurs because the crossing fibers originate from ganglion cells in the nasal halves of each retina. A lesion of the entire optic tract, LGN, optic radiation, or visual cortex on one side causes **homonymous hemianopsia,** which is a loss of vision in the entire contralateral visual field. Partial lesions result in partial visual field defects. For example, a lesion of Meyer's loop causes an upper **homonymous quadrantanopsia,** which is a loss of vision in the contralateral, upper visual field. A lesion of the striate cortex may not destroy all of the neurons that represent the macula, and the result is sometimes a homonymous hemianopsia with **macular sparing.**

Lateral geniculate nucleus. The lateral geniculate nucleus (LGN) is a layered structure (Fig. 8-11). The first two layers, which contain large neurons, are called the magnocellular layers. The other four layers are the parvocellular layers. There is a point-to-point projection from the retina to the LGN. The LGN thus has a retinotopic map. Cells that represent a particular retinal location are aligned along projection lines that can be drawn across the LGN (see Fig. 8-11).

The projection from one eye is distributed to three of the layers of the LGN, to one of the magnocellular layers, and to two parvocellular layers. The contralateral eye projects to layers 1, 4, and 6, whereas the ipsilateral eye projects to layers 2, 3, and 5. Another basis for the diversion of retinal input to different layers of the LGN depends on the subdivision of retinal ganglion cells into P and M cells. M cells innervate layers 1 and 2, whereas P cells supply layers 3 to 6. Furthermore, off-center P cells tend to end in layers 3 and 4 and on-center P cells tend to end in layers 5 and 6.

Each LGN neuron receives an input from only a limited number of retinal ganglion cells. Consequently, the properties of LGN neurons are very similar to those of retinal ganglion cells. For example, LGN neurons can be classified as P or M cells, and they have on-center or off-center receptive fields.

The LGN also receives input from the visual areas of the cerebral cortex, the thalamic reticular nucleus, and several nuclei of the brainstem reticular formation. The activity of LGN projection neurons is inhibited by interneurons both in the LGN and in the thalamic reticular nucleus. These cells use γ-aminobutyric acid (GABA) as their inhibitory neurotransmitter. In addition, the activity of LGN neurons is influenced by corticofugal pathways and by brainstem neurons that use monoamine transmitters. These control systems filter visual information and may be important for selective attention.

Striate cortex. The geniculostriate pathway ends chiefly in layer 4 of the striate cortex. A dense band of axons in this layer forms the **stripe of Gennari.** Axons that represent one eye or the other terminate alternately in patches known as **ocular dominance columns.** Cortical neurons in such a column respond preferentially to input from the appropriate eye. Near the border between two ocular dominance columns, neurons respond about equally to inputs from the two eyes.

Like the LGN, the striate cortex contains a retinotopic map (actually, two interlaced retinotopic maps, one for each eye). The macula is represented by a relatively large region, compared with that of the remainder of the retina. The macular representation extends forward from the occipital pole for about a third of the length of the striate cortex.

The receptive fields of neurons in the striate cortex are more complex than are those of LGN neurons. First, neurons in layer 4 receive direct input from the LGN; such neurons may be activated by stimulation of just one eye. Second, other neurons may respond to stimulation of both eyes, although the input from one eye often dominates (see above). Third, cortical neurons generally have **orientation selectivity,** i.e., they respond best when the stimulus, such as a bar or an edge, is elongated and is oriented in a particular way with respect to the horizontal position (Fig. 8-12). Because neurons in a particular zone of the cortex all tend to have the same orientation selectivity, they are considered to form an **orientation column.** Cortical neurons may also display **direction selectivity,** that is, they may respond when the stimulus is moved in one direction, but not when it is moved in the opposite direction (Fig. 8-12).

Several theories have been proposed to account for these properties of neurons in the visual cortex. One theory holds that the patterns of convergence of neurons at different serial levels of the visual pathway cause the receptive fields to become progressively more complex. **Simple cells** have on- and off-zones in their receptive fields. However, the receptive fields are rectangular and have orientation selectivity. **Complex cells** reflect the convergent input of several simple cells. Their receptive fields also have an orientation preference, but contain no distinct on- and off-zones, and many cells are particularly responsive to movement of the stimulus across the receptive field. **Hypercomplex cells** receive inputs from several complex cells, and thus have even more elaborate receptive fields.

However, this classification does not take into account the P and M cell pathways. Presumably, parallel P and M cell pathways contribute to the complexity of visual cortical organization. Cortical receptive field organization may depend on both serial and parallel processing.

Stereopsis. **Stereopsis** is defined as binocular depth perception. Such perception must be a cortical function,

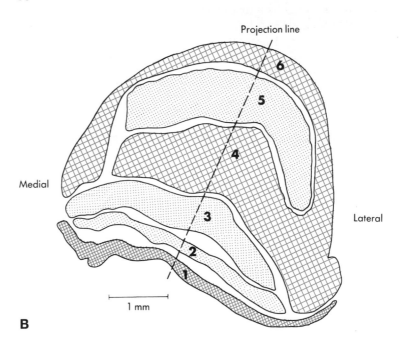

A

■ **Fig. 8-11** Section through the LGN of a human infant. **A,** A micrograph of the Nissl-stained LGN. **B,** A drawing. The layers are numbered *1* to *6*. Cross-hatching indicates the layers innervated by the contralateral eye and the dots the layers supplied by the ipsilateral eye. The projection line shows the location of cells in all the layers that map a point in the visual field. (**A** courtesy of TL Hickey and RW Guillery.)

B

because it depends on convergent inputs from the two eyes. It appears to be caused by slight differences in the retinal images formed in the two eyes. Such disparities give different perspectives that lead to visual cues about depth. Stereopsis is useful only for relatively nearby objects. Depth cues are also available when a single eye is used.

Color vision. As already discussed, color vision may depend on the presence in the retina of three different types of cones, as well as on neurons in the visual pathway that show spectral opposition. Retinal ganglion cells, LGN neurons, visual cortical neurons, and P cells display spectral opponent properties (Fig. 8-13, *A*). Other neurons, the M cells, respond to brightness, but not to spectral opposition. The spectral opponent neurons in the visual cortex are found

in cortical "pegs" or "blobs." The relationships between the ocular dominance and orientation columns and the cortical color pegs are shown in Fig. 8-13, *B*.

Superior colliculus. The **superior colliculus** of the midbrain is a layered structure. The three most superficial layers are exclusively involved in visual processing, whereas the deeper layers have multimodal inputs not only from the visual system, but also from the somatosensory and auditory systems.

Neurons in the superficial layers of the superior colliculus receive a projection from retinal ganglion cells. The axons reach the superior colliculus through the brachium of the superior colliculus. The ganglion cells include both W and M cells (but not P cells), and they are located chiefly in

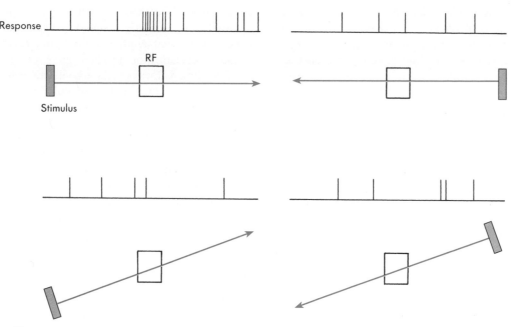

■ **Fig. 8-12** Orientation and direction selectivity. The responses of a neuron in the visual cortex are shown for stimulus oriented vertically *(upper)* or obliquely *(lower)* and moved to the right or to the left *(arrows).*

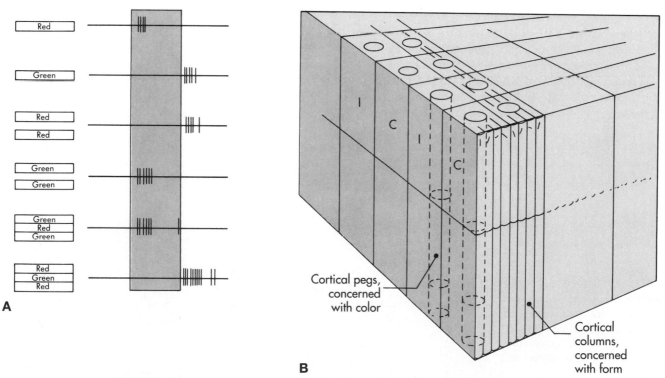

Fig. 8-13 **A,** The responses of a neuron in the striate cortex that responds to various combinations of red and green bars. The best response was to a red bar flanked by two green bars. **B,** A diagram of the columnar arrangement of the visual cortex. Ocular dominance columns are indicated by I (for ipsilateral) and C (for contralateral). Orientation columns are indicated by the short bars at various angles. The cortical pegs contain neurons like that of **A** with spectral opponent receptive fields.

the contralateral nasal retina. Neurons in the superficial layers of the superior colliculus also receive a projection from the visual cortex, including the striate cortex. The cortical loop involves neurons activated by M cells. The superficial layers of the superior colliculus, in turn, project to several thalamic nuclei (pulvinar, LGN), and they are indirectly connected to large areas of the visual cortex.

The superior colliculus contains a retinotopic map. Collicular neurons are particularly sensitive to rapid stimulus motion in a particular direction. Most of the cells have binocular inputs, but they lack orientation selectivity.

Studies on cats demonstrate that the superior colliculus plays an important role in visual perception. Bilateral destruction of the striate cortex of cats impairs visual performance only slightly; some visual acuity is lost. The superior colliculus in cats may be particularly important for determining the location of objects in visual space. How important "collicular vision" is in humans is unclear.

The deep layers of the superior colliculus receive connections from somatosensory and auditory pathways, as well as visual input from the superficial layers. Thus the deep layers of the superior colliculus contain somatotopic and retinotopic maps, as well as a map of sound in space. Corresponding parts of these maps are overlaid. For example, an area that receives information about the contralateral visual field will also receive information about sounds that originate from the contralateral auditory space, and they receive information about somatic stimuli applied to the contralateral surface of the body. In addition, the deep layers of the superior colliculus contain a motor map that controls eye and head position. For instance, activation of neurons in the superior colliculus by a visual target causes movement of the eyes to center the visual target on the fovea. In this way, the superior colliculus is involved in reflex responses to

the sudden appearance of a novel or threatening object in the visual field. Similarly, a sound or a sudden contact with the body will elicit appropriate eye and head movements to enable visualization of the source of the stimulus. The descending pathways include connections to the oculomotor control system through tectoreticular connections and to the spinal cord through the tectospinal tract.

Extrastriate Visual Cortex

In animal studies, at least 25 different visual areas have been identified in the cerebral and striate cortex. The extrastriate areas include several different parallel visual processing pathways. The P pathway originates with P cells and functions in the recognition of form and color. Some of the cortical structures in the P pathway include layer 4Cβ of the striate cortex, area V4, and several areas in the inferotemporal region (Fig. 8-14). The processing of form includes recognition of complex visual patterns, such as faces. Color information is processed separately from form. The M pathway originates with M cells and functions in motion detection and in the control of eye movements. Cortical structures in the M pathway include layers 4B and 4Cα of the striate cortex, and areas MT (middle temporal) and MST (middle superior temporal) on the lateral aspect of the temporal lobe, as well as area 7a of the parietal lobe (Fig. 8-14). Both P and M pathways contribute to depth perception.

> Lesions of the extrastriate visual cortex can produce various deficits. Bilateral lesions of the inferotemporal cortex can result in cortical color blindness (**achromatopsia**) or in the inability to recognize faces, even of close members of the family (**prosopagnosia**). A lesion of area MT or MST can interfere with motion detection and with eye movements.

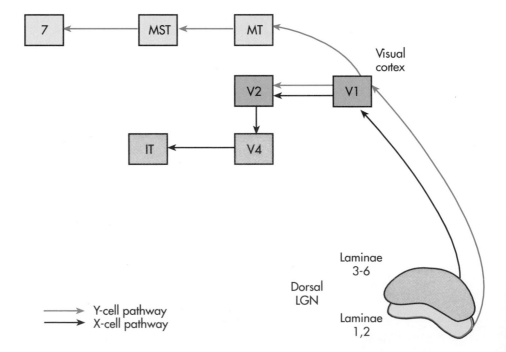

■ **Fig. 8-14** Separation of X and Y cell influences on different areas of visual cortex. *MT*, Medial temporal; *MST*, medial superior temporal; *V1*, striate cortex; *V2, V4,* higher order visual areas; *IT*, inferotemporal area.

Other Visual Pathways

The visual pathways include connections to nuclei that serve functions other than vision. For example, a retinal projection to the **suprachiasmatic nucleus** of the hypothalamus controls circadian rythmicity.

Another retinal projection is to the **pretectum.** This pathway activates parasympathetic preganglionic neurons in the **Edinger-Westphal nucleus,** which in turn causes pupillary constriction in the pupillary light reflex. The pretectal areas are interconnected through the posterior commissure, and thus the reflex causes both ipsilateral (direct) and contralateral (consensual) pupillary constriction.

THE AUDITORY AND VESTIBULAR SYSTEMS

The peripheral parts of the auditory and vestibular systems share components of the bony and membranous labyrinths, use hair cells as mechanical transducers, and transmit information to the central nervous system (CNS) through the eighth cranial nerve. However, the CNS processing and sensory functions of the auditory and vestibular systems are distinct. The function of the auditory system is to transduce sound. This allows us to recognize environmental cues and to communicate with other organisms. The most complex auditory functions are those involved in language. The function of the vestibular system is to provide the CNS with information related to the position and movements of the head in space. The control of eye movements by the vestibular system is discussed in Chapter 9.

Audition

Sound. Sound is produced by compression and decompression waves that are transmitted in air or in other elastic media, such as water. Sound propagates at about 335 m/sec in air. The waves are associated with certain pressure changes, called sound pressure. The unit of sound pressure is N/m², but sound pressure is more commonly expressed as the **sound pressure level (SPL).** The unit of SPL is the **decibel (dB):**

$$SPL = 20 \log P/P_R$$

where P is the sound pressure and P_R is a reference pressure (either 0.0002 dyne/cm², the absolute threshold for human hearing, or 1 dyne/cm²).

Sound frequency is measured in cycles per second, or **Hertz (Hz).** Sound, however, is actually a mixture of pure tones. Each pure tone results from a sinusoidal wave at a particular frequency, and each pure tone is characterized not only by its frequency, but also by its amplitude and phase (Fig. 8-15). Thus, because most sounds are complex mixtures of pure tones, the composition of a particular sound can be broken down into a set of pure tones. Fourier analysis does this breakdown. Conversely, Fourier synthesis permits the construction of a sound by mixing pure tones. **Noise** is sound composed of many unrelated frequencies, and **white noise** is a mixture of all audible frequencies.

The normal human ear is sensitive to pure tones with frequencies that range between about 20 and 20,000 Hz. The threshold for detection of a pure tone varies with its frequency (Fig. 8-16). The lowest thresholds for human hearing are for pure tones of about 1000 to 3000 Hz. By definition, threshold at these frequencies is approximately 0 dB (reference pressure, 0.0002 dynes/cm²). A sound with intensity 10 times greater would be 20 dB; one 100 times greater would be 40 dB.

According to the scale, speech has an intensity of about 65 dB. The main frequencies used in speech fall in the range of 300 to 3500 Hz. Sounds that exceed 100 dB can damage the peripheral auditory apparatus, and those over 120 dB can cause pain. As people age, their ability to hear high frequencies declines, a condition called **presbycusis.**

The ear. The peripheral auditory apparatus is the ear, which can be subdivided into the external ear, the middle ear, and the inner ear (Fig. 8-17).

External ear. The external ear includes the pinna, the external auditory meatus, and the auditory canal. The auditory canal contains glands that secrete **cerumen,** a waxy protective substance. The pinna may help direct sounds into

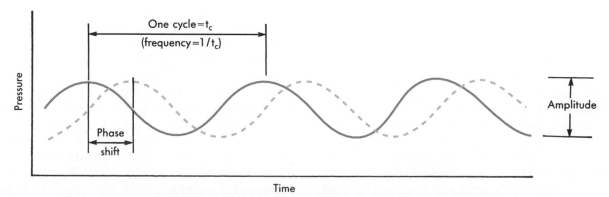

■ **Fig. 8-15** Two pure tones are shown by the solid and dashed lines. Frequency is determined from the wavelength as indicated. Amplitude is the peak-to-peak change in sound pressure. Both of the tones have the same frequency and amplitude but differ in phase.

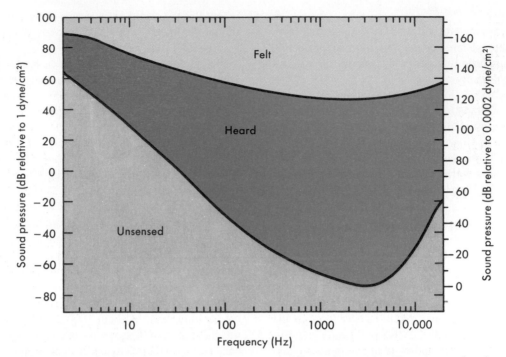

■ **Fig. 8-16** Sound intensities required for hearing at different frequencies. The gray area is subthreshold for hearing. The dark area is the normal range for audition. The light-colored area is the range at which sound is painful.

the auditory canal, at least in animals. The auditory canal transmits sound waves to the tympanic membrane. In humans the auditory canal has a resonant frequency of about 3500 Hz and it limits the frequencies that reach the tympanic membrane.

Middle ear. The external ear is separated from the middle ear by the **tympanic membrane** (Fig. 8-17, *A*). The middle ear contains air. A chain of ossicles connects the tympanic membrane to the oval window, an opening into the inner ear. Adjacent to the oval window is the round window, another membrane-covered opening between the middle and inner ears (Fig. 8-17, *A, B*).

The ossicles include the **malleus,** the **incus,** and the **stapes.** The stapes has a footplate that inserts into the oval window. Beneath the oval window is a fluid-filled component of the **cochlea.** This component is called the **vestibule,** it is continuous with a tubular structure, known as the **scala vestibuli.** Inward movement of the tympanic membrane by a sound pressure wave causes the chain of ossicles to push the footplate of the stapes into the oval window (see Fig. 8-17, *B*). This movement of the stapes footplate in turn displaces the fluid within the scala vestibuli. The pressure wave that ensues within the fluid is transmitted through the **basilar membrane** of the cochlea to the **scala tympani** (see below), and it causes the round window to bulge into the middle ear.

The tympanic membrane and the chain of ossicles serve as an impedance matching device. The ear must detect sound waves traveling in air, but the neural transduction mechanism depends on movements established in the fluid column within the cochlea. Thus, pressure waves in air must be converted into pressure waves in fluid. The acoustic impedance of water is much higher than that of air. Therefore, without a special device for impedance matching, most sound reaching the ear would simply be reflected. Impedance matching in the ear depends on (1) the ratio of the surface area of the tympanic membrane to that of the oval window, and (2) the mechanical advantage of the lever system formed by the ossicle chain. The efficiency of the impedance match is sufficient to improve hearing by 10 to 20 dB.

The middle ear also serves other functions. Two muscles are found in the middle ear: the **tensor tympani** (supplied by the trigeminal nerve) and the **stapedius** (supplied by the facial nerve). These muscles attach, respectively, to the malleus and stapes. When they contract, they dampen movements of the ossicular chain and so decrease the sensitivity of the acoustic apparatus. This action can protect the acoustic apparatus against damaging sounds that can be anticipated. However, a sudden explosion can still damage the acoustic apparatus, because reflex contraction of the middle ear muscles does not occur quickly enough. The middle ear connects to the pharynx through the **eustachian tube.** Pressure differences between the external and middle ears can be equalized through this passage. If fluid collects in the middle ear, such as during an infection, the eustachian tube may become blocked. The resulting pressure difference between the external and middle ears can produce pain by displacement of the

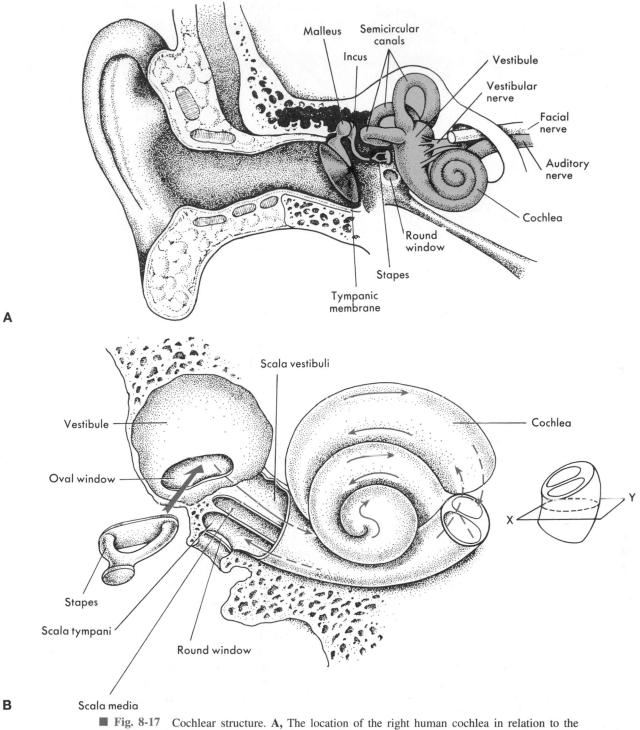

A

B

■ **Fig. 8-17** Cochlear structure. **A,** The location of the right human cochlea in relation to the vestibular apparatus and middle and external ears. **B,** The relationships between the spaces within the cochlea.   *Continued*

tympanic membrane, and, in extreme cases, by rupture of the tympanic membrane. Flying and diving can also cause pressure differences.

Inner ear. The inner ear includes the bony and membranous labyrinths. The cochlea and the vestibular apparatus are formed from these structures.

The cochlea is a spiral-shaped organ (Fig. 8-17, *A, B*). In humans, the spiral consists of $2^3/_4$ turns; it starts from a broad base and extends to a narrow apex. The cochlea forms from the rostral end of the bony and membranous labyrinths. The apex of the cochlea faces laterally (Fig. 8-17, *A*).

The bony labyrinth component of the cochlea includes several chambers. The vestibule is the space facing the oval

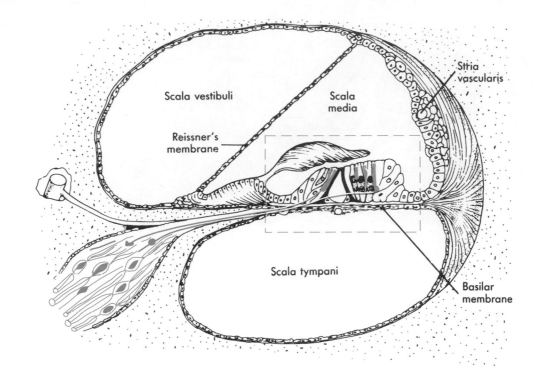

C

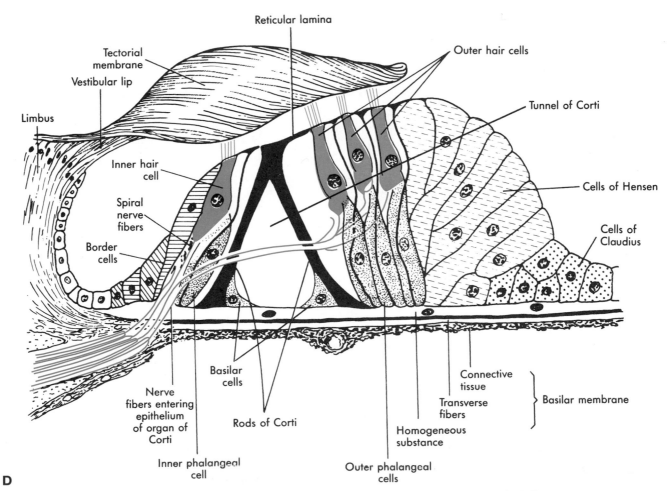

D

■ **Fig. 8-17, cont'd** **C,** A drawing of a cross-section through the cochlea in the plane indicated by the inset to the right of **B. D,** An expanded view of the organ of Corti. (**B** Redrawn from Gulick WL: Hearing: *physiology and psychophysics,* New York, 1971, Oxford University Press; after Maloney.)

window (Fig. 8-17, *B*). Continuous with the vestibule is the scala vestibuli, a spiral-shaped tube that extends to the apex of the cochlea. The scala vestibuli meets the scala tympani at the apex; they merge at the **helicotrema,** the connection between these two components of the bony labyrinth. The scala tympani is another spiral-shaped tube that winds back down the cochlea to end at the round window (Fig. 8-17, *B*). The bony core of the cochlea around which the scalae turn is the **modiolus.**

The membranous labyrinth component of the cochlea is the **scala media,** or **cochlear duct** (Fig. 8-17, *B, C*). The cochlear duct is a membrane-bound spiral tube that extends 35 mm along the cochlea, between the scala vestibuli and scala tympani. One wall of the scala media is formed by the **basilar membrane,** another by **Reissner's membrane,** and the third by the **stria vascularis** (Fig. 8-17, *C*).

The spaces within the cochlea are filled with fluid. The fluid in the scala vestibuli and scala tympani is **perilymph,** which closely resembles cerebrospinal fluid (CSF). The fluid in the scala media is **endolymph,** which is very different from perilymph. Endolymph contains a high concentration of K$^+$ (about 145 mM) and a low concentration of Na$^+$ (about 2 mM); in this respect, it resembles intracellular fluid. Because endolymph has a positive potential (about +80 mV), a large potential gradient (about 140 mV) exists across the membranes of the hair cells found within the cochlea. (These hair cells, which are sensory receptors for sound, are discussed in more detail below.) Endolymph is secreted by the stria vascularis and is drained through the endolymphatic duct into the dural venous sinuses.

The neural apparatus responsible for transduction of sound is the **organ of Corti** (Fig. 8-17, *C, D*), which is located within the cochlear duct. It lies on the basilar membrane and consists of several components, including three rows of **outer hair cells,** a single row of **inner hair cells,** a gelatinous **tectorial membrane,** and a number of types of supporting cells. The organ of Corti in humans contains 15,000 outer and 3500 inner hair cells. The **rods of Corti** and the **reticular lamina** provide a rigid scaffold. Located at the apex of the hair cells are stereocilia, which can be described as non-motile cilia. The stereocilia contact the tectorial membrane.

The organ of Corti is innervated by nerve fibers that belong to the cochlear division of the eighth cranial nerve. The 32,000 auditory afferent fibers in humans originate in sensory ganglion cells in the **spiral ganglion,** which is located within the modiolus. These nerve fibers penetrate the organ of Corti, and they terminate at the base of the hair cells (Fig. 8-17, *C, D*). Those going to the outer hair cells pass through the **tunnel of Corti,** an opening below the rods of Corti.

About 90% of the fibers end on inner hair cells, and the remainder end on outer hair cells. Thus, in this arrangement several afferent fibers converge on each inner hair cell, whereas other afferent fibers diverge to supply many outer hair cells. In addition to afferent fibers, the organ of Corti is supplied by cochlear efferent fibers, which terminate on the outer hair cells and on the afferent fibers that contact the inner hair cells. The cochlear efferent fibers originate in the superior olivary nucleus of the brainstem, and they are often called **olivocochlear fibers.** The efferent fibers that end on cochlear afferent fibers may be inhibitory, and they may help to improve frequency discrimination.

The inner hair cells clearly provide most of the neural information about acoustic signals that the CNS uses for hearing. The function of the outer hair cells is less clear. The length of the outer hair cells varies; this characteristic suggests that changes in outer hair cell length may affect the sensitivity, or "tuning," of the inner hair cells. Cochlear efferent fibers may control outer hair cell length. Such a mechanism could conceivably influence the way the brain recognizes sound.

A common cause of deafness is the destruction of hair cells by loud sounds. Hair cells can be destroyed, for example, by exposure to industrial noise, or by listening to high-intensity rock music. Typically, hair cells in certain parts of the cochlea are selectively damaged, and thus hearing may be lost over a discrete frequency range. Such a selective hearing loss can be diagnosed by **audiometry** (see below).

Sound transduction. Sound waves are transduced by the organ of Corti. Sound waves that reach the ear cause the tympanic membrane to oscillate. These oscillations result in fluid movements within the scala vestibuli and scala tympani (see Fig. 8-17). Part of the hydraulic energy of these fluid movements is used to displace the basilar membrane and, with it, the organ of Corti (Fig. 8-18). Owing to the shear forces set up by the relative displacements of the basilar membrane and the tectorial membrane, the stereocilia of the hair cells bend. When the stereocilia of a hair cell move toward the tallest cilium, the hair cell is depolarized; when the stereocilia bend in the opposite direction, the hair cell is hyperpolarized.

These changes in membrane potential of the hair cells result from changes in cation conductance in membranes at the apical ends of the hair cells. The potential gradient that affects ion movement into the hair cells includes both the resting potential of the hair cells and the positive potential of the endolymph. As noted previously, the total gradient across the membrane of the hair cells is about 140 mV. *Therefore, a change in membrane conductance in the apical membranes of the hair cells results in a large current flow, which produces the receptor potential in these cells. This current flow can be recorded extracellularly as the **cochlear microphonic potential,** an oscillatory event that has the same frequency as the acoustic stimulus. The cochlear microphonic potential represents the sum of the receptor potentials of a number of hair cells.*

Hair cells, like retinal photoreceptors, release an excitatory neurotransmitter (probably glutamate or aspartate) when depolarized. The transmitter produces a generator potential, which excites the cochlear afferent nerve fibers with which the hair cell synapses. In summary, sound is transduced

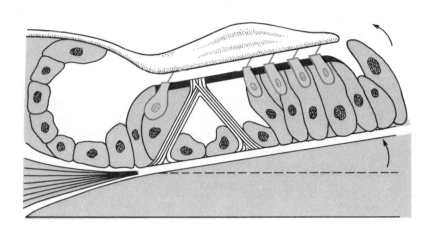

Reticular lamina

Tectorial membrane

Basilar membrane

Rods of Corti

Hair cells

■ **Fig. 8-18**   A demonstration of how a movement of the basilar membrane will cause the stereocilia to bend because of shear forces produced by the relative displacement of the hair cells and the tectorial membrane.

when oscillatory movements of the basilar membrane cause intermittent discharges of cochlear afferent nerve fibers. The activity of a large number of cochlear afferent fibers can be recorded extracellularly as a compound action potential.

However, most cochlear afferent fibers do *not* discharge in response to a particular sound frequency. One factor that influences which afferent fiber discharges is location along the organ of Corti. The location of an afferent fiber is important, because a given sound frequency causes different displacements of the basilar membrane at different locations along the organ of Corti (Fig. 8-19). The location varies because the width and tension along the basilar membrane vary with distance from the base.

On the basis of these differences in width and tension, investigators concluded originally that different parts of the basilar membrane have different resonance frequencies. For example, the basilar membrane is about 100 μm wide at the base and 500 μm wide at the apex. It also has a higher tension at the base. Thus, the base was predicted to vibrate at higher frequencies than the apex, as do the shorter strings of musical instruments. However, experiments have shown that the basilar membrane moves as a whole in traveling waves (see Fig. 8-19). Movements of the basilar membrane are maximal nearer the base of the cochlea during high-frequency tones and maximal nearer the apex during low-frequency tones.

In effect, the basilar membrane serves as a frequency analyzer; it distributes the stimulus along the organ of Corti so that different hair cells will respond to different frequencies of sound. This is the basis of the place theory of hearing. In addition, hair cells located at different places along the organ of Corti are tuned to different frequencies, because of differences in their stereocilia and in their biophysical properties. Because of these factors, the basilar membrane and organ of Corti have a so-called tonotopic map (Fig. 8-20).

Cochlear nerve fibers.   The activity of hair cells in the organ of Corti causes the primary afferent fibers of the cochlear nerve to discharge. The cell bodies of these nerve fibers are in the spiral ganglion; the peripheral processes end on hair cells, and the central processes terminate in the cochlear nuclei of the brainstem. Unlike most other primary afferent neurons, those of the eighth cranial nerve are bipolar cells, with a myelin sheath around the cell bodies as well as around the axons.

Characteristic frequencies.   A cochlear afferent fiber discharges maximally when stimulated by a particular sound frequency, called the **characteristic frequency** of that fiber. The characteristic frequency can be determined from a tuning curve for the fiber (Fig. 8-21). A **tuning curve** plots the threshold for activation of the nerve fiber by different sound frequencies. Typically, tuning curves are sharp near threshold, but they are broad at high sound pressure levels. Both

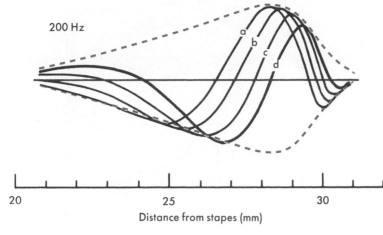

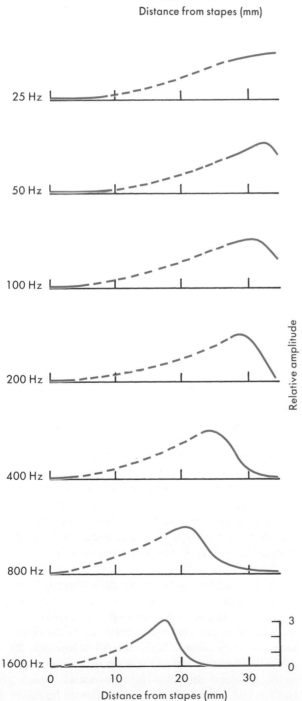

■ **Fig. 8-19** Different frequencies of sound result in different amplitudes of displacement of the basilar membrane at different sites along the organ of Corti. **A,** A traveling wave produced in the basilar membrane by a sound of 200 Hz. The curves at *a, b, c,* and *d* represent the displacements of the basilar membrane at different times, and the dashed line is the envelope formed by the peaks of the wave at different times. The maximum deflection occurs at about 29 mm from the oval window. **B,** The envelopes of traveling waves produced by several frequencies of sound. Note that the maximum displacement varies with frequency and is closest to the oval window when the frequency is highest. (Redrawn from von Bekesy G: *Experiments in hearing,* New York, 1960, McGraw-Hill.)

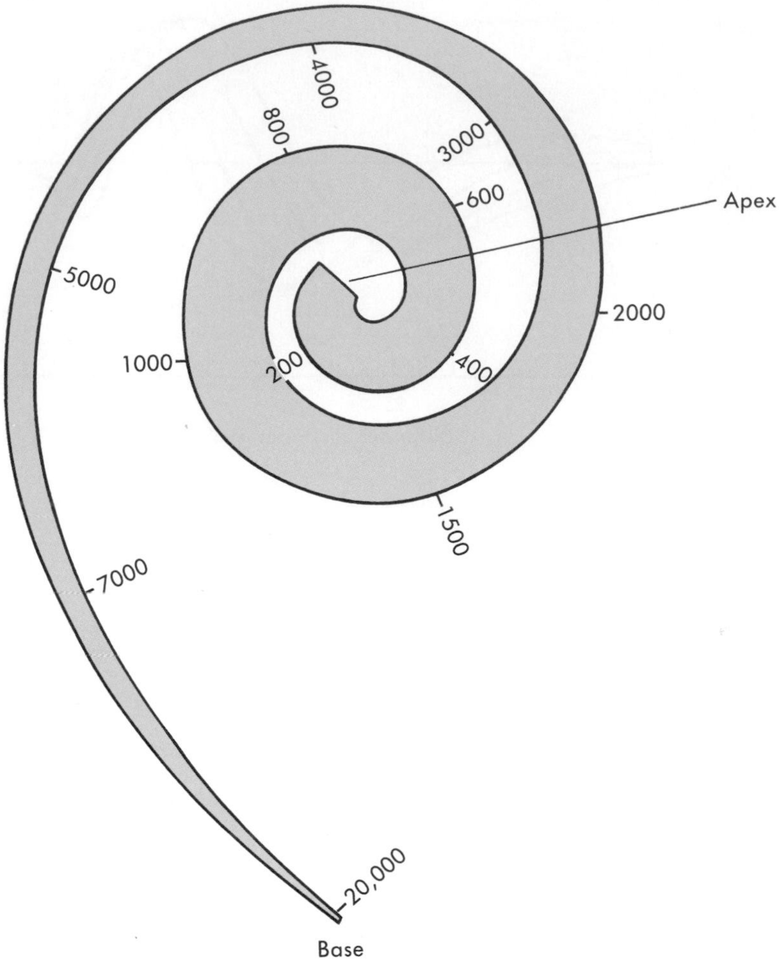

■ **Fig. 8-20**   Layout of the tonotopic map of the cochlea. (Redrawn from Stuhlman O: *An introduction to biophysics,* New York, 1943, John Wiley & Sons.)

excitatory and inhibitory areas can be included in a tuning curve (Fig. 8-21, *A*). The sharpness of some tuning curves may reflect inhibitory processes.

Encoding. The different features of an acoustic stimulus are encoded in the discharges of cochlear nerve fibers. Duration is signaled by the duration of activity; intensity is signaled both by the amount of neural activity and by the number of fibers that discharge. For low-frequency sounds (up to 4000 Hz), the frequency is signaled by the tendency of an afferent fiber to discharge in phase with the stimulus **(phase locking).** Phase locking can occur for sounds with periods shorter than the absolutely refractory period, which limits neural discharges to rates lower than about 500 Hz. Therefore, if the tone is more than 500 Hz, a given fiber cannot discharge during each cycle.

Frequency information can be detected by the CNS, however, from the activity of a population of afferent fibers, each of which discharges in phase with the stimulus. This observation forms the **frequency theory** of hearing. For high-frequency sounds the place theory applies. The CNS interprets sounds that activate afferent fibers that supply hair cells near the base of the cochlea as being of high frequency. Thus, both the place and the frequency theories are required to explain the frequency coding of sound **(duplex theory).**

An important, although relatively uncommon, condition that can interrupt the function of cochlear nerve fibers is an **acoustic neurinoma,** a tumor of the Schwann cells of the eighth nerve. As the tumor grows, irritation of cochlear nerve fibers may cause a ringing sound in the affected ear **(tinnitus).** Eventually, conduction in cochlear nerve fibers is blocked, and the ear becomes deaf. The tumor may be operable while still small; therefore, early diagnosis is important. If the tumor is allowed to enlarge substantially, it could not only interrupt the entire eighth nerve and cause vestibular as well as auditory difficulties, but it could also impinge on or distort neighboring cranial nerves (e.g., V, VII, IX, and X) and it could also produce cerebellar signs by compressing the cerebellar peduncles.

Central auditory pathway.   Cochlear afferent fibers synapse on neurons of the dorsal and ventral cochlear nuclei. These neurons give rise to axons that contribute to the central auditory pathway. Some of the axons cross to the contralateral side, and they ascend in the **lateral lemniscus,** the main ascending auditory tract. Others connect with the ipsilateral or contralateral **superior olivary nuclei,** which project through the ipsilateral and contralateral lemnisci. Each

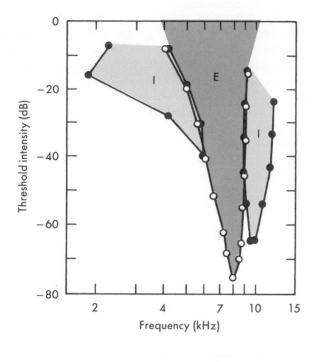

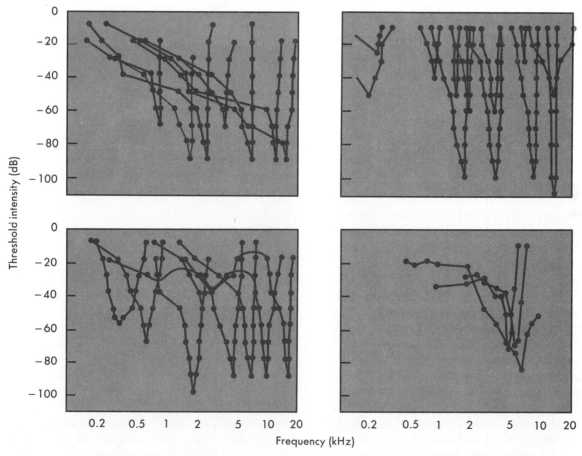

■ **Fig. 8-21**   Tuning curves of neurons in the auditory system. Tuning curves can be considered as receptive field plots. **A,** A tuning curve with excitatory *(E)* and inhibitory *(I)* regions. **B,** Tuning curves for cochlear nerve fibers *(upper left),* neurons in the inferior colliculus *(upper right),* trapezoid body *(lower left),* and medial geniculate nucleus *(lower right).* (**A** Redrawn from Arthur RM et al: *J Physiol [Lond]* 212:593, 1971; **B** Redrawn from Katsui Y: In Rosenblith WA, editor: *Sensory communication,* Cambridge, Mass., 1961, MIT Press.)

lateral lemniscus ends in an **inferior colliculus.** Neurons of the inferior colliculus project to the **medial geniculate nucleus** of the thalamus, which gives rise to the auditory radiation. The auditory radiation ends in the **auditory cortex,** which is located in the transverse temporal gyri in the temporal lobe.

A mixture of ascending auditory system fibers represents both ears at the level of the lateral lemniscus. Thus, the representation of auditory space is complex, even at the brainstem level. Consequently, **unilateral deafness** may occur with isolated lesions of the cochlear nuclei or of more peripheral structures. Central lesions do not cause unilateral deafness, although they may interfere with **sound localization** or **discrimination of tones.**

Functional organization of the central auditory system

Receptive fields and tonotopic maps. The responses of neurons in several structures that belong to the auditory system can be described by **tuning curves** (Fig. 8-21, *B*). By plotting the distribution of the **characteristic frequencies** of neurons within a nucleus or in the auditory cortex, a **tonotopic map** may be revealed. Tonotopic maps have been found in the cochlear nuclei, superior olivary complex, inferior colliculus, medial geniculate nucleus, and auditory cortex. A given auditory structure may, in fact, contain several tonotopic maps.

Binaural interactions. Most auditory neurons at levels above the cochlear nuclei respond to stimulation of either ear, (i.e., they have **binaural receptive fields**). Binaural receptive fields contribute to sound localization. A human can distinguish sounds originating from sources separated by as little as 1 degree. *The auditory system uses certain clues to judge the origin of sounds. These clues include differences in the time (or phase) of sound arrival at the two ears and differences in sound intensity on the two sides of the head.*

These factors provide information about the location of a sound by influencing the activity of neurons in the superior olivary complex. For example, neurons in the medial superior olivary nucleus have medial and lateral dendrites. The synapses on the medial dendrites are largely excitatory, and they originate from the contralateral ventral cochlear nucleus. Those on the lateral dendrites are mostly inhibitory and come from the ipsilateral ventral cochlear nucleus. Differences in the phase of the sound reaching the two ears affect the strength and timing of the excitation and inhibition reaching a particular medial olivary neuron. The activity of that neuron can then provide information about sound localization. The lateral superior olivary nucleus uses differences in the sound intensity that reaches the two ears to provide information about the source of the sound.

Cortical organization. Several features of the primary auditory cortex resemble those of other primary sensory-receiving areas. Not only are sensory maps, in this case tonotopic maps, present in the auditory cortex, but this cor-

tical region also performs feature extractions. For example, some neurons are selective for the direction of frequency modulation. Neurons in the primary auditory cortex form **isofrequency columns** (in which the neurons in the column have the same characteristic frequency), and they also form alternating columns, known as summation and suppression columns. Neurons in **summation columns** are more responsive to binaural than to monaural input. Neurons in **suppression columns** are less responsive to binaural than to monaural stimulation, and accordingly the response to one ear is dominant.

Bilateral lesions of the auditory cortex have little effect on the ability to distinguish the frequencies or intensity of different sounds, but the ability to localize sound and to understand speech is reduced. Unilateral lesions, however, have little effect, especially if the nondominant (for language) hemisphere is involved. Evidently, frequency discrimination depends on the activity at lower levels of the auditory pathway, presumably the inferior colliculus.

As already discussed, unilateral deafness is caused by damage to the peripheral auditory apparatus or to the cochlear nuclei, but not by CNS lesions. A discrete loss of hearing for particular frequencies can result from damage to a part of the organ of Corti (e.g., by exposure to intense sound, such as particularly loud rock music or industrial noise). The degree of deafness can be quantified for different frequencies by **audiometry.** In audiometry, each ear is presented with tones of different frequencies and intensities. An **audiogram** is plotted to show the thresholds of each ear for representative frequencies of sound. Comparison with the audiogram of normal individuals shows the auditory deficit (in decibels). The pattern of deficit aids in the diagnosis of the cause of the hearing loss.

Two simple tests are often used clinically to distinguish the most important types of deafness, *conduction loss and sensorineural loss.* The **Weber test** is used to evaluate the magnitude of a conduction hearing loss. In this test, the base of a vibrating tuning fork is placed against the middle of the forehead and the subject is asked to localize the sound. Normally the sound is not localized to a particular ear. However, if the person has a conductive hearing loss (e.g., because of a punctured tympanic membrane, fluid in the middle ear, otosclerosis, or loss of continuity of the ossicular chain), the sound is localized to the deaf ear because the sound is conducted to the cochlea through bone. Bone-conducted sound can activate the organ of Corti, although not as well as sound conducted normally through the tympanic membrane and ossicle chain. One reason why the sound in the Weber test is not localized to the normal ear may be that hearing in the normal ear is inhibited by the ambient sound level (**auditory masking**).

In the Weber test the localization of sound to the ear deafened by a loss of the normal conduction mechanism can easily be demonstrated in normal subjects, who are asked to place a finger in one ear to impair hearing in that ear. Conversely, in subjects with a sensorineural hearing loss (e.g., because of damage to the organ of Corti, the cochlear nerve, or the cochlear nuclei), the sound is localized to the normal side. In the Rinne test, a vibrating tuning fork is placed against the mastoid process, and the subject is asked to indicate when the sound dies out. The tuning fork is then held near the external auditory meatus. In normal subjects the sound is again heard. If the conduction mechanism is damaged, the sound is not heard. Bone conduction in this case is better than air conduction. If the hearing loss is sensorineural, the sound is heard again.

The Vestibular System

The vestibular system detects angular and linear accelerations of the head. Signals from the vestibular system trigger head and eye movements to provide the retina with a stable visual image and to allow the body to make adjustments in posture in order to maintain balance. The following description of the vestibular system emphasizes the sensory aspects of vestibular function, and it introduces the central vestibular pathways. The role of the vestibular apparatus in motor control is discussed in Chapter 9.

The vestibular apparatus

Structure of the vestibular labyrinth. The vestibular apparatus, like the cochlea, consists of a component of the mem-

branous labyrinth located within the bony labyrinth (Fig. 8-22). The vestibular apparatus on each side is composed of three **semicircular ducts** and two **otolith organs.** These structures are surrounded by **perilymph** and contain **endolymph.** The semicircular ducts include the **horizontal, superior,** and **posterior ducts.** The otolith organs include the **utricle** and the **saccule.** A swelling, called an **ampulla,** is found on each semicircular duct. The semicircular ducts all connect with the utricle. The utricle joins the saccule through the **ductus reuniens.** The **endolymphatic duct** originates from the **ductus reuniens,** and it ends in the **endolymphatic sac.** The saccule connects with the cochlea, through which endolymph (produced by the stria vascularis of the cochlea) can reach the vestibular apparatus.

The three semicircular ducts on one side are matched with corresponding coplanar semicircular ducts on the other side. This arrangement allows the sensory epithelia, in corresponding pairs of ducts on the two sides, to sense movements of the head in all planes. The horizontal ducts on each side of the head correspond, as do the superior duct on one side and the posterior duct on the other side. An important feature of the horizontal ducts is that they are placed in the horizontal plane with respect to the horizon, if the head is first tilted down 30 degrees. The utricle is oriented nearly horizontally; the saccule is oriented vertically.

The ampulla of each of the semicircular ducts contains a sensory epithelium. The sensory epithelium in a semicircular duct is called a **crista ampullaris** or **ampullary crest** (Fig. 8-23). An ampullary crest consists of a ridge that is covered by an epithelium in which vestibular hair cells are

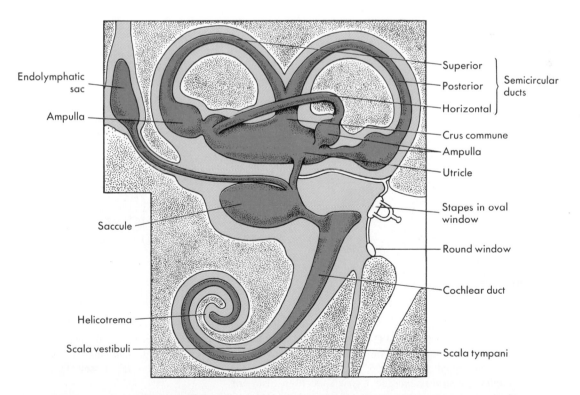

■ Fig. 8-22   Vestibular apparatus. (Redrawn from Kandel ER, Schwartz JH: *Principles of neural science,* New York, 1981, Elsevier.)

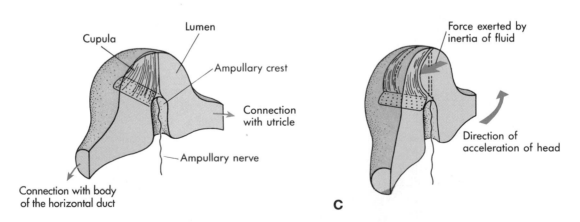

Cupula

Receptor cells

Supporting cells

A

Cupula

Lumen

Ampullary crest

Connection with utricle

Ampullary nerve

Connection with body of the horizontal duct

B

Force exerted by inertia of fluid

Direction of acceleration of head

C

■ **Fig. 8-23** **A,** Drawing of an ampullary crest. The stereocilia and the kinocilium of each hair cell extend into the cupula. **B** and **C** show the distortion of the cupula that is produced when the head is rotated; **B** is before and **C** is during head rotation. (**A** Redrawn from Wersäll J. *Acta Otolaryngol [Stockholm]* suppl 162:1, 1956; **B, C** Redrawn from Kandel ER, Schwartz JH, Jessell TM: *Principles of neural science,* ed 3, New York, 1991, Elsevier.)

embedded. These hair cells are innervated by primary afferent fibers of the vestibular nerve, which is a subdivision of the eighth cranial nerve.

Like cochlear hair cells, each vestibular hair cell contains a set of stereocilia on its apical surface. However, unlike cochlear hair cells, vestibular hair cells also contain a single **kinocilium.** The cilia on ampullary hair cells are embedded in a gelatinous structure, called the **cupula.** The cupula crosses the ampulla and occludes its lumen completely. Movements of endolymph, produced by angular accelerations of the head, deflect the cupula and consequently bend the cilia on the hair cells. The cupula has the same specific gravity as the endolymph, and so it is unaffected by linear acceleratory forces, such as that exerted by gravity.

The sensory epithelia of the otolith organs are called the **macula utriculi** and the **macula sacculi** (Fig. 8-24). Vestibular hair cells are embedded in the epithelium that overlies each macula. As in the ampullary crests, the stereocilia and kinocilia of the macula project into a gelatinous mass. However, the gelatinous mass in the macula contains numerous otoliths ("ear stones"), whilch are composed of calcium carbonate crystals. Together, the gelatinous mass and its otoliths are known as an **otolithic membrane.** The otoliths increase the specific gravity of the otolithic membrane to about twice that of thc cndolymph. Hence, the otolithic membrane tends to move when it is affected by a linear acceleration, such as that produced by gravity. Angular accelerations of the head do not affect the otolithic membranes, which do not protrude substantially into the lumen of the membranous labyrinth.

Innervation of sensory epithelia of vestibular apparatus. The cell bodies of the primary afferent fibers of the vestibular nerve are located in Scarpa's ganglion. The neurons are bipolar, and their cell bodies, as well as axons, are myelinated. The vestibular nerve gives off separate branches to each of the sensory epithelia. The vestibular nerve is accompanied by the cochlear and facial nerves in the internal auditory meatus of the skull.

Vestibular transduction. Like cochlear hair cells, vestibular hair cells are functionally polarized. When the stereocilia are bent toward the longest cilium (in this case, the kinocilium), the conductance of the apical membrane increases for cations and the vestibular hair cell is depolarized (Fig. 8-25). Conversely, when the cilia are bent away from the kinocilium, the hair cell is hyperpolarized. The hair cell releases an excitatory neurotransmitter (either glutamate or aspartate) tonically, so that the afferent fiber on which it synapses has a resting discharge. When the hair cell is depolarized, more transmitter is released, and the discharge rate of the afferent fiber increases. Conversely, when the hair cell is hyperpolarized, less transmitter is released, and the firing rate of the afferent fiber slows or stops.

Semicircular ducts. Angular accelerations of the head produce movements of the endolymph in relation to the head (Figs. 8-23, *B,* 8-26). This happens because the inertia of the endolymph causes it to shift in relation to the fixed wall of the membranous labyrinth. This shift distorts the cupula and causes the cilia to bend. Consequently, the cilia on the hair

cells of the ampullary crests of the semicircular ducts move, and the discharge rates of the vestibular afferent fibers change. All of the cilia in a given ampullary crest are oriented in the same direction. In the horizontal duct, the cilia are oriented toward the utricle, and in the other ampullae they are oriented away from the utricle.

The way in which an angular acceleration of the head affects the discharges of vestibular afferent fibers can be exemplified by the activity that originates from the horizontal ducts. Figure 8-26 shows the horizontal ducts and utricle, as seen from above. The hair cells in these ducts are polarized toward the utricle. Thus, movement of the cilia toward the utricle increases the discharge rates of the afferent fibers that supply the macula utriculi on that side. Conversely, movements of the cilia away from the utricle reduce the discharge rate of the other macula utriculi. In Fig. 8-26, the head is rotated to the left. This left-directed rotation causes the endolymph in the horizontal ducts to shift relatively toward the right. This movement of endolymph bends the cilia on the hair cells of the ampulla of the left horizontal duct toward the utricle, and it bends those cilia of the right duct away from the utricle. These effects on the cilia increase the firing rate in the afferent fibers of the horizontal duct on the left and they decrease the firing rate of the afferent fibers on the right.

Irritation of the vestibular labyrinth, as in **Meniere's disease,** can result in rhythmic conjugate deviations of the eyes, followed by quick return saccades. This condition is known as **nystagmus** (see Chapter 9), These eye movements are accompanied by a sense of **vertigo** and often **nausea.** The brain interprets a difference in the input from the two vestibular systems in terms of head motion. Irritation (or destruction) of one labyrinth produces an asymmetry of input that results in abnormal eye movements and in associated psychological effects.

Otolith organs. The hair cells in the otolith organs, unlike those in the ampullary crests, are not all oriented in the same direction. Instead, they are oriented with respect to a ridge, called the **striola,** along the otolith organ (Fig. 8-27). In the utricle the hair cells on either side of the striola are polarized toward the striola, whereas in the saccule they are polarized away from the striola. Because the striola in each otolith organ is curved, the hair cells have diverse orientations. When the head is tilted so that gravity produces a different linear acceleration, the otolithic membranes shift and the cilia of the hair cells bend in a new way. This bending of the cilia of the hair cells changes the pattern of input from the otolith organs to the CNS. Similarly, a linear acceleration caused by other forces, such as might occur in a space launch or a free fall, will change the output from the otolith organs.

Central Vestibular Pathways

The vestibular afferent fibers project to the brainstem through the vestibular nerve. As previously mentioned, the cell

■ **Fig. 8-24** Structure of the otolith organs. The saccule is shown in **A** and the utricle in **B**. (Redrawn from Lindeman HH: *Adv Otorhinolaryngol* 20:405, 1973.)

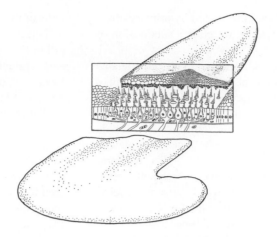

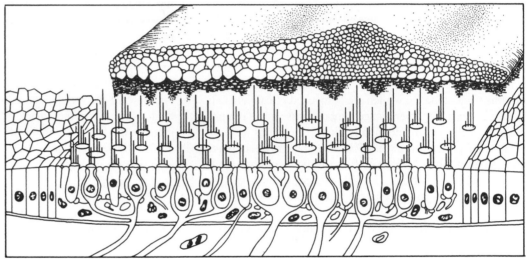

A

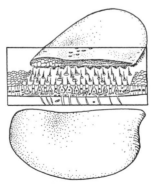

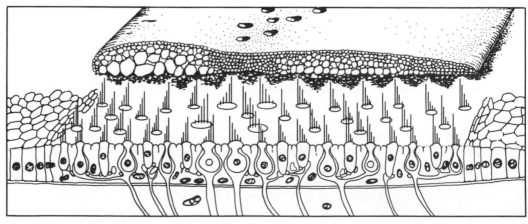

B

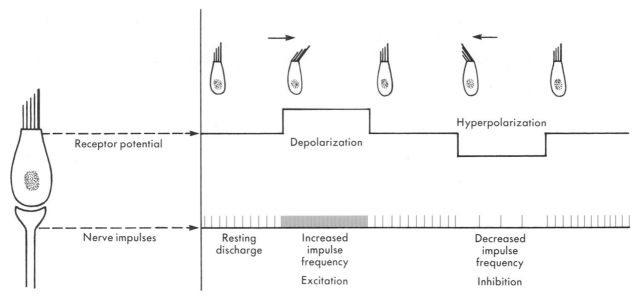

■ **Fig. 8-25**   Functional polarization of vestibular hair cells. When the stereocilia are bent toward the kinocilium, the hair cell is depolarized and the afferent fiber is excited. When the stereocilia are bent away from the kinocilium, the hair cell is hyperpolarized and the afferent discharge slows or stops. (Redrawn from Kandel ER, Schwartz JH: *Principles of neural science,* New York, 1981, Elsevier.)

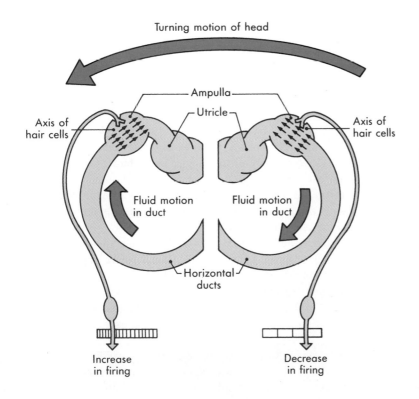

■ **Fig. 8-26**   Effect of head movement to the left on the activity of vestibular afferent fibers supplying hair cells in the horizontal semicircular ducts. Small arrows indicate the functional polarity of the hair cells. The large arrow, *top,* indicates movement of the head; open arrows, relative movements of the endolymph.

bodies of these afferent fibers are located in Scarpa's ganglion. The afferent fibers terminate in the **vestibular nuclei,** which are located in the rostral medulla and caudal pons. Afferent fibers from different parts of the vestibular apparatus end in different vestibular nuclei. The afferent fibers also give off collaterals to the **cerebellum.**

The vestibular nuclei give rise to various projections. These include projections through the **medial longitudinal fasciculus** to the oculomotor nuclei. Therefore, it is not surprising that the vestibular nuclei exert a powerful control over eye movements (the **vestibuloocular reflex**). Other projections give rise to the **lateral** and **medial vestibulospinal**

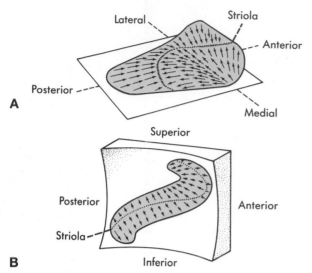

■ Fig. 8-27 Functional polarization of hair cells in the otolith organs. **A,** The utricle. **B,** The saccule. The striola in each case is indicated by the dotted line. (Redrawn from Spoendlin HH: In Wolfson RJ, editor: *The vestibular system and its diseases,* Philadelphia, 1966, University of Pennsylvania Press.)

tracts. These pathways provide, respectively, for the activation of postural and neck muscles and thereby contribute to balance and to head movements (**vestibulocollic reflex).** There are vestibular projections to the cerebellum, the reticular formation, and the contralateral vestibular complex, as well as to the thalamus. The latter mediate conscious sensations related to vestibular activity. The vestibular efferent fibers also originate from the vestibular nuclei.

Vestibular reflexes and clinical tests of vestibular function are described in Chapter 9.

THE CHEMICAL SENSES

The senses of **gustation** (taste) and **olfaction** (smell) depend on chemical stimuli that are present either in food and drink or in the air. In human evolution, these chemical senses do not have the survival value of some of the other senses, but they contribute considerably to the quality of life and are important stimulants of digestion. In other animals, the chemical senses clearly have survival value and their activation evokes a number of social behaviors, including mating, territoriality, and feeding.

Taste

The stimuli that we know as tastes are actually mixtures of four elementary taste qualities: salty, sweet, sour, and bitter. Taste stimuli that are particularly effective in eliciting these sensations include sodium chloride, sucrose, hydrochloric acid, and quinine.

Taste receptors. The sensation of taste depends on the activation of chemoreceptors located in taste buds. A taste bud consists of a group of 50 to 150 receptor cells, as well as supporting cells and basal cells (Fig. 8-28). The chemoreceptor cells synapse at their bases with primary afferent nerve fibers. The two types of chemoreceptor cells can be distinguished by differences in their synaptic vesicle content; one type has dense core vesicles, and the other has clear round vesicles. The apices of the cells have microvilli that extend toward a taste pore.

Chemoreceptor cells live only about 10 days. They are continuously replaced by new chemoreceptor cells that differentiate from basal cells that are located near the base of the taste bud.

Chemoreceptive molecules on the microvilli of chemoreceptor cells detect stimulatory molecules that diffuse into the taste pore from the overlying fluid layer. Part of this fluid originates from glands adjacent to the taste buds. A change in membrane conductance of a chemoreceptor cell leads to a receptor potential and to the release of an excitatory neurotransmitter. The neurotransmitter evokes a generator potential in the primary afferent nerve fiber, and it induces a discharge that is transmitted to the CNS.

Coding for the four primary taste qualities is not based on complete selectivity of the chemoreceptors for the different qualities. Instead, a given chemoreceptor responds to stimuli that evoke several different taste qualities, although perhaps most intensely to one. Recognition of taste quality appears to depend on the patterned input from a population of chemoreceptors. The intensity of the stimulus is reflected in the total amount of evoked activity.

Distribution and innervation of taste buds. Taste buds are located on different types of taste papillae that are found on the tongue, palate, pharynx, and larynx (Fig. 8-29). The types of taste papillae include **fungiform** and **foliate papillae** on the anterior and lateral tongue, and **circumvalate papillae** on the base of the tongue (Fig. 8-29, *C*). The latter may contain several hundred taste buds. The tongue in humans may have several thousand taste buds.

The sensitivity of the tongue for different taste qualities varies with the region of the tongue (Fig. 8-29, *A*). Sweet tastes are detected best at the tip of the tongue, salty and sour tastes originate along the sides, and bitter tastes are sensed best at the base.

The taste buds are innervated by three cranial nerves. The chorda tympani branch of the **facial nerve** supplies taste buds on the anterior two thirds of the tongue, and the **glossopharyngeal nerve** supplies taste buds on the posterior one third of the tongue (Fig. 8-29, *B*). The **vagus nerve** supplies a few taste buds in the larynx and upper esophagus.

Taste is not evaluated in the routine neurological examination. However, a detailed examination can include application of test substances to the anterior two thirds and the posterior one third of the tongue on each side. The tongue must be kept protruded to prevent mixing of the test substances with saliva and to prevent subsequent redistribution to other areas of the tongue. Taste can also be tested by application of a galvanic current to the tongue. Taste sensation can be lost, for example, after damage to a cranial nerve that contains gustatory afferents.

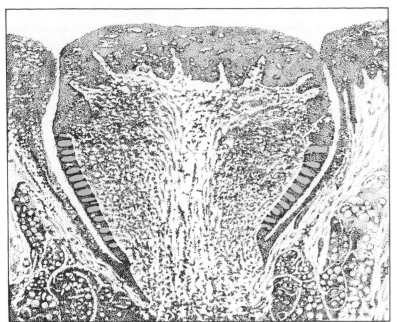

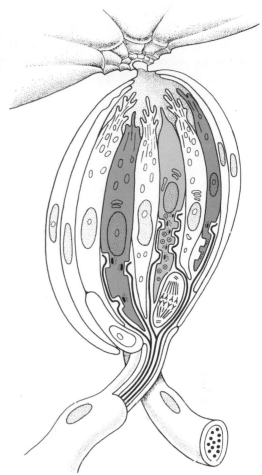

■ **Fig. 8-28**   Taste bud. *Left,* A circumvallate papilla is shown with its taste buds indicated in pink. *Right,* a taste bud is shown with the taste pore at the top and its innervation below. The two types of chemoreceptor cells are shown in color and the supporting cells are uncolored. (Redrawn from Williams PL, Warwick R: *Functional neuroanatomy of man,* Philadelphia, 1975, WB Saunders.)

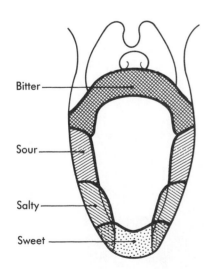

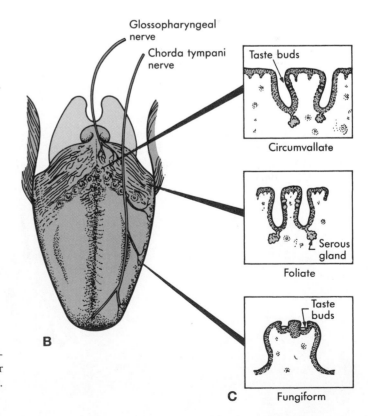

■ **Fig. 8-29**   **A,** Distribution of sensitivity for the four taste qualities. **B,** The innervation of the anterior two thirds and posterior one-third of the tongue by the facial and glossopharyngeal nerves. **C,** The arrangement of taste buds in the three types of papillae.

Central taste pathways. The cell bodies of taste fibers in cranial nerves VII, IX, and X are located in the **geniculate, petrosal,** and **nodose ganglia,** respectively. The central processes of the afferent fibers enter the medulla, join the solitary tract, and synapse in the **nucleus of the solitary tract.** In some animals, including several rodent species, the second-order taste neurons of the solitary nucleus project rostrally to the ipsilateral parabrachial nucleus. The parabrachial nucleus then projects to the small celled (parvocellular) part of the **ventroposterior medial (VPMpc)** nucleus of the thalamus. In monkeys the solitary nucleus projects directly to the VPMpc nucleus. The VPMpc nucleus is connected to two different gustatory areas of the cerebral cortex, one in the face area of the SI cortex and the other in the insula. An unusual feature of the central gustatory pathway is that it is predominantly an uncrossed pathway (unlike the central somatosensory, visual, and auditory pathways, which are predominantly crossed).

Olfaction

The sense of smell is much better developed in animals **(macrosmatic animals)** other than in humans and other primates **(microsmatic animals).** The ability of dogs to track other animals on the basis of odor is legendary, as is the use of **pheromones** by insects to attract mates. However, olfaction contributes to our emotional life, and odors can effectively call up memories.

Olfactory receptors. The olfactory chemoreceptor cells are located in the **olfactory mucosa,** a specialized part of the nasopharynx. Olfactory chemoreceptors are bipolar cells (Fig. 8-30). The apical surface of these chemoreceptor cells contains immobile cilia that detect odorants dissolved in the overlying mucus layer. These cells give off an unmyelinated axon from the basal surface. This axon joins others in **olfactory nerve filaments** that penetrate the base of the skull through openings in the cribriform plate of the ethmoid bone. The olfactory nerves connect synaptically with the **olfactory bulb,** a CNS structure located at the base of the cranial cavity, just below the frontal lobe (Fig. 8-31).

Humans have about 10 million olfactory chemoreceptors. Like taste cells, olfactory chemoreceptors have a short life span (about 60 days), and they are continuously replaced.

Odorant molecules are introduced to the olfactory mucosa by ventilatory air currents or from the oral cavity during feeding. Sniffing increases the influx of odorants. The odorants are temporarily bound in the mucus to an olfactory

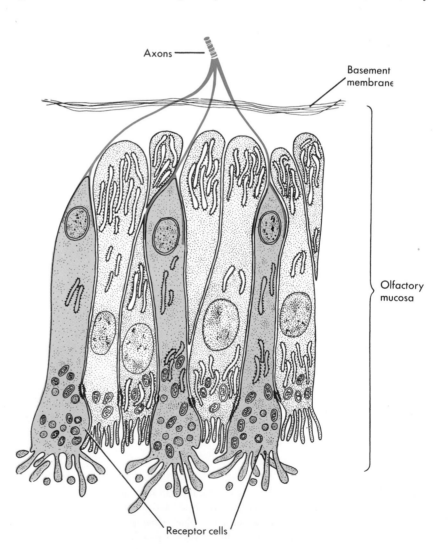

■ **Fig. 8-30**   Olfactory chemoreceptors are shown in color and supporting cells are uncolored. (Redrawn from de Lorenzo AJD: In Zotterman Y, editor: *Olfaction and taste,* Elmsford, NY, 1963, Pergamon Press.)

binding protein, which is secreted by a gland in the nasal cavity.

Odor has more primary qualities than does taste. There are at least six odor qualities: **floral, ethereal, musky, camphor, putrid,** and **pungent.** Natural stimuli with these odors are roses, pears, musk, eucalyptus, rotten eggs, and vinegar, respectively. The olfactory mucosa also contains somatosensory receptors of the trigeminal nerve. When performing clinical tests of olfaction, it is necessary to avoid activating these somatosensory receptors with noxious or thermal stimuli.

A few odorant molecules that reach an olfactory chemoreceptor cell produce a depolarizing receptor potential, which triggers a neural discharge. However, behavioral responses require the activation of a number of olfactory chemoreceptors. The receptor potential probably results from an increased conductance for Na$^+$. However, a G-protein is also activated; therefore, a cascade of second messengers is also involved in olfactory transduction.

Olfactory coding resembles taste coding, in that an individual olfactory chemoreceptor responds to more than one odorant class. Coding for a particular olfactory quality depends on the responses of many olfactory chemoreceptors, and the strength of the odorant is represented by the overall amount of afferent neural activity.

Central Pathways

The initial relay of the olfactory pathway is located in the olfactory bulb, which is a cortical structure. It contains three main cell types: **mitral cells, tufted cells,** and **interneurons (granule cells; periglomerular cells)** (Fig. 8-31). The dendrites of the mitral and tufted cells are long, and they branch to form the postsynaptic components of the olfactory glomeruli. The olfactory afferent fibers that reach the olfactory bulb from the olfactory mucosa ramify as they approach the olfactory glomeruli. These fibers then synapse on the dendrites of the mitral and tufted cells. Olfactory axons converge extensively onto mitral cell dendrites; as many as 1000 afferent fibers synapse on the dendrites of a single mitral cell. The granule and periglomerular cells are inhibitory interneurons. They form **dendrodendritic reciprocal synapses** with the dendrites of the mitral cells. Evidently, activity in a

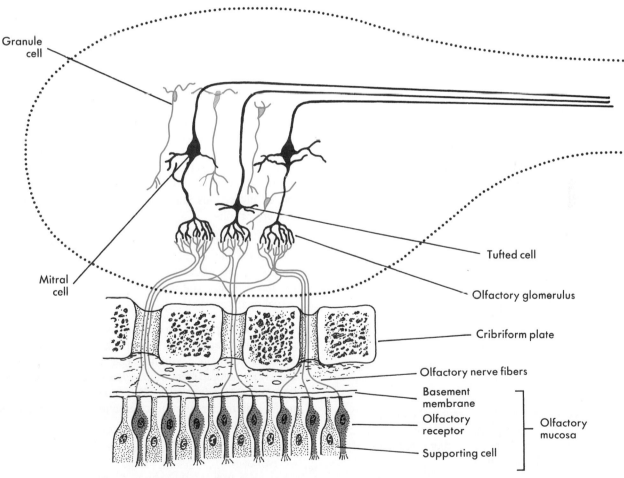

■ **Fig. 8-31** Drawing of a sagittal section through an olfactory bulb, showing the terminations of the olfactory chemoreceptor cells in the olfactory glomerulis and the intrinsic neurons of the olfactory bulb. The axons of the mitral and tufted cells are shown exiting in the olfactory tract to the right. (Redrawn from House EL, Pansky B: *A functional approach to neuroanatomy,* ed 2, New York, 1967, McGraw-Hill.)

mitral cell depolarizes the inhibitory cells that synapse with it. An inhibitory neurotransmitter that acts back on the mitral cell is then released. The olfactory bulb has other inputs besides those formed by the olfactory nerves; these other inputs include a projection from the contralateral olfactory tract via the anterior commissure.

The axons of the mitral and tufted cells leave the olfactory bulb and enter the olfactory tract. From here, the olfactory connections become highly complex. Within the olfactory tract is a nucleus, called the **anterior olfactory nucleus.** Neurons in this structure receive synaptic connections from neurons of the olfactory bulb, and they project to the contralateral olfactory bulb through the **anterior commissure.** As the olfactory tract approaches the anterior perforated substance at the base of the brain, it splits into the **lateral** and **medial olfactory striae.** Axons of the lateral olfactory stria synapse in the primary olfactory receiving area, which includes the prepiriform cortex (and, in many animals, the piriform lobe). The medial olfactory stria includes projections to the **amygdaloid nucleus,** as well as to part of the cortex of the basal forebrain.

Note that the olfactory pathway is the only sensory system that does not have an obligatory synaptic relay in the thalamus. This may reflect the phylogenetic primitiveness of the olfactory system. However, olfactory information does reach the mediodorsal nucleus of the thalamus, and olfactory information is then transmitted to the prefrontal and orbitofrontal cortex.

Olfaction is generally not examined in a routine neurological examination. However, smell can be tested by having the patient inhale and identify an odorant. One nostril should be examined at a time, while the other nostril is occluded. Strong odorants, such as ammonia, should be avoided, because they also activate trigeminal nerve fibers. Smell sensation can be lost (**anosmia**) after a basal skull fracture or after damage to one or both olfactory bulbs or tracts by a tumor (such as an **olfactory groove meningioma**). An aura of a disagreeable odor, often the smell of burning rubber, occurs during **uncinate fits,** which are epileptic seizures that originate in the region of the uncus.

SUMMARY

Vision

1. The surface of the eye has three main layers: (1) the fibrous layer includes the cornea and sclera; (2) the vascular layer includes the choroid, iris, and ciliary body; and (3) the nervous layer includes the retina.

2. The cornea is the most powerful refractive surface, but the lens has a variable power that allows images of near objects to be focused on the retina.

3. Depth of field is adjusted by the iris. Stray light is absorbed by pigment.

4. The retina has 10 layers. The photoreceptor layer absorbs light. Photoreceptors synapse on retinal interneurons, which in turn synapse on other interneurons and on ganglion cells. The ganglion cells project to the brain through the optic nerve.

5. The fovea is specialized for high resolution and color vision, and it contains only cones. The visual fixation point is imaged on the fovea.

6. The optic disk contains no photoreceptors, and therefore it is a blind spot.

7. Photoreceptors transduce visual signals. They are hyperpolarized by light. Pathways through the retina involve relays by retinal interneurons. Bipolar pathways are more direct than amacrine pathways.

8. Horizontal cells mediate lateral inhibition. Bipolar cells and many ganglion cells have receptive fields with an on-center, off-surround, or off-center, on-surround organization. Amacrine cells and some ganglion cells have large, diffuse receptive fields.

9. Many ganglion cells in primates can be classified as P, M, or W cells. P cells with small receptive fields and tonic and linear responses signal fine detail and wavelength. M cells have nonlinear responses and signal motion. Most W cells are difficult to activate.

10. The axons of ganglion cells in the temporal retina project ipsilaterally; those in the nasal retina cross in the optic chiasm. Crossed axons end in layers 1, 4, and 6 of the lateral geniculate nucleus (LGN); uncrossed axons end in layers 2, 3, and 5. Layers 1 and 2, the magnocellular layers, receive M cell projections; the other parvocellular layers receive P cell projections.

11. The LGN projects to the striate cortex through the optic radiation. Some of the axons pass into the temporal lobe in Meyer's loop. These axons carry visual information from the lower retinas and thus represent the contralateral upper visual field quadrants.

12. The LGN projection ends largely in layer 4 of the striate cortex. Information from one or the other eye predominates in ocular dominance columns. The striate cortex contains an orderly retinotopic map. Most striate cortical neurons respond best to bars or edges oriented in a particular way. Cells that prefer a particular stimulus orientation are grouped in orientation columns.

13. Stereopsis involves differences in the retinal images in the two eyes.

14. Color vision depends on wavelength discrimination, based on the three types of cone pigment and also on color opponent neurons.

15. The upper layers of the superior colliculus are involved in visual processing. The deep layers produce eye movements directed at visual targets that move into the field of vision or that are sources of somatosensory or auditory stimuli.

16. The many cortical extrastriate visual areas have different functions. Some in the inferotemporal cortex are influenced chiefly by P cells, and they function in form and color vision. Others in the middle temporal and parietal cortex are activated by M cells, and they function in motion detection and the control of eye movements.

Sound

17. Sound waves are combinations of pure tones, and the composition of a sound can be determined by Fourier analysis. A pure tone is characterized in terms of its amplitude, frequency, and phase.

18. The unit of sound pressure is the decibel. Hearing is most sensitive at about 3000 Hz.

19. The external ear includes the pinna and auditory canal.

20. The middle ear includes the tympanic membrane and a chain of ossicles that ends at the oval window. It is separated from the inner ear by the oval and round windows.

Auditory and vestibular systems

21. The inner ear includes the cochlea and vestibular apparatus. The cochlea has three main compartments: the scala vestibuli and scala tympani, which are parts of the bony labyrinth, and the scala media (cochlear duct), which is part of the membranous labyrinth. The bony labyrinth contains perilymph and the membranous labyrinth, endolymph.

22. The cochlear duct is bounded on one side by the basilar membrane, on which lies the organ of Corti, the sound transduction mechanism. Hair cells of the organ of Corti synapse with cochlear afferent fibers.

23. When the basilar membrane oscillates, the stereocilia of the hair cells are subjected to shear forces at their contacts with the tectorial membrane. This results in a membrane conductance change that induces a generator potential in cochlear afferent fibers.

24. High-frequency sounds activate best the hair cells near the base of the cochlea, and low-frequency sounds activate cells near the apex.

25. A tonotopic organization is also found in central auditory structures, including the cochlear nuclei, superior olivary complex, inferior colliculus, medial geniculate nucleus, and primary auditory cortex.

26. Auditory processing in the central auditory pathway contributes to sound localization, frequency and intensity analysis, and speech recognition.

27. The vestibular apparatus is part of the membranous labyrinth, and it includes three semicircular ducts (horizontal, superior, and posterior) and two otolith organs (utricle and saccule) on each side. These transduce, respectively, angular and linear accelerations of the head.

28. The sensory epithelium, the crista ampullaris, of a semicircular duct is found in a dilatation called the ampulla. Stereocilia and a single kinocilium extend from each hair cell into the cupula. Angular head movements displace the endolymph and distort the cupula, bending the cilia. If the stereocilia bend toward the kinocilium, the hair cell is depolarized; this causes a greater firing rate in the afferent fiber.

29. In the otolith organs, the cilia project into an otolithic membrane. Linear acceleration of the head displaces the otolithic membrane, which is sensitive to gravity because of the otoliths.

30. Central vestibular pathways include afferent connections to the vestibular nuclei, the cerebellum, and the lateral and medial vestibulospinal tracts.

Taste

31. Taste buds detect gustatory stimuli. A population code is used to signal the four elementary qualities of taste: salty, sweet, sour, and bitter.

32. Taste buds are located on several kinds of papillae on the tongue and in the pharynx and larynx. Taste buds contain chemoreceptor cells arranged around a taste pore.

33. The afferent fibers for taste synapse in the nucleus of the solitary tract. The thalamic relay is in the small cell part of the VPM nucleus, and the taste-receiving areas are located in the SI cortex and the insula.

34. Odors are detected by olfactory chemoreceptor cells in the olfactory mucosa. The olfactory chemoreceptor cells project to the olfactory bulb, where they synapse in olfactory glomeruli on the dendrites of mitral and tufted cells.

BIBLIOGRAPHY

Journal articles

Brandt T: Man in motion: historical and clinical aspects of vestibular function: a review, *Brain* 114:2159, 1991.

Burns ME, Baylor DA: Activation, deactivation, and adaptation in vertebrate photoreceptor cells, *Annu Rev Neurosci* 24:779, 2001.

Cumming BG, DeAngelis GC: The physiology of stereopsis, *Annu Rev Neurosci* 24:203, 2001.

Fain GL et al: Adaptation in vertebrate photoreceptors, *Physiol Rev* 81:117, 2001.

Herness MS, Gilbertson TA: Cellular mechanisms of taste transduction, *Annu Rev Physiol* 61:873, 1999.

Hildebrand JG, Shepherd GM: Mechanisms of olfactory discrimination: converging evidence for common principles across phyla, *Annu Rev Neurosci* 20:595,1997.

Hudspeth AJ: How hearing happens, *Neuron* 19:947, 1997.

Kauer JS, White J: Imaging and coding in the olfactory system, *Annu Rev Neurosci* 24:963, 2001.

Lindemann B: Taste reception, *Physiol Rev* 76:719, 1996.

Mombaerts P: Molecular biology of odorant receptors in vertebrates, *Annu Rev Neurosci* 22:487, 1999.

Schild D, Restrepo D: Transduction mechanisms in vertebrate olfactory receptor cells, *Physiol Rev* 78:429, 1998.

Van Essen DC, Gallant JL: Neural mechanisms of form and motion processing in the primate visual system, *Neuron* 13:1, 1994.

Wandell BA: Computational neuroimaging of human visual cortex, *Annu Rev Neurosci* 22:145, 1999.

Zeki S: Localization and globalization in conscious vision, *Annu Rev Neurosci* 24:57, 2001.

Books and monographs

Baloh RW, Honrubia V: *Clinical neurophysiology of the vestibular system,* ed 2, Philadelphia, 1990, FA Davis co.

Hubel DH: *Eye, brain and vision,* New York, 1988, Scientific American Library.

Kaiser PK, Boynton RM: *Human color vision,* ed 2, Washington, DC, 1996, Optical Society of America.

Oyster C: *The human eye: structure and function,* Sunderland, Mass., 1999, Sinauer Associates.

Rodieck RW: *First steps in seeing,* Sunderland, Mass., 1998, Sinauer Associates.

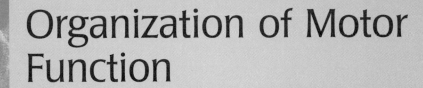

chapter nine

Organization of Motor Function

Movements and posture depend on the coordinated contraction of muscles that operate around joints. Coordination of muscle contractions, in turn, depends on the amount and timing of the discharges of motor neurons to the appropriate muscles and the absence of discharges of motor neurons to inappropriate muscles. Thus, the motor system coordinates muscle actions through control of motor neuronal activity. Although motor control is in part voluntary, it occurs mainly by reflex action and by subconscious mechanisms.

Spinal reflexes are important to motor activity. Many subconscious actions depend largely on simple reflexes that are triggered by the activation of sensory receptors. Activation of sensory receptors then excites interneurons and motor neurons in the spinal cord, and this excitation then triggers the contraction or relaxation of particular muscles. Spinal reflexes can be observed in **spinalized** individuals (i.e., individuals with spinal cord injuries that cause a complete functional transection of the spinal cord). Therefore, these reflexes do not depend on motor commands that originate in the brain and are conveyed to the spinal cord via descending motor pathways.

In addition, many of the motor acts that do originate from motor commands issued by the brain depend on spinal reflex circuitry for their implementation. Only a few of the descending pathways synapse directly on spinal cord motor neurons. Instead, most of the descending projections influence the activity of interneurons that are interposed in reflex circuits and thus alter ongoing spinal reflex activity.

This chapter first describes a number of spinal cord reflex pathways. Motor pathways that descend from the brain will be discussed next. Consideration of the motor control systems of the brain will then follow.

Spinal cord injury is common, especially in young males. Such injuries are caused by automobile collisions, sports accidents, war injuries, or gunshot wounds. Depending on the level and severity of the spinal cord injury, the individual affected may have **paraplegia** (paralysis of both lower extremities) or **quadriplegia** (paralysis of all

four extremities). Much research has focused on ways to ameliorate spinal cord injury. Promising leads include (1) protection against secondary damage by administration of agents such as methylprednisolone shortly after the injury; (2) procedures to assist movement, such as electrical stimulation of muscle nerves of the lower extremities; and (3) treatments to encourage repair of the interrupted descending motor pathways. Recent speculation suggests that transplants of human embryonic stem cells may in the future be helpful in restoring some of the damaged circuitry.

In humans, an abrupt transection of the spinal cord results initially in a condition called **spinal shock,** which is characterized by a flaccid paralysis, areflexia, loss of autonomic function, and loss of all sensation below the level of the transection. In a flaccid paralysis, the joint offers no resistance to passive movement when an examiner bends the joint. This absence of resistance results from the loss of muscle stretch reflexes, which normally cause muscle contractions that oppose changes in the position of the joint. Spinal shock generally lasts 3 to 4 weeks. After spinal shock resolves, reflexes gradually return and then become hyperactive. The hyperactivity of spinal reflexes is demonstrated by greater resistance than normal when an examiner bends the joint. Voluntary movement and sensation never return, and the paralysis changes in character from flaccidity to spasticity. Furthermore, pathological reflexes appear (e.g., the **sign of Babinski;** see page 170), muscle tone increases, and bowel and bladder functions return, but in altered form.

Hyperactivity affects both the muscle stretch reflexes and the flexion reflexes. Hyperactive stretch reflexes are associated not only with an increased resistance to passive stretch, but also often with **clonus** (an alternating contraction of agonist and antagonist muscles around a joint, such as the ankle, after an initial quick passive flexion of the joint). Hyperactive flexion reflexes in response to a noxious stimulus applied to a foot may include not only flexion of one or both lower extremities but also urination, defecation, and sweating. The posture is often one of maintained flexion of the lower extremities.

In animals, spinal transection produces similar changes, but the period of spinal shock is usually brief. Therefore, spinal reflexes can be studied in the absence of descending controls.

DECEREBRATION

Another experimental preparation that has been useful for the study of reflexes is the decerebrate preparation. Surgical decerebration is achieved by transecting the midbrain, often at an intercollicular level. Decerebrate animals no longer have sensation, and their motor control system is profoundly altered. Some descending pathways, such as those that originate in the cerebral cortex, are interrupted, whereas others, such as those that originate in the brainstem, remain intact. In fact, activity in some descending pathways becomes hyperactive because of a change in the balance of excitatory and inhibitory control systems. As a result, some spinal reflexes, such as the flexion reflex, are suppressed, whereas others, such as the stretch reflex, are exaggerated, a condition called **decerebrate rigidity.** Decerebrate rigidity causes decerebrate animals to maintain a posture that has been called **exaggerated standing.** Decerebrate preparations are thus ideal for the study of the stretch reflex, as well as of the inverse myotatic reflex.

Human patients with brainstem damage may also develop a decerebrate state that has many of the same reflex features as animal preparations. The prognosis in such patients is poor if signs of decerebration appear.

SENSORY RECEPTORS RESPONSIBLE FOR ELICITING SPINAL REFLEXES

As noted in the introduction to this chapter, activation of particular sensory receptors triggers simple reflexes that are largely responsible for many subconscious actions. Several important spinal reflexes are activated by muscle stretch receptors, including muscle spindles and Golgi tendon organs. These reflexes are the **muscle stretch reflex** (or **myotatic reflex**) and the **inverse myotatic reflex.** These reflexes are important for the maintenance of posture, and alteration in the activity in the circuits for these reflexes provides an important means by which descending pathways produce movements. Furthermore, abnormalities in the stretch reflexes are prominent in disorders of the motor system. We have already seen how abnormalities in these reflexes contribute to the syndrome associated with complete spinal cord transection.

Another important reflex, the **flexion reflex,** is evoked by various sensory receptors in the skin, muscles, joints, and viscera. Afferents from the different receptors that are able to evoke a flexion reflex are often referred to as flexion reflex afferents (see later in this chapter).

In the following section, the muscle stretch receptors—muscle spindles and Golgi tendon organs—are discussed. These receptors are important both for spinal reflexes and for proprioception (see Chapter 7). Their structure and functional properties are described in detail here because knowledge of their operation is useful for understanding the mechanisms that underlie the spinal reflexes.

The Muscle Spindle

The structure and function of muscle spindles are very complex. Muscle spindles are found in most skeletal muscles, but they are particularly concentrated in muscles that exert fine motor control (e.g., the small muscles of the hand). In large muscles, they are most abundant in those that are rich in slow twitch (type I) muscle fibers.

Structure of the muscle spindle. As its name implies, a muscle **spindle** (or neuromuscular spindle) is a spindle-shaped organ composed of a bundle of modified muscle fibers richly innervated both by sensory and motor axons (Fig. 9-1). The muscle spindle is about 100 μm in diameter and up to 10 mm long. The innervated part of the muscle spindle is

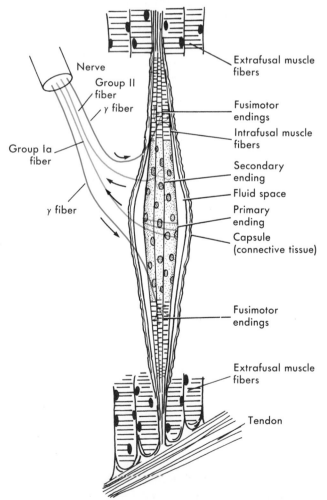

■ Fig. 9-1   Drawing of a muscle spindle. (Redrawn from Brodal A: *Neurological anatomy,* ed 3, New York, 1981, Oxford University Press.)

encased in a connective tissue capsule. Within this capsule, fluid is contained in the so-called lymph space. The muscle spindle lies freely between regular muscle fibers. The distal ends of the spindle are attached to the connective tissue within the muscle **(endomysium).** The muscle spindles lie parallel to the regular muscle fibers. This arrangement has important functional implications, as is made clear below.

Muscle spindles contain modified muscle fibers called **intrafusal muscle fibers** to distinguish them from the regular or **extrafusal muscle fibers.** Individual intrafusal fibers are much narrower than extrafusal fibers and are too weak to contribute to muscle tension. Two types of intrafusal muscle fibers are found within muscle spindles: nuclear bag and nuclear chain fibers (Fig. 9-2). These names are derived from the arrangement of the nuclei in these two kinds of intrafusal fibers. **Nuclear bag fibers** are larger than nuclear chain fibers, and their nuclei are bunched together like a bag of oranges in the central region of the fiber. In **nuclear chain fibers,** the nuclei are arranged in a row.

Muscle spindles receive a complex innervation. The sensory supply includes a single **group Ia afferent** and a variable number of **group II afferent** fibers (see Fig. 9-2). Group Ia fibers belong to the largest diameter class of sensory nerve fibers and conduct at 72 to 120 m/sec; group II fibers are intermediate in size and conduct at 36 to 72 m/sec. A group Ia afferent fiber forms a **primary ending,** which consists of a spiral-shaped terminal composed of branches of the group Ia fiber, on each of the intrafusal muscle fibers. Thus, terminals of primary endings are found on both nuclear bag and nuclear chain fibers, a point that is functionally significant. The group II afferent fiber forms a **secondary ending,** which is found chiefly on the nuclear chain fibers.

The motor supply to the muscle spindle consists of two types of γ-motor axons (Fig. 9-2). **Dynamic γ-motor axons** end on nuclear bag fibers, and **static γ-motor axons** end on nuclear chain fibers. γ-Motor axons are smaller in diameter than the α-motor axons to extrafusal muscle. Hence they conduct more slowly.

Function of the muscle spindle. As the name **stretch receptor** implies, muscle spindles respond to muscle stretch. Figures 9-3 and 9-4, *A* show the changes in the activity of afferent fibers of a muscle spindle when stretching the muscle lengthens the muscle spindle.

The primary and secondary endings respond differently to stretch. The primary ending is sensitive both to the amount of stretch and to its rate, whereas the secondary ending responds chiefly to the amount of stretch (Fig. 9-3, *left*). The difference in the behavior of the two endings is that the activity of the primary ending overshoots during muscle stretch, and the group Ia fiber stops firing when the stretch is first released. These are called **dynamic responses.** The responses in the center of Fig. 9-3 show further examples of dynamic responses of the primary ending. Tapping the muscle or its tendon and sinusoidal stretch are much more effective in causing discharges of the primary than of the secondary ending. Both the primary and the secondary ending display **static responses** to stretch—that is, stretch causes a tonic level of activity in proportion to the amount of stretch. The dynamic response of the primary ending is superimposed on the static response. *These responses show that the primary endings signal both the **length** and the **rate of change in length** of the muscle, whereas the secondary endings signal only the **length** of the muscle.*

The mechanism for these differences between the behavior of primary and secondary endings appears to depend largely on mechanical differences between the nuclear bag and nuclear chain fibers. As stated above, primary endings are found on both nuclear bag and nuclear chain fibers, whereas secondary endings are found chiefly on nuclear chain fibers.

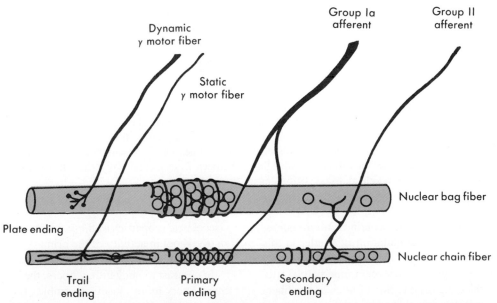

■ **Fig. 9-2** Nuclear bag and nuclear chain fibers and their sensory and motor nerve supply. (Redrawn from Matthews PBC: *Physiol Rev* 44:219, 1964.)

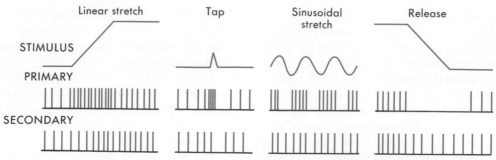

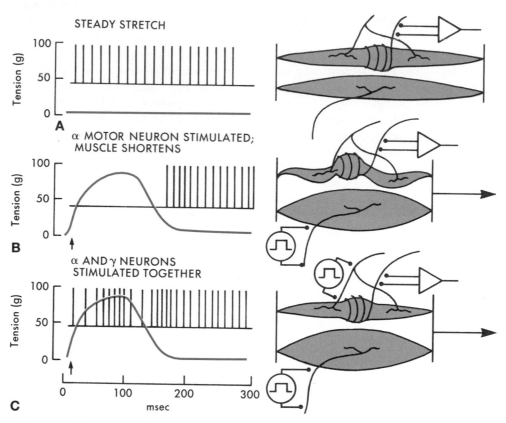

■ **Fig. 9-3** The responses of a primary ending and of a secondary ending to various types of changes in muscle length are shown to illustrate the difference in dynamic and static responsiveness of these endings. The waveforms at the top are the changes in muscle length. The vertical lines in the middle and bottom parts of the figure show the discharges of a primary and of a secondary ending. (Redrawn from Matthews PBC: *Physiol Rev* 44:219, 1964.)

■ **Fig. 9-4** The activity of γ-motor neurons can counteract the effects of unloading on the discharges of a muscle spindle afferent. **A,** The activity of a muscle spindle afferent is shown during steady stretch. **B,** The afferent stops firing when the extrafusal muscle fibers contract, owing to unloading of the muscle spindle. **C,** Activation of a γ-motor neuron causes shortening of the muscle spindle, counteracting the effects of unloading. (Redrawn from Kuffler SW, Nicholls JG: *From neuron to brain,* Sunderland, Mass, 1976, Sinauer Associates.)

Nuclear bag fibers lack contractile protein in their equatorial regions because of the accumulation of nuclei in this region. Therefore, the nuclear bag fibers are readily stretched in their mid-region. However, immediately after they are stretched, the equatorial region of nuclear bag fibers tends to return toward its original length as the polar regions lengthen. This phenomenon, called **creep,** is caused by the

viscoelastic properties of these intrafusal fibers. The result is an overshoot in activity of the primary ending followed by a reduction in activity toward a new static level of firing.

In contrast to nuclear bag fibers, the length of the nuclear chain fibers more closely resembles that of the extrafusal muscle fibers because the nuclear chain fibers contain contractile proteins in their equatorial regions. Hence, they have

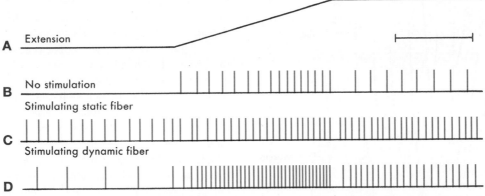

■ **Fig. 9-5** Effects of static and dynamic γ-motor neurons on the responses of a primary ending to muscle stretch. The upper trace, **A,** is the time course of stretch. **B** shows the discharge of the group Ia fiber in the absence of γ-motor neuron activity. In **C,** a static γ-motor axon was stimulated, and in **D** a dynamic γ-motor axon was stimulated. (Redrawn from Crowe A, Matthews PBC: *J Physiol* 174:109, 1964.)

more uniform viscoelastic properties throughout their length. Therefore they do not display creep, and the secondary ending has only a static response.

Contraction of the extrafusal muscle fibers can result in shortening of the muscle spindle because of the parallel arrangement of the muscle spindle described earlier (Fig. 9-4, *B*). This results in cessation of the activity of the muscle spindle afferents, an action known as **unloading.**

Up to this point, we have described only how muscle spindles behave when the γ-motor neurons are not active. However, the efferent innervation of muscle spindles is extremely important, because it determines the sensitivity of muscle spindles to stretch. For example, in Fig. 9-4, *A,* the activity of a muscle spindle afferent is shown during a steady stretch. When the extrafusal part of the muscle contracts (Fig. 9-4, *B*), the muscle spindle is unloaded, and the muscle spindle afferent may stop discharging. However, this effect of muscle unloading can be counteracted if γ-motor neurons are stimulated. This stimulation causes the muscle spindle to shorten along with the extrafusal muscle fibers (Fig. 9-4, *C*). Actually, only the two polar regions of the muscle spindle contract; the equatorial region, where the nuclei are located, does not contract, because it has little contractile protein. As a result, when the polar regions contract, the equatorial region elongates, which stretches and excites the afferent terminals. This mechanism is very important in the normal operation of muscle spindles, because descending motor commands from the brain typically coactivate α- and γ-motor neurons and thus cause cocontraction of both extrafusal and intrafusal muscle fibers.

As previously mentioned, there are two types of γ-motor neurons—dynamic and static γ-motor neurons (see Fig. 9-2). Dynamic γ-motor axons end on nuclear bag fibers and static γ-motor axons synapse on nuclear chain fibers. When a dynamic γ-motor neuron is activated, the dynamic response of the group Ia afferent fiber is enhanced (Fig. 9-5, *D*). When a static γ-motor neuron discharges, the static response

of the group Ia afferent fiber (and also of group II fibers) is increased (Fig. 9-5, *C*); at the same time, the dynamic response of the group Ia fiber may even be reduced. Different descending pathways can preferentially influence dynamic or static γ-motor neurons and thereby alter the nature of reflex activity in the spinal cord.

Golgi Tendon Organ

The other type of stretch receptor found in skeletal muscle is the Golgi tendon organ (Fig. 9-6). A **Golgi tendon organ** is formed from the terminals of a group Ib afferent fiber. The diameter of a Golgi tendon organ is about 100 μm and its length is about 1 mm. The group Ib fiber has a large diameter and conducts in the same velocity range as the group Ia fiber. The terminals are wrapped about bundles of collagen fibers in the tendon of a muscle (or in tendonous inscriptions within the muscle). The sensory ending is arranged in series with the muscle, in contrast to the parallel arrangement of the muscle spindle.

Because of their arrangement in series with muscle, Golgi tendon organs can be activated either by muscle stretch or by contraction of the muscle (Fig. 9-7). However, muscle contraction is a more effective stimulus than muscle stretch. The actual stimulus is the force that develops in the tendon that contains the Golgi tendon organ. Therefore, Golgi tendon organs signal force, unlike muscle spindles, which signal muscle length and rate of change of muscle length.

SPINAL REFLEXES

A reflex is a simple, relatively stereotyped motor response to a specific type of stimulus. A **reflex arc** is the neuronal circuit responsible for a particular reflex. Typically, a reflex arc includes a set of sensory receptors of a particular kind that, when stimulated, elicits the reflex by exciting a set of interneurons and motor neurons. Other interneurons and motor neurons may also be inhibited, so that an appropriate

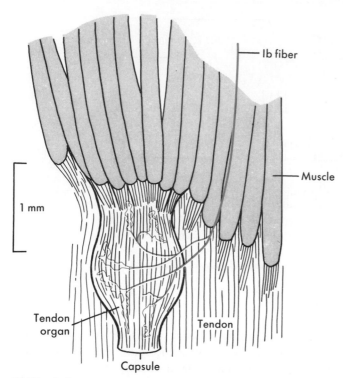

■ **Fig. 9-6** Drawing of a Golgi tendon organ. (Redrawn from Barker D: *Muscle receptors,* Hong Kong, 1962, Hong Kong University Press.)

pattern of muscle contractions occurs about one or more joints.

The Myotatic or Stretch Reflex

The stretch reflex is a key reflex in the maintenance of posture. In addition, changes in this reflex are involved in actions commanded by the brain, and pathological alterations are important signs of neurological disease. This reflex actually has two forms: the phasic stretch reflex and the tonic stretch

reflex. The **phasic stretch reflex** is elicited by primary endings of muscle spindles, whereas the **tonic stretch reflex** depends on both primary and secondary endings.

The phasic stretch reflex. The reflex arc responsible for the phasic stretch reflex is shown in Fig. 9-8. A group Ia afferent fiber from a muscle spindle in the rectus femoris muscle is shown to branch as it enters the spinal cord gray matter. Some branches synapse directly monosynaptically) on α-motor neurons that supply the rectus femoris muscle (and its synergists, such as the vastus intermedius muscle), which extend the leg at the knee. The group Ia fibers produce a monosynaptic excitation of the α-motor neurons. If the excitation is powerful enough, the motor neurons discharge and cause a contraction of the muscle.

Other branches of the group Ia fibers end on group Ia inhibitory interneurons, such as the one shown in black in Fig. 9-8. These inhibitory interneurons end on α-motor neurons that innervate the hamstring muscles, including the semitendinosus muscle, which are antagonists and flex the knee. Activity in the Ia inhibitory interneurons inhibits the motor neurons to the antagonist muscles.

The organization of the stretch reflex arc guarantees that one set of α-motor neurons is activated and the opposing set is inhibited. This arrangement is known as **reciprocal innervation.** Although many reflexes involve such reciprocal innervation, this type of innervation is not the only possible organization of a motor control system. In some instances, a motor command causes co-contraction of synergists and antagonists, for example, when a person makes a fist. The muscles that extend and flex the wrist contract and allow the wrist to resist motion.

Action potentials are elicited in group Ia afferent fibers when a physician taps the tendon of a muscle, such as the quadriceps, with a reflex hammer. The result is normally a brief muscular contraction that is quickly damped.

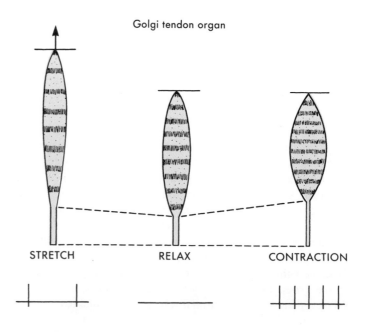

■ **Fig. 9-7** Activation of a Golgi tendon organ by muscle stretch *(left)* or by contraction of the muscle *(right).* (Redrawn from Eyzaguirre C, Fidone SJ: *Physiology of the nervous system,* ed 2, St. Louis, 1975, Mosby.)

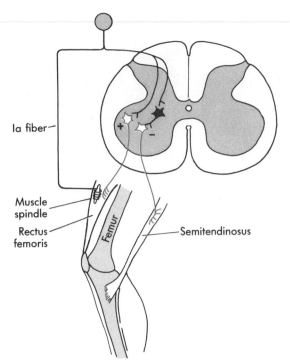

■ **Fig. 9-8** Reflex arc of the stretch reflex. The interneuron shown in black is a group Ia inhibitory interneuron.

When the excitability of the a-motor neurons is altered pathologically, the phasic stretch reflex may become depressed or hyperexcitable. In the past, this type of reflex was termed a **deep tendon reflex.** This term is a misnomer, however, because the receptors responsible for the reflex are in the muscle, not the tendon. The tendon only provides for a quick stretch of the muscle.

The tonic stretch reflex. The other type of stretch reflex, the tonic stretch reflex, is elicited by passively bending a joint. The reflex circuit is the same as that for the phasic stretch reflex (illustrated in Fig. 9-8), except that the receptors involved include both group Ia and group II afferent fibers from muscle spindles. Many group II fibers make monosynaptic excitatory connections with α-motor neurons. Therefore, the tonic stretch reflex is largely a monosynaptic reflex, like the phasic stretch reflex. The tonic stretch reflex contributes to muscle tone, which is judged by the resistance that a joint offers to bending. However, its importance lies in its contribution to posture. When an individual stands, the joints of the leg must maintain a particular position to prevent falling. Any slight extension or flexion will elicit a stretch reflex in the muscles required to oppose the movement, thus helping an individual stand upright. For example, if the knee of a soldier standing at attention begins to flex because of fatigue, the quadriceps muscle will be stretched, a tonic stretch reflex will be elicited, and the quadriceps will contract more, thereby opposing the flexion and restoring the posture.

γ-Motor neurons and stretch reflexes. γ-Motor neurons help set the sensitivity of the stretch reflexes. Muscle spindle afferent fibers have no direct influence on γ-motor neurons, which are instead affected polysynaptically by the flexion reflex afferents at the spinal cord level and by descending commands. Thus, in many clinical disorders of motor control, the activity of γ-motor neurons is inappropriate because of a change, for instance, in the activity of descending pathways. As mentioned, spinal cord transection results initially in spinal shock, with a loss of the stretch reflexes. Spinal shock may be caused in part by the loss of descending excitation of γ-motor neurons. When spinal shock eventually resolves, increased activity in γ-motor neurons may underlie **spasticity,** in which phasic stretch reflexes are hyperactive, and **hypertonia,** in which tonic stretch reflexes are hyperactive.

Testing with a reflex hammer is a common way for a physician to assess the level of excitability of spinal motor neurons. However, another approach is to stimulate the axons of group Ia fibers electrically and to examine changes in the reflex responses to a synchronous volley in muscle spindle afferent fibers. The reflex can be monitored objectively by **electromyography.** The monosynaptic reflex elicited by stimulating the tibial nerve at the popliteal fossa and recorded from the triceps surae muscles is called an **H reflex** (for Hoffmann, who described this technique).

Inverse Myotatic Reflex

Activation of Golgi tendon organs has a reflex effect that seems to oppose the stretch reflex (it actually complements the stretch reflex, as discussed in the next paragraph). This is called the **inverse myotatic reflex,** and its reflex arc is shown in Fig. 9-9. In this example, the receptor organs are Golgi tendon organs located in the rectus femoris muscle. The afferent fibers branch as they enter the spinal cord and end on interneurons. There are no monosynaptic connections to α-motor neurons. Rather, the Golgi tendon organ pathway involves inhibitory interneurons that inhibit α-motor neurons that supply the rectus femoris muscle and excitatory interneurons responsible for activating α-motor neurons to the antagonistic hamstring muscles. Thus, the organization of the inverse myotatic reflex is opposite to that of the stretch reflexes, which explains the name given to this reflex. However, the function of this reflex actually complements that of the stretch reflex. The Golgi tendon organs monitor force in the tendon that they supply. If, during maintained posture, such as standing at attention, the rectus femoris muscle begins to fatigue, the force in the patellar tendon will decline. The decline in force will reduce the activity of Golgi tendon organs in this tendon. Because these receptors normally inhibit the α-motor neurons to the rectus femoris muscle, reduced activity of the Golgi tendon organs will enhance the excitability of the α-motor neurons and increase the force. A coordinated reflex change will then occur, involving both muscle spindle and Golgi tendon organ afferent fibers, that causes a greater

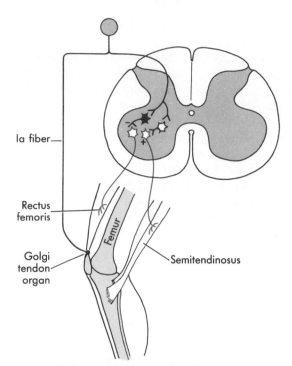

■ **Fig. 9-9** Reflex arc of the inverse myotatic reflex. The interneurons include both excitatory *(clear)* and inhibitory *(black)* interneurons.

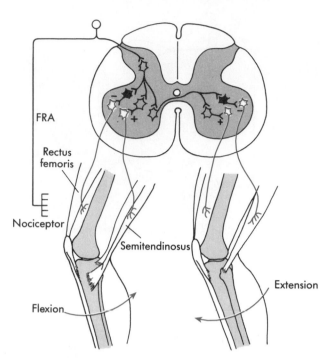

■ **Fig. 9-10**   The reflex arc of the flexion reflex. Black interneurons are inhibitory and clear ones are excitatory. *FRA,* Flexion reflex afferent.

contraction of the rectus femoris muscle and maintenance of the posture.

When reflexes are hyperactive it may be possible to demonstrate a **clasp-knife reflex.** When a joint is passively bent, resistance to the passive movement initially increases. However, if bending continues, the resistance suddenly decreases and the joint movement is readily completed. This change is caused by reflex inhibition. The clasp-knife reflex was once attributed to the activation of Golgi tendon organs, because these receptors were initially thought to have a high threshold to muscle stretch. However, it is now thought that the clasp-knife reflex is caused by activation of other high-threshold muscle receptors that supply the fascia around the muscle.

Flexion Reflexes

The afferent limb of the flexion reflex is furnished by a variety of sensory receptors, called the **flexion reflex afferents (FRAs).** In flexion reflexes, afferent volleys (1) cause excitatory interneurons to activate α-motor neurons that supply flexor muscles in the ipsilateral limb, and (2) cause inhibitory interneurons to prevent the activation of α-motor neurons that supply the antagonistic extensor muscles (Fig. 9-10). This pattern of activity causes one or more joints in the stimulated limb to flex. In addition, commissural interneurons evoke the opposite pattern of activity in the contralateral side of the spinal cord (Fig. 9-10). This opposite pattern results in extension of the opposite limb, the **crossed extension reflex.** The contralateral effect helps in maintaining balance.

There are several different types of flexion reflexes, although they produce similar patterns of muscle contraction. An important part of locomotion is the flexion phase, which involves a pattern of muscle contraction that can be regarded as a flexion reflex. This reflex is controlled predominantly by a neural circuit, called the **locomotor pattern generator,** in the spinal cord. However, afferent input can alter the locomotor pattern so that it can adapt to moment-by-moment changes in the terrain.

The most powerful flexion reflex is the **flexor withdrawal reflex.** This reflex takes precedence over other reflexes, including those associated with locomotion, presumably because flexor withdrawal protects the limb from further damage. This reflex can readily be observed in a dog that holds a hurt paw away from the ground while walking. Nociceptors form the afferent limb of this reflex.

In the flexor withdrawal reflex, a strong noxious stimulus results in withdrawal of the limb from the stimulus. In Fig. 9-10, the neural circuit of the flexion reflex is shown for neurons that affect only the knee joint. Actually, however, considerable divergence of the primary afferent and interneuronal pathways occurs in the flexion reflex. In fact, all of the major joints of a limb (e.g., hip, knee, ankle) may be involved in a strong flexor withdrawal reflex. The details of the flexor withdrawal reflex vary, depending on the nature and location of the stimulus. This variability of the flexion reflex is called the **local sign.** Flexor withdrawal reflexes also occur in areas other than the limbs; for example, visceral disease may cause contractions of the muscles in the chest wall or abdomen, and thereby decrease the mobility of the trunk.

Comparison of the Stretch and Flexion Reflexes

The flexion reflexes have a number of properties that differ strikingly from those of the stretch reflex. The stretch reflex is activated by stimulation of groups Ia and II muscle spindle afferent fibers. The afferent pathway shows some divergence, because it affects all the α-motor neurons that supply the muscle, plus some of those that supply synergistic muscles. In addition, the pathway activates inhibitory interneurons to antagonistic α-motor neurons, an example of reciprocal innervation. The stretch reflex terminates when the afferent volley ceases, and it exerts a graded, specific, and discrete control over the muscles that operate across a joint, such as the knee or the ankle.

By contrast, the flexion reflex can be evoked by various receptor types supplied by the FRAs. The latency is long, because the reflex arc is polysynaptic. Substantial divergence occurs in the reflex pathway, which may involve interneurons that influence α-motor neurons suppling muscles at all of the joints of a limb. In addition, the reflex can activate extensor motor neurons of the opposite limb. Thus the flexion reflex involves double reciprocal innervation. The reflex is nonlinear. Weak stimuli have little or no effect, but when stimuli reach a certain level of intensity, a powerful flexor withdrawal reflex may be elicited, and that dominates other reflexes. The flexion may persist long after the stimulus ends, presumably because of afterdischarges of interneurons in the reflex arc.

PRINCIPLES OF SPINAL ORGANIZATION

As discussed in relation to the stretch reflex, and especially to the flexion reflex, divergence is an important aspect of reflex pathways. Convergence is another important organizational feature of reflex arcs. **Convergence** is defined as the termination of several neurons on one other neuron. For example, all the group Ia afferent fibers from the muscle spindles of a particular hindlimb muscle have convergent monosynaptic terminals on a given α-motor neuron to that muscle. This convergent input accounts for the phenomenon of **spatial facilitation** in the stretch reflex. As noted, the flexion reflex, in contrast, displays considerable divergence. Because of this divergence, the flexion reflex varies in its details, depending on the particular afferent input that triggers it. This variability (the local sign) allows the reflex to withdraw the limb from a noxious stimulus. Only slight variations in the location of the stimulus may alter the nature of the withdrawal response.

An example of spatial facilitation is shown in Fig. 9-11. In that example, a monosynaptic reflex is elicited by electrical stimulation of the group Ia fibers in each of two branches of a muscle nerve (Fig. 9-11, *A*). The reflex is characterized by recording the discharges of α-motor axons from the appropriate ventral root. When muscle nerve branch A is stimulated, a small compound action potential is recorded as reflex A. Similarly, when muscle nerve branch B is stimulated, reflex B is recorded. These reflex discharges have a low electrical threshold, because the group Ia fibers in the muscle nerve are large axons. Also, the latency of the reflex discharge is short, because the reflex pathway is monosynaptic, and the conduction velocities of the afferent and motor axons are high.

Figure 9-11, *B* depicts the motor neurons contained within the motor nucleus. The medium-colored teardrop shapes enclose the α-motor neurons that are activated when each muscle nerve branch is stimulated sequentially. Thus, two α-motor neurons are activated when each muscle nerve branch is stimulated separately. When the two nerves are stimulated at the same time, a much larger reflex discharge is recorded (see recordings at the right of Fig. 9-11, *B*). As the figure demonstates, this reflex represents the discharges of seven α-motor neurons. Thus, three additional α-motor neurons (shown by the dark-colored teardrops) are activated when the two muscle nerves are stimulated simultaneously.

The explanation for this spatial summation is that all the α-motor neurons to the muscle are excited by either muscle afferent volley. However, when only one nerve is stimulated, the excitation is powerful enough to activate only two motor neurons. These motor neurons are in the **discharge zone** (medium-colored area), whereas those that were excited (but not enough to reach threshold) are in the **subliminal fringe** (light-colored area). However, the combined excitation produced by simultaneous volleys in the two nerves reaches threshold in three additional motor neurons (facilitation zone), and a reflex discharge occurs in a total of seven motor neurons.

A similar effect could be elicited by repetitive stimulation of one of the muscle nerves, provided that the stimuli occur close enough together so that some of the excitatory effect of the first volley still persists after the second volley arrives. This effect is called **temporal summation.** Both spatial and temporal summation depend on the properties of the excitatory postsynaptic potentials evoked by the group Ia afferent fibers in α-motor neurons (see Chapter 4).

The number of α-motor neurons that supply each muscle is limited, and not all can be activated, even by a large peripheral input. For these reasons, the availability of motor neurons for summation is limited. If a volley in one of the two muscle nerves of Fig. 9-11 reaches the motor nucleus at a time when the motor neurons are highly excitable, the reflex discharge will be relatively large (Fig. 9-11, *C*). A similar volley in the other muscle nerve might also produce a large reflex response. However, when the two muscle nerves are excited simultaneously, the reflex might be less than the sum of the two independently evoked reflexes. In this case, each muscle nerve activates seven α-motor neurons, but the volleys in the two nerves together cause only 12 motor neurons to discharge. This phenomenon is called **occlusion.**

Reflex testing by the techniques described to demonstrate spatial and temporal summation and occlusion can also be employed to demonstrate **inhibition.** A monosynaptic reflex discharge can be evoked by stimulating the group Ia afferent fibers in a muscle nerve. This tests the reflex excitability of a population of α-motor neurons. The discharges of either extensor or flexor α-motor neurons can be recorded by

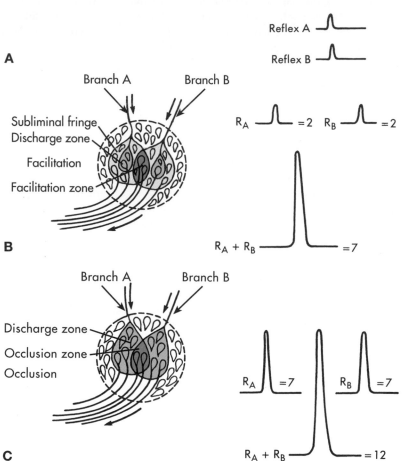

■ **Fig. 9-11** **A,** The arrangement for using electrically evoked afferent volleys and recordings from motor axons in a ventral root to study reflexes. **B,** An experiment in which combined stimulation of two muscle nerves resulted in spatial summation. In **C** the combined volleys caused occlusion. (Redrawn from Eyzaguirre C, Fidone SJ: *Physiology of the nervous system,* ed 2, Chicago, 1975, Mosby-Year Book.)

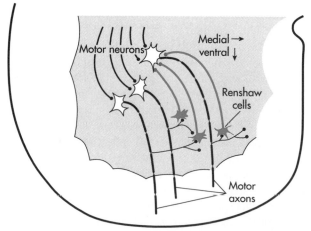

■ **Fig. 9-12**   Recurrent inhibitory pathway. (Redrawn from Eccles JC: *The physiology of synapses,* New York, 1964, Academic Press.)

choosing the proper muscle nerve to be stimulated. Other kinds of afferent fibers can also be stimulated. For example, stimulation of the group Ia afferent fibers in the nerve to the antagonist muscles produces **reciprocal inhibition.** If the small afferent fibers of a cutaneous nerve are stimulated to evoke a flexion reflex, the α-motor neurons to extensor muscles will be inhibited (and those to flexor muscles will be excited). Stimulation of a ventral root causes the excitation of inhibitory interneurons, called **Renshaw cells,** by way of the recurrent collaterals of α-motor axons (Fig. 9-12). The Renshaw cells inhibit monosynaptic reflexes (and also group Ia inhibitory interneurons) and produce recurrent inhibition (or facilitation).

This kind of reflex testing has been used to determine the circuitry involved in the various reflexes described in this

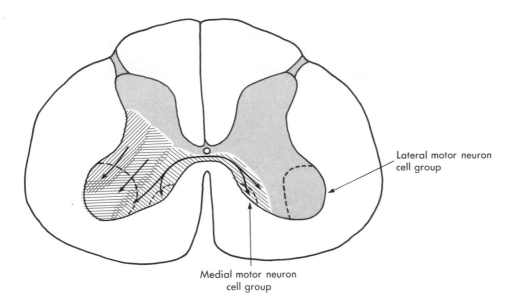

■ **Fig. 9-13** Relationships between interneurons in the intermediate region and ventral horn to the lateral and medial groups of motoneurons. (Redrawn from Sterling P, Kuypers HGJM: *Brain Res* 7:419, 1968.)

Lateral motor neuron cell group

Medial motor neuron cell group

chapter. As previously mentioned, similar reflex testing can be done in human subjects by using the H-reflex to test the excitability of α-motor neurons.

DESCENDING PATHWAYS INVOLVED IN MOTOR CONTROL

Topographic Organization of the Spinal and Cranial Nerve Motor System

Spinal cord motor neurons are organized topographically in the ventral horn. Motor neurons that supply the axial musculature form a column of cells that extends the length of the spinal cord. In the cervical and lumbosacral enlargements, the cells are located in the most medial part of the ventral horn. Motor neurons that supply the limb muscles form columns that extend for one or two segments in the lateral part of the ventral horn in the cervical and lumbosacral enlargements. The motor neurons to the muscles of the distal limb are located most laterally, whereas those that innervate more proximal muscles are located more medially in the lateral ventral horn. Note that the α- and γ-motor neurons to a given muscle are found side by side in the same motor neuron column.

The interneurons that connect with the motor neurons in the enlargements are also topographically organized. In general, interneurons that supply the limb muscles are located mainly in the lateral parts of the deep dorsal horn and intermediate region. Those that supply the axial muscles, however, are located in the medial part of the ventral horn (Fig. 9-13). Because these interneurons receive synaptic connections from primary afferent fibers and from the axons of pathways that descend from the brain, many of these interneurons are found in spinal reflex arcs and in the descending motor control systems.

An important aspect of interneuronal systems is that the laterally placed interneurons project ipsilaterally to motor neurons that supply the distal or the proximal limb muscles, whereas the medial interneurons project bilaterally (see Fig. 9-13). This arrangement of the lateral interneurons allows the limbs to be controlled independently. On the other hand, the bilateral arrangement of the medial interneurons allows bilateral control of motor neurons to the axial muscles to provide postural support to the trunk and neck.

Figure 9-14 shows some of the sites in the reflex circuitry that can be influenced by descending motor control pathways. Descending pathways can synapse on interneurons that (1) cause presynaptic inhibition of primary afferent fibers, or (2) participate in postsynaptic excitation or inhibition of other interneurons or of motor neurons. In addition, some descending pathways make direct excitatory connections to α- or γ-motor neurons.

A similar arrangement is found in cranial nerve motor nuclei. Most of these nuclei are similar to the axial motor nuclei of the spinal cord in that they supply muscles near the midline. For example, facial motor neurons that supply the corrugator muscle of the forehead and the orbicularis oculi muscles, which close the eyes, must operate bilaterally—the blink reflex causes both eyelids to close simultaneously. The head muscles, which function like the distal limb muscles, control facial expression and the tongue. The motor neurons that supply these muscle function independently. Thus, neurons in the facial motor nucleus that supply the lower face can elicit unilateral changes in facial expression, and hypoglossal motor neurons can move the tongue toward one side. The interneuronal systems in the brainstem are organized like those in the spinal cord to support these bilateral or unilateral motor activities.

Classification of Descending Motor Pathways

Pyramidal versus extrapyramidal pathways. Descending motor pathways have traditionally been subdivided into the pyramidal tract and the extrapyramidal pathways. This

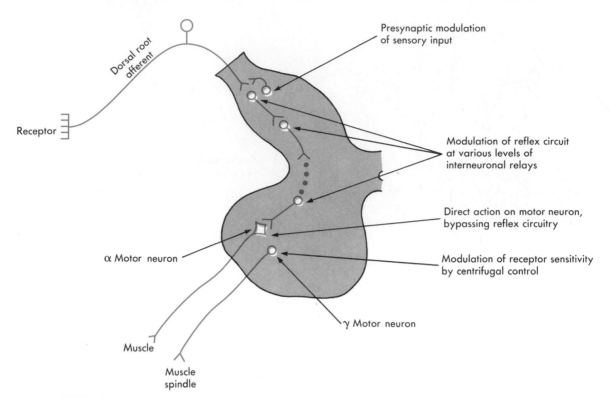

■ Fig. 9-14   Sites in a spinal reflex arc that are potential targets for descending motor control pathways.

terminology reflects the important clinical dichotomy between pyramidal tract disease and extrapyramidal disease. In **pyramidal tract disease,** the corticospinal tract is interrupted. The signs of this disease were originally attributed to the loss of function of the pyramidal tract (so named because the corticospinal tract passes through the medullary pyramid). However, in many cases of pyramidal tract disease, the functions of other pathways are also altered, and pyramidal tract signs are not necessarily caused only by the loss of the corticospinal tract (see page 170).

The term **extrapyramidal** is even more problematic. The extrapyramidal tracts presumably include all descending motor pathways, except the pyramidal tract. The term **extrapyramidal** disease generally signifies one of several diseases of the basal ganglia. However, the main motor pathway involved in basal ganglion diseases is the corticospinal tract. Other extrapyramidal motor pathways, such as the reticulospinal tract, play prominent roles in cerebellar and other motor disorders, as well as in basal ganglion disease. Because the basis for the differences between the pyramidal and extrapyramidal classification system for the descending pathways is not clear, this classification system is not used in this book.

Lateral versus medial motor systems.   Another way of classifying the motor pathways is based on their sites of termination in the spinal cord and on the consequent differences in their roles in the control of manipulation and posture. The **lateral pathways** terminate directly on motor neurons or on the interneuronal groups in the lateral parts of the spinal cord gray matter (Fig. 9-15). The lateral pathways

excite motor neurons directly. They also influence reflex arcs that control the fine movements of the distal limbs, as well as those that activate supporting musculature in the proximal limbs. The **medial pathways** end in the medial ventral horn on the medial group of interneurons (see Fig. 9-15). These interneurons connect bilaterally with motor neurons that control the axial musculature, and thereby contribute to balance and posture. They also contribute to the control of proximal limb muscles. In this book, we use the lateral/medial terminology to classify the descending motor pathways.

The Descending Motor Pathways

The lateral system: lateral corticospinal tract.   The pathway that is most important for control of manipulative ability of the limbs is the **lateral corticospinal tract** (Fig. 9-15). The ventral corticospinal tract belongs to the medial system (see below). The **corticobulbar tract,** which projects to the cranial nerve motor nuclei, has subdivisions that are comparable with the lateral and ventral corticospinal tracts.

Organization of the lateral corticospinal and corticobulbar tracts.   The corticospinal and corticobulbar tracts originate in a wide region of the cerebral cortex. This region includes the motor, premotor, and supplementary motor areas, and the somatosensory cortex. The cells of origin of these tracts include both large and small pyramidal cells of layer V of the cortex and the giant pyramidal cells of Betz. Betz cells are a characteristic feature of the motor cortex.

In the most caudal region of the medulla, about 80% of the axons cross to the opposite side. They then descend in

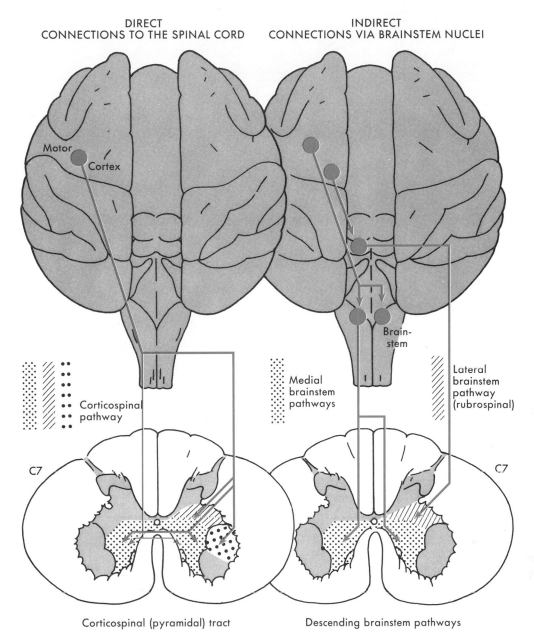

DIRECT
CONNECTIONS TO THE SPINAL CORD

INDIRECT
CONNECTIONS VIA BRAINSTEM NUCLEI

Motor Cortex

Brain-stem

Corticospinal pathway

Medial brainstem pathways

Lateral brainstem pathway (rubrospinal)

C7

C7

Corticospinal (pyramidal) tract

Descending brainstem pathways

■ **Fig. 9-15** Subdivision of the pathways descending from the cerebral cortex and brainstem to the spinal cord into a lateral and a medial system, based on the terminations of these pathways in the spinal cord gray matter. The lateral pathways end on motor neurons to distal muscles *(dots)* and interneurons projecting to these motor neurons *(hatched area).* The medial pathways end on interneurons supplying motor neurons to the axial muscles (stippled area). (Redrawn from Brinkman C: *Split-brain monkeys: cerebral control of contralateral and ipsilateral arm, hand, and finger movements,* doctoral dissertation, Rotterdam, The Netherlands, 1974, Erasmus University.)

the dorsal lateral funiculus, as the lateral corticospinal tract. The remaining axons continue caudally in the ventral funiculus on the same side as the ventral corticospinal tract. The corticobulbar tract terminates in the brainstem at a level near the target nuclei. Part of the corticobulbar tract ends contralaterally in the part of the facial nucleus that supplies muscles of the lower face and in the hypoglossal nucleus. This component of the corticospinal tract is organized like the lateral corticospinal tract. The remainder of the corti-

cobulbar tract ends bilaterally and, in this respect, is organized like the ventral corticospinal tract.

Motor cortex. The motor cortex has a topographic organization that parallels that of the somatosensory cortex (Fig. 9-16, *A*). The face is represented laterally, near the lateral fissure; the hand is represented more medially on the convexity of the cerebrum; and the lower extremity is represented largely on the medial aspect of the hemisphere. The figurine in the illustration is called a **motor homunculus.** The

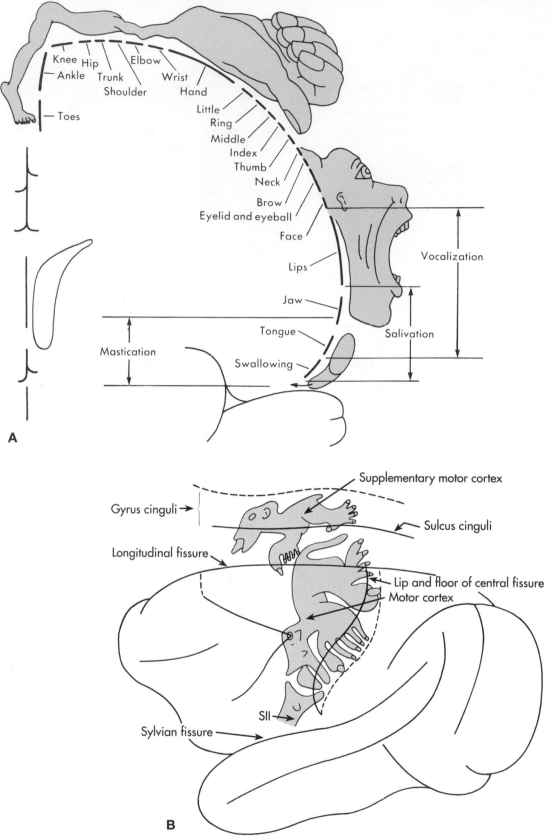

A

Knee Hip Elbow
Ankle Trunk Wrist
Shoulder Hand

Toes

Little
Ring
Middle
Index
Thumb
Neck
Brow
Eyelid and eyeball
Face
Lips
Jaw
Tongue
Swallowing

Vocalization

Salivation

Mastication

B

Supplementary motor cortex

Gyrus cinguli →

Sulcus cinguli

Longitudinal fissure

Lip and floor of central fissure
Motor cortex

Sylvian fissure

SII

■ **Fig. 9-16** Topographic organization of the motor cortex. **A,** The cortex is cut in a coronal section, and the somatotopic map of the body and face is shown as a "motor homunculus." The sizes of different body parts indicate the amount of cortex devoted to motor control of that part. **B,** The somatotopic organization of the motor cortex, supplementary motor cortex, and SII areas of the cerebral cortex of a monkey. (Redrawn from Eyzaguirre C, Fidone SJ: *Physiology of the nervous system,* ed 2, Chicago, 1975, Mosby-Year Book. **A** slightly modified from Penfield W, Rasmussen T: *The cerebral cortex of man,* New York, 1950, The Macmillan Co; **B** slightly modified from Woolsey CN et al: *Res Publ Assoc Res Nerv Ment Dis* 30:238, 1952.)

distortion of the various body parts in the homunculus indicates approximately how much of the cortex is devoted to their motor control.

The other cortical motor areas also contain somatotopic representations. Figure 9-16, *B* shows the motor areas of the cerebral cortex of a monkey. The somatotopic map of the motor cortex is shown along the precentral gyrus. Note how closely this map resembles that of the human (see Fig. 9-16, *A*). Other somatotopic maps exist in the SII cortex, which is located in the roof of the lateral fissure (part of which is shown in Fig. 9-16, *B*), and in the supplementary motor cortex, which is located on the medial aspect of the hemisphere just rostral to the motor cortex. Note that the digital representation in monkeys (and presumably in humans) is directed toward the central sulcus, whereas the proximal limbs are represented more rostrally. This arrangement is significant. Anatomic studies have shown that the caudal part of the precentral gyrus projects to the dorsolateral region of the ventral horn. This locus contains motor neurons that supply the distal musculature of the extremities. The rostral part of the precentral gyrus, however, projects to the intermediate region, which contains interneurons of the lateral group. Thus, the caudal part of the motor cortex can directly influence the activity of motor neurons to the hand and digit muscles.

The motor cortex proper was first identified by electrical stimulation experiments. When an electrical stimulus is applied to the cerebral cortex, the lowest threshold points for a motor response are found to lie in the motor cortex. Such stimuli evoke discrete movements of distal muscles on the contralateral side. For example, when stimuli are applied in the face representation, the contralateral face moves; when the hand representation is stimulated, the contralateral hand moves.

> The motor cortex has been explored in human patients undergoing surgery to remove scar tissue that had caused **posttraumatic epilepsy.** Often, resection of the scar cures the epilepsy. However, the surgeon must be careful not to damage normal areas of the motor cortex, because this will paralyze the affected musculature.

The direct innervation of motor neurons by the lateral corticospinal tract can have important clinical consequences if this pathway is interrupted. The most important function that is lost after interruption of this pathway is fine control of the digits. Similarly, when the corticobulbar tract is interrupted, voluntary movements of the lower face and tongue are lost.

The Medial System

As previously mentioned, the ventral corticospinal tract and much of the corticobulbar tract can be regarded as medial system pathways. These tracts end on the medial group of interneurons in the spinal cord, and on equivalent medial system neurons in the brainstem. The axial muscles are controlled by these pathways. These muscles often contract bilat-

erally to provide postural support or some other bilateral function, such as chewing or wrinkling of the brow.

Other medial system pathways originate in the brainstem. Some of these include the lateral and medial vestibulospinal tracts, the pontine and medullary reticulospinal tracts, and the tectospinal tract.

Lateral and medial vestibulospinal tracts. The lateral vestibulospinal tract originates in the lateral vestibular nucleus. This tract descends ipsilaterally through the ventral funiculus of the spinal cord, and ends on interneurons of the medial group. The lateral vestibulospinal tract excites motor neurons that supply proximal postural muscles. The input to the lateral vestibular nucleus is from both the semicircular ducts and the otolith organs. An important function of the lateral vestibulospinal tract is to assist with postural adjustments after angular and linear accelerations of the head. In decerebrate experimental preparations, the lateral vestibulospinal tract becomes hyperactive, presumably because of the loss of descending inhibitory controls. This hyperactivity is largely responsible for the extensor hypertonus seen in these animals.

The medial vestibulospinal tract originates from the medial vestibular nucleus. This tract descends in the ventral funiculus of the spinal cord to cervical and midthoracic levels, and it ends on the medial group of interneurons. The sensory input to the medial vestibular nucleus from the labyrinth is chiefly from the semicircular ducts. This pathway thus mediates adjustments in head position in response to angular accelerations of the head.

Pontine and medullary reticulospinal tracts. The cells that give rise to the pontine reticulospinal tract are in the medial pontine reticular formation. The tract descends in the ipsilateral ventral funiculus, and it ends on the medial group of interneurons. Its function, like that of the lateral vestibulospinal tract, is to excite motor neurons to the proximal extensor muscles to support posture.

The medullary reticulospinal tracts arise from neurons of the medial medulla. The tracts descend bilaterally in the ventral lateral funiculus, and they end mainly on the medial group of interneurons, although some also end on lateral interneurons. The function of the pathway is mainly inhibitory. Some of the inhibitory connections end directly on motor neurons.

The tectospinal tract. The tectospinal tract originates in the deep layers of the superior colliculus. The axons cross to the contralateral side, just below the periaqueductal gray. They then descend in the ventral funiculus of the spinal cord to terminate on the medial group of interneurons in the upper cervical spinal cord. The tectospinal tract regulates contralateral movements of the head in response to visual, auditory, and somatic stimuli.

Monoaminergic Pathways

In addition to the lateral and medial systems, less specifically organized systems descend from the brainstem to the spinal cord. These include several pathways that use monoamines as synaptic transmitters.

The locus coeruleus and the nucleus subcoeruleus are nuclei located in the rostral pons, and they are composed of norepinephrine-containing neurons. These nuclei project widely to the spinal cord through the lateral funiculi. The terminals are on interneurons and motor neurons. The dominant effect of the pathway is inhibitory.

The raphe nuclei of the medulla give rise to several raphe-spinal projections to the spinal cord. Many of the raphe-spinal cells contain serotonin. Terminals on dorsal horn interneurons are inhibitory, whereas terminals on motor neurons are excitatory. The dorsal horn projection may help reduce nociceptive transmission, whereas the ventral horn projection may enhance motor activity.

In general, the monoaminergic pathways may alter the responsiveness of spinal cord circuits, including the reflex arcs. In this respect, they induce widespread changes in excitability, rather than discrete movements or specific changes in behavior.

A common cause of motor disorder in human patients is interruption of the corticospinal tract as it traverses the internal capsule; such interruptions occur in capsular strokes. The resulting disorder is often termed a **pyramidal tract syndrome,** or **upper motor neuron disease.** The motor changes characteristic of this disorder include (1) increased phasic and tonic stretch reflexes (spasticity); (2) weakness, usually of the distal muscles, especially the finger muscles; (3) pathological reflexes, including the **sign of Babinski** (dorsiflexion of the big toe and fanning of the other toes when the sole of the foot is stroked); and (4) a reduction in superficial reflexes, such as the abdominal and cremasteric reflexes. However, if only the corticospinal tract is interrupted, as can occur with a lesion of the medullary pyramid, most of these signs are absent. In this situation, the most prominent deficits are weakness of the distal muscles, especially of the fingers, and a positive sign of Babinski. Spasticity does not occur, but muscle tone decreases. Evidently, spasticity depends on disordered function of the corticospinal tract and other pathways, such as the reticulospinal tracts.

The effects of interruption of the medial system pathways are quite different from those produced by corticospinal tract lesions. The main deficits of medial system interruption are an initial reduction in the tone of postural muscles and loss of righting reflexes (see page 171). Long-term effects include locomotor impairment and frequent falling. However, manual manipulation of objects is perfectly normal.

BRAINSTEM CONTROL OF POSTURE AND MOVEMENT

The importance of motor control pathways that originate in the brainstem is evident from observations of the extensor hypertonus and the increased phasic stretch reflexes that occur in decerebrate animals. Particular brainstem systems have been identified that influence posture, locomotion, and eye movements.

Postural Reflexes

Several reflex mechanisms are evoked when the head is moved or the neck is bent. There are three types of postural reflexes: vestibular reflexes, tonic neck reflexes, and righting reflexes. The sensory receptors responsible for these reflexes include the vestibular apparatus, which is stimulated by head movements, and stretch receptors in the neck.

The **vestibular reflexes** constitute one class of postural reflexes. Rotation of the head activates sensory receptors of the semicircular ducts (Chapter 8). In addition to eye movements (see page 171), the sensory input to the vestibular nuclei results in postural adjustments. These adjustments are mediated by commands transmitted to the spinal cord through the lateral and medial vestibulospinal tracts and the reticulospinal tracts. The lateral vestibulospinal tract activates extensor muscles that support posture. For instance, if the head is rotated to the left, the postural support is increased on the left side. This increased support prevents the subject from falling to the left as the head rotation continues. Any disease that eliminates labyrinthine function in the left ear will cause the person to tend to fall to the left. Conversely, a disease that irritates the left labyrinth will cause the person to tend to fall to the right. The medial vestibulospinal tract causes contractions of neck muscles that oppose the induced movement (**vestibulocollic reflex).**

Tilting the head changes linear acceleration and activates the otolith organs of the vestibular apparatus. This activation can produce eye movements (see page 171) and postural adjustments. For example, tilting the head and body forward (without bending the neck, and consequently without evoking the tonic neck reflexes) in a quadriped, such as a cat, results in extension of the forelimbs and flexion of the hindlimbs. This vestibular action tends to restore the body toward its original posture. Conversely, if the head and body are tilted backward (without bending the neck), the forelimbs flex and the hindlimbs extend. Otolithic organs also contribute to the **vestibular placing reaction.** If an animal, such as a cat, is dropped, stimulation of the utricles leads to extension of the forelimbs in preparation for landing.

The **tonic neck reflexes** are another type of positional reflex. These reflexes are activated by the muscle spindles found in the neck muscles. These muscles contain the largest concentration of muscle spindles of any muscle in the body. If the neck is bent (without tilting the head), the neck muscle spindles evoke the tonic neck reflexes without interference from the vestibular system. When the neck is extended, the forelimbs extend and the hindlimbs flex (Fig. 9-17). The opposite effects occur when the neck is flexed. Note that these effects are the opposite of those evoked by the vestibular system. Furthermore, if the neck is bent to the left, the extensor muscles in the limbs on the left contract more, and the flexor muscles in the limbs on the right side relax.

The third class of postural reflexes is the **righting reflexes.** These reflexes tend to restore an altered position of

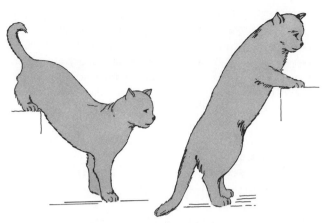

■ Fig. 9-17   Effect of the tonic neck reflexes on limb position. The head is in a normal position in the cat, avoiding vestibular stimulation. Dorsiflexion of the neck causes extension of the forelimbs and flexion of the hindlimbs. Conversely, ventriflexion of the neck results in flexion of the forelimbs and extension of the hindlimbs. (Redrawn from Roberts TDM: *Neurophysiology of postural mechanisms,* London, 1979, Butterworth.)

the head and body toward normal. The receptors responsible for righting reflexes include the vestibular apparatus, the neck stretch receptors, and mechanoreceptors of the body wall.

Locomotion

The spinal cord contains neural circuits that serve as a pattern generator for locomotion. There are actually several pattern generators, one for each limb. These permit independent movements of the limbs. However, all these pattern generators are interconnected to ensure coordination of limb movements. The pattern generator for locomotion is an example of a biological oscillator. Similar oscillators are responsible for activities such as scratching, chewing, and respiration.

The pattern generator for locomotion is normally activated by commands that descend from the brain. The **midbrain locomotor center** is thought to organize commands to initiate locomotion. Voluntary activity that originates in the motor cortex can trigger locomotion by the action of corticobulbar fibers on the midbrain locomotor center. The commands are relayed through the reticular formation and then through the spinal cord via the reticulospinal tracts. Locomotion is also influenced by afferent activity. The afferent influence ensures that the pattern generator adapts to changes in the terrain as locomotion proceeds. Such changes may occur rapidly during running, and locomotion must then be adjusted to ensure proper coordination.

An important requirement for locomotion is adequate postural support. This is normally provided by the postural muscles in response to activity in the reticulospinal tract. Immediately after transection of the spinal cord, postural activity is lost during spinal shock. In humans, locomotion is not recovered, even after spinal shock resolves. However, some locomotion is possible in animals with spinal transec-

tion, especially if postural support is produced by stimulation of afferent fibers or by pharmacological activation of spinal cord interneuronal circuits.

Control of Eye Position

The position of the eyes is controlled by several neural systems. **Conjugate eye movements** are movements of both eyes in the same direction and in an equal amount. Conjugate eye movements are controlled by the vestibuloocular reflex and by the optokinetic, saccadic, and smooth pursuit movement systems. The eyes can also converge or diverge under the control of the vergence system.

Vestibuloocular reflex. The vestibuloocular reflex is designed to maintain a stable image on the retina during rapid head rotation. This reflex causes the eyes to move simultaneously in the direction opposite to, and in an amount equal to, head movement.

Optokinetic reflex. The optokinetic reflex is another means by which the nervous system compensates for head movements to maintain a stable visual target. This reflex maintains a stable image when head movements are slow, and the sensory input for the reflex is provided by the visual system. The optokinetic system can be activated by having a subject view a rotating drum painted with vertical stripes. A more familiar stimulus is provided by viewing telephone poles from a moving car.

Smooth pursuit. In contrast to the vestibuloocular and optokinetic reflexes, which allow the eyes to remain fixated on the visual target during head movements, the smooth pursuit system allows the eyes to remain fixated on a moving visual target, even though the head may be still. Smooth pursuit occurs only when the stimulus is moving; it cannot result from a command.

Saccadic system. A **saccade** is a stereotyped rapid eye movement that allows a visual target to be centered on the fovea of the retina. Saccades can be made voluntarily, or they can be a part of several reflexes. The velocity of a saccade is too rapid for visual processing. Hence, no visual feedback occurs during the movement. Saccades are corrected by smaller saccades that occur after the initial large change in eye position.

Vergence system. The vergence system allows the two eyes to converge or diverge, and thereby permits fixation of the eyes on nearby or distant objects and on objects that approach or move away. During convergence movements, accommodation of the lens for near vision and pupillary constriction also occur (see Chapter 8).

Neural activity in the vestibuloocular reflex. The vestibuloocular reflex is triggered by angular acceleration of the head. The sensory receptors that are involved are the semicircular ducts (Chapter 8). When the head is rotated, for instance to the left, the endolymph distorts the cupulas in the horizontal ducts. Activity in vestibular afferent fibers to the left horizontal duct increases, and that in afferent fibers to the right duct decreases. The increased activity in the vestibular nuclei on the left side activates ascending fibers that excite medial rectus motor neurons on the left side and lateral rectus motor neurons on the right side. The reduced activity in the vestibular nuclei on the right side of the head has the converse effect.

As the head continues to rotate, the eyes reach the limit of their excursion. When this happens the eyes perform a saccade in the same direction as the head rotation. They then fixate a visual target and again begin to rotate in the direction opposite to the head movement. Saccadic eye movements are so rapid that visual images are blurred and therefore the visual process is minimally disrupted.

The alternation of slow and fast eye movements as the head turns is called **vestibular nystagmus.** This process is normal under these conditions of vestibular stimulation. However, vestibular nystagmus can also be produced by diseases that either reduce or increase vestibular afferent discharges. In such cases, the eye movements produce a sense that the environment is spinning, and the subject may report dizziness.

Another reflex that affects eye position and that originates with vestibular signals is **ocular counterrolling.** When the head is tilted, activation of the otolith organs causes rotation of the eyes in the opposite direction. This movement tends to keep the retinal image aligned with the horizon.

When the labyrinth is irritated in one ear, as in **Meniere's disease,** or when a labyrinth is rendered nonfunctional, as may happen as a result of head trauma or disease of the labyrinth, the signals transmitted through the vestibuloocular reflex pathways from the two sides become unbalanced. **Vestibular nystagmus** can then result. For example, irritation of the labyrinth of the left ear can increase the discharges of afferents that supply the left horizontal semicircular duct. The signal produced resembles that normally produced when the head is rotated to the left (which causes a relative shift in endolymph toward the utricle). Thus, the signal elicits a nystagmus with a slow phase to the right and a fast phase to the left. The direction of nystagmus is named according to the fast movement; therefore, this nystagmus is "left-beating." Destruction of the labyrinth in the right ear produces effects similar to those induced by irritation of the left labyrinth.

Clinical testing of labyrinthine function is commonly done either by rotating the patient in a **Bárány chair** to activate the labyrinths in both ears, or by introducing cold or warm water into the external auditory canal of one ear **(caloric test).** When a person is rotated in a Bárány chair, nystagmus develops during the rotation. The direction of the fast phase of the nystagmus is in the same direction as the rotation. When the rotation of the chair is halted, nystagmus develops in the opposite direction (postrotatory nystagmus). If an attempt is made to stand, the person feels dizzy and tends to fall.

The caloric test is more useful, because it can distinguish between malfunction of the labyrinths on the two sides. The head is bent backward about 60 degrees, so that the two horizontal canals are essentially vertical. If warm water is introduced into the left ear, the endolymph in the left semicircular duct tends to rise as the specific gravity of the endolymph decreases because of heating. As a result, the kinocilia of the left ampullary crest hair cells are deflected toward the utricle, the discharge of the afferents that supply this epithelium increases, and a nystagmus occurs with the fast phase toward the left. The nystagmus produces a sense that the environment is spinning to the right, and the subject tends to fall to the right. The opposite effects are produced if cold water is placed in the ear. A mnemonic expression that can help in remembering the direction of the nystagmus in the caloric test is COWS ("cold opposite, warm same"). In other words, cold water results in a fast phase of nystagmus toward the opposite side, and warm water causes a fast phase toward the same side.

Gaze Centers

In addition to the vestibular nuclei, brainstem centers for control of eye movement include the horizontal and vertical gaze centers. The **horizontal gaze center** consists of neurons in the paramedian pontine reticular formation, in the vicinity of the abducens nucleus. The **vertical gaze center** is located in the reticular formation of the midbrain.

The horizontal gaze center. Because the circuitry and operation of the horizontal gaze center are better understood than those of the vertical gaze center, the horizontal gaze center is discussed here in detail. The horizontal gaze center controls both saccadic eye movements and smooth pursuit movements.

Figure 9-18 is an overview of the neural circuitry by which the horizontal gaze center elicits conjugate eye movements, and Fig. 9-19 shows the activity of certain types of neurons that form the circuitry responsible for horizontal eye movements. The right horizontal gaze center has excitatory connections with motor neurons in the ipsilateral abducens nucleus, and with medial rectus motor neurons in the contralateral oculomotor nucleus. It also has inhibitory connections with the left horizontal gaze center by way of the reticular formation.

Burst neurons in one of the horizontal gaze centers may initiate saccadic eye movements (Fig. 9-19). At the same time, pause cells, which are inhibitory interneurons located in the nucleus of the dorsal raphe, stop the discharge of the contralateral burst cells. The activity of burst neurons and the inhibition of pause neurons are triggered by commands that originate elsewhere, such as in the frontal eye field, which is located in the premotor area of the contralateral frontal lobe, or in the superior colliculus. Tonic cells also participate in eye movement control. Tonic cells discharge during smooth pursuit movements, and burst-tonic neurons fire both during saccades and during smooth pursuit movements. Presumably, the burst helps initiate the movement, and the tonic activity maintains the new eye position. Tonic activity may arise as a consequence of activity in a neural integration circuit that is located in a nucleus near the

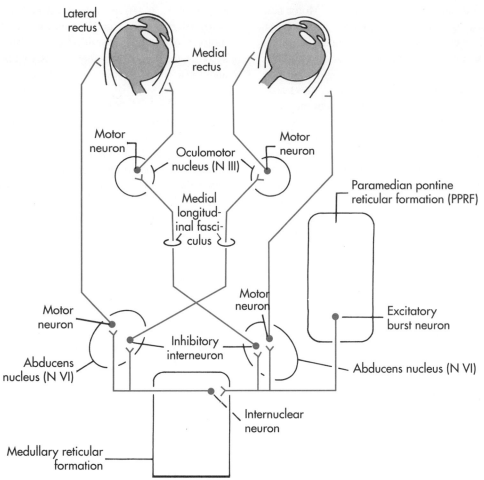

■ **Fig. 9-18** Neural circuit by which the horizontal gaze center elicits conjugate eye movements. Excitation of burst neurons of the right horizontal gaze center causes activation of abducens motor neurons on the right and medial rectus motor neurons on the left. The ascending pathway to the oculomotor nucleus is through the medial longitudinal fasciculus. The left horizontal gaze center is simultaneously inhibited by way of the reticular formation.

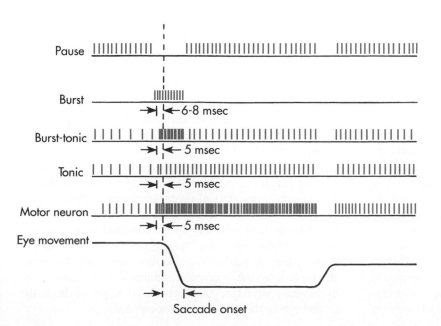

■ **Fig. 9-19** Several types of neurons contribute to the circuitry by which the horizontal gaze center elicits conjugate eye movements. These include pause, burst, burst-tonic, and tonic neurons, in addition to motor neurons.

midline, just rostral to the hypoglossal nucleus. Motor neurons to the eye muscles involved in a saccade have a burst-tonic form of discharge, first to initiate movement, and then to maintain eye position.

A lesion of the brainstem that destroys one of the horizontal gaze centers results in a tonic deviation of the eyes toward the opposite side. This deviation is caused in part by the paralysis of the ipsilateral lateral rectus muscle, but also occurs because the tonic activity of the contralateral horizontal gaze center is no longer compensated for by the destroyed center. If the corticospinal tract is also interrupted on the same side, the limbs on the side of the body opposite to the lesion will be paralyzed.

The role of the cerebellum and the cerebral cortex in the control of eye movements will be discussed later in this chapter.

Superior colliculus. Neurons in the deep layers of the superior colliculus can trigger conjugate eye movements (saccades) that cause the eyes to target novel or threatening visual, auditory, or somatosensory stimuli. The superior colliculus sends impulses to the horizontal or vertical gaze centers to organize the conjugate eye movements.

MOTOR CONTROL BY THE CEREBRAL CORTEX, CEREBELLUM, AND BASAL GANGLIA

Early in this chapter, emphasis was placed on reflexes, which are simple, stereotyped motor acts that occur in response to specific stimuli. The neural basis for voluntary movements will now be emphasized. Voluntary movements are often complex. They may vary when repeated, and they are often initiated as a result of cognitive processes rather than in response to an external stimulus.

The **lateral corticospinal tract** is the most important descending pathway for fine movements that use distal muscles, such as those that control the hand and fingers. A portion of the **corticobulbar tract** is important for the control of facial and tongue movements. However, many other pathways are also engaged to activate more proximal and axial muscles.

Before any movement occurs, commands carried by descending motor pathways must first be organized in the brain. The target of the movement is identified by pooling sensory information in the **posterior parietal cerebral cortex** (Fig. 9-20). This information is then transmitted to the supplementary motor and premotor areas, where a motor plan is developed. The plan includes information about the specific muscles that need to be contracted, the strength of the contraction, and the sequence of contraction. The motor plan is implemented by commands transmitted from the primary motor cortex through the descending pathways. Successful execution of these motor commands, however, depends on feedback provided to the motor cortex through the ascending pathways to the somatosensory

cortex (Fig. 9-20), as well as through the visual pathway. During the planning and execution stages of a movement, motor processing is provided by two major motor control systems, the cerebellum and the basal ganglia (see pages 179 and 183).

Motor Control by the Cerebral Cortex

Cortical motor areas. As previously discussed, the primary motor area in the cerebral cortex was originally mapped on the basis of experiments in which electrical stimuli applied to the cortex evoked discrete, contralateral movements. However, movements can also be evoked when other cortical areas are stimulated more intensely. On the basis of these stimulation studies, the effects produced by lesions, anatomical experiments, electrophysiological recordings, and modern imaging studies in humans, several "motor" areas of the cerebral cortex have been recognized (Fig. 9-20). These include the **primary motor cortex** in the precentral gyrus, the **premotor area** just rostral to the primary motor cortex, the **secondary somatosensory cortex** located in the roof of the lateral fissure (usually called SII), and the **supplementary motor cortex** on the medial aspect of the hemisphere. The **frontal eye fields** are located in a part of the premotor area just rostral to the face representation in the motor cortex.

Stimuli applied to the surface of the **primary motor cortex** evoke discrete contralateral movements that involve several muscles. However, stimulation within the cortex with microelectrodes can elicit contractions of individual muscles. Mapping studies based on microstimulation reveal that the motor cortex consists of a mosaic of motor points related to particular muscles or sets of muscles. These points are called **cortical efferent zones,** which can be regarded as motor columns. They are organized somatotopically, and together they produce the motor homunculus (see Fig. 9-16).

Stimulation of the **supplementary motor cortex** can produce vocalization or complex postural movements. The postural movements can be bilateral. Although stimulation can evoke rhythmic movements from the supplementary motor cortex, it can also have the opposite result, namely a temporary arrest of movement or speech. Removal of the supplementary motor cortex retards movements of the opposite extremities and may evoke forced grasping movements with the contralateral hand. Stimulation of the **premotor cortex** rarely evokes movements unless the stimulus intensity is strong.

Stimulation of the **frontal eye fields** in one hemisphere causes a saccadic conjugate deviation of the eyes toward the contralateral side. Vertical saccades require bilateral stimulation of the frontal eye fields. Removal of the frontal eye field on one side transiently weakens contralateral gaze, and in humans the eyes may deviate toward the side of the lesion. Memory-guided saccades are eliminated, but visually evoked saccades persist. Elimination of all saccadic eye movements would require bilateral lesions of both the frontal eye fields and the superior colliculi.

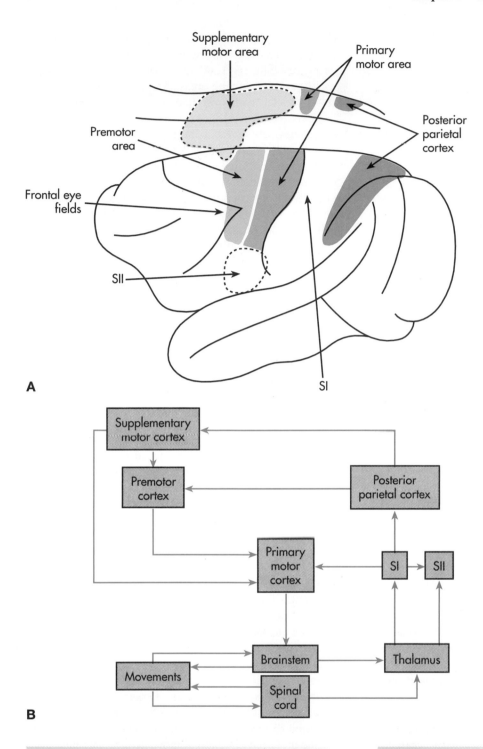

■ Fig. 9-20 **A,** Motor regions of the cerebral cortex of a monkey. The motor cortex, premotor area, SII cortex, and supplementary motor cortex are indicated with different colors. The dashed lines around the SII and the supplementary motor cortex are meant to indicate that these areas are hidden from surface view. **B,** Flow diagram showing the sequence of activity in the voluntary motor and somatosensory feedback pathways. (**A,** Redrawn from Eyzaguirre C, Fidone SJ: *Physiology of the nervous system,* ed 2, St. Louis, 1975, Mosby.)

A lesion of the frontal lobe, which may occur during a stroke, can prevent contralateral conjugate eye movements. Because the frontal eye field on the contralateral side is intact, the eyes tend to deviate toward the side of the lesion. This impairment may be associated with a contralateral hemiplegia. The deficit pattern contrasts with that produced by a brainstem lesion that destroys the horizontal gaze center and interrupts the corticospinal tract in the base of the pons. A lesion of the horizontal gaze center on one side of the pons causes an inability to make conjugate eye movements toward the side of the lesion; the eyes will deviate toward the side contralateral to the lesion. If the corticospinal tract in the base of the pons is also interrupted, contralateral hemiplegia occurs. Thus, a frontal lobe lesion can cause a loss of volitional contralateral conjugate eye movements and cause contralateral hemiplegia, whereas a pontine lesion can cause a loss of volitional ipsilateral conjugate eye movements and cause a contralateral hemiplegia.

Connections of the motor regions of the cortex. The motor areas of the cortex receive input from a number of sources (Fig. 9-20). Ascending pathways that relay in the thalamus provide information about somatosensory events.

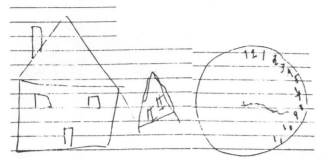

■ **Fig. 9-21** Drawings made by a patient 2 days after damage to the right parietal lobe. The drawing on the left was made by the physician to show a house. The drawing in the middle was made by the patient and was meant to copy the physician's drawing. The drawing of the clock with all of the numbers on the right indicates neglect of the left extrapersonal space by the patient. (From Cotman CW, McGaugh JL: *Behavioral neuroscience,* New York, 1980, Academic Press.)

This information can reach the motor cortex directly from the thalamus, or indirectly by way of the SI somatosensory cortex. Both somatosensory and visual information are conveyed to the motor areas from the posterior parietal cortex. The frontal eye fields receive visual input from the occipital lobe (this connection is not shown in Fig. 9-20). The motor areas of the cortex also receive information through circuits that interconnect with the cerebellum and basal ganglia. In addition, the motor regions of the cortex are interconnected.

The output of the motor regions of the cortex to the spinal cord and brainstem is conducted through several descending pathways. These pathways include not only direct projections through the corticospinal and corticobulbar tracts, but also indirect projections through the reticular formation. The motor regions also contribute to the cerebellar and basal ganglion circuits. The frontal eye fields project to the superior colliculus and to the reticular formation.

Role of supplementary motor and premotor areas in motor programming. The supplementary motor cortex is involved in motor programming and is active during the planning and the execution stages of complex movements. Its actions are partially mediated by direct corticospinal connections, and partly by a relay to the primary motor cortex. Monitoring of the regional blood flow of the cerebral cortex during motor tasks shows that blood flow increases when the individual is merely thinking about a movement, as well as when the movement is actually executed. In contrast, the blood flow in the primary motor cortex increases only when the movement is executed. In addition to its role in motor planning, the supplementary motor cortex may assist in the coordination of posture and voluntary movements.

The premotor cortex receives a major input from the posterior parietal cortex, and its output influences chiefly the medial system of descending pathways. Hence, this region of the cortex appears to control the axial muscles. Neurons in this area may discharge during the preparation for a movement.

The posterior parietal cortex is often called the **parietal association cortex.** This region receives somatosensory, visual, vestibular, and auditory information from the primary sensory receiving areas. A lesion of the left posterior parietal cortex in humans results in language disorders, but when the lesion is on the right side, the subject **neglects** contralateral somatic or visual stimuli. Patients with right parietal lobe lesions have difficulty recognizing or drawing three-dimensional objects and in recognizing spatial relationships (Fig. 9-21). Similar difficulties may be experienced by patients with lesions of the left parietal lobe, but these may be masked by the language disorder.

Preparation for volitional movements requires several hundred milliseconds; the exact time depends on the difficulty of the task. Lesions of the premotor, supplementary motor, and posterior parietal areas can hamper the ability to prepare for voluntary movements. When such lesions are produced experimentally, the results resemble **apraxia,** which represents the failure of patients with frontal or parietal lobe lesions to perform complex movements despite retention of sensation and the ability to make simple movements.

Activity of individual corticospinal neurons. The role of individual corticospinal neurons in the control of movements has been investigated in trained monkeys. In these experiments, discharges from a neuron in the primary motor cortex are recorded during the execution of a simple movement, such as wrist flexion, that the monkey had previously learned (Fig. 9-22). The corticospinal neurons discharge before the onset of the movement. This sequence suggests that these cells induce the movement. Furthermore, analysis of the electrical potentials from the appropriate muscle reveals that a particular corticospinal neuron excites a specific group of motor neurons monosynaptically. The discharges of corticospinal neurons appear to relate either to the contractile force of the muscle that generates the movement, or to the rate of change in force, rather than to the position of the joint.

A given corticospinal neuron may discharge before a movement occurs in any direction. However, a neuron tends to discharge most vigorously when the movement occurs in a preferred direction. Neurons in a motor column all have the same preferred direction of movement. Commands from a population of corticospinal neurons that have somewhat different preferred directions will determine the actual direction of a movement.

Sensory feedback to corticospinal neurons. As already emphasized, the corticospinal neurons of the primary motor cortex receive sensory information through the thalamus, as well as from sensory areas of the cerebral cortex. This information is used by the motor cortex to ensure that the evoked movements are appropriate.

Figure 9-23 shows how somatosensory information influences corticospinal neurons. Cutaneous receptors and proprioceptive receptors, such as muscle spindles, transmit

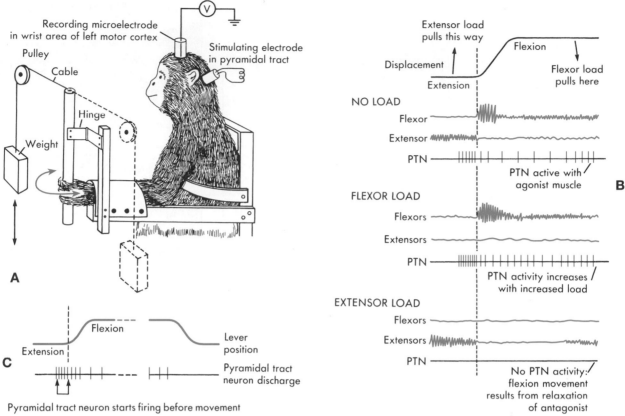

Recording microelectrode in wrist area of left motor cortex

Stimulating electrode in pyramidal tract

Pulley

Cable

Hinge

Weight

A

Extensor load pulls this way

Flexion

Displacement

Extension

Flexor load pulls here

NO LOAD

Flexor

Extensor

PTN

PTN active with agonist muscle

B

FLEXOR LOAD

Flexors

Extensors

PTN

PTN activity increases with increased load

EXTENSOR LOAD

Flexors

Extensors

PTN

No PTN activity: flexion movement results from relaxation of antagonist

Flexion

Extension

Lever position

Pyramidal tract neuron discharge

C

Pyramidal tract neuron starts firing before movement

■ **Fig. 9-22** **A,** Experimental arrangement for recording from a corticospinal neuron during trained movements of the wrist. **B** and **C,** The cell discharges before the movement. With an extensor load (**B,** *lower trace*), the cell fails to discharge, indicating that it encodes force rather than displacement. *PTN,* Pyramidal tract neuron. (Redrawn from Kandel ER, Schwartz JH: *Principles of neural science,* New York, 1981, Elsevier Science Publishing.)

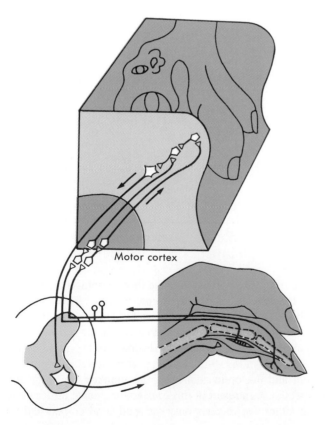

Motor cortex

■ **Fig. 9-23** Sensory input to a corticospinal neuron that causes flexion of a digit. (Redrawn from Asanuma H: *Physiologist* 16:143, 1973.)

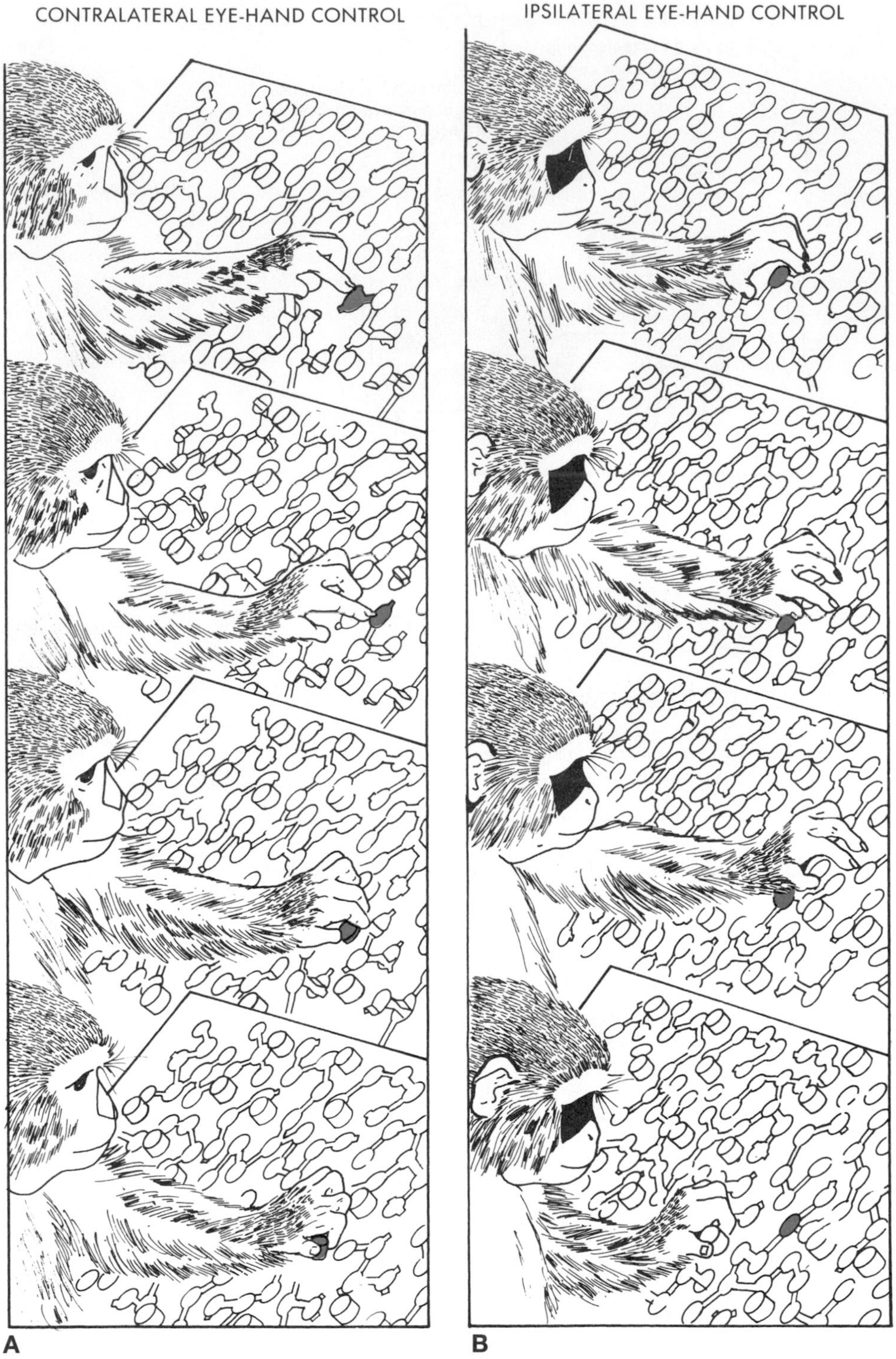

CONTRALATERAL EYE-HAND CONTROL

IPSILATERAL EYE-HAND CONTROL

■ **Fig. 9-24** Drawings showing hand and finger movements by a monkey subjected to a complete commissurotomy. **A,** To retrieve a food pellet from a well, the monkey is able to use a precision grip involving hand and digit muscles. **B,** The task cannot be performed by the left hand when the right eye is masked. (Redrawn from Brinkman C: *Split-brain monkeys: cerebral control of contralateral and ipsilateral arm, hand, and finger movements,* doctoral dissertation, Rotterdam, The Netherlands, 1974, Erasmus University.)

A

B

information about mechanical contact of the fingertip with a surface and the position of the finger joints via the ascending somatosensory pathways (such as the dorsal column–medial lemniscus system). The corticospinal neurons activate motor neurons that flex the finger. As the fingertip moves into contact with the surface, cutaneous receptors in the skin of the ventral surface of the fingertip discharge, and thereby excite the corticospinal neurons through somatosensory projections. Muscle spindle afferent fibers are activated by

stretch of the flexor muscle as the finger contacts the surface and also activates the corticospinal neurons. Thus, sensory feedback from both skin and muscle facilitates the activity of the corticospinal neurons and enhances the movement.

Another example of sensory feedback to the motor cortex is illustrated in Fig. 9-24. In this preparation the corpus callosum and the optic chiasm of the monkey are surgically transected. As a result of this transection, visual information from either eye reaches only the ipsilateral cortex, and no information is transmitted from one hemisphere to the other. The monkey's task is to remove a pellet of food from one of the wells on a board. This task requires fine movements of the digits. Thus, the response involves corticospinal control that originates on the side of the brain contralateral to the hand used. When the right eye is open, the monkey can retrieve the food pellets with its left hand (Fig. 9-24, *A*). However, if the right eye is masked, the monkey can no longer retrieve the food with its left hand (Fig. 9-24, *B*), although it can with its right hand. This movement is possible, because visual information that reaches the left hemisphere through the left eye influences corticospinal neurons in the left motor cortex. Hence, the influence of the corticospinal neurons affects the control of fine movements of the digits in the right hand (Fig. 9-25).

Motor Control by the Cerebellum

Overview of the role of the cerebellum in motor control. The cerebellum helps regulate movements and posture, and it plays a key role in some forms of motor learning. Note that removal of the cerebellum affects neither sensation nor muscle strength. The cerebellum influences the rate, range, force, and direction of movements. Therefore, damage to the cerebellum disturbs the coordination of movements.

The cerebellum helps regulate the vestibuloocular reflex, and it participates in the improvements in motor performances that result from practice of motor skills. Therefore, the cerebellum is thought to be involved in motor learning.

The cerebellum exerts its motor control on a moment-by-moment basis. It uses sensory information from various sources, most prominently from the proprioceptive system, to update its computations of body position, muscle length, and muscle tension. The cerebellum may be able to compare this sensory feedback with neural signals that are transmitted to the cerebellum from the motor areas of the cerebral cortex and that represent the desired motor act. Errors are corrected by output signals from the cerebellum to other components of the motor system.

Cerebellar organization. The cerebellum ("little brain") is located in the posterior fossa of the cranium, just below the occipital lobe, and it is connected to the brainstem. From the cerebellar surface, only the cortex is visible. The cerebellar cortex is subdivided into three rostrocaudally arranged lobes, the **anterior lobe,** the **posterior lobe,** and the **flocculonodular lobe** (Fig. 9-26). The cerebellar lobes are separated by two major fissures, the **primary fissure** and the **posterolateral fissure,** and each lobe is made up of one or more **lobules.** Each lobule of the cerebellar cortex is composed of a series of transverse folds, called **folia.**

In addition to this rostrocaudal organization, the cerebellum also has a sagittal organization. At the midline of the cerebellum is the **vermis** (named for its segmented appearance, which resembles an earthworm). Extending laterally are the **hemispheres.** In the paravermal region, between the hemispheres and vermis, is the **intermediate region.**

Like the cerebrum, the cerebellum has a cortical structure, and white matter is found in both of these parts of the

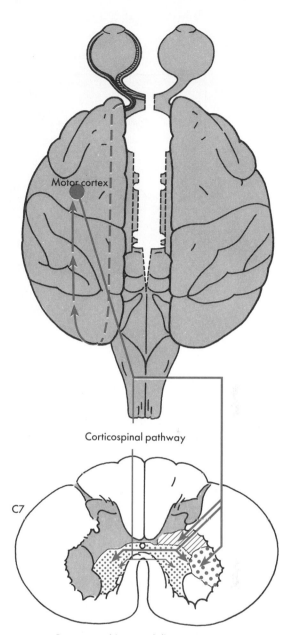

■ **Fig. 9-25**   Split-brain preparation, as in **Fig. 9-24.** Drawing above shows the relationship of pathways carrying visual information to the left hemisphere from the left eye to the corticospinal neurons on the left side that control hand and digit movement on the right. (Redrawn from Brinkman C: *Split-brain monkeys: cerebral control of contralateral and ipsilateral arm, hand, and finger movements,* doctoral dissertation, Rotterdam, The Netherlands, 1974, Erasmus University.)

brain beneath the cortex. When the cerebellum is sectioned, the white matter of the cerebellum can be seen beneath the cortex. Buried in the white matter are the **deep cerebellar nuclei.** The most lateral of these nuclei is the **dentate nucleus.** The other deep nuclei include the **emboliform, globose,** and **fastigial nuclei.**

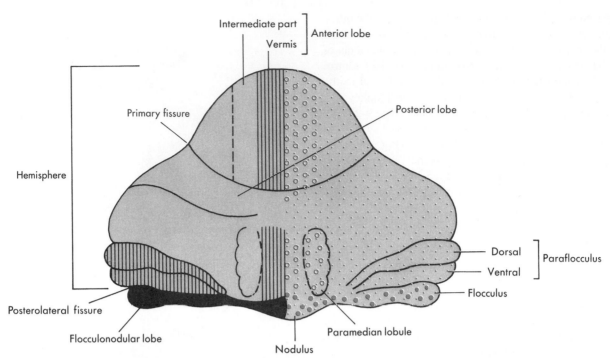

■ **Fig. 9-26**   The subdivision of the cerebellum into archicerebellum, paleocerebellum, and neo-cerebellum is shown by the black, hatched, and gray areas. Terminations of vestibulocerebellar fibers are indicated by the large dots, spinocerebellar fibers by the open circles, and pontocerebellar fibers by the small dots. (Redrawn from Brodal A: *Neurological anatomy,* ed 3, New York, 1981, Oxford University Press.)

Subdivisions of the cerebellum. Phylogenetically, the cerebellum can be subdivided into the archicerebellum, paleocerebellum, and neocerebellum (Fig. 9-26). These subdivisions correspond to regions of the cerebellum that are dominated by vestibular input (the **vestibulocerebellum**), by spinal cord input (the **spinocerebellum**), and by indirect input from the cerebrum by way of the pontine nuclei (the **corticocerebellum**). The vestibulocerebellum consists chiefly of the flocculonodular lobe. However, it also includes a small part of the vermis and intermediate cortex of the posterior lobe. The spinocerebellum is composed of most of the vermis and intermediate region. The corticocerebellum consists of the hemispheres.

Afferent pathways of the cerebellar divisions

Vestibulocerebellum. The afferent pathways of the vestibulocerebellum include direct projections of primary vestibular afferent fibers, and also second-order projections from the vestibular nuclei (Chapter 8). As the vestibular afferent fibers enter the cerebellum, they give off collaterals to the fastigial nuclei before they reach the flocculonodular lobe and parts of the posterior lobe. The vestibulocerebellum regulates eye movements, stance, and gait.

Spinocerebellum. The ascending pathways that convey somatosensory information to the spinocerebellum include several spinocerebellar tracts. These neuronal tracts carry information about the lower extremities, trunk, and upper extremities. Two of the spinocerebellar pathways are respon-

sible for providing discrete, moment-by-moment information to the cerebellum about limb position and muscle actions. The other two spinocerebellar tracts provide less discrete information. They project bilaterally in the cerebellum, and operate under the control of descending systems. There are also indirect projections from the spinal cord to the cerebellum. The spinocerebellum regulates truncal and proximal limb movements.

Corticocerebellum. Wide areas of the cerebral cortex provide input indirectly to the corticocerebellum via connections to the pontine nuclei. The pontine nuclei also receive input from the spinal cord and from brainstem pathways. The pontine nuclei send axons across the midline to enter the cerebellum. The corticocerebellum regulates movements of the distal parts of the limbs, and it participates in motor planning.

Inferior olive. The inferior olivary nucleus is a massive structure located in the rostral medulla. This nucleus receives input from the vestibular system, the spinal cord, and the cerebral cortex through a number of pathways. The cells of the inferior olivary nucleus give rise to the olivocerebellar tract, which crosses the midline and enters the cerebellum. The axons are distributed to all parts of the cerebellum, and they send collaterals to the deep cerebellar nuclei and to the cortex. Their terminals form a special type of cerebellar afferent fibers, called **climbing fibers.** Conversely, all of the other cerebellar afferent pathways terminate as **mossy fibers** in the cerebellar cortex (see Fig. 9-27).

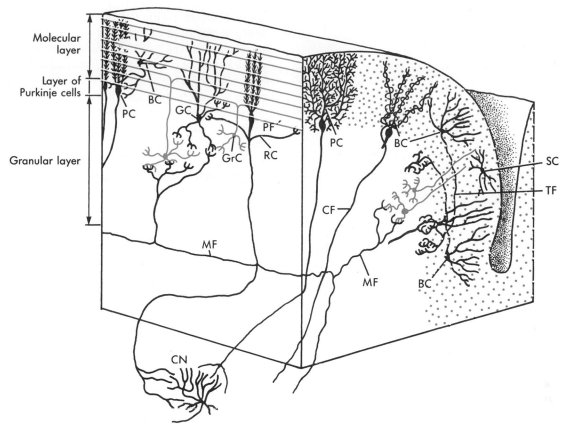

■ Fig. 9-27   Three-dimensional view of the cerebellar cortex. The cut face at the left is along the long axis of the folium; the cut face at the right is at right angles to the long axis. *PC,* Purkinje cell; *BC,* basket cell; *GC,* Golgi cell; *GrC,* granule cell; *PF,* parallel fiber; *RC,* recurrent collateral; *MF,* mossy fiber; *CF,* climbing fiber; *CN,* deep cerebellar nuclear cell; *SC,* stellate cell; *TF,* transverse fiber. (Redrawn from Fox CA: *The structure of the cerebellar cortex.* In Crosby EC, Humphrey TH, Lauer EW, editors: *Correlative anatomy of the nervous system,* New York, 1962, Macmillan.)

Cerebellar cortex

Organization of the cerebellar cortex. The following description of the cerebellar cortex is organized in reference to its output cell, the **Purkinje cell.** The cell bodies of Purkinje cells form the middle of the three layers of the cerebellar cortex. The other two layers are the granular layer and the molecular layer (Fig. 9-27).

The granular layer is adjacent to the white matter, and it contains many interneurons, including **granule cells** and **Golgi cells.** The granule cells comprise about half the neurons in the brain. The mossy fibers form excitatory terminals on the dendrites of granule cells. A given granule cell receives convergent inputs from many mossy fibers. The terminal zones are called **cerebellar glomeruli.** The Golgi cells provide inhibitory projections to the glomeruli.

The axons of the granule cells ascend through the Purkinje cell layer to the molecular layer, where they bifurcate and form **parallel fibers.** The parallel fibers pass along the long axis of the folium, and they form excitatory synapses with the dendrites of the Purkinje cells and the Golgi cells. They also form excitatory synapses with **stellate cells** and **basket cells,** which are interneurons of the molecular layer. A given parallel fiber synapses with about 50 Purkinje cells, and a

given Purkinje cell receives synapses from about 200,000 parallel fibers.

The stellate and basket cells of the molecular layer are inhibitory interneurons that synapse with Purkinje cells. The stellate cells form terminals on the dendrites of the Purkinje cells, and the basket cells form terminals on the cell bodies of the Purkinje cells. The basket cell projections to the Purkinje cells are oriented at right angles to the long axis of the folium. These basket cell axons are called **transverse fibers** (Fig. 9-27).

Activity of Purkinje cells in the cerebellar cortex. As mentioned, the Purkinje cells function as the output cells of the cerebellar cortex. They receive numerous excitatory synapses on their dendrites from the parallel fibers formed by the granule cells. Each Purkinje cell also receives a powerful excitatory connection from a single climbing fiber (Fig. 9-27). The climbing fiber branches repeatedly as it ascends the dendritic tree, and it makes numerous active contacts with the Purkinje cell.

Mossy fiber inputs to the cerebellar cortex cause a Purkinje cell to discharge single action potentials **(simple spikes),** whereas a single climbing fiber causes repetitive discharges of the Purkinje cell **(complex spikes)** (Fig. 9-28). Because

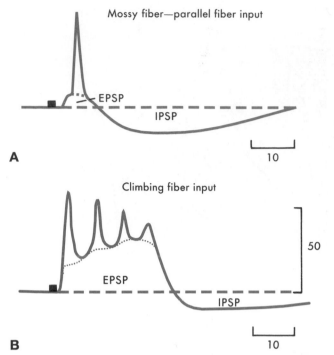

Fig. 9-28   Responses of a Purkinje cell to a mossy fiber input (**A**) and to a climbing fiber input (**B**). *EPSP,* Excitatory postsynaptic potential; *IPSP,* inhibitory postsynaptic potential.

the climbing fibers generate complex spikes at a low frequency, they do not substantially change the average firing rates of Purkinje cells. However, they do alter the responsiveness of Purkinje cells to mossy fiber inputs. These changes can be persistent, and hence they may participate in motor learning. The Purkinje cell also receives inhibitory connections from the basket and stellate cells (see Fig. 9-27). These connections produce inhibitory postsynaptic potentials in Purkinje cells.

The axon of the Purkinje cell descends through the granule layer and enters the cerebellar white matter (see Fig. 9-27). Most Purkinje cell axons terminate in one of the deep cerebellar nuclei. However, some Purkinje cells in the vestibulocerebellum project from the cerebellum to the lateral vestibular nucleus. The discharges of the Purkinje cells inhibit the activity of neurons in the deep cerebellar nuclei and lateral vestibular nucleus. The inhibitory neurotransmitter used by Purkinje cells is γ-aminobutryic acid (GABA).

That the output of the cerebellar cortex is inhibitory may seem paradoxical. However, recall that the input pathways to the cerebellum send collaterals to the deep cerebellar nuclei. It should not be surprising, therefore, that the cells in the deep nuclei are very active. The role of the cerebellar cortex is to modulate this activity appropriately. Thus, the real output of the cerebellum is via the projections of the deep cerebellar nuclei.

The role of cerebellar Purkinje cells in motor learning. As previously mentioned, the climbing fibers may participate in motor learning by influencing the effectiveness of mossy fibers in exciting Purkinje cells. Evidence for this theory comes from experiments on the gain of the vestibuloocular reflex. The "gain" of a reflex describes the direction and amount of the response produced by that reflex. Normally, the gain of this reflex is one: when the head rotates to the left, the eyes will rotate by an equal angle, but in the opposite direction. However, if lenses are used to reverse the visual fields, the eye movements are reversed after a learning period. Thus, the reflex gain is reduced and finally changed in sign. A lesion of the vestibulocerebellum will prevent this alteration in gain.

In monkeys, the frequency of complex spikes recorded from Purkinje cells initially increases as the animals learn to perform a new task. Once the task is learned, the frequency of complex spikes gradually decreases. The increased frequency of complex spikes is thought to change the efficacy of the synapses made by parallel fibers onto Purkinje cells. Such changes are believed to be the basis of motor learning. The cellular mechanism responsible for motor learning in the cerebellum appears to be a form of **long-term depression (LTD).**

Projections of the deep cerebellar nuclei. The deep cerebellar nuclei receive topographically organized projections from the Purkinje cells of the different parasagittal zones of the cerebellum.

Vestibulocerebellum and vermal spinocerebellum. Purkinje cells in the flocculonodular lobe and part of the vermis project to the fastigial nucleus, or directly to the lateral vestibular nucleus. The fastigial nucleus, in turn, projects to the lateral vestibular nucleus and to the reticular formation. Thus the output of these regions of the cerebellum influences axial and proximal limb muscles by way of the lateral vestibulospinal and reticulospinal tracts, which belong to the medial motor projection system (page 169).

Intermediate spinocerebellum. The Purkinje cells of the paravermal region project to the emboliform and globose nuclei. These nuclei connect with brainstem nuclei and also with the contralateral thalamus. The latter pathway resembles that formed by projections from the dentate nucleus (see below). The ascending connections allow the paravermal spinocerebellum to influence the discharges of corticospinal neurons.

Corticocerebellum. Purkinje cells of the cerebellar hemisphere project to the dentate nucleus, which in turn projects to the contralateral thalamus. The thalamic neurons distribute their axons to the premotor and primary motor cortex and influence the planning and initiation of voluntary movements.

Damage to the cerebellum impairs motor function on the ipsilateral side of the body. The reason for this impairment is that the cerebellum gives rise to crossed connections that regulate a contralaterally projecting motor output system, the lateral corticospinal tract. The specific motor deficits that result from cerebellar lesions depend on which functional component of the cerebellum is most affected. If the flocculonodular lobe is damaged, the

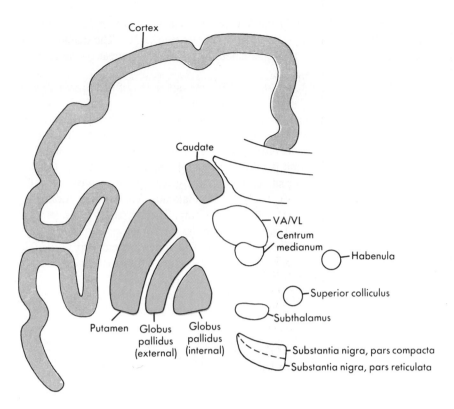

■ Fig. 9-29 Basal ganglia and associated nuclei. *VA/VL,* Ventral anterior and ventral lateral thalamic nuclei. (From Brodal A: *Neurological anatomy,* ed 3, New York, 1981, Oxford University Press.)

motor disorders resemble those produced by a lesion of the vestibular apparatus; the disorders include difficulty in balance and gait, and often in nystagmus. If the vermis is affected, the motor disturbance affects the trunk, and if the intermediate region or hemisphere is involved, motor disorders occur in the limbs. The part of the limbs affected depends on the site of damage; hemispheric lesions affect the distal muscles more than do paravermal lesions.

Types of motor dysfunction in cerebellar disease include disorders of coordination, equilibrium, and muscle tone. Incoordination is called **ataxia** and is often expressed as **dysmetria,** a condition in which errors in the direction and force of movements prevent a limb from being moved smoothly to a desired position. Ataxia may also be expressed as **dysdiadochokinesia,** in which repeated supinations and pronations of the arm are difficult to execute. When more complicated movements are attempted, **decomposition of movement** occurs, in which the movement is accomplished in a series of discrete steps, rather than as a smooth sequence. An **intention tremor** appears when the subject is asked to touch a target; the affected hand (or foot) develops a tremor that increases in magnitude as the target is approached. When equilibrium is disturbed, **impaired balance** may be seen; the individual tends to fall toward the affected side and may walk with a wide-based stance. Speech may be slow and slurred, a defect called **scanning speech.** Muscle tone may be diminished **(hypotonia);** the diminished tone may be associated with a **pendular knee jerk.** This can be demonstrated by eliciting a phasic stretch reflex of

the quadriceps muscle by striking the patellar tendon; the leg continues to swing back and forth because of the hypotonia, in contrast to the highly damped oscillation in a normal person.

Motor Control by the Basal Ganglia

The basal ganglia are the deep nuclei of the cerebrum. In association with other nuclei in the diencephalon and midbrain, the basal ganglia differ from the cerebellum in the way they regulate motor activity. Unlike the cerebellum, the basal ganglia do not receive an input from the spinal cord, but they do receive direct input from the cerebral cortex, unlike the cerebellum. The main action of the basal ganglia is on the motor areas of the cortex by way of the thalamus. In addition to their role in motor control, the basal ganglia contribute to affective and cognitive functions. Lesions of the basal ganglia produce abnormal movements and posture.

Organization of the basal ganglia and related nuclei. The basal ganglia include the **caudate nucleus,** the **putamen,** and the **globus pallidus** (Fig. 9-29). The term **striatum,** derived from the striated appearance of these nuclei, refers only to the caudate nucleus and putamen. The striations are produced by the fiber bundles that are formed by the anterior limb of the internal capsule as it passes between the caudate nucleus and putamen. The globus pallidus has two parts, the **external segment** and the **internal segment.** The combination of putamen and globus pallidus is often referred to as the **lentiform nucleus.**

Associated with the basal ganglia are several thalamic nuclei. These include the **ventral anterior (VA)** and **ventral** lateral (VL) nuclei, and several components of the intralaminar complex. Other associated nuclei are the **subthalamic nucleus** of the diencephalon and the **substantia nigra** of the midbrain. The substantia nigra ("black substance") derives its name from its content of melanin pigment. Many of the neurons in the **pars compacta** of this nucleus contain melanin, a by-product of dopamine synthesis. The other subdivision of the substantia nigra is the **pars reticulata.** This structure can be regarded as an extension of the internal segment of the globus pallidus, because these nuclei have an identical origin and similar connections.

Connections and operation of the basal ganglia. The circuitry of the basal ganglia is very complex, and we still lack a full understanding of the operation of the basal ganglia.

Neurons of the striatum begin to discharge before movements occur. This sequence suggests that these neurons help select the movement that is to be made. Activity in the putamen is related to the occurrence of movements of the body, whereas activity in the caudate nucleus is related to eye movements.

With the exception of the primary visual and auditory cortices, most regions of the cerebral cortex project topographically to the striatum. An important component of the cortical input to the striatum originates in the motor cortex. The corticostriatal projection arises from neurons in layer V of the cortex. The neurons appear to use glutamate as their excitatory neurotransmitter. The striatum then influences neurons in the VA and VL nuclei of the thalamus by two pathways, direct and indirect (Fig. 9-30). The thalamic neurons in turn excite neurons of the motor areas of the cerebral cortex.

Direct pathway. The overall action of the direct pathway through the basal ganglia to the motor areas of the cortex is to enhance motor activity. In the direct pathway, the striatum projects to the internal segment of the globus pallidus (and to the pars reticulata of the substantia nigra; Fig. 9-30). This projection is inhibitory, and the main transmitter is GABA. The internal segment of the globus pallidus projects to the VA and VL nuclei of the thalamus. These connections also use GABA and are inhibitory. The VA and VL nuclei send excitatory connections to the prefrontal, premotor, and supplementary motor cortex. This input to the cortex influences motor planning, and it also affects the discharges of corticospinal and corticobulbar neurons.

The direct pathway appears to function as follows. Neurons in the striatum have little background activity, and during movements they are activated by their inputs from the cortex. In contrast, neurons in the internal segment of the globus pallidus have a high level of background activity. When the striatum is activated, its inhibitory projections to the globus pallidus slow the activity of pallidal neurons. However, the pallidal neurons themselves are inhibitory, and they normally provide a tonic inhibition of neurons in the VA and VL nuclei of the thalamus. Therefore, activation of the striatum causes **disinhibition** of the neurons of the VA and VL nuclei.

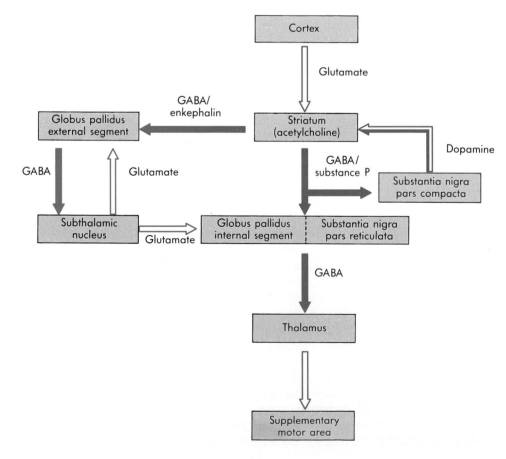

■ **Fig. 9-30**   Direct and indirect pathways through the basal ganglia. The direct pathway is from the cortex to the striatum to the internal segment of the globus pallidus to the thalamus and back to the cortex. The indirect pathway is from the cortex to the striatum to the external segment of the globus pallidus to the subthalamic nucleus to the internal segment of the globus pallidus to the thalamus and back to the cortex. Solid red arrows show inhibitory connections; open arrows show excitatory connections. (Redrawn from Kandel ER, Schwartz JH, Jessell TM: *Principles of neural science,* ed 3, New York, 1991, Elsevier.)

Thus, the disinhibition excites these neurons, and consequently excites their target neurons in the motor areas of the cerebral cortex. Because the motor cortex evokes movements by activating α- and γ-motor neurons in the spinal cord and brainstem, the basal ganglia can regulate movements by enhancing the activity of neurons in the motor cortex.

Indirect pathway. The overall effect of the indirect pathway is to reduce the activity of neurons in the motor areas of the cerebral cortex. The indirect pathway involves inhibitory connections from the striatum to the external segment of the globus pallidus, which in turn sends an inhibitory projection to the subthalamic nucleus. The subthalamic nucleus in turn sends an excitatory projection back to the internal segment of the globus pallidus (Fig. 9-30).

In this pathway, pallidal neurons in the external segment are inhibited by the GABA released from the striatal terminals in the globus pallidus. The external segment of the globus pallidus normally releases GABA in the subthalamic nucleus, and thereby inhibits the subthalamic neurons. Therefore, striatal inhibition of the external segment of the globus pallidus results in the disinhibition of neurons of the subthalamic nucleus. The subthalamic neurons are normally active, and they excite neurons in the external segment of the globus pallidus by releasing glutamate. When the neurons of the subthalamic nucleus become more active because of disinhibition, they release more glutamate in the internal segment of the globus pallidus. This transmitter excites neurons in the internal segment, and consequently activates inhibitory projections that affect the VA and VL thalamic nuclei. The activity of the thalamic neurons consequently decreases, as does the activity of the cortical neurons that they influence.

The direct and indirect pathways thus have opposing actions; an increase in the activity of either one of these pathways might lead to an imbalance in motor control. Such imbalances, which are typical of basal ganglion diseases, may alter the motor output of the cortex.

Actions of neurons in the pars compacta of the substantia nigra on the striatum. Dopamine is the neurotransmitter used by neurons of the pars compacta of the substantia nigra. In the nigrostriatal pathway, the release of dopamine has an overall excitatory action on the direct pathway and an inhibitory action on the indirect pathway. This difference is caused by the action of dopamine on different types of dopamine receptors that are found in the internal segment of the globus pallidus (D1 receptors, which are excitatory) and in the external segment of the globus pallidus (D2 receptors, which are inhibitory). The overall consequence of dopamine release in both cases is a facilitation of activity in the motor areas of the cerebral cortex. Hence, the projection from the substantia nigra affects the mechanisms by which the basal ganglia regulate motor output. A loss of the dopaminergic neurons of the pars compacta of the substantia nigra is a crucial factor in the bradykinesia that is found in Parkinson's disease.

Differences between the basal ganglion and cerebellar motor loops. The organization of the motor loops that connect the basal ganglia and cerebellum with the motor regions of the cerebral cortex differs in several ways. The basal ganglia receive input from most areas of the cerebral cortex, whereas the inputs to the cerebellum from the cerebral cortex are more restricted. The output from the basal ganglia is also more widespread, and reaches the prefrontal cortex, as well as all of the premotor areas. The cerebellar circuit influences only the premotor and motor cortex. Finally, the basal ganglia do not receive somatosensory information from ascending pathways in the spinal cord, and they have few connections with the brainstem. In contrast, the cerebellum is the target of several somatosensory pathways, and it has rich connections with brainstem nuclei.

Subdivision of the striatum into striosomes and matrix. On the basis of the associated neurotransmitters, the striatum has been subdivided into zones, called **striosomes** and **matrix.** The cortical projections related to motor control end in the matrix area. The limbic system projects to the striosomes. The striosomes are thought to synapse in the pars compacta of the substantia nigra and to influence the dopaminergic nigrostriatal pathway.

Role of the basal ganglia in motor control. The basal ganglia mainly influence the motor cortex. Therefore, the basal ganglia has an important influence on the lateral system of motor pathways. Such an influence is consistent with some of the movement disorders observed in diseases of the basal ganglia. However, the basal ganglia also must regulate the medial motor pathways, because diseases of the basal ganglia can also affect posture and tone of the proximal muscles.

The deficits seen in the various basal ganglion diseases include abnormal movements (**dyskinesias**), increased muscle tone (**cogwheel rigidity**), and slowness in initiating movements (**bradykinesia**). Abnormal movements include **tremor, athetosis, chorea, ballism,** and **dystonia.** The tremor of basal ganglion disease is a "pill-rolling" tremor that occurs when the limb is at rest. Athetosis consists of slow, writhing movements of the distal parts of the limbs, whereas chorea is characterized by rapid, flicking movements of the extremities and facial muscles. Ballism is associated with violent, flailing movements of the limbs (ballistic movements). Finally, dystonic movements are slow truncal movements that distort the body positions.

Parkinson's disease is a common disorder that is characterized by tremor, rigidity, and bradykinesia. This disease is caused by loss of neurons in the pars compacta of the substantia nigra. Consequently, the striatum suffers a severe loss of dopamine. Neurons of the locus coeruleus and the raphe nuclei, as well as of other monoaminergic nuclei, are also lost. The loss of dopamine diminishes the activity of the direct pathway and increases the activity of the indirect pathway. The net effect is an increase in the activity of neurons in the internal segment of the globus pallidus. This results in a greater inhibition of the neurons in the VA and VL nuclei, and a less pronounced activation of the motor cortical areas. The consequence is slowed movements (bradykinesia).

Before the dopaminergic neurons are completely lost, administration of L-dopa can relieve some of the motor deficits in Parkinson's disease. L-Dopa is a precursor of dopamine, and it can cross the blood–brain barrier. Currently, the possibility is being explored of transplanting dopamine-synthesizing neurons into the striatum. Future research will no doubt focus on the potential for human embryonic stem cells to play such a therapeutic role.

Another basal ganglion disturbance is **Huntington's disease.** This results from a genetic defect that involves an autosomal dominant gene. This defect leads to the loss of GABAergic and cholinergic neurons of the striatum (and also degeneration of the cerebral cortex, with a resultant dementia). Loss of inhibition of the external globus pallidus presumably diminishes the activity of neurons in the subthalamic nucleus. Hence, the excitation of neurons of the internal segment of the globus pallidus would be reduced. This will disinhibit the neurons in the VA and VL nuclei. The resulting enhancement of activity in neurons in the motor areas of the cerebral cortex may help explain the choreiform movements of Huntington's disease. The rigidity in Parkinson's disease may in a sense be the opposite of chorea, because overtreatment of patients with Parkinson's disease with L-dopa can result in chorea.

Hemiballism is caused by a lesion of the subthalamic nucleus on one side of the brain. In this disorder, involuntary, violent flailing movements of the limbs may occur on the side of the body contralateral to the lesion. Because the subthalamic nucleus excites neurons of the internal segment of the globus pallidus, a lesion of the subthalamic nucleus would reduce the activity of these pallidal neurons. Therefore, the neurons in the VA and VL nuclei of the thalamus would be less inhibited, and the activity of the neurons in the motor cortex would be increased.

In all of these basal ganglia disorders, the motor dysfunction is contralateral to the diseased component. This is understandable, because the main final output of the basal ganglia is mediated by the corticospinal tract.

SUMMARY

1. Muscle spindles are complex sensory receptors found in skeletal muscle. They lie parallel to regular muscle fibers, and they contain nuclear bag and nuclear chain intrafusal muscle fibers.

2. Group Ia afferent fibers form primary endings on nuclear bag and chain fibers, and group II fibers form secondary endings on nuclear chain fibers.

3. Primary endings demonstrate both static and dynamic responses, which signal muscle length and rate of change in muscle length. Secondary endings demonstrate only static responses and signal only muscle length.

4. Golgi tendon organs are located in the tendons of muscles and are arranged in series with the muscle. They are supplied by group Ib afferent fibers and are excited both by stretch and by contraction of the muscle.

5. Reflexes are simple, stereotyped motor responses to a stimulus. A reflex arc includes the afferent fibers, interneurons, and motor neurons responsible for the reflex.

6. The reflex arcs of many reflexes are located in the spinal cord or brainstem.

7. Transection of the spinal cord reveals the reflexes that depend only on spinal cord circuits. These include the stretch (myotatic) reflex, the inverse myotatic reflex, and the flexion reflex.

8. The stretch reflex includes (1) a monosynaptic excitatory pathway from group Ia (and II) muscle spindle afferent fibers to α-motor neurons that supply the same and synergistic muscles, and (2) a disynaptic inhibitory pathway to antagonistic motor neurons.

9. Phasic stretch reflexes are triggered by the dynamic responses of group Ia fibers, and tonic stretch reflexes are triggered by the static responses of group Ia and II afferents.

10. The inverse myotatic reflex is evoked by Golgi tendon organs. Afferent volleys in group Ib fibers from a given muscle cause a disynaptic inhibition of α-motor neurons to the same muscle, and they excite α-motor neurons to antagonist muscles.

11. The flexion reflex is evoked by volleys in afferent fibers that supply various receptors, including nociceptors. In the flexion reflex, ipsilateral flexor motor neurons are excited, and extensor motor neurons are inhibited through polysynaptic pathways. The opposite pattern may occur contralaterally.

12. Spinal reflexes can be studied by electrically stimulating the afferent fibers in nerves and recording volleys in α-motor axons from ventral roots.

13. Spinal cord motor neurons are organized topographically. Those in the lateral ventral horn supply the limb muscles, and those in the medial ventral horn supply the axial muscles.

14. Descending pathways can be subdivided into (1) a lateral system, which ends on motor neurons to limb muscles and on the lateral group of interneurons, and (2) a medial system, which ends on the medial group of inter neurons.

15. The lateral system includes the lateral corticospinal tract and part of the corticobulbar tract. These pathways influence contralateral motor neurons that supply the musculature of

the limbs, especially the digits, and the muscles of the lower face and the tongue.

16. The medial system includes the ventral corticospinal, lateral and medial vestibulospinal, reticulospinal, and tectospinal tracts. These pathways mainly affect posture and provide the motor background for movements of the limbs and digits.

17. Descending monoaminergic pathways affect the general level of excitability of spinal cord reflex circuits and ascending pathways.

18. Pathways that originate in the brainstem influence posture, locomotion, and eye movements. Postural reflexes include several vestibular reflexes (the vestibulocollic reflex, the vestibular placing reaction, and ocular counterrolling), the tonic neck reflexes, and the righting reflexes.

19. Locomotion is triggered by commands relayed through the midbrain locomotor center. However, central pattern generators formed by spinal cord circuits and influenced by afferent input provide for the detailed organization of locomotor activity.

20. Conjugate eye movements are produced by several different control systems (including the vestibuloocular reflex, optokinetic reflex, smooth pursuit system, and saccadic system). Vergent eye movements are controlled by the vergence system.

21. The brainstem centers for control of eye movement include the vestibular nuclei, the horizontal and vertical gaze centers, and the superior colliculi.

22. Voluntary movements depend on interactions among motor areas of the cerebral cortex, the cerebellum, and the basal ganglia.

23. Motor areas of the cerebral cortex include (1) the primary motor cortex, which controls distal muscles of the extremities; (2) the premotor area, which helps control proximal and axial muscles; (3) the supplementary motor cortex, which participates in motor planning and in coordination; and (4) the frontal eye fields, which help initiate saccadic eye movements.

24. Individual corticospinal neurons discharge before voluntary contractions of related muscles occur. The discharges are related to contractile force, rather than to joint position.

25. Corticospinal neurons receive feedback from the sensory systems by way of the somatosensory cortex and the posterior parietal lobe; this feedback helps correct motor commands.

26. The cerebellum influences the rate, range, force, and direction of movements. It also influences muscle tone and posture, as well as eye movements and balance.

27. The vestibulocerebellum connects with the vestibular system and influences eye movements and balance by connections with the vestibulospinal and reticulospinal tracts.

28. The spinocerebellum receives input from spinal cord pathways. It controls (1) the axial musculature, through the medial system of descending pathways, and (2) the proximal limb muscles, through the lateral system.

29. The corticocerebellum receives information from the cerebral cortex by way of the pontine nuclei. It controls the distal muscles of the limbs by connections to the motor cortex (via the thalamus) and to the lateral corticospinal tract.

30. Most of the input to the cerebellum is through pathways that end as mossy fibers. Mossy fibers evoke single action potentials called simple spikes in Purkinje cells.

31. The inferior olive projections to the cerebellum end as climbing fibers. A climbing fiber produces repetitive discharges of a Purkinje cell.

32. The basal ganglia include several deep telencephalic nuclei (including the caudate nucleus, putamen, and globus pallidus). The basal ganglia interact with the cerebral cortex, subthalamic nucleus, substantia nigra, and thalamus.

33. Activity transmitted from the cerebral cortex through the basal ganglia can either facilitate or inhibit thalamic neurons that project to motor areas of the cortex.

34. The basal ganglia regulate the output of the motor cortex. Diseases of the cerebellum and basal ganglia affect motor behavior profoundly.

BIBLIOGRAPHY

Journal articles

Albin RL: The pathophysiology of chorea/ballism and parkinsonism, *Parkinsonism Related Disord* 1:3, 1995.

Brooks DJ: The role of the basal ganglia in motor control: contributions from PET, *J Neurol Sci* 128:1, 1995.

Chesselet MF, Delfs JM: Basal ganglia and movement disorders: an update, *Trends Neurosci* 19:417, 1996.

Gerfen CR: Dopamine receptor function in the basal ganglia, *Clin Neuropharmacol* 18:S162, 1995.

Karni A et al: Functional MRI evidence for adult motor cortex plasticity during motor skill learning, *Nature* 377:155, 1995.

Pearson KG: Proprioceptive regulation of locomotion, *Curr Opin Neurobiol* 5:786, 1995.

Pucard N, Strick PL: Motor areas of the medial wall: a review of their location and functional activation, *Cerebral Cortex* 6:342, 1996.

Robinson FR, Fuchs AF: The role of the cerebellum in voluntary eye movements, *Annu Rev Neurosci* 24:981, 2001.

Tanji J: Sequential organization of multiple movements: involvement of cortical motor areas, *Annu Rev Neurosci* 24:631, 2001.

Thach WT: On the specific role of the cerebellum in motor learning and cognition: clues from PET activation and lesion studies in humans, *Behav Brain Sci* 19:411, 1996.

Wichmann T, DeLong MR: Functional and pathological models of the basal ganglia, *Curr Opin Neurobiol* 6:751, 1996.

Wise SP et al: Premotor and parietal cortex: corticocortical connectivity and combinatorial computations, *Annu Rev Neurosci* 20:25, 1997.

Books and monographs

Dunn RP, Strick PL: The corticospinal system: a structural framework for the central control of movement. In: Rowell LB, Sheperd JT (editors): *Handbook of physiology. Section 12: Exercise: regulation and integration of multiple systems,* New York, Oxford University Press, pp 217–254, 1996.

Jeannnerod M: *The cognitive neuroscience of action.* London, 1997, Blackwell Publishers.

Matthews PBC: *Muscle receptors,* London, 1972, Edward Arnold.

Porter R, Lemon R: *Corticospinal function and voluntary movement,* Oxford, 1993, Clarendon.

Rothwell J: *Control of human voluntary movement,* ed 2, London, 1994, Chapman & Hall.

Sherrington C: *The integrative action of the nervous system,* ed 2, New Haven, 1947, Yale Univeristy Press.

chapter ten

Higher Functions of the Nervous System

Interactions between different parts of the cerebral cortex and between the cerebral cortex and other parts of the brain are responsible for the higher functions that characterize humans. The neural basis for some of these higher functions is discussed in this chapter.

THE CEREBRAL CORTEX

The cerebral cortex in humans occupies a volume of about 600 cm³ and a surface area of 2,500 cm². The surface of the cortex is highly convoluted and is folded into ridges, known as **gyri.** Gyri are separated by grooves called **sulci** (if shallow) and **fissures** (if deep). This folding increases the surface area of the cortex. From the surface, much of the cortex cannot be seen because of the presence of this folding (see Fig. 10-1).

The cerebral cortex can be divided into the left and right hemispheres and subdivided into a number of lobes (Fig. 10-1), including the **frontal, parietal, temporal,** and **occipital lobes.** These lobes are named for the overlying bones of the skull. The frontal and parietal lobes are separated by the central sulcus; they are separated from the temporal lobe by the lateral fissure. The occipital and parietal lobes are separated (on the medial surface of the hemisphere) by the parietooccipital fissure. Buried within the lateral fissure is another lobe, the **insula.** The **limbic lobe** is formed by the cortex on the medial aspect of the hemisphere that borders on the brainstem. Part of the limbic lobe, the **hippocampal formation,** is folded into the temporal lobe and cannot be seen from the surface of the brain. At the base of the brain can be seen an area of **olfactory cortex,** which includes the olfactory tubercle in the anterior perforated substance and the prepiriform lobe (see Chapter 8).

Activity in the two hemispheres of the cerebral cortex is coordinated by interconnections through the cerebral commissures. The bulk of the neocortex on the two sides is connected through the massive **corpus callosum** (see Fig. 10-2). Parts of the temporal lobes connect through the anterior commissure, and the hippocampal formations on the two sides communicate through the hippocampal commissure (which is formed between the fornices on the two sides, as they pass under the corpus callosum).

Functions of the Lobes of the Cerebral Cortex

The specific functions of the cerebral cortex can be associated with the different lobes of the cerebral hemispheres.

Frontal lobe. One of the main functions of the **frontal lobe** is motor behavior. As discussed in Chapter 9, the motor, premotor, and supplementary motor areas are in the frontal lobe, as is the frontal eye field. These areas are responsible for planning and executing voluntary motor acts. In addition, the **motor speech area (Broca's area)** is located in the inferior frontal gyrus, in the dominant hemisphere for human language (almost always the left hemisphere, as explained below). In addition, the prefrontal cortex in the rostral part of the frontal lobe plays a major role in personality and emotional behavior.

Bilateral lesions of this part of the brain may be produced either by disease or by a surgically induced frontal lobotomy. These lesions produce deficits in attention, difficulty in problem solving, and inappropriate social behavior. Aggressive behavior is also reduced, and the motivational-affective component of pain is lost, although pain sensation remains. Frontal lobotomies are rarely performed today, because improved drug therapies have become available for mental illness and for chronic pain.

Parietal lobe. The **parietal lobe** contains the **somatosensory cortex** and the adjacent **parietal association cortex** (see Chapter 7). This lobe is involved in the processing and perception of somatosensory information. Connections with the frontal lobe allow somatosensory information to affect voluntary motor activity. Visual information from the occipital lobe reaches the parietal association cortex and also the frontal lobe, and it assists in visual guidance of voluntary movements. Somatosensory information can also be transferred to the language centers, such as Wernicke's area, in the dominant hemisphere, as described below. The parietal

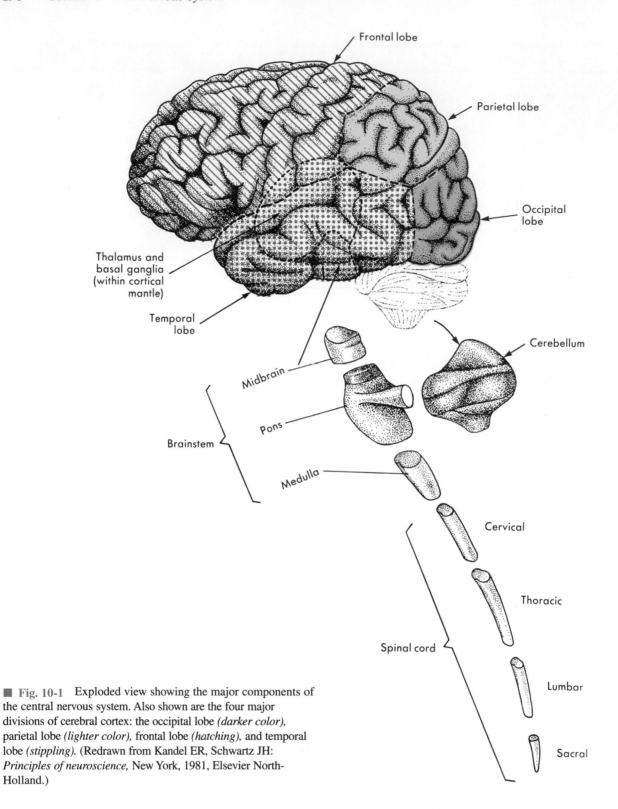

Frontal lobe

Parietal lobe

Occipital lobe

Thalamus and basal ganglia (within cortical mantle)

Temporal lobe

Cerebellum

Midbrain

Pons

Brainstem

Medulla

Cervical

Thoracic

Spinal cord

Lumbar

Sacral

■ **Fig. 10-1** Exploded view showing the major components of the central nervous system. Also shown are the four major divisions of cerebral cortex: the occipital lobe *(darker color)*, parietal lobe *(lighter color)*, frontal lobe *(hatching)*, and temporal lobe *(stippling)*. (Redrawn from Kandel ER, Schwartz JH: *Principles of neuroscience,* New York, 1981, Elsevier North-Holland.)

lobe in the nondominant hemisphere is involved in spatial analysis, as shown by the effects of specific lesions (see Chapters 7 and 9).

Occipital lobe. The primary function of the **occipital lobe** is visual processing and perception (see Chapter 8). Occipital eye fields affect eye movements, and a projection to the midbrain assists in the control of convergent eye

movements, pupillary constriction, and accommodation, all of which occur when the eyes adjust for near vision.

Temporal lobe. The **temporal lobe** has many different functions. One of these is hearing, which depends on the processing and perception of information related to sounds (see Chapter 8). Another function is processing of vestibular information. Several visual areas have been discovered in

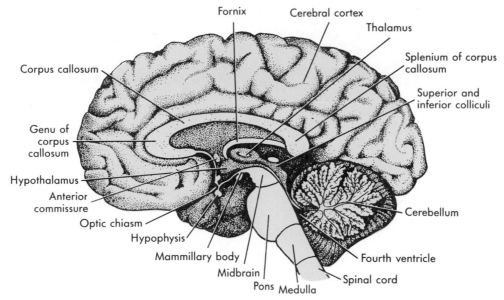

■ Fig. 10-2   Midsagittal section of the brain. Note the relationships among the cerebral cortex, cerebellum, thalamus, and brainstem plus the location of various commissures. (Redrawn from Kandel ER, Schwartz JH: *Principles of neuroscience,* New York, 1981, Elsevier North-Holland.)

the temporal lobe; hence, this lobe is involved in higher-order visual processing (see Chapter 8). For example, the occip-totemporal gyrus is involved in the recognition of faces. In addition, Meyer's loop, which forms part of the optic radiation, passes through the temporal lobe. Therefore, temporal lobe lesions can damage this part of the optic radiation. Similarly, some of Wernicke's area lies in the posterior region of the temporal lobe, as described below; damage to the temporal lobe in the dominant hemisphere can therefore cause language disorders.

The medial temporal lobe belongs to the limbic system, which participates in emotional behavior and regulates the autonomic nervous system (see Chapter 11). The hippocampal formation is involved in learning and memory (see below).

The functions of the different lobes of the cerebral cortex have been defined both from the effects of lesions produced by disease or by surgical interventions to treat disease in humans, and from experiments on animals. In another approach, the physical manifestations of **epileptic seizures** have been correlated with the brain locations that give rise to seizures **(epileptic seizure foci).** For example, epileptic foci in the motor cortex cause movements on the contralateral side; the exact movements relate to the somatotopic location of the seizure focus. Seizures that originate in the somatosensory cortex cause an **epileptic aura,** in which a sensation is experienced. Similarly, seizures that start in the visual cortex cause a visual aura (scintillations, colors), those in the auditory cortex cause an auditory aura (humming, buzzing, ringing), and those in the vestibular cortex cause a feeling of spinning. Complex behaviors result from seizures that

originate in the temporal lobe; in addition, a malodorous aura may be perceived if the olfactory cortex is involved **(uncinate fit).**

Neocortical Layering and Subdivisions

The cerebral cortex can be subdivided phylogenetically into the **archicortex, paleocortex,** and **neocortex.** In humans 90% of the cortex is neocortex.

The different phylogenetic subdivisions of the cerebral cortex can be recognized on the basis of their layering pattern. The neocortex is generally characterized by the presence of six cortical layers (Fig. 10-3). On the other hand, the archicortex has only three layers, and the paleocortex has four to five layers.

Cell types in neocortex.   A number of different cell types have been described in the neocortex (Fig. 10-3). The most abundant cell types are the **pyramidal cells** and the **stellate cells** (various types of nonpyramidal cells). Pyramidal cells have a large triangular cell body, a long apical dendrite, and several basal dendrites. These cells are the main cortical efferent cells. The axon emerges from the cell body opposite the apical dendrite, and it projects into the subcortical white matter. The axon may give off collaterals as it descends through the cortex. Pyramidal cells use an excitatory amino acid (glutamate or aspartate) as their neurotransmitter. Stellate cells, often called **granule cells,** are interneurons. They have a small soma and numerous branched dendrites. Some are excitatory interneurons; these cells are abundant in layer IV of the cortex (see above). Their axons ascend toward the supragranular layers. Other stellate cells are inhibitory interneurons that use γ-aminobutryic acid (GABA) as their neurotransmitter.

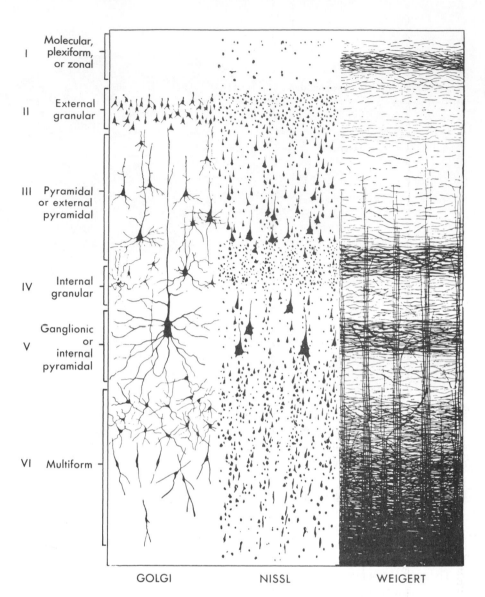

I   Molecular, plexiform, or zonal

II   External granular

III   Pyramidal or external pyramidal

IV   Internal granular

V   Ganglionic or internal pyramidal

VI   Multiform

GOLGI   NISSL   WEIGERT

■ **Fig. 10-3**   Lamination of the neocortex. Neurons in the different layers are demonstrated by the Golgi stain *(left column)* and the Nissl stain *(middle column),* while myelinated fibers are shown by the myelin sheath stain *(right column).* The layers are numbered at the left. (From Brodal A: *Neurological anatomy,* ed 3, London, 1981, Oxford University Press.)

Cytoarchitecture of cortical layers. Each of the six layers of the neocortex has a characteristic cellular content (Fig. 10-3). Layer I (molecular layer) has few neuronal cell bodies; instead it contains mostly axon terminals and synapses on dendrites. Layer II (external granular layer) contains mostly stellate cells, although some pyramidal cells are found in this layer. Layer III (external pyramidal layer) consists mostly of small pyramidal cells. Layer IV (internal granular layer) includes mostly stellate cells, including the excitatory type. Layer V (internal pyramidal layer) is dominated by large pyramidal cells. Layer VI (multiform layer) contains pyramidal, fusiform, and other types of cells.

Myeloarchitecture of cortical layers. The cortex contains concentrations of myelinated axons that are oriented either horizontally or vertically. Prominent horizontal sheets of axons can be found in several layers (Fig. 10-3). In the visual cortex a particularly prominent sheet of axons, known as the stripe of Gennari, gives this part of the cortex the name *striate* cortex. Vertical collections of axons, formed by

cortical afferent and efferent fibers, cross the lower layers of the cortex (Fig. 10-3). These vertical collections of afferent and efferent fibers, and the cortical neurons with which they connect, are presumed to be the morphological basis of cortical columns (see Chapters 7 and 8).

Cortical afferent and efferent fibers. The cortical afferent fibers tend to synapse in particular cortical layers; the site depends on where the fibers originate. Similarly, cortical efferent fibers that originate from particular layers project to particular destinations.

Thalamocortical afferent fibers from thalamic nuclei that have specific cortical projections end chiefly in layers III, IV, and VI. Neurons in other thalamic nuclei project diffusely and terminate in layers I and VI.

Several nonthalamic, diffusely projecting nuclei (including the basal nucleus of Meynert, the locus coeruleus, and the dorsal raphe nucleus) project to all cortical layers. These projections modulate cortical activity globally, perhaps in conjunction with changes in state (e.g., sleep or waking).

The neurotransmitter in the basal nucleus of Meynert is acetylcholine, in the locus coeruleus it is norepinephrine, and in the dorsal raphe nucleus it is serotonin.

The cortical efferent fibers originate from pyramidal cells. Pyramidal cells of layers II and III project to other cortical areas, either ipsilaterally or contralaterally. Pyramidal cells of layer V project in many descending pathways and have synaptic targets in the spinal cord, brainstem, and striatum. They also project to thalamic nuclei that provide diffuse projections back to the cortex. Pyramidal cells of layer VI form corticothalamic projections to thalamic nuclei with specific cortical projections. Reciprocal thalamocortical and corticothalamic interconnections are likely to make important contributions to the electroencephalogram (see below).

Regional variations in neocortical structure. On the basis of differences in the cytoarchitecture, a number of subdivisions of the neocortex can be recognized. Most of the cortex is constructed of six readily distinguishable layers.

The **agranular cortex** of motor areas contains relatively few nonpyramidal cells; the lack of nonpyramidal cells is the basis for the name of this cortex. Instead, pyramidal cells predominate. This kind of cortex appears to specialize in output cells, and thus the presence of this type of cortex in the motor and premotor areas is not surprising.

Another type of cortex has a relatively small number of pyramidal cells and is dominated by nonpyramidal cells. This type of cortex is called the **granular cortex** (or **koniocortex,** for "dustlike"). Evidently, it is specialized for processing afferent input. Therefore, the presence of this kind of cortex in the primary sensory receiving areas, the somatosensory cortex (SI), the primary auditory cortex, and the primary visual (striate) cortex is reasonable.

Most of the other region of cortex show less dramatic variations. These areas have six well-demarcated layers.

The cortex was subdivided further by Brodmann (Fig. 10-4). On the basis of an extensive cytoarchitectural analysis, Brodmann divided the cortex into 52 discrete areas. Important ones include Brodmann's areas 3, 1, and 2, which form the SI cortex; area 4, the primary motor cortex; area 6, the premotor and supplementary motor cortex; areas 41 and 42, the primary auditory cortex; and area 17, the primary visual cortex (striate cortex). Detailed studies have confirmed that the Brodmann areas are in fact distinctly different, both with respect to their interconnections and with respect to their functions.

Archicortex

About 10% of the human cerebral cortex is archicortex and paleocortex. The archicortex has a three-layered structure; the paleocortex has four to five layers. The paleocortex is located at the border between the archicortex and neocortex.

Hippocampal formation. In humans the hippocampal formation forms part of the archicortex. In humans, it is folded into the temporal lobe and can be viewed only when the brain is dissected. The hippocampal formation consists of several parts, including the hippocampus (Ammon's horn or cornu Ammonis), the dentate gyrus, and the subiculum.

These are well demarcated in a cross section through the hippocampal formation (Fig. 10-5).

The hippocampus has three layers: molecular layer, pyramidal cell, and polymorphic. These resemble layers I, V, and VI in the neocortex. The folding of the hippocampus imparts an inverted appearance, because the white matter is at the surface of the lateral ventricle (see Fig. 10-5). The white matter covering the hippocampus is called the *alveus,* which contains hippocampal afferent and efferent fibers. The axons in the alveus continue into a nerve fiber bundle called the *fimbria;* the fimbria is continuous with the fornix.

The dentate gyrus is also a three-layered cortex. However, its middle layer is the granule cell layer instead of the pyramidal layer. The axons of the granule cells do not leave the hippocampal formation. Instead, they project to Ammon's horn.

The hippocampal formation receives its main neural input from the entorhinal cortex of the parahippocampal gyrus through two main projections, the **perforant path** and the **alvear path** (Fig. 10-5, *B*). Important, generally reciprocal, connections are formed between the pyramidal cells of the hippocampus and (1) the septal nuclei and mammillary body by way of the fornix, and (2) the contralateral hippocampal formation by way of the fornix and the hippocampal commissure. The granule cell layer of the dentate gyrus also projects to the hippocampus.

HIGHER FUNCTIONS OF THE NERVOUS SYSTEM

The Electroencephalogram

An **electroencephalogram (EEG)** is a recording of the rhythmic electrical activity that can be made from the cerebral cortex via electrodes placed on the skull. In an **electrocorticogram,** electrical activity of the cortex is recorded via electrodes placed on the surface of the brain. In human studies, the EEG is recorded from a grid of standard recording sites. Thus, EEGs can be recorded from approximately the same sites at different times from one individual or from analogous sites in different subjects (Fig. 10-6). The EEG is an important diagnostic tool in clinical neurology and is particularly useful in patients with epilepsy.

The normal EEG consists of waves of various frequencies. The dominant frequencies depend on several factors, including the state of wakefulness, the age of the subject, the location of the recording electrodes, and the absence or presence of drugs or disease. When a normal awake adult is relaxed with the eyes closed, the dominant frequencies of the EEG recorded over the parietal and occipital lobes are about 8 to 13 Hz, the **alpha rhythm** (see Fig. 10-6). If the subject is asked to open his or her eyes, the EEG becomes less synchronized and the dominant frequency increases to 13 to 30 Hz, which is called the **beta rhythm.** The **delta** (0.5 to 4 Hz) and **theta** (4 to 7 Hz) **rhythms** are observed during sleep (see the following discussion) (Fig. 10-7).

The EEG waves are derived from alternating excitatory and inhibitory synaptic potentials that occur in cortical neurons as a result of thalamocortical and other input. The

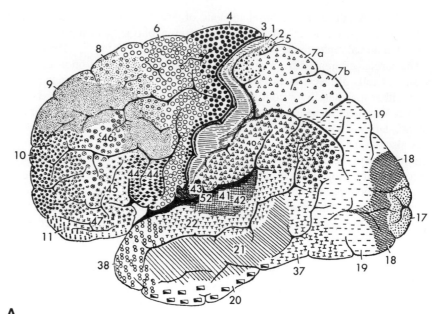

■ **Fig. 10-4** Brodmann's areas in the human cerebral cortex. (Redrawn from Crosby EC et al: *Correlative anatomy of the nervous system,* New York, 1962, Macmillan.)

A

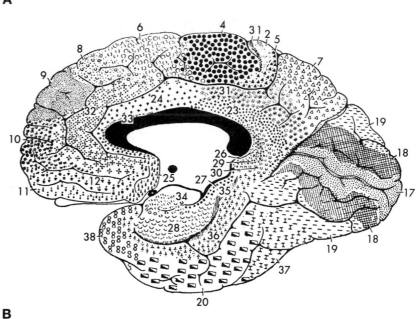

B

potentials are produced chiefly by extracellular currents that flow vertically across the cortex during the generation of synaptic potentials in the pyramidal cells. The extracellular currents associated with action potentials are too small, fast, and asynchronous to be recorded with EEG electrodes.

Although a brief EEG wave is sometimes referred to as a *spike,* this term does not refer to action potentials. The potentials recorded as the EEG are relatively large (around 100 μV). These large potentials reflect the organization of many pyramidal cells, which are arranged with their apical dendrites aligned in parallel to form a dipole sheet. One pole of this sheet is oriented toward the cortical surface and the other toward the subcortical white matter. Note that the sign of an EEG wave does not in itself indicate whether pyramidal cells are being excited or inhibited. For instance, a neg-

ative EEG potential may be generated at the surface of the skull (or cortex) by excitation of apical dendrites or by inhibition near the somas. Conversely, a positive EEG wave can be produced by inhibition of the apical dendrites or by excitation near the somas.

Evoked Potentials

An EEG change, called a **cortical evoked potential,** can be elicited by a stimulus. A cortical evoked potential is best recorded from the part of the skull located over the cortical area being activated. For example, a visual stimulus results in an evoked potential that can be recorded best over the occipital bone, whereas a somatosensory evoked potential is recorded most effectively near the junction of the frontal and

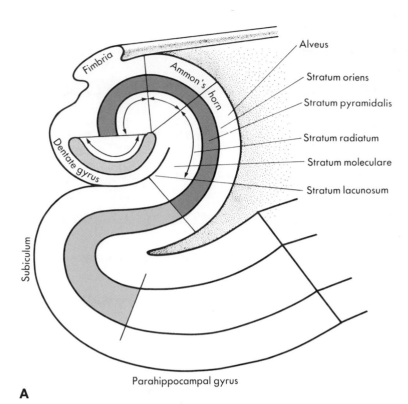

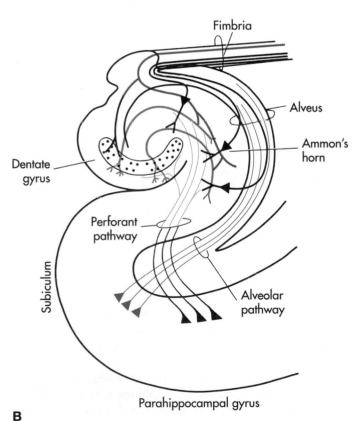

■ **Fig. 10-5** **A,** The main subdivisions of the hippocampal formation. **B,** Some of the connections of the hippocampus. (Redrawn from Williams PL, Warwick R: *Functional neuroanatomy of man,* Philadelphia, 1975, WB Saunders.)

parietal bones. Evoked potentials reflect the synaptic potentials that occur in large numbers of cortical neurons. They may also reflect activity in subcortical structures.

Evoked potentials are small compared with the size of the EEG waves. However, their apparent size can be enhanced by a process called **signal averaging.** In this process, the

stimulation is repeated and EEGs are recorded during each trial. With each repetition of the stimulus, the evoked potential occurs at a fixed interval after the stimulus. However, the underlying EEG may show a positive or a negative deflection on different trials during the time of occurrence of the evoked potential. In signal averaging, evoked potentials are

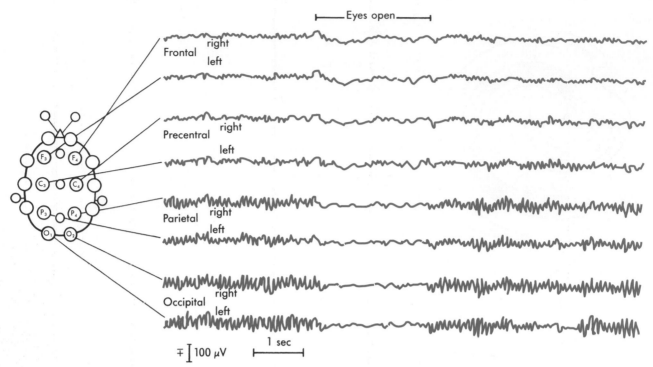

■ **Fig. 10-6** Electroencephalogram (EEG) in a normal, resting, awake human. The recordings were made from eight channels at the same time. The electrode positions are indicated. When the eyes were opened, the alpha rhythm was blocked. (From Schmidt RF, editor: *Fundamentals of neurophysiology,* ed 2, New York, 1978, Springer-Verlag.)

electronically averaged. The EEG waves average out, whereas the evoked potentials sum.

> Evoked potentials are used clinically to assess the integrity of a sensory pathway, at least to the level of the primary sensory receiving area. These potentials can be recorded in comatose individuals, as well as in infants too young to permit a sensory examination. The initial parts of the auditory evoked potential actually reflect activity in the brainstem; therefore, this evoked potential can be used to assess the function of brainstem structures.

Sleep-Wake Cycle

Sleep and wakefulness are among the many functions of the body that show **circadian** (about one day) periodicity. The sleep-wake cycle has an endogenous periodicity of about 25 hours, but it normally becomes entrained to the day-night cycle. However, the entrainment can be disrupted when the subject is isolated from the environment or shifts time zones (jet lag).

Characteristic changes in the EEG can be correlated with the changes in behavioral state during the sleep-wake cycle. **Beta wave** activity dominates in the awake, aroused individual (see Fig. 10-6). The EEG is said to be **desynchronized;** it displays low-voltage, high-frequency activity. In relaxed individuals with eyes closed, the EEG is dominated by **alpha waves** (Figs. 10-6 and 10-7). As the person falls

asleep, he or she passes sequentially through four stages of **slow-wave sleep** (called stages 1 through 4) over a period of 30 to 45 minutes (Fig. 10-7). In stage 1, alpha waves are interspersed with lower frequency waves (3 to 7 Hz) called **theta waves.** In stage 2, the EEG slows further, but the slow-wave activity is interrupted by **sleep spindles,** which are bursts of activity at 12 to 14 Hz, and by large **K complexes** (large, slow potentials). Stage 3 sleep is associated with **delta waves,** which occur at frequencies of 0.5 to 2 Hz, and with occasional sleep spindles. Stage 4 is characterized by delta waves.

During slow-wave sleep the muscles of the body relax, but the posture is adjusted intermittently. The heart rate and blood pressure decrease and gastrointestinal motility increases. The ease with which individuals can be awakened decreases progressively as they pass through these sleep stages. As the person awakens, they pass through the sleep stages in reverse order.

About every 90 minutes slow-wave sleep changes to a different form of sleep, called **rapid eye movement (REM)** sleep. In REM sleep, the EEG again becomes desynchronized. The low-voltage, fast activity of REM sleep resembles that seen in the EEG from an aroused subject (Fig. 10-7, *bottom trace*). The similarity of the EEG to that of an awake individual and the difficulty in awaking the person have suggested the term **paradoxical sleep** for this type of sleep. Muscle tone is completely lost, but phasic contractions occur in a number of muscles, most notably the eye muscles.

Drowsy (8 to 12 cps) alpha waves

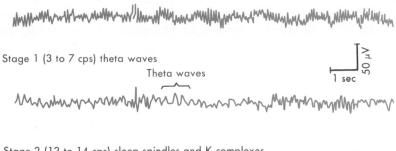

Stage 1 (3 to 7 cps) theta waves

Theta waves

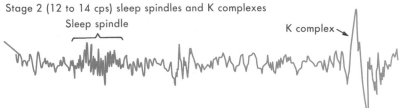

Stage 2 (12 to 14 cps) sleep spindles and K complexes

Sleep spindle

K complex

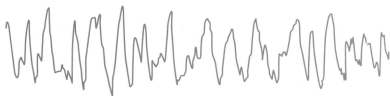

■ **Fig. 10-7** EEG during drowsiness and stages 1, 2, and 4 of slow wave [non-rapid eye movement (non-REM)] sleep and in REM sleep. (Modified from Shepherd GM: *Neurobiology,* London, 1983, Oxford University Press.)

Stage 4 (½ to 2 cps) delta waves

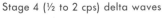

REM sleep—low voltage, fast

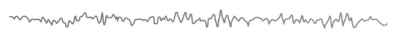

The resulting rapid eye movements are basis of the name for this type of sleep. Many autonomic changes also take place. Temperature regulation is lost, and meiosis occurs. Penile erection may occur during this type of sleep. Heart rate, blood pressure, and respiration change intermittently. Several episodes of REM sleep occur each night. Although it is difficult to arouse a person from REM sleep, internal arousal is common. Most dreams occur during REM sleep.

The proportion of slow-wave (non-REM) to REM sleep varies with age. Newborn children spend about half of their sleep time in REM sleep, whereas the elderly have little REM sleep. About 20% to 25% of the sleep of young adults is REM sleep.

The purpose of sleep is still unclear. However, it must have a high value, because so much of life is spent in sleep and because lack of sleep can be debilitating. Medically important disorders of the sleep-wake cycle include **insomnia, bedwetting, sleepwalking, sleep apnea,** and **narcolepsy.**

The mechanism of sleep is incompletely understood. Stimulation in the brainstem reticular formation in a large region known as the **reticular activating system** causes arousal and low-voltage, fast EEG activity. Sleep was once

thought to be caused by a reduced level of activity in the reticular activating system. However, substantial data, including the observations that anesthesia of the lower brainstem results in arousal and that stimulation in the medulla near the nucleus of the solitary tract can induce sleep, suggest that sleep is an active process. Investigators have tried to relate sleep mechanisms to brainstem networks that use particular neurotransmitters, including serotonin, norepinephrine, and acetylcholine, because manipulations of the levels of these transmitters in the brain can affect the sleep-wake cycle. However, a detailed neurochemical explanation of the neural mechanisms of sleep is not yet available.

The source of circadian periodicity in the brain appears to be the suprachiasmatic nucleus of the hypothalamus. This nucleus receives projections from the retina, and its neurons seem to form a biological clock. Destruction of the suprachiasmatic nucleus disrupts a number of biological rhythms, including the sleep-wake cycle.

The EEG becomes abnormal under a variety of pathological circumstances. For example, during coma the EEG is dominated by delta activity. **Brain death** is defined by a maintained flat EEG.

Epilepsy commonly causes EEG abnormalities. There are several forms of epilepsy, and examples of EEG patterns from some of these are shown in Fig. 10-8. Epileptic seizures can be either partial or generalized.

One form of partial seizures originates in the motor cortex and results in localized contractions of contralateral muscles. The contractions may then spread to other muscles; the spread follows the somatotopic sequence of the motor cortex (see Fig. 9-16). Complex partial seizures (which may occur in **psychomotor epilepsy**) originate in the limbic lobe and result in illusions and semipurposeful motor activity. During and between focal seizures, scalp recordings may reveal EEG spikes (see Fig. 10-8, *C* and *D*).

Generalized seizures involve wide areas of the brain and loss of consciousness. Two major types of seizures are **petit mal** and **grand mal seizures.** In petit mal epilepsy, consciousness is lost transiently, and the EEG displays **spike and wave activity** (see Fig. 10-8, *B*). In grand mal seizures, consciousness is lost for a longer period, and the individual may fall to the ground if he or she is standing when the seizure starts. The seizure begins with a generalized increase in muscle tone **(tonic phase),** followed by a series of jerky movements **(clonic phase).** The bowel and bladder may be evacuated. The EEG shows widely distributed seizure activity (see Fig. 10-8, *A*).

EEG spikes that occur between full-blown seizures are called **interictal spikes.** Similar events can be studied experimentally. These spikes arise from abrupt, long-lasting depolarizations, called **depolarization shifts,** which trigger repetitive action potentials in cortical neurons. These depolarization shifts may reflect several changes in epileptic foci. Such changes include regenerative Ca^{2+}-mediated dendritic action potentials in cortical neurons and a reduction in inhibitory interactions in cortical circuits. Electrical field potentials and the release of K^+ and excitatory amino acids from hyperactive neurons may also contribute to the increased cortical excitability.

Cerebral Dominance and Language

In most people, the left cerebral hemisphere is the **dominant hemisphere** with respect to language. This dominance has been demonstrated (1) by the effects of lesions of the left hemisphere, which may produce deficits in language function **(aphasia);** and (2) by the transient aphasia (inability to speak or write) that results when a short-acting anesthetic is introduced into the left carotid artery. Lesions of the right hemisphere and the injection of anesthetic into the right carotid artery do not usually affect language substantially. The right hemisphere is dominant for functions other than language. For example, left-handedness reflects a dominance of the right hemisphere. However, in most left-handed people the left hemisphere is still dominant for language. Differences in the size of an area called the **planum temporale,** which is located in the floor of the lateral fissure, correlate with language dominance. The left planum temporale is usually larger than that of the right hemisphere.

Several areas in the left hemisphere are involved in language. **Wernicke's area** is a large area centered in the posterior part of the superior temporal gyrus near the auditory cortex. Another important language area, **Broca's area,** is in the posterior part of the inferior temporal gyrus, close to the face representation of the motor cortex. Damage to Wernicke's area results in a **sensory aphasia,** in which the person has difficulty in understanding spoken or written language; however, speech production remains fluent. Conversely, a lesion of Broca's area causes **motor aphasia.** Individuals with motor aphasia have difficulty in speech and in writing, although they can understand language relatively well.

A person with sensory aphasia may not have auditory or visual impairment, and a person with motor aphasia may have normal motor control of the muscles responsible for speech or writing. Thus, aphasia does not depend on an alteration in sensation or in the motor system;

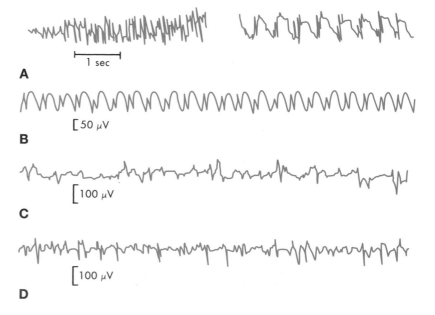

■ **Fig. 10-8** EEG abnormalities in several forms of epilepsy. **A,** EEG during the tonic *(left)* and clonic *(right)* phases of a grand mal seizure. **B,** Spike and wave components of a petit mal seizure. **C,** EEG in temporal lobe epilepsy. **D,** A focal seizure. (Redrawn from Eyzaguirre C, Fidone SJ: *Physiology of the nervous system,* ed 2, St. Louis, 1975, Mosby.)

1 sec

A

$[$ 50 μV

B

$[$ 100 μV

C

$[$ 100 μV

D

rather, it is a deficit in the reception or planning of language expression. However, lesions in the dominant hemisphere may be large enough to result in mixed forms of aphasia, as well as in sensory changes or paralysis of some of the muscles used to express language.

Interhemispheric Transfer

The two cerebral hemispheres can function relatively independently, as in the case of language function. However, information must be transferred between the hemispheres to coordinate activity on the two sides of the body. In other words, each hemisphere must know what the other is doing. Much of the information transferred between the two hemispheres is transmitted through the corpus callosum, although some is transmitted through other commissures (e.g., the anterior commissure or hippocampal commissure).

An experiment that shows the importance of the corpus callosum for interhemispheric transfer of information is illustrated in Fig. 10-9, *A*. An animal with an intact optic chiasm and corpus callosum and with the left eye closed learns a visual discrimination task (Fig. 10-9, *A*). The information is transmitted to both hemispheres through the bilateral connections made by the optic chiasm or through the corpus callosum, or both. When the animal is tested with the left eye open and the right eye closed (Fig. 10-9, *A, center*), the task can still be performed, because both hemispheres have learned the task. If the optic chiasm is transected before the animal is trained, the result is the same (Fig. 10-9, *B*). Information is presumably transferred between the two hemispheres through the corpus callosum. This finding can be confirmed by cutting both the optic chiasm and corpus callosum before training (Fig. 10-9, *C*). Then the information is not transferred, and each hemisphere must learn the task independently.

A similar experiment has been done in human patients who have had a surgical transection of the corpus callosum to prevent the interhemispheric spread of epilepsy (Fig. 10-10). The optic chiasm remained intact. Directing visual information to one or the other hemisphere was possible by having the patient fix his or her vision on a point on a screen. A picture of an object was then projected to one side of the fixation point so that visual information about the picture reached only the contralateral hemisphere. An opening beneath the screen allowed the patient to manipulate objects that could not be seen. The objects included those shown in the projected pictures. Normal individuals would be able to locate the correct object with either hand. However, the patients with a transected corpus callosum could locate the correct object only with the hand ipsilateral to the projected image (contralateral to the hemisphere that received the visual information). The visual information must have had access to the somatosensory and motor areas of the cortex for the hand to explore and recognize the correct object. With the corpus callosum cut, the visual and motor areas are interconnected only on the same side of the brain.

Another test was to ask the patient to identify verbally what object was seen in the picture. The patient would make a correct verbal response to a picture that was projected to the right of the fixation point so that the visual information reached only the left (language dominant) hemisphere. However, the patient could not verbally identify a picture that was presented to the left hemifield so that visual information reached the right hemisphere.

Similar observations can be made in patients with a transected corpus callosum when different forms of stimuli are used. For example, when such patients are given a verbal command to raise the right arm, they will do so without difficulty. The language centers in the left hemisphere send signals to the motor areas on the same side, and these signals produce the movement of the right arm. However, the same patients cannot respond to a command to raise the left arm. The language areas on the left side cannot influence the motor areas on the right unless the corpus callosum is intact. The result is a type of **apraxia** (inability to control voluntary movement).

Somatosensory stimuli applied to the right side of the body can be described by patients with a transected corpus callosum. However, these patients cannot describe the same stimuli applied to the left side of the body. Information that reaches the right somatosensory areas of the cortex cannot reach the language centers if the corpus callosum has been cut.

The functional capabilities of the two hemispheres can be compared by exploring the performance of individuals with a transected corpus callosum. Such patients solve three-dimensional puzzles better with the right than with the left hemisphere, suggesting that the right hemisphere specializes in spatial tasks. Other functions that seem to be more associated with the right than the left hemisphere are facial expression, body language, and speech intonations. The corpus callosum promotes coordination between the two hemispheres. Patients with a transected corpus callosum lack coordination. When they are dressing, for example, one hand may button a shirt while the other tries to unbutton it.

A striking conclusion of experiments on these patients is that the two hemispheres can operate quite independently when they are no longer interconnected. However, one hemisphere can express itself with language, whereas the other communicates only nonverbally.

Learning and Memory

Major functions of the higher levels of the nervous system are learning and memory. *Learning is a neural mechanism by which the individual changes his or her behavior as the result of experience. Memory refers to the storage mechanism for what is learned.*

Types of learning. The two broad classes of learning are **nonassociative** and **associative learning.** Nonassociative

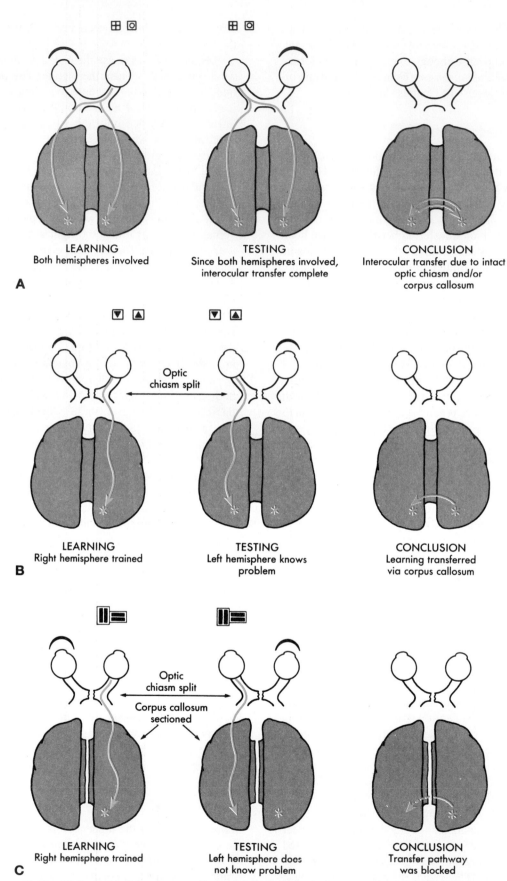

Fig. 10-9 Role of the corpus callosum in the interhemispheric transfer of visual information. **A,** Learning involves one eye. The discrimination depends on distinguishing between a cross and a circle. **B,** Discrimination is between triangles oriented with the apex up or down. **C,** Discrimination is between vertical and horizontal bars.

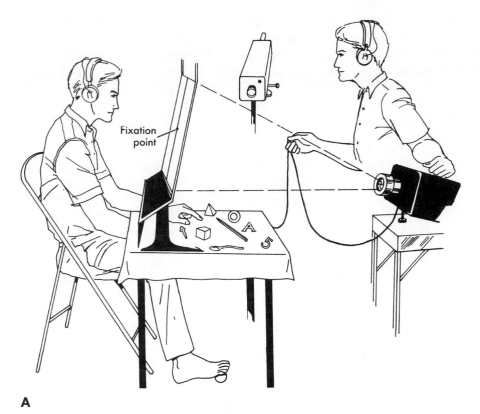

A

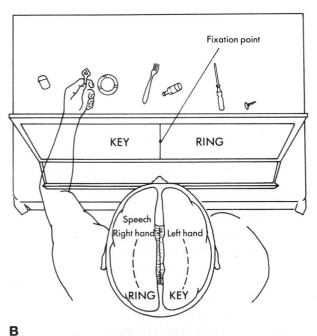

B

■ **Fig. 10-10** Tests in a patient with a transected corpus callosum. **A,** The patient fixes on a point on a rear projection screen, and pictures are projected to either side of the fixation point. The hand can palpate objects that correspond to the projected pictures, but these cannot be seen. **B,** Response by the left hand to a picture of a key in the left field of view. However, the verbal response is that the patient sees a picture of a ring. (Redrawn from Sperry RW: In Schmitt FO, Worden FG, editors: *The neurosciences: third study program,* Cambridge, Mass, 1974, MIT Press.)

learning does not depend on a particular relationship between what is learned and some other stimulus. For example, in a type of nonassociative learning called **habituation,** a repeated stimulus causes a response that gradually diminishes. The responses presumably diminish because the individual learns that the stimulus is not important. A familiar example is the change in attention that typically occurs when a new clock is presented to a subject. At first the ticking noise may be annoying and may cause some

difficulty in sleeping. However, after several nights the clock is no longer noticed. Unfortunately, the response to the clock's morning alarm may also become diminished.

Another type of nonassociative learning is **sensitization.** In sensitization, a strong and consequently threatening stimulus results in a greater probability of a response to later similar stimuli. When the stimulus is first given, the response may be minimal. However, with repetition, the response increases. For example, a spanking can lead to a greater likelihood that a child will obey a parent's admonition. Thus, in sensitization, learning occurs in a direction opposite to that seen in habituation, presumably so that the behavior becomes directed toward escape from the stimulus.

Associative learning occurs when the learning process involves a consistent relationship in the timing between stimuli. In **classic conditioning,** a temporal association is made between a neutral conditioned stimulus and an unconditioned stimulus that elicits an unlearned response. When this combination of stimuli is repeated, provided that the timing relationship is maintained, the association between these stimuli is learned, at which point the conditioned stimulus alone will elicit the unlearned response. An example of classic conditioning is the behavior of dogs in Pavlov's experiments on conditioned reflexes. For example, food presented to a hungry dog elicits an unconditioned response, salivation. If a bell is rung just before the food is presented, the dog learns to associate the bell with the food. Eventually, ringing the bell alone causes salivation. Of course, if the food fails to appear consistently when the bell is rung, the conditioned response fades away, a process called **extinction.**

Another form of associative learning is **instrumental** or **operant conditioning.** In this process, when the response to a stimulus is reinforced, the probability of the response changes. The reinforcement can be either positive or negative. An example of positive reinforcement is giving a fish to a porpoise for jumping out of the water through a hoop. An example of negative reinforcement would be sending a child to his or her room for misbehaving. With positive reinforcement the response probability increases; with negative reinforcement the probability decreases.

Experiments on the mechanisms of learning. The neural circuitry involved in learning in mammals is complex; hence it has been difficult to study these mechanisms. An alternative approach has been to examine the cellular basis of learning in the simpler nervous systems of invertebrates, such as the marine mollusk *Aplysia*. By isolating a connection between a single sensory neuron and a motor neuron responsible for a particular motor response, modeling habituation, sensitization, and even conditioning has been possible.

These examples of learning at a cellular level revealed that the presynaptic endings of the sensory neuron can change the amount of neurotransmitter released during learning. For example, during short-term habituation, the amount of transmitter released in successive responses gradually diminishes. The change involves an alteration in the Ca^{2+} current that triggers neurotransmitter release. The cause of this change is that repeated action potentials lead to a reduction in the number of available Ca^{2+} channels. Long-term habituation can also be produced. In this case the number of synaptic endings and of active zones in the remaining terminals decreases.

Long-term potentiation. Another model of learning is provided by a synaptic phenomenon called **long-term potentiation (LTP).** LTP has been studied most intensively in slices of the hippocampus in vitro. However, LTP has also been described in the neocortex and in other parts of the nervous system. Repetitive activation of an afferent pathway to the hippocampus or of one of the intrinsic connections increases the responses of the pyramidal cells. The increased responses (the LTP) last for hours in vitro (and even days to weeks in vivo). The forms of LTP differ, depending on the particular synaptic system. The mechanism of the enhanced synaptic efficacy seems to involve both pre- and postsynaptic events. The neurotransmitters involved in LTP include excitatory amino acids that act on *N*-methyl-D-aspartate (NMDA) receptors, the responses of which are associated with an influx of Ca^{2+} into the postsynaptic neuron. Second messenger pathways (including G proteins, Ca^{2+}/calmodulin-dependent kinase II, protein kinase G, and protein kinase C) are also involved, and these kinases cause protein phosphorylation and changes in the responsivenss of neurotransmitter receptors. A retrograde messenger, perhaps nitric oxide (or carbon monoxide), may be released from the postsynaptic neurons to act on presynaptic endings in such a way as to enhance transmitter release. Immediate-early genes are also activated during LTP. Hence, changes in gene expression may also be involved.

Another form of synaptic plasticity is **long-term depression (LTD).** LTD has been studied most extensively in the cerebellum, but it also occurs in the hippocampus and in other regions of the central nervous system (CNS). Some of the same factors, such as Ca^{2+} influx and activation of signal transduction mechanism, may account for the induction of LTD, just as for LTP.

Memory. With regard to the stages of memory storage, a distinction between **short-term memory** and **long-term memory** is useful. Recent events appear to be stored in short-term memory by ongoing neural activity, because short-term memory persists for only minutes. Short-term memory is used, for instance, to remember a telephone number after calling the operator. Long-term memory can be subdivided into an intermediate form, which can be disrupted, and a long-lasting form, which is difficult to disrupt. Memory loss can be caused by a disruption of memory per se, or it can be a result of interference with the mechanism for recovering information from memory. Long-term memory may involve structural changes in the nervous system, because this form of memory can remain intact even after events that disrupt short-term memory.

The temporal lobes appear to be particularly important for memory, because bilateral removal of the hippocampal formation severely and permanently disrupts recent memory. Short-term and long-term memories are unaffected, but new long-term memories can no longer be stored.

Neural plasticity. Damage to the nervous system can induce remodeling of neural pathways and thereby alter behavior. Such remodeling is said to reflect the **plasticity** of the nervous system. The CNS is much more plastic than was once believed. For example, the development of neural connections may be altered by certain manipulations, such as by lesions of the brain or by sensory deprivation. Plasticity is greatest in the developing brain, but some degree of plasticity remains in the adult brain.

The capability for developmental plasticity may change for some neural systems at a time referred to as the **critical period.** For example, it may be possible to alter the connections formed in the visual pathways during their development, but only up to a particular developmental period. In visually deprived animals, the visual connections may be abnormal (Fig. 10-11). However, visual deprivation that occurs after several postnatal months does not result in abnormal connections, nor does restoration of vision after this time repair the abnormal connections in previously visually deprived animals. The plastic changes seen in such experiments may reflect a competition between fibers for synaptic connections with postsynaptic neurons in the developing nervous system. If a developing neural pathway "loses" in such a competition, the result may be a neurological deficit in the adult.

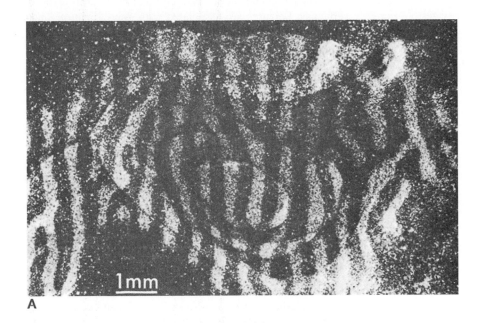

A

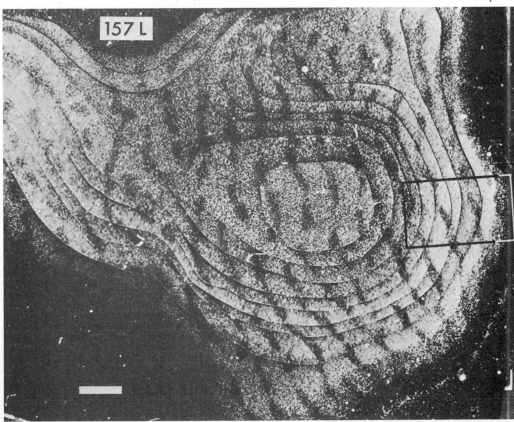

B

■ **Fig. 10-11** Plasticity in the visual pathway as a result of sensory deprivation during development. The ocular dominance columns are demonstrated by autoradiography after injection of a radioactive tracer into one eye. The tracer is transported to the lateral geniculate nucleus and then transneurally transported to the striate cortex. The cortex is labeled in bands that alternate with unlabeled bands whose input is from the uninjected eye. **A,** Normal pattern. **B,** Changed pattern in an animal raised with monocular visual deprivation. The injection was into the nondeprived eye, and the ocular dominance columns for this eye were clearly expanded. In other experiments, it could be shown that the ocular dominance columns for the deprived eye contracted. (**A** from Hubel DH, Wiesel TN: *Proc R Soc Lond B* 198:1, 1977; **B** from LeVay S, Hubel DH, Wiesel TN: *J Comp Neurol* 191:1, 1980.)

A consequence of visual deprivation during development of the visual pathways may be **amblyopia** of the deprived eye. Amblyopia is reduced visual capacity, and it can occur, for example, in children with strabismus (cross-eye) because of a relative weakness of one of the extraocular muscles. Similar effects can be produced by a cataract or by uncorrected myopia.

Plastic changes can also occur after injury to the brain in adults. Sprouting of new axons does occur in the damaged CNS. However, the sprouts do not necessarily restore normal function, and many neural pathways do not appear to sprout. Additional knowledge concerning neural plasticity in the adult nervous system is vital if medical therapy is to be improved for many diseases of the nervous system and after neural trauma. Research is currently being done to explore the potential of human embryonic stem cells for restoring nervous system function.

SUMMARY

1. The cerebral cortex can be subdivided into lobes, based on the pattern of gyri and sulci. Each lobe has special functions, as shown by the effects of lesions or seizures.

2. The cerebral cortex can be subdivided into neocortex, allocortex, and juxtaallocortex. The neocortex typically has six layers, whereas the other types of cortex have fewer layers.

3. The neocortex contains a number of cell types, including pyramidal cells, which serve as the output cells, and several kinds of interneurons. The pyramidal cells release an excitatory amino acid neurotransmitter, whereas the inhibitory interneurons are GABAergic.

4. Specific thalamocortical afferent fibers terminate mainly in the middle layers of the neoocortex; diffuse thalamocortical afferent fibers synapse in layers I and VI.

5. Cortical efferent fibers from layers II and III project to other areas of the cortex; those from layer V project to many subcortical targets, including the spinal cord, brainstem, and striatum, as well as to non-specific thalamic nuclei; and layer VI distributes to the appropriate specific thalamic nucleus.

6. The cortical structure varies in different regions. Agranular cortex is found in the motor areas, whereas granular cortex (koniocortex) occurs in the primary sensory receiving areas. Homotypical cortex is found elsewhere in the neocortex. Brodmann's areas reflect these variations of cortical structure and correlate with functionally discrete areas.

7. The archicortex has three layers, as typified by the hippocampus and dentate gyrus of the hippocampal formation.

8. The electroencephalogram (EEG) varies with the state of the sleep-wake cycle, disease, and other factors. EEG rhythms include alpha, beta, theta, and delta waves.

9. The EEG reflects synaptic activity of pyramidal cells. Cortical evoked potentials are stimulus-triggered changes in the EEG and are useful clinical tests of sensory transmission.

10. Sleep can be divided into slow-wave and rapid eye movement (REM) forms. Slow-wave sleep progresses through stages 1 through 4, each with a characteristic EEG pattern. Most dreams occur in REM sleep. Sleep is produced actively by a brainstem mechanism, and its circadian rhythmicity is controlled by the suprachiasmatic nucleus.

11. The EEG helps in the recognition of the various forms of epilepsy. Seizures are associated with depolarization shifts in pyramidal cells. Such shifts are caused by dendritic Ca^{2+} spikes and a reduction in inhibitory processing.

12. The left cerebral hemisphere is dominant for language in most individuals. Wernicke's area is responsible for the understanding of language and Broca's area for its expression.

13. Information is transferred between the two hemispheres through the corpus callosum. This structure coordinates the two sides of the brain. The right hemisphere is more capable than the left in spatial tasks, facial expression, body language, and speech intonation.

14. Learning includes nonassociative and associative forms. Two kinds of nonassociative learning are habituation and sensitization. Associative learning includes classic and operant conditioning.

15. Long-term potentiation is mediated by an increased synaptic efficacy that lasts hours to weeks and that involves both pre- and postsynaptic changes.

16. Memory includes short-term (minutes), recent, and long-term storage processes, and a retrieval mechanism. The hippocampal formation is important for recent memory.

BIBLIOGRAPHY

Journal articles

Alvarez PS, Zola-Morgan S, Squire LR: Damage limited to the hippocampal region produces long-standing memory impairment in monkeys, *J Neurosci* 15:3796, 1995.

Bear MF, Abraham WC: Long-term depression in hippocampus, *Annu Rev Neurosci* 19:437, 1996.

Best PJ, White AM, Minai A: Spatial processing in the brain: the activity of hippocampal place cells, *Annu Rev Neurosci* 24:459, 2001.

Chen C, Tonegawa S: Molecular genetic analysis of synaptic plasticity, activity-dependent neural development, learning, and memory in the mammalian brain, *Annu Rev Neurosci* 20:157, 1997.

Gage FH: Mammalian neural stem cells, *Science* 287:1433, 2000.

Qiu J, Cai D, Filbin MT: Glial inhibition of nerve regeneration in the mature mammalian CNS, *Glia* 29:166, 2000.

Malenka RC, Nicoll RA: Long-term potentiation: a decade of progress? *Science* 285:1870, 1999.

Martin SJ, Grimwood PD, Morris RGM: Synaptic plasticity and memory: an evaluation of the hypothesis, *Annu Rev Neurosci* 23:649, 2000.

McCormick DA, Bal T: Sleep and arousal: thalamocortical mechanisms, *Annu Rev Neurosci* 20:185, 1997.

Squire LR et al: Activation of the hippocampus in normal humans: A functional anatomical study of memory, *Proc Natl Acad Sci USA* 89:1837, 1995.

Books and monographs

Engel J, Pedley TA: *Epilepsy: a comprehensive textbook*, Philadelphia, 1997, Lippincott-Raven.

Garey LJ: *Brodmann's "Localization in the cerebral cortex,"* London, 1994, Smith-Gordon.

Gazzaniga MS: *The new cognitive neurosciences,* ed 2, Cambridge, Mass., 2000, MIT Press.

Hobson JA: *Sleep,* New York, 1989, Scientific American Library.

McCarley RW: Sleep, dreams and states of consciousness. In Conn PM, editor: *Neuroscience in medicine,* Philadelphia, 1995, JB Lippincott, pp 535–554.

Penfield W, Jasper H: *Epilepsy and the functional anatomy of the human brain,* Boston, 1954, Little, Brown & Co.

chapter eleven

The Autonomic Nervous System and Its Central Control

The **autonomic nervous system** can be regarded as a part of the motor system. However, instead of skeletal muscle, the effectors of the autonomic nervous system are smooth muscle, cardiac muscle, and glands. Because the autonomic nervous system provides motor control of the viscera, it is sometimes called the **visceral motor system.** An older term for this system is the **vegetative nervous system.** This terminology is no longer used, because it does not seem appropriate for a system that is important for all levels of activity, including aggressive behavior.

An important function of the autonomic nervous system is to assist the body in maintaining a constant internal environment **(homeostasis).** When internal stimuli signal that regulation of the body's environment is required, the central nervous system (CNS) and its autonomic outflow issue commands that lead to compensatory actions. For example, a sudden increase in systemic blood pressure activates the baroreceptors, which in turn adjust the autonomic nervous system and restore the blood pressure toward its previous level (see Chapter 21).

The autonomic nervous system also participates in appropriate and coordinated responses to external stimuli. For example, the autonomic nervous system helps regulate pupil size in response to different intensities of ambient light. An extreme example of this regulation is the "fight-or-flight response" that occurs when a threat intensively activates the sympathetic nervous system. This activation causes a variety of responses. Adrenal hormones are released, the heart rate and blood pressure increase, bronchioles dilate, intestinal motility and secretion are inhibited, glucose metabolism increases, pupils dilate, hairs become erect owing to the action of piloerector muscles, cutaneous and splanchnic blood vessels constrict, and blood vessels in skeletal muscle dilate. However, the "fight-or-flight response" is an uncommon event; it does not represent the usual mode of operation of the sympathetic nervous system in daily life.

Accompanying the autonomic motor fibers in peripheral nerves are visceral afferent fibers that originate from sensory receptors in the viscera. Many of these receptors trigger reflexes, but the activity of some receptors evokes sensory experiences, such as pain, hunger, thirst, nausea, and a sense of visceral distension. The chemical senses can also be considered visceral senses (see Chapter 8).

The term autonomic nervous system generally refers to the **sympathetic** and **parasympathetic nervous systems.** In this chapter, the **enteric nervous system** is also included as part of the autonomic nervous system, although it is sometimes considered as a separate entity. In addition, because the autonomic nervous system is under CNS control, the central components of the autonomic nervous system are discussed in this chapter. These central components include the hypothalamus and higher levels of the limbic system, which are associated with emotions and with many visceral behaviors (e.g., feeding, drinking, thermoregulation, reproduction, defense, and aggression) that have survival value.

ORGANIZATION OF THE AUTONOMIC NERVOUS SYSTEM

The primary functional unit of the sympathetic and parasympathetic nervous systems is a two-neuron motor pathway, which consists of a preganglionic neuron, whose cell body is located in the CNS, and a postganglionic neuron, whose cell body is located in one of the autonomic ganglia (Fig. 11-1). The enteric nervous system includes the neurons and nerve fibers in the myenteric and submucosal plexuses, which are located in the wall of the gastrointestinal tract.

The sympathetic preganglionic neurons are located in the thoracic and upper lumbar segments of the spinal cord. For this reason, the sympathetic nervous system is sometimes referred to as the **thoracolumbar division** of the autonomic nervous system. In contrast, the parasympathetic preganglionic neurons are found in the brainstem and in the sacral spinal cord. Hence, this part of the autonomic nervous system is sometimes called the **craniosacral division.** Sympathetic postganglionic neurons are generally found in the paravertebral or the prevertebral ganglia, which are located at some distance from the target organs. Parasympathetic

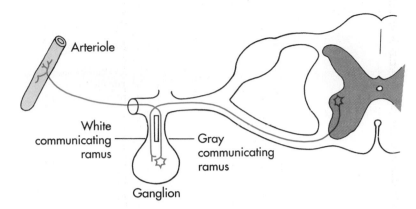

Fig. 11-1 Sympathetic two-neuron motor pathway. A sympathetic preganglionic neuron is shown to have its cell body in the spinal cord gray matter. The axon courses out of the ventral root and enters a sympathetic ganglion through a white communicating ramus. The preganglionic axon synapses on a ganglion cell, and the ganglion cell sends its process, the postganglionic axon, through a gray communicating ramus into the spinal nerve. The postganglionic axon is shown to terminate on an arteriole in the body wall.

postganglionic neurons are found in parasympathetic ganglia near or actually in the walls of the target organs.

The control of the sympathetic and parasympathetic nervous systems of many organs has often been described as antagonistic. This descrption is not entirely correct. It is more appropriate to consider these two parts of the autonomic control system as working in a coordinated way—sometimes acting reciprocally, and sometimes synergistically—to regulate visceral function. Furthermore, not all visceral structures are innervated by both systems. For example, the smooth muscles and glands in the skin and most of the blood vessels in the body receive a sympathetic innervation exclusively; only a small fraction of the blood vessels has a parasympathetic innervation. The parasympathetic nervous system does not innervate the body wall, but only structures in the head and in the thoracic, abdominal, and pelvic cavities.

The Sympathetic Nervous System

Sympathetic preganglionic neurons are concentrated in the **intermediolateral cell column** in the thoracic and upper lumbar segments of the spinal cord (Figs. 11-2 and 11-3). Some neurons may also be found in the C8 segment. In addition to the intermediolateral cell column, groups of sympathetic preganglionic neurons are found in other locations, including the lateral funiculus, the intermediate region, and the part of lamina X dorsal to the central canal.

The axons of the preganglionic neurons are often small myelinated nerve fibers known as B fibers. However, some are unmyelinated C fibers. They leave the spinal cord in the ventral root and enter the paravertebral ganglion at the same segmental level through a white communicating ramus. White rami are found only from T1 to L2. The preganglionic axon may synapse on postganglionic neurons in this ganglion, or they may pass through the ganglion and enter either the sympathetic chain or a splanchnic nerve (see Figs. 11-1 and 11-3).

Preganglionic axons in the paravertebral sympathetic chain of ganglia may travel rostrally or caudally to a nearby or distant paravertebral ganglion and then synapse. If the synapse is in a paravertebral ganglion, the postganglionic axon often passes through a gray communicating ramus to enter a spinal nerve (Fig. 11-1). Each of the 31 pairs of spinal nerves has a gray ramus. Postganglionic axons are distributed through the peripheral nerves to effectors, such as piloerector muscles, blood vessels, and sweat glands, located in the skin, muscle, and joints. Postganglionic axons are generally unmyelinated (C fibers), although some exceptions exist. The distinction between white and gray rami is based on the relative content of myelinated and unmyelinated axons in these rami.

Preganglionic axons in a splanchnic nerve often travel to a prevertebral ganglion and synapse, or they may pass through the ganglion and an autonomic plexus and end in a more distant ganglion. Some preganglionic axons pass through a splanchnic nerve and end directly on cells of the adrenal medulla.

The sympathetic chain extends from cervical to coccygeal levels of the spinal cord. This arrangement serves as a distribution system, enabling preganglionic neurons, which are limited to thoracic and upper lumbar segments, to activate postganglionic neurons that innervate all body segments. However, there are fewer paravertebral ganglia than there are spinal segments, because some of the segmental ganglia fuse during development. For example, the superior cervical sympathetic ganglion represents the fused ganglia of C1 through C4; the middle cervical sympathetic ganglion is the fused ganglia of C5 and C6; and the inferior cervical sympathetic ganglion is the combination of the ganglia at C7 and C8. The term **stellate ganglion** refers to a fusion of the inferior cervical sympathetic ganglion with the ganglion of T1. The superior cervical sympathetic ganglion provides postganglionic innervation to the head and neck; and the middle cervical and stellate ganglia innervate the heart, lungs, and bronchi.

Generally, the sympathetic preganglionic neurons are distributed to ipsilateral ganglia and thus control autonomic function on the same side of the body. One important exception to this is that the sympathetic innervation of the intestine and of the pelvic viscera is bilateral. As with motor neurons to skeletal muscle, sympathetic preganglionic neurons that control a particular organ are spread over several segments. For example, the sympathetic preganglionic neurons that control sympathetic functions in the head and neck region are distributed in C8 to T5, whereas those that control the adrenal gland are in T4 to T12.

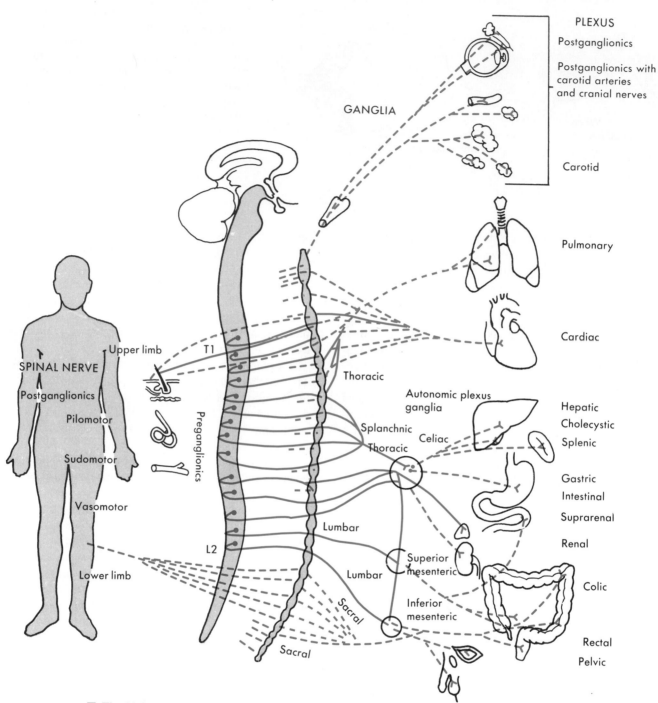

Fig. 11-2 Sympathetic nervous system and its distribution. (Redrawn from Bhagat BD, Young PA, Biggerstaff DE: *Fundamentals of visceral innervation,* Springfield, Ill, 1977, Charles C. Thomas.)

The Parasympathetic Nervous System

The parasympathetic preganglionic neurons are located in several cranial nerve nuclei in the brainstem, as well as in the intermediate region of the S3 and S4 segments of the sacral spinal cord (Fig. 11-4). The cranial nerve nuclei that contain parasympathetic preganglionic neurons are the **Edinger-Westphal nucleus** (cranial nerve III), the **superior** (cranial nerve VII) and **inferior** (cranial nerve IX) **salivatory**

nuclei, and the **dorsal motor nucleus** and **nucleus ambiguus** (cranial nerve X). Postganglionic parasympathetic cells are located in cranial ganglia, including the **ciliary ganglion** (preganglionic input is from the Edinger-Westphal nucleus), the **pterygopalatine** and **submandibular ganglia** (input from the superior salivatory nucleus), and the otic ganglion (input from the inferior salivatory nucleus). The ciliary ganglion innervates the pupillary sphincter and ciliary muscles in the eye. The pterygopalatine ganglion supplies the lacrimal

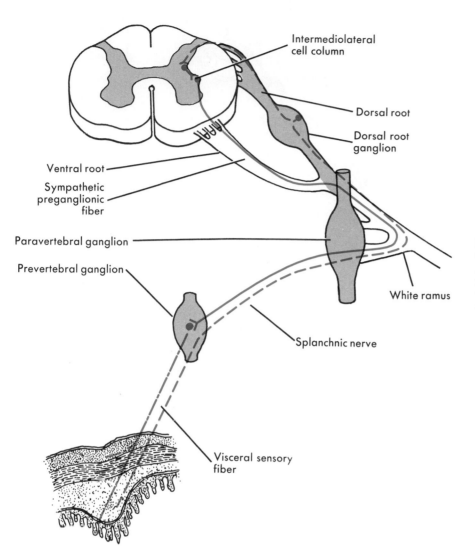

Intermediolateral
cell column

Dorsal root

Dorsal root
ganglion

Ventral root

Sympathetic
preganglionic
fiber

Paravertebral ganglion

Prevertebral ganglion

White ramus

Splanchnic nerve

Visceral sensory
fiber

■ **Fig. 11-3** Simple visceral reflex arc. The postganglionic neuron is shown in a prevertebral ganglion. (Redrawn from Bhagat BD, Young PA, Biggerstaff DE: *Fundamentals of visceral innervation,* Springfield, Ill, 1977, Charles C. Thomas.)

gland, as well as glands in the nasal and oral pharynx. The submandibular ganglion projects to the submandibular and sublingual salivary glands and to glands in the oral cavity. The otic ganglion innervates the parotid salivary gland and glands in the mouth.

Other parasympathetic postganglionic neurons are located near or in the walls of visceral organs in the thoracic, abdominal, and pelvic cavities. Neurons of the enteric plexus include cells that can also be considered parasympathetic postganglionic neurons. These cells receive input from the vagus or pelvic nerves. The vagus nerves innervate the heart, lungs, bronchi, liver, and pancreas, and the gastrointestinal tract from the esophagus to the splenic flexure of the colon. The remainder of the colon and rectum, as well as the urinary bladder and reproductive organs, is supplied by sacral parasympathetic preganglionic neurons that distribute through the pelvic nerves to postganglionic neurons in the pelvic ganglia.

The parasympathetic preganglionic neurons that project to the viscera of the thorax and part of the abdomen are located in the dorsal motor nucleus of the vagus and the nucleus ambiguus. The dorsal motor nucleus is largely

secretomotor (it activates glands), whereas the nucleus ambiguus is **visceromotor** (it modifies the activity of cardiac muscle). The dorsal motor nucleus supplies visceral organs in the neck (pharynx, larynx), thoracic cavity (trachea, bronchi, lungs, heart, esophagus), and abdominal cavity (including much of the gastrointestinal tract, liver, and pancreas). Electrical stimulation of the dorsal motor nucleus results in gastric acid secretion, as well as secretion of insulin and glucagon by the pancreas. Although projections to the heart have been described, their function is uncertain. The nucleus ambiguus contains two groups of neurons: (1) a dorsal group (**branchiomotor**) that activates striated muscle in the soft palate, pharynx, larynx, and esophagus; and (2) a ventrolateral group that innervates and slows the heart (see also Chapter 17).

Visceral Afferent Fibers

The visceral motor fibers in the autonomic nerves are accompanied by visceral afferent fibers. Most of these afferent fibers supply information that originates from sensory receptors in the viscera. The activity of these sensory receptors never reaches the level of consciousness. Instead, these

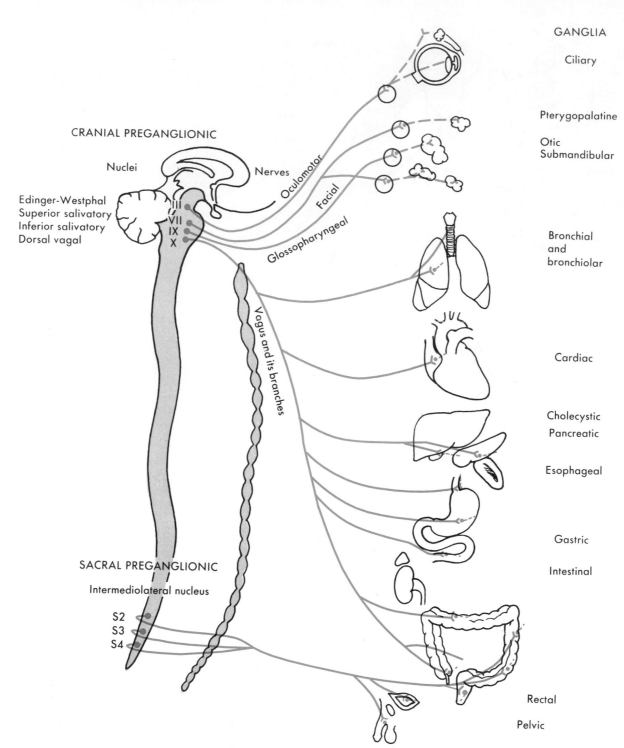

CRANIAL PREGANGLIONIC

Nuclei

Edinger-Westphal
Superior salivatory
Inferior salivatory
Dorsal vagal

Nerves

Oculomotor

Facial

Glossopharyngeal

III
VII
IX
X

Vagus and its branches

SACRAL PREGANGLIONIC

Intermediolateral nucleus

S2
S3
S4

GANGLIA

Ciliary

Pterygopalatine

Otic
Submandibular

Bronchial
and
bronchiolar

Cardiac

Cholecystic

Pancreatic

Esophageal

Gastric

Intestinal

Rectal

Pelvic

■ **Fig. 11-4**   Parasympathetic nervous system. (Redrawn from Bhagat BD, Young PA, Biggerstaff DE: *Fundamentals of visceral innervation,* Springfield, Ill, 1977, Charles C. Thomas.)

afferent fibers form the afferent limb of reflex arcs. Both viscerovisceral and viscerosomatic reflexes are elicited by these afferent fibers. Visceral reflexes operate at a subconscious level, and they are very important for homeostatic regulation and adjustment to external stimuli.

The fast-acting neurotransmitters released by visceral afferent fibers are not well documented, although many of these neurons release an excitatory amino acid transmitter, such as glutamate. However, visceral afferent fibers do contain many neuropeptides, or combinations of these, including angiotensin II, arginine-vasopressin, bombesin, calcitonin gene–related peptide, cholecytstokinin, galanin, substance P, enkephalin, oxytocin, somatostatin, and vasoactive intestinal polypeptide.

Visceral afferent fibers that mediate sensation include nociceptors that travel in sympathetic nerves, such as the splanchnic nerves. Visceral pain is caused by excessive distension of hollow viscera, contraction against an obstruction, or ischemia. The origin of visceral pain is often difficult to identify because of its diffuse nature and its tendency to be referred to somatic structures (see Chapter 7). Visceral nociceptors in sympathetic nerves reach the spinal cord via the sympathetic chain, white rami, and dorsal roots. The terminals of the nociceptive afferent fibers distribute widely in the superficial dorsal horn and also in laminae V and X. They activate not only local interneurons, which participate in reflex arcs, but also projection cells, which include spinothalamic tract cells that signal pain to the brain.

A major visceral nociceptive pathway from the pelvis involves a relay in the lumbosacral spinal cord onto postsynaptic dorsal column neurons that project to the nucleus gracilis. Visceral nociceptive signals are then transmitted to the ventral posterior lateral nucleus of the thalamus, and presumably from there to the cerebral cortex. Interruption of this pathway accounts for the beneficial effects of surgically induced lesions of the dorsal column at lower thoracic levels to relieve pain produced by cancers of the pelvic organs.

Other visceral afferent fibers travel in parasympathetic nerves. These fibers are generally involved in reflexes rather than in sensation (except for the taste afferent fibers; see Chapter 8). For example, the baroreceptor afferent fibers that innervate the carotid sinus are in the glossopharyngeal nerve. They enter the brainstem and pass through the solitary tract to terminate in the nucleus of the solitary tract. These neurons connect with interneurons in the brainstem reticular formation. The interneurons, in turn, project to the autonomic preganglionic neurons that control heart rate and blood pressure (see Chapter 11).

The nucleus of the solitary tract receives information from all visceral organs, except those in the pelvis. This nucleus is subdivided into several areas that receive information from specific visceral organs.

The Enteric Nervous System

The enteric nervous system, which is located in the wall of the gastrointestinal tract, contains about 100 million neurons. The enteric nervous system is subdivided into the myenteric plexus, which lies between the longitudinal and circular muscle layers of the gut, and the submucosal plexus, which lies in the submucosa of the gut. The neurons of the myenteric plexus control gastrointestinal motility (see Chapter 31), whereas those in the submucosal plexus regulate body fluid homeostasis (see Chapter 36).

The types of neurons found in the myenteric plexus include not only excitatory and inhibitory motor neurons (which can be considered as parasympathetic postganglionic neurons), but also interneurons and primary afferent neurons. The afferent neurons supply mechanoreceptors within the wall of the gastrointestinal tract. These mechanoreceptors form the afferent limb of reflex arcs within the enteric plexus. Local excitatory and inhibitory interneurons process these reflexes, and the output is sent through the motor neurons to the smooth muscle cells. *Excitatory motor neurons release acetylcholine and substance P; inhibitory motor neurons release dynorphin and vasoactive intestinal polypeptide.* The circuitry of the enteric plexus is so extensive that it can coordinate the movements of an intestine that has been completely removed from the body. However, normal function requires innervation by the autonomic preganglionic neurons and regulation by the CNS.

Activity in the enteric nervous system is modulated by the sympathetic nervous system. *Sympathetic postganglionic neurons that contain norepinephrine inhibit intestinal motility, those that contain norepinephrine and neuropeptide Y regulate blood flow, and those that contain norepinephrine and somatostatin control intestinal secretion.* Feedback is provided by intestinofugal neurons that project back from the myenteric plexus to the sympathetic ganglia.

The submucosal plexus regulates ion and water transport across the intestinal epithelium and glandular secretion. It also communicates with the myenteric plexus to ensure coordination of the functions of the two components of the enteric nervous system. The neurons and neural circuits of the submucosal plexus are not as well understood as are those of the myenteric plexus, but many of the neurons contain neuropeptides, and the neural networks are well organized.

AUTONOMIC GANGLIA

The main type of neuron in autonomic ganglia is the post ganglionic neuron. These cells receive synaptic connections from preganglionic neurons, and they project to autonomic effector cells. However, many autonomic ganglia also contain interneurons. These interneurons process information within the autonomic ganglia; the enteric plexus can be regarded as an elaborate example of this kind of processing. One type of interneuron found in some autonomic ganglia contains a high concentration of catecholamines. Hence these interneurons have been called **small, intensely fluorescent (SIF) cells.** The SIF cells are believed to be inhibitory.

NEUROTRANSMITTERS
Neurotransmitters in Autonomic Ganglia

The classic neurotransmitter of autonomic ganglia, whether sympathetic or parasympathetic, is acetylcholine. The two classes of acetylcholine receptors in autonomic ganglia are **nicotinic** and **muscarinic receptors,** so named because of their responses to the plant alkaloids, **nicotine** and **muscarine.** Nicotinic acetylcholine receptors can be blocked by such agents as **curare** or **hexamethonium,** and muscarinic receptors can be blocked by atropine. Nicotinic receptors in autonomic ganglia differ somewhat from those on skeletal muscle cells.

■ **Table 11-1**   Responses of effector organs to autonomic nerve impulses

Effector organs	Receptor type	Adrenergic impulses,[1] Responses[2]	Cholinergic impulses,[1] Responses[2]
Eye	α		
Radial muscle, iris		Contraction (mydriasis) ++	—
Sphincter muscle, iris		—	Contraction (miosis) +++
Ciliary muscle	β	Relaxation for far vision +	Contraction for near vision +++
Heart			
SA node	β_1	Increase in heart rate ++	Decrease in heart rate; vagal arrest +++
Atria	β_1	Increase in contractility and conduction velocity ++	Decrease in contractility, and (usually) increase in conduction velocity ++
AV node	β_1	Increase in automaticity and conduction velocity ++	Decrease in conduction velocity; AV block +++
His-Purkinje system	β_1	Increase in automaticity and conduction velocity +++	Little effect
Ventricles	β_1	Increase in contractility, conduction velocity, automaticity, and rate of idioventricular pacemakers +++	Slight decrease in contractility
Arterioles			
Coronary	α,β_2	Constriction +; dilation[3] ++	Dilation +
Skin and mucosa	α	Constriction +++	Dilation[4]
Skeletal muscle	α,β_2	Constriction ++; dilation[3,5] ++	Dilation[6] +
Cerebral	α	Constriction (slight)	Dilation[4]
Pulmonary	α,β_2	Constriction +; dilation[3]	Dilation[4]
Abdominal viscera, renal	α,β_2	Constriction +++; dilation[5] +	—
Salivary glands	α	Constriction +++	Dilation ++
Veins (systemic)	α,β_2	Constriction ++; dilation ++	—
Lung			
Bronchial muscle	β_2	Relaxation +	Contraction ++
Bronchial glands	?	Inhibition (?)	Stimulation +++
Stomach			
Motility and tone	α_2,β_2	Decrease (usually)[7] +	Increase +++
Sphincters	α	Contraction (usually) +	Relaxation (usually) +
Secretion		Inhibition (?)	Stimulation +++
Intestine			
Motility and tone	α_2,β_2	Decrease[7] +	Increase +++
Sphincters	α	Contraction (usually) +	Relaxation (usually) +
Secretion		Inhibition (?)	Stimulation +++
Gallbladder and ducts		Relaxation +	Contraction +
Kidney	β_2	Renin secretion ++	—
Urinary bladder			
Detrusor	β	Relaxation (usually) +	Contraction +++
Trigone and sphincter	α	Contraction +++	Relaxation ++
Ureter			
Motility and tone	α	Increase (usually)	Increase (?)
Uterus	α,β_2	Pregnant: contraction (α); nonpregnant: relaxation (β)	Variable[8]
Sex organs, male	α	Ejaculation +++	Erection +++
Skin			
Pilomotor muscles	α	Contraction ++	—
Sweat glands	α	Localized secretion[9] +	Generalized secretion +++
Spleen capsule	α,β_2	Contraction +++; relaxation +	—
Adrenal medulla		—	Secretion of epinephrine and norepinephrine
Liver	α,β_2	Glycogenolysis, gluconeogenesis[10] +++	Glycogen synthesis +

■ **Table 11-1** Responses of effector organs to autonomic nerve impulses—*Cont'd*

Effector organs	*Receptor type*	*Adrenergic impulses,[1] Responses[2]*	*Cholinergic impulses,[1] Responses[2]*
Pancreas			
Acini	α	Decreased secretion +	Secretion ++
Islets (β cells)	α	Decreased secretion +++	—
	β_2	Increased secretion +	—
Fat cells	α, β_1	Lipolysis[10] +++	—
Salivary glands	α	Potassium and water secretion +	Potassium and water secretion +++
	β	Amylase secretion +	—
Lacrimal glands		—	Secretion +++
Nasopharyngeal glands		—	Secretion +++
Pineal gland	β	Melatonin synthesis	—

From Goodman LS, Gilman A: *The pharmacological basis of therapeutics,* ed 6, New York, 1980, Macmillan.

[1]A long dash—signifies no known functional innervation.

[2]Responses are designated 1+ to 3+ to provide an approximate indication of the importance of adrenergic and cholinergic nerve activity in the control of the various organs and functions listed.

[3]Dilation predominates in situ owing to metabolic autoregulatory phenomena.

[4]Cholinergic vasodilatation at these sites is of questionable physiological significance.

[5]Over the usual concentration range of physiologically released, circulating epinephrine, β-receptor response (vasodilatation) predominates in blood vessels of skeletal muscle and liver, and α-receptor response (vasoconstriction) in blood vessels of other abdominal viscera. The renal and mesenteric vessels also contain specific dopaminergic receptors, activation of which causes dilation, but their physiological significance has not been established.

[6]Sympathetic cholinergic system causes vasodilatation in skeletal muscle, but this is not involved in most physiological responses.

[7]It has been proposed that adrenergic fibers terminate at inhibitory β receptors on smooth muscle fibers and at inhibitory α receptors on parasympathetic cholinergic (excitatory) ganglion cells of Auerbach's plexus.

[8]Depends on stage of menstrual cycle, amount of circulating estrogen and progesterone, and other factors.

[9]Palms of hands and some other sites ("adrenergic sweating").

[10]There is significant variation among species in the type of receptor that mediates certain metabolic responses.

Nicotinic and muscarinic receptors both mediate excitatory postsynaptic potentials (EPSPs), but these potentials have different time courses. Stimulation of preganglionic neurons elicits a fast EPSP, followed by a slow EPSP. The fast EPSP results from activation of nicotinic receptors, which cause the opening of ion channels. The slow EPSP is mediated by muscarinic receptors that inhibit the **M current,** a current that is produced by a potassium conductance.

Neurons in autonomic ganglia also release neuropeptides that act as neuromodulators. Besides acetylcholine, sympathetic preganglionic neurons may release enkephalin, substance P, luteinizing hormone–releasing hormone, neurotensin, or somatostatin.

Catecholamines, such as norepinephrine or dopamine, serve as the neurotransmitters of the SIF cells in autonomic ganglia.

Neurotransmitters between Postganglionic Neurons and Autonomic Effectors

Sympathetic postganglionic neurons. Sympathetic postganglionic neurons typically release norepinephrine, which excites some effector cells, but inhibits other effector cells. The receptors on the target cells may be either α- or β-adrenergic receptors. These receptors are further subdivided into α_1, α_2, β_1, and β_2 receptors. The distribution of these types of receptors and the actions that they mediate when activated by sympathetic postganglionic neurons are listed for various target organs in Table 11-1.

α_1 Receptors are located postsynaptically, but α_2 receptors may be either presynaptic or postsynaptic. Receptors located presynaptically are generally called **autoreceptors;** they usually inhibit transmitter release. The effects of agents that excite α_1 or α_2 receptors can be distinguished by using antagonists to block these receptors specifically. For example, prazosin is a selective α_1 antagonist, and yohimbine is a selective α_2 antagonist. The effects of α_1 receptors are mediated by activation of the inositol trisphosphate/diacylglycerol second messenger system (see Chapter 5). On the other hand, α_2 receptors decrease the rate of synthesis of cAMP through an action on a G protein.

β Receptors are subdivided into β_1 and β_2 receptors on the basis of the ability of antagonists to block them. The proteins that make up the two types of β receptors are similar, with seven membrane-spanning regions connected by intracellular and extracellular domains (see Chapter 5). Agonist drugs that work on β receptors activate a G protein, which stimulates adenylyl cyclase to increase the cAMP concentration. This action is terminated by the build-up of guanosine diphosphate.

β Receptors can also be antagonized by action of α_1 receptors. The number of β receptors can be regulated. If the β receptors are exposed to agonists, they can be desensitized by phosphorylation. Their numbers can also be decreased if they become internalized. β Receptors can also increase in number (upregulation), for example, by denervation. The number of α receptors is also regulated.

In addition to releasing norepinephrine, sympathetic postganglionic neurons release neuropeptides, such as somatostatin and neuropeptide Y. For example, cells that release both norepinephrine and somatostatin supply the mucosa of the gastrointestinal tract, and cells that release both norepinephrine and neuropeptide Y innervate blood vessels in the gut and the limb. Another chemical mediator in sympathetic postganglionic neurons is adenosine triphosphate (ATP).

The endocrine cells of the adrenal medulla are similar in many respects to sympathetic postganglionic neurons (see also Chapter 45). They receive input from sympathetic preganglionic neurons, are excited by acetylcholine, and release catecholamines. However, the cells of the adrenal medulla differ from sympathetic postganglionic neurons in that they release catecholamines into the circulation, rather than synaptically. Also, the main catecholamine released is epinephrine, not norepinephrine. In humans, 80% of the catecholamine released by the adrenal medulla is epinephrine and 20% is norepinephrine.

Some sympathetic postganglionic neurons release acetylcholine, rather than norepinephrine, as their neurotransmitter. For example, sympathetic postganglionic neurons that innervate eccrine sweat glands are cholinergic. The acetylcholine receptors involved are muscarinic, and they are therefore blocked by atropine. Similarly, some blood vessels are innervated by cholinergic sympathetic postganglionic neurons. In addition to releasing acetylcholine, the postganglionic neurons that supply the sweat glands also release neuropeptides, including calcitonin gene-related peptide and vasoactive intestinal polypeptide.

Parasympathetic postganglionic neurons. The neurotransmitter released by parasympathetic postganglionic neurons is acetylcholine. The effects of these neurons on various target organs are listed in Table 11-1. Parasympathetic postganglionic actions are mediated by muscarinic receptors. On the basis of binding studies, the action of selective antagonists, and molecular cloning, several types of muscarinic receptors have now been discovered. At least two types of muscarinic receptors, M_1 and M_2, can be distinguished on the basis of the action of the antagonist, pirenzepine. M_1 receptors have a high affinity for pirenzepine, and their activation enhances the secretion of gastric acid. M_2 receptors have a low affinity for pirenzepine, and their activation slows the heart. A subtype of the M_2 receptor activates glands, such as the lacrimal and submaxillary glands.

Muscarinic receptors, like adrenergic ones, have diverse actions. Some of their effects are mediated by specific second messenger systems. For example, cardiac M_2 muscarinic receptors may act by way of the inositol trisphosphate (IP_3) system, and they may also inhibit adenylyl cyclase and thus cAMP synthesis. Muscarinic receptors also open or close ion channels, particularly K^+ or Ca^{2+} channels. This action on ion channels is likely to occur through activation of G proteins. A third action of muscarinic receptors is to relax vascular smooth muscle by an effect on endothelial cells, which produce endothelium-derived relaxing factor (EDRF). It has recently been shown that EDRF is actually nitric oxide, a gas released when arginine is converted to citrulline by nitric oxide synthase (see Chapter 21). Nitric oxide relaxes vascular smooth muscle by stimulating guanylate cyclase and thereby increasing levels of cGMP, which in turn activates a cGMP-dependent protein kinase (see Chapter 5).

The number of muscarinic receptors is regulated, and exposure to muscarinic agonists decreases the number of receptors by internalization of the receptors.

CENTRAL CONTROL OF AUTONOMIC FUNCTION

The discharges of autonomic preganglionic neurons are controlled by pathways that synapse on autonomic preganglionic neurons. The pathways that influence autonomic activity include spinal cord or brainstem reflex pathways, and also descending control systems that originate at higher levels of the nervous system, such as the hypothalamus.

Examples of Autonomic Control of Particular Organs

The autonomic control of different target organs depends on local reflex circuitry and on signals from parts of the CNS (see Table 11-1).

Pupil. The sphincter and dilator muscles of the iris determine the size of the pupil. Activation of the sympathetic innervation of the eye dilates the pupil (**mydriasis**), which occurs during emotional excitement and also in response to painful stimulation. The neurotransmitter at the sympathetic postganglionic synapses is norepinephrine, which acts at α receptors.

Sympathetic control of the pupil is sometimes affected by disease. For example, interruption of the sympathetic innervation of the head and neck results in **Horner's syndrome.** This syndrome is characterized by pupillary constriction, partial ptosis caused by paralysis of the superior tarsal muscle, loss of sweating on the face, vasodilation of facial skin, and withdrawal of the eye into the orbit (**enophthalmos**). Horner's syndrome can be produced by a lesion that (1) destroys the sympathetic preganglionic neurons in the upper thoracic spinal cord, (2) interrupts the cervical sympathetic chain, or (3) damages the lower brainstem in the region of the reticular formation, through which pathways descend to the spinal cord to activate sympathetic preganglionic neurons.

The parasympathetic nervous system exerts an action on pupillary size opposite to that of the sympathetic nervous system. The sympathetic system elicits pupillary dilation, whereas the parasympathetic system constricts the pupil (**meiosis**). The main neurotransmitter at the postganglionic parasympathetic synapse is acetylcholine, which acts on muscarinic receptors. However, peptides may also serve as neuromodulators for some neurons.

Pupil size is reduced by the pupillary light reflex and during accommodation for near vision. In the **pupillary light**

reflex, light that strikes the retina is processed by retinal circuits that excite W-type retinal ganglion cells (see Chapter 8). These cells respond to diffuse illumination. The axons of some of the W cells project through the optic nerve and tract to the pretectal area, where they synapse in the olivary pretectal nucleus. This nucleus contains neurons that also respond to diffuse illumination. Activity of neurons of the olivary pretectal nucleus causes pupillary constriction by means of bilateral connections with parasympathetic preganglionic neurons in the Edinger-Westphal nuclei. The reflex results in contraction of the pupillary sphincter muscles in both eyes.

In the **accommodation response,** information from M cells of the retina is transmitted to the striate cortex through the geniculostriate visual pathway (see Chapter 8). The stimulus that triggers accommodation is thought to be a blurred retinal image and disparity of the image between the two eyes. After the information is processed in the visual cortex, signals are transmitted directly or indirectly to the middle temporal cortex, where they activate neurons in a visual area known as MT. The MT neurons transmit signals to the midbrain that activate parasympathetic preganglionic neurons in the Edinger-Westphal nuclei bilaterally, which results in pupillary constriction. At the same time signals are transmitted to the ciliary muscle, causing it to contract. This ciliary muscle contraction allows the lens to round up and increase its refractile power.

The pupillary light reflex is sometimes absent in patients with syphilis, which affects the CNS (i.e., in tabes dorsalis). Although the pupil fails to respond to light, it has a normal accommodation response. This condition is known as the **Argyll-Robertson pupil.** The exact mechanism is controversial. One explanation is that fibers that pass through the brachium of the superior colliculus from the optic tract to the pretectal area are interrupted by syphilitic meningitis. The interruption is caused by the presence of spirochetes in the subarachnoid space. Although the input to the olivary pretectal nucleus is interrupted, the optic tract connection to the lateral geniculate nucleus is maintained, and the pupil is able to accommodate.

Urinary bladder. The urinary bladder is controlled by reflex pathways in the spinal cord and also by a supraspinal center (Fig. 11-5). The sympathetic innervation originates from preganglionic sympathetic neurons in the upper lumbar segments of the spinal cord. Postganglionic sympathetic axons act to inhibit the smooth muscle (**detrusor muscle**) throughout the body of the bladder, and they also act to excite the smooth muscle of the trigone region and of the internal urethral sphincter. The detrusor muscle is tonically inhibited during filling of the bladder, and this prevents urine from being voided. The inhibition of the detrusor muscle is mediated by the action of norepinephrine on β receptors, whereas the excitation of the trigone and internal urethral sphincter is elicited by the action of norepinephrine on α receptors.

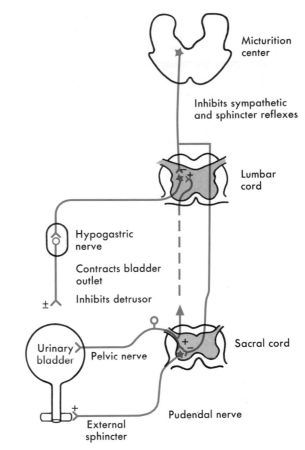

■ Fig. 11-5   The pathway for the reflexes that control the urinary bladder. (Redrawn from de Groat WC, Booth AM: *Autonomic systems to bladder and sex organs.* In Dyck PJ et al, editors: *Peripheral neuropathy,* ed 2, Philadelphia, 1984, WB Saunders.)

The external sphincter of the urethra also helps to prevent voiding. This sphincter is a striated muscle, and it is innervated by motor axons in the pudendal nerves, which are somatic nerves. The motor neurons are located in **Onuf's nucleus,** in the ventral horn of the sacral spinal cord.

The parasympathetic preganglionic neurons that control the bladder are located in the sacral spinal cord (S2 and S3 or S3 and S4 segments). These cholinergic neurons project through the pelvic nerves and are distributed to ganglia in the pelvic plexus and in the bladder wall. Postganglionic parasympathetic neurons in the bladder wall innervate the detrusor muscle, as well as the trigone and sphincter. The parasympathetic activity contracts the detrusor muscle and relaxes the trigone and sphincter. These actions result in **micturition,** or urination. Some of the postganglionic neurons are cholinergic and others are purinergic (they release ATP).

Micturition is normally controlled by the **micturition reflex** (Fig. 11-5). Mechanoreceptors in the bladder wall are excited by both stretch and contraction of the muscles in the bladder wall. Thus, as urine accumulates and distends the bladder, the mechanoreceptors begin to discharge. The pressure in the urinary bladder is low during filling (5 to 10 cm H_2O), but it increases abruptly when micturition begins.

Micturition can be triggered either reflexly or voluntarily. In reflex micturition, bladder afferent fibers excite neurons that project to the brainstem and activate the micturition center in the rostral pons **(Barrington's center)**. The ascending projections also inhibit sympathetic preganglionic neurons that prevent voiding. When a sufficient level of activity occurs in this ascending pathway, micturition is triggered by the micturition center. Commands reach the sacral spinal cord through a reticulospinal pathway. Activity in the sympathetic projection to the bladder is inhibited, and the parasympathetic projections to the bladder are activated. Contraction of the muscle in the wall of the bladder causes a vigorous discharge of the mechanoreceptors that supply the bladder wall and thereby further activate the supraspinal loop. The result is complete emptying of the bladder.

A spinal reflex pathway also exists for micturition. This pathway is operational in the newborn infant. However, with maturation, the supraspinal control pathways take on a dominant role in triggering micturition. After spinal cord injury, human adults lose bladder control during the period of spinal shock (urinary incontinence). As the spinal cord recovers from spinal shock, some degree of bladder function is recovered, because of an enhancement of the spinal cord micturition reflex. However, the bladder has an increased muscle tone, and fails to empty completely. These circumstances frequently lead to urinary infections.

Autonomic Centers in the Brain

An autonomic center consists of a local network of neurons that responds to inputs from a particular source and that influences distant neurons by way of long efferent pathways. The micturition center is the autonomic center in the pons that regulates micturition. Many other autonomic centers with diverse functions are also located in the brain. Vasomotor and vasodilator centers are in the medulla, and respiratory centers are in the medulla and pons. Perhaps the greatest concentration of autonomic centers is in the hypothalamus.

The hypothalamus. The hypothalamus is a part of the diencephalon. Some of the nuclei of the hypothalamus are shown in Fig. 11-6. In the rostrocaudal dimension, the hypothalamus can be subdivided into three regions: **suprachiasmatic, tuberal,** and **mammillary regions.** Some important nuclei include the **supraoptic, paraventricular, tuberal,** and **mammillary nuclei.** Continuing anteriorly from the hypothalamus are telencephalic structures, the preoptic region and septum. Both the preoptic and septal regions help regulate autonomic function. Important fiber tracts that course through the hypothalamus are the **fornix,** the **medial forebrain bundle,** and the **mammillothalamic tract.** The fornix is used as a landmark to divide the hypothalamus into the medial and the lateral hypothalmus.

The hypothalamus has many functions, and its control of autonomic function is emphasized here. See Chapter 45 for a discussion of hypothalamic control of endocrine function.

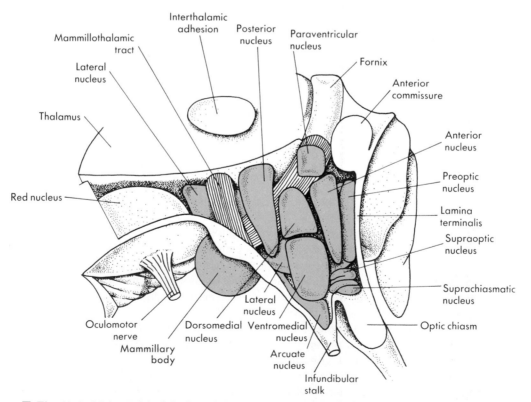

■ Fig. 11-6 Main nuclei of the hypothalamus seen in a view from the third ventricle. (Redrawn from Nauta WJH, Haymaker W: *The hypothalamus,* Springfield, Ill, 1969, Charles C. Thomas.)

Temperature regulation. **Homeothermic animals** are those that are able to regulate their body temperature. When the environmental temperature decreases, the body adjusts by reducing heat loss and by increasing heat production. Conversely, when the temperature rises, the body increases its heat loss and reduces heat production.

Information about the external temperature is provided by thermoreceptors in the skin (and probably other organs, such as muscle). Internal temperature is monitored by central thermoreceptive neurons in the anterior hypothalamus. The central thermoreceptors monitor the temperature of the blood. The system acts as a servomechanism (a control system that uses negative feedback to operate another system) with a set point at the normal body temperature. Error signals, which represent a deviation from the set point, evoke responses that tend to restore body temperature toward the set point. These responses are mediated by the autonomic, somatic, and endocrine systems.

Cooling causes shivering, which consists of asynchronous muscle contractions that increase heat production. Increases in thyroid gland activity and in sympathetic neural activity tend to increase heat production metabolically. Heat loss is reduced by piloerection and by cutaneous vasoconstriction. Piloerection is effective in animals with fur but not in humans; in the latter, the result is goose bumps.

Warming the body causes changes in the opposite direction. The activity of the thyroid gland diminishes, which leads to reduced metabolic activity and less heat production. Heat loss is increased by sweating and cutaneous vasodilation.

The hypothalamus serves as the temperature servomechanism. The heat loss responses are organized by the heat loss center, which is composed of neurons in the preoptic region and anterior hypothalamus. As might be expected, lesions here prevent sweating and cutaneous vasodilation, and they cause **hyperthermia** when the individual is placed in a warm environment. Conversely, electrical stimulation of the heat loss center causes cutaneous vasodilation and inhibits shivering. Heat conservation responses are organized by neurons in the posterior hypothalamus, which form a heat production and conservation center. Lesions in the area that is dorsolateral to the mammillary body interfere with heat production and conservation, and they can cause **hypothermia** when the subject is in a cold environment. Electrical stimulation in this region of the brain evokes shivering.

Thermoregulatory responses are also produced when the hypothalamus is locally warmed or cooled. These responses reflect the presence of central thermoreceptive neurons in the hypothalamus.

In fever, the set point for body temperature is elevated. This can be caused by the release of a pyrogen by microorganisms. The pyrogen changes the set point, leading to increased heat production by shivering and to heat conservation by cutaneous vasoconstriction.

Regulation of food intake. Food intake is also regulated by a servomechanism. However, the set point is affected by many factors. Sensory signals that help regulate food intake operate both on a short-term basis to control ingestion and on a long-term basis to control body weight. Glucoreceptors in the hypothalamus sense blood glucose and use this information to control food intake. Their main action occurs when blood glucose levels decrease. Opioid peptides and pancreatic polypeptide stimulate food intake; cholecystokinin inhibits food intake. Insulin and adrenal glucocorticoids also affect food intake (see Chapters 41 and 45).

Lesions of the lateral hypothalamus suppress food intake **(aphagia),** which can cause starvation and death. Electrical excitation in the lateral hypothalamus stimulates eating. These observations suggest that the lateral hypothalamus contains a **feeding center.** Converse effects are produced by manipulations of the ventromedial nucleus of the hypothalamus. A lesion here causes **hyperphagia,** which is an increased food intake that can result in obesity, whereas electrical stimulation of the same region stops the feeding behavior. This area of the hypothalamus is known as the **satiety center.** The feeding and satiety centers operate reciprocally.

Further work is needed to clarify the role of other parts of the nervous system in feeding behavior.

Regulation of water intake. Water intake also depends on a servomechanism. Fluid intake is influenced by blood osmolality and volume (Fig. 11-7).

With water deprivation, the extracellular fluid becomes hyperosmotic, which in turn causes intracellular fluid to become hyperosmotic. The brain contains neurons that serve as osmoreceptors, which detect increases in the osmotic pressure of the extracellular fluid (see also Chapter 36). The osmoreceptors appear to be located in the organum vasculosum of the lamina terminalis, which is a circumventricular organ. Circumventricular organs surround the cerebral ventricles and lack a blood-brain barrier. The subfornical organ and the organum vasculosum are involved in thirst. The area postrema serves as a chemosensitive zone that triggers vomiting.

Water deprivation also causes a decrease in blood volume, which is sensed by receptors in the low-pressure side of the vasculature, including the right atrium (see also Chapter 17). In addition, decreased blood volume triggers the release of renin by the kidney. Renin breaks down angiotensinogen into angiotensin I, which is then hydrolyzed to angiotensin II (see Chapter 36). This peptide stimulates drinking by an action on angiotensin II receptors in another one of the circumventricular organs, namely, the subfornical organ. Angiotensin II also causes vasoconstriction and release of aldosterone and antidiuretic hormone (ADH).

Insufficient water intake is usually a greater problem than excess water intake. When more water is taken in than is required, it is easily eliminated by inhibition of the release of ADH from neurons in the supraoptic nucleus at their terminals in the posterior pituitary gland (see Chapter 43). As previously mentioned, signals that inhibit ADH release include

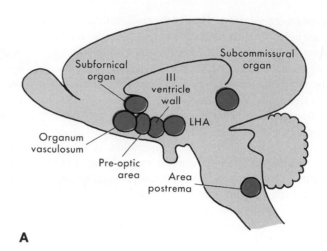

A

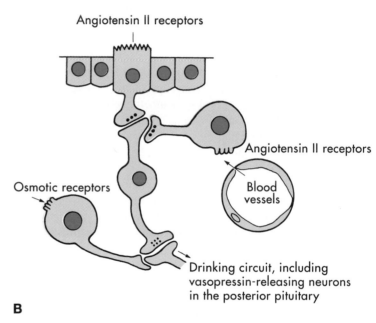

B

■ **Fig. 11-7** **A,** Structures thought to play a role in regulation of water intake in rats. **B,** The neural circuits that signal changes in blood osmolality and volume. (**A,** Redrawn from Shepherd GM: *Neurobiology,* New York, 1983, Oxford University Press.)

an increased blood volume and a decreased osmolality of the extracellular fluid. Other areas of the hypothalamus, particularly the preoptic region and lateral hypothalamus, help regulate water intake, as do several structures outside the hypothalamus.

Other autonomic control structures. Several regions of the forebrain other than the hypothalamus also play a role in autonomic control. These include the central nucleus of the amygdala and bed nucleus of the stria terminalis, as well as a number of areas of the cerebral cortex. Information reaches these higher autonomic centers from viscera through an ascending system that involves the nucleus of the solitary tract, the parabrachial nucleus, the periaqueductal gray, and the hypothalamus. Descending pathways that help control autonomic activity originate in such structures as the paraventricular nucleus of the hypothalamus, the A5 noradrenergic cell group, the rostral ventrolateral medulla, and the raphe nuclei and adjacent structures of the ventromedial medulla.

Neural Influences on the Immune System

Environmental stress can cause immunosuppression, in which the number of helper T cells and the activity of natural killer cells are reduced. Immunosuppression can even be the result of classic conditioning. One mechanism for such an effect involves the release of corticotropin-releasing factor (CRF) from the hypothalamus. CRF causes the release of adrenocorticotropic hormone (ACTH) from the pituitary gland; ACTH release stimulates the secretion of adrenal corticosteroids, which cause immunosuppression (see Chapter 45). Other mechanisms include direct neural actions on lymphoid tissues. The immune system also may influence neural activity.

Emotional Behavior

The limbic system helps control emotional behavior, in part by an influence on the hypothalamus. The limbic lobe is phylogenetically the oldest part of the cerebral cortex. A circuit that connects the limbic lobe with the hypothalamus

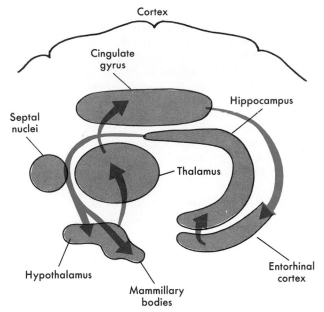

■ Fig. 11-8   The Papez circuit. (From Groves PM, Schlesinger K: *Introduction to biological psychology,* ed 2, Dubuque, Iowa, 1982, Wm C. Brown.)

(the Papez circuit) regulates emotional behavior. The neural components of this circuit were termed the limbic system (Fig. 11-8).

The Papez circuit connects many areas of the neocortex to the hypothalamus. Information passes from the cingulate gyrus to the entorhinal cortex and hippocampus, and from there to the mammillary bodies in the hypothalamus. The mammillothalamic tract then connects the hypothalamus with the anterior thalamic nuclei, which project back to the cingulate gyrus. Other structures included in the limbic system circuitry are the amygdala and the bed nucleus of the stria terminalis.

Bilateral temporal lobe lesions can produce the **Klüver-Bucy syndrome,** which is characterized by loss of the ability to detect and recognize the meaning of objects from visual cues (**visual agnosia,**) a tendency to examine objects orally, attention to irrelevant stimuli, hypersexuality, change in dietary habits, and decreased emotionality. The components of this syndrome can be attributed to damage to different parts of the neocortex and limbic cortex. For instance, the changes in emotional behavior are largely the result of lesions of the amygdala, whereas the visual agnosia is caused by damage to visual areas in the temporal neocortex.

SUMMARY

1. The autonomic nervous system is a motor system that controls smooth muscle, cardiac muscle, and glands. It helps maintain homeostasis and coordinates responses to external stimuli. Its components are the sympathetic, parasympathetic, and enteric nervous systems.

2. Autonomic motor pathways involve preganglionic and postganglionic neurons. Preganglionic neurons reside in the CNS, whereas postganglionic neurons lie in peripheral ganglia.

3. Sympathetic preganglionic neurons are located in the thoracolumbar region of the spinal cord, and sympathetic postganglionic neurons are located in paravertebral and prevertebral ganglia.

4. Parasympathetic preganglionic neurons are located in cranial nerve nuclei or in the sacral spinal cord. Parasympathetic postganglionic neurons reside in ganglia located in or near the target organs.

5. Visceral afferent fibers supply sensory receptors in the viscera. Some have a sensory function, such as visceral pain and taste, but most activate reflexes.

6. The enteric nervous system includes the myenteric and submucosal plexuses in the wall of the gastrointestinal tract. The myenteric plexus regulates motility, and the submucosal plexus regulates ion and water transport and secretion.

7. Neurotransmitters at the synapses of preganglionic neurons in autonomic ganglia include acetylcholine (acting at both nicotinic and muscarinic receptors) and a number of neuropeptides.

8. Interneurons release catecholamines. Sympathetic postganglionic neurons generally release norepinephrine (acting at α_1-, α_2-, β_1-, or β_2-adrenergic receptors) as their neurotransmitter, although neuropeptides are also released. Sympathetic postganglionic neurons that supply sweat glands release acetylcholine. Parasympathetic postganglionic neurons release acetylcholine (acting on M_1 or M_2 muscarinic receptors).

9. The pupil is controlled reciprocally by the sympathetic and parasympathetic nervous systems. Sympathetic activity causes pupillary dilation (mydriasis); parasympathetic activity causes pupillary constriction (meiosis).

10. Emptying of the urinary bladder depends on parasympathetic outflow during the micturition reflex. Sympathetic constriction of the internal sphincter of the urethra prevents voiding. The micturition reflex is triggered by stretch receptors, and it is controlled in normal adults by a micturition center in the pons.

11. The hypothalamus contains several centers that control autonomic and other activities, which include heat loss, heat production and conservation, feeding and satiety, and fluid intake.

12. The limbic system consists of several cortical and other structures. It controls emotional behavior, in part by activation of the autonomic nervous system.

BIBLIOGRAPHY

Journal articles

Adolphs R et al: Fear and the human amygdala, *J Neurosci* 15:5879, 1995.

Brown DA et al: Muscarinic mechanisms in nerve cells, *Life Sci* 60:1137, 1997.

Dampney RAL: Functional organization of central pathways regulating the cardiovascular system, *Physiol Rev* 74:323, 1994.

Jansen ASP et al: Central command neurons of the sympathetic nervous system: basis of the fight or flight response, *Science* 270:644, 1995.

LeDoux JE: Emotion circuits in the brain, *Annu Rev Neurosci* 23:155, 2000.

Watts AG: Neuropeptides and the integration of motor responses to dehydration, *Annu Rev Neurosci* 24:357, 2001.

Books and monographs

Appenzeller O: *The autonomic nervous system: an introduction to basic and clinical concepts,* ed 5, Amsterdam, 1997, Elsevier Biomedical Press.

Blessing WW: *The lower brainstem and bodily homeostasis,* New York, 1997, Oxford University Press.

Brading A: *The autonomic nervous system and its effectors,* 1999, Oxford, Blackwell Science.

Burnstock G, Hoyle CHV, editors: *The autonomic nervous system, Vol. 1. Autonomic neuroeffector mechanisms,* London, 1995, Harwood Academic.

Cannon WB: *The wisdom of the body,* ed 2, New York, 1939, WW Norton & Co.

Gershon M: *The second brain,* New York, 1998, Harper Collins.

Loewy AD, Spyer KM, editors: *Central regulation of autonomic function,* New York, 1990, Oxford University Press.

Mundy AR: Structure and function of the lower urinary tract. In Mundy AR et al, editors: *Scientific basis of urology,* Oxford, 1999, Isis Medical Media Ltd., pp 217-242.

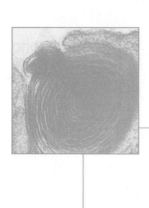

section three

Muscle

James M. Watras

chapter twelve

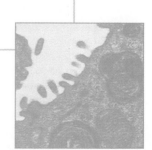

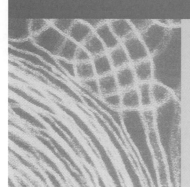

Skeletal Muscle Physiology

Muscle cells are highly specialized cells for the conversion of chemical energy into mechanical energy. Specifically, muscle cells use the energy in adenosine triphosphate (ATP) to generate force or do work. As work can take many forms (such as locomotion, pumping blood, or peristalsis), several types of muscle have evolved. The three basic types of muscle are skeletal muscle, cardiac muscle, and smooth muscle. As shown in Table 12-1, skeletal muscle is a striated muscle that is under voluntary control (i.e., controlled by the central nervous system) and plays a key role in numerous activities such as maintaining posture, locomotion, speech, and respiration. The striations within skeletal muscle cells result from the highly organized arrangement of actin and myosin molecules. The heart is composed of cardiac muscle, and although it is a striated muscle, it is an involuntary muscle (i.e., controlled by an intrinsic pacemaker and modulated by the autonomic nervous system). Smooth muscle, which lacks the striations evident in skeletal and cardiac muscle, is an involuntary muscle typically found lining hollow organs (e.g., urinary bladder, the gastrointestinal tract, and blood vessels). In all three muscle types, force is generated by the interaction of acting and myosin muscles, a process that requires the transient elevation of intracellular Ca^{2+}.

In this chapter, attention will be directed at the molecular mechanisms underlying contraction of skeletal muscle. Mechanisms for regulating the force of contraction will also be addressed. To put this information into perspective, it is important to first examine the basic organization of skeletal muscle.

ORGANIZATION OF SKELETAL MUSCLE

Muscle Fibers

Figure 12-1 illustrates the basic structure of skeletal muscle. Each muscle is composed of numerous cells called **muscle fibers.** A connective tissue layer called the endomysium surrounds each of these fibers. Individual muscle fibers are then grouped together into **fascicles,** which are surrounded by another connective tissue later called the **perimysium.** Within

the perimysium are the blood vessels and nerves that supply the individual muscle fibers. Finally, fascicles are joined together to form the muscle. The connective tissue sheath that surrounds the muscle, which is called the **epimysium,** attaches the muscle to the skeleton. The three connective tissue layers of the muscle are composed mainly of elastin and collagen fibers, and they serve to transmit the movement of the actin and myosin molecules to the skeleton to effect movement.

Individual skeletal muscle cells are narrow (~10 to 80 μm in diameter), but they can be extremely long (up to 25 cm in length). Each skeletal muscle fiber contains bundles of filaments, called **myofibrils,** running along the axis of the cell. The gross striation pattern of the cell results from a repeating pattern in the myofibrils. Specifically, it is the regular arrangement of the thick and thin filaments within these myofibrils coupled with the highly organized alignment of adjacent myofibrils that gives rise to the striated appearance of skeletal muscle.

The myofibril can be subdivided longitudinally into **sarcomeres** (see Fig. 12-2). The sarcomere is demarcated by two dark lines called Z-lines, and represents a repeating contractile unit in skeletal muscle. The average length of a sarcomere is 2 μm. On either side of the Z-line is a light band (I-band), which contains thin filaments composed primarily of the protein actin. The area between two I-bands within a sarcomere is the A band, which contains thick filaments composed primarily of the protein myosin. The thin actin filaments extend from the Z-line toward the center of the sarcomere, overlapping a portion of the tick filaments. The dark area at the end of the A-band represents this region of overlap between thick and thin filaments. A light area is present in the center of the sarcomere, and is called the H-band. This represents the portion of the A-band that contains myosin thick filaments, but no thin actin filaments. Thus, thin actin filaments extend from the Z-line to the edge of the H-band, overlapping a portion of the thick filament in the A-band. A dark line, called the M-line, is evident in the center of the sarcomere, and includes proteins that appear to be critical

■ **Table 12-1**   Basic classification of skeletal muscle fiber types

	Type I: slow oxidative (red)	Type IIB: fast glycolytic (white)	Type IIA*: fast oxidative (red)
Myosin isoenzyme (ATPase rate)	Slow	Fast	Fast
Sarcoplasmic reticular Ca^{2+} pumping capacity	Moderate	High	High
Diameter (diffusion distance)	Moderate	Large	Small
Oxidative capacity: mitochondrial content, capillary density, myoglobin	High	Low	Very high
Glycolytic capacity	Moderate	High	High

*Comparatively infrequent in humans and other primates. In the text a simple designation of type II fiber refers to a fast-glycolytic (type IIB) fiber.

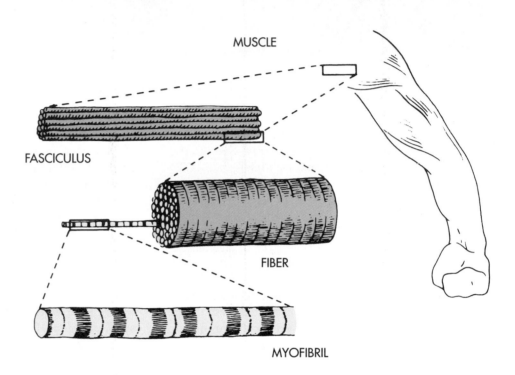

■ **Fig. 12-1**   Skeletal muscle is composed of bundles of muscle fibers called a fasciculus. A muscle fiber represents an individual muscle cell and contains bundles of myofibrils. The striations are due to the arrangement of thick and thin filaments. See text for details. (Redrawn from Bloom W, Fawcett DW: *A textbook of histology,* ed 10, Philadelphia, 1975, WB Saunders.)

for the organization and alignment of the thick filaments in the sarcomere.

As illustrated in Fig. 12-2, each myofibril in the muscle fiber is surrounded by **sarcoplasmic reticulum (SR).** The SR is an intracellular membrane network that plays a critical role in the regulation of intracellular Ca^{2+} concentration. Invaginations of the sarcolemma, called **T-tubules,** pass into the muscle fiber near the ends of the A-band (i.e., close to SR). The SR and the T-tubules, however, are distinct membrane systems. The SR is an intracellular network, whereas the T-tubules are in contact with the extracellular space. A gap (~15 nm in width) separates the T-tubules from the SR. The portion of the SR nearest the T-tubules is called the terminal cisternae, and it is the cite of Ca^{2+} release, which is critical for contraction of skeletal muscle (see below). The longitudinal portions of the SR are continuous with the terminal cisternae, and extend along the length of the sarcomere. This portion of the SR contains a high density of Ca^{2+} pump protein (i.e., Ca^{2+}-ATPase), which is critical for the reaccumulation of Ca^{2+} into the SR, and thereby relaxation of the muscle.

Thick and thin filaments are highly organized in the sarcomere of myofibrils (see Fig. 13-2). As mentioned, thin actin filaments extend from the Z-line toward the center of the sarcomere, whereas the thick myosin filaments are centrally located, and overlap a portion of opposing thin actin filaments. The thick myosin filaments are tethered to the Z-lines by a cytoskeletal protein called titin. **Titin** is a very large, elastic protein (molecular weight in excess of 3000 kDa) that extends from the Z-line to the center of the sarcomere and appears to be important for the organization and alignment of thick filaments in the sarcomere. The thick and thin filaments are oriented such that in the region of overlap within the sarcomere, each thick myosin filament is surrounded by a hexagonal array of thin actin filaments. It is the Ca^{2+}-dependent interaction of the thick myosin and the thin actin filaments that generates the force of contraction following stimulation of the muscle (see below).

A more detailed view of the thin actin filaments is shown in Fig. 12-3. The thin filament is formed by the aggregation of actin molecules (G-actin, or globular actin) into a two stranded helical filament called **F-actin, or filamentous actin.** The elongated cytoskeletal protein nebulin extends along the length of the thin filament and may participate in the

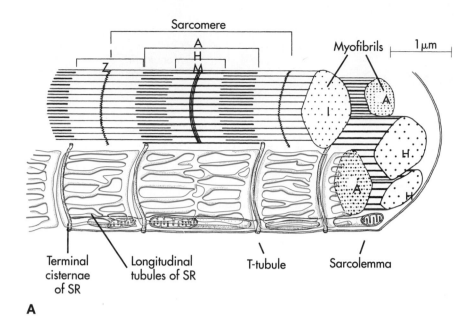

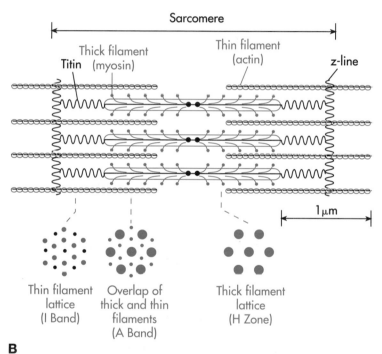

■ Fig. 12-2 **A,** Myofibrils are arranged in parallel within a muscle fiber. Each fibril is surrounded by sarcoplasmic reticulum (SR). Termianl cisternae of the SR are closely associated with T-tubules forming a triad at the juction of the I-bands and A-bands. The Z-lines define the boundary of the sarcomere. The striations are formed by the overlap of the contractile proteins. Three bands can be seen, the A-band, I-band, and H-band. An M-line is seen in the middle of the H-band. **B,** Organization of the proteins within a single sarcomere. The cross-sectional arrangement of the proteins is also illustrated. See text for details.

regulation of the length of the thin filament. Dimers of the protein tropomyosin extend over the entire actin filament covering myosin-binding sites on the actin molecules. Each tropomyosin dimer extends over seven actin molecules, with sequential tropomyosin dimers arranged in a head-to-tail configuration. A troponin complex consisting of three sub-units (**troponin-T, troponin-I,** and **troponin-C**) is present on each tropomyosin dimer and influences the position of the tropomyosin molecule on the actin filament, and hence the ability of tropomyosin to inhibit myosin binding to the actin filament. Troponin-T binds tropomyosin, troponin-I facilitates the inhibition of myosin binding to actin by tropomyosin, and troponin-C binds Ca^{2+}. The binding of Ca^{2+} to troponin-C promotes the movement of tropomyosin on the actin fila-

ment, exposing myosin-binding sites, and thereby the interaction of the myosin and actin filaments and sarcomere contraction (see below). Additional proteins associated with the thin filament include tropomodulin, α-actinin, and capZ protein. Tropomodulin is located at the end of the thin filament, toward the center of the sarcomere, and may participate in setting the length of the thin filament. α-Actinin and capZ protein serve to anchor the thin filament to the Z-line.

Organization of the thick filament is shown in Fig. 12-4. **Myosin** is a large protein (~480 kDa). It consists of six different polypeptides with one pair of large heavy chains (~200 kDa) and two pairs of light chains (~20 kDa). The heavy chains are wound together in an α-helical configuration forming a long rod-like segment, with the N-terminal

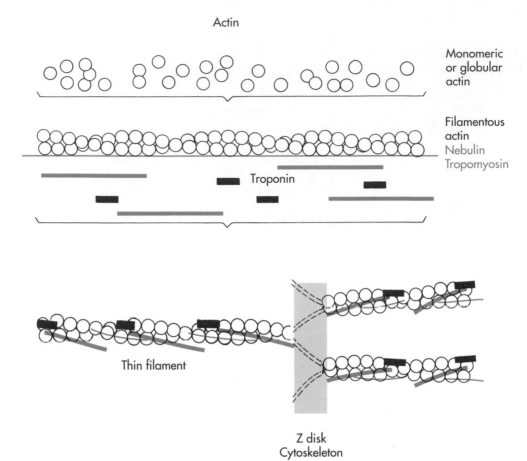

Actin

Monomeric
or globular
actin

Filamentous
actin
Nebulin
Tropomyosin

Troponin

Thin filament

Z disk
Cytoskeleton

■ **Fig. 12-3**   Organization of thin filament. Polymerization of monomeric actin into filamentous actin forms the backbone of the thin filament. The filament contains several other structural/ regulatory proteins such as nebulin, tropomyosin, and troponin.

portion of each heavy chain forming a large globular head. The head region extends away from the thick filament toward the actin thin filament and is the portion of the molecule that can bind to actin. Myosin is also able to hydrolyze ATP, and the ATPase activity is also located in the globular head. The two pairs of light chains are associated with the globular head. One of these pairs of light chains, termed the essential light chains, is critical for the ATPase activity of myosin. The other pair of light chains, sometimes called regulatory light chains, may influence the kinetics of myosin and actin binding under certain conditions. Thus, myosin ATPase activity resides in the globular head of myosin, and requires the preence of light chains (viz. the "essential" light chains).

Myosin filaments form by a tail-to-tail association of myosin molecules, resulting in a bipolar arrangement of the thick filament. The thick filament then extends on either side of the central bare zone by a head-to-tail association of myosin molecules, thus maintaining the bipolar organization of the thick filament centered on the M-line. Such a bipolar arrangement is critical for drawing the Z-lines together (i.e., shortening the length of the sarcomere) during contraction. The mechanisms controlling this highly organized structure of the myosin thick filament are not clear, although the

cytoskeletal protein titin is thought to participate in the formation of a scaffold for the organization and alignment of the thick filament in the sarcomere. Additional proteins found in the thick filaments (e.g., myomesin and C-protein) may also participate in the bipolar organization and/or packing of the thick filament.

The **muscular dystrophies** constitute a group of genetically determined degenerative disorders. **Duchenne muscle dystrophy** (**DMD;** described by G.B. Duchenne in 1861) is the most common of the muscular dystrophies, affecting 1 in 3500 male children (3 to 5 years of age). Severe muscle wasting occurs, with most patient wheelchair bound by age 12, and many dying of respiratory failure in adulthood (30 to 40 years of age). DMD is an X-linked, recessive disease that has been linked to a defect in the dystrophin gene that leads to a deficiency in the dystrophin protein in skeletal muscle, brain, retina, and smooth muscle. Dystrophin is a large (427 kDa) protein that is present in low abundance (0.025%) in skeletal muscle. It is localized on the intracellular surface of the sarcolemma in association with several integral membrane glycoproteins (forming a dystrophin-glycoprotein complex). The function of this dystrophin-glycoprotein

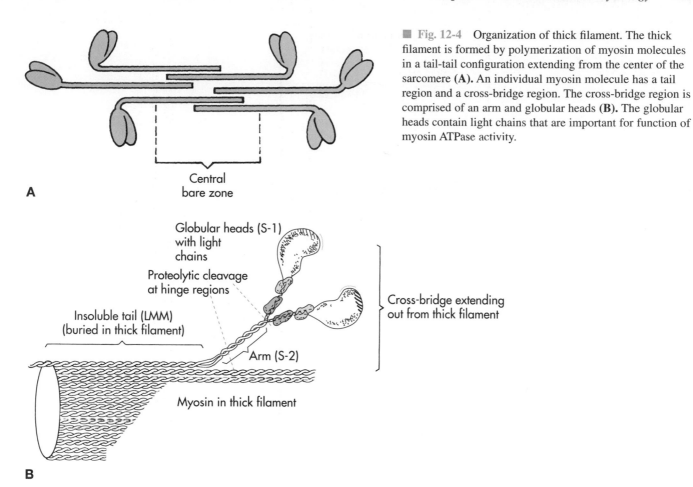

Fig. 12-4 Organization of thick filament. The thick filament is formed by polymerization of myosin molecules in a tail-tail configuration extending from the center of the sarcomere **(A).** An individual myosin molecule has a tail region and a cross-bridge region. The cross-bridge region is comprised of an arm and globular heads **(B).** The globular heads contain light chains that are important for function of myosin ATPase activity.

complex is not known, though mutations in this complex can promote cell death (apoptosis). The dystrophin-glycoprotein complex has been considered to be a structural component of the cell linking actin to the surface membrane, although recent studies suggest that the dystrophin-glycoprotein complex may serve as a scaffold for cell signaling cascades that promote cell survival.

CONTROL OF SKELETAL MUSCLE ACTIVITY

Motor Nerves and Motor Units

Skeletal muscle is controlled by the central nervous system. Specifically, each skeletal muscle is innervated by an α-motor neuron. The cell bodies of the **α-motor neurons** are located in the ventral horn of the spinal cord (see Fig. 12-5). The motor axons exit via the ventral roots and reach the muscle through mixed peripheral nerves. The motor nerves branch in the muscle, with each branch innervating a single muscle fiber. The specialized cholinergic synapse that forms the neuromuscular junction and the neuromuscular transmission process that generates an action potential in the muscle fiber are described in Chapter 4.

A motor unit consists of the motor nerve and all the muscle fibers innervated by the nerve. The motor unit is the functional contractile unit, because all the muscle cells within a motor unit contract synchronously when the motor nerve fires. The size of motor units within a muscle varies depending of the function of the muscle. In the rectus muscles of the eye the motor units are small (i.e., only a small number of muscle fibers are innervated by a motor neuron), and thus the movement of the eye can be precisely controlled. In contrast, the motor units of the muscle of the back are large, which facilitates the maintenance of an erect posture. Activating varying numbers of motor units within a muscle is one way in which the tension developed by a muscle can be controlled (see below).

The neuromuscular junction formed by the α-motor neuron is called an end plate (see Chapter 4 for details). Acetylcholine released from the α-motor neuron at the neuromuscular junction initiates an action potential in the muscle fiber, which rapidly spreads along its length. The duration of the action potential in skeletal muscle is less than 5 msec. This contrasts with the duration of the action potential in cardiac muscle, which is approximately 200 msec in duration. The short duration of the skeletal muscle action potential allows for very rapid contractions of the fiber, and provides yet another mechanism by which the force of contraction can be increased. Increasing tension by repetitive stimulation of the muscle is called tetany (this phenomenon is described in more detail later in this chapter).

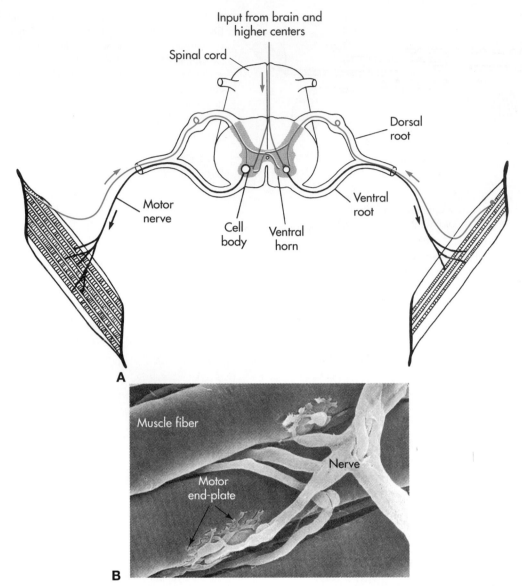

■ Fig. 12-5 Skeletal muscle is a voluntary muscle, controlled by the central nervous system, with efferent signals (i.e., action potentials) passing through an α-motor neuron to muscle fibers. Each motor neuron may innervate many muscle fibers within a muscle, although each muscle fiber is innervated by only one motor neuron (**A**). **B,** Scanning electron micrograph showing innervation of several muscle fibers by a single motor neuron. (**B** from Bloom W, Fawcett DW: *A textbook of physiology,* ed 12, New York, 1994, Chapman & Hall.)

Excitation-Contraction Coupling

When an action potential is transmitted along the sarcolemma of the muscle fiber and then down the T-tubules, Ca^{2+} is released from the terminal cisternae SR into the myoplasm. This release of Ca^{2+} from the SR raises the intracellular Ca^{2+} concentration, which in turn promotes actin-myosin interaction and contraction. The time course for the increase in intracellular Ca^{2+} relative to the action potential and force development is shown in Fig. 12-6. The action potential is extremely short-lived (~5 msec). The elevation of intracellular Ca^{2+} begins slightly after the action potential, and peaks at approximately 20 msec. This increase in intracellular Ca^{2+} initiates a contraction called a twitch.

The mechanism underlying the elevation of intracellular Ca involves an interaction between protein in the T-tubule and the adjacent terminal cisternae of the SR. As previously described (see Fig. 12-2) the T-tubule represents an invagination of the sarcolemma, which extends into the muscle fiber and forms a close association with two terminal cisternae of the SR. The association of a T-tubule with two terminal cisternae is called a triad. Although there is a gap (~15 nm in width) between the T-tubule and the terminal cisternae, proteins bridge this gap. Based on their appearance in electron micrographs these bridging proteins are called feet (see Fig. 12-7). These feet are the Ca^{2+} release channels in the membrane of the terminal cisternae that are responsible for the elevation of intracellular Ca^{2+} in response to their

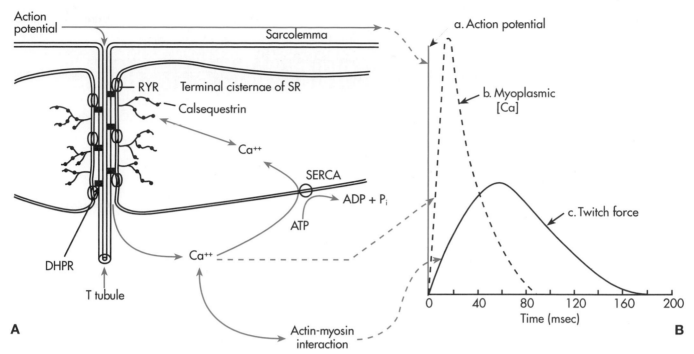

Fig. 12-6   Stimulation of a skeletal muscle fiber initiates an action potential in the muscle, which travels down the T-tubule and induces Ca^{2+} release from the terminal cisternae of the SR **(A)**. The rise in intracellular Ca^{2+} concentration causes contraction. As Ca^{2+} is pumped back into the SR by the Ca^{2+}-ATPase (SERCA) relaxation occurs. **B,** The time courses of the action potential, myoplasmic Ca^{2+} transient, and the force of the twitch contraction.

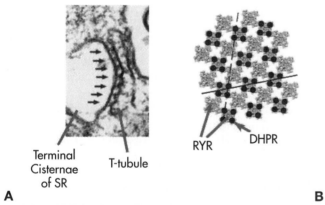

Fig. 12-7   **A,** Electron micrograph of a triad illustrating the "feet" between the T-tubule and the SR, which are thought to be the ryanodine receptors (RYR) in the SR. **B,** Each RTR in the SR is associated with four dihydropyridine receptors (DHPR) in the T-tubule. (From Protasi F, Takekuri H, et al: *Biophys J* 79(5): 2494–2508, 2000.)

action potential. Because this channel binds the drug ryanodine, it is commonly called the **ryanodine receptor (RYR).** The RYR is a large protein (~500 kDa), that exists as a homotetramer. Only a small portion of the RYR molecule is actually imbedded in the SR membrane. Most of the RYR molecule appears to be in the myoplasm, spanning the gap between the terminal cisternae and the T-tubule (see Figs. 12-7 and 12-8).

At the T-tubule membrane, the RYR is thought to interact with a protein called the **dihydropyridine receptor (DHPR).** The DHPR is an L-type voltage-gated Ca^{2+} channel, with five subunits. One of these subunits binds the dihydropyridine class of channel-blocking drugs, and appears to be critical for the ability of the action potential in the T-tubule to induce Ca^{2+} release from the SR. However, Ca^{2+} influx into the cell through the DHPR is not needed for the initiation of Ca^{2+} release from the SR. Indeed, skeletal muscle is able to contract in the absence of extracellular Ca^{2+}, or with a mutated DHPR that does not conduct Ca^{2+}. Instead, the release of Ca^{2+} from the terminal cisternae of the SR is thought to result from a conformational change in the DHPR as the action potential passes down the T-tubule, and this conformational change in the DHPR, by means of a protein-protein interaction, opens the RYR, releasing Ca^{2+} into the myoplasm.

Structural analyses, including the use of freeze fracture techniques, provide evidence for a close physical association of the DHPR with RYR (see Fig. 12-7). DHPR in the T-tubule membrane appears to reside directly opposite the four corners of the underlying homotetrameric RYR channel in the SR membrane. A variety of mutational studies have been done to ascertain the region of the DHPR that is critical for the opening of the RYR. One possible site of interaction (depicted in Fig. 12-8) is the myoplasmic loop between transmembrane domains II

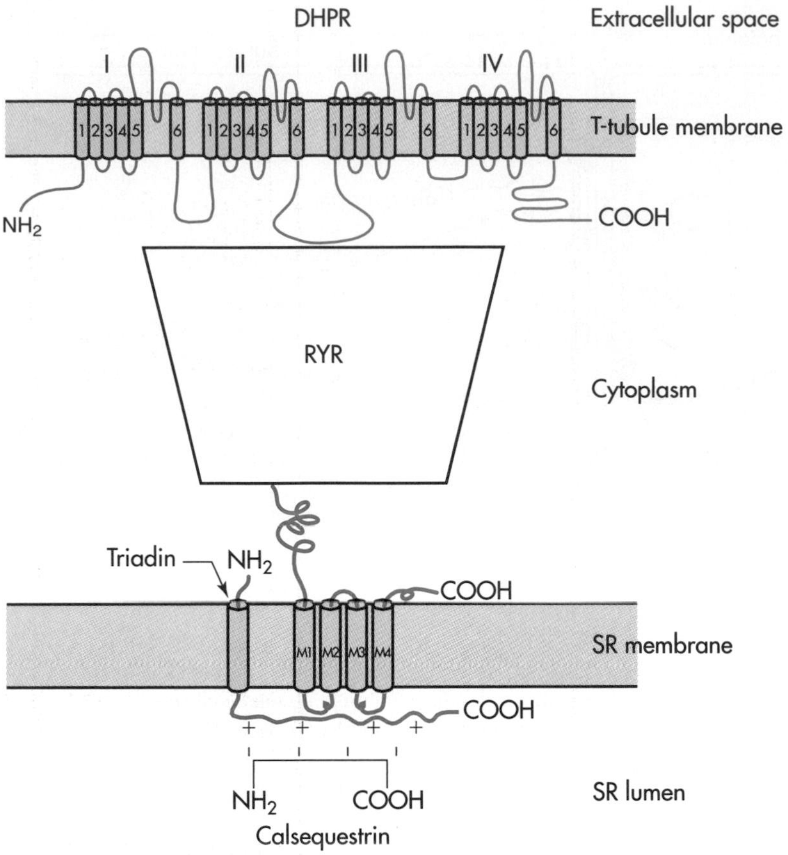

■ **Fig. 12-8** Molecular structure and relationships between the dihydropyridine receptor (DHPR) in the T-tubule membrane and the ryanodine receptor (RYR) in the SR membrane. Triadin is an associated SR protein that may participate in the interaction of the RYR and DHPR. Calsequestrin is a low-affinity Ca^{2+}-binding protein that helps to accumulate Ca^{2+} in the terminal cisternae. See text for details. (From Franzini-Armstrong C, Protasi F: *Physiol Rev* 77(3):699, 1997.)

and III in the α_1-subunit of the DHPR. The voltage-sensing region of the DHPR involved in the intramembranous charge movement is thought to reside in the S4 transmembrane segments of the α_1-subunit. Genetic mutations in the RYR and/or the DHPR have been associated with pathological disturbances in myoplasmic Ca^{2+} concentration. This includes malignant hyperthermia and central core disease, as described at the end of this chapter. These mutations are typically observed in the myoplasmic portion of the RYR, though mutations have also been observed in a myoplasmic loop in the DHPR.

Two other proteins that reside near the RYR are triadin and calsequestrin (see Fig. 12-8). Triadin may participate in the interaction of the RYR with the DHPR. Calsequestrin, on the other hand, is a low-affinity Ca^{2+} binding protein that is present in the lumen of the terminal cisternae. It allows Ca^{2+} to be "stored" at high concentration and thereby establishes a favorable concentration gradient that facilitates the efflux of Ca^{2+} from the SR into the myoplasm when the RYR opens.

Relaxation of the skeletal muscle occurs as intracellular Ca^{2+} is resequestered by the SR. The uptake of Ca^{2+} into the SR is due to the action of a Ca^{2+} pump (i.e., Ca^{2+}-ATPase). This pump is not unique to skeletal muscle and is found in all cells in association with the endoplasmic reticulum. Accordingly, it is named **SERCA,** which stands for **S**arcoplasmic **E**ndoplasmic **R**eticulum **C**alcium **A**TPase.

SERCA is the most abundant protein in the SR of skeletal muscle, and it is distributed throughout the longitudinal tubules and the terminal cisternae as well. It transports two molecules of Ca^{2+} into its lumen for each molecule of ATP hydrolyzed. Thus, the Ca^{2+} transient seen during a twitch contraction (see Fig. 12-6) reflects Ca^{2+} release from the terminal cisternae via the RYR and reuptake primarily into the longitudinal portion of the SR by SERCA. The localization of calsequestrin in the terminal cisternae facilitates the storage of large amounts of Ca^{2+} at its release site.

Genetic disease causing disturbances in Ca homeostasis in skeletal muscle include **malignant hyperthermia (MH), central core disease (CCD),** and **Brody disease (BD).** MH is an autosomal dominant trait that has life-threatening consequences in certain surgical instances. Anesthetics such as halothane or ether and the muscle relaxant succinylcholine can produce uncontrolled release of Ca^{2+} from the SR, resulting in skeletal muscle rigidity, tachycardia, hyperventilation, and hyperthermia. This condition is lethal if not treated immediately. There are currently a series of tests (using contractile responses of muscle biopsies) to assess if a patient has MH. The incidence of MH is approximately 1 in 15,000 children, or 1 in 50,000 adults treated with anesthetics. MH is the result of a defect in the SR Ca^{2+} release channel (RYR), which becomes activated in the presence of the above anesthetics, resulting in the release of Ca^{2+} into the myoplasm,

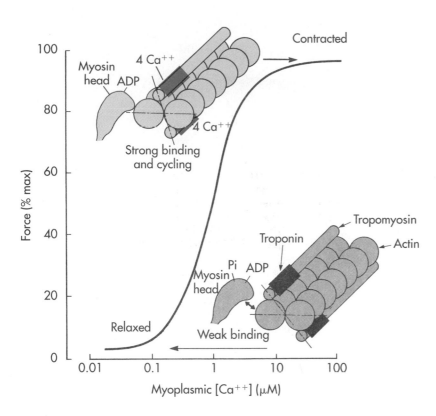

Fig. 12-9 Contractile force of skeletal muscle increases in a Ca^{2+}-dependent manner due to the binding of Ca^{2+} to troponin-C and the subsequent movement of tropomyosin away from myosin-binding sites on the underlying actin molecules. See text for details. (From MacLennan DH, Rice WJ, Green NM: *J Biol Chem* 272(46):28815, 1997.)

and hence prolonged muscle contraction (rigidity). The defect in the RYR is not restricted to a single locus. In some cases, MH has been linked to a defect in the DHPR of the T-tubule.

Central core disease (CCD) is a rare, autosomal dominant trait, which results in muscle weakness, the loss of mitochondria in the core of skeletal muscle fibers, and some disintegration of the contractile filaments. CCD is often closely associated with MH, so CCD patients are treated as MH susceptible in surgical situations. It is hypothesized that central cores devoid of mitochondria represent areas of elevated intracellular Ca^{2+} due to a mutation in the RYR, resulting in mitochondrial Ca^{2+} uptake, which in turn can lead to mitochondrial Ca^{2+} overload and loss of mitochondria.

Brody disease (BD) is characterized by painless muscle cramping and impaired muscle relaxation during exercise. While running upstairs, for example, muscles may stiffen and temporarily cannot be used. This relaxation abnormality is seen in the muscles of the legs, arms, and eyelid, with the response worsened in cold weather. BD can be either autosomal recessive or autosomal dominant and may involved mutations in up to three genes. BD, however, is a rare occurrence (affecting 1 in 10,000,000 births). It appears that BD results from a decreased activity of the SERCA1 Ca^{2+} pump found in fast twitch skeletal muscle. The decreased activity of SERCA1 has been associated with mutation in the SERCA1 gene, though there may also be an accessory factor that contributes to the decreased SR Ca^{2+} uptake in fast twitch skeletal muscle of individuals with BD.

Actin Myosin Interaction: Cross-Bridge Formation

As noted, contraction of skeletal muscle requires an increase in intracellular Ca^{2+}. Moreover, the process of contraction is regulated by the thin filament. As shown in Fig. 12-9, contractile force (i.e., tension) increases in a sigmoidal fashion as intracellular Ca^{2+} concentration is elevated above 0.1 μm, with half-maximal force occurring at less than 1 μm Ca^{2+}. The mechanism by which Ca^{2+} promotes this increase in tension is as follows. Ca^{2+} released from the SR binds to troponin-C. Once bound with Ca^{2+}, troponin-C facilitates the movement of the associated tropomyosin molecule toward the cleft of the actin filament. This movement of tropomyosin exposes the myosin-binding site on the actin filament, allowing a cross-bridge to form, and thereby generate tension (see below). There are four Ca^{2+} binding sites on troponin-C. Two of these sites have a high affinity for Ca^{2+}, but also bind Mg^{2+} at rest. These sites seem to be involved in controlling and enhancing the interaction between the troponin-I and troponin-T subunits. The other two binding sites have a lower affinity and bind Ca^{2+} as its concentration rises following release from the SR. Binding of myosin to the actin filaments appears to cause a further shift in tropomyosin. Although a given tropomyosin molecule extends over seven actin molecules, it is hypothesized that the strong binding of myosin to actin results in movement of an adjacent tropomyosin molecule, perhaps exposing myosin-binding sites on as many as 14 actin molecules. This ability of one tropomyosin molecule to influence the movement of another may be a consequence of the close proximity of adjacent tropomyosin molecules (see Fig. 12-10).

■ **Fig. 12-10** Organization of the thin filament, showing a double helical array of tropomyosin on the actin filament, with sequential tropomyosin molecules arranged in a head-to-tail configuration. Such a configuration may promote the interaction of one tropomyosin unit with an adjacent tropomyosin. Also shown is the troponin complex consisting of its three subunits: troponin-C (TnC), troponin-I (TnI), and troponin-T (TnT). See text for details. (From Gordon AM, Homsher E, Regnier M: *Physiol Rev* 80(2):853, 2000.)

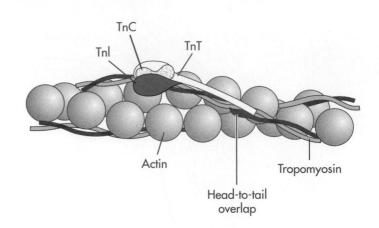

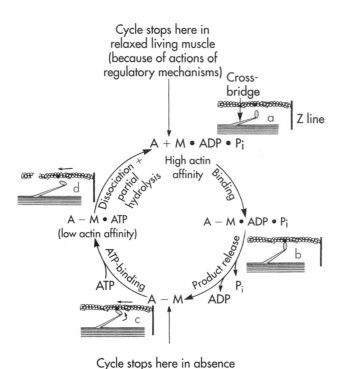

■ **Fig. 12-11**   Cross-bridge cycle. *State a:* In the relaxed state, ATP is partially hydrolyzed (M ADP P_i). *State b:* In the presence of elevated myoplasmic Ca^{2+}, myosin binds to actin. *State c:* Hydrolysis of ATP is completed causing a conformational change in the myosin molecule, which pulls the actin filament toward the center of the sarcomere. *State d:* A new ATP binds to myosin causing release of the cross-bridge. Partial hydrolysis of the newly bound ATP recocks the myosin head, which is now ready to bind again and again. If myoplasmic Ca^{2+} levels are still elevated the cycle repeats. If myoplasmic Ca^{2+} levels are low, relaxation results.

Cross-Bridge Cycling–Sarcomere Shortening

Once myosin and actin have bound, ATP-dependent conformational changes in the myosin molecule result in the movement of the actin filaments toward the center of the sarcomere. This shortens the length of the sarcomere, and thereby contracts the muscle fiber. The mechanism by which myosin produces force and shortens the sarcomere is thought

to involve four basic steps, which collectively are termed the cross-bridge cycle (labeled *a* to *d* in Fig. 12-11). In the resting state, myosin is thought to have partially hydrolyzed ATP (state *a*). When Ca^{2+} is released from the terminal cisternae of the SR, it binds to troponin-C, which in turn promotes the movement of tropomyosin on the actin filament such that myosin-binding sites on actin are exposed. This then allows the "energized" myosin head to bind to the underlying actin (state *b*). Myosin then undergoes a conformational change termed "ratchet action," which pulls the actin filament toward the center of the sarcomere (state *c*). The ATP and P_i are released from myosin for actin, resulting in the release of myosin from the actin filament (state *d*). Myosin then partially hydrolyzes the ATP, which utilizes part of the energy in ATP to recock the head, returning to the resting state. If intracellular Ca^{2+} is still elevated, myosin will undergo another cross-bridge cycle, producing further contraction of the muscle. The ratchet action of the cross-bridge is capable of moving the thin filament approximately 10 nm. The cycle continues until the SERCA pumps Ca^{2+} back into the SR. As the Ca^{2+} levels fall, Ca^{2+} dissociates from troponin-C and the troponin-tropomyosin complex moves and blocks the myosin-binding sites on the actin filament. If the supply of ATP is exhausted, as occurs with death, the cycle stops in state "c" with the formation of permanent actin-myosin complexes (i.e., the rigor state). In this state the muscle is rigid and is termed "rigor mortis."

As already noted, thick filament formation involves the association of myosin molecules in a tail-to-tail configuration producing a bipolar orientation (see Fig. 12-4). Such a bipolar orientation allows myosin to pull the actin filaments toward the center of the sarcomere during the cross-bridge cycle. The myosin molecules are also oriented in a helical array in the thick filament, such that cross-bridges extend toward each of the six thin filaments surrounding the thick filament (see Fig. 12-2). These myosin projections/cross-bridges can be seen in electron micrographs of skeletal muscle (Fig. 12-12), and appear to extend perpendicular from the thick filaments at rest. In the contracted state, the myosin cross-bridges slant toward the center of the sarcomere, consistent with the ratchet action of the myosin head.

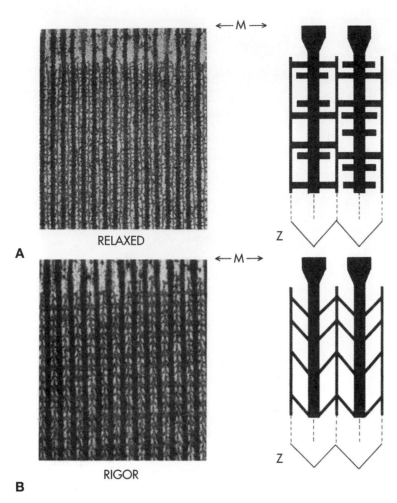

RELAXED

A

M

Z

M

Z

RIGOR

B

■ **Fig. 12-12**   Electron micrograph of skeletal muscle in relaxed and contracted (rigor) states. The direction of the cross-bridges in the contracted state is consistent with a ratchet action of myosin, which pulls actin toward the center of the sarcomere. (Modified from Patton H et al: *Textbook of physiology,* Philadelphia, 1989, WB Saunders.)

The cross-bridge cycling mechanism described above is called the **sliding filament theory,** because the myosin cross-bridge is pulling the actin thin filament toward the center of the sarcomere, resulting in an apparent "sliding" of the thin filament past the thick filament. There is, however, uncertainty as to how many myosin molecules contribute to the generation of force, and/or if both myosin heads in a given myosin molecule are involved. It has been calculated that there may be 600 myosin heads per thick filament, with a stoichiometry of 1 myosin head per 1.8 actin molecules. As a result of steric considerations, it is unlikely that all myosin heads can interact with actin, and calculations suggest that even during maximal force generation, only 20% to 40% of the myosin heads bind to actin.

The conversion of chemical energy (i.e., ATP) into mechanical energy by muscle is highly efficient. In isolated muscle preparations, maximum mechanical efficiency (~65% efficiency) is obtained at a submaximal force of 30% maximal tension. In humans doing steady-state ergometer exercise, mechanical efficiencies range from 40% to 57%.

SKELETAL MUSCLE TYPES

Skeletal muscle can be classified as either **fast twitch** or **slow twitch** muscle. As shown in Fig. 12-13, the lateral rectus muscle of the eye contracts very quickly, attaining peak

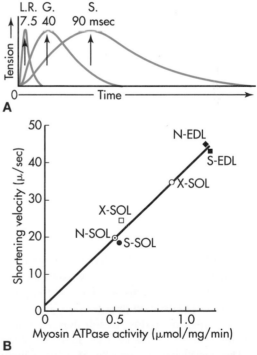

■ **Fig. 12-13**   Muscles vary in terms of the speed of contraction **(A).** The speed of shortening is correlated with the myosin ATPase activity **(B).** *LR,* Lateral rectus muscle of the eye; *G,* gastrocnemius of the leg; *S,* soleus muscle of the leg. (**A** from Best and Taylor: *Physiol basis of medical practice,* ed 12, 1991, Williams & Wilkins. **B** from Barany M, Close RI: *J Physiol* 213(2):455, 1971.)

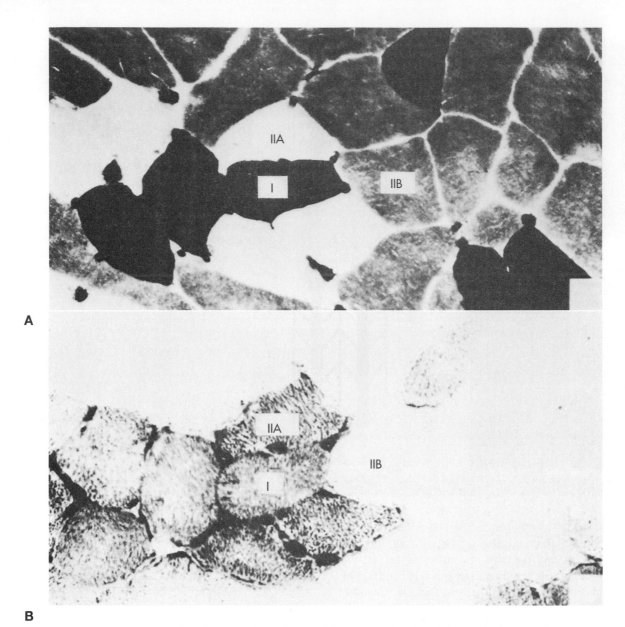

■ Fig. 12-14 Muscles often contain a mixture of fast (IIA and IIB) and slow (I) twitch muscle fibers. **A,** Histochemical staining for the slow twitch myosin isoform. The slow (type I) fibers stain intensely. The fast fibers contain either none of this isoform (type IIA) or a mixture of the slow and fast isoforms (type IIB). **B,** Histochemical staining for enxymes involved in oxidative phosphorylation. Note the high levels in the slow (type I) fibers.

tension with 7.5 msec after stimulation. The gastrocnemius muscle of the leg, on the other, requires 40 msec to develop peak tension. The soleus muscle of the leg requires even longer (~90 msec) to develop peak tension. Thus, the soleus muscle is classified as a slow twitch muscle, whereas the lateral rectus muscle would be classified as a fast twitch muscle. The gastrocnemius muscle contains a mixture of fast and slow twitch fibers, and thus exhibits a weighted average intermediate rate of tension development when the whole muscle is stimulated.

A correlation between speed of contraction and myosin ATPase activity is also seen and reflects the expression of different myosin isoforms in the two muscle fiber types (Fig. 12-13). Although the basic structure of the myosin isoforms in fast twitch and slow twitch muscles is similar (i.e., two heavy chains with two pairs of light chains), they are products of different genes, and thus have different amino acid sequences. Histochemical methods can be used to distinguish the fiber types based on the activity of the myosin ATPase (Fig. 12-14). Typically, **fast fibers** (types IIA and IIB) and **slow fibers** (type I) are intermixed in most mammalian skeletal muscles.

Fast and slow fibers can also be distinguished by the activities of enzymes in the oxidative and glycolytic

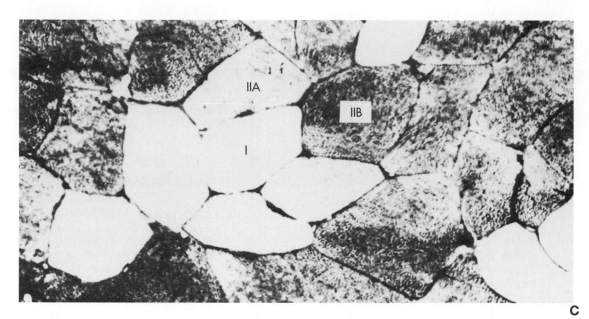

■ **Fig. 12-14, cont'd   C,** Histochemical staining for enzymes involved in glycolysis. Note the low levels in the slow (type I) fibers.

metabolic pathways (Fig. 12-14). In most fast fibers, the activities of glycolytic enzymes are high and the activities of oxidative enzymes are low. These characteristics correlate with the number of mitochondria present in the fiber. Electron micrographs of fast fibers show only a few mitochondria compared to the large number seen in sow fibers. Fast fibers also have a much more extensive SR than do slow fibers.

Because of the dependence of fast fibers on glycolytic metabolism, they fatigue rapidly. Consequently, they are used only occasionally and for brief periods of time. In contrast, the slow fibers meet their metabolic demands with oxidative phosphorylation. Consequently, these muscles fatigue more slowly and therefore are used for more sustained activities (e.g., maintenance of posture). Some fast fibers have both high glycolytic and high oxidative capacities. Such fibers, called **type IIA,** are found in mammals, but are uncommon in humans. The fibers that derive their energy primarily from oxidative phosphoylation (i.e., the slow type I fibers and the fast type IIA fibers) contain numerous mitochondria and high levels of the oxygen-binding protein myoglobin. Because myoglobin is red, these fibers are sometimes called "red fibers." Table 12-2 summarizes some of the differences in the fiber types.

In addition to the differences between fast and slow fibers noted above, other muscle proteins are also expressed in a fiber type specific manner. These include SERCA, the three troponin subunits, tropomyosin, and C-protein. The differential expression of SERCA isoforms (SERCA1 in fast twitch muscle and SERCA2 in slow twitch and cardiac muscle) contributes to the differences in the speed of relaxation between fast and slow twitch muscle. The activity of SERCA1 is greater than that of SERCA2. Therefore, Ca^{2+}

■ **Table 12-2**   Properties of motor units

Characteristics	Motor unit classification	
	Type I	Type II
Properties of nerve		
Cell diameter	Small	Large
Conduction velocity	Fast	Very fast
Excitability	High	Low
Properties of muscle cells		
Number of fibers	Few	Many
Fiber diameter	Moderate	Large
Force of unit	Low	High
Metabolic profile	Oxidative	Glycolytic
Contraction velocity	Moderate	Fast
Fatigability	Low	High

reuptake into the SR occurs more quickly in fast muscles, and as a result, these fibers have a faster relaxation time. Differential expression of troponin and tropomyosin isoforms influences the Ca^{2+} dependency of contraction. Slow fibers begin to develop tension at lower Ca^{2+} concentrations than do fast fibers. This differential sensitivity to Ca^{2+} is related in part to the fact that the troponin-C isoform in slow fibers has only a single low-affinity Ca^{2+}-binding site, whereas troponin-C of fast fibers has two low-affinity binding sites. Changes in the Ca^{2+} dependence of contraction, however, are not restricted to differences in the troponin-C isoforms. Differences in troponin-T and tropomyosin isoforms are also found. Thus, the regulation of the Ca^{2+} dependence of contraction is complex, involving contributions from multiple proteins on the thin filament.

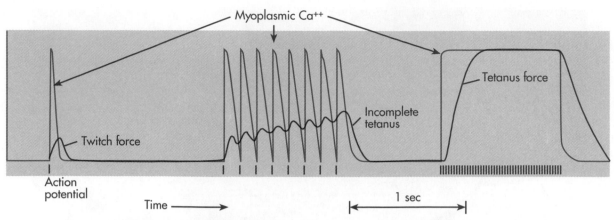

■ **Fig. 12-15**   Increasing the frequence of electrical stimulation of skeletal muscle results in an increase in the force of contraction. This is attributable to a prolongation of the intracellular Ca^{2+} transient and is termed tetany. Incomplete tetany results from initiation of another intracellular Ca^{2+} transient before the muscle has completely relaxed. Thus, there is a summation of twitch forces. See text for details.

MODULATION OF THE FORCE OF CONTRACTION

Recruitment

A simple means of increasing the force of contraction of a muscle is to recruit more muscle fibers. As all of the muscle fibers within a motor unit are activated simultaneously, one recruits more muscle fibers by recruiting more motor units. As already noted, muscle fibers can be classified as fast twitch or slow twitch. The type of fiber is determined by its innervation. Because all fibers in a motor unit are innnervated by a single a-motor neuron, all fibers within a motor unit are of the same type. Slow twitch motor units tend to be small (100 to 500 muscle fibers) and are innnervated by an α-motor neuron that is easily excited. Fast twitch motor units, by contrast, tend to be large (containing 1000 to 2000 muscle fibers) and are innnervated by a-motor neurons that are more difficult to excite. Thus, slow twitch motor units tend to be recruited first. As more and more force is needed, the fast twitch motor units are recruited. The advantage of such a recruitment strategy is that the first muscle fibers recruited are those that have a high resistance to fatigue. Moreover, the small size of slow twitch motor units allows fine motor control at low levels of force. The process of increasing the force of contraction by recruiting additional motor units is termed *spatial summation* because one is "summing" forces from muscle fibers within a larger area of the muscle. This is in contrast to *temporal summation* which is discussed below.

Tetany

Action potentials in skeletal muscles are quite uniform, and these lead to the release of a reproducible pulse of Ca^{2+} from the SR (Fig. 12-15). A single action potential releases sufficient Ca^{2+} to cause a twitch contraction. However, the duration of this contraction is very short, because Ca^{2+} is very rapidly pumped back into the SR. If the muscle is stimulated

a second time before the muscle is fully relaxed, the force of contraction increases (middle panel of Fig. 12-15). Thus, there is a stimulation of the twitch forces as the stimulus frequency increases. At a high level of stimulation, the intracellular Ca^{2+} level increases and is maintained throughout the period of stimulation (right panel of Fig. 12-15), and the level of force developed greatly exceeds that seen during a twitch. The response is termed **tetany.** At intermediate stimulus frequency, intracellular Ca^{2+} levels return to baseline just prior to the next stimulus. However, there is gradual rise in force (middle panel of Fig. 12-15). This phenomenon is termed incomplete tetany. In both cases, the increased frequency of stimulation is said to produce a fusion of twitches.

It is hypothesized that the low force generation during a twitch, compared to that seen during tetany, is due to the presence of a series elastic component in the muscle. Specifically, when the muscle is stretched a small amount shortly after the initiation of the action potential, the muscle generates a twitch force that approximates the maximal tetanic force. This result, coupled with the observation that the size of the intracellular Ca^{2+} transient during a twitch contraction is comparable to that seen during tetany, suggests that enough Ca^{2+} is released into the myoplasm during a twitch to allow the actin-myosin interactions to produce maximal tension. However, the duration of the intracellular Ca^{2+} transient during a twitch is sufficiently short that the contractile elements may not have enough time to fully stretch the series elastic components in the fiber and muscle. As a result, the measured tension is submaximal. Increasing the duration of the intracellular Ca^{2+} transient, as occur with tetany, provides the muscle with sufficient time to completely stretch the series elastic component, resulting in expression of the full contractile force of the actin-myosin interactions (i.e., maximal tension). Partial stretching of the series elastic component (as might be expected during a single twitch), followed by restimulation of the muscle before complete relaxation, on

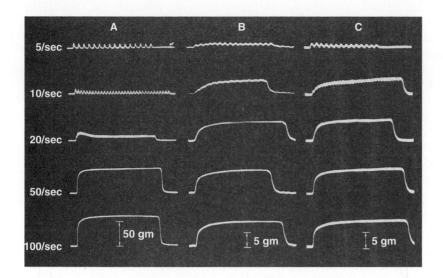

■ **Fig. 12-16** Slow twitch muscles tetanize at a lower stimulation frequency than that required for fast twitch muscles. **A,** Fast twitch motor unit in gastrocnemius muscle. **B,** slow twitch motor unit in gastrocnemius muscle. **C,** slow twitch muscle unit in soleus muscle. The motor units were stimulated at the frequencies indicated on the left. The tension (in grams) generated during concentration is indicated by the vertical arrows. Note the large force generated by the fast twitch motor unit (**A**). (From *Montcastle medical physiology,* ed 12, St. Louis, 1974, Mosby.)

the other hand, would be expected to yield an intermediate level of tension, similar to that seen in incomplete tetany. The location of the series elastic component in skeletal muscle is not known. One potential source is the myosin molecule itself. In addition, it is likely that there are other sources of the series elastic component, such as the connective tissue of the endomysium, perimysium, and epimysium.

The stimulus frequency needed to produce tetany depends on whether the motor unit comprises slow or fast fibers (see Fig. 12-16). Slow fibers can be tetanized at lower frequencies than fast fibers. The ability of slow twitch muscle to tetanize at lower stimulation frequencies reflects, at least in part, the longer duration of contraction seen in slow fibers. As also illustrated in Fig. 12-16, fast fibers develop a larger maximal force than slow fibers. This reflects the fact that fast fibers are larger in diameter than slow fibers, and that there are more fibers in fast motor units than in slow motor units.

MODULATION OF FORCE BY REFLEX ARCS
Stretch Reflex

Skeletal muscles contain sensory fibers (**muscle spindles**— also called **intrafusal fibers**) that run parallel to the skeletal muscle fibers. The muscle spindles assess the degree of stretch of the muscle, as well as the speed of contraction. In the stretch reflex, rapid stretching of the muscle, for example, tapping the tendon lengthens the spindles in the muscle, resulting in an increased frequency of action potentials in the afferent sensory neurons of the spindle. These afferent fibers in turn excite α-motor neurons in the spinal cord, which innervate the stretched muscle. The result is that the reflex arc is a stretch-induced contraction of the muscle, which does not require input from high centers in the brain. It should be noted that as the muscle shortens, efferent output to the spindle also occurs, thereby taking the slack out of the spindle and thus ensuring its ability to respond to stretch at all muscle lengths. By their action, muscle spindles

provide feedback to the muscle in terms of its length, and thus help maintain a joint at a given angle.

Golgi Tendon Organ

The **Golgi tendon organs** (GTO) are located in the tendons of muscles and inhibit muscle contraction when muscle tension becomes high. The GTO reflex thus serves as a protective mechanism, signaling the muscle to drop heavy loads, rather than risk injury of the muscle from the high tension. Like the muscle spindle, the signaling involves a spinal reflex arc (see also Chapter 9). The reflex arc of the GTO differs from that of the muscle spindle in that the afferent fibers from the GTO synapse on interneurons in the cord, rather than directly on α-motor neurons. These interneurons release an inhibitory neurotransmitter, which then stops the α-motor neuron from stimulating the stretched/overloaded muscle.

SKELETAL MUSCLE TONE

The skeletal system supports the body in an erect posture with the expenditure of relatively little energy. However, even at rest, muscles normally exhibit some level of contractile activity. Isolated (i.e., denervated) unstimulated muscles are in a relaxed state and are said to be flaccid. However, relaxed muscles in the body are comparatively firm. This firmness, or tone, is caused by low levels of contractile activity in some of the motor units and is driven by reflex arcs from the muscle spindles. Interruption of the reflex arc by sectioning the sensory afferent fibers will abolish this resting muscle tone. The tone in skeletal muscle is distinct from the "tone" in smooth muscle (see Chapter 13).

ENERGY SOURCES DURING CONTRACTION
ATP

Muscle cells convert chemical energy into mechanical energy. ATP is the energy source used for this conversion. The ATP pool in skeletal muscle is small and capable of supporting only a few contractions, if not replenished. The ATP pool, however, is continually replenished during contraction, as described below, such that even when the muscle fatigues, the ATP stores are only modestly decreased.

Creatine Phosphate

Muscle cells contain creatine phosphate, which is used to convert adenosine diphosphate (ADP) into ATP and thus replenishes the ATP store during muscle contraction. The creatine phosphate store represents the immediate high-energy source for replenishing the ATP supply in skeletal muscle, especially during intense exercise. The enzyme **creatine phosphokinase (CPK)** catalyzes the reaction:

$$ADP + creatine\ phosphate \rightarrow ATP + creatine$$

Although much of the CPK is present in the myoplasm, a small amount is located in the thick filament (near the M-line). The thick filament localized CPK may participate in the rapid resynthesis of ATP near the myosin heads during muscle contraction. The created phosphate store, however, is only about five times the size of the ATP store, and thus cannot support prolonged periods of contraction (less than a minute of maximal muscle activity). Skeletal muscle fatigue during intense exercise is associated with the depletion of the creatine phosphate store, though as described subsequently, this does not necessarily imply that the fatigue is caused by depletion of the creatine phosphate store. As the CPK-catalyzed reaction shown above is reversible, the muscle cell replenishes the creatine phosphate pool during recovery from fatigue by utilizing ATP synthesized through oxidative phosphorylation.

Carbohydrates

Muscle cells contain glycogen, which can be metabolized during muscle contraction to provide glucose for oxidative phosphorylation and glycolysis, both of which will generate ATP to replenish the ATP store. Muscle cells can also take up glucose from the blood, a process that is stimulated by insulin (see Chapter 41). The cystosolic enzyme phosphorylase releases glucose-1-phosphate residues from glycogen, which are then metabolized by a combination of glycolysis (in the cytosol) and oxidative phosphorylation (in the mitochondria) to yield the equivalent of 37 mol of ATP per mol glucose-1-phosphate. Blood glucose yields 36 mol ATP per mol of glucose, since one ATP is used to phosphorylate glucose at the start of glycolysis. These ATP yields, however, are dependent on adequate oxygen supply. Under anaerobic conditions, by contrast, metabolism of glycogen and glucose yield only 3 and 2 mol of ATP per mol of glucose-1-phosphate or glucose, respectively (along with 2 mol of lactate). As discussed below, muscle fatigue during prolonged exercise is associated with depletion of glycogen stores in the muscle.

Fatty Acids and Triglycerides

Fatty acids represent an important source of energy for muscle cells during prolonged exercise. Muscle cells contain fatty acids but can also take up fatty acids from the blood. Muscle cells can also store triglycerides, which can be hydrolyzed when needed to produce fatty acids. The fatty acids are subjected to β-oxidation within the mitochondria. For fatty acids to enter the mitochondria, however, the fatty acid is converted to acyl-carnitine in the cytosol, then transported into the mitochondria where it is converted to acyl-coenzyme A (CoA). Within the mitochondria, the acyl-CoA is subjected to β-oxidation yielding acetyl-CoA, which then enters the citric acid cycle, and ultimately produces ATP.

OXYGEN DEBT

If the energy demands of exercise cannot be met by oxidative phosphorylation, an **oxygen debt** is incurred. After completion of exercise, respiration remains above the resting level in order to "repay" this oxygen debt. The extra oxygen consumption during this recovery phase is used to restore metabolite levels (such as creatine phosphate and ATP) and to metabolize the lactate generated by glycolysis. The increased cardiac and respiratory work during recovery also contributes to the increased oxygen consumption seen at this time and explains why more O_2 has to be "repaid" than was "borrowed." Some oxygen debt occurs even with low levels of exercise, because slow oxidative motor units consume considerable ATP, derived from creatine phosphate or glycolysis, before oxidative metabolism can increase ATP production to meet steady-state requirements. The oxygen debt is much greater with strenuous exercise, when fast glycolytic motor units are used (see Fig. 12-17). The oxygen debt is approximately equal to the energy consumed during exercise minus that supplied by oxidative metabolism (i.e., the dark- and light-colored areas in Fig. 12-17 are roughly equal). As indicated above, the additional oxygen used during recovery from exercise represents the energy requirements for restoring normal cellular metabolite levels.

FATIGUE

The ability of muscle to meet energy needs is a major determinant of the duration of the exercise. However, fatigue is not the result of depletion of energy stores. Instead, metabolic by-products seem to be important factors in the onset of fatigue. Fatigue may potentially occur at any of the points involved in muscle contraction, from the brain to the muscle cells, as well as in the cardiovascular and respiratory systems that maintain energy supplies (i.e., fatty acids and glucose) and O_2 delivery to the exercising muscle.

Several factors have been implicated in **muscle fatigue.** During brief periods of tetany the oxygen supply to the muscle is adequate as long as the circulation is intact. However, the force/stress generated during these brief tetanic periods decays rapidly to a level that can be maintained for long periods (Fig. 12-18). This decay represents the rapid and almost total failure of the fast motor units. This decline in force/stress is paralleled by depletion of glycogen and

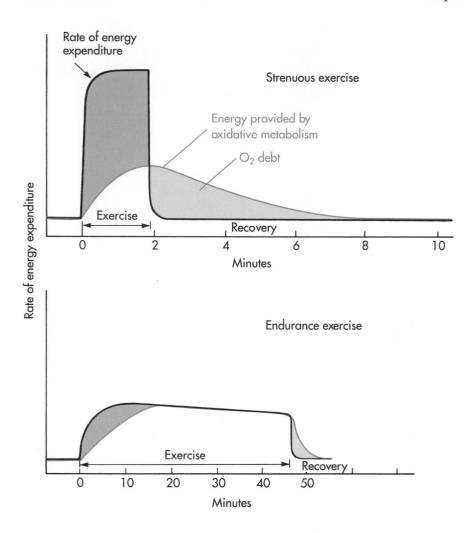

■ **Fig. 12-17**   An oxygen debt is incurred by exercising muscle when the rate of energy expenditure exceeds the rate of energy production by oxidative metabolism. Both strenuous *(upper panel)* and endurance exercise *(lower panel)* are shown. See text for details.

creatine phosphate stores and the accumulation of lactic acid. Importantly, the decline in force/stress occurs when the ATP pool is not greatly reduced, so that the muscle fibers do not go into rigor. In contrast, the slow motor units are able to meet the energy demands of fibers under this condition, and they do not exhibit significant fatigue, even after many hours. Evidently, some factor associated with energy metabolism can inhibit contraction (e.g., in the fast fibers), but this factor has not been clearly identified.

During *intense exercise* accumulation of inorganic phosphate and lactic acid in the myoplasm accounts for muscle fatigue. The accumulation of lactic acid, to levels as high as 15 to 26 mM, decreases myoplasmic pH (from ~7 to ~6.2) and inhibits actin-myosin interactions. This decrease in pH reduces the Ca^{2+} sensitivity of actin-myosin interaction by altering Ca^{2+} binding to troponin-C and by decreasing the maximum number of actin-myosin interactions. Fast twitch fibers appear to be slightly more sensitive to the effects of pH than slow twitch muscle fibers. Inorganic phosphate has also been implicated as an important factor in the development of fatigue during intense exercise, as phosphate concentrations can increased from ~2 mM at rest to nearly 40 mM in the working muscle. Such an elevation in inorganic phosphate concentration can reduce tension by at least the

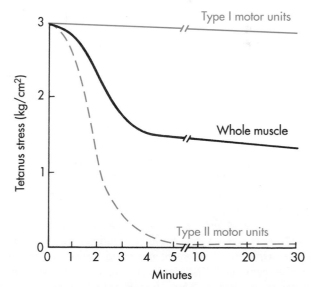

■ **Fig. 12-18**   A series of brief titanic stimulations of skeletal muscle results in a rapid decrease in force (titanic stress; *black line* in plot), which is attributable to fatigue of fast twitch (type II) motor units in the muscle. Under these conditions, however, slow (type I) twitch motor units were fatigue resistant *(upper line)*.

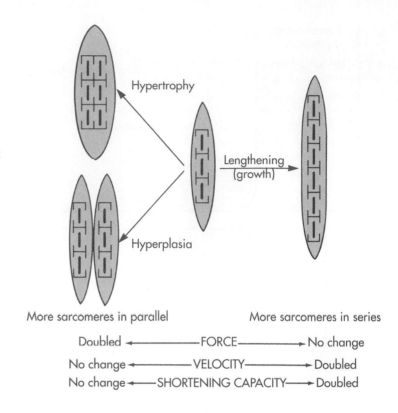

■ **Fig. 12-19**   Effects of growth on the mechanical output of a muscle cell. Typically, skeletal muscle cell growth involves either lengthening (adding more sarcomeres to the ends of the muscle fibers) or increasing muscle fiber diameter (hypertrophy, due to addition of more myofilaments/myofibrils in parallel within the muscle fiber). The formation of new muscle fibers is called hyperplasia, and it is infrequent in skeletal muscle.

following three different mechanisms: (1) inhibition of Ca^{2+} release from the SR, (2) decrease in Ca^{2+} sensitivity of contraction, and (3) alteration in actin-myosin binding. A number of other factors, including glycogen depletion from a specialized compartment, a localized increase in ADP concentration, intracellular elevation of potassium, and generation of oxygen free radicals, have also been implicated in various forms of exercise-induced muscle fatigue. Finally, the central nervous system contributes to fatigue, especially how fatigue is perceived by the individual (see below).

Regardless of whether the muscle fatigued as a consequence of high-intensity exercise or prolonged exercise, the myoplasmic ATP level does not decrease substantially. Given the reliance of all cells on the availability of ATP to maintain viability, fatigue has been described as a protective mechanism to minimize risk of muscle cell injury or death. Consequently, it is likely that skeletal muscle cells have developed redundant systems to ensure that ATP levels do not drop to dangerously low levels and hence risk the viability of the cell.

Most persons tire and cease exercise long before the motor unit fatigues. General physical fatigue may be defined as a homeostatic disturbance produced by work. The basis for the perceived discomfort (or even pain) probably involves many factors. These factors may include a decrease in plasma glucose levels and accumulation of metabolites. Motor system function in the CNS is not impaired. Highly motivated and trained athletes can withstand the discomfort of the fatigue and will exercise to the point at which some motor unit fatigue occurs. Part of the enhanced performance observed after training involves motivational factors.

GROWTH AND DEVELOPMENT

Skeletal muscle fibers differentiate before they are innervated, and some neuromuscular junctions are formed well after birth. Before innervation, the muscle fibers physiologically resemble slow (type I) cells. **Acetylcholine receptors** are distributed throughout the sarcolemma of these uninnervated cells and are supersensitive to that neurotransmitter. An end plate is formed when the first growing nerve terminal establishes contact with a muscle cell. The cell forms no further association with nerves, and the receptors to acetylcholine become concentrated in the end plate membranes. Cells innervated by a small motor neuron form slow oxidative motor units. Fibers innervated by large motor nerves develop all the characteristics of fast (type II) motor units. Innervation produces major cellular changes, including the synthesis of the fast and slow myosin isoforms, which replace embryonic or neonatal variants. Thus, muscle fiber type is determined by the nerves that innervate the fiber.

An increase in muscle strength and size occurs during maturation. As the skeleton grows, the muscle cells lengthen. Lengthening is accomplished by formation of additional sarcomeres at the ends of the muscle cells (Fig. 12-19), a process that is reversible. For example, the length of a cell decreases when terminal sarcomeres are eliminated, which can occur when a limb is immobilized with the muscle in a shortened position, or when an improperly set fracture leads to a shortened limb segment. Changes in muscle length affect the velocity and extent of shortening but do not influence the amount of force that can be generated by the muscle. The gradual increase in strength and diameter of a muscle during growth is achieved mainly by hypertrophy. Doubling the myofibrillar diameter by adding more sarcomeres in parallel (hypertrophy, for example) may double the amount of force generated but has no effect on the maximal velocity of shortening.

Skeletal muscles have a limited ability to form new fibers (**hyperplasia**). These new fibers result from differentiation of satellite cells that are present in the tissues. However, major cellular destruction leads to replacement with scar tissue.

Muscles must not only be used to maintain normal growth and development, but they must also experience a load. Muscles immobilized in a cast lose mass. Also, space flight exposes astronauts to a microgravity environment that mechanically unloads their muscles. This unloading leads to a rapid loss of muscle mass (i.e., atrophy) and weakness. Antigravity muscles that frequently contract to support the body typically have a high number of slow (type I) oxidative motor units. These slow motor units atrophy more rapidly than the fast (type II) motor units during prolonged periods of unloading. This atrophy of slow motor units is associated with a decrease in maximal titanic force but an increase in maximal shortening velocities. The increase in velocity is correlated with the expression of the fast myosin isoform in these fibers. An important aspect of space medicine is the design of exercise programs that minimize such phenotypic changes during prolonged space flight.

Testosterone is a major factor responsible for the greater muscle mass in males, because it has myotrophic actions as well as androgenic (masculinization) effects (see Chapter 46). A variety of synthetic molecules, designated as anabolic steroids, have been designed to enhance muscle growth while minimizing the androgenic actions. These drugs are widely used by body builders and athletes in sports in which strength is important. The doses are typically 10- to 50-fold greater than might be prescribed therapeutically in individuals with impaired hormone production. Unfortunately, none of these compounds lacks androgenic effects. Hence, at the doses used, they induce serious hormone disturbances, including a depression of testosterone production. A major issue is whether these drugs do in fact increase muscle and athletic performance in individuals with normal circulating levels of testosterone. After some four decades of use, the scientific facts remain uncertain, and most experimental studies in animals have no documented significant effects of muscle development. Reports in humans remain controversial. Proponents claim increases in strength that provide the edge in world-class performance. Critics argue that these increases are largely placebo effects associated with expectations and motivational factors. The public debate on abuse of anabolic steroids has led to their designation as controlled substances, along with opiates, amphetamines, and barbiturates.

DENERVATION, REINNERVATION, AND CROSS-INNERVATION

As already noted, **innervation** is critical to the skeletal muscle phenotype. If the motor nerve is cut, muscle fasciculation occurs. **Fasciculation** is characterized by small, irregular contractions caused by the release of acetylcholine from the terminals of the degenerating distal portion of the axon. Several days after denervation, muscle fibrillation begins. **Fibrillation** is characterized by spontaneous, repetitive contractions. At this time, the cholinergic receptors have spread out over the entire cell membrane, in effect reverting to their preinnervation embryonic arrangement. The muscle fibrillations reflect supersensitivity to acetylcholine. Muscles also **atrophy,** with a decrease in the size of the muscle and of it cells. Atrophy is progressive in humans, with degeneration of some cells 3 or 4 months after denervation. Most of the muscle fibers are replaced by fat and connective tissue after 1 to 2 years. These changes can be reversed if reinnervation occurs within a few months. **Reinnervation** is normally achieved by growth of the peripheral stump of the motor nerve axons along the old nerve sheath.

Reinnervation of formerly fast (type II) fibers by a small motor axon causes that cell to redifferentiate into a slow (type I) fiber, and vice versa. This suggests that large and small motor nerves differ qualitatively, and that the nerves have specific "trophic" effects on the muscle fibers. It is likely that this "trophic" effect reflects the rate of fiber stimulation. For example, stimulation, via electrodes implanted in the muscle can lessen denervation atrophy. More strikingly, chronic low-frequency stimulation of fast motor units causes fast motor units to be converted to slow units. Some conversion toward a typical fast-fiber phenotype can occur when the frequency of contraction in slow units is greatly decreased by reducing the excitatory input. The excitatory input can be reduced by sectioning the appropriate spinal or dorsal root or by severing the tendon, which functionally inactivates peripheral mechanoreceptors.

Frequency of contraction determines fiber development and phenotype through changes in gene expression and protein synthesis. Fibers that undergo frequent contractile activity form many mitochondria and synthesize the slow isoform of myosin. Fibers innervated by large, less excitable axons contract infrequently. Such relatively inactive fibers typically form few mitochondria and have large concentrations of glycolytic enzymes. The fast isoform of myosin is synthesized in such cells.

Intracellular Ca^{2+} concentration may also play an important role in the expression of the slow myosin isoform. Slow twitch muscle fibers have a higher resting level of intracellular Ca^{2+} compared to fast twitch muscle. Also, chronic electrical stimulation of fast twitch muscle is accompanied by a 2.5-fold increase in resting myoplasmic Ca^{2+} concentration that precedes the increase expression of slow twitch myosin and decreased expression of fast twitch myosin. Similarly, chronic elevation of intracellular Ca^{2+} (~5-fold) in muscle cells expressing fast twitch myosin induces a change in gene expression from the slow muscle myosin isoform to the fast twitch myosin isoform within 8 days. An increase in citrate synthetase activity (an indicator of oxidative capacity) and a decrease in lactate dehydrogenase activity (an indicator for glycolytic capacity) accompanies this Ca^{2+}-dependent transition from fast twitch to slow twitch myosin. These

■ Table 12-3   Effects of exercise

Type of training	Example	Major adaptive response
Learning/coordination	Typing	Increased rate and accuracy of motor skills (central nervous system)
Endurance (submaximal, sustained efforts)	Marathon running	Increased oxidative capacity in all involved motor units with limited cellular hypertrophy
Strength (brief, maximal efforts)	Weight lifting	Hypertrophy and enhanced glycolytic capacity of motor units employed

Ca^{2+}-dependent change are reversible by lowering the intracellular Ca^{2+} concentration.

RESPONSE TO EXERCISE

Exercise physiologists identify three categories of training regimens and responses: **learning, endurance,** and **strength training** (Table 12-3). Typically, most athletic endeavors involve elements of all three. The learning aspect of training involves motivational factors as well as neuromuscular coordination. This aspect of training does not involve adaptive changes in the muscle fibers per se. However, motor skills can persist for years without regular training, unlike the responses of muscle cells to exercise.

All healthy persons can maintain some level of continuous muscular activity that is supported by oxidative metabolism. This level can be greatly increased by a regular exercise regimen that is sufficient to induce adaptive responses. The adaptive response of skeletal muscle fibers to endurance exercise is mainly the result of an increase in the oxidative metabolic capacity of the motor units involved. This demand places an increased load on the cardiovascular and respiratory systems and increases the capacity of the heart and respiratory muscles. The latter effects are responsible for the principal health benefits associated with endurance exercise.

Muscle strength can be increased by regular massive efforts that involve most motor units. Such efforts recruit fast glycolytic motor units as well as slow oxidative motor units. During these efforts, blood supply to the working muscles may be interrupted as tissue pressures rise above the intravascular pressures. The reduced blood flow limits the duration of the contraction. Regular maximal strength exercise, such as weight lifting, induces synthesis of more myofibrils and hence hypertrophy of the active muscle cells. The increased stress also induces growth of tendons and bones.

Endurance exercise does not cause fast motor units to become slow, not does maximal muscular effort produce a shift from slow to fast motor units. Thus, any practical exercise regimen, when superimposed on normal daily activities, probably does not alter muscle fiber phenotype.

DELAYED-ONSET MUSCLE SORENESS

Activities, such as hiking or particularly downhill running, in which contracting muscles are stretched and lengthened too vigorously, are followed by more pain and stiffness than follows comparable exercise that does not involve vigorous muscle stretching and lengthening (e.g., cycling). The resultant dull, aching pain develops slowly and reaches its peak within 24 to 48 hours. The pain is associated with a reduced range of motion, stiffness, and weakness of the affected muscles. The prime factors that cause the pain are swelling and inflammation that result from injury to muscle cells, most commonly near the myotendinous junction. Fast type II motor units are more affected than are type I motor units, because the maximal forces are highest in large cells, where the loads imposed are some 60% greater than the maximal force the cells can develop. Recovery is slow and depends of regeneration of the injured sarcomeres.

BIOPHYSICAL PROPERTIES OF SKELETAL MUSCLE

The molecular mechanisms of muscle contraction described above underlie, and are responsible for, the biophysical properties of muscle. Historically, these biophysical properties were well described prior to the elucidation of the molecular mechanisms of contraction. They remain important ways of describing muscle function

Length-Tension Relationship

When muscles contract they generate force (often measured as tension or stress) and decrease in length. When studying the biophysical properties of muscle, one of these parameters is usually held constant, while the other is measured following an experimental maneuver. Accordingly, an **isometric contraction** is one in which muscle length is held constant, and the force generated during the contraction is measured. An isotonic contraction is one in which force (or tone) is constant, and the change in the length of the muscle is measured.

When a muscle at rest is stretched, it resists stretch by a force that increases slowly at first, but then more rapidly as the extent of stretch increases (Fig. 12-20). This purely passive property is due to the elastic tissue in the muscle. If the muscle is stimulated to contract at these various lengths, a different relationship is obtained. Specifically, contractile force increases as the muscle length is increased up to a point (designated L_0 to indicate optimal length). As the muscle is stretched beyond L_0, contractile force decreases. This length-tension curve is consistent with the sliding filament theory. At a very long sarcomere length (3.7 μm), actin filaments no longer overlap with the myosin filaments, so there is no contraction. As the muscle length is decreased toward

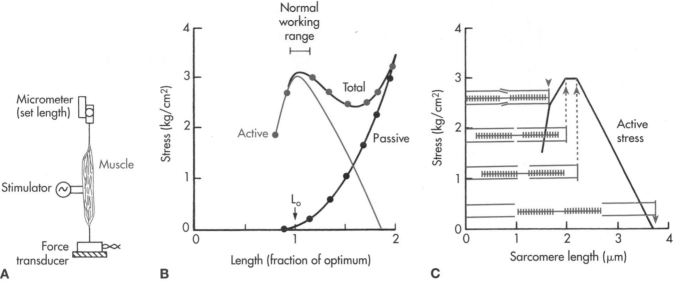

■ **Fig. 12-20** Length-tension relationship in skeletal muscle. **A,** The experimental setup, where maximal isometric tetanic tensions are measured at various muscle lengths. **B,** How active tension was calculated at various muscle lengths (i.e., by subtracting passive tension from total tension at each muscle length). **C,** A plot of active tension as a function of muscle length, with the predicted overlap of thick and thin filaments at selected points.

L_0, the amount of overlap increases, resulting in a progressive increase in contractile force. As sarcomere length decreases below 2 µm, the thin filaments collide in the middle of the sarcomere, disturbing actin-myosin interaction, and hence decreasing contractile force. Note that for the construction of the length-tension curves, muscles were maintained at a given length, and then contractile force was measured (i.e., isometric contraction). Thus, the length-tension relationship supports the sliding filament theory of muscle contraction described previously.

Force-Velocity Relationship

The velocity at which a muscle shortens is strongly dependent on the amount of force that the muscle must develop (Fig. 12-21). In the absence of any load, the shortening velocity of the muscle is maximal (denoted as V_0). V_0 corresponds to the maximal cycling rate of the cross-bridges [i.e., it is proportional to the maximal rate of energy turnover (ATPase activity) by myosin]. Thus, V_0 for fast twitch muscle is higher than that for slow twitch muscle. Increasing the load decreases the velocity of muscle shortening until, at maximal load, the muscle cannot lift the load and hence cannot shorten (zero velocity). Further increases in load result in stretching the muscle (negative velocity). The maximal isometric tension (i.e., force where shortening velocity was zero) is proportional to the number of active cross-bridges between actin and myosin, and it is usually greater for fast twitch motor units (given the larger diameter of fast twitch muscle fibers and greater number of muscle fibers in a typical fast twitch motor unit). The red curve (labeled power-stress curve) reflects the rate of work done at each load and shows that maximal rate of work was done at a submaximal load (viz. when the force of contraction was approximately

30% of the maximal tetanic tension). The latter curve was simply calculated by multiplying the x and y coordinates, then plotting the product as a function of the x coordinate.

SUMMARY

1. Skeletal muscle is composed of numerous muscle cells (muscle fibers), which are typically 10 to 80 µm in diameter and up to 25 cm in length. Striations are apparent in skeletal muscle and are due to the highly organized arrangement of thick and thin filaments in the myofibrils of the skeletal muscle fibers. The sarcomere is a contractile unit in skeletal muscle. Each sarcomere is approximately 2 µm in length at rest and is bounded by two Z-lines. Sarcomeres are arranged in series along the length of the myofibril. Thin filaments, containing actin, extend from the Z-line toward the center of the sarcomere. Thick filaments, containing myosin, are positioned in the center of the sarcomere and overlap the actin thin filaments. Muscle contraction results from the Ca^{2+}-dependent interaction of myosin and actin, with myosin pulling the thin filaments toward the center of the sarcomere.

2. Contraction of skeletal muscle is under the control of the central nervous system (i.e., voluntary). Motor centers in the brain control the activity of α-motor neurons in the ventral horns of the spinal cord. These α-motor neurons, in turn, synapse on skeletal muscle fibers. Although each skeletal muscle fiber is innervated by only one motor neuron, a motor neuron innervates several muscle fibers within the muscle. A motor unit refers to all muscle fibers innervated by a single motor neuron.

3. The motor neuron initiates contraction of skeletal muscle by producing an action potential in the muscle fiber. As the

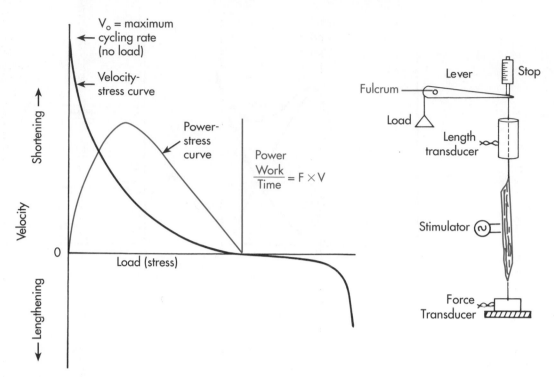

■ **Fig. 12-21**   Force-velocity relationship of skeletal muscle. The experimental setup is shown on the right. The initial muscle length was constant, but the amount of weight that the muscle had to lift during tetanic stimulation varied. Muscle shortening velocity while lifting these various amounts of weight was measured. See text for details.

action potential passes down the T-tubules of the muscle fiber, dihydropyridine receptors (DHPR) in the T-tubules undergo conformational changes that result in the opening of neighboring SR Ca^{2+} channels called ryanodine receptors (RYR), which then release Ca^{2+} to the myoplasm from the SR. The increase in myoplasmic Ca^{2+} promotes muscle contraction by exposing myosin-binding sites on the actin thin filaments (a process that involves Ca^{2+} binding to troponin-C, followed by movement of tropomyosin toward the groove in the thin filament). Myosin cross-bridges then appear to undergo a ratchet action, pulling the thin filaments toward the center of the sarcomere, contracting the skeletal muscle fiber. Relaxation of the muscle follows, as myoplasmic Ca^{2+} is resequestered by Ca^{2+}-ATPase (SERCA) in the SR.

4. The force of contraction can be increased by activating more motor neurons (i.e., recruiting more muscle fibers), and/or by increasing the frequency of action potentials in the muscle fiber, which produces tetany. The increased force during tetanic contractions is due to prolonged elevation of intracellular Ca^{2+} concentration.

5. There are two basic types of skeletal muscle fibers, distinguished on the basis of their speed of contraction (i.e., fast twitch vs. slow twitch). The difference in speed of contraction is attributed to the expression of different myosin isoforms, which differ in myosin ATPase activity. In addition to the difference in myosin ATPase activity, fast and slow twitch muscle also differ in metabolic activity, fiber diameter, motor unit size, sensitivity to tetany, and recruitment pattern.

6. Typically, slow twitch muscles are recruited before fast twitch muscle fibers due to the greater excitability of motor neurons innervating slow twitch muscles. The high oxidative capacity of slow twitch muscle fiber supports sustained contractile activity. Fat twitch muscle fibers, on the other hand, tend to be large, and typically have low oxidative capacity and high glycolytic capacity. The fast twitch motor units are thus best suited for short periods of activity when high levels of force are required.

7. Fast twitch muscle fibers can be converted into slow twitch muscle fibers (and vice versa), depending on the stimulation pattern. Chronic electrical stimulation of a fast twitch muscle results in the expression of slow twitch myosin and decreased expression of the fast twitch myosin, along with an increase in oxidative capacity. The mechanism(s) underlying this change in gene expression is unknown, but may be secondary to an elevation in resting intracellular Ca^{2+} concentration.

8. Skeletal muscle fibers atrophy after denervation. Muscle fibers depend on the activity of their motor nerves for maintenance of the differentiated phenotype. Reinnervation by axon growth along the original nerve sheath can reverse these changes. Skeletal muscle has a limited capacity to replace cells lost as a result of trauma or disease.

9. Skeletal muscle exhibits considerable phenotypic plasticity. Normal growth is associated with cellular hypertrophy caused by the addition of more myofibrils and more

sarcomeres at the ends of the cell to match skeletal growth. Strength training induces cellular hypertrophy, whereas endurance training increases the oxidative capacity of all involved motor units. Training regimens are not able to alter fiber type or the expression of myosin isoforms.

10. Muscle fatigue during exercise is not due to depletion of ATP. The mechanism(s) underlying exercise-induced fatigue is not known, although the accumulation of various metabolic products (lactate, inorganic phosphate, ADP) has been implicated. Given the importance of preventing depletion of myoplasmic ATP, which would affect the viability of the cell, it is likely that multiple mechanisms may have been developed to induce fatigue, and hence lower the rate of ATP hydrolysis before risking injury/death of the skeletal muscle cell.

11. When the energy demands of an exercising muscle cannot be met by oxidative metabolism, an oxygen debt is incurred. Increased breathing during the recovery period after exercise reflects this oxygen debt. The greater the reliance on anaerobic metabolism to meet the energy requirements of muscle contraction, the greater the oxygen debt.

BIBLIOGRAPHY

Journal articles

Allen DG, Westerblad H: Role of phosphate and calcium stores in muscle fatigue, *J Physiol* 536:657, 2001.

Carroll S, Nicotera P, Pette D: Calcium transients in single fibers of low-frequency stimulated fast-twitch muscle of rat, *Am J Physiol* 277:C1122, 1999.

Cooke R: Actomyosin interaction in striated muscle, *Physiol Rev* 77:671, 1997.

Dirksen RT, Beam KG: Role of calcium permeation in dihydropyridine receptor function. Insights into channel gating and excitation-contraction coupling, *J Gen Physiol* 114:393, 1999.

Franzini-Armstrong C, Protasi F: Ryanodine receptors of striated muscles: a complex channel capable of multiple interactions, *Physiol Rev* 77:699, 1997

Gordon AM, Homsher E, Regnier M: Regulation of contraction in striated muscle, *Physiol Rev* 80:853, 2000.

Huxley AF: Mechanics and models of the myosin motor, *Philos Trans F Soc Lond B Biol Sci* 355:433, 2000.

Jurkat-Rott K, McCarthy T, Lehmann-Horn F: Genetics and pathogenesis of malignant hyperthermia, *Muscle Nerve* 23:4, 2000.

Kubis HP, Haller EA, Wetzel P, Gros G: Adult fast myosin patter and Ca^{2+} induced slow myosin pattern in primary skeletal muscle culture, *Proc Natl Acad Sci USA* 94:4205, 1997.

Littlefield R, Fowler VM: Defining actin filament length in striated muscle: rulers and caps of dynamic stability? *Annu Rev Cell Dev Biol* 14:487, 1998.

MacLennan DH: Ca^{2+} signalling and muscle disease, *Eur J Biochem* 267:5291, 2000.

MacLennan DH, Rice WJ, Green NM: The mechanism of Ca^{2+} transport by sarco(endo)plasmic reticulum Ca^{2+}-ATPases, *J Biol Chem* 272:28815, 1997.

McElhinny AS et al: The N-terminal end of nebulin interacts with tropomodulin at the pointed ends of the thin filaments, *J Biol Chem* 276:583, 2001.

Obermann WB et al: Molecular structure of the sarcomeric M band: mapping of titin and myosin binding in myomesin and the identification of a potential regulatory phosphorylation site in myomesin, *EMBO J* 16:211, 1997.

O'Brien KF, Kunkel LM: Dystrophin and muscular dystrophy: past present, and future, *Mol Genet Metab* 74:75, 2001.

Pette D, Staron RS: Myosin isoforms, muscle fiber types, and transitions, *Microsc Res Tech* 50:500, 2000.

Rall JA: Sense and nonsense about the Fenn effect, *Am J Physiol* 242:I11, 1982.

Rando TA: The dystrophin-glycoprotein complex, cellular signaling, and the regulation of cell survival in the muscular dystrophies, *Muscle Nerve* 24:1575, 2001.

Sahlin K, Tonkonogi M, Soderlund K: Energy supply and muscle fatigue in humans, *Acta Physiol Scand* 162:261, 1998.

Schiaffino S, Reggiani C: Molecular diversity of myofibrillar proteins: gene regulation and functional significance, *Physiol Rev* 76:371, 1996.

Sugi H et al: Evidence for the load-dependent mechanical efficiency of individual myosin heads in skeletal muscle fibers activated by laser flash photolysis of caged calcium in the presence of a limited amount of ATP, *Proc Natl Acad Sci USA* 95:2273, 1998.

Van der Ven PF et al: Thick filament assembly occurs after the formation of a cytoskeletal scaffold, *J Muscle Res Cell Motil* 20:569, 1999.

chapter thirteen

Smooth Muscle Physiology

Nonstriated, or smooth, muscle cells are a major component of the airways, vasculature, alimentary canal, urogenital tract, and other systems. Smooth muscle must develop force or shorten to provide motility, or to alter the dimensions of an organ. Smooth muscle must also be capable of economical [i.e., minimal adenosine triphosphate (ATP) consumption] sustained, or tonic contractions, to maintain organ dimensions against imposed loads. For example, the blood vessels must be able to withstand the blood pressure. In hollow organs, smooth muscle cells are mechanically coupled, allowing them to function in a highly coordinated fashion. In this chapter the structure and function of smooth muscle are reviewed. Where appropriate, differences between smooth and skeletal muscle are highlighted.

OVERVIEW OF SMOOTH MUSCLE

Types of Smooth Muscle

Smooth muscle has been subdivided into two groups: **single-unit** and **multiunit**. In single-unit smooth muscle, the smooth muscle cells are electrically coupled, such that electrical stimulation of one cell is followed by stimulation of adjacent smooth muscle cells This results in a wave of contraction as in peristalsis. Moreover, this wave of electrical activity, and hence contraction, in single-unit smooth muscle may be initiated by a pacemaker cell (i.e., a smooth muscle cell that exhibits a spontaneous depolarization). On the other hand, multiunit smooth muscle cells are not electrically coupled, so that stimulation of one cell does not necessarily result in activation of the adjacent smooth muscle cell. Examples of multiunit smooth muscle include the vas deferens of the male genital tract and the iris of the eye. Smooth muscle, however, is even more diverse, with single-unit and multiunit classification representing ends of a spectrum. Moreover, the terms *single-unit* and *multiunit* represent an oversimplification, because most smooth muscles are modulated by a combination of neural elements, with at least some degree of cell-to-cell coupling, and by locally produced activators or inhibitors, which also promote a somewhat coordinated response of smooth muscles.

A second consideration when discussing types of smooth muscle is the activity pattern (see Fig. 13-1). In some organs, the smooth muscle cells contract rhythmically or intermittently, whereas in other organs, the smooth muscle cells are continuously active maintaining a level of "tone." Smooth muscle exhibiting rhythmic or intermittent activity is termed **phasic smooth muscle** and includes smooth muscles in the walls of the gastrointestinal and urogenital tracts. Such phasic smooth muscle corresponds to the single-unit category described above because the smooth muscle cells contract in response to action potentials that propagate from cell to cell. Smooth muscle that is continuously active, on the other hand, is termed **tonic smooth muscle.** Vascular smooth muscle, respiratory smooth muscle, and some sphincters are continuously active. The continuous partial activation of tonic smooth muscle is not associated with action potentials, although it is proportional to the membrane potential. Tonic smooth muscle would thus correspond to the multiunit smooth muscle described above. Phasic and tonic contractions of smooth muscle result from interactions of actin and myosin filaments, although as will be discussed later in this chapter, there is a change in the cross-bridge cycling kinetics during tonic contraction such that the smooth muscle can maintain force at low energy cost.

STRUCTURE OF SMOOTH MUSCLE CELLS

Smooth muscle cells typically form layers around hollow organs (see Fig. 13-2). Blood vessels and airways exhibit a simple tubular structure where the smooth muscle cells are arranged circumferentially, so that contraction reduces the diameter of the tube. This contraction increases the resistance to the flow of blood or air, but has little effect on the length of the organ. Smooth muscle cell organization is more complex in the gastrointestinal tract. Layers of smooth muscle in both circumferential and longitudinal orientations provide the mechanical actions for mixing food, and also propelling the luminal contents from the mouth to the anus. Coordination between these layers depends on a complex system of autonomic nerves linked by plexuses. These

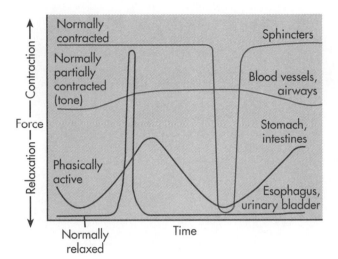

■ **Fig. 13-1**   Some contractile activity patterns exhibited by smooth muscles. Tonic smooth muscles are normally contracted and generate a variable steady-state force. Examples are sphincters, blood vessels, and airways. Phasic smooth muscles commonly exhibit rhythmic contractions (e.g., peristalsis in the gastrointestinal tract), but may contract intermittently in physiological activities under voluntary control (e.g., voiding of urine and swallowing).

plexuses are located between the two muscle layers. The smooth muscle in the walls of sacular structures, such as the urinary bladder or rectum, allows the organ to increase in size with the accumulation of urine or feces. The varied arrangement of cells in the walls of these organs contributes to their ability to reduce the internal volume almost to zero

during urination or defecation, respectively. Smooth muscle cells in hollow organs occur in a spectrum of forms, depending on their function and the mechanical loads.

In all hollow organs, the smooth muscle is separated from the contents of the organ by other cellular elements, which may be as simple as the vascular endothelium or as complex as the mucosa of the digestive tract. The walls of hollow organs also contain large amounts of connective tissue that bear an increasing share of the wall stress as the organ volume increases.

The following sections describe the structural components that enable smooth muscle to set or alter hollow organ volumes. These include the contractile and regulatory proteins, force-transmitting systems such as the cytoskeleton, linkages between cells and to the extracellular matrix, and membrane systems that transduce extracellular signals into changes in the myoplasmic Ca^{2+} concentration.

Cell-to-Cell Contacts

A variety of specialized contacts exist between smooth muscle cells. These contacts allow mechanical linkage and communication between the cells (Fig. 13-3). In contrast to skeletal muscle cells, which are normally attached at either end to a tendon, smooth (and cardiac) muscle cells are connected to each other. Because smooth muscle cells are anatomically arranged in series, they must not only be mechanically linked, but must also be activated simultaneously and to the same degree. This mechanical and functional linkage is crucial to smooth muscle function. If such linkages did not exist, contraction in one region would

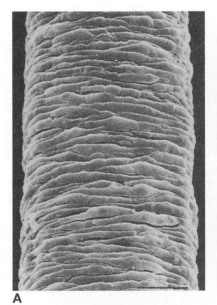

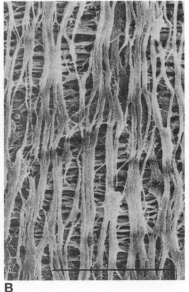

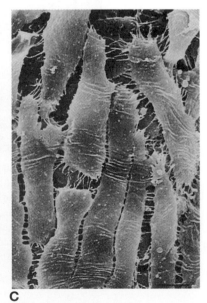

A   **B**   **C**

■ **Fig. 13-2**   Scanning electron micrographs of smooth muscle. **A,** Muscular arteriole with fusiform smooth muscle cells in a circular orientation (bar: 20 μm). **B,** Superimposed images of circular *(below)* and longitudinal *(above)* layers of intestinal smooth muscle sandwiching neural components of the myenteric plexus *(asterisks)* (bar: 50 mm). **C,** Rectangular smooth muscle cells with thin projections to adjacent cells in a small testicular duct (bar: 5 μm). (From Uehara Y et al. In Motta PM, editor: *Ultrastructure of smooth muscle*, Norwell, Mass, 1990, Kluwer Academic.)

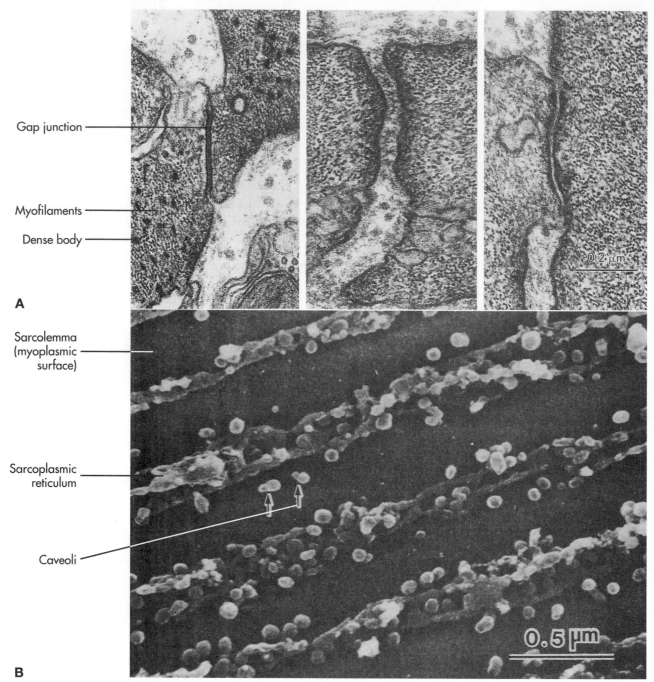

Gap junction

Myofilaments

Dense body

A

Sarcolemma
(myoplasmic
surface)

Sarcoplasmic
reticulum

Caveoli

B

■ **Fig. 13-3** Junctions and membranes in smooth muscle. **A,** Transmission electron micrograph of junctions between intestinal smooth muscle cells. **B,** Scanning electron micrograph of the inner surface of the sarcolemma of an intestinal smooth muscle cell. Longitudinal rows of caveoli project into the myoplasm *(small, light-colored spheres)* surrounded by darker elements of the tubular sarcoplasmic reticulum. The attachments of thin filaments to the sarcolemma between the rows of membrane elements were removed during specimen preparation. (**A** from Gabella G and **B** from Inoué T. In Motta PM, editor: *Ultrastructure of smooth muscle,* Norwell, Mass, 1990, Kluwer Academic.)

simply stretch another region without a substantial decrease in radius or increase in pressure. The mechanical connections are provided by attachments to sheaths of connective tissue and by specific junctions between muscle cells.

Several types of junctions are found in smooth muscle (Fig. 13-4). Functional linkage of the cells is provided by **gap junctions.** Gap junctions form low-resistance pathways between cells. They also allow chemical communication by diffusion of low-molecular-weight compounds. In certain

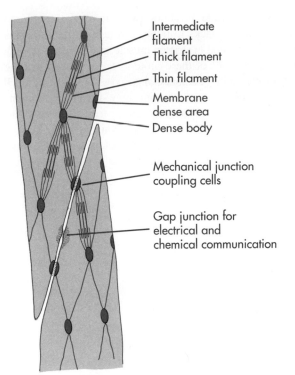

Intermediate
filament
Thick filament
Thin filament
Membrane
dense area
Dense body
Mechanical junction
coupling cells
Gap junction for
electrical and
chemical communication

■ **Fig. 13-4** Apparent organization of cell-to-cell contacts, cytoskeleton, and myofilaments in smooth muscle cells. Small contractile elements functionally equivalent to a sarcomere underlie the similarities in mechanics between smooth and skeletal muscles. Linkages consisting of specialized junctions or interstitial fibrillar material functionally couple the contractile apparatus of adjacent cells.

tissues, such as the outer longitudinal layer of smooth muscle in the intestine, large numbers of such junctions exist. Action potentials are readily propagated from cell to cell through such tissues.

Adherens junctions (also called dense plaques or attachment plaques) provide mechanical linkages between smooth muscle cells. As depicted in Fig. 13-4, the adherens junction appears as thickened regions of opposing cell membranes, which are separated by a small gap (~60 nm). A dense, granular material is present in this gap (perhaps serving to mechanically link the two cells). Thin filaments extend into the adherens junction, allowing contractile force generated in one smooth muscle cell to be transmitted to adjacent smooth muscle cells.

Figure 13-3 also shows the presence of **caveoli,** which represent invaginations of the smooth muscle membrane (analogous to the T-tubules in striated muscle). The **sarcoplasmic reticulum (SR)** extends throughout the smooth muscle cell, although as depicted in Fig. 13-3, there are junctional regions of the SR where it abuts regions of the sarcolemma and/or caveoli. As will be discussed in a subsequent section, these subsarcolemmal regions of the SR play an important role in the regulation of intracellular Ca^{2+} and hence smooth muscle tone.

Cells and Membranes

Embryonic smooth muscle cells do not fuse, and each differentiated cell has a single, centrally located nucleus (Fig. 13-5). Although dwarfed by skeletal muscle cells, smooth muscle cells are nevertheless quite large (typically 40 to 600 μm long). These cells are 2 to 10 μm in diameter in the region of the nucleus, and most taper toward their ends. Contracting cells become quite distorted as a result of forces exerted on the cell by attachments to other cells or to the extracellular matrix, and cross sections of these cells are often very irregular.

Smooth muscle cells lack T-tubules, the invaginations of the skeletal muscle sarcolemma that provide electrical links to the SR. However, the sarcolemma of smooth muscle has longitudinal rows of tiny saclike inpocketings called caveoli (Figs. 13-3 and 13-5). Caveoli increase the surface-to-volume ratio of the cells. They may be sites where Ca^{2+} enters the cell because the sarcolemma contains voltage-gated Ca^{2+} channels. The resting membrane potential of some smooth muscles is in the range of –60 to –40 mV, which is sufficient to allow some Ca^{2+} to enter the cell through these voltage-gated Ca^{2+} channels.

Smooth muscle also has an intracellular membrane network of SR, that serves as an intracellular reservoir for Ca^{2+} (Figs. 13-3 and 13-5). Calcium can be released from the SR into the myoplasm when stimulatory neurotransmitters, hormones, or drugs bind to receptors on the sarcolemma. Importantly, intracellular Ca^{2+} channels in SR of smooth muscle include the **ryanodine receptor (RYR),** which is similar to that found in skeletal muscle SR, and the **inositol 1,4,5-trisphosphate (IP$_3$)**-gated Ca^{2+} channel. The RYR is typically activated by a rise in intracellular Ca^{2+} (i.e., Ca^{2+}-induced Ca^{2+} release in response to an influx of Ca^{2+} through the sarcolemma). The IP$_3$-gated Ca^{2+} channel is activated by IP$_3$, which is produced when hormone(s) bind to various Ca^{2+}-mobilizing receptors on the sarcolemma. Intracellular Ca^{2+} is lowered through the action of an **SR Ca^{2+}-ATPase (SERCA),** and Ca^{2+} extrusion from the cell via a $3Na^+/Ca^{2+}$ antiporter and a sarcolemmal Ca^{2+}-ATPase. The amount of sarcoplasmic reticulum in smooth muscle cells varies from 2% to 6% of cell volume), and approximates that of skeletal muscle. As mentioned above, chemical signals such as IP$_3$, or a localized increase in intracellular Ca^{2+} functionally link the sarcolemma and the SR.

Smooth muscle cells contain a prominent rough endoplasmic reticulum and Golgi apparatus, which are located centrally at each end of the nucleus. These structures reflect significant protein synthetic and secretory functions. The scattered mitochondria (Fig. 13-5) are sufficient for oxidative phosphorylation to generate the increased ATP consumed during contraction.

Contractile Apparatus

Thick and thin filaments of smooth muscle cells are about 10,000 times longer than their diameter and are tightly packed. Therefore, the probability of observing an intact filament by electron microscopy is extremely low. Whereas the thick and thin filaments of skeletal muscle are easy to localize because of their precise transverse alignment, which appears as striations, the cytoskeletal and contractile filaments in smooth muscle are not in uniform transverse alignment, and therefore striations are absent. The lack of striations in smooth muscle does not imply a lack of order. The thick and thin filaments are organized in contractile units that are analogous to sarcomeres.

The thin filaments of smooth muscle have an actin and tropomyosin composition and structure similar to skeletal muscle. However, the cellular content of actin and tropomyosin in smooth muscle is about twice that of striated muscle. Smooth muscle lacks troponin and nebulin, but contains two proteins not found in striated muscle: caldesmon and calponin. The precise roles of these proteins are unknown, but they do not appear to be fundamental to cross-bridge cycling. It has been suggested that calponin may inhibit the binding of unphosphorylated myosin to actin. Most of the myoplasm is filled with thin filaments that are roughly aligned along the long axis of the cell. The myosin content of smooth muscle is only one-fourth that of striated muscle. Small groups of three to

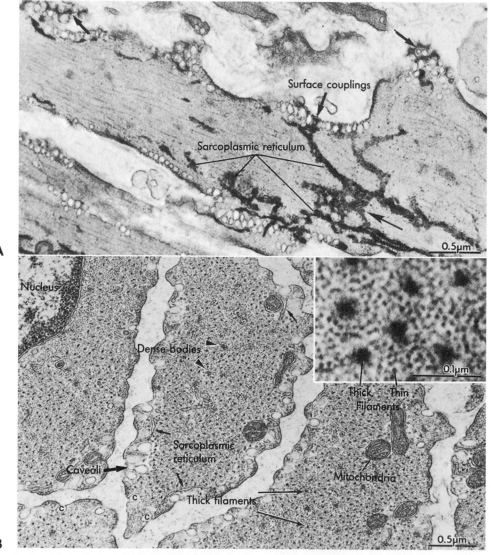

■ **Fig. 13-5 A,** Longitudinal view of a pulmonary artery smooth muscle cell. The sarcoplasmic reticulum is stained with osmium ferricyanide and appears to form a continuous network throughout the cell consisting of tubules, fenestrated sheets *(long arrows)*, and surface couplings at the cell membrane *(short arrows)*. **B,** Transverse section of a bundle of venous smooth muscle cells illustrating the regular spacing of thick filaments *(long arrows)* and the relatively large number of surrounding thin *(actin)* filaments *(inset)*. Dense bodies *(arrowheads)* are sites of attachment for the thin actin filaments and equivalent to the Z-lines of striated muscles. Elements of sarcoplasmic reticulum *(short arrows)* occur at the periphery of these cells. (From Somlyo AP, Somlyo AV: Smooth muscle structure and function. In Fozzard HA et al, editors: *The heart and cardiovascular system*, ed 2, New York, 1992, Raven Press.)

five thick filaments are aligned and are surrounded by many thin filaments. These groups of thick filaments with interdigitating thin filaments are connected to dense bodies or areas (Fig. 13-4), and represent the equivalent of the sarcomere. The contractile apparatus of adjacent cells is mechanically coupled by the links between membrane-dense areas (Fig. 13-4).

Cytoskeleton

The cytoskeleton in smooth muscle cells serves as attachment points for the thin filaments and permits force transmission to the ends of the cell. In contrast to skeletal muscle, the contractile apparatus in smooth muscle is not organized into myofibrils, and Z-lines are lacking. The functional equivalents of the Z-lines in smooth muscle cells are ellipsoidal **dense bodies** in the myoplasm and **dense areas** that form bands along the sarcolemma (Figs. 13-3, 13-4, and 13-5). These structures serve as attachment points for the thin filaments and contain α-actinin, a protein also found in the Z-lines of striated muscle. **Intermediate filaments** with diameters between those of thin filaments (7 nm) and thick

filaments (15 nm) are prominent in smooth muscle. These filaments link the dense bodies and areas into a cytoskeletal network (Fig. 13-4). The intermediate filaments consist of protein polymers of **desmin** or **vimentin.**

CONTROL OF ACTIVITY OF SMOOTH MUSCLE

The contractile activity of smooth muscle can be controlled by numerous factors, including hormones, autonomic nerves, pacemaker activity, and a variety of drugs. Like skeletal muscle or cardiac muscle, the contraction of smooth muscle is Ca^{2+}-dependent, and the agents listed above cause smooth muscle contraction by increasing intracellular Ca^{2+} concentration. However, in contrast to skeletal or cardiac muscle, action potentials in smooth muscle are highly variable and not always needed to initiate contraction. Moreover, several agents can increase the intracellular Ca^{2+} concentration, and hence contract smooth muscle, without changing the membrane potential. Fig. 13-6 shows various types of action

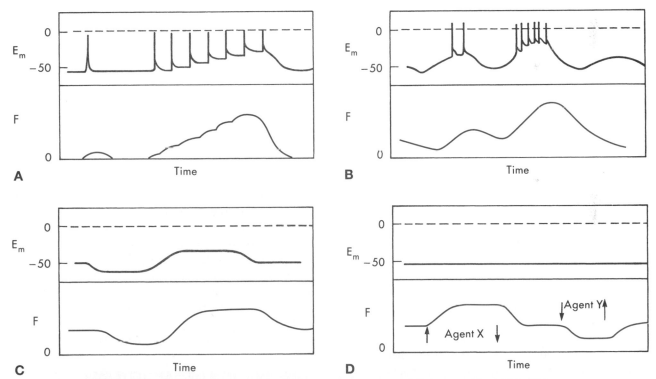

■ **Fig. 13-6** Relationships between membrane potential (E_m) and force generation *(F)* in different types of smooth muscle. **A,** Action potentials may be generated and lead to a twitch or larger summed mechanical responses. Action potentials are characteristic of single-unit smooth muscles (many viscera). Gap junctions permit the spread of action potentials throughout the tissue. **B,** Rhythmic activity produced by slow waves that trigger action potentials. The contractions are usually associated with a burst of action potentials. Slow oscillations in membrane potential usually reflect the activity of electrogenic pumps in the cell membrane. **C,** Tonic contractile activity may be related to the value of the membrane potential in the absence of action potentials. Graded changes in E_m are common in multiunit smooth muscles (e.g., vascular), where action potentials are not generated and propagated from cell to cell. **D,** Pharmacomechanical coupling; changes in force produced by the addition or removal *(arrows)* of drugs or hormones that have no significant effect on the membrane potential.

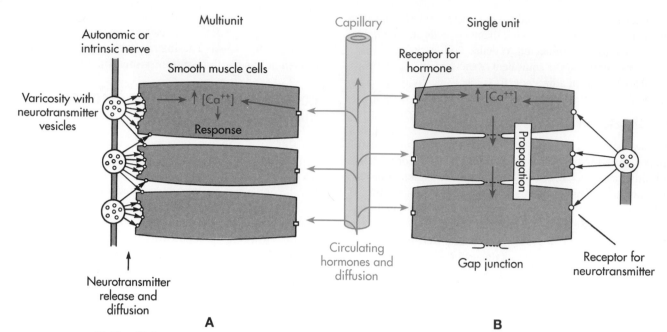

■ Fig. 13-7 Control systems of smooth muscle. Contraction (or inhibition of contraction) of smooth muscles can be initiated by (1) intrinsic activity of pacemaker cells, (2) neurally released transmitters, or (3) circulating or locally generated hormones or signaling molecules. The combination of a neurotransmitter, hormone, or drug with specific receptors activates contraction by increasing cell Ca^{2+}. The response of the cells depends on the concentration of the transmitters or hormones at the cell membrane and the nature of the receptors present. Hormone concentrations depend on diffusion distance, release, reuptake, and catabolism. Consequently, cells lacking close neuromuscular contacts will have a limited response to neural activity unless they are electrically coupled so that depolarization is transmitted from cell to cell. **A,** Multiunit smooth muscles resemble striated muscles in that there is no electrical coupling, and neural regulation is important. **B,** Single-unit smooth muscles are like cardiac muscle, and electrical activity is propagated throughout the tissue. Most smooth muscles probably lie between the two ends of the single unit–multiunit spectrum.

potentials in smooth muscle, and the corresponding changes in force. An action potential in smooth muscle can be associated with a slow twitch-like response, and the twitch forces can summate (i.e., similar to tetany in skeletal muscle) during periods of repetitive action potentials. Such a pattern of activity is characteristic of single-unit smooth muscles in many viscera.

Periodic oscillations in membrane potential can occur as a result of changes in the activity of the Na^+,K^+-ATPase in the sarcolemma. These oscillations in membrane potential can trigger multiple action potentials in the cell. Alternatively, the contractile activity of smooth muscle may not be associated with the generation of action potentials, or even a change in the membrane potential. As already noted, the resting membrane potential of smooth muscle is sufficiently depolarized (–60 to –40 mV) such that a small decrease in membrane potential can significantly inhibit Ca^{2+} influx through voltage-gated Ca^{2+} channels in the sarcolemma. By decreasing Ca^{2+} influx the force developed by smooth muscle decreases. Such a graded response to slight changes in the resting membrane potential is common among multiunit smooth muscles that maintain a constant tension (e.g., vascular smooth muscle).

The contraction of smooth muscle in response to an agent that does not produce a change in membrane potential is termed "pharmacomechanical coupling" and typically reflects the ability of the agent to increase the level of the intracellular second messenger IP_3. Other agents result in a decrease in tension, also without a change in membrane potential. These agents typically increase levels of the intracellular second messengers cGMP or cAMP. The molecular mechanisms by which IP_3, cGMP, cAMP, and Ca^{2+} alter contractile force of smooth muscle are presented below.

INNERVATION OF SMOOTH MUSCLE

Neural regulation of contraction of smooth muscle depends on the type of innervation and neurotransmitters released, the proximity of the nerves to the muscle cells, and the type and distribution of the neurotransmitter receptors on the muscle cell membranes (Fig. 13-7). In general, smooth muscle is innervated by the autonomic nervous system. The smooth muscle in arteries is innervated primarily by sympathetic fibers. Smooth muscle in other tissues can have both sympathetic and parasympathetic innervation. In the gastrointestinal tract, smooth muscle is innervated by nerve

■ **Table 13-1** Modulation of smooth muscle activity by neurotransmitters, hormones, and local factors

Agonist	Response	Receptor	Second messenger
Norepinephrine and epinephrine from sympathetic stimulation	Contraction* (predominant)	α_1-AR	IP$_3$
	Relaxation†	β_2-AR	cAMP
Acetylcholine from parasympathetic stimulation	Contraction‡ (direct)	Muscarinic receptor on SMC	
	Relaxation‡ (indirect)	Muscarinic receptor on EC	
Angiotensin II	Contraction§	ATII receptor	IP$_3$
Vasopressin	Contraction§	Vasopressin receptor	IP$_3$
Endothelin	Contraction§	Endothelin receptor	IP$_3$
Adenosine	Relaxation‖	Adenosine receptor	cAMP

*The predominant effect of sympathetic stimulation is smooth muscle contraction due to the abundance of α_1-AR relative to β_2-AR in smooth muscle.
†Activation β_2-AR on smooth muscle modulates the degree of smooth muscle contraction during sympathetic stimulation. Therapeutic β_2-AR agonists are important for the relaxation of bronchial smooth muscle during asthmatic attacks.
‡Vascular smooth muscles are poorly innervated by the parasympathetic system. During vagal stimulation, however, acetylcholine (ACh) can become elevated in the coronary circulation, resulting in coronary relaxation (mediated by ACh binding to endothelial cells). Note this effect of ACh is indirect, as ACh binding to endothelial cells results in the release of the smooth muscle relaxant nitric oxide from the endothelial cells. In regions of the coronary circulation with a damaged endothelium, ACh binding to coronary smooth muscle could promote contraction (vasospasm; direct effect).
§A variety of hormones can elevate IP$_3$ in smooth muscle, resulting in smooth muscle contraction. These include angiotensin II, vasopressin, and endothelin, along with the neurotransmitters norepinephrine and acetylcholine. As noted above, however, each hormone/transmitter binds to a specific receptor type.
‖During periods of intense muscular activity, adenosine can be released from the working muscle, diffuse to the neighboring vasculature, and promote vasodilation. Thus, adensoine is acting as a local factor to increase blood flow to a specific region (i.e., working muscle).

plexuses that comprise the enteric nervous system. The smooth muscle cells of some tissues, such as the uterus, have no innervation.

The neuromuscular junctions and neuromuscular transmission in smooth muscle are functionally comparable with skeletal muscle, but structurally less complex. Autonomic nerves that supply smooth muscle have a series of swollen areas or varicosities that are spaced at intervals along the axon. These varicosities contain the vesicles of neurotransmitter (Fig. 13-7). The postsynaptic membrane of smooth muscle exhibits little specialization compared to that of skeletal muscle (see Chapter 4). The synaptic cleft is typically ~80–120 nm wide, but can be as narrow as 6 to 20 nm, or even greater than 120 nm. In those where a wide synaptic cleft is found, neurotransmitter release can affect multiple smooth muscle cells. There are a large number of neurotransmitters that affect smooth muscle activity. A partial listing is provided in Table 13-1.

The enteric nervous system controls many aspects of gastrointestinal function, including motility. Some children are born without enteric nerves in the distal portion of the colon. The absence of nerves is caused by mutant genes that disrupt the signals necessary for the embryonic nerves to migrate to the colon. In these children normal motility of the colon does not occur, and severe constipation results. This condition is called **Hirschsprung's disease**. It can be corrected by surgically removing the portion of the colon that does not contain the enteric nerves.

REGULATION OF CONTRACTION

Like skeletal muscle, contraction of smooth muscle occurs in response to an elevation of intracellular Ca^{2+}. However, in contrast to skeletal muscle, where the rise in intracellular [Ca^{2+}] affects actin (i.e., contraction is regulated by actin), the increase in intracellular [Ca^{2+}] in smooth muscle affects myosin (i.e., contraction is regulated by myosin). Specifically, the rise in intracellular Ca^{2+} activates a Ca^{2+}-calmodulin-dependent protein kinase, which phosphorylates a regulatory light chain in myosin, allowing it to then interact with actin, and thus develop force. As depicted in Fig. 13-8, four Ca^{2+} molecules bind to the protein calmodulin, then the Ca^{2+}-calmodulin complex activates **myosin light chain kinase (MLCK)**, which phosphorylates the regulatory light chain of myosin. This phosphorylation step is critical for the interaction of smooth muscle myosin with actin. In addition to this phosphorylation step, an ATP molecule is also needed to energize the myosin cross-bridge for the development of force.

The myosin cross-bridge cycle in smooth muscle is similar to that in striated muscle, in that following attachment to the actin filament, the cross-bridge undergoes a ratchet action pulling the thin filament toward the center of the thick filament, and generating force. Adenosine diphosphate (ADP) and P$_i$ are released from the myosin head at this time, allowing ATP to bind. ATP decreases the affinity of myosin for actin, allowing the release of myosin from actin. Energy from the newly bound ATP is then used to produce a conformational change in the myosin head (i.e., recocking the head), so the cross-bridge is ready for another contraction cycle. The cross-bridge cycle continues as long as the myosin cross-bridge remains phosphorylated. Note that although the basic steps of the cross-bridge cycle appear to be the same for striated and smooth muscle, the kinetics of cross-bridge cycling is much slower for smooth muscle.

Cross-bridge cycling continues, with the hydrolysis of one ATP per cycle, until the myoplasmic [Ca^{2+}] falls. With the decrease in [Ca^{2+}] the MLCK becomes inactive, and the cross-bridges are dephosphorylated by myosin phosphatase (Fig. 13-8).

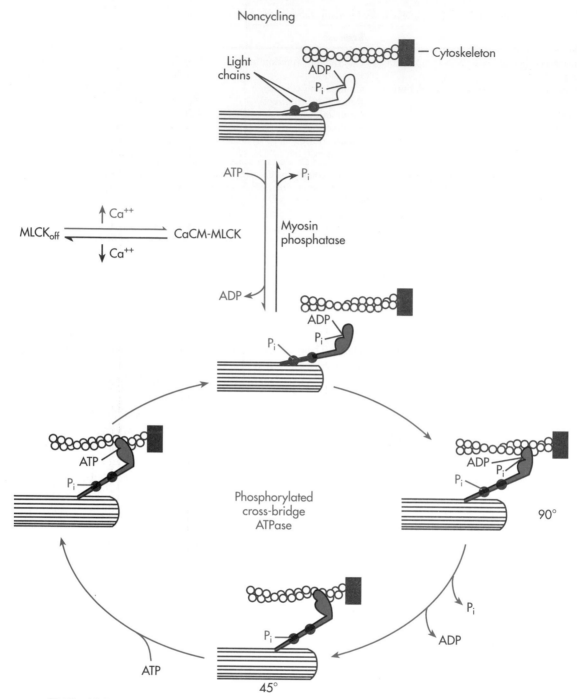

■ Fig. 13-8 Regulation of smooth muscle myosin interactions with actin by Ca^{2+}-stimulated phosphorylation. In the relaxed state cross-bridges are present as a high-energy myosin-ADP-P_i complex in the presence of ATP. Attachment to actin depends on phosphorylation of the cross-bridge by a Ca^{2+}-calmodulin-dependent myosin light chain kinase (MLCK). Phosphorylated cross-bridges *(color)* cycle until they are dephosphorylated by myosin phosphatase. Note that cross-bridge phosphorylation at a specific site on a myosin regulatory light chain requires ATP in addition to that used in each cyclic interaction with actin. *CM,* Calmodulin.

As indicated in Fig. 13-4, the thin filaments in smooth muscle are attached to dense bodies, and the myosin thick filaments appear to reside between two dense bodies, overlapping a portion of the thin filaments much like the overlap of thick and thin filaments in the sarcomere of striated muscle. A bipolar arrangement of myosin molecules within the thick filament is thought to allow the myosin cross-bridges to pull the actin filaments toward the center of the thick filament, thus contracting the smooth muscle and hence developing force.

From a structural standpoint, smooth muscle myosin is similar to striated muscle myosin in that they both contain a

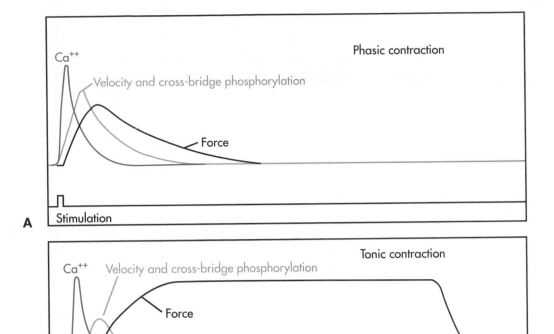

■ **Fig. 13-9**   Time course of events in cross-bridge activation and contraction in smooth muscle. **A,** A brief period of stimulation is associated with Ca^{2+} mobilization followed by cross-bridge phosphorylation and cycling to produce a brief phasic, twitchlike contraction. **B,** In a sustained tonic contraction produced by prolonged stimulation, the Ca^{2+} and phosphorylation levels typically fall from an initial peak. Force is maintained during tonic contractions at a reduced Ca^{2+} concentration (and hence a low level of myosin light chain phosphorylation), with lower cross-bridge cycling rates manifested by lower shortening velocities and ATP consumption.

pair of heavy chains and two pairs of light chains. Despite this similarity, they represent different gene products, and thus have different amino acid sequences. As noted, smooth muscle myosin, unlike skeletal muscle myosin, is unable to interact with the actin thin filament unless the regulatory light chain of myosin is phosphorylated. Moreover, the thin filament in smooth muscle lacks troponin, which plays a critical role in the thin filament regulation of contraction in striated muscle (see Chapter 12).

Phasic Versus Tonic Contraction

During a phasic contraction, myoplasmic $[Ca^{2+}]$, cross-bridge phosphorylation, and force reach a peak and then return to baseline (Fig. 13-9). In contrast, during a tonic contraction, myoplasmic $[Ca^{2+}]$ and cross-bridge phosphorylation decline after an initial spike, but do not return to baseline levels. During this later phase force slowly increases and is sustained at a high level (Fig. 13-9). This sustained force is maintained with only 20% to 30% of the cross-bridges phosphorylated, and thus ATP utilization is reduced. The term "latch state" refers to this state of tonic

contraction during which force is maintained at low energy expenditure.

The latch state is thought to reflect dephosphorylation of the myosin light chain (Fig. 13-10). When the myosin light chain is phosphorylated the cross-bridges recycle as long as myoplasmic $[Ca^{2+}]$ is elevated (red pathway in Fig. 13-10). However, if an attached cross-bridge is dephosphorylated by myosin phosphatase, the rate of cross-bridge recycling is decreased (black pathway in Fig. 13-10). This decreased rate of cross-bridge recycling results from slower detachment of cross-bridges, and because the myosin light chain must be rephosphorylated before another cycle can begin. When the myoplasmic $[Ca^{2+}]$ is high, most of the cross-bridges will be phosphorylated (i.e., the MLCK-to-myosin phosphatase activity ratio is high) and shortening velocities or rates of force development will be relatively high. When the myoplasmic $[Ca^{2+}]$ falls during tonic contractions, the likelihood that a cross-bridge will be dephosphorylated and spend more time in an attached, force-generating conformation increases. However, a low rate of Ca^{2+}-dependent phosphorylation of myosin light chains is essential for contraction.

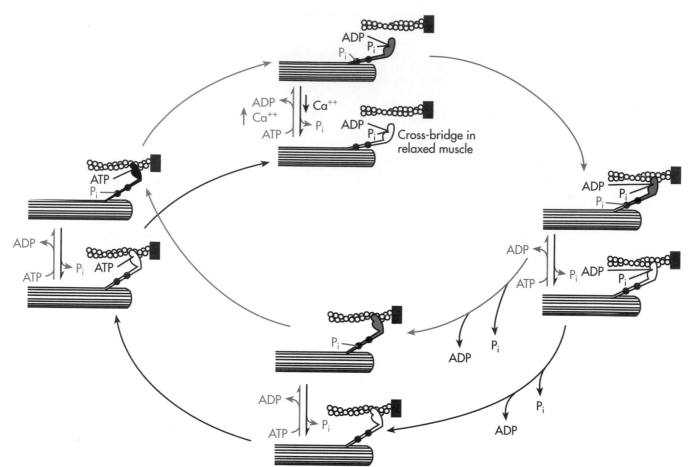

Fig. 13-10 Covalent regulation allows eight cross-bridge states in smooth muscle. Phosphorylation by MLCK *(vertical colored arrows)* is obligatory for cross-bridge attachment. Phosphorylated cross-bridges *(color)* cycle comparatively rapidly. Dephosphorylation of a cross-bridge during a cycle by a constitutively active myosin phosphatase *(vertical black arrows)* slows cycling rates and produces the latch state. Calcium regulates cross-bridge cycling by determining phosphorylation rates. Note that ATP is required for both regulation *(vertical arrows)* and cycling *(curved arrows)*.

The muscle will relax if the $[Ca^{2+}]$ falls below that required for binding to calmodulin and activation of myosin light chain kinase (about 0.1 μM).

Inappropriate contraction of smooth muscle is associated with many pathological situations. One example is a **sustained vasospasm of a cerebral artery** that develops several hours after a subarachnoid hemorrhage. It is thought that free radicals generated as a result of the hemorrhage raise the myoplasmic $[Ca^{2+}]$ in surrounding arterial smooth muscle cells. The rise in myoplasmic $[Ca^{2+}]$ activates MLCK, which leads to cross-bridge phosphorylation and contraction. The vasoconstriction deprives other areas of the brain of oxygen and may lead to permanent injury or death of surrounding neurons. For a few days the cerebral artery remains sensitive to vasoactive agents, and therefore treatment with vasodilators may restore flow. However, after several days the smooth muscle cells cease to respond to the vasodilators, and they lose con-

tractile proteins and secrete extracellular collagen. The lumen of the artery remains constricted as a result of structural and mechanical changes that do not involve active contraction.

Energetics and Metabolism

As already noted, ATP consumption is reduced during the latch state. Under this condition, smooth muscle utilizes 300-fold less ATP than would be required by skeletal muscle to generate the same force. Smooth muscle, like skeletal muscle, requires ATP for ion transport to maintain the resting membrane potential, to sequester Ca^{2+} in the SR, and to extrude Ca^{2+} from the cell. All of these metabolic needs are readily met by oxidative phosphorylation. Fatigue of smooth muscle does not occur unless the cell is deprived of oxygen. However, aerobic glycolysis with lactic acid production normally supports membrane ion pumps even when oxygen is plentiful.

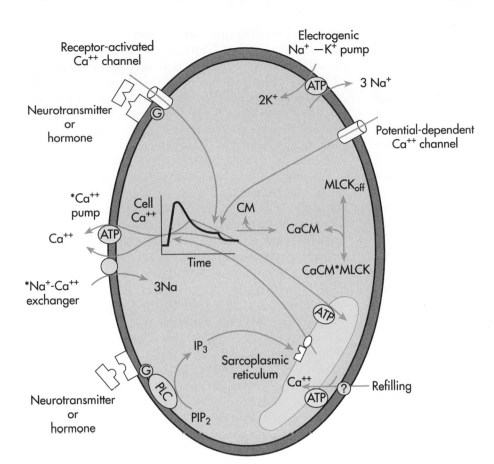

■ **Fig. 13-11** Principal mechanisms determining the myoplasmic [Ca^{2+}] in smooth muscle. Ca^{2+} release from the sarcoplasmic reticulum is a rapid initial event in activation, whereas both the sarcoplasmic reticulum and the sarcolemma participate in the subsequent stimulus-dependent regulation of myoplasmic [Ca^{2+}]. The sarcolemma integrates many simultaneous excitatory and inhibitory inputs to govern the cellular response. Higher-order regulatory mechanisms can alter the activity of various pumps, exchangers, or enzymes (the asterisks designate well-established instances). *G*, Guanine nucleotide binding proteins; *ATP*, process requires ATP hydrolysis; *PL C*, phospholipase C; *PIP$_2$*, phosphatidylinositol bisphosphate; IP$_3$, inositol 1,4,5-trisphosphate; *CM*, calmodulin; *MLCK*, myosin light chain kinase.

REGULATION OF MYOPLASMIC CA^{2+} CONCENTRATION

The mechanisms that couple activation to contraction in smooth muscle involve two Ca^{2+} pools, one in the sarcolemma and the other in the SR. The sarcolemma regulates Ca^{2+} influx and efflux from the extracellular Ca^{2+} pool (i.e., the extracellular fluid). The SR membranes determine Ca^{2+} movements between the myoplasm and the intracellular pool. Skeletal muscle contraction does not require extracellular Ca^{2+} (see Chapter 12). In contrast, extracellular Ca^{2+} is important for smooth muscle contraction. Thus, the regulation of myoplasmic [Ca^{2+}] involves not only the SR, but also the sarcolemma (Fig. 13-11). A number of factors can alter the myoplasmic [Ca^{2+}] of smooth muscle (Fig. 13-11). This is in contrast to skeletal muscle where the action potential-induced release of Ca^{2+} from the SR fully activates the contractile apparatus.

Sarcoplasmic Reticulum

The role of the smooth muscle SR in regulating myoplasmic [Ca^{2+}] is comparable with skeletal muscle. Stimulation of the cell opens SR Ca^{2+} channels, and the myoplasmic [Ca^{2+}] rapidly increases. This release is not linked to voltage sensors, as is the case in skeletal muscle, but to binding of the second messenger, IP$_3$ to receptors in the SR. IP$_3$ is generated by a stimulus that acts on sarcolemmal receptors that are

coupled via a guanine nucleotide binding protein (**G-protein**) to activate **phospholipase C.** Phospholipase C hydrolyzes the membrane phospholipid phosphatidylinositol bisphosphate (PIP2) into IP$_3$ and diacyl glycerol. The IP$_3$ then diffuses to the SR, opening the IP$_3$-gated Ca^{2+} channel, resulting in a release of Ca^{2+} from the SR into the myoplasm. This complex process may permit a graded Ca^{2+} release from the SR and also enable many different neurotransmitters and hormones to effect smooth muscle contraction. Ca^{2+} is reaccumulated by the SR through the activity of the SERCA, although, as indicated below, Ca^{2+} extrusion from the smooth muscle cell also contributes to the reduction in myoplasmic [Ca^{2+}]. Refilling of the sarcoplasmic reticulum with Ca^{2+} involves not only the reaccumulation of cytosolic Ca^{2+}, but also depends on the extracellular Ca^{2+}. The dependence on extracellular Ca^{2+} is thought to reflect the operation of a "store-operated" Ca^{2+} channel present in the sarcolemma at points near underlying SR called "junctional SR."

A variety of hormones and neurotransmitters elevate myoplasmic [Ca^{2+}] by stimulating IP$_3$ production. Vascular smooth muscle, for example, is innervated by sympathetic fibers of the autonomic nervous system. These fibers use norepinephrine as a neurotransmitter, which when released binds to α_1-adrenergic receptors on the vascular smooth muscle cells resulting in a G-protein dependent activation of phospholipase C. Activation of phospholipase C results in the production of IP_3, which activates the IP_3-gated Ca^{2+} channel in the SR, thereby elevating the myoplasmic $[Ca^{2+}]$ and thereby causing vasoconstriction. Other agents that promote vasoconstriction by activating the IP_3 cascade include **angiotensin II** and **vasopressin.** The development of drugs that block the production of angiotensin II (e.g., angiotensin-converting enzyme inhibitors: ACE inhibitors) provides a means of promoting vasodilation, which is important for individuals with hypertension and/or congestive heart failure. As mentioned previously, a variety of agents can produce contraction of smooth muscle without altering membrane potential (i.e., pharmacomechanical coupling). Agonist-induced activation of the IP_3 cascade represents an example of pharmacomechanical coupling.

In addition to the IP_3 receptor, the SR also contains the Ca^{2+}-gated Ca^{2+} channel, also called the ryanodine receptor (RYR), which may be activated during periods of Ca^{2+} influx through the sarcolemma. Short-lived, spontaneous openings of the RYR resulting in localized elevations of myoplasmic Ca^{2+} occurs in many cells including smooth muscle. When observed with Ca^{2+}-sensitive fluorescent dyes, these spontaneous localized elevations of myoplasmic $[Ca^{2+}]$ produce brief light flashes, and as a result are named "Ca^{2+} sparks." In smooth muscle, an increase in cyclic adenosine monophosphate (cAMP) has been associated with an increase in the frequency of Ca^{2+} sparks, particularly where the SR is in close proximity to the sarcolemma (i.e., junctional SR). An increase in the frequency of these sparks hyperpolarizes vascular smooth muscle by activation of a large conductance Ca^{2+}-gated K channel in the sarcolemma This hyperpolarization then decreases overall myoplasmic $[Ca^{2+}]$ and relaxation occurs.

Sarcolemma

Calcium extrusion from the smooth muscle cell occurs by the activity of the sarcolemmal Ca^{2+}-ATPase, and by a $3Na^+/Ca^{2+}$ antiporter (i.e., three Na^+ enter the cell for each Ca^{2+} extruded). Extrusion of Ca^{2+} from the cell competes with Ca^{2+} sequestration in the SR by SERCA, and thus reduces the accumulation of Ca^{2+} in the SR. It is thought that a decrease in SR Ca^{2+} content results in the release of a calcium influx factor (CIF) from the SR, which then activates a "store-operated" Ca^{2+} channel in the sarcolemma near the junctional SR, allowing the SR to completely refill with Ca^{2+} from the extracellular fluid. The identity of this CIF and the identity of the store-operated Ca^{2+} channel are not yet known. Nevertheless it is clear that sustained contraction of smooth muscle requires extracellular Ca^{2+}.

In addition to the stimulatory effects of various agents on sarcolemma Ca^{2+} channels and IP_3 cascades, there are several inhibitory factors that lower myoplasmic $[Ca^{2+}]$, and thereby relax smooth muscle. For example, the dihydropyridine class of Ca^{2+} channel-blocking drugs decreases the influx of Ca^{2+} through sarcolemmal L-type voltage-gated Ca^{2+} channels, and reduces vasomotor tone. Similarly, drugs that open potassium channels in the sarcolemma (e.g., hydralazine)

promote relaxation (e.g., vasodilation) by hyperpolarizing the membrane potential, which reduces Ca^{2+} influx through voltage-gated Ca^{2+} channels. Conversely, agents that decrease the potassium permeability of the sarcolemma may promote vasoconstriction by causing membrane depolarization, which then increases Ca^{2+} influx through these same voltage-gated Ca^{2+} channels. Smooth muscle also contains receptor-activated Ca^{2+} channels. The conductance of these receptor-activated Ca^{2+} channels is linked to receptor occupancy.

A variety of drugs and hormones relax smooth muscles by increasing the cellular concentrations of cAMP or cyclic guanosine monophosphate (cGMP). Nitric oxide (NO) is produced by nerves and vascular endothelial cells, and it relaxes smooth muscle by increasing cGMP. Acetylcholine released from parasympathetic fibers causes vasodilation in some vascular beds as a result of stimulating the production of nitric oxide by vascular endothelial cells. The molecular mechanism(s) underlying the cGMP-dependent relaxation of vascular smooth muscle are complex and may involve activation of a myosin light chain phosphatase, stimulation of a sarcolemma Ca^{2+}-ATPase pump, and/or stimulation of SR Ca^{2+} uptake. Similarly, elevation of cAMP in vascular smooth muscle by stimulation of β-adrenergic receptors or activation of adenosine receptors promotes vasodilation through cAMP-dependent phosphorylations. In particular, cAMP-dependent phosphorylation of MLCK has been proposed to attenuate the Ca^{2+}-dependent increase in MLCK activity, thereby reducing the ability of MLCK to phosphorylate the regulatory light chain of myosin. cAMP may also promote relaxation of smooth muscle through an increase in the frequency of Ca^{2+} sparks, which, as described above, hyperpolarizes the membrane potential by activation of a Ca^{2+}-gated K^+ channels. Relaxation of smooth muscle by elevation of cAMP has afforded asthmatics a means of reversing bronchiolar constriction through the use of $β_2$-adrenergic agonists. The local vasodilatory effect of adenosine produced in working muscle during periods of intense exercise has also been attributed, at least in part, to elevation of cAMP in the vascular smooth muscle secondary to adenosine stimulation of purigenic receptors on the sarcolemma of the vascular smooth muscle. Adenosine may also activate a sarcolemmal K^+ channel, resulting in membrane hyperpolarization, which as already noted will decrease Ca^{2+} influx through voltage-gated Ca^{2+} channels, and thereby cause vasodilation. Thus, regulation of smooth muscle tone may be under the influence of not only the autonomic nervous system and circulating hormones but also neighboring endothelial cells and skeletal muscle cells using diffusible substances such as NO and adenosine.

DEVELOPMENT AND HYPERTROPHY

During development and growth, the number of smooth muscle cells increases (Fig. 13-12). Smooth muscle tissue mass also increases if an organ is subjected to a sustained increase in mechanical work. This increase in mass is called

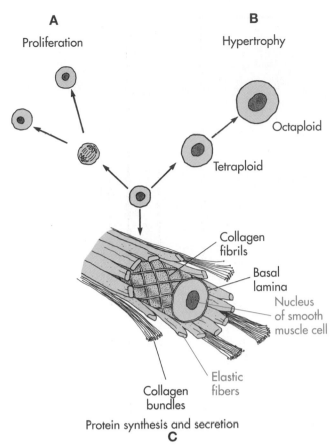

A Proliferation

B Hypertrophy

Octaploid

Tetraploid

Collagen
fibrils

Basal
lamina

Nucleus
of smooth
muscle cell

Collagen
bundles

Elastic
fibers

Protein synthesis and secretion
C

■ **Fig. 13-12** Smooth muscle cells carry out many activities. **A,** They retain the capacity to divide during normal growth or in certain pathological responses such as formation of atherosclerotic plaques. **B,** Cells may also hypertrophy in response to increased loads. Chromosomal replication, not followed by cell division, yields cells with a greater content of contractile proteins. **C,** Smooth muscle cells also synthesize and secrete the constituents of the extracellular matrix.

Although smooth muscle is involved in the physiological adjustments to exercise, sustained changes in the mechanical loading that induce cellular adaptations are usually the result of a pathological condition (e.g., hypertension). A fairly common example in men is **urinary bladder hypertrophy** caused by benign or cancerous enlargement of the prostate gland, which obstructs the bladder outlet. The clinical result is difficulty in urination, distension of the bladder, and impaired emptying. In this situation, the ability of the bladder smooth muscle to contract and develop stress is diminished. The reasons for this remain unexplained, but phenotypic modulation of the smooth muscle cells with altered contractile protein isoform expression and gross anatomical distortion of the bladder wall occurs. Neuromuscular changes also affect myoplasmic Ca^{2+} mobilization and cross-bridge phosphorylation. Fortunately, normal structure and function are usually restored after the obstruction is alleviated.

SYNTHETIC AND SECRETORY FUNCTIONS

The growth and development of tissues that contain smooth muscles are associated with increases in the connective tissue matrix. Smooth muscle cells can synthesize and secrete the materials that make up this matrix. These components include collagen, elastin, and proteoglycans (Fig. 13-12). The synthetic and secretory capacities are evident when smooth muscle cells are isolated and placed in tissue culture. The cells rapidly lose thick myosin filaments and much of the thin filament lattice, and there is expansion of the rough endoplasmic reticulum and Golgi apparatus. The phenotypically altered cells multiply and lay down connective tissue. This process is reversible, and some degree of redifferentiation with formation of thick filaments occurs after cell replication ceases. The determinants of the smooth muscle cell phenotype are largely unknown, but hormones and growth factors in the blood, as well as the mechanical loads on the cells, are implicated in the control of phenotypic modulation.

Atherosclerosis is a disease characterized by lesions located in the wall of blood vessels. The lesions are induced by disorders such as hypertension, diabetes, and smoking that injure the endothelium. Three formed elements (monocytes, T lymphocytes, and platelets) that circulate in the bloodstream act on the damaged vascular endothelium. There, they generate chemotactic factors and mitogens that modify the structure of the surrounding smooth muscle cells. The latter lose most of their thick and thin filaments, and develop an extensive rough endoplasmic reticulum and Golgi complex. These cells migrate to the subendothelial space (the arterial intima), proliferate, and participate in formation of the fatty lesions or the fibrous plaques that characterize atherosclerosis.

compensatory hypertrophy. A striking example occurs in the arterial media in hypertension. The increased mechanical load on the muscle cells appears to be the common factor that induces this hypertrophy. Chromosomal replication can result in significant numbers of polyploid muscle cells. The polyploid cells contain multiple sets of the normal number of chromosomes. They synthesize more contractile proteins and thus increase the size of the cell (Fig. 13-12).

The myometrium, which is the smooth muscle component of the uterus, undergoes hypertrophy as parturition (birth) approaches. Hormones play an important role in this response. The smooth muscle is quiescent during pregnancy (when the hormone progesterone predominates), and few gap junctions that electrically couple the smooth muscle cells are present. At term, under the dominant influence of estrogen, the myometrium undergoes marked hypertrophy. Large numbers of gap junctions form just before birth and convert the myometrium into a single-unit tissue to coordinate contraction during parturition.

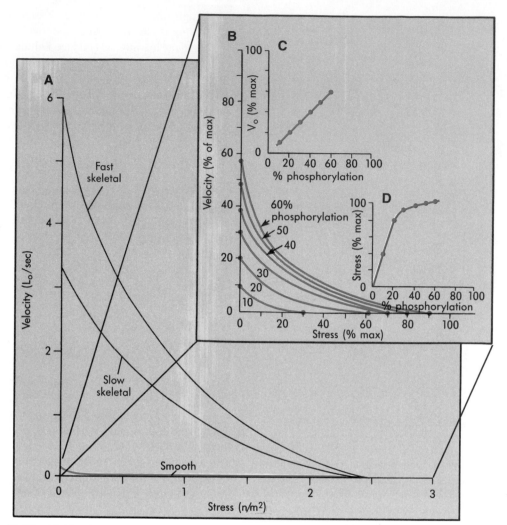

■ Fig. 13-13   A, Force-velocity curves for fast and slow human skeletal muscle cells and smooth muscle. **B,** Smooth muscles have variable force-velocity relationships that are determined by the level of Ca^{2+}-stimulated cross-bridge phosphorylation. **C,** Maximal shortening velocities with no load (intercepts on the ordinate in **B**) are directly dependent on cross-bridge phosphorylation by MLCK. **D,** Active force/stress (abscissa intercepts in **B**) rises rapidly with phosphorylation, and near maximal stress may be generated with only 20% to 30% of the cross-bridges in the phosphorylated state. (From Berne RM, Levy MN, editors: *Principles of physiology*, St Louis, 1990, Mosby.)

BIOPHYSICAL PROPERTIES OF SMOOTH MUSCLE

Length-Tension Relationship

Smooth muscle contains large amounts of connective tissue, which is composed of **extensible elastin fibrils** and **inextensible collagen fibrils.** Because this extracellular matrix can withstand high distending forces or loads, it is responsible for the passive length-tension curve measured in relaxed tissues. This ability of the matrix also limits organ volume. The active force developed on stimulation depends on tissue length. When lengths are normalized to the optimal length for force development (i.e., L_0), the **length-tension curves** for smooth and skeletal muscle are very similar (see Chapter 12). However, the length-tension curves of the two muscle types differ quantitatively. For example, smooth muscle cells shorten more than do

skeletal muscle cells. Also, smooth muscle is characteristically only partially activated, and the peak isometric force attained varies with the stimulus. In skeletal muscle, the stimulus (i.e., action potential) always produces a full twitch contraction. Smooth muscles can generate active forces comparable to that of skeletal muscle. However, smooth muscle contains only about one-fourth of the myosin, and thus cross-bridge content of skeletal muscles. This does not imply that cross-bridges in smooth muscle have a greater force-generating capacity. Instead, active cross-bridges in smooth muscle are much more likely to be in the attached, force-generating configuration, because of their slow cycling kinetics.

Force-Velocity Relationship

Smooth and striated muscles both exhibit a hyperbolic dependence of shortening velocity on load. However, contraction velocities are far slower in smooth muscle than in striated muscle. One factor that underlies these slow velocities is that the myosin isoform in smooth muscle cells has a low ATPase activity.

Skeletal muscle cells have a **force-velocity curve** in which shortening velocities are determined only by load and the myosin isoform (see Chapter 12). In contrast, both forces and shortening velocity, which reflect the numbers of cycling cross-bridges and their cycling rates, vary in smooth muscle. When activation of smooth muscle is altered, for example, by different frequencies of nerve stimulation or changing hormone concentrations, a "family" of velocity-stress curves can be derived (Fig. 13-13). This implies that both cross-bridge cycling rates and the number of active cross-bridges in smooth muscle are regulated in some way, which is in marked contrast to striated muscle. This difference is conferred by a regulatory system that depends on the phosphorylation of cross-bridges, which in turn depends on the concentration of Ca^{2+} in the myoplasm. Because myosin light chain phosphorylation is required for actin-myosin interaction in smooth muscle, a dependence of maximal force on degree of myosin phosphorylation is expected (i.e., phosphorylation of more myosin molecules results in more actin myosin interactions and hence more force generated). The variation in maximal shortening velocity as a function of degree of myosin phosphorylation may reflect dephosphorylation of the myosin light chain while the myosin is still attached to the actin, thus slowing the rate of detachment (i.e., latch state) at low levels of phosphorylation. At higher levels of phosphorylation, the likelihood of latch states would be reduced, allowing the myosin cross-bridges to release more quickly from actin, thereby yielding a higher shortening velocity at all loads (Fig. 13-13, *B*).

SUMMARY

1. Smooth muscle in hollow organs has two roles: (1) to develop force or shorten like skeletal muscle, and (2) to contract tonically to maintain organ dimensions against imposed loads.

2. Smooth muscle cells are linked by a variety of junctions that serve both mechanical and communication roles. These linkages are essential in cells that must contract uniformly.

3. Smooth muscle cells have a high ratio of surface area to volume, and the sarcolemma plays an important role in Ca^{2+} exchange between the extracellular fluid and the myoplasm. The sarcoplasmic reticulum contains an intracellular Ca^{2+} pool that can be mobilized to transiently increase the myoplasmic concentration of Ca^{2+}.

4. Smooth muscles contain contractile units that consist of small groups of thick myosin filaments that interdigitate with large numbers of thin filaments attached to Z-line equivalents, termed dense bodies or membrane-dense areas. No striations are evident. Contraction is caused by a sliding filament–cross-bridge mechanism.

5. Smooth muscle activity is controlled by nerves (principally autonomic), circulating hormones, locally generated signaling substances, junctions with other smooth muscle cells, and even junctions with other non-smooth muscle cells.

6. The contraction of smooth muscle is dependent upon both Ca^{2+} release from the SR and Ca^{2+} entry across the sarcolemma. Smooth muscle lacks troponin. Phosphorylation of cross-bridges by a Ca^{2+}-dependent myosin light chain kinase (MLCK) is necessary for attachment to the thin filament. Dephosphorylation of an attached cross-bridge by myosin phosphatase slows its cycling rates. Higher myoplasmic Ca^{2+} concentrations increase the ratio of MLCK to myosin phosphatase activities, with the result that more of the cross-bridges remain phosphorylated throughout a cycle. This increases shortening velocities.

7. The myoplasmic $[Ca^{2+}]$ is dependent upon extracellular Ca^{2+}. Transporters in the sarcolemma that regulate the myoplasmic $[Ca^{2+}]$ include receptor-mediated Ca^{2+} channels, voltage-gated Ca^{2+} channels, Ca^{2+}-ATPase, and $3Na^+$-Ca^{2+} antiporter.

8. The SR also regulates the myoplasmic $[Ca^{2+}]$. The Ca^{2+} channels in the sarcoplasmic reticulum open in response to a chemical rather than an electrical signal. Neurotransmitters or hormones that act via receptors in the sarcolemma can activate phospholipase C, followed by generation of the second messenger, IP_3. IP_3 then activates IP_3-gated Ca^{2+} channels on the sarcoplasmic reticulum. Smooth muscle SR also contains Ca^{2+}-gated Ca^{2+} channels (RYR). Ca^{2+} is reaccumulated into the SR by SERCA.

9. The response to sustained or tonic stimulation is a rapid contraction followed by sustained force maintenance with reduced cross-bridge cycling rates and ATP consumption. This behavior, called the latch state, is advantageous for muscles that may need to withstand continuous external forces, such as blood vessels that must be able to withstand blood pressure. ATP consumption during the latch state consumes less than 1/300th of the ATP needed to maintain the same force in skeletal muscle.

10. The length-tension relationships, hyperbolic velocity-load relationships, power output curves, and the ability to resist imposed loads are comparable with those of skeletal muscle. Shortening velocities and ATP consumption rates are very low in smooth muscle, in keeping with expression of a myosin isoform with low activity. Uniquely, smooth muscles have variable velocity-stress relationships that reflect regulation of both the numbers of active cross-bridges (determining force) and their average cycling rates for a given load (determining velocity).

11. Smooth muscle is also a synthetic and secretory cell with a major role in the formation of the extensive extracellular matrix that surrounds and links the cells. Cellular hypertrophy occurs in response to physiological needs, and smooth muscle cells retain the potential to divide.

BIBLIOGRAPHY

Journal articles

Berridge MJ: Inositol trisphosphate and calcium signaling, *Nature* 361:315, 1993.

Carl A, Lee HK, Sanders KM: Regulation of ion channels in smooth muscles by calcium, *Am J Physiol* 271(*Cell Physiol* 40):C9, 1996.

Chen Q, van Breemen C: Function of smooth muscle sarcoplasmic reticulum, *Adv Second Messenger Phosphoprotein Res* 26:335, 1992.

Christ GJ et al: Gap junctions in vascular tissues, *Circ Res* 79:631, 1996.

Huizinga JD et al: Intercellular communication in smooth muscle, *Experientia* 48:932, 1992.

Karaki H et al: Calcium movements, distribution, and functions in smooth muscle, *Pharmacol Rev* 49:157, 1997.

Lincoln TM, Cornwell TL: Towards an understanding of the mechanism of action of cyclic AMP and cyclic GMP in smooth muscle relaxation, *Blood Vessels* 28:129, 1991.

Malmqvist U et al: Slow cycling of unphosphorylated myosin is inhibited by calponin, thus keeping smooth muscle relaxed, *Proc Natl Acad Sci USA* 94:7655, 1997.

Mecham RP, Stenmark KR, Parks WC: Connective tissue production by vascular smooth muscle in development and disease, *Chest* 99(suppl):43S, 1991.

Miriel VA et al: Local and cellular Ca^{2+} transients in smooth muscle of pressurized rat resistance arteries during myogenic and agonist stimulation, *J Physiol* 518:815, 1999.

Missiaen L et al: Calcium ion homeostasis in smooth muscle, *Pharmacol Ther* 56:191, 1992.

Murphy RA: What is special about smooth muscle? The significance of covalent crossbridge regulation, *FASEB J* 8:311, 1994.

Nelson MT et al: Relaxation of arterial smooth muscle by calcium sparks, *Science* 270:633, 1995.

Owens GK: Regulation of differentiation of vascular smooth muscle cells, *Physiol Rev* 75:487, 1995.

Putney JW Jr: Cell biology. Channelling calcium, *Nature* 410:648, 2001.

Raeymaekers L, Wuytack F: Ca^{2+} pumps in smooth muscle cells, *J Muscle Res Cell Motil* 14:141, 1993.

Sanders KM: Ionic mechanisms of electrical rhythmicity in gastrointestinal smooth muscles, *Annu Rev Physiol* 54:439, 1992.

Shmigol AV, Eisner DA, Wray S: Simultaneous measurements of changes in sarcoplasmic reticulum and cytosolic [Ca^{2+}] in rat uterine smooth muscle cells, *J Physiol* 531:707, 2001.

Somlyo AP, Somlyo AV: Signal transduction and regulation in smooth muscle, *Nature* 372:231, 1994.

Trybus KM: Regulation of smooth muscle myosin, *Cell Motil Cytoskeleton* 18:81, 1991.

Wellman GC et al: Role of phospholamban in the modulation of arterial Ca(2+)-activated K(+) channels by cAMP, *Am J Physiol Cell Physiol* 281:C1029, 2001.

Books and monographs

Bárány M, editor: *Biochemistry of smooth muscle contraction*, San Diego, Calif, 1996, Academic Press.

Moreland RS, editor: *Regulation of smooth muscle contraction*, New York, 1991, Plenum.

Motta PM, editor: *Ultrastructure of smooth muscle*, Lancaster, England, 1990, Kluwer Academic.

Sperelakis N, Wood JD: *Frontiers in smooth muscle research* (*Prog Clin Biol Res* 327), New York, 1990, Wiley-Liss.

Wood JD, editor: *Handbook of physiology: the gastrointestinal system*, section 6, vol I, *Motility and circulation*, Bethesda, Md, 1989, American Physiological Society.

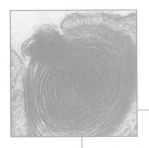

section four

The Cardiovascular System

Matthew N. Levy

chapter fourteen

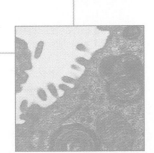

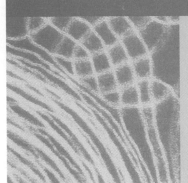

Overview of the Heart, Blood Vessels, and Blood

The circulatory system transports and distributes essential substances to tissues and removes by-products of metabolism. This system also participates in homeostatic mechanisms such as the regulation of body temperature and maintenance of fluid, and the adjustment of oxygen and nutrient supply under various physiological states. The cardiovascular system that accomplishes these tasks is composed of a pump (the heart), a series of distributing and collecting tubes (the blood vessels), and an extensive system of thin vessels (the capillaries) that permit rapid exchange between the tissues and the vascular channels. The blood vessels throughout the body are filled with a heterogeneous fluid (the blood), which is essential for implementing the transport processes performed by the heart and blood vessels. This chapter is a general, functional overview of the heart, the blood vessels, and the blood. The characteristics and functions of the blood are discussed later in this chapter, whereas the functions of the heart and blood vessels are analyzed in much greater detail in subsequent chapters.

THE HEART

The heart consists of two pumps in series: one pump propels blood through the lungs for exchange of oxygen and carbon dioxide (the **pulmonary circulation**) and the other pump propels blood to all other tissues of the body (the **systemic circulation**). The flow of blood through the heart is one-way (unidirectional). Unidirectional flow through the heart is achieved by the appropriate arrangement of flap valves. Although the cardiac output is intermittent, continuous flow to the body tissues (periphery) occurs by distension of the aorta and its branches during ventricular contraction (**systole**) and by elastic recoil of the walls of the large arteries with forward propulsion of the blood during ventricular relaxation (**diastole**).

BLOOD VESSELS

Blood moves rapidly through the aorta and its arterial branches. These branches narrow and their walls become thinner as they approach the periphery. They also change histologically. The aorta is a predominantly elastic structure, but the peripheral arteries become more muscular until at the arterioles the muscular layer predominates (Fig. 14-1).

In the large arteries, frictional resistance is relatively small and pressures are only slightly less than in the aorta. The small arteries, on the other hand, offer moderate resistance to blood flow. This resistance reaches a maximal level in the arterioles, which are sometimes referred to as the stopcocks of the vascular system. *Hence, the pressure drop is greatest across the terminal segment of the small arteries and the arterioles* (Fig. 14-2). Adjustment in the degree of contraction of the circular muscle of these small vessels permits regulation of tissue blood flow and aids in the control of arterial blood pressure.

In addition to the reduction in pressure along the arterioles, there is a change from a pulsatile to a steady blood flow (Fig. 14-3). *The **pulsatile arterial blood flow**, caused by the intermittent ejection of blood from the heart, is damped at the capillary level by a combination of two factors: distensibility of the large arteries and frictional resistance in the small arteries and arterioles.*

In a patient with hyperthyroidism (**Graves' disease**), the basal metabolism is elevated and is often associated with arteriolar vasodilation. This reduction in arteriolar resistance diminishes the damping effect on the pulsatile arterial pressure and is manifested as pulsatile flow in the capillaries, as observed in the finger nailbed of patients with this ailment.

Many capillaries arise from each arteriole. The total cross-sectional area of the capillary bed is very large, despite the fact that the cross-sectional area of each capillary is less than that of each arteriole. As a result, blood flow velocity becomes quite slow in the capillaries, analogous to the decrease in velocity of flow (Fig. 14-3) in the wide regions of a river. Because capillaries consist of short tubes with walls that are only one cell thick and because flow velocity is low,

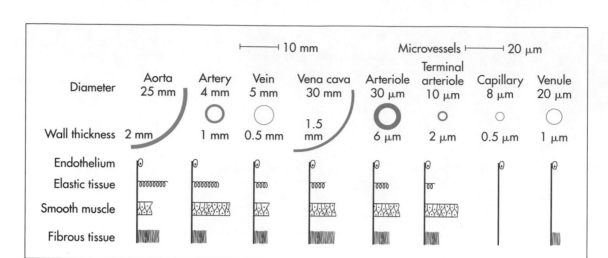

■ **Fig. 14-1** Internal diameter, wall thickness, and relative amounts of the principal components of the vessel walls of the various blood vessels that compose the circulatory system. Cross sections of the vessels are not drawn to scale because of the huge range from aorta and venae cavae to capillary. (Redrawn from Burton AC: *Physiol Rev* 34:619, 1954.)

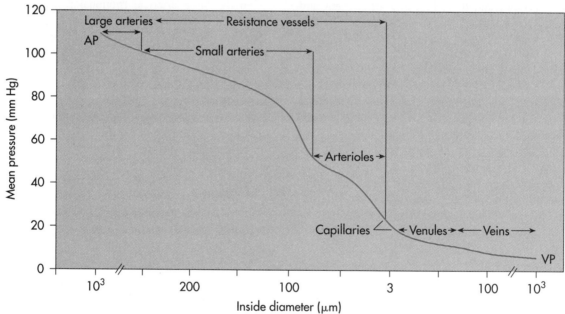

■ **Fig. 14-2** Pressure drop across the vascular system in the hamster cheek pouch. *AP*, Mean arterial pressure; *VP*, venous pressure. (Redrawn from David MJ et al: *Am J Physiol* 250:H291, 1986.)

conditions in the capillaries are ideal for the exchange of diffusible substances between blood and tissue.

On its return to the heart from the capillaries, blood passes through venules and then through veins of increasing size. Pressure within these vessels progressively decreases until the blood reaches the right atrium (Fig. 14-2). Near the heart, the number of veins decreases, the thickness and composition of the vein walls change (Fig. 14-1), the total cross-sectional area of the venous channels diminishes, and the **velocity of blood flow** increases (Fig. 14-3). Note that the velocity of blood flow and the cross-sectional area at each level of the vasculature are essentially mirror images (Fig. 14-3).

Data from a 20-kg dog (Table 14-1) indicate that between the aorta and the capillaries the number of vessels increases about 3 billion-fold, and the total cross-sectional area increases about 500-fold. The volume of blood in the systemic vascular system is greatest in the veins and venules (67%). Only 5% of total blood volume exists in the capillaries, and 11% of total blood volume is found in the aorta, arteries, and arterioles. In contrast, blood volume in the

■ Table 14-1   Vascular dimensions in a 20-kg dog

Vessels	No.	Total cross-sectional area (cm2)	Total blood volume (%)
Systemic			
Aorta	1	2.8	
Arteries	40-110,000	40	11
Arterioles	2.8 × 106	55	
Capillaries	2.7 × 109	1357	5
Venules	1 × 107	785	
Veins	660,000-110	631	67
Venae cavae	2	3.1	
Pulmonary			
Arteries and arterioles	1-1.5 × 106	137	3
Capillaries	2.7 × 109	1357	4
Venules and veins	1 × 106-4	210	5
Heart			
Atria	2		
Ventricles	2		5

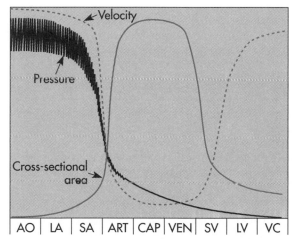

■ **Fig. 14-3** Phasic pressure, velocity of flow, and cross-sectional area of the systemic circulation. The important features are the inverse relationship between velocity and cross-sectional area, the major pressure drop across the small arteries and arterioles, and the maximal cross-sectional area and minimal flow rate in the capillaries. *AO*, Aorta; *LA*, large arteries; *SA*, small arteries; *ART*, arterioles; *CAP*, capillaries; *VEN*, venules; *SV*, small veins; *LV*, large veins; *VC*, venae cavae.

pulmonary vascular bed is about equally divided among the arterial, capillary, and venous vessels. The cross-sectional area of the venae cavae is larger than that of the aorta. Therefore, the velocity of flow is slower in the venae cavae than that in the aorta (Fig. 14-3).

THE CARDIOVASCULAR CIRCUIT

Blood entering the right ventricle via the right atrium is pumped through the pulmonary arterial system at a mean pressure about one-seventh that in the systemic arteries. The blood then passes through the lung capillaries, where carbon dioxide in the blood is released and oxygen is taken up. The O_2-rich blood returns via the pulmonary veins to the left atrium, where it is pumped from the ventricle to the periphery, thus completing the cycle.

In the normal, intact circulation, the total volume of blood is constant, and an increase in the volume of blood in one area must be accompanied by a decrease in another. However, the distribution of the circulating blood to the different regions of the body is determined by the output of the left ventricle and by the contractile state of the resistance vessels (arterioles) of these regions. The circulatory system is composed of conduits arranged in series and in parallel (Fig. 14-4). This arrangement, which is discussed in subsequent chapters, has important implications in terms of resistance, flow, and pressure in the blood vessels.

BLOOD

Blood performs many functions in the body. The main function of the circulating blood is to carry oxygen and nutrients to the tissues and to remove carbon dioxide and waste products from the tissues. In addition, blood transports other substances (e.g., hormones) from their sites of production to their sites of action and it transports white blood cells and platelets to where they are needed. Blood also aids in the distribution of water, solutes, and heat, and thus it contributes to **homeostasis,** the maintenance of a constant internal body environment.

Blood consists of red blood cells, white blood cells, and platelets, all suspended in a complex solution (**plasma**) of gases, salts, proteins, carbohydrates, and lipids. The circulating blood volume accounts for about 7% of body weight. Approximately 55% of the blood is plasma; the protein content is 7 g/dl (about 4 g/dl of albumin and 3 g/dl of plasma globulins).

Blood Components

Erythrocytes. The erythrocytes (red blood cells) are flexible, biconcave disks that transport oxygen to the body

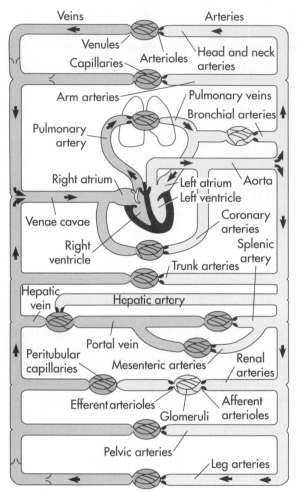

■ **Fig. 14-4** Schematic diagram of the parallel and series arrangement of the vessels composing the circulatory system. The capillary beds are represented by thin lines connecting the arteries (on the right) with the veins (on the left). The crescent-shaped thickenings proximal to the capillary beds represent the arterioles (resistance vessels). (Redrawn from Green HD: In Glasser O, editor: *Medical physics*, vol 1, Chicago, 1944, Mosby–Year Book.)

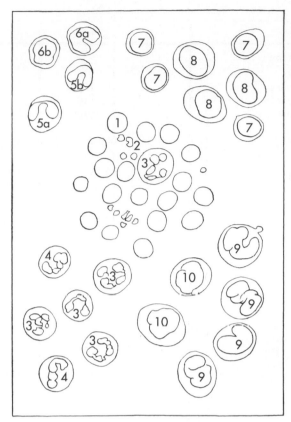

■ **Fig. 14-5** The morphology of blood cells. *1,* Normal red cells; *2,* platelets; *3,* neutrophils; *4,* neutrophil, band form; *5a,* eosinophil, two lobes; *5b,* eosinophil, band form; *6a,* basophil, band form; *6b,* metamyelocyte, basophilic; *7,* lymphocyte, small; *8,* lymphocyte, large; *9,* monocyte, mature; *10,* monocyte, young. (From Daland GA: *A color atlas of morphologic hematology,* Cambridge, Mass, 1951, Harvard University Press.)

tissues (Fig. 14-5). Erythrocytes are unusual in that they lack a nucleus. The average erythrocyte is 7 μm in diameter. Erythrocytes arise from stem cells in the bone marrow. During maturation, they lose their nuclei before entering the circulation, where their average lifespan is 120 days. Approximately 5 million erythrocytes are present per microliter of blood.

The main protein in erythrocytes is hemoglobin (about 15 g/dl of blood). Hemoglobin consists of **heme,** an iron-containing tetrapyrrole, linked to **globin,** a protein composed of four polypeptide chains (two α and two β chains in the normal adult). The iron moiety of hemoglobin binds loosely and reversibly to oxygen to form **oxyhemoglobin.** The affinity of hemoglobin for oxygen is affected by pH, temperature, and the 2,3-diphosphoglycerate concentration. These factors facilitate O_2 uptake in the lungs and its release in the tissues (see Chapter 28). Changes in the polypeptide sub-

units of globin can also affect the affinity of hemoglobin for O_2. For example, fetal hemoglobin has two γ chains instead of two β chains. This substitution increases its affinity for O_2. Changes in the polypeptide subunits of globin can also result in disease states, such as **sickle cell anemia** and **thalassemia.**

The number of circulating red cells remains fairly constant under normal conditions. The production of erythrocytes (**erythropoiesis**) is regulated by the glycoprotein **erythropoietin,** which is secreted mainly by the kidneys. Erythropoietin regulates erythrocyte production by accelerating the differentiation of stem cells in the bone marrow.

Anemia and chronic hypoxia (e.g., as a result of living at high altitudes) stimulate erythrocyte production and can produce **polycythemia,** an increased number of red blood cells. When the hypoxic stimulus is removed in subjects with altitude polycythemia, the high red blood cell concentration in the blood inhibits erythropoiesis. The red

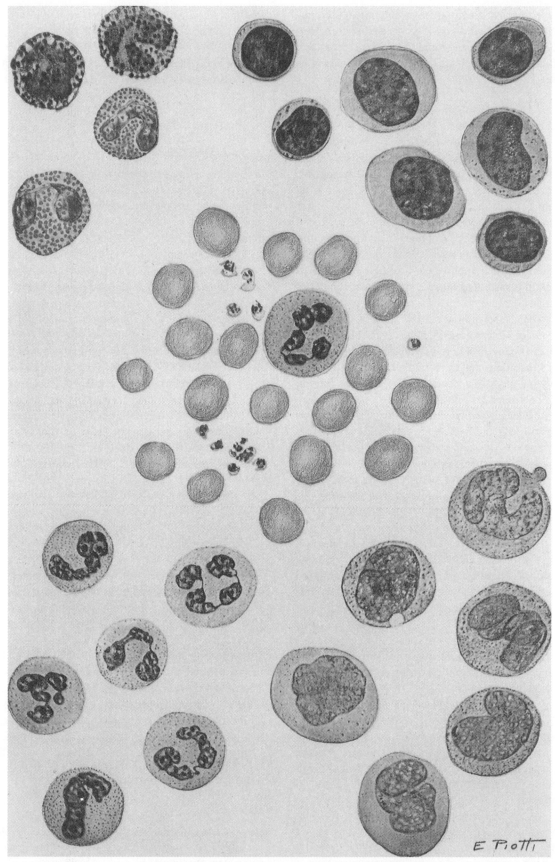

■ **Fig. 14-5, cont'd**   For legend see opposite page.

blood cell count is also greatly increased in **polycythemia vera,** a disease of unknown cause. The elevated erythrocyte concentration in this disease can increase blood viscosity, and therefore the flow to vital tissues may be impaired (see Chapter 18).

Leukocytes. Normally about 4000 to 10,000 leukocytes (white blood cells) are present per microliter of blood. The leukocytes include **granulocytes** (65%), **lymphocytes** (30%), and **monocytes** (5%). Of the granulocytes, about 95% are **neutrophils,** 4% **eosinophils,** and 1% **basophils.** During fetal development, white blood cells arise from primitive stem cells in the bone marrow (Fig. 14-5). After birth, granulocytes and monocytes continue to be produced in the bone marrow, whereas lymphocytes are produced in lymph nodes, spleen, and thymus.

The granulocytes and monocytes are motile, nucleated cells that contain **lysosomes,** which in turn contain enzymes capable of digesting foreign materials, such as microorganisms, damaged cells, and cellular debris. Thus, the leukocytes constitute a major defense mechanism against infections. Microorganisms or the products of cell destruction release **chemotactic substances** that attract granulocytes and monocytes. When the migrating leukocytes reach the foreign agents, they engulf them **(phagocytosis),** and then they destroy them by the action of enzymes that form **oxygen-derived free radicals** and **hydrogen peroxide.**

Lymphocytes vary in size and have large nuclei. Most lymphocytes lack cytoplasmic granules (Fig. 14-5). The two main types are **B lymphocytes,** which are responsible for humoral immunity, and **T lymphocytes,** which are responsible for cell-mediated immunity. When stimulated by an **antigen** (a foreign protein on the surface of a microorganism or allergen), the B lymphocytes are transformed into **plasma cells,** which synthesize and release antibodies (gamma globulin). Antibodies are carried by the bloodstream to the site of infection, where they "tag" foreign invaders for destruction by other components of the immune system.

The main T lymphocytes are cytotoxic and are responsible for long-term protection against some viruses, bacteria, and cancer cells. They are also responsible for the rejection of transplanted organs.

Other T lymphocytes are **helper T cells,** which activate B cells, and **suppressor T cells,** which inhibit B cell activity. Special B and T lymphocytes, called **memory cells,** "remember" specific antigens. These cells can quickly generate an immune response when subsequently exposed to the same antigen.

Protection against several infectious diseases has been achieved by injection of the appropriate antigen. Also, **vaccines** have been developed for the prevention or treatment of certain diseases. Such treatments involve the injection of killed or attenuated organisms (antigens) into suitable hosts (horses, sheep). Vaccines work by stimulating the production of specific antibodies against a particular microorganism.

Platelets. Platelets are small (3-μm) nuclear cell fragments of **megakaryocytes.** The megakaryocytes reside in the bone marrow. When the megakaryocytes mature, they break up into platelets, which enter the circulation. The platelets are important in hemostasis, as discussed below.

Blood Groups

In humans, there are four principal blood groups, designated O, A, B, and AB. These blood groups differ in the types of antigens that are present on the erythrocytes. Persons with type A blood have A antigens; those with type B, B antigens; those with type AB, both A and B antigens; and those with type O, neither antigen. In addition, the plasma of group O blood contains antibodies to A, B, and AB. Group A plasma contains antibodies to B antigens, and group B plasma contains antibodies to A antigens. Group AB plasma has no antibodies to O, A, or B antigens. In blood transfusions, cross-matching is necessary to prevent agglutination of donor red cells by antibodies in the plasma of the recipient. Because plasma of groups A, B, and AB has no antibodies to group O erythrocytes, people with group O blood are called **universal donors.** Conversely, persons with AB blood are called **universal recipients,** because their plasma has no antibodies to the antigens of the other three groups.

In addition to the ABO blood grouping, there are **Rh (Rhesus factor)-positive** and **RH-negative groups.**

An Rh-negative person can develop antibodies to Rh-positive red blood cells if that person is exposed to Rh-positive blood. For example, during pregnancy, a mother who is Rh negative can make antibodies for Rh-positive cells if the fetus is Rh positive (inherited from the father). Rh-positive red cells from the fetus can enter the maternal bloodstream at the time of placental separation and induce Rh-positive antibodies in the mother's plasma. The Rh-positive antibodies from the mother can also reach the fetus via the placenta, and agglutinate and hemolyze fetal red cells. This condition is known as **erythroblastosis fetalis,** a hemolytic disease of the newborn. Red blood cell destruction can also occur in Rh-negative individuals who have previously been transfused with Rh-positive blood and have developed Rh antibodies. If these individuals are given a subsequent transfusion of Rh-positive blood, the transfused red blood cells will be destroyed by the Rh antibodies in their plasma.

Hemostasis

Hemostasis is defined as the arrest of bleeding. When blood vessels are damaged bleeding occurs. Three processes then act to stem the flow of blood: vasoconstriction, platelet aggregation, and blood coagulation.

Vasoconstriction. Physical injury to a blood vessel elicits a contractile response **(vasoconstriction)** of the vascular smooth muscle and thus a narrowing of the vessel. Vasoconstriction in severed small arteries or arterioles can completely close the lumen of the vessel and stop the flow of blood. The contraction of the vascular smooth muscle is probably caused by direct mechanical stimulation by the penetrating object, as well as by mechanical stimulation of the perivascular nerves.

Platelet aggregation. Damage to the endothelium of a blood vessel causes platelets to adhere to the site of injury. The adherent platelets release **adenosine diphosphate** and **thromboxane A$_2$,** which cause additional platelets to adhere. The aggregation of platelets may continue in this manner until some of the small blood vessels become blocked by the mass of aggregated platelets. Platelets are prevented from aggregating along the length of a normal vessel by the anti-aggregation action of **prostacyclin.** This substance is released from the normal endothelial cells in the adjacent, uninjured part of the vessel. Platelets also release **serotonin (5-hydroxytryptamine),** which enhances vasoconstriction, and **thromboplastin,** which hastens blood coagulation.

Bleeding is an important clinical problem and trauma is the most common cause of bleeding. Gastrointestinal bleeding can also occur and cause severe anemia or even cardiovascular shock, and occult blood in the stools can be the first sign of cancer of the bowel or peptic ulcer.

When the platelet count is low, as in **thrombolytopenic purpura,** tiny hemorrhages (**petechiae**) or larger hemorrhages (**ecchymoses**) may appear in the skin and mucous membranes.

Bleeding occurs into the tissues (especially joints) in hemophilia, a hereditary disease. The disease occurs only in males, but the genetic abnormality is carried by females.

Blood coagulation. Blood clotting is a complex process consisting of sequential activation of various factors that are present in the blood. The cascade of reactions in which one activated factor activates another is depicted in Fig. 14-6. Several of the factors are synthesized in the liver, as is vitamin K, which is essential for synthesis of these liver-derived clotting factors.

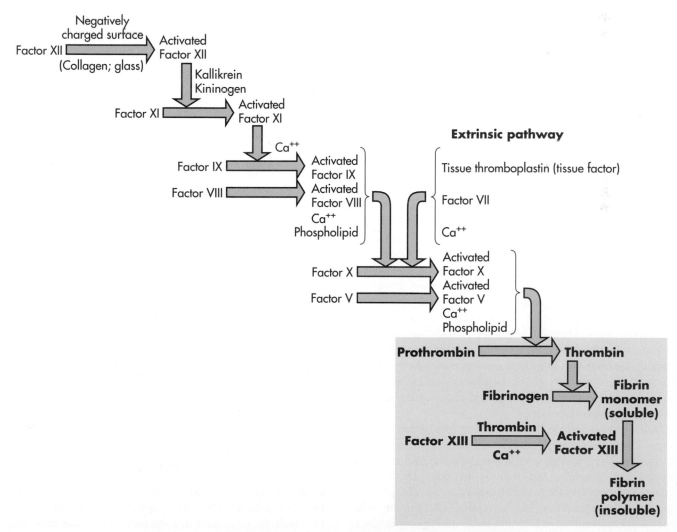

■ **Fig. 14-6** The intrinsic and extrinsic pathways in the formation of a fibrin clot.

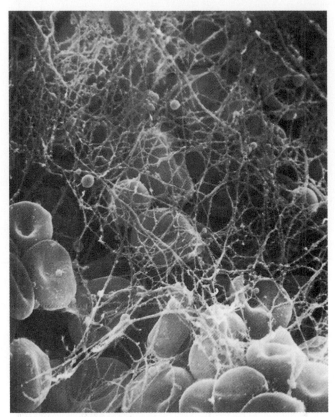

■ **Fig. 14-7** Human blood clot showing red blood cells immobilized within a network of fibrin threads. The small spheres are platelets. Scanning electron micrograph (×9000). (From Shelly WB: *JAMA* 249:3089, 1983.)

The key step in blood clotting is the conversion of fibrinogen to fibrin by thrombin. The clot formed by this reaction consists of a dense network of fibrin strands in which blood cells and plasma are trapped (Fig. 14-7). The two blood coagulation pathways, the **extrinsic** and the **intrinsic pathways,** converge on the activation of factor X, which catalyzes the cleavage of prothrombin to thrombin (Fig. 14-6). Blood clotting via the extrinsic pathway is initiated by tissue damage and the release of tissue thromboplastin. Blood clotting via the intrinsic pathway is initiated by exposure of the blood to a damaged endothelium or a negatively charged surface. When the endothelium of blood vessels is damaged, blood comes into contact with collagen. Outside the body, clotting can occur when blood comes into contact with negatively charged surfaces, such as glass. If blood is carefully drawn into a syringe coated with silicone, clotting is greatly delayed.

After a clot is formed, the actin and myosin of the platelets trapped in the fibrin mesh interact in a manner similar to that in muscle. The resultant contraction pulls the fibrin strands toward the platelets, and thereby extrudes the **serum** (plasma without fibrinogen) and shrinks the clot. This process is called **clot retraction**. The function of clot retraction is not clear, but it may serve to approximate the edges of severed small blood vessels.

Several cofactors are required for blood coagulation (Fig. 14-6); the most important is calcium. If the calcium ions in blood are removed or bound, coagulation will not occur.

Clot lysis. Blood clots may be liquefied (**fibrinolysis**) by a proteolytic enzyme called **plasmin.** Normal blood contains **plasminogen,** an inactive precursor of plasmin. Activators of the conversion of plasminogen to plasmin are found in tissues, plasma, and urine (urokinase).

Exogenous plasminogen activators, such as streptokinase and tissue plasminogen activator (tPA), are used clinically to dissolve intravascular clots. This treatment is used especially to dissolve clots in the coronary arteries of patients with acute myocardial infarction (damage to the heart muscle, most frequently caused by a clot in a major coronary artery).

Anticoagulants. Blood coagulation can be prevented in vitro by the addition of citrate or oxalate, which removes the calcium ions from solution. For rapid in vivo anticoagulation, **heparin,** a sulfated polysaccharide produced by mast cells, is injected intravenously.

Heparin is used in artificial perfusion circuits during open heart surgery and for prevention of intravascular clot extension. For prolonged anticoagulation, **dicumarol** is used. This drug inhibits the synthesis of vitamin K-dependent factors and is used in treating such conditions as **thrombophlebitis** (inflammation of a vein associated with an intravascular blood clot).

SUMMARY

1. The circulatory system consists of a pump (the heart), a series of distributing and collecting tubes (blood vessels), and an extensive system of thin vessels that permit rapid exchange of substances between the tissues and blood.

2. The greatest resistance to blood flow, and hence the greatest pressure drop, in the arterial system occurs at the level of the small arteries and the arterioles.

3. Pulsatile pressure is progressively damped by the elasticity of the arteriolar walls and the frictional resistance of the small arteries and arterioles, so that capillary blood flow is essentially nonpulsatile.

4. Velocity of blood flow is inversely related to the cross-sectional area at any point along the vascular system.

5. Most of the blood in the systemic vascular bed is located in the venous side of the circulation.

6. Blood consists of red blood cells (erythrocytes), white blood cells (leukocytes and lymphocytes), and platelets, all of which are suspended in a solution containing salts, proteins, carbohydrates, and lipids.

7. The four major blood groups are O, A, B, and AB. Type O blood can be given to persons in any of the blood groups because the plasma of all the blood groups lacks antibodies to group O erythrocytes. Hence, people with type O blood are referred to as universal donors. People with AB blood are referred to as universal recipients because their plasma lacks antibodies to erythrocytes of all the blood groups. In addition to O, A, B, and AB blood groups, there are Rh-positive and Rh-negative blood groups.

8. A cascade of reactions that constitute the intrinsic and extrinsic pathways is involved in blood coagulation. The final steps where the two pathways join are (a) the conversion of prothrombin to thrombin and (b) the conversion of fibrinogen to fibrin, a reaction catalyzed by thrombin.

9. Blood clots may be liquefied by plasmin, a proteolytic enzyme whose formation from plasminogen is catalyzed by tissue activators or by exogenous activators [e.g., streptokinase, tissue plasminogen activator (tPA)].

BIBLIOGRAPHY

Journal articles

Butenas S et al: Antiplatelet agents in tissue factor-induced blood coagulation, *Blood* 97:2314, 2001.

Dormann D, Clemetson KJ, Kehrel BE: The GPIb thrombin-binding site is essential for thrombin-induced platelet procoagulant activity, *Blood* 97:2469, 2000.

Hoyer LW: Hemophilia, *N Engl J Med* 330:38, 1994.

Mosesson MW, Siebenlist KR, Meh DA: The structure and biological features of fibrinogen and fibrin, *Ann N Y Acad Sci* 936:11, 2001.

Ross JM, McIntire LV: Molecular mechanisms of mural thrombosis under dynamic flow conditions, *New Physiol Sci* 10:117, 1995.

Taka T et al: Inhibitory effect of various thrombin inhibitors on shear-induced platelet function and dynamic coagulation, *Eur J Pharmacol* 406:181, 2000.

Triplett DA: Coagulation and bleeding disorders: review and update, *Clin Chem* 46:1260, 2000.

White JG: EDTA-induced changes in platelet structure and function: clot retraction, *Platelets* 11:49, 2000.

chapter fifteen

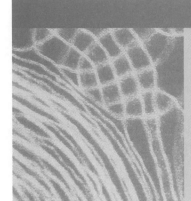

Electrical Activity of the Heart

Two centuries ago, Galvani and Volta demonstrated that electrical phenomena were involved in the spontaneous contractions of the heart. In 1855, Kölliker and Müller found that when they placed the nerve of an innervated skeletal muscle preparation in contact with the surface of a beating frog's heart, the skeletal muscle twitched with each cardiac contraction. These researchers concluded that the spontaneous excitation of the heart had generated sufficient electrical activity to excite the motor nerve fibers and stimulate the skeletal muscle.

The electrical events that normally take place in the heart initiate cardiac contraction. Disorders in electrical activity can induce serious and sometimes lethal disturbances in the cardiac rhythm.

TRANSMEMBRANE POTENTIALS

To investigate the electrical behavior of single cardiac cells, researchers insert a microelectrode into the interior of the cell. The microelectrode is attached to a device that measures the strength of an electrical current. The potential changes recorded from a typical ventricular muscle fiber are illustrated in Fig. 15-1, *A*. When two electrodes are placed in an electrolyte solution near a strip of quiescent cardiac muscle, no potential difference (point *a*) is measurable between the two electrodes. When one of the electrodes is inserted into the interior of a cardiac muscle fiber (point *b*), the galvanometer immediately records a potential difference (V_m) across the cell membrane. The potential of the interior of the cell becomes about 90 mV lower than that of the surrounding medium. This electronegativity of the interior of the resting cell with respect to the exterior is also characteristic of skeletal and smooth muscle, nerves, and most cells within the body (see also Chapter 2).

At point *c*, the ventricular cell is excited by an electronic stimulator, and the cell membrane rapidly depolarizes. During depolarization, the potential difference is actually reversed, such that the potential of the interior of the cell exceeds that of the exterior by about 20 mV. The rapid **upstroke** of the

action potential is designated **phase 0.** The upstroke is followed immediately by a brief period of partial, **early repolarization (phase 1),** and then by a **plateau (phase 2)** that persists for about 0.1 to 0.2 second. The membrane then repolarizes **(phase 3)** until the resting state of polarization **(phase 4)** is again attained (at point *e*). **Final repolarization** (phase 3) develops more slowly than does depolarization (phase 0).

The relationships between the electrical events in the cardiac muscle and actual contraction of the cardiac muscle are shown in Fig. 15-2. Rapid depolarization (phase 0) occurs before force develops, and completion of repolarization coincides approximately with peak force. The relaxation of the muscle takes place mainly during phase 4 of the action potential. The duration of contraction usually parallels the duration of the action potential.

Principal Types of Cardiac Action Potentials

Two main types of action potentials take place in the heart and are shown in Fig. 15-1. One type, the **fast response,** occurs in normal atrial and ventricular myocytes and in the specialized conducting fibers (**Purkinje** fibers of the heart). The other type of action potential, the **slow response,** occurs in the **sinoatrial (SA) node,** which is the natural pacemaker region of the heart, and in the **atrioventricular (AV) node,** which is the specialized tissue that conducts the cardiac impulse from atria to ventricles.

Fast responses may change to slow responses under certain pathological conditions. For example, in coronary artery disease, a region of cardiac muscle may be deprived of its normal blood supply. As a result, the K^+ concentration in the interstitial fluid that surrounds the affected muscle cells rises because K^+ is lost from the inadequately perfused (or *ischemic*) cells. The action potentials in some of these cells may then be converted from fast to slow responses. An experimental conversion from a fast to a slow response is illustrated in Fig. 15-14.

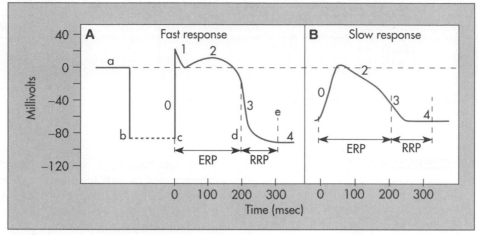

■ **Fig. 15-1** Changes in transmembrane potential recorded from a fast-response and a slow-response cardiac fiber in isolated cardiac tissue immersed in an electrolyte solution. **A,** At time *a* the microelectrode was in the solution surrounding the cardiac fiber. At time *b* the microelectrode entered the fiber. At time *c* an action potential was initiated in the impaled fiber. Time *c* to *d* represents the effective refractory period *(ERP)*, and time *d* to *e* represents the relative refractory period *(RRP)*. **B,** An action potential recorded from a slow-response cardiac fiber. Note that compared with the fast-response fiber, the resting potential of the slow fiber is less negative, the upstroke (phase *0*) of the action potential is less steep, the amplitude of the action potential is smaller, phase *1* is absent, and the relative refractory period *(RRP)* extends well into phase *4* after the fiber has fully repolarized.

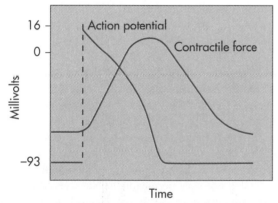

■ **Fig. 15-2** Time relationships between the developed force and the changes in transmembrane potential in a thin strip of ventricular muscle. (Redrawn from Kavaler F, Fisher VJ, Stuckey JH: *Bull NY Acad Med* 41:592, 1965.)

As shown in Fig. 15-1, not only is the resting membrane potential (phase 4) of the fast response considerably more negative than that of the slow response, but also the slope of the upstroke (phase 0), the amplitude of the action potential, and the extent of the overshoot are greater in the fast response than in the slow response. The amplitude of the action potential and the steepness of the upstroke are important determinants of how fast the action potential is propagated along the myocardial fibers. In slow-response cardiac tissue, the action potential is propagated more slowly than in fast-response cardiac tissue. In addition, the conduction is more likely to be blocked in slow-response cardiac tissue

than in fast-response tissue. Slow conduction and a tendency toward conduction block increase the likelihood of some rhythm disturbances (see section on Reentry, page 294).

IONIC BASIS OF THE RESTING POTENTIAL

The various phases of the cardiac action potential are associated with changes in the permeability of the cell membrane, mainly to sodium, potassium, and calcium ions. Changes in cell membrane permeability alter the movement of these ions across the membrane. The permeability of the membrane to a given ion, its transmembrane concentration difference, and the transmembrane potential difference define the net quantity of the ion that will diffuse across the membrane. Changes in permeability are accomplished by the opening and closing of ion channels that are specific for the individual ions.

As with all other cells in the body (see also Chapter 2), the concentration of potassium ions inside a cardiac muscle cell ($[K^+]_i$) is far greater than the concentration outside the cell ($[K^+]_o$) (Fig. 15-3). The reverse concentration gradient exists for sodium and calcium ions. Estimates of the extracellular and intracellular concentrations of Na^+, K^+, and Ca^{2+} and the equilibrium potentials (defined below) for these ions are compiled in Table 15-1.

The resting cell membrane is relatively permeable to K^+ but much less so to Na^+ and Ca^{2+}. Hence, K^+ tends to diffuse from the inside to the outside of the cell in the direction of the K^+ concentration gradient, as shown on the right side of the cell in Fig. 15-3.

■ Table 15-1   Intracellular and extracellular ion concentrations and equilibrium potentials in cardiac muscle cells

Ion	Extracellular concentrations (mM)	Intracellular concentrations (mM)*	Equilibrium potential (mV)
Na^+	145	10	70
K^+	4	135	–94
Ca^{2+}	2	10-4	132

Modified from Ten Eick RE, Baumgarten CM, Singer DH: *Prog Cardiovasc Dic* 24:157, 1981.
*The intracellular concentrations are estimates of the free concentrations in the cytoplasm.

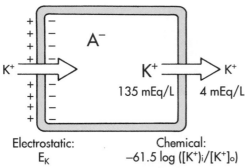

Electrostatic: Chemical:
E_K $-61.5 \log ([K^+]_i/[K^+]_o)$

■ **Fig. 15-3**   The balance of chemical and electrostatic forces acting on a resting cardiac cell membrane. The estimations are based on a 34:1 ratio of the intracellular to extracellular K^+ concentrations and the existence of a nondiffusible anion (A^-) inside, but not outside, the cell.

Any flux of K^+ that occurs during phase 4 takes place mainly through specific **K^+ channels.** Several types of K^+ channels exist in cardiac cell membranes. The opening and closing of some of these channels are regulated by the transmembrane potential, whereas others are regulated by a chemical signal (e.g., the extracellular acetylcholine concentration). One of the specific K^+ channels through which K^+ passes during phase 4 is a voltage-regulated channel that conducts the **inwardly rectifying K^+ current.** This current is symbolized i_{K1} and is discussed in more detail below (Fig. 15-8). For now, it is only necessary to know how this current is established. Many of the anions (labeled A^-), such as the proteins, inside the cell, are not free to diffuse out with the K^+ (Fig. 15-3). Therefore, the K^+ diffuses out of the cell and leaves the impermeant A^- behind. The deficiency of cations then causes the interior of the cell to become electronegative (see also Chapter 2). As a result, the positively charged K^+ ions are attracted to the interior of the cell by the negative potential that exists there, as shown on the left side of the cell in Fig. 15-3.

Therefore, two opposing forces are involved in the movement of K^+ across the cell membrane. A chemical force, based on the concentration gradient, results in net outward diffusion of K^+. The counterforce is based on electrostatic differences between the interior and exterior of the cell. If the system came into equilibrium, the chemical and the electrostatic forces would be equal. As explained in Chapter 2, this equilibrium is expressed by the **Nernst equation** for potassium:

$$E_K = 61.5 \log([K^+]_i/[K^+]_o)$$

The right-hand term represents the chemical potential difference, and the left-hand term, E_K, represents the electrostatic potential difference that would exist across the cell membrane if K^+ were the only diffusible ion. E_K is called the **potassium equilibrium potential.**

When the measured concentrations of $[K^+]_i$ and $[K^+]_o$ for mammalian myocardial cells are substituted into the Nernst equation, the calculated value of E_K equals about –95 mV (Table 15-1). This value is close to, but slightly more negative than, the resting potential actually measured in myocardial cells. Therefore, the potential that tends to drive K^+ out of the resting cell is small. The actual resting potential is slightly less negative than the predicted potential because the cell membrane is slightly permeable to other ions, notably to Na^+. The balance of the forces acting on Na^+ is opposite to the balance of forces acting on K^+ in resting cardiac cells. The intracellular Na^+ concentration, $[Na^+]_i$ is much lower than the extracellular concentration, $[Na^+]_o$. The sodium equilibrium potential, E_{Na}, expressed by the Nernst equation, is about 70 mV (Table 15-1).

At equilibrium, therefore, an electrostatic force of about 70 mV, oriented with the inside of the cell more positive than the outside, is necessary to counterbalance the chemical potential for Na^+. However, as we have seen, the actual resting membrane potential of myocytes is about –90 mV. Hence, both chemical and electrostatic forces act to pull extracellular Na^+ into the cell. The influx of Na^+ through the membrane is small, however, because the membrane of the resting cell is not very permeable to Na^+. Nevertheless, this small inward current of Na^+ is sufficient to cause the potential (V_m) on the inside of the resting cell membrane to be slightly less negative than the value (E_K) predicted by the Nernst equation for K^+ (Fig. 15-4).

The dependence of V_m on the conductances and on the intracellular and extracellular concentrations of K^+, Na^+, and other ions is described by the **chord conductance equation,** as explained in Chapter 2. This equation reveals that relative—not absolute—membrane conductances to Na^+ and K^+ determine the resting potential. In the resting cardiac cell, the conductance (g_K) to K^+ is about 100 times greater than the conductance (g_{Na}) to Na^+. Therefore, the chord conductance equation reduces essentially to the Nernst equation for K^+. Because gNa is so small in the resting cell, changes in external Na^+ concentration do not significantly affect V_m (Fig. 15-5).

When the ratio $[K^+]_i/[K^+]_o$ is decreased experimentally by raising $[K^+]_o$ in a suspension of myocytes, the measured

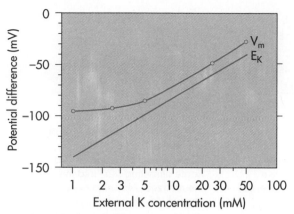

■ **Fig. 15-4**   Transmembrane potential (V_m) of a cardiac muscle fiber varies inversely with the potassium concentration of the external medium. The straight line (E_K) represents the change in transmembrane potential predicted by the Nernst equation for potassium. (Redrawn from Page E: *Circulation* 26:582, 1962.)

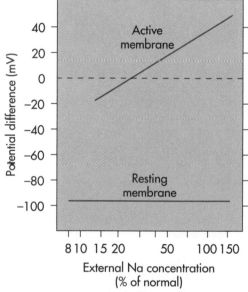

■ **Fig. 15-5**   Concentration of sodium in the external medium is a critical determinant of the amplitude of the action potential in cardiac muscle *(upper line)* but it has very little influence on the resting membrane potential *(lower line)*. (Redrawn from Weidmann S: *Elektrophysiologie der Herzmuskelfaser,* Bern, 1956, Verlag Hans Huber.)

value of V_m approximates the value of EK predicted by the Nernst equation (Fig. 15-4). For extracellular K^+ concentrations greater than about 5 mM, the measured values correspond closely with the predicted values. The measured levels are only slightly less than those predicted by the Nernst equation because g_K is so much greater than g_{Na}. However, for values of $[K^+]_o$ below about 5 mM, g_K decreases as $[K^+]_o$ is diminished. As g_K decreases, the effect of g_{Na} on the transmembrane potential becomes relatively more significant, as

predicted by the chord conductance equation. This change in g_K accounts for the greater deviation of the measured V_m from the value predicted by the Nernst equation for K^+ at low levels of $[K^+]_o$.

IONIC BASIS OF THE FAST RESPONSE

Phase 0: Genesis of the Upstroke

Any stimulus that abruptly changes the resting membrane potential to a critical value (called the threshold) results in an action potential. The characteristics of fast response action potentials are shown in Fig. 15-1, *A*. The rapid depolarization (phase 0) is related almost exclusively to the influx of Na^+ into the myocyte due to a sudden increase in g_{Na}. The **amplitude** of the action potential (the potential change during phase 0) varies linearly with the logarithm of $[Na^+]_o$, as shown in Fig. 15-5. When $[Na^+]_o$ is reduced from its normal value of about 140 mM to about 20 mM, the cell is no longer excitable.

The physical and chemical forces responsible for these transmembrane movements of Na^+ are diagrammed in Fig. 15-6. When the resting membrane potential, V_m, is suddenly changed from –90 mV (Fig. 15-6, *A*) to the threshold level of about –65 mV (Fig. 15-6, *B*) by some external electrical stimulus, the properties of the cell membrane change dramatically. Na^+ enters the myocyte through specific **fast Na^+ channels** that exist in the membrane (see also Chapter 3). These channels can be blocked by the puffer fish toxin, **tetrodotoxin.** Also, many of the drugs used to treat certain cardiac rhythm disturbances (**cardiac arrhythmias**) act by blocking these fast Na^+ channels.

The manner in which Na^+ moves through these fast channels suggests that the flux is controlled by two types of **gates** in each channel. One of these, the **m gate,** tends to open (that is, to *activate*) the channel as V_m becomes less negative. This is therefore called an **activation gate.** The other gate, the **h gate,** tends to close the channel as V_m becomes less negative and hence is called an **inactivation gate.** The "m" and "h" designations were originally employed by Hodgkin and Huxley in their mathematical model of impulse conduction in nerve fibers.

As we have seen, the V_m of a resting cell is about –90 mV. The m gates are closed and the h gates are wide open, as shown in Fig. 15-6, *A*. Because the Na^+ concentration (145 mM) outside the cell is greater than the Na^+ concentration inside the cell (10 mM), the interior of the cell is electrically negative with respect to the exterior. Hence, both chemical and electrostatic forces are oriented to draw Na^+ into the cell.

The electrostatic force in Fig. 15-6, *A*, is a potential difference of 90 mV, and it is represented by the white arrow. The chemical force, based on the difference in Na^+ concentration between the outside and inside of the cell, is represented by the black arrow. For an Na^+ concentration difference of about 130 mM, a potential difference of 60 mV (with the inside more positive than outside) is necessary to counterbalance the chemical, or diffusional, force, according to the

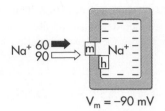

$V_m = -90$ mV

During phase 4, the chemical (60 mV) and electrostatic (90 mV) forces favor influx of Na⁺ from the extracellular space. Influx is negligible, however, because the activation *(m)* gates are closed.
A

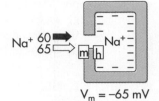

$V_m = -65$ mV

If V_m is brought to about −65 V, the *m* gates begin to swing open, and Na⁺ begins to enter the cell. This reduces the negative charge inside the cell, and thereby opens still more Na⁺ channels, which accelerates the influx of Na⁺. The change in V_m also initiates the closure of inactivation *(h)* gates, which operate more slowly than the *m* gates.
B

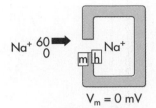

$V_m = 0$ mV

The rapid influx of Na⁺ sharply decreases the negativity of V_m. As V_m approaches 0, the electrostatic force attracting Na⁺ into the cell is neutralized. Na⁺ continues to enter the cell, however, because of the substantial concentration gradient, and V_m begins to become positive.
C

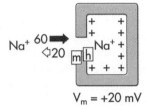

$V_m = +20$ mV

When V_m is positive by about 20 mV, Na⁺ continues to enter the cell, because the diffusional forces (60 mV) exceed the opposing electrostatic forces (20 mV). The influx of Na⁺ is slow, however, because the net driving force is small, and many of the inactivation gates have already closed.

D

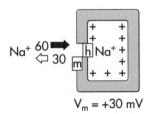

$V_m = +30$ mV

When V_m reaches about 30 mV, the *h* gates have now all closed, and Na⁺ influx ceases. The *h* gates remain closed until the first half of repolarization, and thus the cell is absolutely refractory during this entire period. During the second half of repolarization, the *m* and *h* gates approach the state represented by panel A, and thus the cell is relatively refractory.
E

■ **Fig. 15-6**   The gating of a sodium channel in a cardiac cell membrane during phase 4 (**A**) and during various stages of the action potential upstroke (**B** to **E**). The positions of the m and h gates in the fast Na⁺ channels are shown at the various levels of V_m. The electrostatic forces are represented by the white arrows and the chemical (diffusional) forces by the black arrows.

Nernst equation for Na⁺ (see Chapter 2). Therefore, the net chemical force that favors the inward movement of Na⁺ in Fig. 15-6 *(black arrows)* is equivalent to a potential difference of 60 mV. In the resting cell, the total electrochemical force that favors the inward movement of Na⁺ is 150 mV (A). The m gates are closed, however, and the conductance of the resting cell membrane to Na⁺ is low. Therefore, when the cell is in the resting state, virtually no Na⁺ moves into the cell.

Any stimulus that makes V_m less negative tends to open the m gates, and thereby tends to activate the fast Na⁺ channels. The precise potential required to open the m gates and thus activate the Na⁺ channels varies somewhat from one channel to another in the cell membrane. As V_m becomes progressively less negative, more and more m gates swing open, and the influx of Na⁺ accelerates (Fig. 15-6, *B*). The entry of Na⁺ into the interior of the cell neutralizes some of the negative charges within the cell, and thereby makes V_m still less negative. The consequent change in V_m then opens

more m gates and augments the inward Na⁺ current. This process is called **regenerative.** As V_m approaches about −65 mV, the remaining m gates rapidly swing open in the fast Na⁺ channels until virtually all the m gates are open (Fig. 15-6, *B*).

The rapid opening of the m gates in the fast Na⁺ channels is responsible for the large and abrupt increase in Na⁺ conductance (g_{Na}) that occurs in phase 0 (the upstroke) of the action potential (Fig. 15-7). The rapid influx of Na⁺ accounts for the steepness of the upstroke of the action potential. The maximal rate of change of V_m varies from 100 to 200 V/sec in myocardial cells and from 500 to 1000 V/sec in Purkinje fibers. Although the Na⁺ that enters the cell during one action potential alters V_m by more than 100 mV, the actual quantity of Na⁺ that enters the cell is so small that the change in the intracellular Na⁺ concentration cannot be measured. Hence, the chemical force remains virtually constant, and only the electrostatic force changes throughout the action potential. In Fig. 15-6, note that the lengths of the

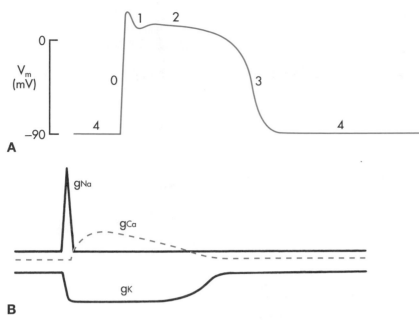

■ **Fig. 15-7**   Changes in the conductances of Na$^+$ (g$_{Na}$), Ca^{2+} (g$_{Ca}$), and K$^+$ (g$_K$) during the various phases of the action potential **(A)** of a fast-response cardiac cell. The conductance diagram **(B)** shows directional changes only.

black arrows remain constant (denoting a chemical force of 60 mV), whereas the white arrows change in magnitude and direction.

As Na$^+$ rushes into the cardiac cell during phase 0, the negative charges inside the cell are neutralized, and V$_m$ becomes progressively less negative. When V$_m$ reaches zero (Fig. 15-6, *C*), an electrostatic force no longer exists to pull Na$^+$ into the cell. As long as the fast Na$^+$ channels are open, however, Na$^+$ continues to enter the cell because of the large concentration gradient. This continuation of the inward Na$^+$ current causes the inside of the cell to become positively charged (Fig. 15-6, *D*). This reversal of the membrane polarity is the so-called **overshoot** of the cardiac action potential. Such a reversal of the electrostatic gradient would, of course, tend to repel the entry of additional Na$^+$ (Fig. 15-6, *D*). However, as long as the inwardly directed chemical forces exceed the outwardly directed electrostatic forces, the net flux of Na$^+$ is directed inward, although the rate at which Na$^+$ enters the cell diminishes.

The inward Na$^+$ current finally stops when the h (inactivation) gates close (Fig. 15-6, *E*). Like the activity of the m gates, the activity of the h gates is governed by the value of V$_m$. However, the m gates open very rapidly (in about 0.1 msec), whereas the closure of the h gates requires several milliseconds. Phase 0 is finally terminated when all of the h gates have closed, thereby inactivating the fast Na$^+$ channels. The closure of the h gates so soon after the opening of the m gates accounts for the quick return of g$_{Na}$ from its maximum to its resting value (Fig. 15-7).

The h gates then remain closed until the cell has partially repolarized during phase 3 (at about time *d* in Fig. 15-1, *A*). From time *c* to time *d* the cell is in its **effective refractory period** and will not respond to further excitation. This mechanism prevents a sustained, tetanic contraction of cardiac muscle. *Tetanic contraction of the ventricular myocytes would retard ventricular relaxation and therefore interfere with the normal intermittent pumping action of the heart.*

About midway through phase 3 (time *d* in Fig. 15-1, *A*), the m and h gates in some of the fast Na$^+$ channels have resumed the states shown in Fig. 15-6, *A*. Such channels are said to have **recovered from inactivation.** The cell can begin to respond (but weakly at first) to further excitation (Fig. 15-15). Throughout the remainder of phase 3 the cell completes its recovery from inactivation. By time e in Fig. 15-1, *A*, the h gates have reopened and the m gates have reclosed in all the fast Na$^+$ channels; that is, they have resumed the status depicted in Fig. 15-6, *A*.

Phase 1: Genesis of Early Repolarization

In many cardiac cells that have a prominent plateau, phase 1 constitutes an early, brief period of limited repolarization. In Fig. 15-1, this brief repolarization is represented by a notch between the end of the upstroke and the beginning of the plateau. Repolarization occurs briefly owing to the activation of a **transient outward current (i$_{to}$)**, carried mainly by K$^+$. Activation of K$^+$ channels during phase 1 causes a brief efflux of K$^+$ from the cell, because the interior of the cell is positively charged and because the internal K$^+$ concentration greatly exceeds the external K$^+$ concentration (Fig. 15-8). As a result of this transient efflux of positively charged ions, the cell is briefly and partially repolarized (phase 1).

The phase 1 notch is prominent in myocytes located in the the epicardial and midmyocardial regions of the left ventricular wall (Fig. 15-9) and in ventricular Purkinje fibers (Fig. 15-13). However, the notch is negligible in myocytes from the endocardial region of the left ventricle (Fig. 15-9). The cycle length of depolarization also affects the prominence of phase 1. When the basic cycle length at which the epicardial and midmyocardial fibers are depolarized is increased from 300 to 8000 msec, the phase 1 notch becomes more pronounced and the action potential duration is increased substantially. In endocardial fibers, the same increase in basic cycle length has no effect on phase 1 and only a small effect on the action potential duration (Fig. 15-9). In the

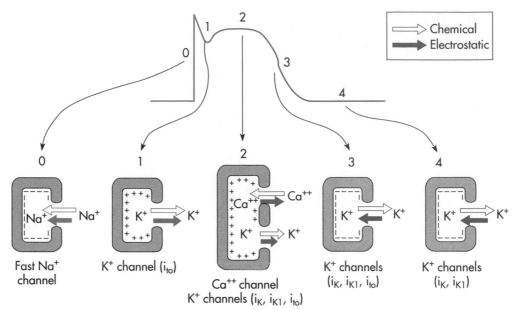

■ **Fig. 15-8**   The principal ionic currents and channels that generate the various phases of the action potential in a cardiac cell. Phase 0: The chemical and electrostatic forces both favor the entry of Na^+ into the cell through fast Na^+ channels to generate the upstroke. Phase 1: The chemical and electrostatic forces both favor the efflux of K^+ through i_{to} channels to generate early, partial repolarization. Phase 2: During the plateau, the net influx of Ca^{2+} through Ca^{2+} channels is balanced by the efflux of K^+ through i_K, i_{K1}, and i_{to} channels. Phase 3: The chemical forces that favor the efflux of K^+ through i_K, i_{K1}, and i_{to} channels predominate over the electrostatic forces that favor the influx of K^+ through these same channels. Phase 4: The chemical forces that favor the efflux of K^+ through i_K and i_{K1} channels exceed very slightly the electrostatic forces that favor the influx of K^+ through these same channels.

presence of 4-aminopyridine, which blocks the K^+ channels that carry i_{to}, the phase 1 notch becomes much less prominent in the action potentials recorded from the epicardial and midmyocardial regions of the ventricles.

Phase 2: Genesis of the Plateau

During the plateau of the action potential, Ca^{2+} enters the myocardial cells through **calcium channels,** which activate and inactivate much more slowly than do the fast Na^+ channels. During the flat portion of phase 2 (Fig. 15-8), this influx of positive charge carried by Ca^{2+} is counterbalanced by the efflux of positive charge carried by K^+. K^+ exits through channels that conduct mainly the i_{to}, i_K, and i_{K1} currents. The i_{to} current is responsible for phase 1, as described previously, but it is not completely inactivated until after phase 2 has expired. The i_K and i_{K1} currents are described later in this chapter.

Ca^{2+} **conductance during the plateau.** The Ca^{2+} channels are voltage-regulated channels that are activated as V_m becomes progressively less negative during the upstroke of the action potential. Various types of Ca^{2+} channels have been identified in cardiac tissues (see Chapter 3), but this discussion concentrates on the predominant channel, the so-called L-type Ca^{2+} channel. Some of the important characteristics of this channel are illustrated in Fig. 15-10, which also shows the Ca^{2+} currents generated by voltage-clamping an isolated atrial myocyte. Note that when V_m is suddenly

increased to $+30$ mV from a holding potential of -30 mV, an inward Ca^{2+} current is activated. Note also that after the inward current reaches its maximal value (in the downward direction), it returns toward zero only very gradually (i.e., the channel inactivates very slowly). Thus, because the current that passes through these channels is long-lasting, the channels are designated "L-type."

Opening of the Ca^{2+} channels is reflected by an increase in Ca^{2+} conductance (g_{Ca}) immediately after the upstroke of the action potential (Fig. 15-7). At the beginning of the action potential, the intracellular Ca^{2+} concentration is much less than the extracellular concentration (Table 15-1). Consequently, the increase in g_{Ca} promotes an influx of Ca^{2+} into the cell throughout the plateau. *This influx of Ca during the plateau is involved in excitation-contraction coupling*, as described in Chapters 12 and 16.

Various factors, such as neurotransmitters and drugs, may substantially influence g_{Ca}. The adrenergic neurotransmitter **norepinephrine,** the β-adrenergic receptor agonist **isoproterenol,** and various other **catecholamines** may enhance Ca^{2+} conductance, whereas the parasympathetic neurotransmitter, **acetylcholine,** may decrease Ca^{2+} conductance. The enhancement of Ca^{2+} conductance by catecholamines is the principal mechanism by which they enhance cardiac muscle contractility.

To enhance Ca^{2+} conductance, catecholamines first interact with **β-adrenergic receptors** in the cardiac cell

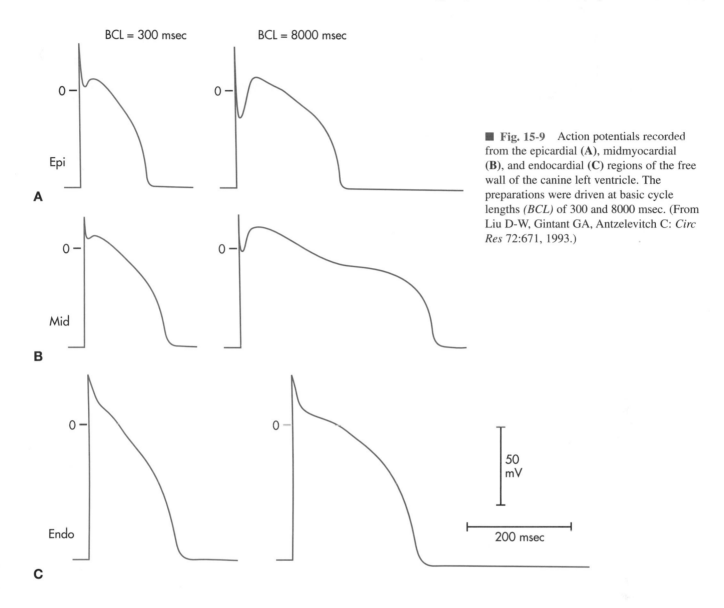

■ **Fig. 15-9** Action potentials recorded from the epicardial (**A**), midmyocardial (**B**), and endocardial (**C**) regions of the free wall of the canine left ventricle. The preparations were driven at basic cycle lengths *(BCL)* of 300 and 8000 msec. (From Liu D-W, Gintant GA, Antzelevitch C: *Circ Res* 72:671, 1993.)

membrane. This interaction stimulates the membrane-bound enzyme, **adenylyl cyclase,** which raises the intracellular concentration of **cyclic adenosine monophosphate (cAMP)** (see also Chapter 5). The rise in the level of cAMP enhances the activation of the L-type Ca^{2+} channels in the cell membrane (Fig. 15-10), and thus augments the influx of Ca^{2+} into the cells from the interstitial fluid. Conversely, acetylcholine interacts with **muscarinic receptors** in the cell membrane to inhibit adenylyl cyclase. In this way, acetylcholine antagonizes the activation of Ca^{2+} channels, and thereby diminishes g_{Ca}.

The **Ca^{2+} channel antagonists** are substances that block Ca^{2+} channels. Examples include the drugs **verapamil** and **diltiazem.** These drugs decrease g_{Ca}, and thereby impede the influx of Ca^{2+} into myocardial cells. The Ca^{2+} channel antagonists decrease the duration of the action potential plateau and diminish the strength of the cardiac contraction (Fig. 15-11). Although the Ca^{2+} channel antagonists diminish the contractile strength of the heart,

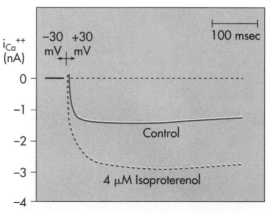

■ **Fig. 15-10** Effect of isoproterenol on the Ca^{2+} current conducted by L-type Ca^{2+} channels in voltage-clamped, canine atrial myocytes when the potential was changed from −30 to +30 mV. (Redrawn from Bean BP: *J Gen Physiol* 86:1, 1985.)

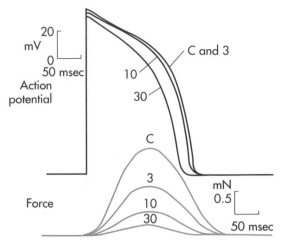

■ **Fig. 15-11**   Effects of diltiazem, a Ca^{2+} channel antagonist, on the action potentials (in millivolts) and isometric contractile forces (in millinewtons) recorded from an isolated papillary muscle of a guinea pig. The tracings were recorded under control conditions *(C)* and in the presence of diltiazem, in concentrations of 3, 10, and 30 μmol/L. (Redrawn from Hirth C, Borchard U, Hafner D: *J Mol Cell Cardiol* 15:799, 1983.)

these agents are used widely in the treatment of **congestive heart failure,** a common clinical condition in which the contractile performance of the heart is already compromised. As a result, the heart cannot generate enough blood flow to meet the needs of the tissues. The Ca^{2+} channel antagonists weaken the cardiac contraction and depress the contraction of the vascular smooth muscle, and thereby induce generalized vasodilation. This diminished vascular resistance reduces the counterforce **(afterload)** that opposes the propulsion of blood from the ventricles into the arterial system, as explained in Chapters 18 and 19. Hence, vasodilator drugs, such as the Ca^{2+} channel antagonists, are often referred to as **afterload-reducing drugs.** This ability to diminish the counterforce leads to a more adequate cardiac output, despite the direct depressant effect of these drugs on the heart muscle.

K^+ conductance during the plateau. During the plateau (phase 2) of the action potential, the concentration gradient for K^+ across the cell membrane is virtually the same as it is during phase 4. However, V_m is positive during phase 2. Therefore, both the chemical and the electrostatic forces favor the efflux of K^+ from the cell during phase 2 (Fig. 15-8). If g_K were the same during the plateau as it is during phase 4, the efflux of K^+ during phase 2 would greatly exceed the influx of Ca^{2+}, and a sustained plateau could not be achieved. However, as V_m approaches and then attains positive values near the peak of the action potential upstroke, g_K suddenly decreases (Fig. 15-7). *The diminished K^+ current associated with the reduction in g_K prevents an excessive loss of K^+ from the cell during the plateau.*

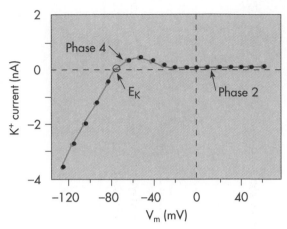

■ **Fig. 15-12**   Inwardly rectified K^+ currents recorded from a rabbit ventricular myocyte when the potential was changed from a holding potential of −80 mV to various test potentials. Positive values along the vertical axis represent outward currents; negative values represent inward currents. The V_m coordinate of the point *(open circle)* at which the curve intersects the X axis is the reversal potential; it denotes the Nernst equilibrium potential, at which point the chemical and electrostatic forces are equal. (Redrawn from Giles WR, Imaizumi Y: *J Physiol [Lond]* 405:123, 1988.)

This reduction in g_K at both positive and low negative values of V_m is called **inward rectification.** Inward rectification is a characteristic of several K^+ currents, including the i_{K1} current. The current-voltage relationship of the K^+ channels that conduct i_{K1} has been determined by voltage-clamping cardiac cells (Fig. 15-12). Note that for the cell depicted in the figure, the current-voltage curve intersects the voltage axis at a V_m of about −70 mV. The absence of ionic current flow at the point of intersection indicates that the electrostatic forces were equal to the chemical (diffusional) forces (Fig. 15-3) at this potential. Therefore, in the ventricular cell preparation, depicted in Fig. 15-12, the Nernst equilibrium potential (E_K) for K^+ was −70 mV. This value reflects the ratio of intracellular to extracellular K^+ concentration that prevails in this particular experimental preparation.

When the membrane potential is clamped at levels negative to −70 mV in this same isolated cardiac cell (Fig. 15-12), the electrostatic forces exceeded the chemical forces and an inward K^+ current was induced (as denoted by the negative values of K^+ current over this range of voltages). Note also that for V_m more negative than −70 mV, the curve has a steep slope, even at the point of intersection (at which $V_m = E_K$). Thus when V_m equals or is negative to E_K, a small change in V_m induces a substantial change in K^+ current; that is, g_K is large. During phase 4, the V_m of a myocardial cell is slightly less negative than E_K (Fig. 15-4). The substantial g_K that prevails during phase 4 of the cardiac action potential (Fig. 15-7) is accounted for mainly by the i_{K1} channels.

When the transmembrane potential is clamped at levels less negative than −70 mV (Fig. 15-12), the chemical forces exceed the electrostatic forces. Therefore, the net K^+ currents are directed outward (as denoted by the corresponding positive values of the K^+ current). Note that for V_m values less negative than –70 mV the curve is relatively flat, and for V_m values less negative than about –30 mV the K^+ current is virtually zero. Thus, at V_m values (about +10 mV) that prevail during the action potential plateau, the efflux of K^+ through the i_{K1} channels is negligible. Conversely, as we have seen, the inwardly directed K^+ current is substantial for those values of V_m (about –90 mV) that prevail during phase 4. Thus, the i_{K1} current is **inwardly rectified**; that is, this K^+ current is substantial when V_m is negative to about –70 mV, whereas this K^+ current is negligible when V_m is positive to about –30 mV.

The characteristics of another K^+ channel, the **delayed rectifier (i_K)** channel, also contribute to the low g_K that prevails during the plateau. These K^+ channels are closed during phase 4, but they are activated by the potentials that prevail toward the end of phase 0. However, activation proceeds very slowly during the plateau. Hence, activation of these channels tends to increase g_K very gradually during phase 2. Thus, these channels play only a minor role during phase 2, but they do contribute to the process of final repolarization (phase 3), as described below. Two types of i_K channels exist, depending on their rates of activation. The more slowly activating channel is designated as the i_{Ks} channel, whereas the more rapidly activating channel is designated as the i_{Kr} channel. The action potential duration in myocytes in various regions of the ventricular myocardium is determined in part by the relative distributions of these i_{Ks} and i_{Kr} channels.

The action potential plateau persists as long as the efflux of charge carried mainly by K^+ is balanced by the influx of charge carried mainly by Ca^{2+}. The effects of altering this balance are demonstrated by the action of the calcium channel antagonist, diltiazem, in an isolated papillary muscle preparation. Figure 15-11 shows that with increasing concentrations of diltiazem, the voltage of the plateau becomes progressively less positive and the duration of the plateau diminishes. Similarly, administration of certain K^+ channel antagonists prolongs the plateau substantially.

Phase 3: Genesis of Final Repolarization

The process of final repolarization (phase 3) starts at the end of phase 2, when the efflux of K^+ from the cardiac cell begins to exceed the influx of Ca^{2+}. As we have noted, at least three outward K^+ currents (i_{to}, i_K, and i_{K1}) contribute to the final repolarization (phase 3) of the cardiac cell (Fig. 15-8).

The transient outward (i_{to}) and the delayed rectifier (i_K) currents help initiate repolarization. These currents are therefore important determinants of the duration of the plateau. For example, the plateau duration is substantially less in atrial than in ventricular myocytes (Fig. 15-19). Electrophysiological experiments have shown that the magnitude of the outward K^+ current during the plateau is greater in atrial than in ventricular myocytes. When the outward K^+ current starts to exceed the inward Ca^{2+} current, repolarization begins. Hence, the greater the K^+ current during phase 2, the earlier repolarization begins. The greater intensity of the K^+

current in atrial than in ventricular myocytes accounts for the shorter action potentials in atrial than in ventricular myocytes.

The action potential duration in ventricular myocytes varies considerably with the locations of these myocytes in the ventricular walls (Fig. 15-9). The delayed rectifier (i_K) current mainly accounts for these differences. In endocardial myocytes, where the action potential duration is least, the magnitude of i_K is greatest. The converse applies to the midmyocardial myocytes. The magnitude of i_K and the action potential duration are intermediate for the epicardial myocytes.

The inwardly rectified K^+ current, i_{K1}, does not participate in the initiation of repolarization, because the conductance of these channels is very small over the range of V_m values that prevail during the plateau. However, *the i_{K1} channels do contribute substantially to the rate of repolarization once phase 3 has been initiated.* As the net efflux of cations causes V_m to become increasingly negative during phase 3, the conductance of the channels that carry the i_{K1} current progressively increases. In Fig. 15-12, the hump in the flat portion of the current-voltage curve reflects the increase in i_{K1} conductance as V_m changes from about –20 to about –60 mV. Thus, as V_m passes through this range of values positive to the Nernst equilibrium potential (open circle in Fig. 15-12), the outward K^+ current increases and thereby accelerates repolarization.

Phase 4: Restoration of Ionic Concentrations

The excess Na^+ that enters the cell rapidly during phase 0 and more slowly throughout the cardiac cycle is eliminated by the action of the enzyme Na^+,K^+-ATPase. This enzyme ejects three Na^+ ions in exchange for two K^+ ions that had exited from the cell mainly during phases 2 and 3. Similarly, most of the excess Ca^{2+} ions that had entered the cell mainly during phase 2 is eliminated principally by a Na^+/Ca^{2+} exchanger, which exchanges three Na^+ ions for one Ca^{2+} ion. However, some of the Ca^{2+} ions are eliminated by an ATP-driven Ca^{2+} pump (Fig. 16-5).

IONIC BASIS OF THE SLOW RESPONSE

Fast-response action potentials (Fig. 15-1, *A*) consist of four principal components: an upstroke (phase 0); an early, partial repolarization (phase 1); a plateau (phase 2); and a final repolarization (phase 3). However, in the slow response (Fig. 15-1, *B*), the upstroke is much less steep, early repolarization (phase 1) is absent, the plateau is less prolonged and not as flat, and the transition from the plateau to the final repolarization is less distinct.

Blocking fast Na^+ channels with tetrodotoxin in a fast-response fiber can generate slow responses under appropriate conditions. The Purkinje fiber action potentials shown in Fig. 15-13 clearly exhibit the two response types. In the control tracing *(A)*, the typical fast-response action potential displays a prominent notch, which separates the upstroke from the plateau. In action potentials *B* to *E*, progressively

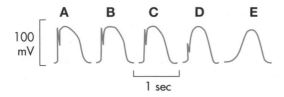

■ **Fig. 15-13** Effect of tetrodotoxin on the action potentials recorded in a calf Purkinje fiber perfused with a solution containing epinephrine and K^+ (10.8 mM). The concentration of tetrodotoxin was 0 M in **A,** 3×10^{28} M in **B,** 3×10^{27} M in **C,** and 3×10^{26} M in **D** and **E**; **E** was recorded later than **D**. (Redrawn from Carmeliet E, Vereecke J: *Pflugers Arch* 313:300, 1969.)

larger quantities of tetrodotoxin are added to the bathing solution to produce a graded blockade of the fast Na^+ channels. The upstroke and notch become progressively less prominent in action potentials *B* to *D*. In action potential *E*, the notch has disappeared and the upstroke is very gradual; this action potential resembles a typical slow response.

Certain cells in the heart, notably those in the SA and AV nodes, are normally slow-response fibers. In such fibers, depolarization is achieved mainly by the influx of Ca^{2+} through the Ca^{2+} channels instead of the influx of Na^+ through fast Na^+ channels. Repolarization is accomplished in these fibers by the inactivation of the Ca^{2+} channels and by the increased K^+ conductance through i_K channels (Fig. 15-8). (Note: i_{K1} channels are not found in SA or AV nodal cells – they are in Purkinje fibers and cardiac myocytes.)

CONDUCTION IN CARDIAC FIBERS

An action potential traveling along a cardiac muscle fiber is propagated by local circuit currents, much as it does in nerve and skeletal muscle fibers (see Chapter 3). The characteristics of conduction differ in fast- and slow-response fibers.

Conduction of the Fast Response

In fast-response fibers, the fast Na^+ channels are activated when the transmembrane potential of one region of the fiber suddenly changes from a resting value of about –90 mV to the threshold value of about –70 mV. The inward Na^+ current then rapidly depolarizes the cell at that site. This portion of the fiber then becomes part of the depolarized zone, and the border is displaced accordingly. The same process then begins at the new border. This process is repeated again and again, and the border moves continuously down the fiber as a wave of depolarization (see Fig. 3-12).

The conduction velocity along the fiber varies directly with the amplitude of the action potential and the rate of change of potential (dV_m/dt) during phase 0. The amplitude of the action potential equals the difference in potential between the fully depolarized and the fully polarized regions of the cell interior. The magnitude of the local currents is proportional to this potential difference (see Chapter 3). Because these local currents shift the potential of the resting zone toward the threshold value, they act as the local stimuli that depolarize the adjacent resting portion of the fiber to its thresh-

old potential. *The greater the potential difference between the depolarized and polarized regions (i.e., the greater the amplitude of the action potential), the more effective are the local stimuli in depolarizing adjacent parts of the membrane and the more rapidly is the wave of depolarization propagated down the fiber.*

The rate of change of potential during phase 0 is also an important determinant of the conduction velocity. If the active portion of the fiber depolarizes gradually, the local currents between the resting region and the neighboring depolarizing region are small. The resting region adjacent to the active zone is depolarized gradually, and consequently more time is required for each new section of the fiber to reach threshold.

The level of the resting membrane potential is also an important determinant of conduction velocity. This factor operates by influencing the amplitude of the action potential and the slope of the upstroke. The transmembrane potential just prior to depolarization may vary for the following reasons: (1) the external K^+ concentration has changed (Fig. 15-4); (2) in cardiac fibers that are intrinsically automatic, V_m becomes progressively less negative during phase 4 (Fig. 15-19, *B*); and (3) if the cell is excited prematurely, the cell membrane has not repolarized fully from the preceding excitation (Fig. 15-15). In general, the less negative the level of V_m, the less is the velocity of impulse propagation, regardless of the reason for the change in V_m.

The V_m level affects conduction velocity because the inactivation, or h, gates (Fig. 15-6) in the fast Na^+ channels are voltage dependent. The less negative the V_m, the greater is the number of h gates that tend to close. During the normal process of excitation, depolarization proceeds so rapidly during phase 0 that the comparatively slow h gates do not close until the end of that phase. However, if partial depolarization is produced by a more gradual process, such as by an elevation of the level of external K^+, the gates have ample time to close and thereby inactivate some of the Na^+ channels. When the cell is partially depolarized, many of the Na^+ channels are already inactivated; thus, only a fraction of the Na^+ channels is available to conduct the inward Na^+ current during phase 0.

Figure 15-14 shows an experiment in which the resting V_m of a bundle of Purkinje fibers is closed by altering the value of $[K^+]_o$. When $[K^+]_o$ is 3 mM (Fig. 15-14, *A* and *F*), the resting V_m is –82 mV and the slope of phase 0 is steep. At the end of phase 0, the overshoot attains a value of 30 mV. Hence, the amplitude of the action potential is 112 mV. The tissue is stimulated at some distance from the impaled cell, and the stimulus artifact *(St)* appears as a diphasic deflection just before phase 0. The distance from this artifact to the beginning of phase 0 is inversely proportional to the conduction velocity.

When $[K^+]_o$ is increased gradually to 16 mM (Fig. 15-14, *B* to *E*), the resting V_m becomes progressively less negative. At the same time, the amplitudes and durations of the action potentials and the steepness of the upstrokes all diminish. As a consequence, the conduction velocity diminishes

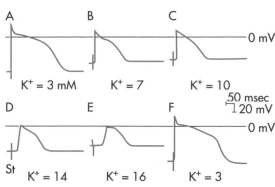

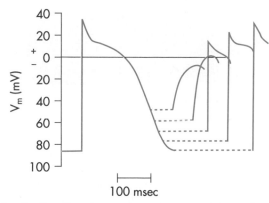

■ **Fig. 15-14** Effect of changes in external potassium concentration on the transmembrane action potentials recorded from a Purkinje fiber. The stimulus artifact *(St)* appears as a biphasic spike to the left of the upstroke of the action potential. The horizontal lines near the peaks of the action potentials denote 0 mV. (From Myerburg RJ, Lazzara R: In Fisch E, editor: *Complex electrocardiography,* Philadelphia, 1973, FA Davis.)

■ **Fig. 15-15** The changes in action potential amplitude and upstroke slope as action potentials are initiated at different stages of the relative refractory period of the preceding excitation. (Redrawn from Rosen MR, Wit AL, Hoffman BF: *Am Heart J* 88:380, 1974.)

progressively. At $[K^+]_o$ levels of 14 and 16 mM (Fig. 15-14, *D* and *E*), the resting V_m attains levels sufficient to inactivate all the fast Na^+ channels. The action potentials in Fig. 15-14, *D* and *E*, are characteristic slow responses.

Most of the experimentally induced changes in transmembrane potential shown in Fig. 15-14 also take place in the cardiac tissue of patients with **coronary artery disease.** When blood flow to a region of the myocardium is diminished, the supply of oxygen and metabolic substrates delivered to the ischemic tissues is insufficient. The Na^+,K^+-ATPase in the membrane of the cardiac myocytes requires considerable metabolic energy to maintain the normal transmembrane exchanges of Na^+ and K^+. When blood flow is inadequate, the activity of the Na^+,K^+-ATPase is impaired, and the ischemic myocytes gain excess Na^+ and lose K^+ to the surrounding interstitial space. Consequently, the K^+ concentration in the extracellular fluid surrounding the ischemic myocytes is elevated. Hence, the myocytes are affected by the elevated K^+ concentration in much the same way as is the myocyte depicted in Fig. 15-14. Such changes in K^+ concentration may disturb cardiac rhythm and conduction critically.

Conduction of the Slow Response

Local circuits (see Fig. 3-12) are also responsible for propagation of the slow response. However, the characteristics of the conduction process differ quantitatively from those of the fast response. The threshold potential is about –40 mV for the slow response, and conduction is much slower than for the fast response. The conduction velocities of the slow responses in the SA and AV nodes are about 0.02 to 0.1 m/sec. The fast-response conduction velocities are about 0.3 to 1 m/sec for myocardial cells and 1 to 4 m/sec for the specialized conducting (Purkinje) fibers in the ventricles. Slow responses are more likely to be blocked than are fast

responses; that is, conduction ceases before the impulse reaches the end of the myocardial fiber. Also, fast-response fibers can respond at repetition rates that are much greater than the repetition rates of slow-response fibers.

CARDIAC EXCITABILITY

Owing to the rapid development of artificial pacemakers and other electrical devices for correcting cardiac rhythm disturbances, detailed knowledge of cardiac excitability is essential. The excitability characteristics of various types of cardiac cells differ considerably, depending on whether the action potentials are fast or slow responses.

Fast Response

Once the fast response has been initiated, the depolarized cell is no longer excitable until the cell has partially repolarized (Fig. 15-1, *A*). The interval from the beginning of the action potential until the fiber is able to conduct another action potential is called the **effective refractory period.** In the fast response, this period extends from the beginning of phase 0 to a point in phase 3 at which repolarization has reached about –50 mV (time *c* to time *d* in Fig. 15-1, *A*). At about this value of V_m, the electrochemical m and h gates for many of the fast Na channels have been reset.

However, the cardiac fiber is not fully excitable until it has been completely repolarized (time *e* in Fig. 15-1, *A*). Before complete repolarization (period *d* to *e* in Fig. 15-1, *A*), an action potential may be evoked only when the stimulus is stronger than a stimulus that could elicit a response during phase 4. Period *d* to *e* is called the **relative refractory period.**

When a fast response is evoked during the relative refractory period of a previous excitation, its characteristics vary with the membrane potential that exists at the time of stimulation (Fig. 15-15). The later in the relative refractory period the fiber is stimulated, the greater is the increase in the amplitude of the response and in the slope of the upstroke.

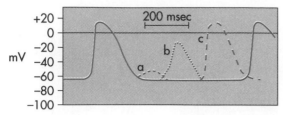

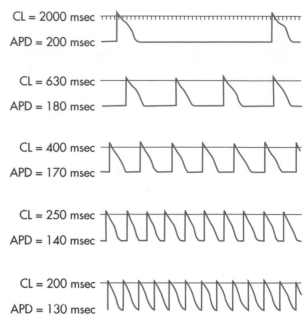

■ Fig. 15-16 Effects of excitation at various times after the initiation of an action potential in a slow-response fiber. In this fiber, excitation very late in phase 3 (or early in phase 4) induces a small, nonpropagated (local) response *(a)*. Later in phase 4, a propagated response *(b)* can be elicited, but its amplitude is small and the upstroke is not very steep; this response is conducted very slowly. Still later in phase 4, full excitability is regained, and the response *(c)* displays normal characteristics. (Modified from Singer DH et al: *Prog Cardiovasc Dis* 24:97, 1981.)

■ Fig. 15-17 Effect of changes in cycle length *(CL)* on the action potential duration *(APD)* of canine Purkinje fibers. (Modified from Singer D, Ten Eick RE: *Am J Cardiol* 28:381, 1971.)

Presumably, the number of fast Na^+ channels that have recovered from inactivation increases as repolarization proceeds during phase 3. As a consequence of the greater amplitude and upstroke slope of the evoked response, the propagation velocity also increases the later in the relative refractory period that the fiber is stimulated. Once the fiber is fully repolarized, the response is constant no matter what time in phase 4 the stimulus is applied.

> In a patient who has occasional **premature depolarizations** (see Fig. 15-39), the timing of these early beats may determine their clinical consequence. If they occur late in the relative refractory period of the preceding depolarization, or after full repolarization, the premature depolarization is probably inconsequential. However, if the premature depolarizations originate early in the relative refractory period of the ventricles, conduction of the premature impulse from the site of origin will be slow, and hence reentry is more likely to occur. If that reentry is irregular (i.e., if **ventricular fibrillation** ensues), the consequence may be grave (see Fig. 15-41).

Slow Response

In slow-response fibers, the relative refractory period frequently extends well beyond phase 3 (Fig. 15-1, *B*). Even after the cell has completely repolarized, it may be difficult to evoke a propagated response for some time. This characteristic of slow-response fibers is called **postrepolarization refractoriness.**

Action potentials evoked early in the relative refractory period are small and the upstrokes are not very steep (Fig. 15-16). The amplitudes and upstroke slopes progressively improve as action potentials are elicited later in the relative refractory period. The recovery of full excitability is much slower than in the fast response. Impulses that arrive early in the relative refractory period are conducted much more slowly than those that arrive late in that period. The lengthy refractory periods also lead to conduction blocks. Even

when slow responses recur at a low repetition rate, the fiber may be able to conduct only a fraction of those impulses; for example, under certain conditions only alternate impulses may be propagated (see Fig. 15-38, *B*).

EFFECTS OF CYCLE LENGTH

Changes in cycle length alter the duration of action potentials in cardiac cells (see Figs. 15-9 and 15-17) and thus change their refractory periods. Consequently, changes in cycle length are often important factors in the initiation or termination of certain arrhythmias (irregular heat rhythms).

The changes in action potential durations produced by stepwise reductions in cycle length from 2000 to 200 msec in a Purkinje fiber are shown in Fig. 15-17. Note that as the cycle length diminishes, the action potential duration decreases. The direct correlation between action potential duration and cycle length is mediated by g_K changes that involve at least two types of K^+ channels, namely, those that conduct the delayed rectifier K^+ current, i_K, and those that conduct the transient outward K^+ current, i_{to}.

The i_K current is activated at values of V_m near zero, but the current activates slowly and remains activated for hundreds of milliseconds. The i_K current also inactivates very slowly. Consequently, as the basic cycle length diminishes, each action potential tends to occur earlier in the inactivation period of the i_K current initiated by the preceding action potential. Therefore, the shorter the basic cycle length, the greater is the outward K^+ current during phase 2, and hence the shorter the duration of the action potential.

The i_{to} current also influences the relationship between cycle length and action potential duration. The i_{to} current is also activated at near zero potentials, and its magnitude varies inversely with the cardiac cycle length. Therefore, as cycle length decreases, the consequent increase in the outward K$^+$ current shortens the plateau. The relative contributions of i_K and of i_{to} to the relationship between action potential duration and cardiac cycle length vary from species to species.

NATURAL EXCITATION OF THE HEART

The nervous system controls various aspects of cardiac behavior, such as the heart rate and the strength of each contraction. However, cardiac function does not require an intact innervation. Indeed, a cardiac transplant patient, whose heart is completely denervated, may still adapt well to stressful situations. The ability of the denervated, transplanted heart to adapt to changing conditions lies in certain intrinsic properties of cardiac tissue, especially its automaticity.

The properties of **automaticity** *(the ability to initiate its own beat) and* **rhythmicity** *(the regularity of such pacemaking activity) allow a perfused heart to beat even when it is completely removed from the body.* If the coronary vasculature of an excised heart is artificially perfused with blood or an oxygenated electrolyte solution, rhythmic cardiac contractions may persist for many hours. At least some cells in the atria and ventricles can initiate beats; such cells mainly reside in the nodal tissues or specialized conducting fibers of the heart.

The region of the mammalian heart that ordinarily generates impulses at the greatest frequency is the **sinoatrial (SA) node;** it is the main **pacemaker** of the heart. Detailed mapping of the electrical potentials on the surface of the right atrium reveals that two or three sites of automaticity, located 1 or 2 cm from the SA node itself, serve along with the SA node as an **atrial pacemaker complex.** At times, all of these loci initiate impulses simultaneously. At other times, the site of earliest excitation shifts from locus to locus, depending on certain conditions, such as the level of autonomic neural activity.

> Regions of the heart other than the SA node may initiate beats under special circumstances. Such sites are called **ectopic foci,** or **ectopic pacemakers.** Ectopic foci may become pacemakers when (1) their own rhythmicity becomes enhanced, (2) the rhythmicity of the higher-order pacemakers becomes depressed, or (3) all conduction pathways between the ectopic focus and those regions with greater rhythmicity become blocked. Ectopic pacemakers may act as a safety mechanism when normal pacemaking centers fail. However, if an ectopic center fires while the normal pacemaking center still functions, the ectopic activity may induce either sporadic rhythm disturbances, such as **premature depolarizations** (see Fig. 15-39), or continuous rhythm disturbances, such as **paroxysmal tachycardias** (see Fig. 15-40).

When the SA node or other components of the atrial pacemaker complex are excised or destroyed, pacemaker cells in

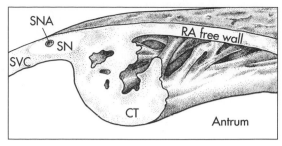

■ Fig. 15-18 Location of the sinoatrial *(SA)* node near the junction between the superior vena cava *(SVC)* and the right atrium *(RA)*. *SN,* SA node; *SNA,* sinoatrial artery; *CT,* crista terminalis. (Redrawn from James TN: *Am J Cardiol* 40:965, 1977.)

the AV junction usually take over the pacemaker function for the entire heart. After some time, which may vary from minutes to days, automatic cells in the atria usually become dominant. Purkinje fibers in the specialized conduction system of the ventricles also display automaticity. Characteristically, these fibers fire at a very slow rate. When the AV junction cannot conduct cardiac impulses from the atria to the ventricles (see Fig. 15-38, *C*), these **idioventricular pacemakers** in the Purkinje fiber network initiate the ventricular contractions, but at a frequency of only 30 to 40 beats/min.

Sinoatrial Node

In humans, the SA node is about 8 mm long and 2 mm thick, and it lies posteriorly in the groove at the junction between the superior vena cava and the right atrium (Fig. 15-18). The sinus node artery runs lengthwise through the center of the node. The SA node contains two principal types of cells: (1) small, round cells, which have few organelles and myofibrils; and (2) slender, elongated cells, which are intermediate in appearance between the round and "ordinary" atrial myocardial cells. The round cells are probably the pacemaker cells, whereas the slender, elongated cells probably conduct the impulses within the node and to the nodal margins.

A typical transmembrane action potential recorded from a cell in the SA node is depicted in Fig. 15-19, *B*. Compared with the transmembrane potential recorded from a ventricular myocardial cell (Fig. 15-19, *A*), the resting potential of the SA node cell is usually less negative, the upstroke of the action potential (phase 0) is less steep, the plateau is not sustained, and repolarization (phase 3) is more gradual. These attributes are all characteristic of the slow response. Again, as in cells that exhibit the slow response, tetrodotoxin (which blocks the fast Na$^+$ current) has no influence on the SA nodal action potential. Thus, the upstroke of the action potential is not produced by an inward current of Na$^+$ through fast channels.

The transmembrane potential during phase 4 is much less negative in SA (and AV) nodal automatic cells than in atrial or ventricular myocytes, because the i_{K1} (inward rectifying) type of K$^+$ channel is sparse in the nodal cells. Therefore, the ratio of g_K to g_{Na} during phase 4 is much less in the nodal

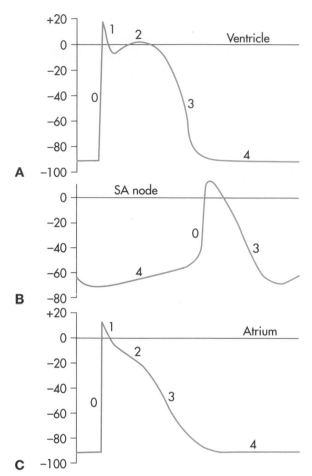

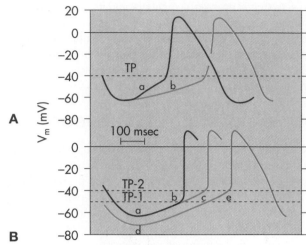

■ **Fig. 15-19** Typical action potentials (in millivolts) recorded from cells in the ventricle **(A)**, SA node **(B)**, and atrium **(C)**. Sweep velocity in **B** is one-half that in **A** or **C**. (From Hoffman BF, Cranefield PF: *Electrophysiology of the heart*, New York, 1960, McGraw-Hill.)

■ **Fig. 15-20** Mechanisms involved in the changes in frequency of pacemaker firing. In **A,** a reduction in the slope (from *a* to *b*) of slow diastolic depolarization diminishes the firing frequency. In **B,** an increase in the threshold potential (from *TP-1* to *TP-2*) or an increase in the magnitude of the resting potential (from *a* to *d*) also diminishes the firing frequency. (From Hoffman BF, Cranefield PF: *Electrophysiology of the heart*, New York, 1960, McGraw-Hill.)

cells than in the myocytes. Hence, during phase 4, V_m deviates much more from the K^+ equilibrium potential (E_K) in nodal cells than it does in myocytes.

However, the principal feature of a pacemaker fiber that distinguishes it from the other fibers we have discussed resides in phase 4. In nonautomatic cells, the potential remains constant during this phase, whereas *a pacemaker fiber is characterized by a slow diastolic depolarization throughout phase 4*. Depolarization proceeds at a steady rate until a threshold is attained, and an action potential is triggered.

The discharge frequency of pacemaker cells may be varied by a change in (1) the rate of depolarization during phase 4, (2) the maximal negativity during phase 4, or (3) the threshold potential (Fig. 15-20). When the rate of slow diastolic depolarization is increased (from *b* to *a* in Fig. 15-20, *A*), the threshold potential is attained earlier, and therefore the heart rate increases. A rise in the threshold potential (from TP-1 to TP-2 in Fig. 15-20, *B*) delays the onset of phase 0 (from time *b* to time *c*), and the heart rate is reduced accordingly. Similarly, when the maximal negative potential is increased (from *a* to *d* in Fig. 15-20, *B*),

more time is required to reach threshold potential TP-2 when the slope of phase 4 remains unchanged, and the heart rate therefore diminishes.

Ordinarily, the frequency of pacemaker firing is controlled by the activity of both divisions of the autonomic nervous system. Increased sympathetic nervous activity, through the release of norepinephrine, raises the heart rate principally by increasing the slope of the slow diastolic depolarization. This mechanism of increasing heart rate occurs during physical exertion, anxiety, or certain illnesses, such as **febrile infectious diseases.**

Increased vagal activity, through the release of acetylcholine, diminishes the heart rate by hyperpolarizing the pacemaker cell membrane and reducing the slope of the slow diastolic depolarization (Fig. 15-21). These mechanisms of decreasing heart rate occur when vagal activity is predominant over sympathetic activity. An extreme example is **vasovagal syncope,** a brief period of lightheadedness or loss of consciousness caused by an intense burst of vagal activity. This type of syncope is a reflex response to pain or to certain psychological stimuli.

Changes in autonomic neural activity usually do not change heart rate by altering the threshold level of V_m in the nodal pacemaker cells. However, certain antiarrhythmic drugs, such as **quinidine** and **procainamide,** do raise the threshold potential of the automatic cells to less negative values.

Ionic basis of automaticity. Several ionic currents contribute to the slow diastolic depolarization that characteristically occurs in the automatic cells in the heart. In the pacemaker cells of the SA node, at least three ionic currents

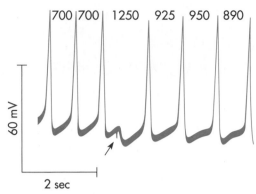

Fig. 15-21 Effect of a brief vagal stimulus *(arrow)* on the transmembrane potential recorded from an SA node pacemaker cell in an isolated cat atrium preparation. The cardiac cycle lengths, in milliseconds, are denoted by the numbers at the top of the figure. (Modified from Jalife J, Moe GK: *Circ Res* 45:595, 1979.)

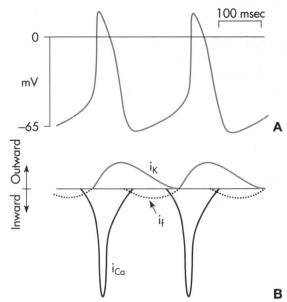

Fig. 15-22 The transmembrane potential changes **(A)** that occur in SA node cells are produced by three principal currents **(B)**: (1) an inward Ca^{2+} current, iCa; (2) a hyperpolarization-induced inward current, i_f; and (3) an outward K^+ current, i_K.

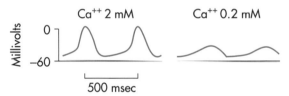

Fig. 15-23 Transmembrane action potentials recorded from an SA node pacemaker cell in an isolated rabbit atrium preparation. The concentration of Ca^{2+} in the bath was reduced from 2 mM to 0.2 mM. (Modified from Kohlhardt M, Figulla HR, Tripathi O: *Basic Res Cardiol* 71:17, 1976.)

mediate the slow diastolic depolarization: (1) an inward current, i_f, induced by hyperpolarization; (2) an inward Ca^{2+} current, i_{Ca}; and (3) an outward K^+ current, i_K (Fig. 15-22).

The inward current, i_f, is activated near the end of repolarization. This "funny" current is carried mainly by Na^+ through specific channels that differ from the fast Na^+ channels. The current was dubbed "funny" because its discoverers had not expected to detect an inward Na^+ current in pacemaker cells at the end of repolarization. This current is activated as the membrane potential becomes more negative than about –50 mV. The more negative the membrane potential at this time, the greater is the activation of the i_f current.

The second current responsible for diastolic depolarization is the Ca^{2+} current, i_{Ca}. This current is activated toward the end of phase 4, as the transmembrane potential reaches a value of about –55 mV (Fig. 15-15). Once the Ca^{2+} channels are activated, influx of Ca^{2+} into the cell increases. This influx accelerates the rate of diastolic depolarization, which then leads to the upstroke of the action potential. A decrease in the external Ca^{2+} concentration (Fig. 15-23) or the addition of calcium channel antagonists (Fig. 15-24) diminishes the amplitude of the action potential and the slope of the slow diastolic depolarization in SA node cells.

The progressive diastolic depolarization mediated by the two inward currents, i_f and i_{Ca}, is opposed by an outward current, the delayed rectifier K^+ current, i_K. This efflux of K^+ tends to repolarize the cell after the upstroke of the action potential. K^+ continues to move out well beyond the time of maximal repolarization, but its efflux diminishes throughout phase 4 (Fig. 15-15). As the current diminishes, its opposition to the depolarizing effects of the two inward currents (i_{Ca} and i_f) also gradually decreases.

The ionic basis for automaticity in the AV node pacemaker cells resembles that in the SA node cells. Similar mechanisms also account for automaticity in ventricular Purkinje fibers, except that the Ca^{2+} current is not involved. In other words, the slow diastolic depolarization is mediated principally by the imbalance between the effects of the

hyperpolarization-induced inward current, i_f, and the gradually diminishing outward K^+ current, i_K.

The autonomic neurotransmitters affect automaticity by altering the ionic currents across the cell membranes. The adrenergic transmitters increase all three currents involved in SA nodal automaticity. To increase the slope of diastolic depolarization, the augmentations of i_f and i_{Ca} by the adrenergic transmitters must exceed the enhancement of i_K by these same transmitters.

The hyperpolarization (Fig. 15-21) induced by the acetylcholine released at the vagus nerve endings in the heart is achieved by an increase in g_K. This change in conductance is mediated through activation of specific K^+ channels, the **acetylcholine-regulated K^+** channels. Acetylcholine also depresses the i_f and i_{Ca} currents. The autonomic neural effects on cardiac cells are described in greater detail in Chapter 17.

Overdrive suppression. The automaticity of pacemaker cells diminishes after these cells had been excited at a high

■ **Fig. 15-24**   Effects of nifedipine (5.6×10^{27} M), a Ca^{2+} channel antagonist, on the transmembrane potentials recorded from an SA node cell in a rabbit. (From Ning W, Wit AL: *Am Heart J* 106:345, 1983.)

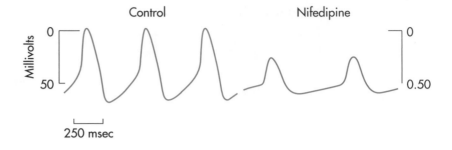

frequency. This phenomenon is known as **overdrive suppression.** Because the intrinsic rhythmicity of the SA node is greater than that of the other latent pacemaking sites in the heart, the firing of the SA node tends to suppress the automaticity in the other loci.

If an ectopic focus in one of the atria suddenly began to fire at a high rate (e.g., 150 impulses/min) in an individual with a normal heart rate of 70 beats/min, the ectopic site would become the pacemaker for the entire heart. If that rapid ectopic focus suddenly stopped firing, the SA node might remain briefly quiescent because of overdrive suppression. The interval from the end of the period of overdrive until the SA node resumes firing is called the **sinus node recovery time.** In patients with **sick sinus syndrome,** the sinus node recovery time is prolonged. The consequent period of **asystole** (absence of a heartbeat) may cause the patient to lose consciousness.

Overdrive suppression results from the activity of the membrane pump, Na^+,K^+-ATPase, which extrudes three Na^+ from the cardiac cell in exchange for two K^+. Normally, a certain amount of Na^+ enters the cardiac cell during each depolarization. The more frequently the cell is depolarized, therefore, the more Na^+ enters the cell per minute. At high excitation frequencies, the activity of the Na^+,K^+-ATPase increases to extrude this larger amount of Na^+ from the cell interior. Because the amount of Na^+ extruded by the pump exceeds the amount of K^+ that enters the cell, the activity of the Na^+,K^+-ATPase hyperpolarizes the cell. Therefore, the slow diastolic depolarization requires more time to reach the firing threshold, as shown in Fig. 15-20, *B.* Furthermore, when the overdrive suddenly ceases, the activity of the Na^+,K^+-ATPase does not slow down instantaneously, but it remains overactive temporarily. This excessive extrusion of Na^+ opposes the gradual depolarization of the pacemaker cell during phase 4, and thereby it temporarily suppresses the cell's intrinsic automaticity.

Atrial Conduction

From the SA node, the cardiac impulse spreads radially throughout the right atrium (Fig. 15-25) along ordinary atrial myocardial fibers, at a conduction velocity of approximately 1 m/sec. A special pathway, the anterior interatrial myocardial band (or Bachmann's bundle), conducts the impulse

from the SA node directly to the left atrium. The wave of excitation that proceeds inferiorly through the right atrium ultimately reaches the AV node (Fig. 15-25), which is normally the sole route of entry of the cardiac impulse to the ventricles.

The configuration of the atrial transmembrane potential is depicted in Fig. 15-19, *C.* Compared with the potential recorded from a typical ventricular fiber (Fig. 15-19, *A*), the atrial plateau (phase 2) is briefer and less developed, and repolarization (phase 3) is slower. The action potential duration in atrial myocytes is shorter than that in ventricular myocytes because the efflux of K^+ is greater during the plateau in atrial myocytes than in ventricular myocytes.

Atrioventricular Conduction

The atrial excitation wave reaches the ventricles via the AV node. In adult humans, this node is approximately 15 mm long, 10 mm wide, and 3 mm thick. The node is situated posteriorly on the right side of the interatrial septum near the ostium of the coronary sinus. The AV node contains the same two cell types as the SA node, but the round cells in the AV node are less abundant and the elongated cells predominate.

The AV node is made up of the following three functional regions: (1) the AN region, the transitional zone between the atrium and the remainder of the node; (2) the N region, the midportion of the AV node; and (3) the NH region, the zone in which nodal fibers gradually merge with the bundle of His (Fig. 15-25), which is the upper portion of the specialized conducting system for the ventricles. Normally, the AV node and bundle of His are the only pathways along which the cardiac impulse travels from atria to ventricles.

Some people have accessory AV pathways. Because these pathways often serve as a part of a reentry loop (Fig. 15-30), they can be associated with serious cardiac rhythm disturbances. **Wolff-Parkinson-White syndrome,** a congenital disturbance, is the most common clinical disorder in which a bypass tract of myocardial fibers serves as an accessory pathway between atria and ventricles. Ordinarily, the syndrome causes no functional abnormality. The disturbance is easily detected in the electrocardiogram (ECG) because a portion of the ventricular myocardium is excited via the bypass tract before the

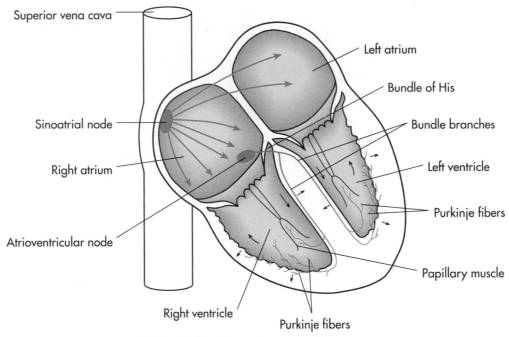

Superior vena cava

Left atrium

Bundle of His

Sinoatrial node

Bundle branches

Right atrium

Left ventricle

Purkinje fibers

Atrioventricular node

Papillary muscle

Right ventricle

Purkinje fibers

■ **Fig. 15-25**   The cardiac conduction system.

remainder of the ventricular myocardium is excited via the AV node and His-Purkinje system. This preexcitation can be seen as a bizarre configuration in the ventricular (QRS) complex of the ECG. Occasionally, however, a reentry loop develops in which the atrial impulse travels to the ventricles via one of the two AV pathways (AV node or bypass tract), and then back to the atria through the other of these two pathways. Continuous circling around the loop leads to a very rapid rhythm (**supraventricular tachycardia**). This rapid rhythm may be incapacitating because it may not allow sufficient time for ventricular filling. Transient block of the AV node by injecting **adenosine** intravenously or by increasing vagal activity reflexly (by pressing on the neck over the **carotid sinus region**) usually abolishes the tachycardia and restores a normal sinus rhythm.

Several features of AV conduction are of physiological and clinical significance. The principal delay in the passage of the impulse from the atria to the ventricles occurs in the AN and N regions of the AV node. The conduction velocity is actually less in the N region than in the AN region. However, the path length is substantially greater in the AN than in the N region. The conduction times through the AN and N zones account for the delay between the start of the **P wave** (the electrical manifestation of the spread of atrial excitation) and the **QRS complex** (the electrical manifestation of the spread of ventricular excitation) on an ECG (Fig. 15-33). *Functionally, the delay between atrial and ventricular excitation permits optimal ventricular filling during atrial contraction.*

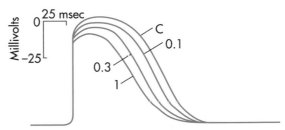

■ **Fig. 15-26**   Transmembrane potentials recorded from a rabbit atrioventricular (AV) node cell under control conditions *(C)* and in the presence of the calcium channel antagonist diltiazem, in concentrations of 0.1, 0.3, and 1 μmol/L. (Redrawn from Hirth C, Borchard U, Hafner D: *J Mol Cell Cardiol* 15:799, 1983.)

In the N region, slow-response action potentials prevail. The resting potential is about –60 mV, the upstroke velocity is low (about 5 V/sec), and the conduction velocity is about 0.05 m/sec. Tetrodotoxin, which blocks the fast Na^+ channels, has virtually no effect on the action potentials in this region (or on any other slow-response fibers). Conversely, Ca^{2+} channel antagonists decrease the amplitude and duration of the action potentials (Fig. 15-26) and depress AV conduction. The shapes of the action potentials in the AN region are intermediate between those in the N region and those in the atria. Similarly, the action potentials in the NH region are transitional between those in the N region and those in the bundle of His.

Like other slow-response action potentials, the relative refractory period of cells in the N region extends well beyond the period of complete repolarization; that is, these cells

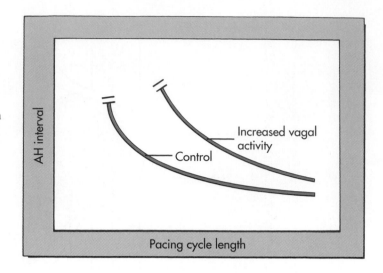

■ **Fig. 15-27** Changes in atrium-His *(A-H)* intervals induced by pacing the atria at various cycle lengths in a group of human subjects under control conditions and during a reflexly induced increase in vagal activity produced by the intravenous infusion of phenylephrine. (Redrawn from Page RL et al: *Circ Res* 68:1614, 1991.)

display **postrepolarization refractoriness** (Fig. 15-16). As the time between successive atrial depolarizations is decreased, conduction through the AV junction slows (Fig. 15-27). An abnormal prolongation of the AV conduction time is called **first-degree AV block** (Fig. 15-38, *A*). Most of the prolongation of AV conduction induced by a decrease in atrial cycle length takes place in the N region of the AV node.

Impulses tend to be blocked in the AV node at stimulation frequencies that are easily conducted in other regions of the heart. If the atria are depolarized at a high repetition rate, only a fraction (e.g., one half) of the atrial impulses might be conducted through the AV junction to the ventricles. The conduction pattern in which only a fraction of the atrial impulses are conducted to the ventricles is called **second-degree AV block** (Fig. 15-38, *B*). This type of block may protect the ventricles from excessive contraction frequencies, wherein the filling time between contractions might be inadequate.

Retrograde conduction can occur through the AV node. However, the propagation time is significantly longer and the impulse is blocked at lower repetition rates when the impulse is conducted in the retrograde instead of in the antegrade direction. Finally the AV node is a common site for reentry; the underlying mechanisms are explained on page 294.

The autonomic nervous system regulates AV conduction. Weak vagal activity may simply prolong the AV conduction time. Thus, for any given atrial cycle length, the atrium to His (A-H) or atrium to ventricle (A-V) conduction time will be prolonged by vagal stimulation (Fig. 15-27). Stronger vagal activity may cause some or all of the impulses arriving from the atria to be blocked in the node. The conduction pattern in which none of the atrial impulses reaches the ventricles is called **third-degree**, or **complete, AV block** (Fig. 15-38, *C*). The vagally induced delay or absence of conduction through the AV junction occurs mainly in the N region of the node.

Acetylcholine released by the vagal nerve fibers hyperpolarizes the conducting fibers in the N region (Fig. 15-28).

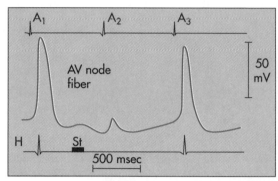

■ **Fig. 15-28** Effects of a brief vagal stimulus *(St)* on the transmembrane potential recorded from an AV nodal fiber from a rabbit. Note that shortly after vagal stimulation, the membrane of the fiber was hyperpolarized. The atrial excitation *(A₂)* that arrived at the AV node when the cell was hyperpolarized failed to be conducted, as denoted by the absence of a depolarization in the His electrogram *(H)*. The atrial excitations that preceded *(A₁)* and followed *(A₃)* excitation A₂ were conducted to the His bundle region. (Redrawn from Mazgalev T et al: *Am J Physiol* 251:H631, 1986.)

The greater the hyperpolarization at the time of arrival of the atrial impulse, the more impaired is the AV conduction. In the experiment shown in Fig. 15-28, vagus nerve fibers are stimulated intensely (at *St*) shortly before the second atrial depolarization *(A₂)*. That atrial impulse arrives at the AV node cell when its cell membrane is maximally hyperpolarized in response to the vagal stimulus. The absence of a corresponding depolarization of the bundle of His shows that the vagal stimulus prevents the conduction of the second atrial impulse through the AV node. Only a small, nonpropagated response to the second atrial impulse is evident in the recording from the conducting fiber.

The cardiac sympathetic nerves, on the other hand, facilitate AV conduction. They decrease the AV conduction time and enhance the rhythmicity of the latent pacemakers in the AV junction. The norepinephrine released at the

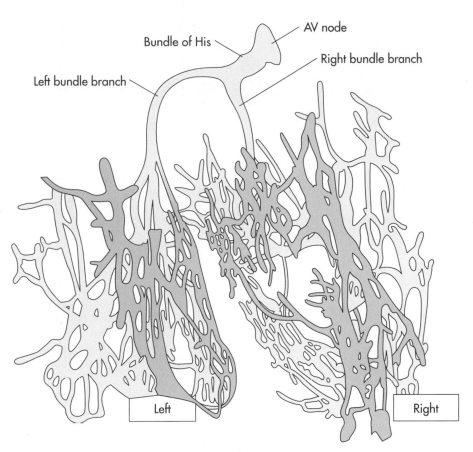

■ **Fig. 15-29** Atrioventricular and ventricular conduction system of the calf heart. (Redrawn from DeWitt LM: *Anat Rec* 3:475, 1909.)

postganglionic sympathetic nerve terminals increases the amplitude and slope of the upstroke of the AV nodal action potentials, principally in the AN and N regions of the node.

Ventricular Conduction

The bundle of His passes subendocardially down the right side of the interventricular septum for about 1 cm and then divides into the right and left **bundle branches** (Figs. 15-25 and 15-29). The right bundle branch, which is a direct continuation of the bundle of His, proceeds down the right side of the interventricular septum. The left bundle branch, which is considerably thicker than the right, arises almost perpendicularly from the bundle of His and perforates the interventricular septum. On the subendocardial surface of the left side of the interventricular septum, the left bundle branch splits into a thin anterior division and a thick posterior division.

Impulse conduction in the right or left bundle branch or in either division of the left bundle branch may be impaired. Conduction blocks may develop in one or more of these conduction pathways as a consequence of **coronary artery disease** or degenerative processes associated with aging, and they give rise to characteristic ECG patterns. Block of either of the main bundle branches is known as right or left **bundle branch block.** Block of either division of the left bundle branch is called left anterior or left posterior **hemiblock.**

The right bundle branch and the two divisions of the left bundle branch ultimately subdivide into a complex network of conducting fibers, called **Purkinje fibers,** which spread out over the subendocardial surfaces of both ventricles. In certain mammalian species, such as cattle, the Purkinje fiber network is arranged in discrete, encapsulated bundles (Fig. 15-29).

Purkinje fibers have abundant, linearly arranged sarcomeres, as do myocytes. However, the T-tubular system is absent in the Purkinje fibers of many species, although the T-tubular system is well developed in the myocytes. Purkinje fibers are the broadest cells in the heart: they are 70 to 80 μm in diameter, compared with diameters of 10 to 15 μm for ventricular myocytes. Partly because of the large diameter of the Purkinje fibers, conduction velocity (1 to 4 m/sec) in these fibers exceeds that in any other fiber type within the heart. The increased conduction velocity permits a rapid activation of the entire endocardial surface of the ventricles.

The action potentials recorded from Purkinje fibers resemble those of ordinary ventricular myocardial fibers (Figs. 15-9 and 15-19, *A*). In general, phase 1 is prominent in Purkinje fiber action potentials (Fig. 15-13) and the duration of the plateau (phase 2) is intermediate between those of epicardial and midmyocardial myocytes (Fig. 15-9).

Because of the long refractory period of Purkinje fiber action potentials, many premature excitations of the atria are conducted through the AV junction but are blocked by the Purkinje fibers. Blockage of these atrial excitations prevents premature contraction of the ventricles. This function of protecting the ventricles against the effects of premature atrial depolarizations is especially pronounced at slow heart rates, because the action potential duration, and hence the effective refractory period of the Purkinje fibers, varies inversely with the heart rate (Fig. 15-17). At slow heart rates, the effective refractory period of the Purkinje fibers is especially prolonged; as the heart rate increases, the refractory period diminishes.

Similar directional changes in the refractory period occur also in ventricular myocytes in response to changes in rate (Fig. 15-9). However, in the AV node, the effective refractory period does not change appreciably over the normal range of heart rates, and it actually increases at very rapid heart rates (Fig. 15-27). Therefore, *when the atrium is excited at high repetition rates, it is the AV node that protects the ventricles from these excessively high frequencies.*

The first portions of the ventricles to be excited by impulses arriving from the AV node are the interventricular septum (except the basal portion) and the papillary muscles. The wave of activation spreads into the substance of the septum from both its left and right endocardial surfaces. Early contraction of the septum tends to make it more rigid and allows it to serve as an anchor point for the contraction of the remaining ventricular myocardium. Also, early contraction of the papillary muscles prevents eversion of the AV valves into the atria during ventricular systole.

The endocardial surfaces of both ventricles are activated rapidly, but the wave of excitation spreads from endocardium to epicardium at a slower velocity (about 0.3 to 0.4 m/sec). Because the right ventricular wall is appreciably thinner than the left, the epicardial surface of the right ventricle is activated earlier than that of the left ventricle. Also, apical and central epicardial regions of both ventricles are activated somewhat earlier than their respective basal regions. The last portions of the ventricles to be excited are the posterior basal epicardial regions and a small zone in the basal portion of the interventricular septum.

Reentry

Under certain conditions, a cardiac impulse may reexcite some myocardial region through which it had passed previously. This phenomenon, known as **reentry**, is responsible for many clinical **arrhythmias** (disturbances of cardiac rhythm). The reentry may be **ordered** or **random.** In the ordered variety the impulse traverses a fixed anatomical path, whereas in the random type the path continues to change.

The conditions necessary for reentry are illustrated in Fig. 15-30. In each of the four panels a single bundle *(S)* of cardiac fibers splits into a left *(L)* and right *(R)* branch. A connecting bundle *(C)* runs between the two branches. Normally the impulse moving down bundle *S* is conducted along the *L* and *R* branches (Fig. 15-30, *A*). As the impulse reaches connecting link *C*, it enters from both sides and

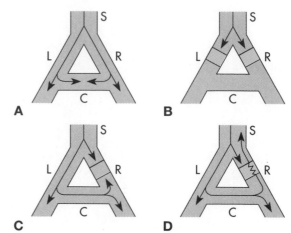

■ **Fig. 15-30**   The role of unidirectional block in reentry. In **A,** an excitation wave traveling down a single bundle *(S)* of fibers continues down the left *(L)* and right *(R)* branches. The depolarization wave enters the connecting branch *(C)* from both ends and is extinguished at the zone of collision. In **B,** the wave is blocked in the L and R branches. In **C,** bidirectional block exists in branch R. In **D,** unidirectional block exists in branch R. The antegrade impulse is blocked, but the retrograde impulse is conducted through and reenters bundle *S.*

becomes extinguished at the point of collision. The impulse from the left side cannot proceed farther because the tissue beyond is absolutely refractory; it has just been depolarized from the other direction. The impulse also cannot pass through bundle *C* from the right, for the same reason.

Figure 15-30, *B*, shows that the impulse cannot complete the circuit if antegrade block exists in the *L* and *R* branches of the fiber bundle. Furthermore, if bidirectional block exists at any point in the loop (e.g., branch R in Fig. 15-30, *C*), the impulse also cannot reenter.

A necessary condition for reentry is that at some point in the loop the impulse can pass in one direction but not in the other. This phenomenon is called **unidirectional block.** As shown in Fig. 15-30, *D*, the impulse may travel down branch *L* normally and become blocked in the antegrade direction in branch *R*, because of some pathological change in the myocardial fibers in the branch. The impulse that was conducted down branch *L* and through the connecting branch *C* may be able to penetrate the depressed region in branch *R* from the retrograde direction, even though the antegrade impulse had been blocked previously at this same site. Why is the antegrade impulse blocked but not the retrograde impulse? The reason is that the antegrade impulse arrives at the depressed region in branch *R* earlier than the retrograde impulse, because the path length of the antegrade impulse is very short, whereas the retrograde impulse traverses a much longer path. Therefore, the antegrade impulse may be blocked simply because it arrives at the depressed region during its effective refractory period. If the retrograde impulse is delayed sufficiently, the refractory period may have ended in the affected region, and the impulse can then be conducted back through this region and return to bundle *S.*

Although unidirectional block is a necessary condition for reentry, it alone cannot cause reentry. *For reentry to occur, the effective refractory period of the reentered region must be shorter than the propagation time around the loop.* In Fig. 15-30, *D*, if the tissue just beyond the depressed zone in branch *R* is still refractory from the antegrade depolarization, the retrograde impulse will not be conducted into branch S. Therefore the conditions that promote reentry are those that prolong conduction time or shorten effective refractory period.

The functional characteristics of the various components of the reentry loops responsible for specific cardiac arrhythmias are diverse. Some loops are large and involve entire specialized conduction bundles, whereas others are microscopic. The loop may include myocardial fibers, specialized conducting fibers, nodal cells, and junctional tissues in almost any conceivable arrangement. Also, the various cardiac cells in the loop may be normal or deranged.

The propagation velocity along a multicellular cardiac conduction fiber is normally facilitated by the **gap junctions** (see Figs. 16-1 and 16-3) that lie between consecutive conduction fibers. Variations in the protein structure of the **connexins** in the gap junctions can affect the propagation velocity along these fibers. The chemical structure of the specific connexins can vary locally in cardiac tissues, and thereby establish local variations in propagation velocity. Such topical variations in velocity might include regions of unidirectional block and thereby induce reentrant rhythm disturbances.

Triggered Activity

Triggered activity is so named because it is always coupled to a preceding action potential. Because reentrant activity is also coupled to a preceding action potential, the arrhythmias induced by triggered activity are usually difficult to distinguish from those induced by reentry. Triggered activity is caused by **afterdepolarizations.** Two types of afterdepolarizations are recognized: **early (EAD)** and **delayed (DAD).** EADs may appear either at the end of the action potential plateau (phase 2) or about midway through repolarization (phase 3), whereas DADs occur near the very end of repolarization or just after full repolarization (phase 4).

Early afterdepolarizations. EADs tend to appear near the end of the action potential plateau or during repolarization, but before the cell has fully repolarized. They are more likely to occur when the prevailing heart rate is slow; a rapid heart rate suppresses EADs.

In the experiment shown in Fig. 15-31, EADs are induced by adding cesium to an isolated Purkinje fiber preparation. No afterdepolarizations are evident when the preparation is driven at a cycle length of 2 seconds. When the cycle length is increased to 4 seconds, however, EADs appear. Most of the EADs are subthreshold *(first two arrows),* but the third EAD reaches threshold and triggers an action potential. When the cycle length is increased to 6 seconds, each driven action potential generates an EAD that triggers a second action potential. Furthermore, when the cycle length is increased to 10 seconds, each driven action potential triggers a salvo of four or five additional action potentials.

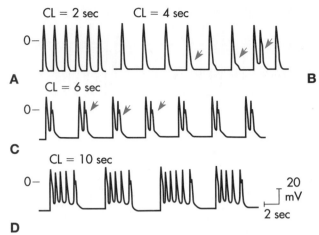

D

■ **Fig. 15-31** Effect of pacing at different cycle lengths *(CL)* on cesium-induced early afterdepolarizations (EADs) in a canine Purkinje fiber. **A,** EADs not evident. **B,** EADs first appear *(arrows).* Third EAD reaches threshold and triggers an action potential *(third arrow).* **C,** EADs that appear after each driven depolarization trigger an action potential. **D,** Triggered action potentials occur in salvos. (Modified from Damiano BP, Rosen M: *Circulation* 69:1013, 1984.)

EADs are more likely to occur in cardiac cells with prolonged action potentials than in cells with shorter action potentials. For example, EADs can be induced more readily in myocytes from the midmyocardial region of the ventricular walls than in myocytes from the endocardial or epicardial regions, owing to the disparity in these cells' action potential durations (Fig. 15-9). Furthermore, EADs may be produced experimentally by interventions that prolong the action potential. As we have seen, in the experiment shown in Fig. 15-31, EADs are more prevalent as the basic cycle length is increased. Such increases in basic cycle length do, of course, prolong the action potential (Fig. 15-17), and this prolongation undoubtedly contributes to the generation of the EADs. Certain antiarrhythmic drugs, such as **quinidine,** act to prolong the action potential. Consequently, these drugs increase the likelihood that EADs may occur. Hence, *antiarrhythmic drugs are also frequently proarrhythmic.*

The direct correlation between a cell's action potential duration and its susceptibility to EADs is probably related to the time required for the Ca^{2+} channels in the cell membranes to recover from inactivation. When action potentials are sufficiently prolonged, those Ca^{2+} channels that were activated at the beginning of the plateau have sufficient time to recover from inactivation and thus may be reactivated before the cell fully repolarizes. This secondary activation could then trigger an early afterdepolarization.

Delayed afterdepolarizations. In contrast to EADs, DADs are more likely to occur when the heart rate is high. The most important characteristics of DADs are shown in Fig. 15-32. In the experiment depicted in this figure, transmembrane potentials are recorded from Purkinje fibers exposed to a high concentration of acetylstrophanthidin, a

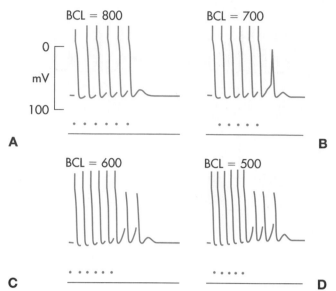

■ **Fig. 15-32** Transmembrane action potentials recorded from isolated canine Purkinje fibers. Acetylstrophanthidin, a digitalis-like agent, was added to the bath, and sequences of six driven beats (denoted by the dots) were produced at basic cycle lengths *(BCL)* of 800 **(A)**, 700 **(B)**, 600 **(C)**, and 500 **(D)** msec. Note that delayed afterpotentials occurred after the driven beats, and that these after-potentials reached threshold after the last driven beat in **B** to **D**. (From Ferrier GR, Saunders JH, Mendez C: *Circ Res* 32:600, 1973.)

digitalis-like substance. In the absence of any driving stimuli, these fibers are quiescent.

In each panel of Fig. 15-32, a sequence of six driven depolarizations is induced at a specific basic cycle length. When the cycle length is 800 msec (Fig. 15-32, *A*), the last driven depolarization is followed by a brief, partial depolarization (DAD) that does not reach threshold. Once that after-depolarization subsides, the transmembrane potential remains constant until another driving stimulus is given. The upstroke of a DAD can be detected after each of the first five driven depolarizations.

When the basic cycle length is reduced to 700 msec (Fig. 15-32, *B*), the DAD that followed the last driven beat does reach threshold, and a nondriven depolarization (or extrasystole) ensues. This extrasystole is itself followed by an after-potential that is subthreshold. Reducing the basic cycle length to 600 msec (Fig. 15-32, *C*) also evokes an extrasystole after the last driven depolarization. The afterpotential that follows the extrasystole does reach threshold, however, and a second extrasystole occurs. When the six driven depolarizations are separated by intervals of 500 msec (Fig. 15-32, *D*), a sequence of three extrasystoles follows. Slightly shorter basic cycle lengths or slightly greater concentrations of acetylstrophanthidin evoke a long sequence of nondriven beats; such a sequence resembles a paroxysmal tachycardia (Fig. 15-40).

DADs are associated with elevated intracellular Ca^{2+} concentrations. The amplitudes of the DADs are increased by interventions that raise intracellular Ca^{2+} concentrations. Such interventions include increasing the extracellular Ca^{2+}

concentration and administering toxic amounts of digitalis glycosides. The elevated levels of intracellular Ca^{2+} provoke the oscillatory release of Ca^{2+} from the sarcoplasmic reticulum. Hence, in myocardial cells, DADs are accompanied by small, rhythmic changes in developed force. The high intracellular Ca^{2+} concentrations also activate certain membrane channels that permit the passage of Na^+ and K^+. The net flux of these cations constitutes a **transient inward current, i_{ti},** that contributes to the appearance of afterdepolarizations. The elevated intracellular Ca^{2+} concentration may also activate Na^+, Ca^{2+} exchange (see Chapter 1). This electrogenic exchanger, which pumps three Na^+ ions into the cell for each Ca^{2+} ion it ejects, also creates a net inward current of cations that contributes to the appearance of DADs.

ELECTROCARDIOGRAPHY

The ECG enables the physician to infer the course of the cardiac impulse by recording the variations in electrical potential at various loci on the surface of the body. By analyzing the details of these fluctuations of electrical potential, the physician gains valuable insight into (1) the anatomical orientation of the heart; (2) the relative sizes of its chambers; (3) various disturbances of rhythm and conduction; (4) the extent, location, and progress of ischemic damage to the myocardium; (5) the effects of altered electrolyte concentrations; and (6) the influence of certain drugs (notably digitalis, antiarrhythmic agents, and Ca^{2+} channel antagonists). Because electrocardiography is an extensive and complex discipline, only elementary principles are considered in this section.

Scalar Electrocardiography

In electrocardiography a **lead** is the electrical connection from the patient's skin to the recording device (electrocardiograph). The leads are connected to a **galvanometer** (a device that measures the strength of an electrical current) within the electrocardiograph. The systems of leads used to record routine ECGs are oriented in certain planes of the body. The diverse electromotive forces that exist in the heart at any moment can be represented by a three-dimensional **vector** (a quantity with magnitude and direction). A system of recording leads oriented in a given plane detects only the projection of the three-dimensional vector on that plane. The potential difference between two recording electrodes represents the **projection** of the vector on the line between the two leads. Components of vectors projected on such lines are not vectors but **scalar quantities** (having magnitude, but not direction). Hence, a recording of changes of the differences of potential between two points on the surface of the skin over time is called a **scalar ECG.**

The scalar ECG detects temporal changes of the electrical potential between some point on the surface of the skin and an indifferent electrode, or between pairs of points on the skin surface. The cardiac impulse progresses through the heart in a complex, three-dimensional pattern. Hence, the precise configuration of the ECG varies from individual to

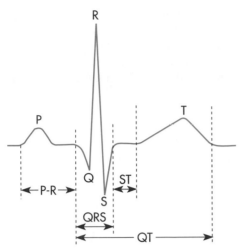

■ **Fig. 15-33** The important deflections and intervals of a typical scalar electrocardiogram.

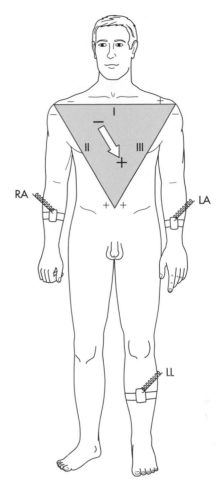

■ **Fig. 15-34** Einthoven triangle, illustrating the galvanometer connections for standard limb leads I, II, and III.

individual, and in any given individual the pattern varies with the anatomical location of the leads. The graphic display of the electrical impulse recorded by an ECG is called a **tracing.**

In general, a tracing consists of P, QRS, and T waves (Fig. 15-33). The PR interval (or more precisely, the PQ interval) is a measure of the time from the onset of atrial activation to the onset of ventricular activation; it normally ranges from 0.12 to 0.20 second. A considerable fraction of this time involves passage of the impulse through the AV conduction system. *Pathological prolongations of the PR interval are associated with disturbances of AV conduction. Such disturbances may be produced by inflammatory, circulatory, pharmacologic, or nervous mechanisms.*

The configuration and amplitude of the QRS complex vary considerably among individuals. The duration is usually between 0.06 and 0.10 second. An abnormally prolonged QRS complex may indicate a block in the normal conduction pathways through the ventricles (such as a block of the left or right bundle branch). During the ST interval, the entire ventricular myocardium is depolarized. Therefore, the ST segment normally lies on the **isoelectric line.** *Any appreciable deviation of the ST segment from the isoelectric line may indicate ischemic damage of the myocardium.* The QT interval is sometimes referred to as the period of "electrical systole" of the ventricles; the QT interval is closely correlated with the mean action potential duration of the ventricular myocytes. The QT interval duration is about 0.4 second, but it varies inversely with heart rate, mainly because the myocardial cell action potential duration varies inversely with heart rate (Fig. 15-17).

In most leads, the T wave is deflected in the same direction from the isoelectric line as is the major component of the QRS complex, although biphasic (that is, oppositely directed) T waves are perfectly normal in certain leads. Deviation of the T wave and QRS complex in the same direction from the isoelectric line indicates that the repolar-

ization process proceeds in a direction counter to that of the depolarization process. *T waves that are abnormal either in direction or in amplitude may indicate myocardial damage, electrolyte disturbances, or cardiac hypertrophy.*

Standard Limb Leads

The original ECG lead system was devised by Einthoven about one century ago. In his lead system, the vector sum of all cardiac electrical activity at any moment is called the **resultant cardiac vector.** This directional electrical force is considered to lie in the center of an equilateral triangle whose apices are located in the left and right shoulders and the pubic region (Fig. 15-34). This triangle, called **Einthoven's triangle,** is oriented in the frontal plane of the body. Hence, only the projection of the resultant cardiac vector on the frontal plane is detected by this system of leads. For convenience, the electrodes are connected to the right and left forearms rather than to the corresponding shoulders, because electrically the arms represent simple extensions of the leads from the shoulders. Similarly, the leg represents an extension of the lead system from the pubis, and thus the third electrode is usually connected to an ankle (usually the left one).

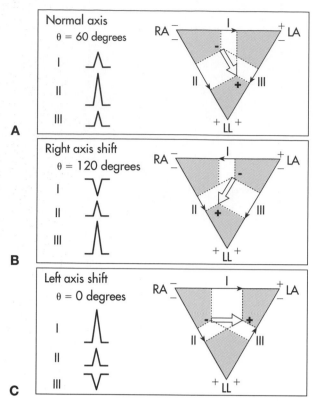

Fig. 15-35 Magnitude and direction of the QRS complexes in limb leads I, II, and III, when the mean electrical axis (Q) is 60 degrees (**A**), 120 degrees (**B**), and 0 degrees (**C**).

Certain conventions dictate the manner in which these standard limb leads are connected to the galvanometer. Lead I records the potential difference between the left arm *(LA)* and the right arm *(RA)*. The galvanometer connections are such that when the potential at *LA* (V_{LA}) exceeds the potential at *RA* (V_{RA}), the galvanometer stylus is deflected upward from the isoelectric line. In Figs. 15-34 and 15-35, this arrangement of the galvanometer connections for lead I is designated by a (+) at *LA* and by a (−) at *RA*. Lead II records the potential difference between *RA* and *LL* (left leg), and the stylus is deflected upward when V_{LL} exceeds V_{RA}. Finally, lead III registers the potential difference between *LA* and *LL*, and the stylus is deflected upward when V_{LL} exceeds V_{LA}. *These galvanometer connections were arbitrarily chosen so that the QRS complexes are upright in all three standard limb leads in most normal individuals.*

Let the frontal projection of the resultant cardiac vector at some moment be represented by an arrow (tail negative, head positive), as in Fig. 15-34. The potential difference, $V_{LA}-V_{RA}$, recorded in lead I is represented by the component of the vector projected along the horizontal line between *LA* and *RA*, also shown in Fig. 15-34. If the vector makes an angle, Θ, of 60 degrees with the horizontal line (as in Fig. 15-35, *A*), the magnitude of the potential recorded by lead I equals the vector magnitude times cosine 60 degrees. The deflection recorded in lead I is upward because the positive arrowhead lies closer to *LA* than to *RA*. The deflection in lead II is also upright because the arrowhead lies closer to

LL than to *RA*. The magnitude of the lead II deflection is greater than that in lead I because in this example the direction of the vector parallels that of lead II; therefore, the magnitude of the projection on lead II exceeds that on lead I. Similarly, in lead III, the deflection is upright and its magnitude equals that in lead I.

If the vector in Fig. 15-35, *A*, is the result of electrical events that occur during the peak of the QRS complex, the orientation of this vector is said to represent the **mean electrical axis** of the heart in the frontal plane. The positive rotatory direction of this axis is taken to be in the clockwise direction from the horizontal plane (contrary to the usual mathematical convention). In normal individuals, the average mean electrical axis is approximately +60 degrees (as in Fig. 15-35, *A*). Therefore, the QRS complexes are usually upright in all three leads and largest in lead II.

Changes in the mean electrical axis may occur if the anatomic position of the heart is altered or if the relative mass of the right and left ventricles is abnormal, as it is in certain cardiovascular disturbances. For example, the axis tends to shift toward the left (more horizontal) in short, stocky individuals and toward the right (more vertical) in tall, thin persons. Also, in left or right **ventricular hypertrophy** (increased myocardial mass of either ventricle), the axis shifts toward the hypertrophied side.

If the mean electrical axis shifts substantially to the right (as in Fig. 15-35, *B*, where Θ = 120 degrees), the projections of the QRS complexes on the standard leads change considerably. In this case, the largest upright deflection is in lead III, and the deflection in lead I is inverted because the arrowhead is closer to *RA* than to *LA*. When the axis shifts to the left (Fig. 15-35, *C*, where Θ = 0 degrees), the largest upright deflection is in lead I, and the QRS complex in lead III is inverted.

In addition to limb leads I, II, and III, other limb leads that are also oriented in the frontal plane are routinely recorded in patients. The axes of such **unipolar limb leads** form angles of +90, −30, and −150 degrees with the horizontal axis. Furthermore, the **precordial leads** are also recorded to determine the projections of the cardiac vector on the sagittal and transverse planes of the body. These precordial leads are recorded from six selected points on the anterior and lateral surfaces of the chest in the vicinity of the heart. The unipolar and precordial lead systems are described in all textbooks on electrocardiography and are not considered further here.

ARRHYTHMIAS

Cardiac arrhythmias reflect disturbances of either **impulse initiation** or **impulse propagation.** Disturbances of impulse initiation include those that arise from the SA node and those that originate from various ectopic foci. The principal disturbances of impulse propagation are conduction blocks and reentrant rhythms.

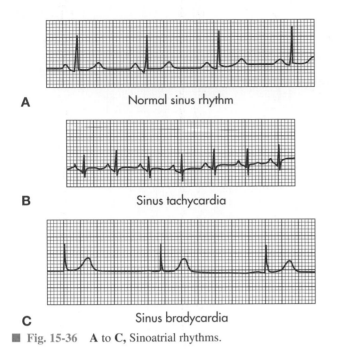

A Normal sinus rhythm

B Sinus tachycardia

C Sinus bradycardia

■ **Fig. 15-36** **A** to **C,** Sinoatrial rhythms.

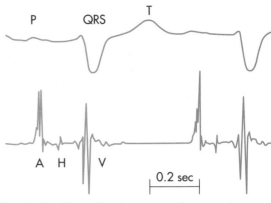

■ **Fig. 15-37** His bundle electrogram (*lower tracing,* retouched) and lead II of the scalar electrocardiogram *(upper tracing)*. The deflection, *H,* which represents the impulse conduction over the bundle of His, is clearly visible between the atrial *(A)* and the ventricular *(V)* deflections. The conduction time from the atria to the bundle of His is denoted by the A-H interval; that from the bundle of His to the ventricles, by the H-V interval. (Courtesy of Dr. J. Edelstein.)

Altered Sinoatrial Rhythms

Mechanisms that vary the firing frequency of cardiac pacemaker cells were described above (Fig. 15-20). Changes in the firing rate of the SA node are usually produced by the cardiac autonomic nerves. Examples of ECGs of **sinus tachycardia** and **sinus bradycardia** are shown in Fig. 15-36. The P, QRS, and T deflections are all normal, but the cardiac cycle duration (the PP interval) is altered. Characteristically, cardiac frequency changes gradually. A rhythmic variation of the PP interval at the respiratory frequency (i.e., a respiratory sinus arrhythmia) is a normal, common occurrence (see Fig. 17-10).

Atrioventricular Conduction Blocks

Various physiological, pharmacological, and pathological processes can impede impulse transmission through the AV conduction tissue. The site of block can be localized more precisely by recording the **His bundle electrogram** (Fig. 15-37). To obtain such tracings, an electrode catheter is introduced into a peripheral vein and threaded centrally into the right side of the heart until the electrode lies in the AV junctional region. When the electrode is properly positioned, a distinct deflection (*H* in Fig. 15-37) is registered as the cardiac impulse passes through the bundle of His. The time intervals required for propagation from the atrium to the bundle of His (A-H interval) and from the bundle of His to the ventricles (H-V interval) may be measured accurately. Abnormal prolongation of the A-H or H-V interval indicates block above or below the bundle of His, respectively.

Three degrees of AV block can be distinguished, as shown in Fig. 15-38. **First-degree AV block** is charac-

terized by a prolonged P-R interval. In Fig. 15-38, *A,* the P-R interval is 0.28 second; an interval greater than 0.20 second is abnormal. In most cases of first-degree block, the A-H interval is prolonged and the H-V interval is normal. Hence, the delay in a first-degree AV block is located above the His bundle (i.e., in the AV node).

In **second-degree AV block,** all QRS complexes are preceded by P waves, but not all P waves are followed by QRS complexes. The ratio of P waves to QRS complexes is usually the ratio of two small integers (such as 2:1, 3:1, or 3:2). Figure 15-38, *B,* illustrates a typical 2:1 block. The site of block may be located above or below the His bundle. A block below the bundle is usually more serious than one above the bundle, because the former is more likely to evolve into a third-degree block. An artificial pacemaker is frequently implanted when the block is below the bundle.

Third-degree AV block is often referred to as **complete heart block** because the impulse is completely unable to traverse the AV conduction pathway from atria to ventricles. The most common sites of complete block are distal to the bundle of His. In complete heart block, the atrial and ventricular rhythms are entirely independent, as shown in Fig. 15-38, *C.* Because of the slow ventricular rhythm (32 beats/min in this example), the volume of blood pumped by the heart is often inadequate, especially during muscular exercise. Third-degree block is often associated with **syncope** (pronounced lightheadedness), which is caused principally by insufficient cerebral blood flow. Third-degree block is one of the most common conditions that require artificial pacemakers.

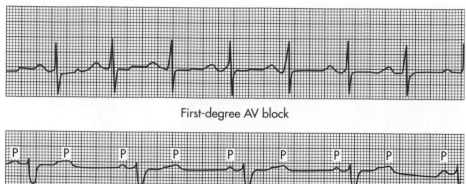

A   First-degree AV block

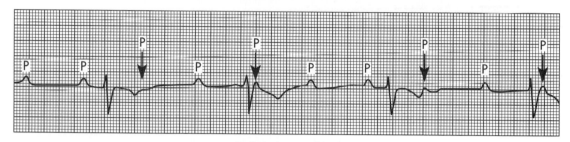

B   Second-degree AV block (2:1)

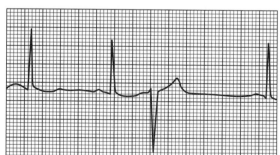

C   Third-degree AV block

■ **Fig. 15-38**   AV blocks. **A,** First-degree block; PR interval is 0.28 second. **B,** Second-degree block (2:1). **C,** Third-degree block; note the dissociation between the P waves and the QRS complexes.

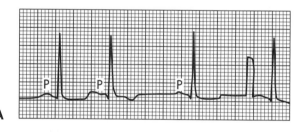

A

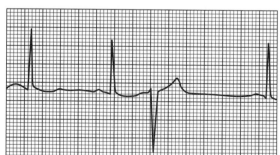

B

■ **Fig. 15-39**   A premature atrial depolarization (**A**) and a premature ventricular depolarization (**B**). The premature atrial depolarization (the second beat in the top tracing) is characterized by an inverted P wave and normal QRS and T waves. The interval after the premature depolarization is not much longer than the usual interval between beats. The brief rectangular deflection just before the last depolarization is a standardization signal. The premature ventricular depolarization is characterized by bizarre QRS and T waves and is followed by a compensatory pause.

Premature Depolarizations

Premature depolarizations occur occasionally in most normal individuals, but they arise more commonly under certain abnormal conditions. Such depolarizations may originate in the atria, AV junction, or ventricles. One type of premature depolarization follows a normally conducted depolarization after a constant time interval (the **coupling interval**). If the normal depolarization is suppressed in some way (e.g., by vagal stimulation), the premature depolarization is also abolished. Such premature depolarizations are called **coupled extrasystoles,** or simply **extrasystoles,** and they usually reflect a reentry phenomenon (Fig. 15-30). A second type of premature depolarization occurs as the result of enhanced automaticity in some ectopic focus. This ectopic center may fire regularly, and a zone of tissue that conducts unidirectionally may protect this center from being depolarized by the normal cardiac impulse. If this premature depolarization occurs at a regular interval or at an integer multiple of that interval, the disturbance is called **parasystole.**

A **premature atrial depolarization** is shown in Fig. 15-39, *A*. In the tracing, the normal interval between beats is 0.89 second (heart rate, 68 beats/min). The premature atrial depolarization (second P wave in the figure) follows the preceding P wave by only 0.56 second. The configuration of the premature P wave differs from the configuration of the other, normal P waves because the course of atrial excitation, which originates at some ectopic focus in the atrium, differs

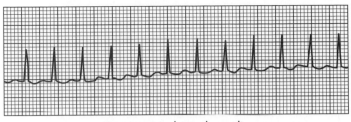

A Supraventricular tachycardia

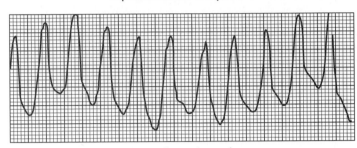

B Ventricular tachycardia

■ **Fig. 15-40** **A** and **B,** Paroxysmal tachycardias.

from the normal spread of excitation, which originates at the SA node. The configuration of the QRS complex of the premature depolarization is usually normal because the ventricular excitation spreads over the usual pathways.

A **premature ventricular depolarization** appears in Fig. 15-39, *B*. Because the premature excitation originates at some ectopic focus in the ventricles, the impulse propagation is abnormal and the configurations of the QRS and T waves are entirely different from the normal ventricular deflections. The premature QRS complex follows the preceding normal QRS complex by only 0.47 second. The interval after the premature excitation is 1.28 seconds, which is considerably longer than the normal interval between beats (0.89 second). The interval (1.75 seconds) from the QRS complex just before the premature excitation to the QRS complex just after it is virtually equal to the duration of two normal cardiac cycles (0.89 + 0.89 = 1.78 seconds).

The prolonged interval that usually follows a premature ventricular depolarization is called a **compensatory pause.** This pause occurs because the ectopic ventricular impulse does not disturb the natural rhythm of the SA node, either because the ectopic ventricular impulse is not conducted retrograde through the AV conduction system or because the SA node had already fired at its natural interval before the ectopic impulse could have reached it and depolarized it prematurely. Likewise, the SA nodal impulse generated just before or after the ventricular extrasystole usually does not affect the ventricle, because the AV junction and perhaps also the ventricles are still refractory from the premature ventricular excitation. In Fig. 15-39, *B*, the P wave associated with the extrasystole occurs synchronously with the T wave of the premature ventricular depolarization, and therefore it cannot easily be identified in the tracing.

Ectopic Tachycardias

In contrast to the gradual rate changes that characterize sinus tachycardia, tachycardias that originate from an ectopic focus typically begin and end abruptly. Hence, such ectopic tachycardias are usually called **paroxysmal tachycardias.** Episodes of paroxysmal tachycardia may persist for only a few beats or for many hours or days, and episodes often recur. Paroxysmal tachycardias may result from (1) the rapid firing of an ectopic pacemaker, (2) triggered activity secondary to afterpotentials that reach threshold, or (3) an impulse that circles a reentry loop repetitively.

Paroxysmal tachycardias that originate either in the atria or in the AV junctional tissues (Fig. 15-40, *A*) are usually indistinguishable, and therefore both are included in the term **paroxysmal supraventricular tachycardia.** In this tachycardia, the impulse often circles a reentry loop that includes atrial and AV junctional tissue. The QRS complexes are often normal, because ventricular activation proceeds over the usual pathways.

As its name implies, **paroxysmal ventricular tachycardia** originates from an ectopic focus in the ventricles. The ECG is characterized by repeated, bizarre QRS complexes that reflect the abnormal intraventricular impulse conduction (Fig. 15-40, *B*). Paroxysmal ventricular tachycardia is much more ominous than supraventricular tachycardia, because the former is frequently a precursor of ventricular fibrillation, a lethal arrhythmia described in the next section.

Fibrillation

Under certain conditions, cardiac muscle undergoes an irregular type of contraction that is entirely ineffectual in propelling blood. Such an arrhythmia is termed **fibrillation,** and the disturbance may involve either the atria or the ventricles. Fibrillation probably represents a reentry phenomenon, in which the reentry loop fragments into multiple, irregular circuits.

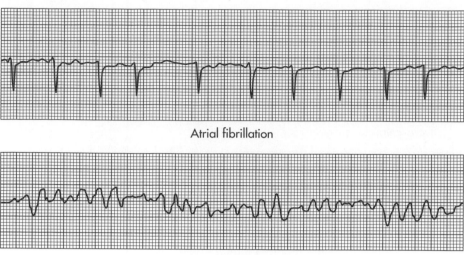

Atrial fibrillation

Ventricular fibrillation

■ **Fig. 15-41** Atrial and ventricular fibrillation.

The ECG changes in **atrial fibrillation** are shown in Fig. 15-41, *A*. This arrhythmia occurs in various types of chronic heart disease. The atria do not contract and relax sequentially during each cardiac cycle, and thus they do not contribute to ventricular filling. Instead, the atria undergo a continuous, uncoordinated, rippling motion. P waves do not appear in the ECG; they are replaced by continuous irregular fluctuations of potential, called **f waves.** The AV node is activated at intervals that may vary considerably from cycle to cycle. Hence, no constant interval occurs between successive QRS complexes or between successive ventricular contractions. Because the strength of ventricular contraction depends on the interval between beats (see Figure 17-20), the volume and rhythm of the pulse are irregular. In many patients, the atrial reentry loop and the pattern of AV conduction are more regular than they are in atrial fibrillation. The rhythm is then referred to as atrial flutter.

Atrial fibrillation and flutter are usually not life threatening; some people with these disturbances can function normally. However, because the atria do not contract and relax rhythmically, blood clots tend to form in the atria. Such clots may then travel to the pulmonary or systemic vascular beds. Hence, patients with atrial fibrillation or flutter are usually treated with anticoagulant drugs, such as **dicumarol.**

Ventricular fibrillation, on the other hand, leads to loss of consciousness within a few seconds. The irregular, continuous, uncoordinated twitchings of the ventricular muscle fibers pump no blood. Death ensues unless immediate effective resuscitation is achieved or unless the rhythm spontaneously reverts to normal, which rarely occurs. Ventricular fibrillation may supervene when the entire ventricle, or some portion of it, is deprived of its normal blood supply. It may also occur as a result of electrocution or in response to certain drugs and anesthetics.

In the ECG (Fig. 15-41, *B*), the fluctuations of potential are high irregular.

Ventricular fibrillation is often initiated when a premature impulse arrives during the **vulnerable period** of the cardiac cycle. This period coincides with the downslope of the T wave of the ECG. During this period, the excitability of the cardiac cells varies spatially. Some fibers are still in their effective refractory periods; others have almost fully recovered their excitability; and still others are able to conduct impulses but only at very slow conduction velocities. Consequently, the action potentials are propagated over the chambers in many irregular wavelets that travel along circuitous paths and at various conduction velocities. As a region of cardiac cells becomes excitable again, it is ultimately reentered by one of the wave fronts traveling around the chamber. Hence, the process is self-sustaining.

Several congenital forms of the long QT syndrome (Fig. 15-42) have been identified in human subjects. Two genes that have been identified as the basis for this syndrome are the HERG gene (a putative potassium gene), located on chromosome 7, and the SCN5A gene (a putative sodium gene), located on chromosome 3. Patients with the congenital form of the long QT syndrome may have periodic episodes of syncope (fainting), and about 10% of pediatric subjects with this disorder may die suddenly, without any preceding symptoms.

Atrial fibrillation may be changed to a normal sinus rhythm by drugs that prolong the refractory period. As the cardiac impulse completes the reentry loop, it may then encounter refractory myocardial fibers. When atrial fibrillation does not respond adequately to drugs, electrical defibrillation may be used to correct this condition.

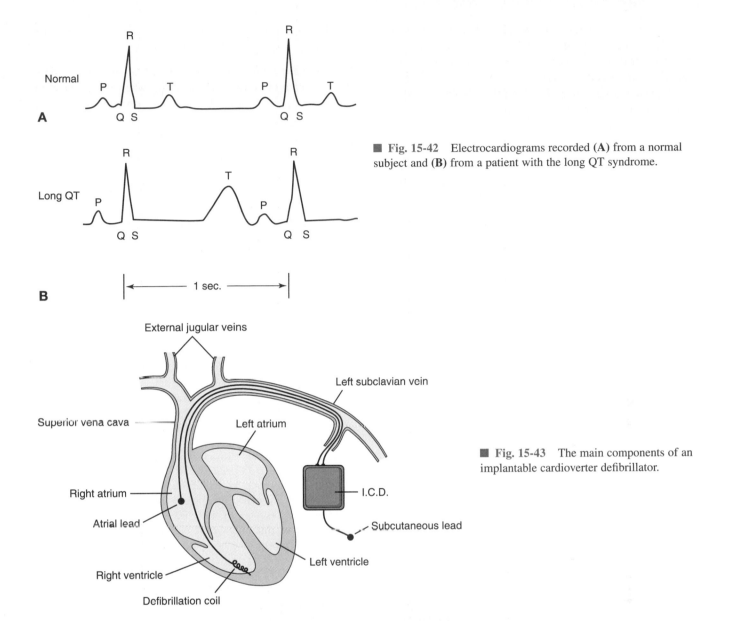

■ **Fig. 15-42** Electrocardiograms recorded (**A**) from a normal subject and (**B**) from a patient with the long QT syndrome.

■ **Fig. 15-43** The main components of an implantable cardioverter defibrillator.

Dramatic therapy is required in ventricular fibrillation. Conversion to a normal sinus rhythm is accomplished by means of a strong electrical current that places the entire myocardium briefly in a refractory state. Techniques have been developed to administer the current safely through the intact chest wall. In successful cases, the SA node again takes over the normal pacemaker function for the entire heart.

Implantable cardioverter defibrillator (ICD) devices (Fig. 15-43) have recently been developed to prevent death in patients who have suddenly developed either ventricular fibrillation or paroxysmal ventricular tachycardia. The former is lethal unless it is treated immediately, and the latter often leads to ventricular fibrillation and sudden death. The ICD device is implanted subcutaneously in the left subclavicular region of the chest wall. Atrial and ventricular leads permit the recording of the right atrial and right ventricular electrograms and provide the ability for right atrial or right ventricular pacing, or

both. The defibrillation coil in the right atrium permits the application of a strong electrical current to the ventricle, and thereby usually terminates the lethal arrythmia.

SUMMARY

1. The transmembrane action potentials that can be recorded from cardiac myocytes contain the following five phases:

Phase 0: The action potential upstroke is initiated when a suprathreshold stimulus rapidly depolarizes the membrane by activating the fast Na^+ channels.

Phase 1: The notch is an early partial repolarization that is achieved by the efflux of K^+ through transmembrane channels that conduct the transient outward current, i_{to}.

Phase 2: The plateau represents a balance between the influx of Ca^{2+} through transmembrane Ca^{2+} channels and the efflux of K^+ through several types of K^+ channels.

Phase 3: Final repolarization is initiated when the efflux of K^+ exceeds the influx of Ca^{2+}. The resultant partial repolarization rapidly increases the K^+ conductance and rapidly restores full repolarization.

Phase 4: The resting potential of the fully repolarized cell is determined by conductance of the cell membrane to K^+ mainly through i_{K1} channels.

2. Fast-response action potentials are recorded from atrial and ventricular myocardial fibers and from ventricular specialized conducting (Purkinje) fibers. The action potential is characterized by a large amplitude, a steep upstroke, and a relatively long plateau.

3. The effective refractory period of fast-response fibers begins at the upstroke of the action potential and persists until midway through phase 3. The fiber is relatively refractory during the remainder of phase 3, and it regains full excitability when it is fully repolarized (phase 4).

4. Slow-response action potentials are recorded from normal SA and AV nodal cells and from abnormal myocardial cells that have been partially depolarized. The action potential is characterized by a less negative resting potential, a smaller amplitude, a less steep upstroke, and a shorter plateau than is typical of the fast-response action potential. The upstroke in slow response fibers is produced by the activation of Ca^{2+} channels.

5. Slow-response fibers become absolutely refractory at the beginning of the upstroke, and partial excitability may not be regained until very late in phase 3 or until after the fiber is fully repolarized.

6. Automaticity is characteristic of certain cells in the SA and AV nodes and in the ventricular specialized conducting system. Slow depolarization of the membrane during phase 4 is the hallmark of automaticity.

7. Normally the SA node initiates the impulse that induces cardiac contraction. This impulse is propagated from the SA node to the atrial tissues and ultimately reaches the AV node. After a delay in the AV node, the cardiac impulse is propagated throughout the ventricles.

8. Ectopic foci in the atrium, AV node, or His-Purkinje system may initiate propagated cardiac impulses if the normal pacemaker cells in the SA node are suppressed or if the rhythmicity of the ectopic automatic cells is abnormally enhanced.

9. Under certain abnormal conditions, afterdepolarizations may appear early in phase 3 of a normally initiated heart beat, or the afterdepolarizations may be delayed until near the end of phase 3 or the beginning of phase 4. Such after-depolarizations may themselves trigger propagated impulses.

10. Early afterdepolarizations are more likely to occur when the basic cycle length of the initiating beats is very long and when the cardiac action potentials are abnormally prolonged. Delayed afterdepolarizations are more likely to occur when the basic cycle length of the initiating beats is short and when cardiac cells are overloaded with Ca^{2+}.

11. Simple conduction block is the retardation or failure of impulse propagation in a cardiac fiber.

12. A cardiac impulse may traverse a loop of cardiac fibers and reenter previously excited tissue when the impulse is conducted slowly around the loop, and when the impulse is blocked unidirectionally in some section of the loop.

13. The electrocardiogram (ECG), which is recorded from the surface of the body, traces the conduction of the cardiac impulse throughout the heart.

14. The ECG may be used to detect and analyze certain cardiac arrhythmias, such as altered sinoatrial rhythms, AV conduction blocks, premature depolarizations, ectopic tachycardias, and atrial and ventricular fibrillation.

BIBLIOGRAPHY

Journal articles

Baker JC et al: Enhanced dispersion of repolarization and refractoriness in transgenic mouse hearts promotes reentrant ventricular tachycardia, *Circ Res* 86:396, 2000.

Demir SS et al: Parasympathetic modulation of sinoatrial node pacemaker activity in rabbit heart: a unifying model, *Am J Physiol* 276:H2221, 1999.

Irisawa H, Brown HF, Giles W: Cardiac pacemaking in the sinoatrial node, *Physiol Rev* 73:197, 1993.

Priori SG: Long QT and Brugada syndromes: from genetics to clinical management, *J Cardiovasc Electrophysiol* 11:1174, 2000.

Roden DM, George AL Jr, Bennett PB: Recent advances in understanding the molecular mechanisms of the long QT syndrome, *J Cardiovasc Electrophysiol* 6:1023, 1995.

Rogers JM et al: Incidence, evolution, and spatial distribution of functional reentry during ventricular fibrillation in pigs, *Circ Res* 84:945, 1999.

Sanguinetti MC, Keating MT: Role of delayed rectified potassium channels in cardiac repolarization and arrhythmias, *New Physiol Sci* 12:152, 1997.

Schuessler RB, Boineau JP, Bromberg BI: Origin of the sinus impulse, *J Cardiovasc Electrophysiol* 7:263, 1996.

Sicouri S, Antzelevitch C: Electrophysiologic characteristics of M cells in the canine left ventricular free wall, *J Cardiovasc Electrophysiol* 6:591, 1995.

Tamaddon HS et al: High resolution optical mapping of the right bundle branch in connexin40 knockout mice reveals slow conduction in the specialized conduction system, *Circ Res* 87:929, 2000.

Trépanier-Boulay V et al: Gender-based differences in cardiac repolarization in mouse ventricle, *Circ Res* 89:437, 2001.

Van Waggoner DR et al: Atrial L-type Ca^{2+} currents and human atrial fibrillation, *Circ Res* 85:428, 1999.

Books and monographs

Levy MN, Schwartz PJ: *Vagal control of the heart: experimental basis and clinical implications,* Armonk, NY, 1994, Futura Publishing.

Mazgalev T, Tchou PJ: *Atrial-AV nodal electrophysiology: a view from the millenium,* Armonk, NY, 2000, Futura Publishing.

Saoudi N, Schoels W, El-Sherif N: *Atrial flutter and fibrillation: from basis to clinical applications,* Armonk NY, 1998, Futura Publishing.

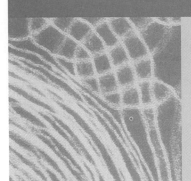

chapter sixteen

The Cardiac Pump

The staggering amount of work performed by the heart over an individual's lifetime is impressive. A useful way to understand how the heart accomplishes its important task is to consider the relationships between the structure and function of its components.

RELATION OF THE HEART STRUCTURE TO FUNCTION

The Myocardial Cell

Many important morphological and functional differences exist between myocardial and skeletal muscle cells. Despite these differences, the contractile elements within the two types of cells are quite similar. Each skeletal and cardiac muscle cell is composed of **sarcomeres** (from Z-line to Z-line) containing thick and thin filaments. Thick filaments are composed of myosin (in the band), whereas thin filaments contain actin. The thin filaments extend from the point at which they are anchored to the Z-line (through the I-band) to interdigitate with the thick filaments. As in skeletal muscle, shortening of cardiac muscle filaments occurs by the **sliding filament mechanism.** Actin filaments slide along adjacent myosin filaments by cycling of the intervening cross-bridges and thereby bring the Z-lines closer together (see Chapter 12).

Skeletal and cardiac muscle show similar length-force relationships. The developed force is maximal when the muscle begins its contractions at resting sarcomere lengths of 2 to 2.4 μm. At this resting length, the overlap of thick and thin filaments is optimal, and the number of cross-bridge attachments is maximal. Stretch of the myocardium by increases in load enhances the affinity of troponin C for Ca^{2+}. How an increase in sarcomere length increases the sensitivity of the myofilaments to calcium is not known. One hypothesis is that the thick and thin filaments are brought closer to each other as the diameter of the muscle fiber decreases during stretch. When sarcomeres are stretched beyond the optimal length, the developed force of cardiac muscle drops to less than the maximal value owing to less overlap of the filaments and hence less cycling of the cross-bridges (see Chapter 12). At resting sarcomere lengths shorter than the optimal value, the thin filaments overlap, which diminishes contractile force.

In general, the fiber length-force relationship for the isolated papillary muscle also holds true for fibers in the intact heart. This relationship may be expressed graphically, as in Fig. 16-1, by substituting ventricular systolic pressure for force, and end-diastolic ventricular volume for resting myocardial fiber (and hence sarcomere) length. The lower curve in Fig. 16-1 represents the increment in pressure produced by each increment in volume when the heart is in diastole. The upper curve represents the peak pressure developed by the ventricle during systole as a function of the filling pressure. This curve illustrates the **Frank-Starling relationship** (also called *Starling's law of the heart*).

Note that the pressure-volume curve during diastole is initially quite flat, which indicates that large increases in volume can be accommodated with only small increases in pressure. In contrast, systolic pressure development is considerable at the lower filling pressures. However, the ventricle becomes much less distensible with greater filling, as evidenced by the sharp rise of the diastolic curve at large intraventricular volumes.

In the normal intact heart, peak force may be attained at a filling pressure of about 12 mm Hg. At this intraventricular diastolic pressure, which is near the upper limit observed in the normal heart, the sarcomere length is 2.2 μm. However, developed force peaks at filling pressures as high as 30 mm Hg in the isolated heart. At even higher diastolic pressures (>50 mm Hg), the sarcomere length is not greater than 2.6 μm. This ability of the myocardium to resist stretch at high filling pressures probably resides in the noncontractile constituents of the heart tissue (connective tissue), and it may serve as a safety factor against overloading of the heart in diastole. Usually, ventricular diastolic pressure is about 0 to 7 mm Hg, and the average diastolic sarcomere length is about 2.2 μm. Thus, *the normal heart operates on the ascending portion of the Frank-Starling curve* depicted in Fig. 16-1.

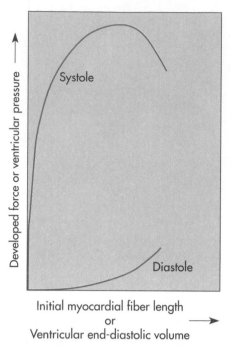

■ Fig. 16-1   Relationship of myocardial resting fiber length (sarcomere length) or end-diastolic volume to developed force or peak systolic ventricular pressure during ventricular contraction in the intact dog heart. (Redrawn from Patterson SW, Piper H, Starling EH: *J Physiol* 48:465, 1914.)

If the heart becomes greatly distended with blood during diastole, as may occur in **cardiac failure,** it functions less efficiently. More energy is required (greater wall tension) for the distended heart to eject a given volume of blood per beat than is required for the normal undilated heart. The less efficient pumping of the distended heart is an example of Laplace's law (see Chapter 20), which states that the tension in the wall of a vessel or chamber (in this case the ventricles) equals the transmural pressure (pressure across the wall, or distending pressure) times the radius of the vessel or chamber. The Laplace relationship ordinarily applies to infinitely thin-walled vessels, but it can be applied to the heart if correction is made for wall thickness. The equation is $\tau = Pr/w$, where τ = wall stress, P = transmural pressure, r = radius, and w = wall thickness.

The Cardiac Pump

Functional anatomy of cardiac muscle. A striking difference between the cardiac and skeletal muscle is that cardiac muscle fibers possess branching interconnections, whereas skeletal muscle does not (Figs. 16-2 and 16-3). Laterally, the myocardial fibers are separated from adjacent fibers by their respective sarcolemmas, and the end of each fiber is separated from its neighbor by dense structures, **intercalated disks,** that are continuous with the sarcolemma (Figs. 16-2 to 16-4). Nevertheless, *cardiac muscle functions as a syncytium;* that is, a stimulus applied to any one part of the cardiac muscle results in the contraction of the entire muscle. A wave of depolarization followed by contraction of the entire myocardium (an *all-or-none response*) occurs when a suprathreshold stimulus is applied to any one focus.

As the wave of excitation approaches the end of a cardiac cell, the spread of excitation to the next cell depends on the level of the electrical conductance of the boundary between the two cells. **Gap junctions (nexi)** with high conductances are present in the intercalated disks between adjacent cells (Figs. 16-2 to 16-4). These gap junctions, which facilitate the conduction of the cardiac impulse from one cell to the next, are made up of **connexons,** hexagonal structures that connect the cytosol of adjacent cells. Each connexon consists of six polypeptides that surround a core channel approximately 1.6 to 2.0 mm wide. Each channel thus serves as a low-resistance pathway for cell-to-cell conductance (see Chapter 4).

Impulse conduction in cardiac tissues progresses more rapidly in a direction parallel to the long axes of the constituent fibers than in a direction perpendicular to the long axes of those fibers. Gap junctions exist in the borders between myocardial fibers that are in contact with each other longitudinally; they are sparse or absent in the borders between myocardial fibers that lie side by side.

Another difference between cardiac and fast skeletal muscle fibers is in the number of mitochondria (**sarcosomes)** in the two tissues. Fast skeletal muscle is called on for relatively short periods of repetitive or sustained contraction, and it can metabolize anaerobically and build up a substantial oxygen debt. Fast skeletal muscle fibers contain relatively few mitochondria. In contrast, cardiac muscle contracts repetitively for a lifetime, and hence it requires a continuous supply of oxygen. Cardiac muscle is therefore very rich in mitochondria (Figs. 16-2 to 16-4). The large number of mitochondria—which contain the enzymes necessary for oxidative phosphorylation—permits the rapid oxidation of substrates and the synthesis of adenosine triphosphate (ATP) and thus sustains the myocardial energy requirements.

To provide adequate oxygen and substrate for its metabolic machinery, the myocardium is also endowed with a rich capillary supply, about one capillary per fiber. Thus, diffusion distances are short, and oxygen, carbon dioxide, substrates, and waste material can move rapidly between the myocardial cell and capillary. A structure called the **transverse (T)-tubular system** within myocardial cells participates in this exchange of substances between the capillary blood and the myocardial cells. In electron micrographs of myocardium, the T-tubular system appears as deep invaginations of the sarcolemma into the fiber at the Z-lines (Figs. 16-2 to 16-4). The lumina of these T-tubules are continuous with the bulk interstitial fluid, and they play a key role in excitation-contraction coupling.

In mammalian ventricular cells, adjacent T-tubules are interconnected by longitudinal or axial tubules, and thus form an extensively interconnected lattice of "intracellular" tubules (Fig. 16-4). This T-tubule system is open to the interstitial fluid, it is lined with a basement membrane continuous

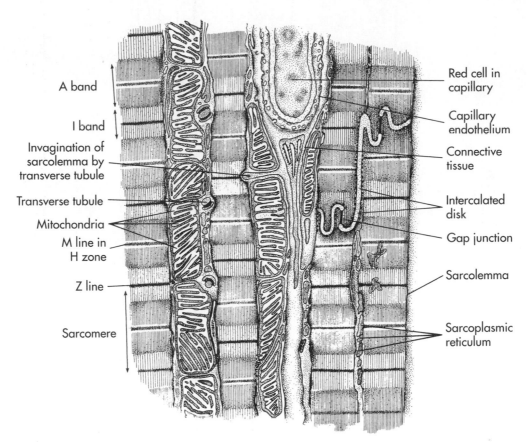

A band
I band
Invagination of sarcolemma by transverse tubule
Transverse tubule
Mitochondria
M line in H zone
Z line
Sarcomere

Red cell in capillary
Capillary endothelium
Connective tissue
Intercalated disk
Gap junction
Sarcolemma
Sarcoplasmic reticulum

■ **Fig. 16-2** Diagram of an electron micrograph of cardiac muscle showing large numbers of mitochondria and the intercalated disks with nexi (gap junction), transverse tubules, and longitudinal tubules.

with that of the surface sarcolemma, and it contains micropinocytotic vesicles. Thus, in ventricular cells, the T-tubular system provides the myofibrils and mitochondria with ready access to the interstitial fluid. The T-tubular system is absent or poorly developed in atrial cells of many mammals.

A network of **sarcoplasmic reticulum** (Fig. 16-4), consisting of small-diameter sarcotubules, also surrounds the myofibrils. These sarcotubules appear to be "closed," because colloidal tracer particles (2 to 10 nm in diameter) do not enter them. They do not contain basement membrane. Flattened elements of the sarcoplasmic reticulum are often close to the T-tubular system and to the surface sarcolemma, and they form **diads.**

Excitation-contraction coupling. The earliest studies on isolated hearts perfused with isotonic saline solutions indicated that optimal concentrations of Na^+, K^+, and Ca^{2+} are necessary for cardiac muscle contraction. Without Na^+, the heart is not excitable and will not beat. In contrast, the resting membrane potential is independent of the Na ion gradient across the membrane (see Fig. 15-5). Under normal conditions, the extracellular K^+ concentration is about 4 mM. A reduction in extracellular K^+ has little effect on myocardial excitation and contraction. However, increases in extracellular K^+, if great enough, produce depolarization, loss of excitability of the myocardial cells, and cardiac arrest in diastole. Ca^{2+} is also essential for cardiac contraction.

Removal of Ca^{2+} from the extracellular fluid results in decreased contractile force and eventual arrest in diastole. Conversely, an increase in extracellular Ca^{2+} enhances contractile force, and very high Ca^{2+} concentrations induce cardiac arrest in systole (rigor). *The free intracellular Ca^{2+} concentration is the factor principally responsible for the contractile state of the myocardium.*

Cardiac muscle is excited when a wave of excitation spreads rapidly along the myocardial sarcolemma from cell to cell via gap junctions. Excitation also spreads into the interior of the cells via the T-tubules (Figs. 16-2 to 16-4), which invaginate into the cardiac fibers at the Z-lines. Electrical stimulation at the Z-line or the application of Ca^{2+} to the Z-lines in the skinned (sarcolemma removed) cardiac fiber elicits a localized contraction of the adjacent myofibrils. During the plateau (phase 2) of the action potential, Ca^{2+} permeability of the sarcolemma increases. Ca^{2+} flows down its electrochemical gradient and enters the cell through Ca^{2+} channels in the sarcolemma and in the T-tubules (see also Chapters 12 and 15).

Opening of the Ca^{2+} channels is initiated by phosphorylation of the channel proteins by a cyclic adenosine monophosphate (cAMP)-dependent protein kinase. The primary source of extracellular Ca^{2+} is the interstitial fluid (10^{-3} M Ca^{2+}). Some Ca^{2+} may also be bound to the sarcolemma and to the **glycocalyx,** a mucopolysaccharide that covers the sarcolemma. The amount of calcium that enters the cell

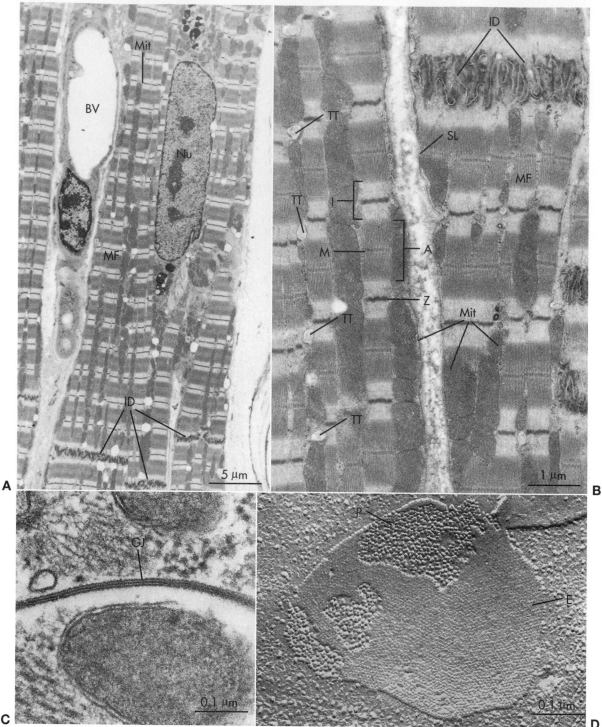

■ **Fig. 16-3** **A,** Low-magnification electron micrograph of a monkey heart (ventricle). Typical features of myocardial cells include the elongated nucleus *(Nu)*, striated myofibrils *(MF)* with columns of mitochondria *(Mit)* between the myofibrils, and intercellular junctions (intercalated disks, *ID*). A blood vessel *(BV)* is located between two myocardial cells. **B,** Medium-magnification electron micrograph of monkey ventricular cells showing details of the ultrastructure. The sarcolemma *(SL)* is the boundary of the muscle cells and is thrown into multiple folds where the cells meet at the intercalated disk region *(ID)*. The prominent myofibrils *(MF)* show distinct banding patterns, including the A-band *(A)*, dark Z-lines *(Z)*, I-band regions *(I)*, and M-lines *(M)* at the center of each sarcomere unit. Mitochondria *(Mit)* occur either in rows between myofibrils or in masses just underneath the sarcolemma. Regularly spaced transverse tubules *(TT)* appear at the Z-line levels of the myofibrils. **C,** High-magnification electron micrograph of a specialized intercellular junction between two myocardial cells of the mouse. Called a gap junction *(GJ)* or nexus, this attachment consists of very close apposition of the sarcolemmal membranes of the two cells and appears in thin section to consist of seven layers. **D,** Freeze-fracture replica of mouse myocardial gap junction, showing distinct arrays of characteristic intramembranous particles. Large particles *(P)* belong to the inner half of the sarcolemma of one myocardial cell, whereas the "pitted" membrane face *(E)* is formed by the outer half of the sarcolemma of the cell above.

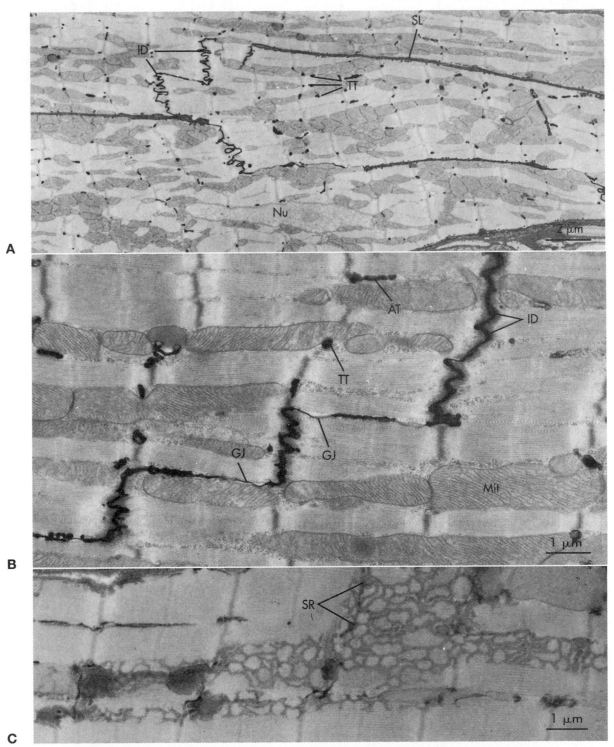

■ **Fig. 16-4** **A,** Low-magnification electron micrograph of the right ventricular wall of a mouse heart. Tissue was fixed in a phosphate-buffered glutaraldehyde solution and postfixed in ferro-cyanide-reduced osmium tetroxide. This procedure has resulted in the deposition of electron-opaque precipitate in the extracellular space, thus outlining the sarcolemmal borders *(SL)* of the muscle cells and delineating the intercalated disks *(ID)* and transverse tubules *(TT)*. *Nu,* Nucleus of the myocar-dial cell. **B,** Mouse cardiac muscle in longitudinal section, treated as in **A.** The path of the extracel-lular space is traced through the intercalated disk region *(ID)*, and sarcolemmal invaginations that are oriented transverse to the cell axis (transverse tubules, *TT*) or parallel to it (axial tubules, *AT*) are clearly identified. Gap junctions *(GJ)* are associated with the intercalated disk. Mitochondria are large and elongated and lie between the myofibrils. **C,** Mouse cardiac muscle. Tissue was treated with ferrocyanide-reduced osmium tetroxide to identify the internal membrane system (sarcoplasmic reticulum, *SR*). Specific staining of the SR reveals its architecture as a complex network of small-diameter tubules that are closely associated with the myofibrils and mitochondria.

interior from the extracellular space is not sufficient to induce contraction of the myofibrils. Instead, it acts as a trigger (**trigger Ca²⁺**) to release Ca²⁺ from the sarcoplasmic reticulum, where the intracellular Ca²⁺ is stored (Fig. 16-5). The concentration of free Ca²⁺ in the cytoplasm increases from a resting level of about 10^{-7} M to levels of about 10^{-5} M during excitation. This Ca²⁺ then binds to the protein, troponin C. The Ca²⁺-troponin complex interacts with tropomyosin to unblock active sites between the actin and myosin filaments. This unblocking initiates cross-bridge cycling and hence contraction of the myofibrils (see Chapter 12).

Mechanisms that raise the cytosolic Ca²⁺ concentration increase the developed force, and those that lower the cystolic Ca²⁺ concentration decrease the developed force. For example, catecholamines increase the movement of Ca²⁺ into the cell by phosphorylation of the channels via a cAMP-dependent protein kinase (see also Chapters 12 and 15). In addition, catecholamines, like other agonists, enhance myocardial contractile force by increasing the sensitivity of the contractile machinery to Ca²⁺. Increasing the extracellular concentration of Ca²⁺ or decreasing the Na⁺ gradient across

the sarcolemma also results in an increase in the cytosolic concentration of Ca²⁺.

The sodium gradient can be reduced by increasing the intracellular concentration of Na⁺ or by decreasing the extracellular concentration of Na⁺. Cardiac glycosides increase intracellular Na⁺ concentration by inhibiting the Na⁺,K⁺-ATPase, and thereby raise the concentration of Na⁺ in the cells. The elevated cytosolic Na⁺ reverses the direction of the Na⁺,Ca²⁺ exchanger, and therefore less Ca²⁺ is removed from the cell. A lowered extracellular Na⁺ concentration causes less Na⁺ to enter the cell, and hence less Na⁺ is exchanged for Ca²⁺ (Fig. 16-5).

Developed tension in myocardial fibers is diminished by a reduction in extracellular Ca²⁺ concentration, by an increase in the Na⁺ gradient across the sarcolemma, or by the administration of a Ca²⁺ channel antagonist that prevents Ca²⁺ from entering the myocardial cell (see Fig. 15-11).

A patient in **heart failure** usually has a dilated heart, low cardiac output, fluid retention, high venous pressure, an enlarged liver, and peripheral edema, and he or she is

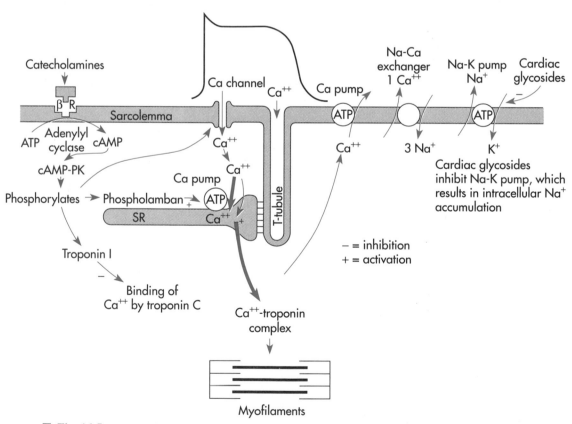

■ **Fig. 16-5**   Schematic diagram of the movements of calcium in excitation-contraction coupling in cardiac muscle. The influx of Ca²⁺ from the interstitial fluid during excitation triggers the release of Ca²⁺ from the saroplasmic reticulum *(SR)*. The free cytosolic Ca²⁺ activates contraction of the myofilaments (systole). Relaxation (diastole) occurs as a result of uptake of Ca²⁺ by the sarcoplasmic reticulum, by extrusion of intracellular Ca²⁺ by Na⁺-Ca²⁺ exchange, and to a limited degree by the Ca pump. bR, β-Adrenergic receptor; *cAMP*, cyclic adenosine monophosphate; *cAMP-PK*, cyclic AMP-dependent protein kinase.

often treated with digitalis and a diuretic. The digitalis increases cardiomyocyte intracellular calcium, and thereby enhances contractile force. The diuretic reduces extracellular fluid volume, and thereby decreases the volume load (preload) on the heart and the venous pressure, liver congestion, and edema.

At the end of systole, the Ca^{2+} influx stops, and the sarcoplasmic reticulum is no longer stimulated to release Ca^{2+}. In fact, the sarcoplasmic reticulum avidly takes up Ca^{2+} by means of an ATP-energized calcium pump. This pump is stimulated by the protein, **phospholamban,** after the phospholamban has been phosphorylated by cAMP-dependent protein kinase. In addition, phosphorylation of troponin I inhibits the binding of Ca^{2+} to troponin C. This process permits tropomyosin to again block the sites for interaction between the actin and myosin filaments, and relaxation (diastole) occurs (see also Chapter 12).

Cardiac contraction and relaxation are both accelerated by catecholamines and adenylyl cyclase activation. The resulting increase in cAMP activates the cAMP-dependent protein kinase, which phosphorylates the Ca channel in the sarcolemma. These events cause more Ca^{2+} to move into the cell, and hence they accelerate contraction. However, these events also accelerate *relaxation* (1) by phosphorylating phospholamban, which enhances Ca^{2+} uptake by the sarcoplasmic reticulum, and (2) by phosphorylating troponin I, which inhibits the Ca^{2+} binding of troponin C. Thus, the phosphorylations by cAMP-dependent protein kinase increase the speeds of contraction and of relaxation.

Mitochondria also take up and release Ca^{2+}, but the process is too slow to affect normal excitation-contraction coupling. Only at pathologically high intracellular Ca^{2+} levels do the mitochondria take up a significant amount of Ca^{2+}.

The Ca^{2+} that enters the cell to initiate contraction must be removed during diastole. The removal is primarily accomplished by the exchange of three Na^+ ions for one Ca^{2+} ion (Fig. 16-5). Ca^{2+} is also removed from the cell by an electrogenic pump that uses ATP to transport Ca^{2+} across the sarcolemma (Fig. 16-5).

Myocardial contractile machinery and contractility. The sequence of events that occur during the contraction of a preloaded and afterloaded papillary muscle is shown in Fig. 16-6. In Fig. 16-6, *A*, the muscle is relaxed and bears no extra weight. For the intact left ventricle,[*] this situation is analogous to the time in the cardiac cycle when the ventricle has relaxed after ejection, the aortic valve is closed, and the mitral valve is about to open (the end of isovolumic relaxation—see Fig. 16-10). In Fig. 16-6, *B*, the resting muscle is stretched by a preload, which in the intact heart represents the end of filling of the left ventricle during ventricular diastole (in other words, it represents the **end-diastolic volume**). In Fig. 16-6, *C*, the resting muscle is still stretched by the preload, but a supported afterload has been added without allowing the muscle to be stretched further. In the intact heart, this condition is analogous to the point in the cardiac cycle when ventricular contraction has started and the mitral valve has closed. However, the aortic valve has not yet opened, because the ventricle has not developed enough intraventricular pressure to open it (isovolumic contraction phase—see Fig. 16-10). In Fig. 16-6, *D*, the ventricle has contracted and lifted the afterload. In the intact heart, this condition represents left ventricular ejection into the aorta. During ejection, the afterload is represented by aortic and intraventricular pressures, which are virtually equal to each other.

---

[*]The left ventricle has been chosen because it supplies the entire body except the lungs, and thus faces the larger afterload. However, the principles of preload and afterload apply equally well to the right ventricle.

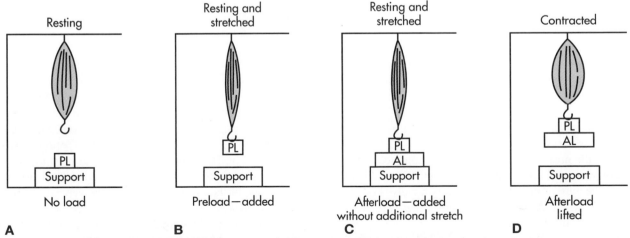

■ **Fig. 16-6** Preload and afterload in a papillary muscle. **A,** Resting stage—in the intact heart just before opening of the AV valves. **B,** Preload—in the intact heart at the end of ventricular filling. **C,** Supported preload plus afterload—in the intact heart just before opening of the aortic valve. **D,** Lifting preload plus afterload—in the intact heart ventricular ejection with a decrease in ventricular volume. *PL,* Preload; *AL,* afterload; *PL + AL* = total load.

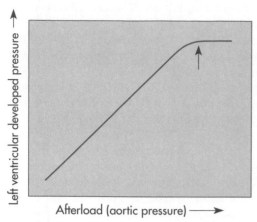

■ **Fig. 16-7**   Effect of increasing afterload on developed pressure at constant preload. At the arrow, maximal developed pressure is reached. Further increments in afterload prevent opening of the aortic valve.

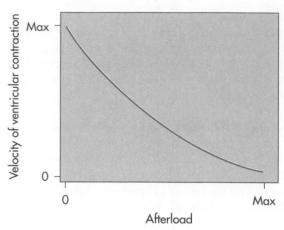

■ **Fig. 16-8**   Effect of increasing afterload on the velocity of contraction at constant preload.

The preload can be increased by greater filling of the left ventricle during diastole (Fig. 16-1). At lower end-diastolic volumes, incremental increases in filling pressure during diastole elicit a greater systolic pressure during the subsequent contraction. Systolic pressure increases until a maximal systolic pressure is reached at the optimal preload (Fig. 16-1). If diastolic filling continues beyond this point, no further increase in developed pressure will occur. At very high filling pressures, peak pressure development in systole is actually reduced.

At a constant preload, a higher systolic pressure can be reached during ventricular contractions by raising the afterload (e.g., increasing aortic pressure by restricting the runoff of arterial blood to the periphery). Incremental increases in afterload produce progressively higher peak systolic pressures (Fig. 16-7). If the afterload increases continue, the afterload becomes so great that the ventricle can no longer generate enough force to open the aortic valve (Fig. 16-7). At this point, ventricular systole is totally isometric; there is no ejection of blood, and thus no change in volume of the ventricle during systole. The maximal pressure developed by the left ventricle under these conditions is the maximal isometric force the ventricle is capable of generating at a given preload. At preloads below the optimal filling volume, an increase in preload can yield a greater maximal isometric force (Fig. 16-1).

When an isolated strip of cardiac muscle, such as that shown in Fig. 16-6, is subjected to a series of increasing afterloads, the maximum velocity of each contraction varies inversely with the afterload. Thus, when the afterload is minimal, the muscle strip can shorten very rapidly (Fig. 16-8). Conversely, when the afterload is great, the muscle strip shortens much more slowly.

In the intact animal, preloads and afterloads depend on certain characteristics of the vascular system and the behavior of the heart. With respect to the vasculature, the degree of venomotor tone and peripheral resistance influence preload and afterload. With respect to the heart, a change in rate

or stroke volume can also alter preload and afterload. Hence, cardiac and vascular factors interact with each other to affect preload and afterload (see Chapter 22 for a full explanation).

Contractility defines the performance of the heart at a given preload and afterload. Contractility determines the change in peak isometric force (isovolumic pressure) at a given initial fiber length (end-diastolic volume). Contractility can be augmented by certain drugs, such as norepinephrine or digitalis, or by an increase in contraction frequency (**tachycardia**). The increase in contractility (**positive inotropic effect**) produced by any of these interventions is reflected by incremental increases in developed force and in the velocity of contraction.

In rare instances, patients have received excessive doses of epinephrine subcutaneously in the treatment of severe asthmatic attacks. Such patients develop marked tachycardia and increases in myocardial contractility, cardiac output, and total peripheral resistance. The result of this treatment is dangerously high blood pressure.

Indices of contractility.   A reasonable index of myocardial contractility can be derived from the contour of ventricular pressure curves (Fig. 16-9). A hypodynamic heart is characterized by an elevated end-diastolic pressure, a slowly rising ventricular pressure, and a somewhat reduced ejection phase (curve *C*, Fig. 16-9). A hyperdynamic heart (curve *B*, Fig. 16-9) shows a reduced end-diastolic pressure, a fast-rising ventricular pressure, and a brief ejection phase. The slope of the ascending limb of the ventricular pressure curve indicates the maximal rate of force development by the ventricle. The maximal rate of change in pressure with time, that is, the maximum dP/dt, is illustrated by the tangents to the steepest portion of the ascending limbs of the ventricular pressure curves in Fig. 16-9. The slope of the ascending limb is maximal during the isovolumic phase of systole (Fig. 16-10). At any given degree of ventricular

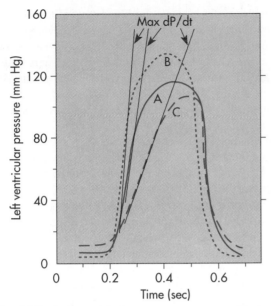

■ **Fig. 16-9** Left ventricular pressure curves with tangents drawn to the steepest portions of the ascending limbs to indicate maximal dP/dt values. *A,* Control; *B,* hyperdynamic heart, as with norepinephrine administration; *C,* hypodynamic heart, as in cardiac failure.

filling, the slope provides an index of the initial contraction velocity, and hence of contractility.

A similar indication of the contractile state of the myocardium can be obtained from the velocity of blood flow that occurs initially in the ascending aorta during the cardiac cycle (Fig. 16-10). Also, the **ejection fraction,** which is the ratio of the volume of blood ejected from the left ventricle per beat (**stroke volume**) to the volume of blood in the left ventricle at the end of diastole (**end-diastolic volume**), is widely used clinically as an index of contractility.

Cardiac chambers. The atria are thin-walled, low-pressure chambers that function more as large-reservoir conduits of blood for their respective ventricles than as important pumps for the forward propulsion of blood. The ventricles comprise a continuum of muscle fibers originating from the fibrous skeleton at the base of the heart (chiefly around the aortic orifice). These fibers sweep toward the cardiac apex at the epicardial surface. They pass toward the endocardium and gradually undergo a 180-degree change in direction to lie parallel to the epicardial fibers and to form the endocardium and papillary muscles (Fig. 16-11).

At the apex of the heart, the fibers twist and turn inward to form papillary muscles. At the base of the heart and around the valve orifices, these myocardial fibers form a thick, powerful muscle mass that not only decreases the ventricular circumference to implement the ejection of blood, but also narrows the atrioventricular (AV) valve orifices as an aid to valve closure. Ventricular ejection is also accomplished by decreasing the longitudinal axis as the heart begins to narrow toward the base. The early contraction of the apical part of the ventricles, coupled with the approximation of the

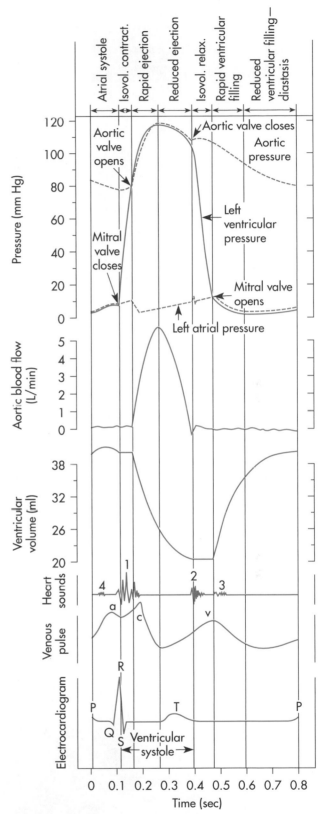

■ **Fig. 16-10** Left atrial, aortic, and left ventricular pressure pulses correlated in time with aortic flow, ventricular volume, heart sounds, venous pulse, and the electrocardiogram for a complete cardiac cycle in the dog.

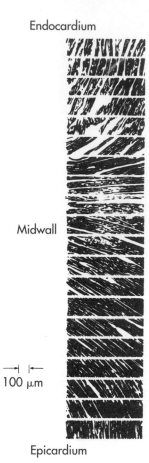

Endocardium

Midwall

100 μm

Epicardium

■ **Fig. 16-11** Sequence of photomicrographs showing fiber angles in successive sections taken from the middle of the free wall of the left ventricle from a heart in systole. The sections are parallel to the epicardial plane. The fiber angle is 90 degrees at the endocardium, running through 0 degrees at the midwall to –90 degrees at the epicardium. (From Streeter DD Jr et al: *Circ Res* 24:339, 1969.)

ventricular walls, propels the blood toward the ventricular outflow tracts. The right ventricle, which develops a mean pressure that is about one seventh of that developed by the left ventricle, is considerably thinner than the left ventricle.

Cardiac valves. The cardiac valve leaflets consist of thin flaps of flexible, tough, endothelium-covered fibrous tissue that are firmly attached at the base to the fibrous valve rings. Movements of the valve leaflets are essentially passive, and the orientation of the cardiac valves is responsible for the unidirectional flow of blood through the heart. There are two types of valves in the heart: the **atrioventricular** and the **semilunar valves** (Figs. 16-12 and 16-13).

Atrioventricular valves. The AV valve (**tricuspid valve**) located between the right atrium and the right ventricle is made up of three cusps, whereas the **mitral valve** that lies between the left atrium and the left ventricle has two cusps. The total area of the cusps of each AV valve is approximately twice that of the respective AV orifice, so that considerable overlap of the leaflets occurs when the valves are in the closed position (Figs. 16-12 and 16-13). Attached to the free edges of these valves are fine, strong ligaments (**chordae tendineae),** which arise from the powerful papillary muscles of the respective ventricles. These ligaments prevent the valves from becoming everted during ventricular systole.

In the normal heart, the valve leaflets remain relatively close together during ventricular filling. The partial approximation of the valve surfaces during diastole is caused by eddy currents that prevail behind the leaflets and by tension that is exerted by the chordae tendineae and papillary muscles.

Movements of the mitral valve leaflets throughout the cardiac cycle are shown in an **echocardiogram** (Fig. 16-14).

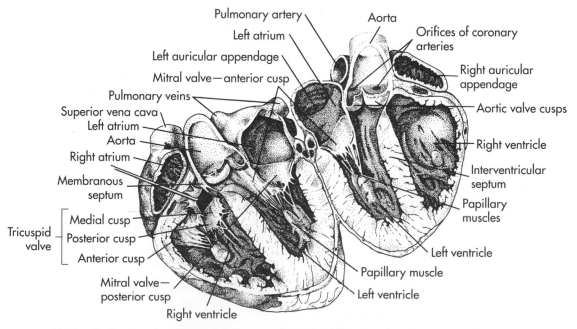

Pulmonary artery
Left atrium
Left auricular appendage
Mitral valve—anterior cusp
Pulmonary veins
Superior vena cava
Left atrium
Aorta
Right atrium
Membranous septum
Tricuspid valve — Medial cusp / Posterior cusp / Anterior cusp
Mitral valve—posterior cusp
Right ventricle

Aorta
Orifices of coronary arteries
Right auricular appendage
Aortic valve cusps
Right ventricle
Interventricular septum
Papillary muscles
Left ventricle
Papillary muscle
Left ventricle

■ **Fig. 16-12** Drawing of a heart split perpendicular to the interventricular septum to illustrate the anatomic relationships of the leaflets of the atrioventricular and aortic valves.

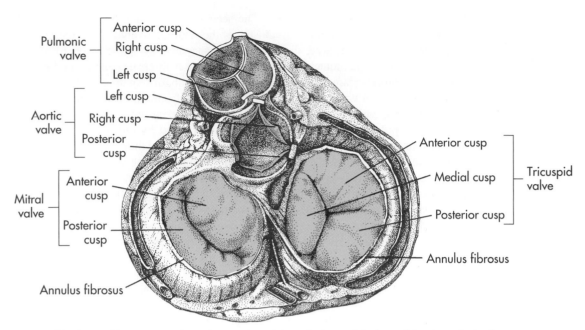

■ **Fig. 16-13** Four cardiac valves as viewed from the base of the heart. Note how the leaflets overlap in the closed valves.

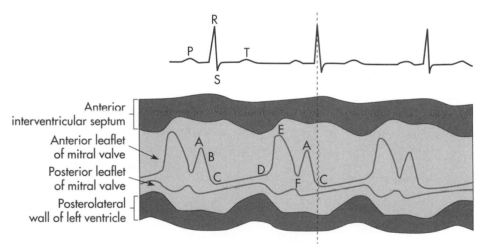

■ **Fig. 16-14** Drawing made from an echocardiogram showing movements of the mitral valve leaflets (particularly the anterior leaflet) and the changes in the diameter of the left ventricular cavity and the thickness of the left ventricular walls during cardiac cycles in a normal person. *D* to *C*, Ventricular diastole; *C* to *D*, ventricular systole; *D* to *E*, rapid filling; *E* to *F*, reduced filling (diastasis); *F* to *A*, atrial contraction. The mitral valve closes at *C* and opens at *D*. Simultaneously recorded electrocardiogram at top.

Echocardiography is achieved by sending short pulses of high-frequency sound waves (ultrasound) through the chest tissues and the heart and by recording the echoes reflected from the various cardiac structures. The timing and pattern of the reflected waves provide such information as the diameter of the heart, the ventricular wall thickness, and the magnitude and direction of the movements of various components of the heart.

In Fig. 16-14, the echocardiogram depicts the movement of the anterior leaflet of the mitral valve. The posterior leaflet moves in a pattern that is a mirror image of the anterior leaflet, but in the projection shown in Fig. 16-14 its movements appear to be smaller. At point *D*, the mitral valve opens, and during rapid filling (*D* to *E*) the anterior leaflet moves toward the ventricular septum. During the reduced

filling phase (*E* to *F*), the valve leaflets float toward each other, but the valve does not close. The ventricular filling contributed by atrial contraction (*F* to *A*) forces the leaflets apart. This motion is followed by a second approximation of the leaflets (*A* to *C*). At point C the valve is closed by ventricular contraction. The valve leaflets, which bulge toward the atrium, stay pressed together during ventricular systole (*C* to *D*).

Semilunar valves. The semilunar valves are located between the right ventricle and the pulmonary artery and between the left ventricle and the aorta. These valves consist of three cuplike cusps that are attached to the valve rings (Figs. 16-12 and 16-13). At the end of the reduced ejection phase of ventricular systole, blood flow briefly reverses toward the ventricles. This flow appears as a negative flow in the phasic aortic flow curve in Fig. 16-10. This reversal of blood flow snaps the cusps together and prevents regurgitation of blood into the ventricles. During ventricular systole, the cusps do not lie back against the walls of the pulmonary artery and aorta, but instead float in the bloodstream at a point approximately midway between the vessel walls and their closed position. Behind the semilunar valves are small outpocketings (**sinuses of Valsalva**) of the pulmonary artery and aorta. In these sinuses, eddy currents develop that tend to keep the valve cusps away from the vessel walls. Furthermore, the orifices of the right and left coronary arteries are behind the right and the left cusps, respectively, of the aortic valve. Were it not for the presence of the sinuses of Valsalva and of the eddy currents developed therein, the coronary ostia could be blocked by the valve cusps. Hence, coronary blood flow would cease.

The pericardium. The pericardium is an epithelialized fibrous sac. It closely invests the entire heart and the cardiac portion of the great vessels, and it is reflected onto the cardiac surface as the epicardium. The sac normally contains a small amount of fluid, which provides lubrication for the continuous movement of the enclosed heart. The pericardium is not very distensible, and therefore it strongly resists a large, rapid increase in cardiac size. Hence, the pericardium prevents sudden overdistention of the chambers of the heart. However, in congenital absence of the pericardium or after its surgical removal, cardiac function is not seriously affected. Nevertheless, with the pericardium intact, an increase in diastolic pressure in one ventricle increases the pressure and decreases the compliance of the other ventricle.

Heart sounds. Four sounds are usually generated by the heart, but only two are ordinarily audible through a stethoscope. With electronic amplification, the less intense sounds can be detected and recorded graphically as a **phonocardiogram.** This means of registering faint heart sounds helps to delineate the precise timing of the heart sounds relative to other events in the cardiac cycle.

The first heart sound is initiated at the onset of ventricular systole (Fig. 16-10) and it consists of a series of vibrations of mixed, unrelated, low frequencies (a noise). It is the loudest and longest of the heart sounds, it has a crescendo-decrescendo quality, and it is heard best over the apical region of the heart. The tricuspid valve sounds are heard best in the fifth intercostal space, just to the left of the sternum; the mitral sounds are heard best in the fifth intercostal space at the cardiac apex.

The first heart sound is chiefly caused by oscillation of blood in the ventricular chambers and vibration of the chamber walls. The vibrations are engendered in part by the abrupt rise of ventricular pressure and the acceleration of blood back toward the atria. However, the main cause of the first heart sound is the sudden tension and recoil of the AV valves and adjacent structures, with deceleration of the blood as the AV valves close. The vibrations of the ventricles and the contained blood are transmitted through surrounding tissues and they reach the chest wall (where they may be heard or recorded).

The second heart sound, which occurs with the abrupt closure of the semilunar valves (Fig. 16-10), is composed of higher-frequency vibrations (higher pitch), and it is of shorter duration and lower intensity. The second heart sound has a more snapping quality than does the first heart sound. Semilunar valve closure initiates oscillations of the columns of blood and of the tensed vessel walls. The portion of the second sound caused by closure of the pulmonic valve is heard best in the second thoracic interspace just to the left of the sternum, whereas that caused by closure of the aortic valve is heard best in the same intercostal space but to the right of the sternum. The aortic valve sound is usually louder than the pulmonic, but in cases of pulmonary hypertension the reverse is true.

A normal phonocardiogram taken simultaneously with an electrocardiogram (ECG) is illustrated in Fig. 16-15. The first sound starts just beyond the peak of the R waves of the electrocardiogram. Note that this sound is composed of irregular waves and is of greater intensity and duration than the second sound, which appears at the end of the T wave. A third and fourth heart sound do not appear on this record.

The third heart sound is sometimes heard in children with thin chest walls or in patients with left ventricular failure. It consists of a few low-intensity, low-frequency vibrations heard best in the region of the cardiac apex. The vibrations occur in early diastole and are caused by the abrupt cessation of ventricular distention and by the deceleration of blood entering the ventricles.

In overloaded hearts, as in congestive heart failure, when the ventricular volume is very large and the ventricular walls are stretched to the point where distensibility is minimal, a third heart sound may be heard. A third heart sound in patients with heart disease is usually a grave sign.

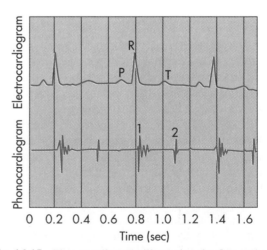

■ **Fig. 16-15** Phonocardiogram illustrating the first and second heart sounds and their relationship to the P, R, and T waves of the electrocardiogram. Time lines = 0.04 second.

A fourth, or atrial, sound consists of a few low-frequency oscillations. This sound is occasionally heard in normal individuals. It is caused by oscillation of blood and cardiac chambers created by atrial contraction (Fig. 16-10).

Mitral insufficiency and **mitral stenosis** produce, respectively, systolic and diastolic murmurs that are heard best at the cardiac apex. **Aortic insufficiency** and **aortic stenosis,** on the other hand, produce, respectively, diastolic and systolic murmurs that are heard best in the second intercostal space just to the right of the sternum. The characteristics of the murmurs serve as an important guide in the diagnosis of valvular disease.

When the third and fourth (atrial) sounds are accentuated, as occurs in certain abnormal conditions, triplets of sounds (called **gallop rhythms**) may occur, resembling the sound of a galloping horse.

THE CARDIAC CYCLE

Ventricular Systole

Isovolumic contraction. The onset of ventricular contraction coincides with the peak of the R wave on an ECG and with the initial vibration of the first heart sound. It is indicated on the ventricular pressure curve as the earliest rise in ventricular pressure after atrial contraction. The time between the start of ventricular systole and the opening of the semilunar valves (when ventricular pressure rises abruptly) is called the **isovolumic** (literally, "same volume") **contraction period.** This term is appropriate because ventricular volume remains constant during this brief period (Fig. 16-10).

Ejection. Opening of the semilunar valves marks the onset of the ventricular ejection phase, which may be subdivided into an earlier, shorter phase (**rapid ejection**) and a later, longer phase (**reduced ejection**). The rapid ejection phase is distinguished from the reduced ejection phase by three characteristics. (1) A sharp rise in ventricular and aortic pressures that terminates at the peak ventricular and aortic pressures, (2) an abrupt decrease in ventricular volume, and (3) a pronounced increase in aortic blood flow (Fig. 16-10). The sharp decrease in the left atrial pressure at the onset of ventricular ejection results from the descent of the base of the heart and the consequent stretch of the atria. During the reduced ejection period, runoff of blood from the aorta to the peripheral blood vessels exceeds the rate of ventricular output, and therefore aortic pressure declines. Throughout ventricular systole, the blood returning from the peripheral veins to the atria produces a progressive increase in atrial pressure.

Note that during the rapid ejection period, left ventricular pressure slightly exceeds aortic pressure and the aortic blood flow accelerates (continues to increase), whereas during the reduced ventricular ejection phase, the reverse holds true. This reversal of the ventricular-aortic pressure gradient in the presence of the continuous flow of blood from the left ventricle to the aorta is the result of storage of potential energy in the stretched arterial walls. This stored potential energy decelerates blood flow from the left ventricle into the aorta. The peak of the flow curve coincides with the point at which the left ventricular pressure curve intersects the aortic pressure curve during ejection. Thereafter, flow decelerates (continues to decrease) because the pressure gradient has been reversed.

The effect of ventricular systole on left ventricular diameter is shown in an echocardiogram (Fig. 16-14). During ventricular systole (Fig. 16-14, *C* to *D*), the septum and the free wall of the left ventricle become thicker and move closer to each other.

Figure 16-10 shows a tracing of a venous pulse curve recorded from a jugular vein. The c wave in this tracing is caused by the impact of the common carotid artery with the adjacent jugular vein and to some extent by the abrupt closure of the tricuspid valve in early ventricular systole. Note that except for the c wave, the venous pulse closely follows the left atrial pressure curve.

At the end of ventricular ejection, a volume of blood approximately equal to that ejected during systole remains in the ventricular cavities. This **residual volume** is fairly constant in normal hearts. However, the residual volume decreases somewhat when heart rate increases or when peripheral vascular resistance has diminished.

An increase in myocardial contractility, as produced by catecholamines or by digitalis in a patient with a failing heart, may decrease residual ventricular volume and increase the stroke volume and ejection fraction. With severely hypodynamic and dilated hearts, the residual volume can become much greater than the stroke volume.

Ventricular Diastole

Isovolumic relaxation. Closure of the aortic valve produces the characteristic **incisura** (notch) on the descending limb of the aortic pressure curve and it also produces the second heart sound (with some vibrations evident on the atrial pressure curve). The incisura marks the end of ventricular systole. The period between closure of the semilunar valves and opening of the AV valves is termed **isovolumic relaxation.** It is characterized by a precipitous fall in ventricular pressure without a change in ventricular volume.

Rapid filling phase. The major part of ventricular filling occurs immediately after the opening of the AV valves. At this point the blood that had returned to the atria during the previous ventricular systole is abruptly released into the relaxing ventricles. This period of ventricular filling is called the **rapid filling phase.** In Fig. 16-10 the onset of the rapid filling phase is indicated by the decrease in left ventricular pressure below left atrial pressure. This pressure reversal opens the mitral valve. The rapid flow of blood from atria to relaxing ventricles produces a transient decrease in atrial and ventricular pressures and a sharp increase in ventricular volume.

Diastasis. The rapid ventricular filling phase is followed by a phase of slow ventricular filling called **diastasis.** During diastasis, blood returning from the peripheral veins flows into the right ventricle, and blood from the lungs flows into the left ventricle. This small, slow addition to ventricular filling is indicated by a gradual rise in atrial, ventricular, and venous pressures and in ventricular volume (Fig. 16-10).

Atrial systole. The onset of atrial systole occurs soon after the beginning of the P wave (curve of atrial depolarization) of the ECG. The transfer of blood from atrium to ventricle achieved by the atrial contraction completes the period of ventricular filling. Atrial systole is responsible for the small increases in atrial, ventricular, and venous pressures, as well as in ventricular volume, as shown in Fig. 16-10. Throughout ventricular diastole, atrial pressure barely exceeds ventricular pressure. This small pressure difference indicates that the pathway through the open AV valves during ventricular filling has a low resistance.

Because there are no valves at the junctions of the venae cavae and right atrium or of the pulmonary veins and left atrium, atrial contraction may force blood in both directions. Actually, little blood is pumped back into the venous tributaries during the brief atrial contraction, mainly because of the inertia of the inflowing blood.

> Atrial contraction is not essential for ventricular filling, as can be observed in patients with atrial fibrillation or complete heart block. In atrial fibrillation, the atrial myofibers contract in a continuous uncoordinated fashion and therefore cannot pump blood into the ventricles. In complete heart block, the atria and ventricles beat independently of each other. However, ventricular filling may be normal in patients with these two arrhythmias.

The contribution of atrial contraction to ventricular filling is governed to a great extent by the heart rate and the position of the AV valves. At slow heart rates, filling practically ceases toward the end of diastole, and atrial contraction contributes little additional filling. During tachycardia, however, diastasis is abbreviated and the atrial contribution can become substantial. Should tachycardia become so great that the rapid filling phase is encroached on, atrial contraction assumes great importance in rapidly propelling blood into the ventricle during this brief period of the cardiac cycle. Of course, if the period of ventricular relaxation is so brief that filling is seriously impaired, even atrial contraction cannot provide adequate ventricular filling. The consequent reduction in cardiac output may result in syncope (fainting).

Pressure-volume relationship. The changes in left ventricular pressure and volume throughout the cardiac cycle are summarized in Fig. 16-16. Diastolic filling starts at *A*, when the mitral valve opens, and it terminates at *C*, when the mitral valve closes. The initial decrease in left ventricular pressure (*A* to *B*), despite the rapid inflow of blood from the left atrium, is attributed to progressive ventricular relaxation and distensibility. During the remainder of diastole (*B* to *C*), the increase in ventricular pressure reflects ventricular

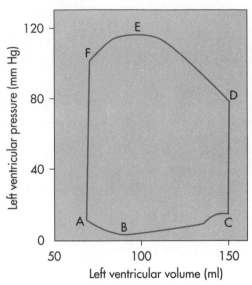

■ **Fig. 16-16** Pressure-volume loop of the left ventricle for a single cardiac cycle *(ABCDEF).*

filling and the changes in the passive elastic characteristics of the ventricle. Note that only a small increase in pressure accompanies the substantial increase in ventricular volume during diastole (*B* to *C*). The small pressure increase reflects the compliance of the left ventricle during diastole. The small increase in pressure just to the left of *C* is caused by the contribution of atrial contraction to ventricular filling. With isovolumic contraction (*C* to *D*), pressure rises steeply, but ventricular volume does not change because the mitral and aortic valves are both closed. At *D*, the aortic valve opens, and during the first phase of ejection (rapid ejection, *D* to *E*), the large reduction in volume is associated with a steady increase in ventricular pressure. This volume reduction is followed by reduced ejection (*E* to *F*) and a small decrease in ventricular pressure. The aortic valve closes at *F*, and this event is followed by isovolumic relaxation (*F* to *A*), which is characterized by a sharp drop in pressure. Ventricular volume does not change during the interval from *F* to *A* because the mitral and aortic valves are both closed. The mitral valve opens at A to complete one cardiac cycle.

> In certain disease states, the AV valves may be markedly narrowed (**stenotic**). Under such conditions, atrial contraction plays a much more important role in ventricular filling than it does in the normal heart.

MEASUREMENT OF CARDIAC OUTPUT
Fick Principle

In 1870 the German physiologist Adoph Fick contrived the first method for measuring cardiac output in intact animals and people. The basis for this method, called the **Fick principle,** is simply an application of the law of conservation of mass. The principle is derived from the fact that the quantity

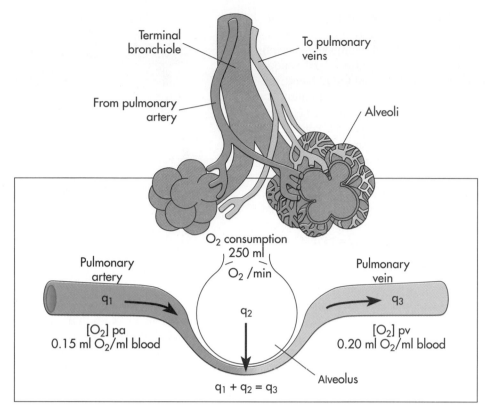

■ **Fig. 16-17**   Schema illustrating the Fick principle for measuring cardiac output. The change in color from pulmonary artery to pulmonary vein represents the change in color of the blood as venous blood becomes fully oxygenated.

of oxygen (O_2) delivered to the pulmonary capillaries via the pulmonary artery, plus the quantity of O_2 that enters the pulmonary capillaries from the alveoli, must equal the quantity of O_2 that is carried away by the pulmonary veins.

The Fick principle is depicted schematically in Fig. 16-17. The rate, q_1, of O_2 delivery to the lungs equals the O_2 concentration in the pulmonary arterial blood, $[O_2]_{pa}$, times the pulmonary arterial blood flow, Q, which equals the cardiac output; that is

$$q_1 = Q[O_2]_{pa} \qquad (16\text{-}1)$$

Let q_2 be the net rate of O_2 uptake by the pulmonary capillaries from the alveoli. At equilibrium, q_2 equals the O_2 consumption of the body. The rate, q_3, at which O_2 is carried away by the pulmonary veins equals the O_2 concentration in the pulmonary venous blood, $[O_2]_{pv}$, times the total pulmonary venous flow, which is virtually equal to the pulmonary arterial blood flow, Q; that is,

$$q_3 = Q[O_2]_{pv} \qquad (16\text{-}2)$$

From conservation of mass,

$$q_1 + q_2 = q_3 \qquad (16\text{-}3)$$

Therefore,

$$Q[O_2]_{pa} + q_2 = Q[O_2]_{pv} \qquad (16\text{-}4)$$

Solving for cardiac output,

$$Q = q_2/([O_2]_{pv} - [O_2]_{pa}) \qquad (16\text{-}5)$$

Equation 16-5 is the statement of the Fick principle.

The clinical determination of cardiac output requires three values: (1) the O_2 consumption of the body, (2) the O_2 concentration in the pulmonary venous blood ($[O_2]_{pv}$, and (3) the O_2 concentration in the pulmonary arterial blood ($[O_2]_{pa}$). O_2 consumption is computed from measurements of the volume and O_2 content of expired air over a given interval of time. Because the O_2 concentration of peripheral arterial blood is essentially identical to that in the pulmonary veins, $[O_2]_{pv}$ is determined on a sample of peripheral arterial blood withdrawn by needle puncture. The compositions of pulmonary arterial blood and of mixed systemic venous blood are virtually identical to one another. Samples for O_2 analysis are obtained from the pulmonary artery or right ventricle through a catheter. In the past, a relatively stiff catheter had to be introduced into the pulmonary artery under fluoroscopic guidance. Today, a very flexible catheter with a small balloon near the tip can be inserted into a peripheral vein. As the flexible tube is advanced, it is carried by the flowing blood toward the heart. By following the pressure changes, the physician is able to advance the catheter tip into the pulmonary artery without the aid of fluoroscopy.

An example of the calculation of cardiac output in a normal, resting adult is illustrated in Fig. 16-17. With an O_2 consumption of 250 ml/min, an arterial (pulmonary venous) O_2 content of 0.20 ml O_2/ml blood, and a mixed venous (pulmonary arterial) O_2 content of 0.15 ml O_2/ml blood, the cardiac output equals 250/(0.20 − 0.15) = 5000 ml/min.

The Fick principle is also used for estimating the O_2 consumption of organs when blood flow and the O_2 contents of the arterial and venous blood can be determined. Algebraic rearrangement reveals that O_2 consumption equals the blood flow times the arteriovenous O_2 concentration difference. For example, if the blood flow through one kidney is 700 ml/min, arterial O_2 content is 0.20 ml O_2/ml blood, and renal venous O_2 content is 0.18 ml O_2/ml blood, the rate of O_2 consumption by that kidney must be 700 (0.2 × 0.18) = 14 ml O_2/min.

Indicator Dilution Techniques

The indicator dilution technique for measuring cardiac output is also based on the law of conservation of mass and is illustrated by the model in Fig. 16-18. In this model, a liquid flows through a tube at a rate of Q ml/sec, and q mg of dye is injected as a slug into the stream at point A. Mixing of the liquid and the dye occurs at some point downstream. If a small sample of liquid is continually withdrawn from point B farther downstream and passed through a densitometer, a curve of the dye concentration, c, may be recorded as a function of time, t, as shown in the lower half of Fig. 16-18.

If no dye is lost between points A and B, the amount of dye, q, passing point B between times t_1 and t_2 will be

$$q = \bar{c}Q(t_1 - t_2) \qquad (16\text{-}6)$$

where $\bar{c}$ is the mean concentration of dye. The value of $\bar{c}$ may be computed by dividing the area of the dye concentration by the duration $(t_2 - t_1)$ of the curve; that is

$$\bar{c} = \int_{t_1}^{t_2} c\, dt/(t_2 - t_1) \qquad (16\text{-}7)$$

Substituting this value of $\bar{c}$ into equation 16-6 and solving for Q yields

$$Q = \frac{q}{\int_{t_1}^{t_2} c\, dt} \qquad (16\text{-}8)$$

Thus, flow may be measured by dividing the amount of indicator (the dye) injected upstream by the area under the downstream concentration curve.

This technique has been widely used to estimate cardiac output in humans. A measured quantity of some indicator (a dye or isotope that remains within the circulation) is injected rapidly into a large central vein or into the right side of the heart through a catheter. Arterial blood is continuously drawn through a detector (densitometer or isotope rate counter), and a curve of indicator concentration is recorded as a function of time.

Currently, the most popular indicator dilution technique is **thermodilution.** The indicator used in this method is cold saline. The temperature and volume of the saline are measured accurately before injection. A flexible catheter is intro-

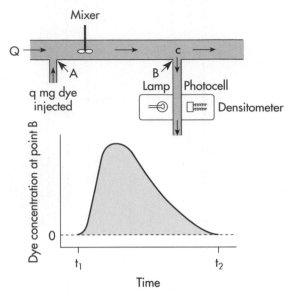

■ **Fig. 16-18**   Indicator dilution technique for measuring cardiac output. In this model, in which there is no recirculation, q mg of dye is injected instantaneously at point A into a stream flowing at Q ml/min. A mixed sample of the fluid flowing past point B is withdrawn at a constant rate through a densitometer; C is concentration of dye in the fluid. The resultant dye concentration curve at point B has the configuration shown in the lower section of the figure.

duced into a peripheral vein and advanced so that the tip lies in the pulmonary artery. A small thermistor at the catheter tip records the changes in temperature. The opening in the catheter lies a few inches proximal to the catheter tip. When the tip is in the pulmonary artery, the opening lies in or near the right atrium. The cold saline is injected rapidly into the right atrium through the catheter and flows out through the opening in the catheter. The change in temperature downstream is recorded by the thermistor in the pulmonary artery.

The thermodilution technique has the following advantages: (1) an arterial puncture is not necessary; (2) the small volumes of saline used in each determination are innocuous, and thus repeated determinations can be made; and (3) recirculation of the small volume of cold saline has a neglible effect on the recorded temperature. Equilibration takes place as the cooled blood flows through the pulmonary and systemic capillary beds, before it flows by the thermistor in the pulmonary artery the second time.

SUMMARY

1. An increase in myocardial fiber length, as occurs with augmented ventricular filling (preload) during diastole, produces a more forceful ventricular contraction. This relation between fiber length and strength of contraction is known as the Frank-Starling relationship or Starling's law of the heart.

2. Although the myocardium is made up of individual cells with discrete membrane boundaries, the cardiac myocytes that make up the ventricles contract almost in unison, as do

those of the atria. The myocardium functions as a syncytium with an all-or-none response to excitation. Cell-to-cell conduction occurs through gap junctions that connect the cytosol of adjacent cells.

3. On excitation, voltage-gated calcium channels open to admit extracellular Ca^{2+} into the cell. The influx of Ca^{2+} triggers the release of Ca^{2+} from the sarcoplasmic reticulum. The elevated intracellular $[Ca^{2+}]$ elicits contraction of the myofilaments. Relaxation is accomplished via restoration of the resting cytosolic Ca^{2+} level by pumping Ca^{2+} back into the sarcoplasmic reticulum and exchanging it for extracellular Na^+ across the sarcolemma.

4. Velocity and force of contraction are functions of the intracellular concentration of free calcium ions. Force and velocity are inversely related, so that with no load, velocity is maximal. In an isovolumic contraction, no external shortening occurs.

5. In ventricular contraction, the preload is the stretch of the fibers by the blood during ventricular filling. The afterload is the arterial pressure against which the ventricle ejects the blood.

6. Contractility is an expression of cardiac performance at a given preload and afterload.

7. Simultaneous recording of the left atrial, left ventricular, and aortic pressures, ventricular volume, heart sounds, and the electrocardiogram graphically portray the sequential and parallel electrical and cardiodynamic events throughout a cardiac cycle.

8. The first heart sound is caused mainly by abrupt closure of the AV valve; the second heart sound is caused by the abrupt closure of the semilunar valves.

9. Cardiac output can be determined, according to the Fick principle, by measuring the oxygen consumption of the body (q_2) and the oxygen content of arterial $[O_2]_a$ and mixed venous $[O_2]_v$ blood. Cardiac output = $q_2/([O_2]_a [O_2]_v)$. It can also be measured by dye dilution or thermodilution techniques.

BIBLIOGRAPHY

Journal articles

Alvarex BV et al: Mechanisms underlying the increase in force and Ca^{++} transient that follow stretch of cardiac muscle: a possible explanation of the Anrep effect, *Circ Res* 85:716, 1999.

Blaustein MP, Lederer WJ: Sodium/calcium exchange: its physiological implications, *Physiol Rev* 79:763, 1999.

Cannell MB, Cheng H, Lederer WJ: The control of calcium release in heart muscle, *Science* 268:1045, 1995.

Gaughan JP et al: Sodium/calcium exchange contributes to contraction and relaxation in failed humed ventricular myocytes, *Am J Physiol* 277:H714, 1999.

Landesberg A, Sideman S: Mechanical regulation of cardiac muscle by coupling calcium kinetics with crossbridge cycling: a dynamic model, *Am J Physiol* 267:H779, 1994.

Lorenz JN, Kranias EG: Regulatory effects of phosphlamban on cardiac function in intact mice, *Am J Physiol* 273: H2826, 1997.

Niggi E: Ca^{++} sparks in cardiac muscle: is there life without them? *News Physiol Sci* 14:129, 1999.

Pieske B et al: Ca^{++} handling and sarcoplasmic reticulum Ca^{++} content in isolating failing and nonfailing human myocardium, *Circ Res* 85:38, 1999.

Wier WG, Balke CW: Ca^{++} release mechanisms, Ca^{++} sparks, and local control of excitation-contraction coupling in normal heart muscle, *Circ Res* 85:770, 1999.

Zhang R et al: Cardiac troponin I phosphorylation increases the rate of cardiac muscle relaxation, *Circ Res* 76:1028, 1995.

chapter seventeen

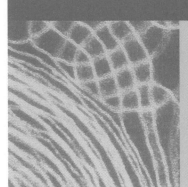

Regulation of the Heartbeat

Cardiac output (CO) is defined as the quantity of blood pumped by the heart each minute. Cardiac output may be varied by changing the frequency of the heartbeat [i.e., the **heart rate** (HR)] or the volume of blood ejected from either ventricle with each heartbeat; this volume is called the **stroke volume** (SV). In mathematical terms, cardiac output can be expressed as the product of heart rate and stroke volume:

$$CO = HR \times SV$$

As this equation demonstrates, an understanding of how cardiac activity is controlled can be gained by considering how heart rate and stroke volume are regulated. Heart rate is regulated through the activity of the cardiac pacemaker, and stroke volume is directly related to myocardial performance. These two determinants cannot be considered independently, however. A change in one of these determinants of cardiac output almost invariably alters the other determinant.

NERVOUS CONTROL OF HEART RATE

Although certain local factors, such as temperature changes and tissue stretch, can affect the heart rate, the autonomic nervous system is the principal means by which heart rate is controlled.

The average resting heart rate is approximately 70 beats per minute in normal adults, and it is significantly greater in children. During sleep, the heart rate diminishes by 10 to 20 beats per minute, and during emotional excitement or muscular activity it may accelerate to rates considerably above 100. In well-trained, resting athletes, the rate is usually only about 50 beats per minute.

Both divisions of the autonomic nervous system tonically influence the cardiac pacemaker, which normally is the SA node. The sympathetic system enhances automaticity, whereas the parasympathetic system inhibits it. Changes in heart rate usually involve a reciprocal action of these two divisions of the autonomic nervous system. Thus the heart rate ordinarily increases with a combined decrease in parasympathetic activity and an increase in sympathetic activity; the heart rate decreases with the opposite changes in autonomic neural activity.

Parasympathetic tone usually predominates in healthy, resting individuals. When a resting individual is given **atropine,** a muscarinic receptor antagonist that blocks parasympathetic effects, heart rate usually increases substantially. If a resting individual is given **propranolol,** a β-adrenergic receptor antagonist that blocks sympathetic effects, heart rate usually decreases only slightly (Fig. 17-1). When both divisions of the autonomic nervous system are blocked, the heart rate of young adults averages about 100 beats per minute. The rate that prevails after complete autonomic blockade is called the **intrinsic heart rate.**

Parasympathetic Pathways

The cardiac parasympathetic fibers originate in the medulla oblongata, in cells that lie in the **dorsal motor nucleus of the vagus** or in the **nucleus ambiguus** (see Chapter 11). The precise location of the parasympathetic fibers varies from species to species. In humans, centrifugal vagal fibers (Fig. 17-2) pass inferiorly through the neck close to the common carotid arteries and then through the mediastinum to synapse with postganglionic vagal cells. These cells are located either on the epicardial surface or within the walls of the heart. Most of the vagal ganglion cells are located in epicardial fat pads near the SA and AV nodes.

The right and left vagi are distributed to different cardiac structures. The right vagus nerve affects the SA node predominantly. Stimulation of this nerve slows SA nodal firing and can even stop the firing for several seconds. The left vagus nerve mainly inhibits AV conduction tissue to produce various degrees of AV block (see Chapter 15). However, the distribution of the efferent vagal fibers is overlapping. As a result of this overlap, left vagal stimulation also depresses the SA node, and right vagal stimulation impedes AV conduction.

The SA and AV nodes are rich in **cholinesterase,** an enzyme that breaks down the neurotransmitter acetylcholine.

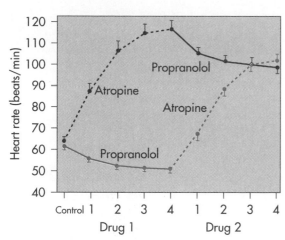

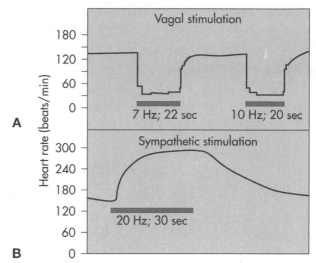

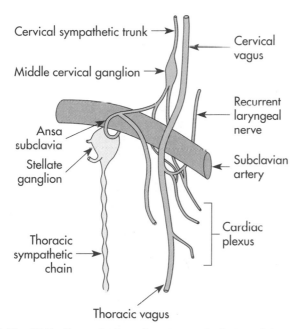

■ **Fig. 17-2** Sympathetic and parasympathetic (vagal) innervation of the heart on the right side of the body in humans.

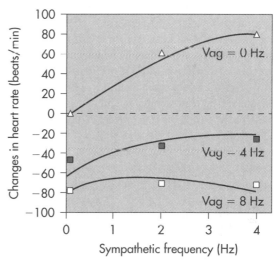

Acetylcholine released at the nerve terminals is thus rapidly hydrolyzed. Owing to this rapid breakdown of acetylcholine, the effects of any given vagal stimulation decay very quickly (Fig. 17-3, *A*) when vagal stimulation is discontinued. Furthermore, the effects of vagal activity on SA and AV nodal function have a very short latency (about 50 to 100 msec), because the released acetylcholine quickly activates special acetylcholine-regulated K^+ channels in the cardiac cells. The reason these channels open so quickly is that the response to acetylcholine does not require an intermediate second messenger system, such as the adenylyl cyclase

system (see Chapter 5). The combination of these two features of the vagus nerves—brief latency and the rapid decay of the response—permits these nerves to exert a beat-by-beat control of SA and AV nodal function.

Parasympathetic influences usually preponderate over sympathetic effects at the SA node. The experiment shown in Fig. 17-4 shows that as the frequency of sympathetic stimulation increases from 0 to 4 Hz in an anesthetized dog, the heart rate increases by about 80 beats per minute in the absence of vagal stimulation (*Vag* = 0 Hz). However, when the vagi are stimulated at 8 Hz, increasing the sympathetic stimulation frequency from 0 to 4 Hz has only a negligible influence on heart rate.

Sympathetic Pathways

The cardiac sympathetic fibers originate in the **intermediolateral columns** of the upper five or six thoracic and lower one or two cervical segments of the spinal cord (see Chapter 11). These fibers emerge from the spinal column through the white communicating branches and enter the paravertebral chains of ganglia (Fig. 17-2). The preganglionic and postganglionic neurons synapse mainly in the stellate or middle cervical ganglia, depending on the species. In the mediastinum, the postganglionic sympathetic fibers and preganglionic parasympathetic fibers join to form a complicated plexus of mixed efferent nerves to the heart.

The postganglionic cardiac sympathetic fibers in this plexus approach the base of the heart along the adventitial surface of the great vessels. On reaching the base of the heart, these fibers are distributed to the various chambers as an extensive epicardial plexus. They then penetrate the myocardium, usually accompanying the coronary vessels.

As with the vagus nerves, the left and right sympathetic fibers are distributed to different areas of the heart. In the dog, for example, the fibers from the left side of the body have more pronounced effects on myocardial contractility than do fibers from the right side, whereas the fibers from the left side of the body exert much less effect on heart rate than do the fibers from the right side (Fig. 17-5). In some dogs, left cardiac sympathetic nerve stimulation may not affect heart rate at all. This bilateral asymmetry probably also exists in humans.

In contrast to the abrupt termination of the response after vagal activity, the effects of sympathetic stimulation decay only gradually after stimulation is stopped (Fig. 17-3, *B*). Nerve terminals take up most of the norepinephrine released during sympathetic stimulation, and much of the remainder is carried away by the bloodstream. These processes are slow. Furthermore, at the beginning of sympathetic stimulation, the facilitatory effects on the heart attain steady-state values much more slowly than do the inhibitory effects of vagal stimulation. The onset of the cardiac response to sympathetic stimulation is slow for two main reasons. First, norepinephrine appears to be released slowly from the cardiac sympathetic nerve terminals. Second, the cardiac effects of the neurally released norepinephrine are mediated mainly via a relatively slow second messenger system, principally the adenylyl cyclase system (see Chapter 5). Hence, sympathetic activity alters heart rate and AV conduction much more slowly than does vagal activity. Consequently, although vagal activity can exert beat-by-beat control of cardiac function, sympathetic activity cannot.

Control by Higher Centers

Stimulation of various regions of the brain can have significant effects on cardiac rate, rhythm, and contractility (see Chapter 11). In the cerebral cortex, the centers that regulate

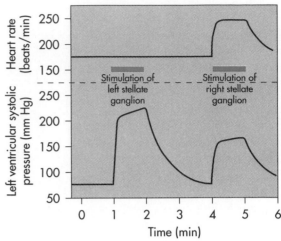

■ Fig. 17-5   In the dog, stimulation of the left stellate ganglion has a greater effect on ventricular contractility than does right-sided stimulation, but it has a lesser effect on heart rate. In this example, traced from an original record, left stellate ganglion stimulation had no detectable effect on heart rate but had a considerable effect on ventricular performance in an isovolumic left ventricle preparation. (From Levy MN: Unpublished tracing.)

cardiac function are located mostly in the anterior half of the brain, principally in the frontal lobe, the orbital cortex, the motor and premotor cortex, the anterior part of the temporal lobe, the insula, and the cingulate gyrus. Stimulation of the midline, ventral, and medial nuclei of the thalamus elicits tachycardia. Stimulation of the posterior and posterolateral regions of the hypothalamus can also change the heart rate. Stimuli applied to the H2 fields of Forel in the diencephalon evoke various cardiovascular responses, including tachycardia; these changes resemble those observed during muscular exercise. Undoubtedly the cortical and diencephalic centers initiate the cardiac reactions that occur during excitement, anxiety, and other emotional states. The hypothalamic centers also initiate the cardiac response to alterations in environmental temperature. Experimentally induced temperature changes in the preoptic anterior hypothalamus alter heart rate and peripheral resistance.

Stimulation of the parahypoglossal area of the medulla reciprocally activates cardiac sympathetic pathways and inhibits cardiac parasympathetic pathways. In certain dorsal regions of the medulla, distinct cardiac accelerator and augmentor sites have been detected in animals with transected vagi. Stimulation of accelerator sites increases heart rate, whereas stimulation of augmentor sites increases cardiac contractility. The accelerator regions are more abundant on the right side, whereas the augmentor sites are more prevalent on the left side. A similar distribution also exists in the hypothalamus. Therefore, the sympathetic fibers mainly descend ipsilaterally through the brainstem.

Baroreceptor Reflex

Sudden changes in arterial blood pressure initiate a reflex that evokes an inverse change in heart rate (Fig. 17-6).

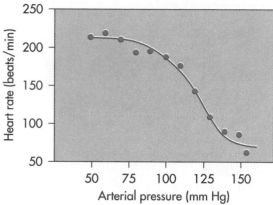

■ **Fig. 17-6** Heart rate as a function of mean arterial pressure in a group of five conscious, chronically instrumented monkeys. The mean control arterial pressure was 114 mm Hg. Pressure was increased above the control value by infusing phenylephrine and was decreased below the control value by infusing nitroprusside. (Adapted from Cornish KG et al: *Am J Physiol* 257:R595, 1989.)

Baroreceptors located in the aortic arch and carotid sinuses (see Chapter 21) are responsible for this reflex. The inverse relationship between heart rate and arterial blood pressure is usually most pronounced over an intermediate range of arterial blood pressures. In experiments conducted on conscious, chronically instrumented monkeys (Fig. 17-6), this range varied from about 70 to about 160 mm Hg. Below this intermediate range of pressures, the heart rate maintains a constant, high value; above this pressure range, the heart rate maintains a constant, low value.

The effects of these changes in carotid sinus pressure on the activity in the cardiac autonomic nerves of an anesthetized dog are shown in Fig. 17-7. This experiment shows that over an intermediate range of carotid sinus pressures (100 to 180 mm Hg), reciprocal changes are evoked in vagal and sympathetic neural activity. Below this range of carotid sinus pressures, sympathetic activity is intense and vagal activity is virtually absent. Conversely, above the intermediate range of carotid sinus pressures, vagal activity is intense and sympathetic activity is minimal.

Bainbridge Reflex, Atrial Receptors, and Atrial Natriuretic Peptide

In 1915, Bainbridge reported that infusing blood or saline into dogs accelerated their heart rate. This increase did not seem to be tied to arterial blood pressure—the heart rate rose regardless of whether the arterial blood pressure did or did not rise. However, Bainbridge also noted that the heart rate did increase whenever central venous pressure rose sufficiently to distend the right side of the heart. Bilateral transection of the vagi abolished this response.

Numerous investigators have confirmed Bainbridge's observations and have noted that the magnitude and direction of the response depended on the prevailing heart rate. When the heart rate was slow, intravenous infusions usually accelerated the heart. At more rapid heart rates, however, infusions ordinarily slowed the heart. What accounts for

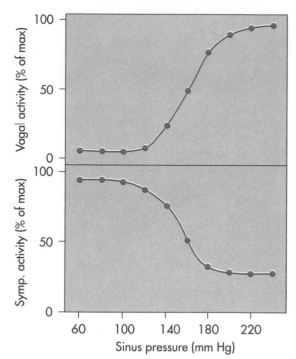

■ **Fig. 17-7** Effects of changes in pressure in the isolated carotid sinuses on the neural activity in cardiac vagal and sympathetic nerve fibers in an anesthetized dog. (Adapted from Kollai M, Koizumi K: *Pflugers Arch* 413:365, 1989.)

these different responses? Increases in blood volume not only evoke the so-called **Bainbridge reflex,** but they also activate other reflexes (notably the baroreceptor reflex). These other reflexes tend to elicit opposite changes in the heart rate. Therefore, changes in heart rate evoked by an alteration of blood volume are the result of these antagonistic reflex effects (Fig. 17-8).

The antagonistic effects of the Bainbridge and baroreceptor reflexes can be seen in the experiment shown in Fig. 17-9. In a group of unanesthetized dogs, volume loading with blood increased heart rate and cardiac output proportionately. Consequently, stroke volume remain virtually constant. Conversely, reductions in blood volume diminished the cardiac output but increased heart rate. Undoubtedly, the Bainbridge reflex predominates over the baroreceptor reflex when the blood volume rises, but the baroreceptor reflex prevails over the Bainbridge reflex when the blood volume diminishes.

Both atria have receptors that are affected by changes in blood volume and that influence heart rate. These receptors are located principally in the venoatrial junctions: in the right atrium at its junctions with the venae cavae and in the left atrium at its junctions with the pulmonary veins. Distension of these atrial receptors sends impulses centripetally in the vagi. The efferent impulses are carried by fibers from both autonomic divisions to the SA node.

The cardiac response to these changes in autonomic neural activity is highly selective. Even when the reflex increase in heart rate is large, changes in ventricular contractility are usually negligible. Furthermore, the neurally

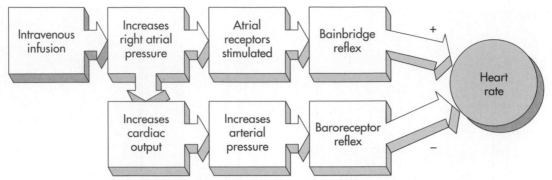

■ **Fig. 17-8** Intravenous infusions of blood or electrolyte solutions tend to increase heart rate via the Bainbridge reflex and to decrease heart rate via the baroreceptor reflex. The actual change in heart rate induced by such infusions is the result of these two opposing effects.

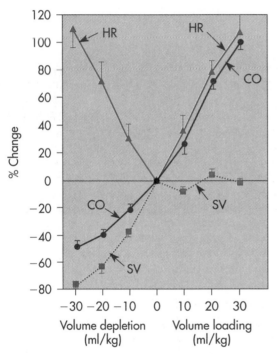

■ **Fig. 17-9** Effects of blood transfusion and of bleeding on cardiac output *(CO),* heart rate *(HR),* and stroke volume *(SV)* in unanesthetized dogs. (From Vatner SF, Boettcher DH: *Circ Res* 42:557, 1978.)

induced increase in heart rate is usually not accompanied by an increase of sympathetic activity to the peripheral arterioles.

Not only does stimulation of the atrial receptors increase heart rate, but it also increases urine volume. Reduced activity in the renal sympathetic nerve fibers may be partially responsible for this diuresis. However, the principal mechanism appears to be a neurally mediated reduction in the secretion of **vasopressin** (antidiuretic hormone) by the posterior pituitary gland (see Chapter 43).

Stretch of the atrial walls also releases atrial natriuretic peptide (ANP) from the atrial tissues. ANP exerts potent diuretic and natriuretic effects on the kidneys (see also

Chapter 36) and vasodilator effects on the resistance and capacitance blood vessels. Thus, ANP is an important regulator of blood volume and blood pressure.

> In **congestive heart failure,** NaCl and water are retained, mainly because stimulation by the renin-angiotensin system increases the release of aldosterone from the adrenal cortex. The plasma level of ANP is also increased in congestive heart failure. By enhancing the renal excretion of NaCl and water, this peptide gradually reduces the fluid retention and the consequent elevations of central venous pressure and cardiac preload.

Respiratory Sinus Arrhythmia

Rhythmic variations in heart rate, occurring at the frequency of respiration, are detectable in most individuals and tend to be more pronounced in children. The heart rate typically accelerates during inspiration and decelerates during expiration (Fig. 17-10).

Recordings from the autonomic nerves to the heart reveal that neural activity increases in the sympathetic fibers during inspiration, whereas neural activity in the vagal fibers increases during expiration (Fig. 17-11). As previously noted, the heart rate response to cessation of vagal stimulation is very quick, because the acetylcholine released from the vagus nerves is rapidly broken down by cholinesterase. It is this short latency that permits the heart rate to vary rhythmically at the respiratory frequency. Conversely, the norepinephrine released periodically at the sympathetic endings is removed very slowly. Therefore, the rhythmic variations in sympathetic activity do not induce any appreciable oscillatory changes in heart rate. Hence, this **respiratory sinus arrhythmia** is almost entirely accomplished by changes in vagal activity. In fact, respiratory sinus arrhythmia is exaggerated when vagal tone is enhanced.

Both reflex and central factors help initiate respiratory cardiac arrhythmia (Fig. 17-12). Stretch receptors in the lungs are stimulated during inspiration, and this action leads to a reflex increase in heart rate. The afferent and efferent

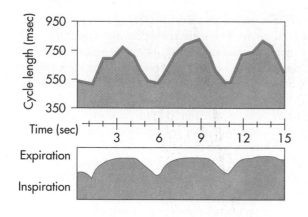

■ **Fig. 17-10** Respiratory sinus arrhythmia in a resting, unanesthetized dog. Note that the cardiac cycle length increases during expiration and decreases during inspiration. (Modified from Warner MR et al: *Am J Physiol* 251:H1134, 1986.)

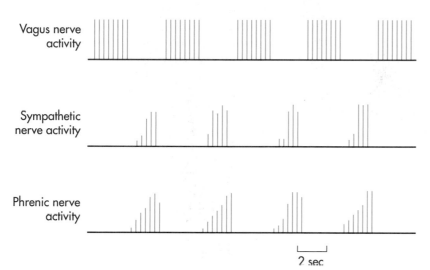

■ **Fig. 17-11** The respiratory fluctuations in efferent activity in the cardiac nerves of an anesthetized dog. Note that the sympathetic nerve activity occurs synchronously with the phrenic nerve discharges (which initiate diaphragmatic contraction), whereas the vagus nerve activity occurs between the phrenic nerve discharges. (From Kollai M, Koizumi K: *J Auton Nerv Syst* 1:33, 1979.)

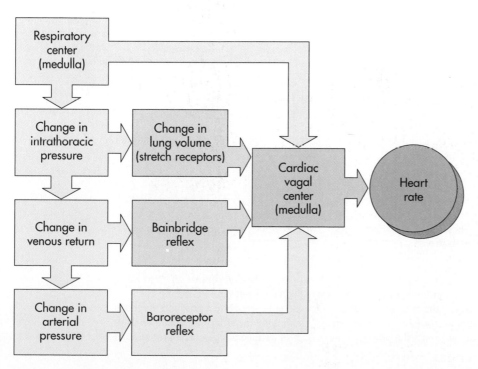

■ **Fig. 17-12** Respiratory sinus arrhythmia is generated by a direct interaction between the respiratory and cardiac centers in the medulla, as well as by reflexes that originate from stretch receptors in the lungs, stretch receptors in the right atrium (Bainbridge reflex), and baroreceptors in the carotid sinuses and aortic arch.

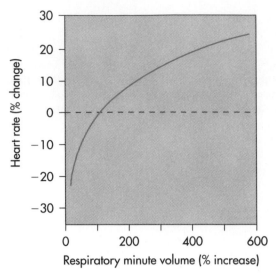

Fig. 17-13 Relationship between the change in heart rate and the change in respiratory minute volume during carotid chemoreceptor stimulation in spontaneously breathing cats and dogs. When respiratory stimulation was relatively slight, heart rate usually diminished; when respiratory stimulation was more pronounced, heart rate usually increased. (From Daly MdeB, Scott MJ: *J Physiol* 144:148, 1958.)

limbs of this reflex are located in the vagus nerves. Intrathoracic pressure also decreases during inspiration, and thereby increases venous return to the right side of the heart (see Chapter 22). The consequent stretch of the right atrium elicits the Bainbridge reflex (Fig. 17-12). After the time delay required for the increased venous return to reach the left side of the heart, left ventricular output increases and raises arterial blood pressure. This rise in blood pressure in turn reduces heart rate through the baroreceptor reflex (Fig. 17-12).

Central factors are also responsible for respiratory cardiac arrhythmia. The respiratory center in the medulla directly influences the cardiac autonomic centers (Fig. 17-12). In heart-lung bypass experiments conducted in animals, the chest is open, the lungs are collapsed, venous return is diverted to a pump-oxygenator, and arterial blood pressure is maintained at a constant level. In such experiments, rhythmic movements of the rib cage attest to the activity of the medullary respiratory centers. These movements of the rib cage are often accompanied by rhythmic changes in heart rate at the respiratory frequency. This respiratory cardiac arrhythmia is almost certainly induced by a direct interaction between the respiratory and cardiac centers in the medulla.

Chemoreceptor Reflex

The cardiac response to peripheral chemoreceptor stimulation merits special consideration, because it illustrates the complex interactions that may ensue when one stimulus excites two organ systems simultaneously. In intact animals, stimulation of the carotid chemoreceptors consistently

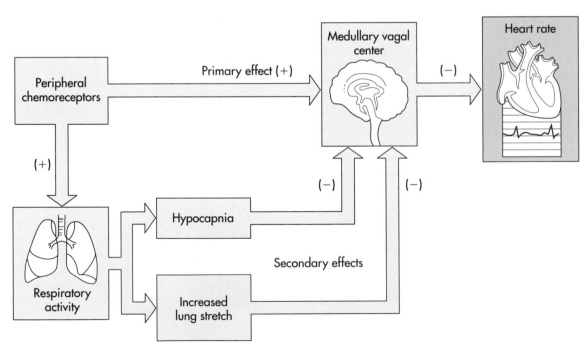

Fig. 17-14 The primary effect of stimulation of the peripheral chemoreceptors on heart rate is to excite the cardiac vagal center in the medulla and thus to decrease heart rate. Peripheral chemoreceptor stimulation also excites the respiratory center in the medulla. This effect produces hypocapnia and increases lung inflation, both of which secondarily inhibit the medullary vagal center. Thus, these secondary influences attenuate the primary reflex effect of peripheral chemoreceptor stimulation on heart rate.

increases ventilatory rate and depth (see Chapter 29), but ordinarily it changes heart rate only slightly. The magnitude of the ventilatory response determines whether the heart rate increases or decreases as a result of carotid chemoreceptor stimulation, as shown in Fig. 17-13. Mild respiratory stimulation decreases heart rate moderately; more pronounced stimulation increases heart rate only slightly. If the pulmonary response to chemoreceptor stimulation is blocked, the heart rate response may be greatly exaggerated, as described below.

The cardiac response to peripheral chemoreceptor stimulation is the result of primary and secondary reflex mechanisms (Fig. 17-14). The principal effect of this primary stimulation is to excite the medullary vagal center and thereby to decrease heart rate. Secondary reflex effects are mediated by the respiratory system. The respiratory stimulation by the arterial chemoreceptors tends to inhibit the medullary vagal center. This inhibitory effect varies with the level of concomitant stimulation of respiration; small increases in respiration inhibit the vagal center slightly, whereas greater increases in ventilation inhibit the vagal center more profoundly.

An example of this primary inhibitory influence is shown in Fig. 17-15. In this experiment on an anesthetized dog, the lungs were completely collapsed and blood oxygenation was accomplished by an artificial oxygenator. When the carotid chemoreceptors were stimulated, an intense bradycardia and some degree of AV block ensued. Such effects are mediated primarily by efferent vagal fibers.

The identical primary inhibitory effect also operates in humans. The electrocardiogram in Fig. 17-16 was recorded

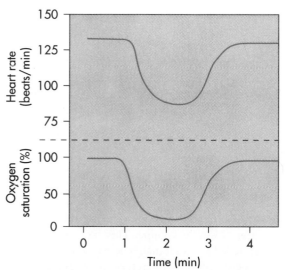

■ **Fig. 17-15** Changes in heart rate during carotid chemoreceptor stimulation in an anesthetized dog on total heart bypass. The lungs remain deflated and respiratory gas exchange is accomplished by an artificial oxygenator. The lower tracing represents the oxygen saturation of the blood perfusing the carotid chemoreceptors. The blood perfusing the remainder of the animal, including the myocardium, was fully saturated with oxygen throughout the experiment. (Modified from Levy MN, DeGeest H, Zieske H: *Circ Res* 18:67, 1966.)

from a **quadriplegic patient** who could not breathe spontaneously, but required tracheal intubation and artificial respiration. When the tracheal catheter was briefly disconnected (near the beginning of the top strip in the figure) to permit nursing care, the patient quickly developed a profound bradycardia. His heart rate was 65 beats per minute just before the tracheal catheter was disconnected. In less than 10 seconds after cessation of artificial respiration, his heart rate dropped to about 20 beats per minute. This bradycardia could be prevented by blocking the effects of efferent vagal activity with atropine, and its onset could be delayed considerably by hyperventilating the patient before disconnecting the tracheal catheter.

The pulmonary hyperventilation that is ordinarily evoked by carotid chemoreceptor stimulation influences heart rate secondarily, both by initiating more pronounced pulmonary inflation reflexes and by producing hypocapnia (Fig. 17-14). Both influences tend to depress the primary cardiac response to chemoreceptor stimulation and thereby accelerate the heart. Hence, when pulmonary hyperventilation is not prevented, the primary and secondary effects neutralize each other, and carotid chemoreceptor stimulation affects heart rate only moderately (Fig. 17-13).

Ventricular Receptor Reflexes

Sensory receptors located near the endocardial surfaces of the ventricular walls initiate reflex effects similar to those elicited by the arterial baroreceptors. Excitation of these endocardial receptors diminishes the heart rate and peripheral resistance. Other sensory receptors have been identified in the epicardial regions of the ventricles. Although it is known that all these ventricular receptors are excited by various mechanical and chemical stimuli, their exact physiological functions remain unclear.

Ventricular receptors have been implicated in the initiation of **vasovagal syncope,** which is a feeling of lightheadedness or brief loss of consciousness that may be triggered by psychological or by orthostatic stress. The ventricular receptors are believed to be stimulated by a reduced ventricular filling volume combined with a vigorous ventricular contraction. In a person standing quietly, ventricular filling is diminished because blood tends to pool in the veins in the abdomen and legs, as explained in Chapter 15. Consequently, the reduction in cardiac output and arterial blood pressure leads to a generalized increase in sympathetic neural activity via the baroreceptor reflex (Fig. 17-7). The enhanced sympathetic activity to the heart evokes a vigorous ventricular contraction, which thereby stimulates the ventricular receptors. Excitation of the ventricular receptors is believed to initiate the autonomic neural changes that evoke the vasovagal syncope, namely, a combination of a profound, vagally mediated bradycardia and a generalized arteriolar vasodilation mediated by a reduction in sympathetic neural activity.

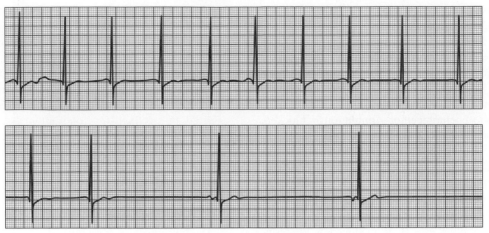

■ **Fig. 17-16**   Electrocardiogram of a 30-year-old quadriplegic man who could not breathe spontaneously and required tracheal intubation and artificial respiration. The two strips are continuous. (Modified from Berk JL, Levy MN: *Eur Surg Res* 9:75, 1977.)

REGULATION OF MYOCARDIAL PERFORMANCE

Intrinsic Regulation of Myocardial Performance

Just as the heart can initiate its own beat in the absence of any nervous or hormonal control, so also can the myocardium adapt to changing hemodynamic conditions by means of mechanisms that are intrinsic to cardiac muscle itself. Experiments on denervated hearts reveal that this organ adjusts remarkably well to stress. For example, racing greyhounds with denervated hearts perform almost as well as do those with intact innervation. Their maximal running speed was found to decrease only 5% after complete cardiac denervation. In these dogs, the threefold to fourfold increase in cardiac output during a race was achieved principally by an increase in stroke volume. In normal dogs, the increase of cardiac output with exercise is accompanied by a proportionate increase of heart rate; stroke volume does not change much (see Chapter 17). It is unlikely that the cardiac adaptation in the denervated animals is achieved entirely by intrinsic mechanisms; circulating catecholamines undoubtedly contribute. If β-adrenergic receptor antagonists are given to greyhounds with denervated hearts, their racing performance is severely impaired.

The heart is partially or completely denervated in various clinical situations: (1) the surgically transplanted heart is totally decentralized, although the intrinsic, postganglionic parasympathetic fibers persist; (2) atropine blocks vagal effects on the heart, and propranolol blocks sympathetic β-adrenergic influences; (3) certain drugs, such as reserpine, deplete cardiac norepinephrine stores and thereby restrict or abolish sympathetic control; and (4) in chronic congestive heart failure, cardiac norepinephrine stores are often severely diminished, and therefore any sympathetic influences are attenuated.

Two principal intrinsic mechanisms, namely the **Frank-Starling mechanism** and **rate-induced regulation,** enable the myocardium to adapt to changes in hemodynamic conditions. The Frank-Starling mechanism (also referred to as **Starling's law of the heart**) is invoked in response to changes in the resting length of the myocardial fibers. The physiological basis of this mechanism is explained in Chapter 16. Rate-induced regulation is invoked in response to changes in the frequency of the heartbeat. The physiological basis of this mechanism is explained in relation to Fig. 17-20. How these two mechanisms allow the heart to adapt to alterations in hemodynamic conditions is explained below.

Frank-Starling mechanism. About one century ago, the German physiologist Otto Frank and the English physiologist Ernest Starling independently studied the responses of isolated hearts to changes in preload and afterload (see Chapter 16). When the ventricular filling pressure (the preload) was increased (e.g., by raising a blood reservoir connected to the right atrium), the ventricular volume initially increased progressively. After several beats, however, the ventricles attained a constant, larger volume. At equilibrium, the volume of blood ejected by the ventricles (the stroke volume) with each heartbeat had increased to equal the greater quantity of venous return to the right atrium with each heartbeat.

The increased ventricular volume had somehow facilitated ventricular contraction and had enabled the ventricles to pump a greater stroke volume. This increase in the stroke volume achieved an exact match between the cardiac output and the increased venous return at equilibrium. Other researchers noted subsequently that the increased ventricular volume was associated with an increase in the length of the individual myocardial fibers that make up the ventricular chambers. On the basis of this observation, they concluded that the increase in fiber length altered cardiac performance mainly by altering the number of myofilament cross-bridges that could interact. However, more recent evidence indicates that the principal mechanism involves a

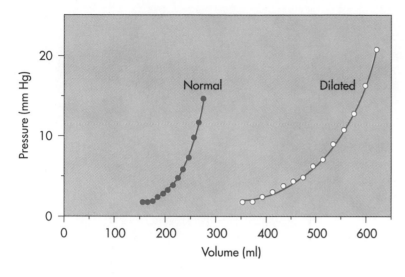

■ **Fig. 17-17** Pericardial pressure-volume relations in a normal dog and in a dog with experimentally induced chronic cardiac hypertrophy. (Modified from Freeman GL, Le Winter MM: *Circ Res* 54:294, 1984.)

stretch-induced change in the sensitivity of the cardiac myofilaments to calcium (see Chapter 16). An optimal fiber length exists, however. Excessively high filling pressures that overstretch the myocardial fibers may depress rather than enhance the pumping capacity of the ventricles.

Starling also showed that isolated heart preparations could adapt to changes in the counterforce to the ventricular ejection of blood during systole. As the left ventricle contracts, it does not eject blood into the aorta until the ventricle has developed a pressure that just exceeds the prevailing aortic pressure (see Chapter 16). The aortic pressure during ventricular ejection essentially constitutes the left ventricular afterload. In Starling's experiments, the arterial pressure was controlled by a hydraulic device in the tubing that led from the ascending aorta to the right atrial blood reservoir. Venous return to the right atrium was held constant by maintaining the hydrostatic level of the blood reservoir. As Starling raised the arterial pressure to a new, constant level, the left ventricle responded at first to the increased afterload by pumping a diminished stroke volume. Because venous return was held constant, the diminution of stroke volume was attended by a rise in ventricular diastolic volume as well as by an increase in the length of the myocardial fibers. This change in end-diastolic fiber length finally enabled the ventricle to pump a normal stroke volume against the greater peripheral resistance. As stated above, a change in the number of cross-bridges between the thick and thin filaments probably contributes to this adaptation, but the major factor appears to be a stretch-induced change in the sensitivity of the contractile proteins to calcium.

Changes in ventricular volume are also involved in the cardiac adaptation to alterations in heart rate. During bradycardia, for example, the increased duration of diastole permits greater ventricular filling. The consequent increase in myocardial fiber length increases stroke volume. Therefore, the reduction in heart rate may be fully compensated by the increase in stroke volume, and the cardiac output may therefore remain constant (see Fig. 15-16).

When cardiac compensation involves ventricular dilation, it is necessary to consider how the increased size of the ventricle affects the generation of the intraventricular pressure. If the ventricle enlarges, the force required by each myocardial fiber to generate a given intraventricular systolic pressure must be appreciably greater than that developed by the fibers in a ventricle of normal size. The Laplace relationship between wall tension and cavity pressure for the cardiac ventricles resembles that for cylindrical tubes (see Chapter 20), in that for a constant internal pressure, wall tension varies directly with the radius. As a consequence, more energy is required for the dilated heart to perform a given amount of external work than for the normal-sized heart. Hence, in the computation of the afterload on the contracting myocardial fibers in the walls of the ventricles, the dimensions of the ventricles must be considered along with the intraventricular (and aortic) pressure.

The relatively rigid pericardium that encloses the heart determines the pressure-volume relationship at high levels of pressure and volume. The pericardium exerts this limitation of volume even under normal conditions, when an individual is at rest and the heart rate is slow. In patients with chronic **congestive heart failure,** the sustained cardiac dilation and hypertrophy may stretch the pericardium considerably. In such patients, the pericardial limitation of cardiac filling is exerted at pressures and volumes entirely different from those in normal individuals (Fig. 17-17).

The major problem in assessing the role of the Frank-Starling mechanism in intact animals and humans is the difficulty of measuring end-diastolic volume or end-diastolic myocardial fiber length. In intact subjects, the Frank-Starling mechanism has been represented graphically by plotting some index of ventricular performance along the ordinate and some index of end-diastolic ventricular volume or fiber length along the abscissa. The most commonly used indices of ventricular performance have been cardiac output, stroke volume, and stroke work; stroke work is the product of stroke volume and mean arterial pressure. The indices of end-diastolic ventricular volume and fiber length have been end-diastolic ventricular pressure and mean atrial pressure.

To assess changes in ventricular performance, the Frank-Starling mechanism is often represented by a family of

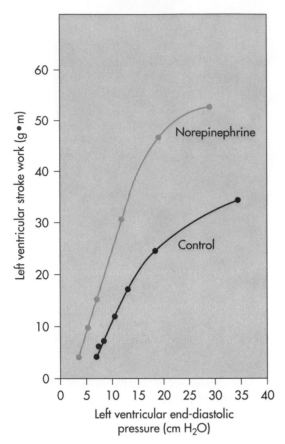

■ **Fig. 17-18**   A constant infusion of norepinephrine in a dog shifts the ventricular function curve to the left. This shift signifies an enhancement of ventricular contractility. (Redrawn from Sarnoff SJ et al: *Circ Res* 8:1108, 1960.)

so-called **ventricular function curves.** To construct a control ventricular function curve, for example, blood volume is altered over a range of values, and stroke work and end-diastolic ventricular pressure are measured at each step. Similar observations are then made during the desired experimental intervention, such as an intravenous infusion of norepinephrine. For example, the ventricular function curve obtained during a norepinephrine infusion in an anesthetized dog lies above and to the left of the control ventricular function curve (Fig. 17-18). It is evident that for a given level of left ventricular end-diastolic pressure (an index of the preload), the left ventricle performs more work during the norepinephrine infusion than during control conditions. Hence, a shift of the ventricular function curve upward and to the left signifies an improvement of ventricular **contractility** (see Chapter 16). Conversely, a shift downward and to the right indicates an impairment of contractility, and a consequent tendency toward **cardiac failure.**

Disparities between right and left ventricular outputs. The Frank-Starling mechanism is ideally suited to matching the cardiac output to the venous return. Any sudden, excessive output by one ventricle soon causes an increase in the venous return to the second ventricle. The consequent increase in diastolic fiber length in the second ventricle augments the

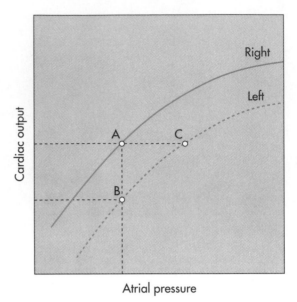

■ **Fig. 17-19**   Relationships between the outputs of the right and left ventricles and the mean pressures in the right and left atria, respectively. At any given level of cardiac output, mean left atrial pressure (e.g., point *C*) exceeds mean right atrial pressure (point *A*).

output of that ventricle to correspond with the output of its mate. In this way, the Frank-Starling mechanism maintains a precise balance between the outputs of the right and left ventricles. Because the two ventricles are arranged in series in a closed circuit, any small, but maintained, imbalance in the outputs of the two ventricles would otherwise be catastrophic.

The curves that relate cardiac output to mean atrial pressure for the two ventricles do not coincide; the curve for the left ventricle usually lies below that for the right ventricle (Fig. 17-19). At equal right and left atrial pressures (points *A* and *B*), right ventricular output would exceed left ventricular output. Hence, venous return to the left ventricle (a function of right ventricular output) would exceed left ventricular output, and left ventricular diastolic volume and pressure would rise. By the Frank-Starling mechanism, left ventricular output would therefore increase (from *B* toward *C*). Only when the outputs of both ventricles are identical (points *A* and *C*) would equilibrium be reached. Under such conditions, however, left atrial pressure *(C)* would exceed right atrial pressure *(A)*, and this is precisely the relationship that ordinarily prevails.

This greater left than right atrial pressure accounts for the observation that in individuals with **congenital atrial septal defects,** in which the two atria communicate with each other via a **patent foramen ovale,** the direction of the shunt flow is usually from left to right.

Rate-induced regulation. Myocardial performance is also regulated by changes in the frequency at which the myocardial fibers contract. The effects of changes in the frequency of contraction on the force developed in an

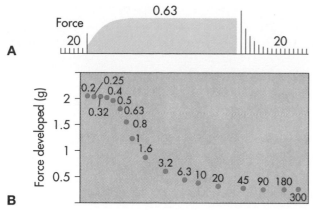

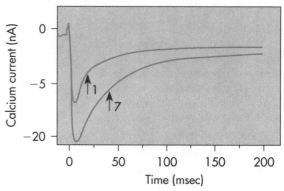

■ **Fig. 17-20** Changes in force development in an isolated papillary muscle from a cat as the interval between contractions is varied from 20 seconds to 0.63 second, and then back to 20 seconds (**A**). In **B**, the points represent the steady-state forces developed by the same papillary muscle at each of the indicated intervals (in seconds). (Redrawn from Koch-Weser J, Blinks JR: *Pharmacol Rev* 15:601, 1963.)

■ **Fig. 17-21** Calcium currents induced in a guinea pig myocyte during the first and seventh depolarizations in a consecutive sequence of depolarizations. The arrows indicate the half-times of inactivation. Note that during the seventh depolarization, the maximal inward Ca^{2+} current and the half-time of inactivation were greater than the respective values for the first depolarization. (Modified from Lee KS: *Proc Natl Acad Sci USA* 84:3941, 1987.)

isometrically contracting cat papillary muscle are shown in Fig. 17-20. Initially the strip of cardiac muscle was stimulated to contract only once every 20 seconds (Fig. 17-20, *A*). When the muscle was suddenly made to contract once every 0.63 second, the developed force increased progressively over the next several beats. At the new steady state, the developed force was more than five times as great as it was at the larger contraction interval. A return to the larger interval (20 seconds) had the opposite influence on developed force.

The effects of a wide range of contraction intervals on the steady-state levels of developed force are shown in Fig. 17-20, *B*. As the contraction interval was diminished from 300 seconds down to about 20 seconds, little change occurred in developed force. As the interval was reduced further, to a value of about 0.5 second, force increased sharply. Further reduction of the interval to 0.2 second had little additional effect on developed force.

The initial progressive rise in developed force when the contraction interval was suddenly decreased (e.g., from 20 seconds to 0.63 second in Fig. 17-20, *B*) is caused by a gradual increase in intracellular Ca^{2+} concentration. Two mechanisms contribute to the rise in Ca^{2+} concentration: (1) an increase in the number of depolarizations per minute and (2) an increase in the inward Ca^{2+} current per depolarization.

In the first mechanism, Ca^{2+} enters the myocardial cell during each action potential plateau (see Fig. 15-8). As the interval between beats is diminished, the number of plateaus per minute increases. Although the duration of each action potential (and of each plateau) decreases as the interval between beats is reduced (see Fig. 15-17), the overriding effect of the increased number of plateaus per minute on the influx of Ca^{2+} prevails, and the intracellular concentration of Ca^{2+} increases.

In the second mechanism, as the interval between beats is suddenly diminished, the inward Ca^{2+} current (i_{Ca}) progres-

sively increases with each successive beat until a new steady state is attained at the new basic cycle length. Figure 17-21 shows that in an isolated ventricular myocyte subjected to repetitive depolarizations, the influx of Ca^{2+} into the myocyte increased on successive beats. For example, the maximal i_{Ca} was considerably greater during the seventh depolarization than it was during the first depolarization. Furthermore, the decay of that current (i.e., its rate of inactivation) was substantially slower during the seventh depolarization than during the first depolarization. Both of these characteristics of the i_{Ca} would result in a greater influx of Ca^{2+} into the myocyte during the seventh depolarization than during the first depolarization. The greater influx of Ca^{2+} would, of course, strengthen the myocyte's contraction.

Transient changes in the intervals between beats also profoundly affect the strength of contraction. When the left ventricle contracts prematurely (Fig. 17-22, beat *A*), the premature contraction (extrasystole) itself is feeble, whereas contraction *B* (postextrasystolic contraction) after the compensatory pause is very strong. In the intact circulatory system, this response depends partly on the Frank-Starling mechanism. Inadequate time for ventricular filling just before the premature beat accounts partly for the weak premature contraction. Subsequently, the exaggerated degree of filling associated with the long compensatory pause (see Fig. 17-22) explains in part the vigorous postextrasystolic contraction.

Although the Frank-Starling mechanism is certainly involved in the usual ventricular adaptation to a premature beat, it is not the exclusive mechanism. Figure 17-22 shows the ventricular pressure curves recorded from an isovolumic left ventricle preparation, in which the ventricle neither fills nor ejects during the cardiac cycle. Although the left ventricular volume remained constant throughout the entire tracing, the premature beat *(A)* was feeble and the postextrasystolic contraction *(B)* was supernormal. Such enhanced contractility in the postextrasystolic contraction

■ **Fig. 17-22** In an isovolumic canine left ventricle preparation, a premature ventricular systole (beat *A*) is typically feeble, whereas the postextrasystolic contraction (beat *B*) is characteristically strong, and the enhanced contractility may diminish over a few beats (e.g., contraction *C*). (From Levy MN: Unpublished tracing.)

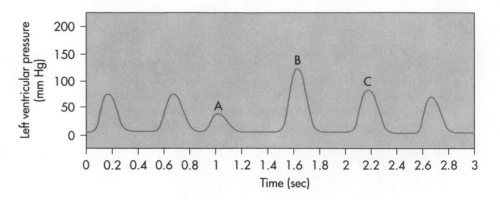

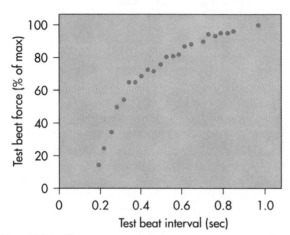

■ **Fig. 17-23** Force generated during premature contractions in an isolated ventricular muscle preparation from a guinea pig. The muscle was stimulated to contract once per second. Periodically the muscle was stimulated prematurely. The scale along the X axis denotes the time between the driven and the premature beat. The Y axis denotes the ratio of the contractile force of the premature beat to that of the driven beat. (Modified from Seed WA, Walker JM: *Cardiovasc Res* 22:303, 1988.)

is an example of **postextrasystolic potentiation,** and it may persist for one or more additional beats (e.g., contraction C).

The weakness of the premature beat is directly related to its degree of prematurity. In other words, the earlier the premature beat occurs, the weaker is its force of contraction. Conversely, as the time (**coupling interval**) between the premature beat and the preceding beat increases, the premature beat gains strength. The curve that relates the strength of contraction of a premature beat to the coupling interval is called a **mechanical restitution curve.** Figure 17-23 shows the restitution curve obtained by varying the coupling intervals of test beats in an isolated ventricular muscle preparation from a guinea pig.

The restitution of the force of contraction probably depends on the time course of the intracellular circulation of Ca^{2+} in the cardiac myocytes during the contraction and relaxation process. During relaxation, the Ca^{2+} that dissociates from the contractile proteins is taken up by the sarcoplasmic reticulum for subsequent release. However, there is a lag of about

500 to 800 msec before this Ca^{2+} becomes available for release from the sarcoplasmic reticulum in response to the next depolarization.

If we examine once again the experiment depicted in Fig. 17-22 (beat *A*), the premature beat itself was feeble. The time during the preceding relaxation was probably insufficient to allow much of the Ca^{2+} taken up by the sarcoplasmic reticulum to become available for release during the premature beat. The postextrasystolic beat *(B),* conversely, was considerably stronger than normal. The increase in contraction force developed in beat B was probably so great because a relatively large quantity of Ca^{2+} was taken up by the sarcoplasmic reticulum during the substantial time that had elapsed from the end of the last regular beat until the beginning of the postextrasystolic beat. This large quantity of Ca^{2+} would have been available for release during beat *B*.

Extrinsic Regulation of Myocardial Performance

Although the completely isolated heart can adapt well to changes in preload and afterload, various extrinsic factors also influence the heart in the intact animal. Under many natural conditions, these extrinsic regulatory mechanisms may overwhelm the intrinsic mechanisms. The extrinsic regulatory factors may be subdivided into nervous and chemical components.

Nervous control

Sympathetic influences. Sympathetic nervous activity enhances atrial and ventricular contractility. Effects of increased cardiac sympathetic activity on the ventricular myocardium are asymmetric laterally. As shown in Fig. 17-5, the cardiac sympathetic nerves on the left side of the body usually have a much greater effect on ventricular contraction than do those on the right side.

The alterations in ventricular contraction evoked by electrical stimulation of the left stellate ganglion in a canine isovolumic left ventricle preparation are shown in Fig. 17-24. The peak pressure and the maximal rate of pressure rise (dP/dt) during systole are markedly increased by sympathetic stimulation. Also, the duration of systole is reduced and the rate of ventricular relaxation is increased during the early phases of diastole; both of these responses assist ventricular

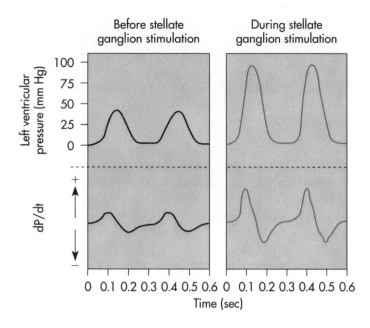

Before stellate ganglion stimulation | During stellate ganglion stimulation

■ **Fig. 17-24** In an isovolumic left ventricle preparation, stimulation of cardiac sympathetic nerves evokes a substantial rise in peak left ventricular pressure and in the maximal rates of intraventricular pressure rise and fall *(dP/dt)*. (From Levy MN: Unpublished tracing.)

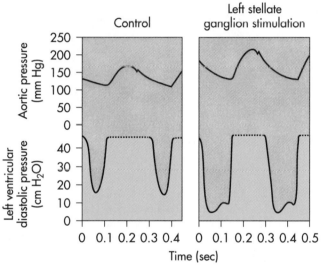

■ **Fig. 17-25** Stimulation of the left stellate ganglion of a dog increases arterial pressure, stroke volume, and stroke work but decreases the ventricular end-diastolic pressure. Note also the abridgement of systole, which allows more time for ventricular filling; the heart was paced at a constant rate. In the ventricular pressure tracings the pen excursion is limited at 45 mm Hg; actual ventricular pressures during systole can be estimated from the aortic pressure tracings. (Redrawn from Mitchell JH, Linden RJ, Sarnoff SJ: *Circ Res* 8:1100, 1960.)

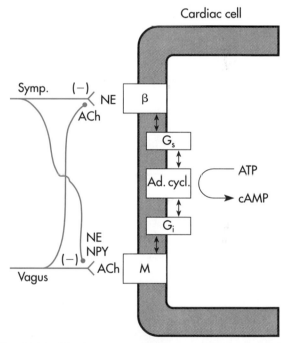

■ **Fig. 17-26** The interneuronal and intracellular mechanisms responsible for the interactions between the sympathetic and parasympathetic systems in the neural control of cardiac function. *NE*, Norepinephrine; *ACh*, acetylcholine; *NPY*, neuropeptide Y; β, β-adrenergic receptor; *M*, muscarinic receptor; *Gs* and *Gi*, stimulatory and inhibitory G proteins; *Ad. cycl.*, adenylyl cyclase; *ATP*, adenosine triphosphate; *cAMP*, cyclic adenosine monophosphate. (From Levy MN. In Kulbertus HE, Franck G, editors: *Neurocardiology*, Mt. Kisco, NY, 1988, Futura.)

filling. For any given cardiac cycle length, the abbreviation of systole allows more time for diastole and hence for ventricular filling. In the experiment shown in Fig. 17-25, for example, the animal's heart was paced at a constant rapid rate. Sympathetic stimulation *(right panel)* shortened systole. The consequent lengthening of diastole allowed substantially more time for ventricular filling.

Sympathetic nervous activity also enhances myocardial performance by activating calcium channels in myocardial

cell membranes. Neurally released norepinephrine or circulating catecholamines interact with β-adrenergic receptors on the cardiac cell membranes (Fig. 17-26). This interaction activates adenylyl cyclase, which raises the intracellular levels of cyclic AMP (see Chapter 5). Consequently, protein kinases that promote the phosphorylation of various proteins are activated within the myocardial cells. Phosphorylation of specific sarcolemmal proteins activates the calcium channels in the membranes of myocardial cells.

Activation of the calcium channels increases the influx of Ca^{2+} during the action potential plateau, and more Ca^{2+} is released from the sarcoplasmic reticulum in response to each cardiac excitation. The contractile strength of the heart is thereby increased. Figure 17-27 shows the correlation between the contractile force in a thin strip of ventricular muscle and the Ca^{2+} concentration (as reflected by the aequorin light signal) in the myocytes as the concentration of isoproterenol (a β-adrenergic agonist) was increased in the tissue bath.

The overall effect of increased cardiac sympathetic activity in intact animals can best be appreciated in terms of families of ventricular function curves. When stepwise increases in the frequency of electrical stimulation are applied to the left stellate ganglion, the ventricular function curves shift progressively to the left. The changes parallel those produced by norepinephrine infusions (Fig. 17-18). Hence, for any given left ventricular end-diastolic pressure, the ventricle can perform more work as the level of sympathetic nervous activity is increased.

During cardiac sympathetic nerve stimulation, the increase in work is usually accompanied by a reduction in left ventricular end-diastolic pressure. An example of the response to stellate ganglion stimulation in a heart paced at a constant frequency is shown in Fig. 17-25. In this experiment, stroke work increased by about 50%, despite a reduction in left ventricular end-diastolic pressure. The reason for the reduction in ventricular end-diastolic pressure is explained in Chapter 22.

Parasympathetic influences. The vagus nerves inhibit the cardiac pacemaker, atrial myocardium, and AV conduction tissue (see Chapter 17). The vagus nerves also depress the ventricular myocardium, but the effects are less pronounced

in the ventricles than in the atria. In an isovolumic left ventricle preparation, vagal stimulation decreased the peak left ventricular pressure, the maximal rate of pressure development (dP/dt), and the maximal rate of pressure decline during diastole (Fig. 17-28). In pumping heart preparations, the ventricular function curve shifts to the right during vagal stimulation.

At least two mechanisms are responsible for the vagal effects on the ventricular myocardium. In one mechanism, acetylcholine *(ACh)* released from the vagus nerve endings can interact with muscarinic *(M)* receptors in the cardiac cell membrane (Fig. 17-26). This interaction leads to the inhibition of adenylyl cyclase. The consequent diminution in the

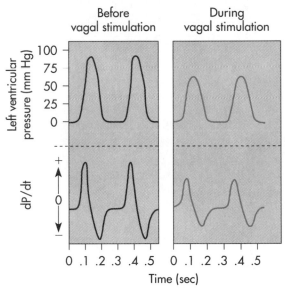

■ **Fig. 17-28**   In an isovolumic left ventricle preparation, when the ventricle is paced at a constant frequency, vagal stimulation decreases the peak left ventricular pressure and diminishes the maximal rates of pressure rise and fall *(dP/dt)*. (From Levy MN: Unpublished tracing.)

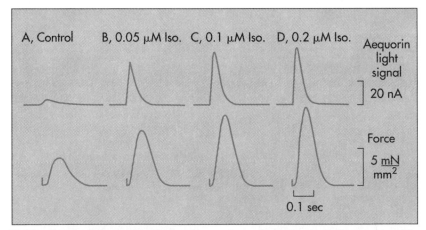

■ **Fig. 17-27**   Effects of various concentrations of isoproterenol *(Iso)* on aequorin light signal (in *nA*) and contractile force (in *mN/mm²*) in a rat ventricular muscle injected with aequorin. The aequorin light signal reflects the instantaneous changes in intracellular Ca^{2+} concentration. (Modified from Kurihara S, Konishi M: *Pflugers Arch* 409:427, 1987.)

intracellular concentration of cyclic AMP leads to a reduction in Ca²⁺ conductance of the cell membrane, and hence to a decrease in myocardial contractility.

In another mechanism, ACh released from the vagal endings can also inhibit the release of norepinephrine from neighboring sympathetic nerve endings (Fig. 17-26). The experiment illustrated in Fig. 17-29 demonstrates that stimulation of the cardiac sympathetic nerves *(S)* causes a substantial overflow of norepinephrine into the coronary sinus blood. Concomitant vagal stimulation *(SV)* reduces the overflow of norepinephrine by about 30%. The amount of norepinephrine that enters the coronary sinus blood probably parallels the amount released at the sympathetic terminals in the myocardium. Thus, vagal activity can decrease ventricular contractility partly by antagonizing any stimulatory effects that concomitant sympathetic activity may be exerting on ventricular contractility. Similarly, sympathetic

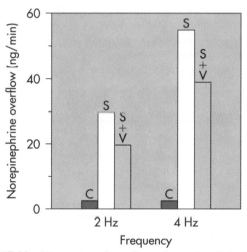

■ **Fig. 17-29**   Mean rates of overflow of norepinephrine into the coronary sinus blood in a group of seven dogs under control conditions *(C)*, during cardiac sympathetic stimulation *(S)* at 2 or 4 Hz, and during combined sympathetic and vagal stimulation *(S + V)*. The combined stimulus consisted of sympathetic stimulation at 2 or 4 Hz and vagal stimulation at 15 Hz. (Redrawn from Levy MN, Blattberg B: *Circ Res* 38:81, 1976.)

nerves release norepinephrine and certain neuropeptides, including neuropeptide Y (NPY). Norepinephrine and NPY both inhibit the release of acetylcholine from neighboring vagal fibers (Fig. 17-26).

Chemical control

Hormones

Adrenomedullary hormones. The adrenal medulla is essentially a component of the autonomic nervous system (see Chapters 11 and 45). The principal hormone secreted by the adrenal medulla is epinephrine, although some norepinephrine is also released. The rate of secretion of these catecholamines by the adrenal medulla is regulated by mechanisms that resemble those that control the activity of the sympathetic nervous system. The concentrations of catecholamines in the blood rise under the same conditions that activate the sympathoadrenal system. However, the cardiovascular effects of circulating catecholamines are probably minimal under normal conditions.

The changes in myocardial contractility induced by norepinephrine infusions have been tested in resting, unanesthetized dogs. The maximal rate of rise of left ventricular pressure (dP/dt), an index of myocardial contractility, varies directly with the norepinephrine concentration in the blood (Fig. 17-30). In these same animals, moderate exercise increased the maximum dP/dt by almost 100%, but it raised the circulating catecholamines by only 0.5 ng/ml. By itself, such a rise in blood norepinephrine concentration would have had only a negligible effect on left ventricular dP/dt (Fig. 17-30). Therefore, the pronounced change in dP/dt observed during exercise must have been mediated mainly by the norepinephrine released from the cardiac sympathetic nerve fibers rather than by the catecholamines released from the adrenal medulla.

Adrenocortical hormones. Information about the influence of adrenocortical steroids on myocardial contractility is sketchy and controversial. Cardiac muscle removed from adrenalectomized animals and placed in a tissue bath is more likely to fatigue in response to stimulation than is cardiac muscle obtained from normal animals. In some species,

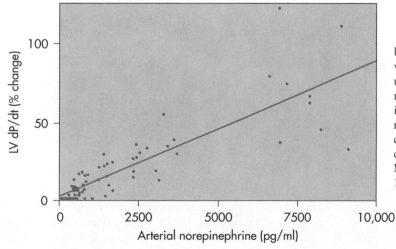

■ **Fig. 17-30**   Effect of norepinephrine infusions on ventricular contractility in a group of resting, unanesthetized dogs. The plasma concentrations of norepinephrine *(pg/ml)* plotted along the abscissa are the increments above the control values. The maximal rate of rise of left ventricular pressure *(LV dP/dt)*, an index of contractility, is plotted along the ordinate as percentage change from the control value. (Redrawn from Young MA, Hintze TH, Vatner SF: *Am J Physiol* 178:H82, 1985.)

however, the adrenocortical hormones enhance contractility. Furthermore, hydrocortisone potentiates the cardiotonic effects of catecholamines. This potentiation may be mediated in part by the ability of the adrenocortical steroids to inhibit the catecholamine uptake mechanisms.

> Cardiovascular problems are common in adrenocortical insufficiency (**Addison's disease**). The blood volume tends to fall, which may lead to severe hypotension and cardiovascular collapse, the so-called **addisonian crisis** (see Chapter 45).

Thyroid hormones. Numerous studies in intact animals and humans have demonstrated that thyroid hormones enhance myocardial contractility. The rates of adenosine triphosphate (ATP) hydrolysis and of Ca^{2+} uptake by the sarcoplasmic reticulum are increased in experimental hyperthyroidism, and the opposite effects occur in hypothyroidism. Thyroid hormones increase protein synthesis in the heart, and this response leads to cardiac hypertrophy. These hormones also affect the composition of myosin isoenzymes in cardiac muscle. By increasing those isoenzymes with the greatest ATPase activity, thyroid hormones enhance myocardial contractility.

The cardiovascular changes in thyroid dysfunction also depend on indirect mechanisms. Thyroid hyperactivity increases the body's metabolic rate, which in turn results in arteriolar vasodilation. The consequent reduction in the total peripheral resistance increases cardiac output, as explained in Chapter 22.

> Cardiac activity is sluggish in patients with inadequate thyroid function (**hypothyroidism**). The converse is true in patients with overactive thyroid glands (**hyperthyroidism**). Characteristically, hyperthyroid patients exhibit tachycardia, high cardiac output, palpitations, and arrhythmias, such as atrial fibrillation (see Chapter 44). In hyperthyroid subjects, sympathetic neural activity may be increased, or the sensitivity of the heart to such activity may be enhanced. Studies have shown that thyroid hormone increases the density of β-adrenergic receptors in cardiac tissue (see also Chapter 44). In experimental animals, the cardiovascular manifestations of hyperthyroidism may be simulated by the administration of thyroxine.

Insulin. Insulin has a positive inotropic effect on the heart (see Chapter 41). The effect of insulin is evident even when hypoglycemia is prevented by glucose infusions and when the β-adrenergic receptors are blocked. In fact, the positive inotropic effect of insulin is potentiated by β-adrenergic receptor antagonists. The enhancement of contractility cannot be explained satisfactorily by the concomitant augmentation of glucose transport into the myocardial cells.

Glucagon. Glucagon has potent positive inotropic and chronotropic effects on the heart (see Chapter 40). This endogenous hormone is probably not important in the normal regulation of the cardiovascular system, but it has been used clinically to enhance cardiac performance. The effects of glucagon on the heart closely resemble those of the catecholamines, and certain metabolic effects are similar. Both glucagon and catecholamines activate adenylyl cyclase to increase the myocardial tissue levels of cyclic AMP. The catecholamines activate adenylyl cyclase by interacting with β-adrenergic receptors, but glucagon activates this enzyme through a different mechanism. Nevertheless, the consequent rise in cyclic AMP increases Ca^{2+} influx through the Ca^{2+} channels in the sarcolemma and facilitates Ca^{2+} release and reuptake by the sarcoplasmic reticulum, just as do the catecholamines.

Anterior pituitary hormones. The cardiovascular derangements in hypopituitarism are related principally to the associated deficiencies in adrenocortical and thyroid function (see Chapter 43). Growth hormone does affect the myocardium, at least in combination with thyroxine. In hypophysectomized animals, growth hormone alone has little effect on the depressed heart, whereas thyroxine by itself restores adequate cardiac performance under basal conditions. However, when blood volume or peripheral resistance is increased, thyroxine alone does not restore adequate cardiac function, but the combination of growth hormone and thyroxine does reestablish normal cardiac performance. In certain animal models of heart failure, administration of growth hormone alone does increase cardiac output and myocardial contractility.

Blood gases

Oxygen. Changes in oxygen tension (Pao_2) of the blood perfusing the brain and the peripheral chemoreceptors affect the heart through nervous mechanisms, as described earlier in this chapter. These indirect effects of hypoxia are usually prepotent. When a subject is exposed to moderate degrees of hypoxia, heart rate, cardiac output, and myocardial contractility are usually enhanced. These changes are largely abolished by β-adrenergic receptor antagonists.

The Po_2 of the arterial blood perfusing the myocardium also influences myocardial performance directly. The effect of hypoxia is biphasic: mild hypoxia is stimulatory, but more severe hypoxia is depressant, because oxidative metabolism is limited.

Carbon dioxide and acidosis. Changes in $Paco_2$ may also affect the myocardium directly and indirectly. The direct effects on the heart elicited by changes of Pco_2 in the coronary arterial blood are illustrated in Fig. 17-31. In this experiment on an isolated left ventricle preparation, the control $Paco_2$ was 45 mm Hg *(arrow A)*. Decreasing the Pco_2 to 34 mm Hg *(arrow B)* was stimulatory, whereas increasing Pco_2 to 86 mm *(arrow C)* was depressant.

The indirect, neurally mediated effects produced by an increased Pco_2 in the systemic arterial blood are similar to those evoked by a decrease in Pao_2. An increase in systemic arterial Pco_2 stimulates the central and peripheral chemoreceptors, which then leads to a generalized increase in sympathetic neural activity. The effect of moderate increases in systemic arterial Pco_2 on the cardiovascular system is to

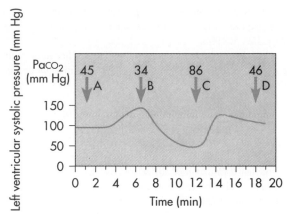

■ **Fig. 17-31** Decrease in Paco₂ increases left ventricular systolic pressure *(arrow B)* in an isovolumic left ventricle preparation; a rise in Paco₂ *(arrow C)* has the reverse effect. When the Paco₂ is returned to the control level *(arrow D),* left ventricular systolic pressure returns to its original value *(arrow A).* (From Levy MN: Unpublished tracing.)

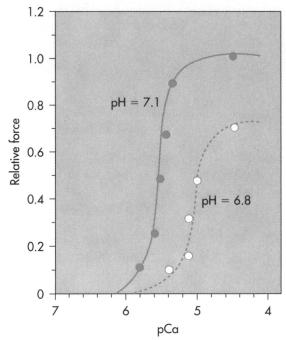

■ **Fig. 17-32** Effect of pH on the relationship between relative force and pCa (negative logarithm of the Ca concentration) in a "skinned" ventricular fiber from a rat. Relative force is the force developed by the preparation at various combinations of pH and pCa, expressed as a percentage of the maximal force developed by the preparation when the intracellular pH was 7.1 and the pCa was less than 4.6. The "skinned" fiber was prepared by treating the preparation with a detergent to solubilize the cell membranes, and thereby to expose the contractile proteins in the fiber to the concentrations of H^+ and of Ca^{2+} that prevailed in the bathing solution. (Modified from Mayoux E et al: *Am J Physiol* 266:H2051, 1994.)

increase heart rate, cardiac output, and arterial blood pressure. Thus, in intact animals, the activation of the sympathoadrenal system by moderate increases in systemic arterial Pco_2 tends to prevail over the direct depressant effect on the heart imposed by the increased arterial Pco_2 in the coronary arterial blood.

Neither the arterial Pco_2 nor the blood pH is a primary determinant of myocardial behavior; the associated change in intracellular pH is the critical factor. The reduced intracellular pH diminishes the amount of Ca^{2+} released from the sarcoplasmic reticulum in response to excitation. The diminished pH also decreases the sensitivity of the myofilaments to Ca^{2+}. The effect of this acidosis on the sensitivity to Ca^{2+} is reflected by a shift in the relationship between developed force and pCa (the negative logarithm of the intracellular Ca^{2+} concentration). Increases in intracellular pH have the opposite effect; that is, they enhance the sensitivity to Ca^{2+}.

Figure 17-32 illustrates such a shift in sensitivity to Ca^{2+} in an experiment on isolated ventricular fibers immersed in a tissue bath. When the pH of the bath was changed from 7.1 to 6.8, the curve of contractile force as a function of pCa was shifted substantially to the right (the normal intracellular pH is about 7.1). Furthermore, in this same preparation, at high intracellular Ca^{2+} concentrations (i.e., at values of pCa below about 4.6), a reduction in pH diminished the maximal developed force. This reduction in maximal force suggests that the low pH depresses the actomyosin interactions.

SUMMARY

1. Cardiac function is regulated by a number of intrinsic and extrinsic mechanisms.

2. Heart rate is regulated mainly by the autonomic nervous system. Sympathetic nervous activity increases heart rate, whereas parasympathetic (vagal) activity decreases heart

rate. When both systems are active, the vagal effects usually dominate.

3. The following reflexes regulate heart rate: the baroreceptor, chemoreceptor, pulmonary inflation, atrial receptor (Bainbridge), and ventricular receptor reflexes.

4. The principal intrinsic mechanisms that regulate myocardial contraction are the Frank-Starling mechanism and rate-induced regulation.

   a. The Frank-Starling mechanism is the process by which a change in the resting length of the myocardial fiber influences subsequent contraction by altering the affinity of the myofilaments for calcium and by altering the number of interacting cross-bridges between the thick and thin filaments.

   b. Rate-induced regulation is the process by which a sustained change in contraction frequency affects the strength of contraction by altering the rate of influx of Ca^{2+} into the cell. Conversely, a transient change in contraction frequency alters contractile strength because an appreciable delay exists between the time that Ca^{2+} is taken up by the sarcoplasmic reticulum and the time that it becomes available again for release.

5. The autonomic nervous system regulates myocardial performance mainly by varying the Ca^{2+} conductance of the cell membrane via the adenylyl cyclase system.

6. Certain hormones, such as epinephrine, adrenocortical steroids, thyroid hormones, insulin, glucagon, and anterior pituitary hormones, regulate myocardial performance.

7. Changes in the arterial blood concentrations of O_2, CO_2, and H^+ directly alter cardiac function and indirectly alter it via the chemoreceptor.

BIBLIOGRAPHY

Journal articles

Bers DM: Calcium fluxes involved in control of cardiac myocyte contraction, *Circ Res* 87:275, 2000.

Dampney RAL: Functional organization of central pathways regulating the cardiovascular system, *Physiol Rev* 74:323, 1994.

Hool LC: Hypoxia increases the sensitivity of the L-type Ca^{2+} current to the β-andrenergic receptor stimulation via a C_2 region-containing protein kinase C isoform, *Circ Res* 87:1164, 2000.

Khoury SF et al: Effects of thyroid hormone of left ventricular performance and regulation of contractile and Ca^{2+}-cycling proteins in the baboon, *Circ Res* 79:727, 1996.

Kowallik P, Meesman M: Independent autonomic modulation of the human sinus and AV nodes: evidence from beat-to-beat measurements of PR and PP intervals during sleep, *J Cardiovasc Electrophysiol* 6:993, 1995.

Löhn M et al: Ignition of calcium sparks in arterial and cardiac muscle through caveolae, *Circ Res* 87:1034, 2000,

Lolska BM et al: Correlation between myofilament response to Ca^{2+} and altered dynamics of contraction and relaxation in transgenic cardiac cells that express β-tropomyosin, *Circ Res* 84:745, 1999.

Marshall JM: Peripheral chemoreceptors and cardiovascular regulation, *Physiol Rev* 74:543, 1994.

Onishi K et al: Decrease in oxygen cost of contractility during hypocapnic alkalosis in canine hearts, *Am J Physiol* 270:H1905, 1996.

Pachucki J, Burmeister LA, Larsen PR: Thyroid hormone regulates hyperpolarization-activated cyclic nucleotide-gated channel (HCN2) mRNA in the rat heart, *Circ Res* 85:498, 1999.

Perez NG et al: Reverse mode of the Na^+-Ca^{2+} exchange after myocardia stretch: underlying mechanism of the slow force response, *Circ Res* 88:376, 2001.

Protas L, Shen J-B, Pappano AJ: Carbachol increases contractions and intracellular Ca^{++} transients in guinea pig ventricular myocytes, *J Pharmacol Exp Ther* 284:66, 1998.

Sauvadet A et al: Synergistic actions of glucagon and miniglucagon on Ca^{2+} mobilization in cardiac cells, *Circ Res* 78:102, 1996.

Shigekawa M, Iwamoto T: Cardiac Na^+-Ca^{2+} exchange: molecular and pharmacological aspects, *Circ Res* 88:864, 2001.

Simmerman HKB, Jones LR: Phospholamban: protein structure, mechanism of action, and role in cardiac function, *Physiol Rev* 78:921, 1998.

Solaro RJ, Rarick HM: Troponin and tropomyosin: proteins that switch on and tune in the activity of cardiac myofilaments, *Circ Res* 83:471, 1998.

Wier WG, Balke CW: Ca^{2+} release mechanisms, Ca^{2+} sparks, and local control of excitation-contraction coupling in normal heart muscle, *Circ Res* 85:770, 1999.

Books and monographs

Armour JA, Ardell JL, editors: *Neurocardiology,* New York, 1994, Oxford University Press.

Levy MN, Schwartz PJ, editors: *Vagal control of the heart: experimental basis and clinical implications,* Armonk, NY, 1994, Futura Publishing.

Share L, editor: *Hormones and the heart in health and disease,* Totawa, NJ, 1999, Humana Press.

Shepherd JT, Vatner SF, editors: *Nervous control of the heart,* Amsterdam, 1996, Harwood Academic.

chapter eighteen

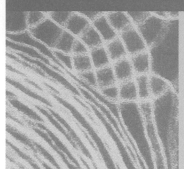

Hemodynamics

The precise analysis of the pulsatile flow of blood through the cardiovascular system is difficult. The heart is a complicated pump, and many physical and chemical factors affect its behavior. The blood vessels are multibranched, and their elasticity ensures complex variations in their dimensions. The blood itself is not a simple, homogeneous solution but instead it is a complex suspension of red and white blood corpuscles, platelets, and lipid globules dispersed in a colloidal solution of proteins.

Despite this complexity, one can gain insight into the dynamics of the cardiovascular system by applying the elementary principles of fluid mechanics as they pertain to simple hydraulic systems. These principles are invoked in this chapter to explain the interrelationships among velocity of blood flow, blood pressure, and the dimensions of the various components of the systemic circulation.

VELOCITY OF THE BLOODSTREAM

Before the variations in blood flow in different vessels are described, one must distinguish between the terms **velocity** and **flow.** Velocity refers to the rate of displacement of a particle of fluid with respect to time, and it is expressed in units of distance per unit time (e.g., cm/sec). Flow refers to the rate of displacment of a volume of fluid, and it is expressed in units of volume per unit time (e.g., cm³/sec). In a tube with varying cross-sectional dimensions, velocity (v), flow (Q), and cross-sectional area (A) are related by the equation:

$$v = Q/A \qquad (18\text{-}1)$$

The interrelationships among velocity, flow, and area are shown in Fig. 18-1. The principle of conservation of mass requires that the flow of an incompressible fluid past successive cross sections of a rigid tube must be constant. For a given flow, the velocity of the fluid varies inversely with the cross-sectional area. Thus, as fluid flows from section *a* into section *b*, where the cross-sectional area is five times greater, the velocity diminishes to one fifth of its previous value, because the area of section *b* is five times greater than that

of section *a* (Fig. 18-1). Conversely, when the fluid flows from section *b* to section *c*, where the cross-sectional area is one tenth as great as that of section *b*, the velocity of each particle of fluid increases 10-fold.

The velocity of the fluid at any point in the system depends not only on the area, but also on the flow, Q. Flow, in turn, depends on the pressure gradient, properties of the fluid, and dimensions of the entire hydraulic system, as discussed in the following section. For any given flow, however, the ratio of the velocity past one cross section relative to that past a second cross section depends only on the inverse ratio of the respective areas, that is,

$$v_1/v_2 = A_2/A_1 \qquad (18\text{-}2)$$

This rule applies whether the system is composed of a single large tube or of several smaller tubes in parallel.

As shown in Fig. 14-3, velocity decreases progressively as the blood traverses the aorta, its larger primary branches, the smaller secondary branches, and the arterioles. Finally, at the capillaries, the velocity decreases to a minimal value. As the blood then passes through the venules and continues centrally toward the venae cavae, the velocity progressively increases again. The relative velocities in the various components of the circulatory system are related only to the respective cross-sectional areas. Thus, each point on the cross-sectional area curve is inversely proportional to the corresponding point on the velocity curve (see Fig. 14-3).

RELATIONSHIP BETWEEN VELOCITY AND PRESSURE

In the specific portions of a hydraulic system in which the total energy remains virtually constant, changes in velocity may be accompanied by appreciable changes in measured pressure. Consider three sections (*A, B,* and *C*) of the hydraulic system depicted in Fig. 18-2. Six pressure probes, or **Pitot tubes,** have been inserted at various points in the system. The openings at the bottoms of three of these tubes (*2, 4,* and *6*) are tangential to the direction of flow, and hence

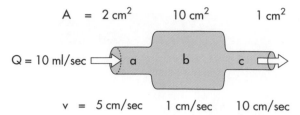

$$A = 2\ cm^2 \qquad 10\ cm^2 \qquad 1\ cm^2$$

$$Q = 10\ ml/sec$$

$$v = 5\ cm/sec \qquad 1\ cm/sec \qquad 10\ cm/sec$$

■ **Fig. 18-1** As fluid flows through a tube of variable cross-sectional area, *A,* the linear velocity, *v,* varies inversely as the cross-sectional area.

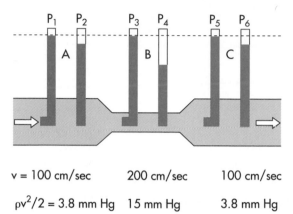

$$v = 100\ cm/sec \qquad 200\ cm/sec \qquad 100\ cm/sec$$

$$\rho v^2/2 = 3.8\ mm\ Hg \quad 15\ mm\ Hg \qquad 3.8\ mm\ Hg$$

■ **Fig. 18-2** In a narrow section, *B,* of a tube, the linear velocity, v, and hence the dynamic component of pressure, $\rho v^2/2$, are greater than in the wide sections, *A* and *C,* of the same tube. If the total energy is virtually constant throughout the tube (i.e., if the energy loss because of viscosity is negligible), the total pressures (*P*₁, *P*₃, and *P*₅) will not be detectably different from each other, but the lateral pressure, *P*₄, in the narrow section will be less than the lateral pressures (*P*₂ and *P*₆) in the wide sections of the tube.

they measure the lateral, or static, pressure within the tube. The openings at the bottoms of the remaining three Pitot tubes (*1, 3,* and *5*) face upstream. These Pitot tubes detect the total pressure, which is the lateral pressure plus a dynamic pressure component that reflects the kinetic energy of the flowing fluid. This dynamic component, P_d, of the total pressure may be calculated from the following equation:

$$P_d = \rho v^2/2 \qquad (18\text{-}3)$$

where ρ is the density of the fluid (in g/cm³) and v is the velocity of the fluid (in cm/sec). If the midpoints of segments *A, B,* and *C* are at the same hydrostatic level, then the corresponding total pressures, P_1, P_3, and P_5, will be equal, provided that the energy loss from viscosity in these segments is negligible (in other words, this fluid is an "ideal fluid"). However, because of the differences in cross-sectional area along the system, the concomitant velocity changes alter the dynamic component, as defined by equation 18-3.

In tube sections *A* and *C,* let ρ equal 1 g/cm³ and let v equal 100 cm/sec; note also that 1 mm Hg equals 1330 dynes/cm². From equation 18-3

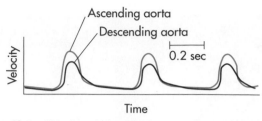

■ **Fig. 18-3** Velocity of blood in the ascending and descending aorta of a dog. (From Falsetti HL et al: *Circ Res* 31:328, 1972.)

$$P_d = 5000\ dynes/cm^2, = 3.8\ mm\ Hg$$

In the narrow section, *B,* of the tube, let the velocity be twice as great as in sections *A* and *C.* In the narrow section, therefore,

$$P_d = 20,000\ dynes/cm^2, = 15\ mm\ Hg$$

Hence, in the wide sections of the tube (*A* and *C*), the lateral pressures (P_2 and P_6) will be only 3.8 mm Hg less than the respective total pressures (P_1 and P_5), whereas in the narrow section *(B),* the lateral pressure (P_4) is 15 mm Hg less than the total pressure (P_3).

We can make two generalizations from these calculations. First, as velocity decreases, the dynamic component becomes a smaller fraction of the total pressure. Second, in narrowed sections of a tube, the dynamic component increases significantly, because the flow velocity is associated with a large kinetic energy. For example, the peak velocity of flow in the ascending aorta of a normal dog is about 150 cm/sec. Because the dynamic component is a significant fraction of the total pressure, the measured pressure may vary significantly, depending on the orientation of the pressure probe. In the descending thoracic aorta, the peak velocity is substantially less than that in the ascending aorta (Fig. 18-3), and lesser velocities have been recorded in still more distal arterial sites. In most arterial locations, the dynamic component will be a negligible fraction of the total pressure, and the orientation of the pressure probe will not materially influence the pressure recorded. At the site of an arterial constriction, however, the high flow velocity is associated with a large kinetic energy, and therefore the dynamic pressure component may increase significantly. Hence, the lateral pressure would be reduced correspondingly.

The pressure tracings shown in Fig. 18-4 were obtained from two pressure transducers inserted into the left ventricle of a patient with aortic stenosis, a condition in which the aortic orifice is narrow. The transducers were located on the same catheter and were 5 cm apart. When both transducers were well within the left ventricular cavity (Fig. 18-4, *A*), they both recorded the same pressures. However, when the proximal transducer was positioned in the aortic valve orifice (Fig. 18-4, *B*), the lateral pressure recorded during ejection was much less than that recorded by the transducer in the ventricular cavity. This pressure difference was associated almost entirely with

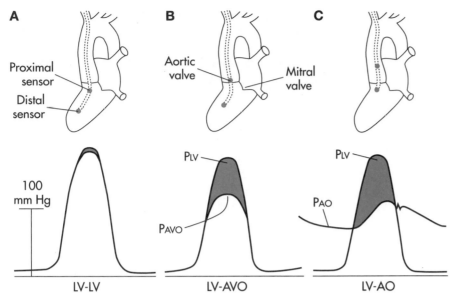

■ **Fig. 18-4** Pressures *(P)* recorded by two transducers in a patient with aortic stenosis. **A,** Both transducers were in the left ventricle *(LV-LV).* **B,** One transducer was in the left ventricle and the other was in the aortic valve orifice *(LV-AVO).* **C,** One transducer was in the left ventricle and the other in the ascending aorta *(LV-AO).* (Redrawn from Pasipoularides A et al: *Am J Physiol* 246:H542, 1984.)

the much greater velocity of flow in the narrowed valve orifice than in the ventricular cavity. The pressure difference reflects mainly the conversion of some potential energy to kinetic energy. When the catheter was withdrawn still farther, so that the proximal transducer was in the aorta (Fig. 18-4, *C*), the pressure difference was even more pronounced, because substantial energy was lost through friction (viscosity) as blood flowed rapidly through the narrow orifice.

The reduction of lateral pressure in the region of the narrowed aortic valve orifice may influence the coronary blood flow in patients with aortic stenosis. The orifices of the right and left coronary arteries are located in the sinuses of Valsalva, just behind the valve leaflets. The initial segments of these vessels are thus oriented at right angles to the direction of blood flow through the aortic valves. Therefore, the lateral pressure is that component of the total pressure that propels the blood through the two major coronary arteries. During the ejection phase of the cardiac cycle, the lateral pressure is diminished by the conversion of potential energy to kinetic energy.

Angiographic studies in patients with aortic stenosis have revealed that the direction of flow often reverses in the large coronary arteries toward the end of the ejection phase of systole (i.e., blood flows toward the aorta rather than toward the myocardial capillaries). The decreased lateral pressure in the aorta in aortic stenosis is undoubtedly an important factor in causing this reversal of coronary blood flow. An important feature that aggravates this condition is that the demands of the heart muscle for oxygen are greatly increased. Therefore, the pronounced drop in lateral pressure during cardiac ejection may contribute to the tendency for patients with severe aortic stenosis to experience **angina pectoris** (anterior chest pain associated with inadequate blood supply to the heart muscle), which can lead to sudden death.

RELATIONSHIP BETWEEN PRESSURE AND FLOW

The most fundamental law that governs the flow of fluids through cylindrical tubes was derived empirically by the French physiologist, Poiseuille. He was primarily interested in the physical determinants of blood flow, but he substituted various simpler liquids for blood in his measurements of flow through glass capillary tubes. His work was so precise and important that his observations have been designated Poiseuille's law. Subsequently, this same law has been derived mathematically.

Application of Poiseuille's Law

Poiseuille's law applies to the steady, laminar flow of newtonian fluids through cylindrical tubes. The term **newtonian fluid** applies to a fluid whose viscosity remains constant over a substantial range of shear rate and shear stress, as described in more detail below. The term steady flow signifies the absence of variations of flow in time (i.e., a nonpulsatile flow). **Laminar flow** is the type of motion in which the fluid moves as a series of individual layers, with each layer moving at a different velocity from its neighboring layers (Fig. 18-5). In the case of laminar flow through a tube, the fluid consists of a series of infinitesimally thin concentric tubes sliding past one another. Laminar flow is described in greater detail below, where it is distinguished from turbulent flow. For the present discussion, laminar flow is considered a homogeneous fluid, such as water, in contrast to a suspension, such as blood.

At the most basic level, Poiseuille's law describes the flow of fluids through cylindrical tubes in terms of flow, pressure, the dimensions of the tube, and the viscosity of liquid in the tube. These terms will first be explained individually and then will be related to each other to yield Poiseuille's law.

Pressure is one of the principal determinants of the rate of flow. The pressure, P, in dynes/cm², at a distance h centimeters below the surface of a liquid is

$$P = h\rho g \qquad (18\text{-}4)$$

where r is the density of the liquid, in g/cm³, and g is the acceleration of gravity, in cm/sec². For convenience, however,

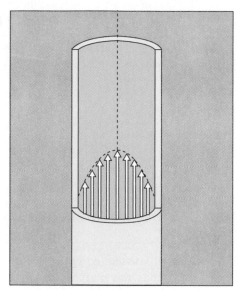

Fig. 18-5 When flow is laminar, all elements of the fluid move in streamlines that are parallel to the axis of the tube; the fluid does not move in a radial or circumferential direction. The layer of fluid in contact with the wall is motionless; the fluid that moves along the axis of the tube has the maximal velocity.

pressure is frequently expressed simply in terms of the height (h) of the column of liquid above some arbitrary reference point.

Consider the tube that connects reservoirs R_1 and R_2 in Fig. 18-6, *A*. Reservoir R_1 is filled with liquid to height h_1, and reservoir R_2 is empty. The outflow pressure, P_o, is therefore equal to the atmospheric pressure, which shall be designated as the zero, or reference, level. The inflow pressure, P_i, is then equal to the same reference level plus the height, h_1, of the column of liquid in reservoir R_1. Under these conditions, let the flow (Q) through the tube be 5 ml/sec.

In Fig. 18-6, *B*, reservoir R_1 is filled to height h_2, which is twice h_1, and reservoir R_2 is again empty. The flow in Fig. 18-6, *B* is twice as great (i.e., 10 ml/sec) as that in Fig. 18-6, *A*. Thus, when the outflow pressure (P_o) in reservoir R_2 equals zero, the flow is directly proportional to the inflow pressure, P_i. If reservoir R_2 is now allowed to fill to height h_1, and the fluid level in R_1 is maintained at h_2 (as in Fig. 18-6, *C*), the flow will again become 5 ml/sec. Thus, flow is directly proportional to the difference between the inflow and outflow pressures:

$$Q \propto P_i - P_o \qquad (18\text{-}5)$$

If the fluid level in R_2 attains the same height as in R_1, flow will cease (Fig. 18-6, *D*).

Now, consider how the dimensions of a tube affect flow. For any given pressure difference between the two ends of a tube, the flow depends on the dimensions of the tube. Consider the horizontal tube connected to the reservoir in Fig. 18-7, *A*. With length l_1 and radius r_1, the flow Q_1 is 10 ml/sec. The horizontal tube connected to the reservoir in

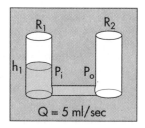

A, When R_2 is empty, fluid flows from R_1 to R_2 at a rate proportional to the pressure in R_1.

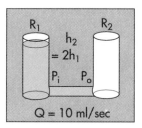

B, When the fluid level in R_1 is increased twofold, the flow increases proportionately.

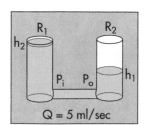

C, Flow from R_1 to R_2 is proportional to the difference between the pressures in R_1 and R_2.

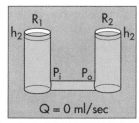

D, When pressure in R_2 rises to equal the pressure in R_1, flow ceases in the connecting tube.

■ **Fig. 18-6** **A to D,** The flow, *Q*, of fluid through a tube connecting two reservoirs, R_1 and R_2, is proportional to the difference between the pressure, P_i, at the inflow end and the pressure, P_o, at the outflow end of the tube.

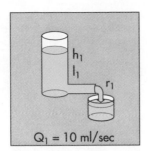

A, Reference condition: for a given pressure, length, radius, and viscosity, let the flow (V_1) equal 10 ml/sec.

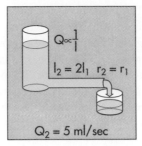

B, If tube length doubles, flow decreases by 50%.

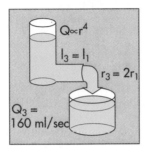

C, If tube radius doubles, flow increases 16-fold.

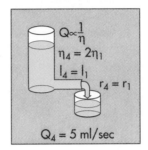

D, If viscosity doubles, flow decreases by 50%.

■ Fig. 18-7   **A** to **D,** The flow, Q, of fluid through a tube is inversely proportional to the length, l, and the viscosity, η, and is directly proportional to the fourth power of the radius, r.

Fig. 18-7, *B* has the same radius but is twice as long as the horizontal tube in Fig. 18-7, *A*. Under these conditions, the flow Q_2 is 5 ml/sec, or only half as great as Q_1. Conversely, for a horizontal tube half as long as l_1, the flow would be twice as great as Q_1. In other words, *flow is inversely proportional to the length of the tube:*

$$Q \propto 1/l \tag{18-6}$$

The horizontal tube connected to the reservoir in Fig. 18-7, *C,* is the same length as l_1, but the radius, r_3, is twice as great as r_1. Under these conditions the flow Q_3 is found to increase to 160 ml/sec, which is 16 times greater than Q_1. The precise measurements of Poiseuille revealed that *flow varies directly as the fourth power of the radius:*

$$Q \propto r^4 \tag{18-7}$$

Thus, in the example above, because $r_3 = 2r_1$, Q_3 will be proportional to $(2r_1)^4$, or $16r_1^4$; therefore, Q_3 will equal $16Q_1$.

Finally, for a given pressure difference and for a cylindrical tube of given dimensions, the flow varies as a function of the nature of the fluid itself. This flow-determining property of fluids is termed **viscosity**, η, which has been defined by Newton as the ratio of **shear stress** to the **shear rate** of the fluid.

These terms can be understood most clearly by considering the flow of a homogeneous fluid between parallel plates.

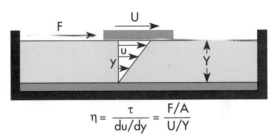

$$\eta = \frac{\tau}{du/dy} = \frac{F/A}{U/Y}$$

■ Fig. 18-8   For a newtonian fluid, the viscosity, η, is defined as the ratio of shear stress, τ, to shear rate, du/dy. For a plate of contact area, A, moving across the surface of a liquid, τ equals the ratio of the force, F, applied in the direction of motion to the contact area, A, and du/dy equals the ratio of the velocity of the plate, U, to the depth of the liquid, Y.

In Fig. 18-8, the bottom plate (the bottom of a large basin) is stationary, and the upper plate moves along the upper surface of the fluid. The **shear stress,** τ, is defined as the ratio of F:A, where F is the force applied to the upper plate in the direction of its motion along the upper surface of the fluid, and A is the area of the upper plate that is in contact with the fluid. The **shear rate** is du/dy, where u is the velocity of a minute fluid element in the direction parallel to the motion of the upper plate, and y is the distance of that fluid element above the bottom, stationary plate.

For a plate that travels with constant velocity, U, across the surface of a homogeneous fluid, the velocity profile of the fluid will be linear. The fluid layer in contact with the upper plate will adhere to it and therefore will move at the same velocity, U, as the plate. Each minute element of fluid between the plates will move at a velocity, u, that is proportional to its distance, y, from the lower plate. Therefore, the shear rate will be U/Y where Y is the distance between the two plates. Because viscosity, h, is defined as the ratio of shear stress, t, to the shear rate, du/dy, in the example illustrated in Fig. 18-8,

$$\eta = (F/A)/(U/Y) \qquad (18\text{-}8)$$

Thus, the dimensions of viscosity are dynes/cm² divided by (cm/sec)/cm, or dyne • sec/cm². In honor of Poiseuille, 1 dyne • sec/cm² has been termed a **poise.** The viscosity of water at 20°C is approximately 0.01 poise, or 1 centipoise. In the case of certain nonhomogeneous fluids, notably suspensions such as blood, the ratio of the shear stress to the shear rate is not constant; that is, the fluid does not possess a characteristic viscosity. Such fluids are said to be **non-newtonian.** *With regard to the flow of newtonian fluids through cylindrical tubes, the flow varies inversely with the viscosity.*

$$Q \propto 1/\eta \qquad (18\text{-}9)$$

Looking back at the example of flow from the reservoir in Fig. 18-6, *D,* if the viscosity of the fluid in the reservoir were doubled, the flow would be halved (5 ml/sec instead of 10 ml/sec).

In summary, *for the steady, laminar flow of a newtonian fluid through a cylindrical tube, the flow, Q, varies directly as the pressure difference, $P_i - P_o$, and the fourth power of the radius, r, of the tube, and it varies inversely as the length, l, of the tube and the viscosity, η, of the fluid.* The full statement of Poiseuille's law is

$$Q = \pi(P_i - P_o) \, r^4/8\eta l \qquad (18\text{-}10)$$

where $\pi/8$ is the constant of proportionality.

Resistance to Flow

In electrical theory, **Ohm's law** states that the resistance, R, equals the ratio of voltage drop, E, to current flow, I. Similarly, in fluid mechanics, *the hydraulic resistance, R, may be defined as the ratio of pressure drop, Pi – Po, to flow, Q.* P_i and P_o are the pressures at the inflow and outflow ends, respectively, of the hydraulic system. For the steady, laminar flow of a newtonian fluid through a cylindrical tube, the physical components of hydraulic resistance may be appreciated by rearranging Poiseuille's law to give the **hydraulic resistance equation:**

$$R = (P_i - P_o)/Q = 8\eta \, l/\pi \, r^4 \qquad (18\text{-}11)$$

Thus, when Poiseuille's law applies, the resistance to flow depends only on the dimensions of the tube and on the characteristics of the fluid.

Because *resistance varies inversely as the fourth power of the radius of the tube,* the principal determinant of the resis-

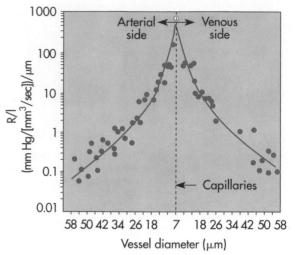

■ **Fig. 18-9** The resistance per unit length *(R/l)* for individual small blood vessels in the cat mesentery. The capillaries, diameter 7 µm, are denoted by the vertical dashed line. Resistances of the arterioles are plotted to the left and resistances of the venules to the right of the vertical dashed line. The solid circles represent the actual data. The two curves through the data represent the following regression equations for the arteriole and venule data, respectively: (a) arterioles, $R/l = 1.02 \times 10^6 \, D^{-4.04}$, and (b) venules, $R/l = 1.07 \times 10^6 \, D^{-3.94}$. Note that for both types of vessels, the resistance per unit length is inversely proportional to the fourth power (within 1%) of the vessel diameter *(D).* (Redrawn from Lipowsky HH, Kovalcheck S, Zweifach BW: *Circ Res* 43:738, 1978.)

tance to blood flow through any individual vessel within the circulatory system is the caliber of the vessel. In Fig. 18-9, the resistance to flow through small blood vessels in the cat mesentery was measured and the resistance per unit length of vessel (R/l) was plotted against the vessel diameter. The resistance is highest in the capillaries (diameter 7 µm), and it diminishes as the vessels increase in diameter on the arterial and venous sides of the capillaries. The values of R/l are virtually proportional to the fourth power of the diameter (or radius) of the larger vessels on both sides of the capillaries.

Changes in vascular resistance induced by natural stimuli occur when the caliber of vessels changes. The most important factor that leads to a change in vessel caliber is the contraction of the circular smooth muscle cells in the vessel wall. However, changes in internal pressure also alter the caliber of the blood vessels, and therefore alter the resistance to blood flow through those vessels. The blood vessels are elastic tubes. Hence, the greater the **transmural pressure** (i.e., the difference between internal and external pressures) across the wall of a vessel, the greater is the caliber of the vessel and the less is its hydraulic resistance.

It is apparent from Fig. 14-2 that the greatest upstream-to-downstream drop in internal pressure occurs in the very small arteries and arterioles. Because the total flow is the same through each of the various series components of the circulatory system, it follows that the greatest resistance to flow resides in the small arteries and arterioles. For example, if R_a represents the resistance of all these small arterial vessels and R_x represents the resistance of any other group of vessels that is in series with these high-resistance vessels, then by the definition of hydraulic resistance (equation 18-11), the resistance of all the small arterial vessels is

$$R_a = (P_i - P_o)/Q_a \qquad (18\text{-}12)$$

Similarly, the resistance of any other group of vessels in series with the group of high resistance small arterial vessels is

$$R_x = (P_i - P_o)/Q_x \qquad (18\text{-}13)$$

However, at equilibrium, the flow, Q_a, through all the small arterial vessels must equal the flow, Q_x, through each of the other groups of vessels in series with these small arterial vessels. Because Q_a equals Q_x, division of equation 18-11 by equation 18-12 yields the following relationship between relative resistances and relative pressure drops:

$$R_a/R_x = (P_i - P_o)_a/(P_i - P_o)_x \qquad (18\text{-}14)$$

That is, *the ratio of the pressure drop across the length of the small arterial vessels to the pressure drop across the length of any other vascular component in series equals the ratio of the hydraulic resistances of these two vascular components.*

With regard to individual vessels, capillaries that have a mean diameter of about 7 μm (Fig. 18-9) have the greatest resistance to blood flow. Nevertheless, it is the arterioles, not the capillaries, that have the greatest resistance of all the different varieties of blood vessels that lie in series with one another (as in Fig. 14-2). This seeming paradox is related to the relative numbers of parallel capillaries and parallel arterioles, as explained below. A simple explanation is that there are far more capillaries than arterioles in the systemic circulation, and total resistance across the many capillaries is much less than the total resistance across the fewer arterioles. Furthermore, arterioles have a thick coat of circularly arranged smooth muscle fibers, that can vary the lumen radius. Even small changes in radius alter resistance greatly, as we can see from the hydraulic resistance equation (equation 18-11), wherein R varies inversely with r^4.

Resistances in Series and in Parallel

In the cardiovascular system, the various types of vessels listed along the horizontal axis in Fig. 14-3 lie in series with one another. Furthermore, the individual members of each category of vessels are ordinarily arranged in parallel with one another (see Fig. 14-4). For example, the capillaries throughout the body are in most instances parallel elements, except for the renal vasculature (in which the peritubular capillaries are in series with the glomerular capillaries) and the splanchnic vasculature (in which the intestinal and hepatic capillaries are aligned in series with each other). Formulas for the total hydraulic resistance of components arranged in series or in parallel have been derived in the same manner as those for analogous combinations of electrical resistances.

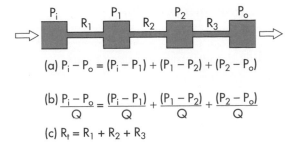

(a) $P_i - P_o = (P_i - P_1) + (P_1 - P_2) + (P_2 - P_o)$

(b) $\dfrac{P_i - P_o}{Q} = \dfrac{(P_i - P_1)}{Q} + \dfrac{(P_1 - P_2)}{Q} + \dfrac{(P_2 - P_o)}{Q}$

(c) $R_t = R_1 + R_2 + R_3$

■ **Fig. 18-10** For resistances (R_1, R_2, and R_3) arranged in series, the total resistance, R_t, equals the sum of the individual resistances. *P*, Pressure; *Q*, flow.

Resistance of vessels in series. Three hydraulic resistances, R_1, R_2, and R_3, are arranged in series in the system depicted in Fig. 18-10. The pressure drop across the entire system—that is, the difference between inflow pressure, P_i, and outflow pressure, P_o—consists of the sum of the pressure drops across each of the individual resistances (equation *a* in Fig. 18-10). Under steady-state conditions, the flow, Q, through any given cross section must equal the flow through any other cross section. By dividing each component in equation *a* by Q (equation *b* in Fig. 18-10), it becomes evident from the definition of resistance (equation 18-11, above) that *for resistances in series, the total resistance, R_t, of the entire system equals the sum of the individual resistances,* that is,

$$R_t = R_1 + R_2 + R_3 \qquad (18\text{-}15)$$

Resistance of vessels in parallel. For resistances in parallel, as illustrated in Fig. 18-11, the inflow and outflow pressures are the same for all tubes. Under steady-state conditions, the total flow, Q_t, through the system equals the sum of the flows through the individual parallel elements (equation *a*). Because the pressure gradient ($P_i - P_o$) is identical for all parallel elements, each term in equation *a* may be divided by that pressure gradient to yield equation *b*. From the definition of resistance, equation *c* may be derived. This equation states that *for resistances in parallel, the reciprocal of the total resistance, R_t, equals the sum of the reciprocals of the individual resistances*, that is,

$$1/R_t = 1/R_1 + 1/R_2 + 1/R_3 \qquad (18\text{-}16)$$

A simpler way of stating this relation is to use the term hydraulic **conductance,** which can be defined as the reciprocal of resistance. It then becomes evident that *for tubes in parallel, the total conductance is the sum of the individual conductances; that is $C_t = C_1 + C_2 + C_3$.*

By considering a few simple illustrations, some of the fundamental properties of parallel hydraulic systems become apparent. For example, if the resistances of the three parallel elements in Fig. 18-11 were all equal, then

$$R_1 = R_2 = R_3 \qquad (18\text{-}17)$$

Therefore, from equation 18-16:

$$1/R_t = 3/R_1 \qquad (18\text{-}18)$$

By equating the reciprocals of these terms:

$$R_t = R_1/3 \qquad (18\text{-}19)$$

Thus, the total resistance is less than the individual resistances. In other words, *for any parallel arrangement, the total resistance must be less than that of any individual component.* For example, consider a system in which a very-high-resistance tube is added in parallel to a low-resistance tube. The total resistance of the system must be less than that of the low-resistance component by itself, because the high-resistance component affords an additional pathway, or conductance, for fluid flow.

As a physiological illustration of these principles, consider the relationship between the total peripheral resistance (TPR) of the entire systemic vascular bed and the resistance of one of its components, such as the renal vasculature. TPR is the ratio of the arteriovenous pressure

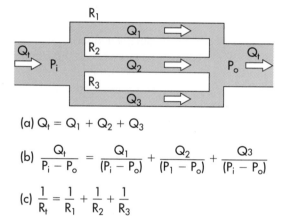

(a) $Q_t = Q_1 + Q_2 + Q_3$

(b) $\dfrac{Q_t}{P_i - P_o} = \dfrac{Q_1}{(P_i - P_o)} + \dfrac{Q_2}{(P_1 - P_o)} + \dfrac{Q_3}{(P_i - P_o)}$

(c) $\dfrac{1}{R_t} = \dfrac{1}{R_1} + \dfrac{1}{R_2} + \dfrac{1}{R_3}$

■ **Fig. 18-11**   For resistances (R_1, R_2, and R_3) arranged in parallel, the reciprocal of the total resistance, R_t, equals the sum of the reciprocals of the individual resistances. *P,* Pressure; *Q,* flow.

difference ($P_a - P_v$) to the flow through the entire systemic vascular bed (i.e., the cardiac output, Q_t). The renal vascular resistance (R_r) would be the ratio of the same arteriovenous pressure difference ($P_a - P_v$) to the renal blood flow (Q_r).

In an individual with an arterial pressure of 100 mm Hg, a peripheral venous pressure of about 0 mm Hg, and a cardiac output of 5000 ml/min, TPR will be 0.02 mm Hg/ml/min, or 0.02 PRU (peripheral resistance units). Normally, blood flow through one kidney would be approximately 600 ml/min. Renal resistance would therefore be 100 mm Hg ÷ 100 ml/min, or 0.17 PRU, which is 8.5 times greater than the TPR. One might be surprised initially that an organ such as the kidney, which weighs only about 1% as much as the whole body, has a vascular resistance much greater than that of the entire systemic circulation. But consider that the entire systemic circulation possesses many more alternate pathways for blood to flow than just one kidney. Hence, it is not surprising that the resistance to flow would be greater for a component organ, such as the kidney, than for the entire systemic circulation.

In examining Fig. 14-2, it may seem paradoxical that the resistance to flow through the small arteries and arterioles (as manifested by the pressure drop from the arterial to the capillary ends of these vessels) is considerably greater than that through certain other vascular components, such as the large arteries, despite the fact that the total cross-sectional area of the small arterial vessels exceeds that for the large arteries.

Consideration of simple models of tubes in parallel will help resolve this apparent paradox. In Fig. 18-12 the resistance to flow through one wide tube of cross-sectional area Aw is compared with that through four narrower tubes in parallel, each of area An. The total cross-sectional area of the parallel system of four narrow tubes equals the area of the wide tube; that is,

$$A_w = 4A_n \qquad (18\text{-}20)$$

■ **Fig. 18-12**   When four narrow tubes, each of area A_n, are connected in parallel, the total cross-sectional area equals the area, A_w, of a wide tube of area such that $A_w = 4A_n$. Although the total areas are equal, he total resistance, R_p to flow through the parallel narrow tubes is four times as great as the resistance, R_w, through the single wide tube. R_n is the resistance of one narrow tube; k is a constant of proportionality.

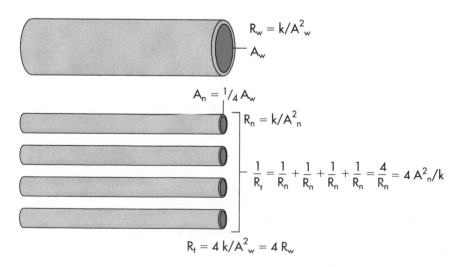

$$R_w = k/A^2_w$$

$$A_w$$

$$A_n = {}^1\!/_4 A_w$$

$$R_n = k/A^2_n$$

$$\frac{1}{R_t} = \frac{1}{R_n} + \frac{1}{R_n} + \frac{1}{R_n} + \frac{1}{R_n} = \frac{4}{R_n} = 4 A^2_n/k$$

$$R_t = 4 k/A^2_w = 4 R_w$$

For a cylindrical tube,

$$A = \pi r^2 \qquad (18\text{-}21)$$

From equation (18-11), resistance, R, is inversely proportional to the fourth power of the radius, r. It follows from equation 18-21, therefore, that

$$R = k/A^2 \qquad (18\text{-}22)$$

The proportionality constant, k, is related to tube length and fluid viscosity, both of which will be held constant in this example. From equation 18-22, the resistances of the wide tube, R_w, and a single narrow tube, R_n, are

$$R_w = k/A_w^2 \qquad (18\text{-}23)$$
$$R_n = k/A_n^2 \qquad (18\text{-}24)$$

From equation 18-16,

$$1/R_t = 1/R_n + 1/R_n + 1/R_n + 1/R_n = 4/R_n \qquad (18\text{-}25)$$

Substituting the value of Rn in equation 18-24 into equation 18-25, and rearranging,

$$R_t = k/4A_n^2 \qquad (18\text{-}26)$$

From equations 18-20 and 18-23,

$$R_t = 4k/A_w^2 = 4\ R_w \qquad (18\text{-}27)$$

Hence, the total resistance, Rt, of four such narrow tubes in parallel is four times as great as the resistance, Rw, of a single wide tube of equal total cross-sectional area.

If a similar calculation is made for eight such tubes in parallel, with each tube having one- fourth the cross-sectional area of the single wide tube, it will be found that the total resistance equals $2R_w$. In this circumstance, the resistance to flow through eight such narrow tubes in parallel will still be twice as great as that through the single tube, despite the fact that the total cross-sectional area for the eight narrow tubes is twice as great as for the single wide tube. This relationship is analogous to the relationship that exists between resistance and area in the circulatory system when the small arteries and arterioles are compared with the large arteries. Although the total cross-sectional area of all the small arterial vessels greatly exceeds that of all the large arteries (see Fig. 14-3), the resistance to flow through the small arterial vessels is considerably greater than that through the large arteries (see Fig. 14-2).

If we expand this example still further, we would find that 16 such narrow tubes in parallel, now with four times the total cross-sectional area of the single wide tube, would exert a resistance to flow just equal to the resistance through the wide tube. Any number of these narrow tubes in excess of 16, then, would have a resistance lower than that of the single wide tube. This situation is analogous to the comparison of the arterioles and capillaries that we encountered in Fig. 14-2. The resistance to flow through a single capillary is much greater than that through a single arteriole (Fig. 18-9), yet the number of capillaries so greatly exceeds the number of

arterioles, as reflected by the relative difference in total cross-sectional areas (see Fig. 14-3), that the pressure drop across the arterioles is considerably greater than the pressure drop across the capillaries (see Fig. 14-2).

Laminar and Turbulent Flow

Under certain conditions, the flow of a fluid in a cylindrical tube will be laminar (sometimes called streamlined), as illustrated in Fig. 18-5. As the fluid moves through the tube, a thin layer of fluid in contact with the tube wall adheres to the wall and hence is motionless. The layer of fluid just central to this external lamina must shear against this motionless layer, and therefore the layer moves slowly, but with a finite velocity. Similarly, the next more central layer moves still more rapidly; the longitudinal velocity profile is that of a paraboloid (Fig. 18-5). The fluid elements in any given lamina remain in that lamina as the fluid progresses longitudinally along the tube. The velocity at the center of the stream is maximal and equal to twice the mean velocity of flow across the entire cross section of the tube.

Irregular motions of the fluid elements may develop in the flow of fluid through a tube; such flow is called turbulent. Under such conditions, fluid elements do not remain confined to definite laminae, but rapid, radial mixing occurs (Fig. 18-13). A considerably greater pressure is required to force a given flow of fluid through the same tube when the flow is turbulent than when it is laminar. In turbulent flow, the pressure drop is approximately proportional to the square of the flow rate, whereas in laminar flow the pressure

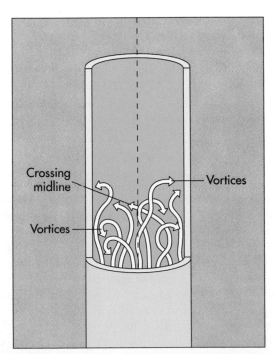

■ **Fig. 18-13** In turbulent flow the elements of the fluid move irregularly in axial, radial, and circumferential directions. Vortices frequently develop.

drop is proportional to the first power of the flow rate. Hence, to produce a given flow, a pump such as the heart must do considerably more work if turbulence develops.

Whether turbulent or laminar flow will exist in a tube under given conditions may be predicted on the basis of a dimensionless number, called **Reynold's number, N_R.** This number represents the ratio of inertial to viscous forces. For a fluid flowing through a cylindrical tube,

$$N_R = \rho D v / \eta \qquad (18\text{-}28)$$

where r is the fluid density, D is the tube diameter, v is the mean velocity, and η is the viscosity. For N_R less than 2000, the flow will usually be laminar; for N_R greater than 3000, the flow will be turbulent; and for N_R between 2000 and 3000, the flow will be transitional between laminar and turbulent. Equation 18-28 indicates that high fluid densities, large tube diameters, high flow velocities, and low fluid viscosities predispose to turbulence. In addition to these factors, abrupt variations in tube dimensions or irregularities in the tube walls may produce turbulence.

Turbulence is usually accompanied by audible vibrations. When turbulent flow exists within the cardiovascular system, it may be detected through a stethoscope during a physical examination as a **murmur.** The factors listed above that predispose to turbulence may account for murmurs heard during the physical examination. In severe anemia, **functional cardiac murmurs** (murmurs not caused by structural abnormalities) are frequently detectable. The physical basis for such murmurs resides in (1) the reduced viscosity of blood in anemia and (2) the high flow velocities associated with the high cardiac output that usually prevails in anemic patients.

Blood clots, or **thrombi,** are much more likely to develop in turbulent than in laminar flow. One of the problems with the use of artificial valves in the surgical treatment of **valvular heart disease** is that thrombi may occur in association with the prosthetic valve. The thrombi may be dislodged and occlude a crucial blood vessel. It is thus important to design such valves to avert turbulence.

Shear Stress on the Vessel Wall

In Fig. 18-8, an external force is applied to a plate floating on the surface of a liquid in a large basin. This force, directed parallel to the surface, exerts a shearing stress on the liquid below, and thus it produces a differential motion of each layer of liquid relative to the adjacent layers. At the bottom of the basin, the flowing liquid exerts a shearing stress on the surface of the basin in contact with the liquid. Rearranging the equation for viscosity shown in Fig. 18-8 discloses that the shear stress, t, equals h (du/dy) (i.e., the shear stress equals the product of the viscosity and the shear rate). Hence, the greater the rate of flow, the greater is the shear stress (i.e., the **viscous drag**) that the liquid exerts on the walls of the container in which it flows.

For precisely the same reasons, the rapidly flowing blood in a large artery tends to pull the endothelial lining of the artery along with it. This force, the viscous drag, is proportional to the shear rate (du/dy) of the layers of blood near the wall. For a flow regimen that obeys Poiseuille's law,

$$\tau = 4\eta Q / \rho r^3 \qquad (18\text{-}29)$$

The greater the rate of blood flow (Q) in the artery, the greater is the shear rate (du/dy) near the arterial wall, and therefore the greater the viscous drag (τ).

In certain types of arterial disease, particularly in patients with hypertension, the subendothelial layers of vessels tend to degenerate locally, and small regions of the endothelium may lose their normal support. The viscous drag on the arterial wall may cause a tear between a normally supported and an unsupported region of the endothelial lining. Blood may then flow from the vessel lumen through the rift in the lining and dissect between the various layers of the artery. Such a lesion is called a dissecting aneurysm. It occurs most often in the proximal portions of the aorta and is extremely serious. One reason for its predilection for this site is the high velocity of blood flow, with the associated large values of du/dy at the endothelial wall. The shear stress at the vessel wall also influences many other vascular functions, such as the permeability of the vascular walls to large molecules, the biosynthetic activity of the endothelial cells, the integrity of the formed elements in the blood, and the coagulation of the blood. An increase in shear stress on the endothelial wall is also an effective stimulus for the release of nitric oxide (NO) from the vascular endothelial cells; NO is a potent vasodilator (see Chapter 21).

RHEOLOGIC PROPERTIES OF BLOOD

The viscosity of a newtonian fluid, such as water, may be determined by measuring the steady, laminar flow of the fluid at a given pressure gradient through a cylindrical tube of known length and radius. The viscosity is then computed by substituting these values into Poiseuille's equation. The viscosity of a given newtonian fluid at a specified temperature will be constant over a wide range of tube dimensions and flows. However, for a non-newtonian fluid, the viscosity calculated by substituting into Poiseuille's equation may vary considerably as a function of tube dimensions and flows. Therefore, in considering the rheologic properties of a suspension such as blood, the term **viscosity** does not have a unique meaning. The term apparent viscosity is frequently applied to the derived value of viscosity obtained for blood under the particular conditions of measurement.

Rheologically, blood is a suspension of formed elements, principally erythrocytes, in a relatively homogeneous liquid, the blood plasma. Because blood is a suspension, the apparent viscosity of blood varies as a function of the **hematocrit ratio** (ratio of the volume of red blood cells to the volume of whole blood). In Fig. 18-14, the upper curve represents the ratio of the apparent viscosity of whole blood relative to that of plasma over a range of hematocrit ratios from 0% to 80%; the measurements were made in a tube 1 mm in diameter. The viscosity of plasma is 1.2 to 1.3 times that of water. The upper curve in Fig. 18-14 shows that blood, with a normal hematocrit ratio of 45%, has an apparent viscosity 2.4 times that of plasma. In severe anemia (in which the concentration of erythrocytes is low), blood viscosity is low. With greater hematocrit ratios, the slope of the curve increases progressively; it is especially steep at the upper range of erythrocyte concentrations.

A rise in hematocrit ratio from 45% to 70% (such as occurs in the blood disease polycythemia vera) increases the apparent viscosity more than twofold. This change in viscosity tends to exert a proportionate effect on the resistance to blood flow. The change in peripheral resistance that occurs with an increase in blood viscosity may be appreciated when it is recognized that even in the most severe cases of essential hypertension, which is the most common type of arterial hypertension, the total peripheral resistance rarely increases by more than a factor of two. In this type of hypertension, the increase in peripheral resistance is achieved by arteriolar vasoconstriction.

For any given hematocrit ratio, the apparent viscosity of blood, relative to that of water, depends on the dimensions of the tube employed in estimating the viscosity. Fig. 18-15 demonstrates that the apparent viscosity of blood diminishes progressively as the tube diameter decreases below a value

of about 0.3 mm. The diameters of the highest-resistance blood vessels, the arterioles, are considerably less than this critical value. This phenomenon therefore reduces the resistance to flow in the blood vessels that possess the greatest resistance.

The apparent viscosity of blood, when measured in living tissues, is considerably less than the apparent viscosity of that same blood when it is measured in a conventional capillary tube viscometer with a diameter greater than 0.3 mm. In the lower curve of Fig. 18-14, the apparent viscosity of blood was assessed by using the hind leg of an anesthetized dog as a biological viscometer. Over the entire range of hematocrit ratios, the apparent viscosity was less when it was measured in the living tissue than in the capillary tube viscometer (upper curve). Furthermore, the disparity was greater the higher the hematocrit ratio.

The influence of tube diameter on apparent viscosity is explained in part by the actual change in composition of the blood as it flows through small tubes. The composition changes because the red blood cells tend to accumulate in the faster axial stream, whereas plasma tends to flow in the slower marginal layers. To illustrate this phenomenon, a reservoir such as R_1 in Fig. 18-6, *C*, has been filled with blood with a given hematocrit ratio. The blood in R_1 was constantly agitated to prevent settling and the blood was permitted to flow through a narrow capillary tube into reservoir R_2. As long as the tube diameter was substantially greater than the diameter of the red blood cells, the hematocrit ratio of the blood in R_2 was not detectably different from that in R_1. Surprisingly, however, the hematocrit ratio of the blood contained within the tube was found to be considerably lower than the hematocrit ratio of the blood in either reservoir.

In Fig. 18-16, the **relative hematocrit** is defined as the ratio of the hematocrit in the tube to that in the reservoir at either end of the tube. For tubes 300 μm in diameter or greater, the relative hematocrit ratio was close to 1; that is, the hematocrit ratio in the tube was virtually equal to the

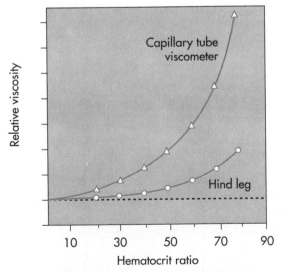

Fig. 18-14 The apparent viscosity of whole blood, relative to that of plasma, increases at a progressively greater rate as the hematocrit ratio increases. For any given hematocrit ratio, the apparent viscosity of blood is less when measured in a biological viscometer (such as the blood vessels in the hind leg of a dog) than in a conventional capillary tube viscometer. (Redrawn from Levy MN, Share L: *Circ Res* 1:247, 1953.)

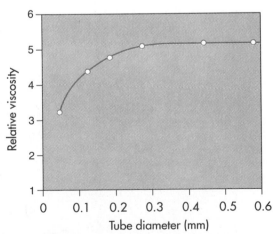

Fig. 18-15 Viscosity of blood, relative to that of water, increases as a function of tube diameter up to a diameter of about 0.3 mm. (Redrawn from Fåhraeus R, Lindqvist T: *Am J Physiol* 96:562, 1931.)

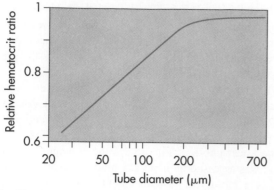

■ **Fig. 18-16** The relative hematocrit ratio of blood flowing from a feed reservoir through capillary tubes of various calibers as a function of the tube diameter. The relative hematocrit ratio equals the hematocrit ratio of the blood in the tubes divided by that of the blood in the feed reservoir. (Redrawn from Barbee JH, Cokelet GR: *Microvasc Res* 3:6, 1971.)

hematocrit ratio in the reservoirs. However, as the tube diameter was diminished below 300 μm, the relative hematocrit ratio progressively diminished; for a tube diameter of 30 μm, the relative hematocrit ratio was only 0.6; that is, *the erythrocyte content of a given volume of blood in the capillary tube was 40% less than that in the blood reservoirs at either end of the tube.*

That this situation results from a disparity in the relative velocities of the red cells and plasma can be appreciated in the following analogy. Consider the flow of automobile traffic across a bridge that is 3 miles long. Let the cars move in one lane at a speed of 60 mph and the trucks in another lane at 20 mph, as illustrated in Fig. 18-17. If one car and one truck start out across the bridge each minute, then except for the initial few minutes of traffic flow across the bridge, one car and one truck will arrive at the other end each minute. Yet if one counts the actual number of cars and trucks on the bridge at any moment, three times as many slower-moving trucks will be on the bridge than will be rapidly traveling cars.

Because the axial portions of the bloodstream contain a greater proportion of red cells and this axial portion will

■ **Fig. 18-17** When the car velocity is three times as great as the truck velocity, the ratio of the number of cars to trucks on the bridge will be 1:3 after 9 minutes, even though one of each type of vehicle enters and leaves the bridge each minute.

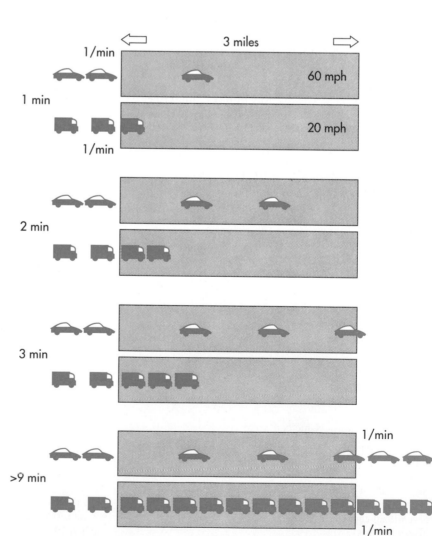

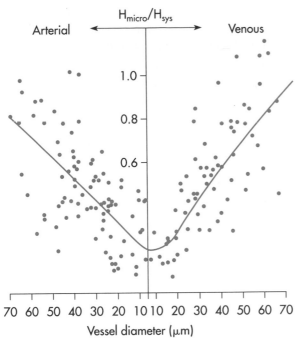

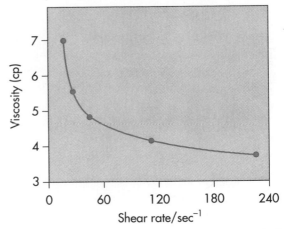

■ **Fig. 18-19** Decrease in the viscosity of blood (centipoise) at increasing rates of shear (s⁻¹). The shear rate refers to the velocity of one layer of fluid relative to that of the adjacent layers and is directionally related to the rate of flow. (Redrawn from Amin TM, Sirs JA: *Q J Exp Physiol* 70:37, 1985.)

■ **Fig. 18-18** The hematocrit ratio (H_{micro}) of the blood in various-sized arterial and venous microvessels in the cat mesentery, relative to the hematocrit ratio (H_{sys}) in the large systemic vessels. The hematocrit ratio is least in the capillaries and tiny venules. (Modified from Lipowsky HH, Usami S, Chien S: *Microvasc Res* 19:297, 1980.)

move with a greater velocity, the red cells tend to traverse the tube in less time than does the plasma. Therefore, the red cells correspond to the rapidly moving cars in the analogy, and the plasma corresponds to the slowly moving trucks. Measurement of transit times of the different blood constituents through the vascular beds of various organs has shown that red cells do travel faster through these vascular beds than does the plasma. Furthermore, the hematocrit ratios of the blood contained in the small blood vessels of various tissues are lower than those in blood samples withdrawn from large arteries or veins in the same animal (Fig. 18-18).

The physical forces responsible for the drift of the erythrocytes toward the axial stream and away from the vessel walls when blood is flowing at normal rates are not fully understood. One factor is the great flexibility of the red blood cells. At low flow rates, comparable with those in the microcirculation, rigid particles do not migrate toward the axis of a tube, whereas flexible particles do migrate. The concentration of flexible particles near the tube axis is enhanced by increasing the shear rate.

The apparent viscosity of blood diminishes as the flow rate is increased (Fig. 18-19), a phenomenon called **shear thinning.** The greater the flow, the greater the rate that one lamina of fluid shears against an adjacent lamina. The greater tendency for the erythrocytes to accumulate in the axial laminae at higher flow rates is partly responsible for this non-newtonian behavior. However, a more important

factor is that at very slow flow rates, the suspended cells tend to form aggregates, which would increase the blood viscosity. As the flow is increased, this aggregation decreases and so also does the apparent viscosity of the blood (Fig. 18-19).

The tendency for the erythrocytes to aggregate at low flows depends on the concentration in the plasma of the larger protein molecules, especially fibrinogen. For this reason, the changes in blood viscosity with flow rate are much more pronounced when the concentration of fibrinogen is high. Also, at low flow rates, leukocytes tend to adhere to the endothelial cells of the microvessels and thereby increase the apparent viscosity of the blood.

The deformability of the erythrocytes is also a factor in shear thinning, especially when hematocrit ratios are high. The mean diameter of human red blood cells is about 7 µm, yet they are able to pass through openings with a diameter of only 3 µm. As blood with densely packed erythrocytes flows at progressively greater rates, the erythrocytes become more and more deformed. Such deformation diminishes the apparent viscosity of the blood. The flexibility of human erythrocytes is enhanced as the concentration of fibrinogen in the plasma increases (Fig. 18-20). If the red blood cells become hardened, as they are in certain **spherocytic anemias,** shear thinning may diminish.

SUMMARY

1. The vascular system is composed of two major subdivisions: the systemic circulation and the pulmonary circulation. These subdivisions are in series with each other.

2. Each subdivision comprises a number of types of vessels (e.g., arteries, arterioles, capillaries) that are aligned in series with one another. In general, the vessels of a given type are arranged in parallel with each other.

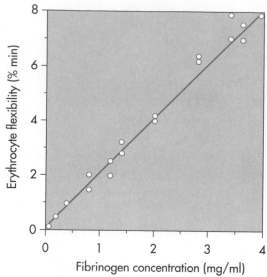

Fig. 18-20   Effect of the plasma fibrinogen concentration on the flexibility of human erythrocytes. (Redrawn from Amin TM, Sirs JA: *Q J Exp Physiol* 70:37, 1985.)

3. The mean velocity (v) of blood flow in a given type of vessel is directly proportional to the total blood flow (Q_t) being pumped by the heart, and it is inversely proportional to the cross-sectional area (A) of all the parallel vessels of that type (i.e., $v = Q_t/A$).

4. The laterally directed pressure in the bloodstream decreases as the flow velocity increases; the decrement in lateral pressure is proportional to the square of the velocity. The changes are insignificant, however, except when flow is very great.

5. When blood flow is steady and laminar in vessels larger than arterioles, the flow (Q) is proportional to the pressure drop down the vessel ($P_i - P_o$) and to the fourth power of the radius (r), and it is inversely proportional to the length (l) of the vessel and to the viscosity (η) of the fluid; that is, $Q = \rho(P_i - P_o)r^4/8\eta l$ (Poiseuille's law).

6. For resistances aligned in series, the total resistance equals the sum of the individual resistances.

7. For resistances aligned in parallel, the reciprocal of the total resistance equals the sum of the reciprocals of the individual resistances.

8. Flow tends to become turbulent when (1) flow velocity is high, (2) fluid viscosity is low, (3) fluid density is great, (4) tube diameter is large, or (5) the wall of the vessel is irregular.

9. Blood flow is non-newtonian in very small blood vessels (i.e., Poiseuille's law is not applicable).

10. The apparent viscosity of the blood diminishes as shear rate (flow) increases and as the tube dimensions decrease.

BIBLIOGRAPHY

Journal articles

Alonso C et al: Transient rheological behavior of blood in low-shear tube flow: velocity profiles and effective viscosity, *Am J Physiol* 268:H25, 1995.

Davis ME et al: Shear stress regulates endothelial nitric oxide synthase expression through c-Src by divergent signaling pathways, *Circ Res* 89:1073, 2001.

Hoeks APG et al: Noninvasive determination of shear-rate distribution across the arterial wall, *Hypertension* 26:26, 1995.

Lee RT, Kamm RD: Vascular mechanics for the cardiologist, *J Am Coll Cardiol* 23:1289, 1994.

Maeda N, Shiga T: Velocity of oxygen transfer and erythrocyte rheology, *News Physiol Sci* 9:22, 1994.

Melkumyants AM et al: Control of arterial lumen by shear stress on endothelium, *News Physiol Sci* 10:204, 1995.

Morita T et al: Role of Ca^{2+} and protein kinase C in shear stress-induced actin depolymerization and endothelin 1 gene expression, *Circ Res* 75:630, 1994.

Mullen MJ et al: Heterogeneous nature of flow-mediated dilatation in human conduit arteries in vivo, *Circ Res* 88:145, 2001.

Pries AR et al: Resistance to blood flow in microvessels in vivo, *Circ Res* 75:904, 1994.

Pries AR, Secomb TW, Gaetgens P: Design principles of vascular beds, *Circ Res* 77:1017, 1995.

Reinhart WH et al: Influence of endothelial surface on flow velocity in vitro, *Am J Physiol* 265:H523, 1993.

White KC et al: Hemodynamics and wall shear rate in the abdominal aorta of dogs: effects of vasoactive agents, *Circ Res* 75:637, 1994.

Yamamoto K et al: Fluid shear stress activates Ca^{2+} influx into human endothelial cells via P2X4 purinoceptors, *Circ Res* 87:385, 2000.

chapter nineteen

The Arterial System

The principal function of the systemic and pulmonary arterial systems is to distribute blood to the capillary beds throughout the body. The arterioles, the terminal components of this system, are high-resistance vessels that regulate the distribution of flow to the various capillary beds. Because of their elasticity, the aorta, the pulmonary artery, and their major branches form a system of channels capable of handling a considerable volume. These two features of the arterial system—its elastic conduits and high-resistance terminals—are also shared by certain mechanical fluid systems, called **hydraulic filters,** which tend to dampen fluctuations in flow. Thus, the body's arterial system constitutes a hydraulic filter; these filters are analogous to the resistance-capacitance filters of electrical circuits.

The main advantage of hydraulic filtering in the arterial system is that it *converts the intermittent output of the heart to a steady flow through the capillaries.* This important function of the large elastic arteries has been likened to the Windkessels of antique fire engines. The Windkessel contained a large volume of trapped air. The compressibility of the air that remained trapped above the water in the Windkessel converted the intermittent inflow of water from the water source to a steady outflow of water at the nozzle of the fire hose. Without the Windkessel, water would flow only in spurts, making firefighting inefficient at best and dangerous at worst.

OVERVIEW OF THE HYDRAULIC FILTER

The role that the large elastic arteries play in the hydraulic filtering is illustrated in Fig. 19-1. Because the heart pumps intermittently, the entire stroke volume is discharged into the arterial system during systole. Systole usually occupies only about one-third of the cardiac cycle. In fact, most of the stroke volume is actually pumped during the rapid ejection phase, which constitutes about half of systole (see Chapter 16). A small part of the energy of cardiac contraction is dissipated as forward capillary flow during systole; the remainder is stored as potential energy, as much of the stroke

volume is retained by the distensible arteries (Fig. 19-1, *A* and *B*). During diastole, the elastic recoil of the arterial walls converts this potential energy into capillary blood flow. If the arterial walls were rigid, capillary flow would not occur during diastole (Fig. 19-1, *C* and *D*).

Hydraulic filtering minimizes the workload of the heart. More work is required to pump a given flow intermittently than steadily. The more effective the hydraulic filtering, the less the work that is required. A simple example illustrates this point.

Consider first the steady flow of a fluid at a rate of 100 ml/sec through a hydraulic system with a resistance of 1 mm Hg/ml/sec. This combination of flow and resistance would result in a constant pressure of 100 mm Hg, as shown in Fig. 19-2, *A*. If we neglect any inertial effect, the hydraulic work, W, may be defined as

$$W = \int_{t_1}^{t_2} P\,dV \qquad (19\text{-}1)$$

That is, each small increment of volume that is pumped, dV, is multiplied by the associated pressure, P, and the products (PdV) are integrated over the time interval of interest, $t_2 - t_1$, to give the total work, W. For steady flow,

$$W = PV \qquad (19\text{-}2)$$

In the example in Fig. 19-2, *A*, the work done in pumping the fluid for 1 second would be 10,000 mm Hg • ml (or 1.33×10^7 dyne • cm).

Next, consider an intermittent pump that puts out the same volume per second but pumps the entire volume at a steady rate over 0.5 second and then pumps nothing during the next 0.5 second. Hence, it pumps at the rate of 200 ml/sec for 0.5 second, as shown in Fig. 19-2, *B* and *C*. In Fig. 19-2, *B*, the conduit is rigid and the fluid is incompressible, but the hydraulic system has the same resistance as in Fig. 19-2, *A*. During the pumping phase of the cycle (systole), the flow of 200 ml/sec through a resistance of 1 mm Hg/ml/sec would produce a pressure of 200 mm Hg. During the filling phase of the pump (diastole), the

Compliant

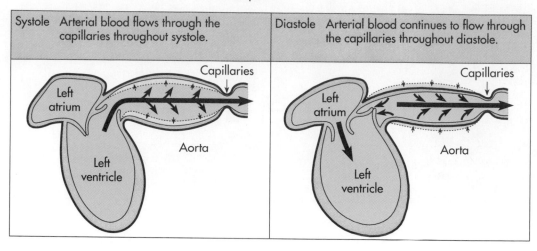

| Systole   Arterial blood flows through the capillaries throughout systole. | Diastole   Arterial blood continues to flow through the capillaries throughout diastole. |

A, When the arteries are normally compliant, a substantial fraction of the stroke volume is stored in the arteries during ventricular systole. The arterial walls are stretched.

B, During ventricular diastole the previously stretched arteries recoil. The volume of blood that is displaced by the recoil furnishes continuous capillary flow throughout diastole.

Rigid arteries

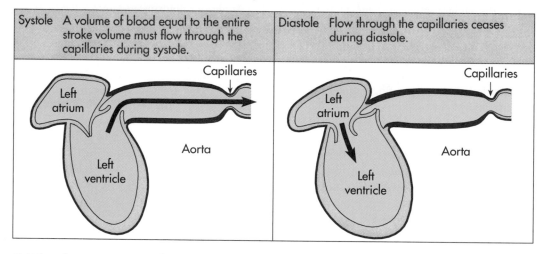

| Systole   A volume of blood equal to the entire stroke volume must flow through the capillaries during systole. | Diastole   Flow through the capillaries ceases during diastole. |

C, When the arteries are rigid, virtually none of the stroke volume can be stored in the arteries.

D, Rigid arteries cannot recoil appreciably during diastole.

■ Fig. 19-1   **A** to **D,** When the arteries are normally compliant, blood flows through the capillaries throughout the cardiac cycle. When the arteries are rigid, blood flows through the capillaries during systole, but flow ceases during diastole.

pressure would be 0 mm Hg in this rigid system. The work done during systole would be 20,000 mm Hg • ml, which is twice that required in the example shown in Fig. 19-2, *A*.

The more distensible the system, the more efficient is the hydraulic filtering. The reason for this increased efficiency is that in a very distensible system, the pressure remains virtually constant throughout the entire cycle (Fig. 19-2, *C*). Of the 100 ml of fluid pumped during the 0.5 second of systole, only 50 ml would be emitted

through the high-resistance outflow end of the system during systole. The remaining 50 ml would be stored by the distensible conduit during systole and would flow out during diastole. Hence, the pressure would be virtually constant at 100 mm Hg throughout the cycle. The fluid pumped during systole would be ejected at only half the pressure that prevailed in Fig. 19-2, *B*, and therefore the work would be only half as great. With nearly perfect filtering, as in Fig. 19-2, *C*, the work would be identical to that for steady flow (Fig. 19-2, *A*).

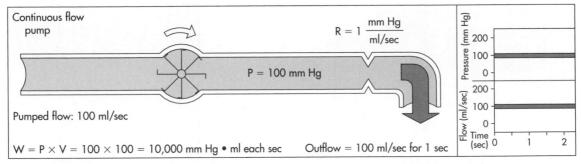

A The flow is steady, and pressure will remain constant regardless of the distensibility of the conduit.

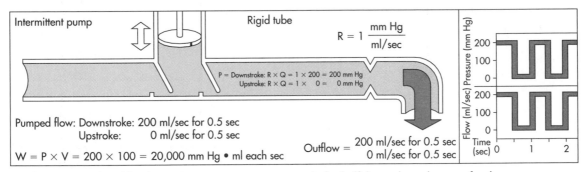

The flow (Q) produced by the pump is intermittent; it is steady for half the cycle and ceases for the remainder of the cycle. The conduit is rigid, and therefore the flow produced by the pump during its downstroke must exit through the resistance during the same 0.5 second that elapses during the **B** downstroke. The pump must do twice as much work as the pump in **A**.

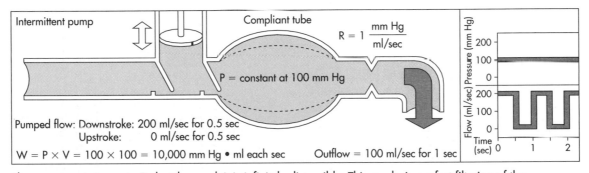

The pump operates as in **B,** but the conduit is infinitely distensible. This results in perfect filtering of the pressure; that is, the pressure is steady, and the flow through the resistance is also steady. The work equals **C** that in **A**.

■ Fig. 19-2 **A to C,** Relationships between pressure and flow for three hydraulic systems. In each the overall flow is 100 ml/sec, and the resistance is 1 mm Hg/(ml/sec).

The filtering accomplished by the systemic and pulmonic arterial systems is intermediate between the system with rigid conduits shown in Fig. 19-2, *B*, and the system with infinitely distensible conduits in Fig. 19-2, *C*. Ordinarily, the additional work imposed by intermittency of pumping, in excess of that for steady flow, is about 35% for the right ventricle and about 10% for the left ventricle. These fractions change, however, with variations in heart rate, peripheral resistance, and arterial distensibility.

Rigid conduits in a hydraulic system create the need for more energy to pump fluid through the system. The increased cardiac energy requirements imposed by a rigid arterial system are illustrated by the experimental results shown in Fig. 19-3. In a group of anesthetized dogs, the cardiac output pumped by the left ventricle could be allowed to flow through the natural route (the aorta), or it could be diverted into a stiff plastic tube attached to the peripheral arteries. The total peripheral resistances were found to be virtually identical, regardless of which pathway was selected. The data (Fig. 19-3) from a representative animal show that for any given stroke volume, the myocardial oxygen consumption was substantially greater when the blood was diverted

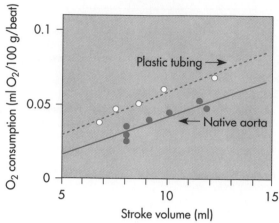

■ **Fig. 19-3** Relationship between myocardial oxygen consumption *(ml/100 g/beat)* and stroke volume *(ml)* in an anesthetized dog whose cardiac output could be pumped by the left ventricle either through the aorta or through a stiff plastic tube to the peripheral arteries. (Modified from Kelly RP, Tunin R, Kass DA: *Circ Res* 71:490, 1992.)

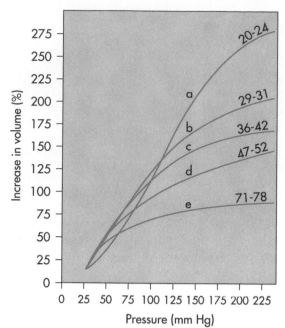

■ **Fig. 19-4** Pressure-volume relationships for aortas obtained at autopsy from humans in different age-groups (denoted by the numbers at the right end of each of the curves). (Redrawn from Hallock P, Benson IC: *J Clin Invest* 16:595, 1937.)

through the plastic tubing than when it flowed through the aorta. This increase in oxygen consumption indicates that the left ventricle had to expend more energy to pump blood through a less compliant conduit than through a more compliant conduit.

ARTERIAL ELASTICITY

A good way to appreciate the elastic properties of the arterial wall is to consider the **static pressure-volume relationship** for the aorta. To obtain the curves shown in Fig. 19-4, aortas were obtained at autopsy from people in different age-groups. All branches of the aorta were tied off, and successive volumes of liquid were injected into this closed elastic system, just as successive amounts of water might be introduced into a balloon. After each increment of volume had been introduced, the internal pressure was measured. In Fig. 19-4, the curve that relates pressure to volume for the youngest age-group (curve *a*) is sigmoidal. Although the curve is nearly linear over most of its extent, the slope decreases at the upper and lower ends. The aortic compliance at any point on the curve is represented by the slope, dV/dP, at that point. Thus, in young individuals, the aortic **compliance** is least at both very high and very low pressures and it is greatest over the pressure range (75 to 140 mm Hg) that prevails in healthy people. This sequence of compliance changes induced by increasing fluid volumes resembles the familiar compliance changes encountered when one inflates a balloon. The greatest difficulty in introducing air into the balloon is encountered at the beginning of inflation and again when the volume is near maximum, just before the balloon is about to rupture. At intermediate fluid volumes the balloon is relatively easy to inflate; that is, it is very compliant.

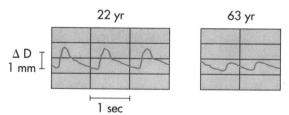

■ **Fig. 19-5** Pulsatile changes in diameter, measured ultrasonically, in a 22-year-old and a 63-year-old man. (Modified from Imura T et al: *Cardiovasc Res* 20:208, 1986.)

As people age, the pressure-volume curves of their arterial systems shift downward, and the slopes of these curves diminish (Fig. 19-4). Thus, for any pressure above about 80 mm Hg, the compliance decreases with age. This change in compliance is a manifestation of the increased rigidity (**atherosclerosis**) of the system caused by progressive changes in the collagen and elastin contents of the arterial walls.

The effects of the subject's age on the elastic characteristics of the arterial system, as shown in Fig. 19-4, were derived from aortas removed at autopsy. Age-related changes have also been confirmed in living subjects by ultrasound imaging techniques. These studies show that the increase in the diameter of the aorta produced by each cardiac contraction is much less in elderly persons than in young persons (Fig. 19-5). The effects of aging on the **elastic modulus** of the aorta in healthy subjects are shown in Fig. 19-6. The elastic modulus, E_p, is defined as

$$E_p = \Delta P/(\Delta D/D) \qquad (19\text{-}3)$$

where ΔP is the aortic pulse pressure (i.e., the change in aortic pressure during a cardiac cycle; Fig. 19-7), D is the mean aortic diameter during the cardiac cycle, and ΔD is the maximal change in aortic diameter during the cardiac cycle.

The fractional change in diameter ($\Delta D/D$) of the aorta during the cardiac cycle reflects the change in aortic volume as the left ventricle ejects its stroke volume into the aorta with each systole. Thus, E_p is **inversely** related to compliance, which is the ratio of ΔV to ΔP. Consequently, the **increase** in elastic modulus with aging (Fig. 19-6) and the **decrease** in compliance with aging (Fig. 19-4) both reflect the stiffening of the arterial walls as individuals age.

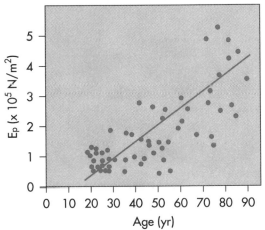

■ **Fig. 19-6**   Effects of age on the elastic modulus (E_p) of the abdominal aorta in a group of 61 human subjects. (Modified from Imura T et al: *Cardiovasc Res* 20:208, 1986.)

DETERMINANTS OF ARTERIAL BLOOD PRESSURE

The determinants of arterial blood pressure cannot be evaluated precisely. However, arterial blood pressure is routinely measured in patients, and it provides a useful estimate of their cardiovascular status. We therefore present a simplified explanation of the principal determinants of arterial blood pressure. First, we will analyze the determinants of **mean arterial pressure,** which is the pressure averaged over time (Fig. 19-7). The **systolic** (maximal) and **diastolic** (minimal) **arterial pressures** within the cardiac cycle (Fig. 19-7) will then be considered as the upper and lower limits of periodic oscillations about this mean pressure. Finally, the changes in arterial pressure as the pulse wave progresses from the origin of the aorta toward the capillaries will be discussed.

In our discussion, we arbitrarily divide the determinants of the arterial blood pressure into "physical" and "physiological" factors (Fig. 19-8). The physical factors relate to the fluid mechanical characteristics, whereas the physiological factors relate to certain features of the cardiovascular system of living subjects. Because we will assume that the arterial system is a static, elastic system, the only two physical factors that we will consider are **fluid volume** (i.e., blood volume) within the arterial system and the **elastic characteristics** (compliance) of the system. Certain physiological factors will be considered, namely, **cardiac output** (which equals **heart rate × stroke volume**) and **peripheral resistance.** Such physiological factors will be shown to operate through one or both of the physical factors.

Mean Arterial Pressure

The mean arterial pressure, $\bar{P}_a$, may be estimated from an arterial blood pressure tracing by measuring the area under the pressure curve and dividing this area by the time interval involved, as shown in Fig. 19-7. Alternatively, $\bar{P}_a$ can usually be approximated satisfactorily from the measured values of the systolic (P_s) and diastolic (P_d) pressures by means of the following formula:

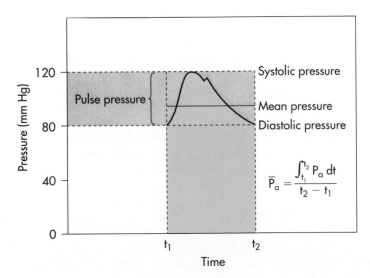

$$\bar{P}_a = \frac{\int_{t_1}^{t_2} P_a\, dt}{t_2 - t_1}$$

■ **Fig. 19-7**   Arterial systolic, diastolic, pulse, and mean pressures. The mean arterial pressure ($\bar{P}_a$) represents the area under the arterial pressure curve *(shaded area)* divided by the cardiac cycle duration $(t_2 - t_1)$.

■ **Fig. 19-8** The arterial blood pressure is determined directly by two major physical factors, the arterial blood volume and the arterial compliance. These physical factors are affected in turn by certain physiological factors, namely, heart rate, stroke volume, cardiac output (heart rate × stroke volume), and peripheral resistance.

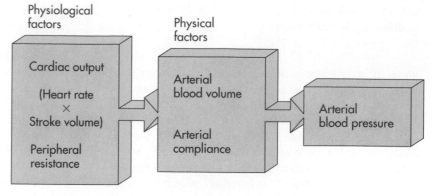

$$P_a = P_d + (P_s - P_d)/3 \qquad (19\text{-}4)$$

As noted previously, in this discussion we consider that the mean arterial pressure depends on only two physical factors: the mean blood volume in the arterial system and the arterial compliance (Fig. 19-8). The arterial volume, V_a, in turn depends on the rate of inflow, Q_h, into the arteries from the heart (cardiac output) and on the rate of outflow, Q_r, from the arteries through the resistance vessels (peripheral runoff). These relationships can be expressed mathematically as

$$dV_a/dt = Q_h - Q_r \qquad (19\text{-}5)$$

This equation expresses the law of conservation of mass. It states that the change in arterial blood volume per unit time (dV_a/dt) represents the difference between the rate at which blood is pumped into the arterial system by the heart (Q_h) and the rate at which it leaves the arterial system through the resistance vessels (Q_r). If arterial inflow exceeds outflow, arterial volume increases, the arterial walls are stretched further, and pressure rises. The converse happens when arterial outflow exceeds inflow. When inflow equals outflow, arterial pressure remains constant.

The change in pressure in response to an alteration of cardiac output can be better appreciated by considering the simple example in the box below.

Under control conditions, let cardiac output be 5 L/min and mean arterial pressure ($\bar{P}_a$) be 100 mm Hg (Fig. 19-9, *A*). From the definition of total peripheral resistance

$$R \equiv (\bar{P}_a - P_{ra})/Q_r \qquad (19\text{-}6)$$

If $\bar{P}_{ra}$ (mean right atrial pressure) is negligible in comparison with $\bar{P}_a$, then

$$R \equiv \bar{P}_a/Q_r \qquad (19\text{-}7)$$

In this example, therefore, R is 100/5, or 20 mm Hg/L/min.

Now let cardiac output, Q_h, suddenly increase to 10 L/min (Fig. 19-9, *B*). Instantaneously, $\bar{P}_a$ will be unchanged. Because the outflow, Q_r, from the arteries depends on P_a and R, Q_r will also remain unchanged at first. Therefore, Q_h, now 10 L/min, will exceed Q_r, still only 5 L/min. This will increase the mean arterial blood

volume (V_a). From equation 19-5, when $Q_h > Q_r$, then $d\bar{V}_a/dt > 0$; that is, volume is increasing.

Because $\bar{P}_a$ depends on the mean arterial blood volume, $\bar{V}_a$, and the arterial compliance, C_a, an increase in $\bar{V}_a$ will increase $\bar{P}_a$ By definition,

$$C_a \equiv dV_a/d\bar{P}_a \qquad (19\text{-}8)$$

After rearranging this equation, and dividing both sides by dt,

$$dV_a/dt = C_a \, dP_a/dt \qquad (19\text{-}9)$$

From equation 19-5, we can substitute $Q_h - Q_r$ for $d\bar{V}_a/dt$ in equation 19-9. Therefore,

$$d\bar{P}_a/dt = (Q_h - Q_r)/C_a \qquad (19\text{-}10)$$

Hence, $\bar{P}_a$ will rise when $Q_h > Q_r$, will fall when $Q_h < Q_r$, and will remain constant when $Q_h = Q_r$.

In this example, in which cardiac output (Q_h) is suddenly increased to 10 L/min, mean arterial pressure ($\bar{P}_a$) continues to rise as long as cardiac output exceeds arterial outflow (Q_r). Equation 19-7 indicates that arterial outflow will not reach 10 L/min until the mean arterial pressure reaches a level of 200 mm Hg and as long as peripheral resistance (R) remains constant at 20 mm Hg/L/min. Hence, as the mean arterial pressure approaches 200, arterial outflow will almost equal cardiac output, and mean arterial pressure will rise very slowly. When cardiac output is first raised, however, it greatly exceeds arterial outflow, and therefore mean arterial pressure rises sharply. The pressure-time tracing in Fig. 19-10 indicates that regardless of the value of arterial compliance (C_a), the slope gradually diminishes as pressure rises and approaches its final asymptotic value (equilibrium).

Furthermore, the *height* that mean arterial pressure will attain at equilibrium is independent of the elastic characteristics of the arterial walls (Fig. 19-10). We have seen that at equilibrium, mean arterial pressure must rise to a level such that arterial outflow equals cardiac output. Equation 19-6 indicates that cardiac output depends only on pressure gradient and resistance to flow. Hence, compliance determines only the rate at which the new equilibrium value of mean arterial pressure will be approached, as illustrated in Fig. 19-10. When compliance is small (rigid vessels), a

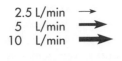

2.5 L/min →
5   L/min ⇒
10   L/min ⇒

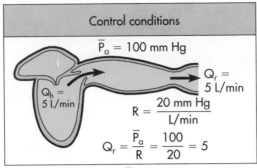

A, Under control conditions Q_h = 5 L/min, $\bar{P}_a$ = 100 mm Hg, and R = 20 mm Hg/L/min. Q_r must equal Q_h, and therefore the mean blood volume ($\bar{V}_a$) in the arteries will remain constant from heartbeat to heartbeat.

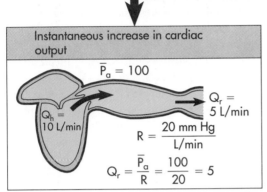

B, If Q_h suddenly increases to 10 L/min, Q_h will initially exceed Q_r, and therefore $\bar{P}_a$ will begin to rise rapidly.

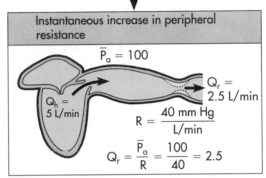

D, If R abruptly increases to 40 mm Hg/L/min, Q_r suddenly decreases and therefore Q_h exceeds Q_r. Thus $\bar{P}_a$ will rise progressively.

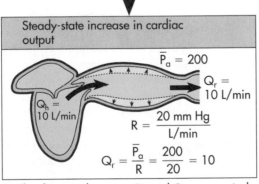

C, The disparity between Q_h and Q_r progressively increases arterial blood volume. The volume continues to increase until $\bar{P}_a$ reaches a level of 200 mm Hg.

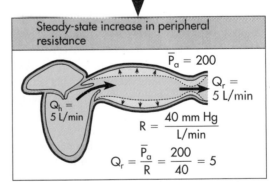

E, The excess of Q_h over Q_r accumulates blood in the arteries. Blood continues to accumulate until $\bar{P}_a$ rises to a level of 200 mm Hg.

■ **Fig. 19-9**   Relationship of mean arterial blood pressure ($\bar{P}_a$) to cardiac output (Q_h), peripheral runoff (Q_r), and peripheral resistance (R) under control conditions (**A**), in response to an increase in cardiac output (**B** and **C**), and in response to an increase in peripheral resistance (**D** and **E**).

relatively slight increment in mean arterial blood volume (caused by a transient excess of cardiac output over arterial outflow) greatly increases mean arterial pressure. Hence, mean arterial pressure attains its new equilibrium level quickly. Conversely, when compliance is large, considerable volumes can be accommodated with relatively small pressure changes.

Therefore, the new equilibrium value of mean arterial pressure is reached at a slower rate.

Peripheral Resistance

Similar reasoning may now be used to explain the changes in mean arterial pressure that accompany alterations in peripheral

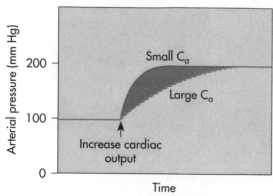

■ **Fig. 19-10** When cardiac output is suddenly increased, the arterial compliance *(C_a)* determines the rate at which the mean arterial pressure will attain its new, elevated value, but it does not determine the *magnitude* of the new pressure.

resistance. Let the control conditions be identical with those of the preceding example; that is, let $Q_h = 5$, $\bar{P}_a = 100$, and $R = 20$ (Fig. 19-9, *A*). Then, let R suddenly be increased to 40 (Fig. 19-9, *D*). Instantaneously, $\bar{P}_a$ will be unchanged. With $\bar{P}_a = 100$ and $R = 40$, $Q_r = \bar{P}_a/R = 2.5$ L/min. If Q_h remained constant at 5 L/min, $Q_h > Q_r$, and therefore $\bar{V}_a$ would increase. Hence, $\bar{P}_a$ would rise, and it would continue to rise until it reached 200 mm Hg (Fig. 19-9, *E*). At this level $Q_r = 200/40 = 5$ L/min, which equals Q_h. $\bar{P}_a$ would then remain at this new elevated equilibrium level as long as Q_h and R did not change again.

These examples indicate, therefore, that *the level of the mean arterial pressure depends on two physiological factors: cardiac output and peripheral resistance* (Fig. 19-11). It does not matter whether changes in cardiac output are accomplished by an alteration of heart rate, stroke volume, or both. Any change in heart rate that is balanced by an opposite change in stroke volume would not alter cardiac output. Hence, mean arterial pressure would not be affected.

Arterial Pulse Pressure

Arterial pulse pressure is defined as the difference between systolic and diastolic pressures. The following discussion will show that *the arterial pulse pressure is principally a function of just one physiological factor, namely, stroke volume,* which would determine the change in arterial blood volume (a physical factor) during ventricular systole. This physical factor, plus the second physical factor (arterial compliance), would determine the arterial pulse pressure (Fig. 19-11).

Stroke volume. The effect of a change in stroke volume on pulse pressure may be analyzed under conditions in which arterial compliance (C_a) remains virtually constant over a substantial range of pressures. In the example described below and illustrated in Fig. 19-12, we assume that C_a remains constant over the range of pressures and volumes that prevail in the example.

Under steady-state conditions, the arterial blood pressure of a subject oscillates about some mean value (e.g., $\bar{P}_A$ in Fig. 19-12) that, as previously explained, depends entirely on cardiac output and peripheral resistance. This mean arterial pressure corresponds to some mean arterial blood volume, $\bar{V}_A$. The coordinates, $\bar{P}_A$, $\bar{V}_A$ (point $\bar{A}$ on the graph), represent the mean arterial pressure and volume that prevail for the existing cardiac output and peripheral resistance. During the period of ventricular diastole, peripheral runoff from the arterial system occurs. At the same time, no blood is ejected from the ventricles into the arterial system. As a result, P_A and V_A diminish to minimal values, P_1 and V_1, just before the next ventricular ejection. P_1 is then, by definition, the **diastolic pressure.**

During the rapid ejection phase of systole, the volume of blood introduced into the arterial system exceeds the volume that exits the system through the arterioles (see Chapter 23). Arterial pressure and volume therefore rise from point A_1 toward point A_2 in Fig. 19-12. The maximal arterial volume, V_2, is reached at the end of the rapid ejection phase (see Fig. 16-10), and this volume corresponds to a peak pressure, P_2, which is the **systolic pressure.**

The **pulse pressure** is the difference between systolic and diastolic pressures ($P_2 - P_1$ in Fig. 19-12). Pulse pressure can also be understood in terms of a concept called the **arterial volume increment,** $V_2 - V_1$. *This increment equals the volume of blood discharged into the aorta by the left ventricle*

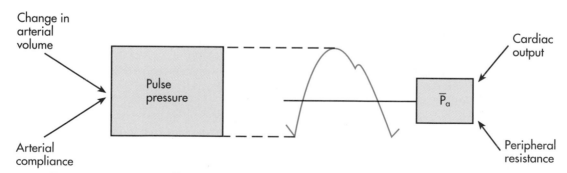

■ **Fig. 19-11** The two physiological determinants of the mean arterial pressure *(P_a)* are the cardiac output and the total peripheral resistance. The two physical determinants of the pulse pressure are the arterial compliance *(C_a)* and the change in arterial volume.

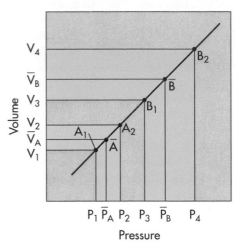

■ **Fig. 19-12**   Effect of a change in stroke volume on pulse pressure in a system in which arterial compliance remains constant over the prevailing range of pressures and volumes. A larger volume increment [$(V_4 - V_3) > (V_2 - V_1)$] results in a greater mean pressure ($\overline{P}_B > \overline{P}_A$) and a greater pulse pressure [$(P_4 - P_3) > (P_2 - P_1)$].

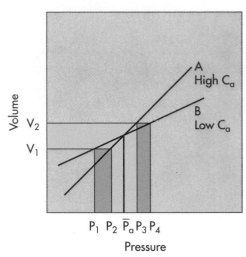

■ **Fig. 19-13**   For a given volume increment ($V_2 - V_1$), a reduced arterial compliance (compliance B < compliance A) results in an increased pulse pressure [$(P_4 - P_1) > (P_3 - P_2)$].

during the rapid ejection phase minus the volume that has run off from the arteries and through the microcirculation during this same phase of the cardiac cycle. Pulse pressure corresponds to this volume increment. For instance, when a normal heart beats at a normal frequency, the volume increment during the rapid ejection phase constitutes a large part of the stroke volume (about 80%). It is this increment that raises arterial volume rapidly from V_1 to V_2, and hence that causes the arterial pressure to rise from the diastolic to the systolic level (P_1 to P_2 in Fig. 19-12). During the remainder of the cardiac cycle, peripheral runoff greatly exceeds cardiac ejection. During ventricular diastole, of course, cardiac ejection equals zero. The resultant decrement in the arterial blood volume thus causes volumes and pressures to fall from point A_2 back to point A_1.

If stroke volume is now doubled while heart rate and peripheral resistance remain constant, the mean arterial pressure doubles, to in Fig. 19-12. The arterial pressure will now oscillate each heartbeat about this new $\overline{P}_B$ value of the mean arterial pressure. A normal, vigorous heart ejects this greater stroke volume mainly during the rapid ejection phase of the cardiac cycle; the duration of this phase is approximately equal to the duration of this phase that prevailed at the lower stroke volume. Therefore, the arterial volume increment, $V_4 - V_3$, will be a large fraction of the new stroke volume, and hence the volume increment will be approximately twice as great as the previous volume increment ($V_2 - V_1$). If compliance remains constant, the greater volume increment will be reflected by a pulse pressure ($P_4 - P_3$) approximately twice as great as the original pulse pressure ($P_2 - P_1$). Inspection of Fig. 19-12 reveals that when both mean pressure and pulse pressure increase, the rise in systolic pressure (from P_2 to P_4) exceeds the rise in diastolic pressure (from P_1 to P_3).

The arterial pulse pressure affords valuable clues about a person's stroke volume, provided that the arterial compliance is essentially normal. Patients who have severe **congestive heart failure** or who have had a severe hemorrhage are likely to have very small arterial pulse pressures, because their stroke volumes are abnormally small. Conversely, individuals with large stroke volumes, as in **aortic valve regurgitation,** are likely to have increased arterial pulse pressures. Similarly, well-trained athletes at rest tend to have large stroke volumes because their heart rates are usually low. The prolonged ventricular filling times in these individuals induce the ventricles to pump a large stroke volume, and hence their pulse pressures are large.

Arterial compliance.   Arterial compliance also affects pulse pressure. To illustrate this relationship, let us compare the relative effects of a given volume increment ($V_2 - V_1$ in Fig. 19-13) in a young person (curve A) with that in an elderly person (curve B). Let cardiac output and total peripheral resistance be the same in both people; therefore, $\overline{P}_a$ will be the same. Figure 19-13 shows that the same volume increment ($V_2 - V_1$) will generate a greater pulse pressure ($P_4 - P_1$) in the less compliant arteries of the elderly individual than in the more compliant arteries of the young person ($P_3 - P_2$). The reason for this discrepancy is shown in Fig. 19-2. Diminished arterial compliance imposes a greater workload on the left ventricle of the elderly person than on that of the young person, even if the stroke volumes, total peripheral resistances, and mean arterial pressures are equal in the two individuals.

We can also see this same effect on pulse pressure in Fig. 19-14, which shows how changes in arterial compliance and

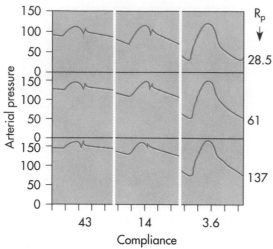

■ **Fig. 19-14** Changes in aortic pressure induced by changes in arterial compliance and peripheral resistance *(R_p)* in an isolated cat heart preparation. (Modified from Elizinga G, Westerhof N: *Circ Res* 32:178, 1973.)

peripheral resistance, R_p, affect the arterial pressure in an isolated cat heart preparation. As the compliance was reduced from 43 to 14 to 3.6 units, the pulse pressure increased significantly. However, in contrast to our human example, in which stroke volume was held at a constant value, the stroke volume decreased in the cat heart preparation as the compliance was diminished (not shown). This change in stroke volume accounts for the failure of the mean arterial pressure to remain constant in the cat heart preparation at different levels of arterial compliance. The effects of changes in peripheral resistance on the arterial pulse pressure are described in the next section.

Total peripheral resistance and arterial diastolic pressure. Clinicians have often proclaimed that the total peripheral resistance (TPR) affects the level of the diastolic arterial pressure much more profoundly than it affects the systolic

arterial pressure, but is this true? To investigate this assertion, first let TPR be increased in an individual whose arterial system has a $P_a:V_a$ curve that is virtually linear over a wide range of pressures and volumes, as depicted in Fig. 19-15, *A*. If heart rate and stroke volume remain constant, then an increase in TPR will increase mean arterial pressure $(\overline{P}_a)$ proportionately (from $\overline{P}_2$ to $\overline{P}_5$). If the arterial volume increments $(V_2 - V_1$ and $V_4 - V_3)$ are equal at both levels of TPR, the pulse pressures $(P_3 - P_1$ and $P_6 - P_4)$ will also be equal. Hence, systolic (P_6) and diastolic (P_4) pressures will have been elevated by exactly the same amounts from their respective control levels $(P_3$ and $P_1)$. Therefore, we can assert confidently that the above assertion is not true, because in the absence of a pressure-induced change in arterial compliance, an increase in peripheral resistance will not have a differential effect on the levels of systolic and diastolic arterial pressures.

In chronic **hypertension,** a condition characterized by a persistent elevation of TPR, the $P_a:V_a$ curve resembles that shown in Fig. 19-15, *B*. The changing slope of the curve in Fig. 19-15, *B*, reveals that the arteries are less compliant at higher than at lower arterial pressures. Any given arterial volume increment will produce a greater pressure increment (i.e., a greater pulse pressure) when the arteries are more rigid than when they are more compliant. Hence, the rise in arterial systolic pressure $(P_6 - P_3)$ will exceed the increase in arterial diastolic pressure $(P_4 - P_1)$. Thus, if the arteries become substantially less compliant when arterial pressure rises, an increase in peripheral resistance will elevate systolic pressure more than it will elevate diastolic pressure.

These hypothetical changes in arterial pressure closely resemble those actually seen in patients with hypertension. Diastolic pressure is indeed elevated in such individuals, but ordinarily not more than 10 to 40 mm Hg above the average normal level of 80 mm Hg. Not uncommonly, however, systolic pressures are elevated by 50 to 100 mm

■ **Fig. 19-15** Comparison of the effects of a given change in peripheral resistance on pulse pressure when the pressure-volume curve for the arterial system is either rectilinear **(A)** or curvilinear **(B).** The arterial volume increment is the same for both conditions: $[(V_4 - V_3) = (V_2 - V_1)]$.

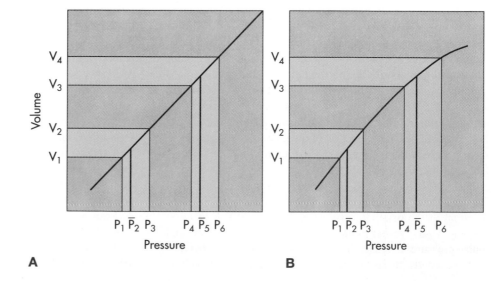

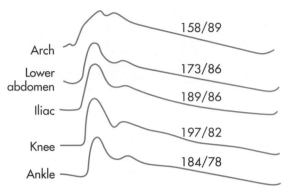

Arch 158/89

Lower abdomen 173/86

Iliac 189/86

Knee 197/82

Ankle 184/78

■ **Fig. 19-16** Arterial pressure curves recorded from various sites in an anesthetized dog. (From Remington JW, O'Brien LJ: *Am J Physiol* 218:437, 1970.)

Hg above the average normal level of 120 mm Hg. The combination of increased resistance and diminished arterial compliance would be represented in Fig. 19-14 by a shift in direction from the top left panel to the bottom right panel; that is, both the mean pressure and the pulse pressure would be increased significantly. These results also coincide with the systolic and diastolic arterial pressure changes predicted by Fig. 19-15, *B*.

Peripheral Arterial Pressure Curves

The radial stretch of the ascending aorta brought about by left ventricular ejection initiates a pressure wave that is propagated down the aorta and its branches. The pressure wave travels much faster than does the blood itself. This pressure wave is the "pulse" that can be detected by palpating a peripheral artery.

The velocity of the pressure wave varies inversely with the arterial compliance. Accurate measurement of the transmission velocity has provided valuable information about the elastic characteristics of the arterial tree. In general, transmission velocity increases with age, confirming the observation that the arteries become less compliant with advancing age (Figs. 19-4 and 19-6). Velocity also increases progressively as the pulse wave travels from the ascending aorta toward the periphery. This increase in velocity reflects the decrease in vascular compliance in the more distal than in the more proximal portions of the arterial system. This spatial change in compliance has been confirmed by direct measurement.

The arterial pressure contour becomes distorted as the wave is transmitted down the arterial system. This distortion in the pressure wave contour is demonstrated by changes in configuration of the pulse at distant sites; these changes are shown in Fig. 19-16. Aside from the increasing delay in the onset of the initial pressure rise, three major changes occur in the arterial pulse contour as the pressure wave travels distally. First, the systolic portions of the pressure wave

become narrowed and elevated. In the curves shown in Fig. 19-16, the systolic pressure at the level of the knee was 39 mm Hg greater than that recorded in the aortic arch. Second, the high-frequency components of the pulse, such as the incisura (i.e., the notch that appears at the end of ventricular ejection), are damped out and soon disappear. Third, a hump may appear on the diastolic portion of the pressure wave, at a point in the pressure wave just beyond the locus at which the incisura had initially appeared. These changes in contour are pronounced in young individuals, but they diminish with age. In elderly patients, the pulse wave may be transmitted virtually unchanged from the ascending aorta to the periphery.

The damping of the high-frequency components of the arterial pulse is largely caused by the viscoelastic properties of the arterial walls. Several factors, including wave reflection and resonance, vascular tapering, and pressure-induced changes in transmission velocity, contribute to the peaking of the arterial pressure wave.

BLOOD PRESSURE MEASUREMENT IN HUMANS

In hospital intensive care units, needles or catheters may be introduced into peripheral arteries of patients, and arterial blood pressure can then be measured **directly** by means of strain gauges. Ordinarily, however, blood pressure is estimated **indirectly** by means of a **sphygmomanometer.** This instrument consists of a noncompliant cuff that contains an inflatable bag. The cuff is wrapped around an extremity (usually an arm); the inflatable bag lies between the cuff and the skin, directly over the artery to be compressed. The artery is occluded by inflating the bag, by means of a rubber squeeze bulb, to a pressure in excess of the arterial systolic pressure. The pressure in the bag is measured by means of a mercury or an aneroid manometer. Pressure is released from the bag at a rate of 2 or 3 mm Hg per second by means of a needle valve in the inflating bulb (Fig. 19-17).

When blood pressure readings are taken from the arm, the systolic pressure may be estimated by palpating the radial artery at the wrist (**palpatory method**). While pressure in the bag exceeds the systolic level, no pulse is perceived. As the pressure falls just below the systolic level (Fig. 19-17, *A*), a spurt of blood passes through the brachial artery under the cuff during the peak of systole, and a slight pulse will be felt at the wrist.

The **auscultatory method** is a more sensitive and therefore more precise method for measuring systolic pressure, and it also permits the diastolic pressure level to be estimated. The practitioner listens with a stethoscope applied to the skin of the antecubital space over the brachial artery. While the pressure in the bag exceeds the systolic pressure, the brachial artery is occluded and no sounds are heard (Fig. 19-17, *B*). When the inflation pressure falls just below the systolic level (120 mm Hg in Fig. 19-17, *A*), a small spurt of blood escapes the occluding pressure of the cuff, and slight tapping sounds (called **Korotkoff sounds**) are heard with each heartbeat. The pressure at which the first sound is

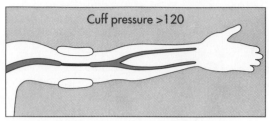

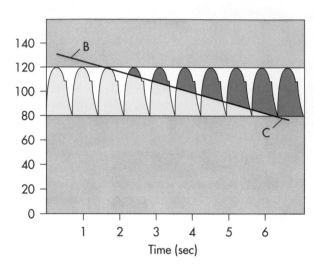

A, Consider that the arterial blood pressure is being measured in a patient whose blood pressure is 120/80 mm Hg. The pressure (represented by the *oblique line*) in a cuff around the patient's arm is allowed to fall from greater than 120 mm Hg (point *B*) to below 80 mm Hg (point *C*) in about 6 seconds.

B, When the cuff pressure exceeds the systolic arterial pressure (120 mm Hg), no blood progresses through the arterial segment under the cuff, and no sounds can be detected by a stethoscope bell placed on the arm distal to the cuff.

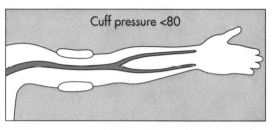

C, When the cuff pressure falls below the diastolic arterial pressure, arterial flow past the region of the cuff is continuous, and no sounds are audible. When the cuff pressure is between 120 and 80 mm Hg, spurts of blood traverse the artery segment under the cuff with each heartbeat, and the Korotkoff sounds are heard through the stethoscope.

■ **Fig. 19-17**   **A** to **C,** Measurement of arterial blood pressure with a sphygmomanometer.

detected represents the **systolic pressure.** It usually corresponds closely with the directly measured systolic pressure.

As the inflation pressure of the cuff continues to fall, more blood escapes under the cuff per beat and the sounds become louder. When the inflation pressure approaches the diastolic level, the Korotkoff sounds become muffled. When the inflation pressure falls just below the diastolic level (80 mm Hg in Fig. 19-17, *A*), the sounds disappear; the pressure reading at this point indicates the **diastolic pressure.** The origin of the Korotkoff sounds is related to the discontinuous spurts of blood that pass under the cuff and meet a static column of blood beyond the cuff; the impact and turbulence generate audible vibrations. Once the inflation pressure is less than the diastolic pressure, flow is continuous in the brachial artery, and sounds are no longer heard (Fig. 19-17, *C*).

SUMMARY

1. The arteries not only conduct blood from the heart to the capillaries but also store some of the ejected blood during each cardiac systole. Hence, blood flow continues through the capillaries during cardiac diastole.

2. The aging process diminishes the compliance of the arteries.

3. The less compliant the arteries, the more work the heart must do to pump a given cardiac output.

4. The mean arterial pressure varies directly with the cardiac output and total peripheral resistance.

5. The arterial pulse pressure varies directly with the stroke volume, but inversely with the arterial compliance.

6. The contour of the systemic arterial pressure wave is distorted as it travels from the ascending aorta to the periphery. The high-frequency components of the pulse wave are damped, the pressure components of the wave during ventricular systole are elevated, and a hump appears in the early diastolic component of the wave.

7. When blood pressure is measured by a sphygmomanometer, (a) the systolic pressure is manifested by a tapping sound that is produced by the spurts of blood that pass through the compressed artery as the cuff pressure falls below the peak arterial pressure, and (b) the diastolic pressure is manifested by the disappearance of the sound as the flow through the artery becomes continuous when the cuff pressure falls below the minimal arterial pressure.

BIBLIOGRAPHY

Journal articles

Armentano RL et al: Arterial wall mechanics in conscious dogs: assessment of viscous, inertial, and elastic moduli to characterize aortic wall behavior, *Circ Res* 76:468, 1995.

Burattini R, Campbell KB: Effective distributed compliance of the canine descending aorta estimated by modified T-tube model, *Am J Physiol* 194:H1977, 1993.

Cernadas MR et al: Expression of constitutive and inducible nitric oxide synthases in the vascular wall of young and aging rats, *Circ Res* 83:279, 1998.

Folkow B, Svanborg A: Physiology of cardiovascular aging, *Physiol Rev* 73:725, 1993.

Frasch HF, Kresh JY, Noordergraaf A: Two-port analysis of microcirculation: an extension of Windkessel, *Am J Physiol* 270:H376, 1996.

Kingwell BA et al: Arterial compliance may influence baroreflex function in athletes and hypertensives, *Am J Physiol* 198:H411, 1995.

Lee RT, Kamm RD: Vascular mechanics for the cardiologist, *J Am Coll Cardiol* 23:1289, 1994.

Loscalzo J: Nitric oxide insufficiency, platelet activation, and arterial thrombosis, *Circ Res* 88:756, 2001

Mulvany MJ, Aalkjaer C: Structure and function of small arteries, *Physiol Rev* 70:921, 1990.

O'Rourke M: Mechanical principles in arterial disease, *Hypertension* 19:2, 1995.

Perloff D et al: Human blood pressure determination by sphygmomanometry, *Circulation* 88:2460, 1993.

Rose WC, Schwaber JS: Analysis of heart rate-based control of arterial blood pressure, *Am J Physiol* 271:H812, 1996.

Stergiopulos N, Meister J-J, Westerhof N: Determinants of stroke volume and systolic and diastolic aortic pressure, *Am J Physiol* 270:H2050, 1996.

Van Gorp A et al: Technique to assess aortic distensibility and compliance in anesthetized and awake rats, *Am J Physiol* 270:H780, 1996.

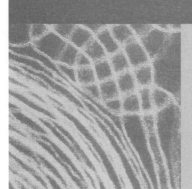

chapter twenty

The Microcirculation and Lymphatics

The circulatory system is geared to supply the tissues with blood in amounts that meet the body's requirements for oxygen and nutrients. The capillaries, whose walls consist of a single layer of endothelial cells, permit the rapid exchange of gases, water, and solutes with interstitial fluid. The muscular arterioles, which are the major **resistance vessels,** regulate regional blood flow to the capillary beds. The venules and veins serve primarily as collecting channels and storage vessels.

The lymphatic system is composed of lymphatic vessels, nodes, and lymphoid tissue. This system collects the fluid and proteins that have escaped from the blood and transports them back into the veins for recirculation in the blood. In this chapter, the network of the smallest blood vessels of the body, as well as the lymphatic vessels, is explored in detail.

THE MICROCIRCULATION

The microcirculation is defined as the circulation of blood through the smallest vessels of the body—the arterioles, capillaries, and venules. Arterioles, which range in diameter from about 5 to 100 μm, have a thick smooth muscle layer, a thin adventitial layer, and an endothelial lining (see Fig. 14-1). The arterioles give rise directly to the capillaries (5 to 10 μm in diameter) or in some tissues to metarterioles (10 to 20 μm in diameter), which then give rise to capillaries (Fig. 20-1). The metarterioles can either bypass the capillary bed and thus serve as thoroughfare channels to the venules, or serve as direct conduits to the capillary bed. Cross-connections are often made between small vessels of similar diameters. Arterioles that give rise directly to capillaries regulate flow through these capillaries by constriction or dilation. The capillaries form an interconnecting network of tubes with an average length of 0.5 to 1 mm.

Functional Properties of Capillaries

Capillary distribution varies from tissue to tissue. In metabolically active tissues, such as cardiac, skeletal, muscle, and glandular tissues, capillary density is high. In less active tissues, such as subcutaneous tissue or cartilage, capillary density is low.

Capillary diameter also varies. Some capillaries have diameters less than those of erythrocytes. Passage through these tiny capillaries requires the erythrocytes to become temporarily deformed. Fortunately, normal erythrocytes are quite flexible.

Blood flow in the capillaries depends chiefly on the contractile state of the arterioles. The average velocity of blood flow in the capillaries is approximately 1 mm/sec; however, it can vary from zero to several millimeters per second in the same vessel within a brief period. These changes in capillary blood flow may be random or rhythmic. The rhythmic oscillatory behavior of capillaries is caused by contraction and relaxation (**vasomotion**) of the precapillary vessels (i.e., the arterioles and small arteries).

Vasomotion is an intrinsic contractile behavior of the vascular smooth muscle and is independent of external input. In addition, changes in **transmural pressure** (intravascular minus extravascular pressure) influence the contractile state of the precapillary vessels. An increase in transmural pressure, whether produced by an increase in venous pressure or by dilation of arterioles, results in contraction of the terminal arterioles. A decrease in transmural pressure causes precapillary vessel relaxation (see "Myogenic Response" in Chapter 20). Humoral and possibly neural factors also affect vasomotion. For example, when the precapillary vessels contract in response to increased transmural pressure, the contractile response can be overridden and vasomotion abolished. This effect is accomplished by metabolic (humoral) factors (see Chapter 20) when the oxygen supply becomes too low to meet the requirements of the parenchymal tissue, as occurs in skeletal muscle during exercise.

Although reduction of transmural pressure relaxes the terminal arterioles, blood flow through the capillaries cannot increase if the reduction in intravascular pressure is caused by severe constriction of the miscrovessels upstream. Large arterioles and metarterioles also exhibit vasomotion. However, their contraction does not usually completely occlude the lumen of the vessel and arrest blood flow, whereas contraction

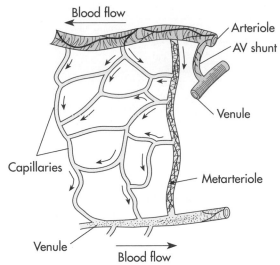

Blood flow

Arteriole
AV shunt

Venule

Capillaries

Metarteriole

Venule

Blood flow

■ **Fig. 20-1** Composite schematic drawing of the microcirculation. The circular structures on the arteriole and venule represent smooth muscle fibers, and the branching solid lines represent sympathetic nerve fibers. The arrows indicate the direction of blood flow.

of the terminal arterioles may arrest blood flow (Fig. 20-2). *Thus, flow rate in the capillaries may be altered by contraction and relaxation of small arteries, arterioles, and metarterioles.*

Because blood flow through the capillaries provides for exchange of gases and solutes between blood and tissue, it has been called **nutritional flow.** Conversely, blood flow that bypasses the capillaries as it travels from the arterial to the venous side of the circulation has been termed **nonnutritional,** or **shunt, flow** (Fig. 20-1). In some areas of the body (e.g., fingertips, ears), true **arteriovenous shunts** exist (see Chapter 23). However, in many tissues, such as muscle, anatomic shunts are lacking. Even in the absence of these shunts, nonnutritional flow can occur; this flow has been called **physiological shunting.** In tissues that have metarterioles, nonnutritional flow may be continuous from arteriole to venule during low metabolic activity, when many precapillary vessels are closed. When metabolic activity increases in these tissues, more precapillary vessels open. Blood passing through the metarterioles is then readily available for capillary perfusion.

True capillaries are devoid of smooth muscle and are therefore incapable of active constriction. Nevertheless, the endothelial cells that form the capillary wall contain actin and myosin and they can alter their shape in response to certain chemical stimuli.

Because of their narrow lumens, the thin-walled capillaries can withstand high internal pressures without bursting. This property can be explained in terms of the **law of Laplace,** which is illustrated in the following comparison of wall tension of a capillary with that of the aorta (Table 20-1). The Laplace equation is

$$T = Pr \qquad (20\text{-}1)$$

where

T = tension in the vessel wall
P = transmural pressure
r = radius of the vessel

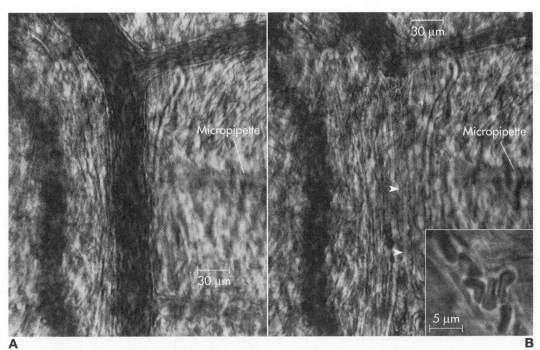

A

30 µm

Micropipette

Micropipette

30 µm

5 µm

B

■ **Fig. 20-2** **A,** Arterioles of a hamster cheek pouch before microinjection of norepinephrine. **B,** After injection of norepinephrine. Note the complete closure of the arteriole between the arrows, and the narrowing of a branch arteriole at the upper right. Inset: Capillary with red cells during a period of complete closure of the feeding arteriole. Scale in **A** and **B,** 30 µm; in inset, 5 µm. (Courtesy David N. Damon.)

■ **Table 20-1**   Vessel wall tension in the aorta and a capillary

	Aorta	*Capillary*
Radius (r)	1.5 cm	5×10^{-4} cm
Height of Hg column (h)	10 cm Hg	2.5 cm Hg
ρ	13.6 g/cm^3	13.6 g/cm^3
g	980 cm/sec^2	980 cm/sec^2
P	$10 \times 13.6 \times 980 = 1.33 \times 10^5$ dyne/cm	$2.5 \times 13.6 \times 980 = 3.33 \times 10^4$ dyne/cm
w	0.2 cm	1×10^{-4} cm
T = Pr	$(1.33 \times 10^5)(1.5) = 2 \times 10^5$ dyne/cm	$(3.33 \times 10^4)(5 \times 10^{-4}) = 16.7$ dyne/cm
σ = Pr/w	$2 \times 10^5/0.2 = 1 \times 10^6$ dyne/cm^2	$16.7/1 \times 10^{-4} = 1.67 \times 10^5$ dyne/cm^2

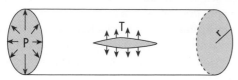

■ **Fig. 20-3**   Diagram of a small blood vessel to illustrate the law of Laplace: T = Pr, where *P* = intraluminal pressure, *r* = radius of the vessel, and *T* = wall tension as the force per unit length tangential to the vessel wall. Wall tension acts to pull apart a theoretical longitudinal slit in the vessel.

Wall tension (T) is the force per unit length of a thin-walled vessel. The Laplace equation applies to very thin-walled vessels, such as capillaries. Wall tension opposes the distending force (Pr) that tends to pull apart a theoretical longitudinal slit in the vessel (Fig. 20-3). Transmural pressure of a blood vessel in vivo is essentially equal to intraluminal pressure, because extravascular pressure is usually negligible.

Wall thickness must be taken into consideration when the equation is applied to thick-walled vessels, such as the aorta. To account for wall thickness of the aorta, P_r (pressure × radius) is divided by wall thickness (w).

The equation now becomes

$$\sigma \text{ (wall stress)} = Pr/w \qquad (20\text{-}2)$$

Pressure in mm Hg is converted to dynes per square centimeter according to the equation P = hρg, where h is the height of a Hg column in centimeters, ρ is the density of Hg in g/cm^3, g is gravitational acceleration in cm/s^2, and wall stress (σ) is force per unit area within the vascular wall.

Thus, at normal aortic and capillary pressures, the wall tension of the aorta is about 12,000 times greater than that of the capillary (Table 20-1). In a person standing quietly, capillary pressure in the feet may reach 100 mm Hg. Under such conditions, capillary wall tension increases to 66.5 dyne/cm, a value that is still only one three-thousandth that of the wall tension in the aorta at the same internal pressure. However, σ (wall stress), which takes wall thickness into account, is only about 10-fold greater in the aorta than in the capillary.

In addition to providing an explanation for the ability of capillaries to withstand large internal pressures, the above calculations also point out that as vessels dilate, wall stress increases if internal pressure remains constant.

> **Syphilitic aortic aneurysm,** which is now rare, and **abdominal aneurysm** (caused by atherosclerotic degeneration of the aortic wall) are characterized by a dilated segment of the aorta. The diseased part of the aorta is under severe stress because of its increased radius and thin wall. Unless treated surgically, the aneurysm can rupture and cause immediate death. Treatment consists of resection of the aneurysm and replacement with a Dacron graft.

The diameter of the resistance vessels (arterioles) is determined by the balance between the contractile force of the vascular smooth muscle and the distending force produced by the intraluminal pressure. The greater the contractile activity of the vascular smooth muscle of an arteriole, the smaller is its diameter. In small arterioles, contraction can continue to the point where the vessel is completely occluded. Occlusion is caused by infolding of the endothelium and by trapping of the blood cells in the vessel.

With progressive reduction in the intravascular pressure, vessel diameter decreases (as does tension in the vessel wall—law of Laplace) and blood flow eventually ceases, although pressure within the arteriole is still greater than the tissue pressure. The pressure that causes flow to cease has been referred to as the **critical closing pressure,** and its mechanism is still controversial. This critical closing pressure is low when vasomotor activity is reduced by inhibition of sympathetic nerve activity to the vessel, and is increased when vasomotor tone is enhanced by activation of the vascular sympathetic nerve fibers.

> If the heart becomes greatly dilated, as may occur in heart failure caused by **idiopathic cardiomyopathy,** the combination of a weakened myocardium and increased left ventricular wall stress (predicted by the Laplace equation) may result in a dangerously low cardiac output. Recently, a small number of patients with severely dilated hearts have been treated successfully by resection of the myocardium (a remodeling procedure called **ventriculotomy**) to reduce the diastolic volume of the left ventricle and thereby enhance its efficiency.

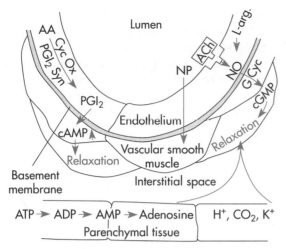

■ **Fig. 20-4** Endothelium- and nonendothelium-mediated vasodilation. Prostacyclin *(PGI₂)* is formed from arachidonic acid *(AA)* by the action of cyclooxygenase *(Cyc Ox)* and prostacyclin synthase *(PGi₂ Syn)* in the endothelium, and elicits relaxation of the adjacent vascular smooth muscle via increases in cyclic adenosine monophosphate *(cAMP)*. Stimulation of the endothelial cells with acetylcholine *(ACh)* or other agents (see text) results in the formation and release of an endothelium-derived relaxing factor *(EDRF)*, identified as nitric oxide *(NO)*. The NO stimulates guanylyl cyclase *(G Cyc)* to increase cyclic guanosine monophosphate *(cGMP)* in the vascular smooth muscle to produce relaxation. The vasodilator agent nitroprusside *(NP)* acts directly on the vascular smooth muscle. Substances such as adenosine, hydrogen ions *(H⁺)*, CO₂, and potassium ions *(K⁺)* can arise in the parenchymal tissue and elicit vasodilation by direct action on the vascular smooth muscle.

Vasoactive Role of the Capillary Endothelium

For many years, the endothelium of capillaries was thought to be an inert single layer of cells that served solely as a passive filter to permit passage of water and small molecules across the blood vessel wall, and to retain blood cells and large molecules (proteins) within the vascular compartment. However, the endothelium is now recognized as an important source of substances that cause contraction or relaxation of the vascular smooth muscle.

Onc of these substances is **prostacyclin.** As shown in Fig. 20-4, prostacyclin can relax vascular smooth muscle via an increase in the cyclic adenosine monophosphate (cAMP) concentration. Prostacyclin is formed in the endothelium from arachidonic acid, and the process is catalyzed by prostacyclin synthase. The mechanism by which prostacyclin synthesis is triggered is not known. However, prostacyclin may be released by an increase in shear stress caused by an accelerated blood flow. The primary function of prostacyclin is to inhibit platelet adherence to the endothelium and platelet aggregation, and thus prevent intravascular clot formation.

Of far greater importance in endothelium-mediated vascular dilation is the formation and release of **nitric oxide**

(NO) (Fig. 20-4). When endothelial cells are stimulated by acetylcholine or other vasodilator agents [adenosine triphosphate (ATP), bradykinin, serotonin, substance P, histamine], NO is released. In blood vessels from which the endothelium has been mechanically removed, these agents do not cause vasodilation. NO (synthesized from L-arginine) activates guanylyl cyclase in the vascular smooth muscle to increase the cyclic guanosine monophosphate (cGMP) concentration, which produces relaxation by decreasing the cytosolic free Ca^{2+} concentration. NO release can be stimulated by the shear stress of blood flow on the endothelium. The drug nitroprusside also increases cGMP, but it acts directly on the vascular smooth muscle and is not endothelium-mediated (Fig. 20-4). Vasodilator agents such as adenosine, hydrogen ions, CO_2, and potassium may be released from parenchymal tissue and act locally on the resistance vessels (Fig. 20-4).

The endothelium can also synthesize **endothelin,** a potent vasoconstrictor peptide. Endothelin can affect vascular tone and blood pressure in humans and may be involved in such pathological states as atherosclerosis, pulmonary hypertension, congestive heart failure, and renal failure.

Passive Role of the Capillary Endothelium

Transcapillary exchange. Solvent and solute move across the capillary endothelial wall by three processes: diffusion, filtration, and pinocytosis. *Diffusion is the most important process for transcapillary exchange and pinocytosis is the least important.*

Diffusion. Under normal conditions, only about 0.06 ml of water per minute moves back and forth across the capillary wall per 100 g of tissue as a result of filtration and absorption. In contrast, 300 ml of water per minute per 100 g of tissue moves across the capillary wall by diffusion, a 5000-fold difference.

When filtration and diffusion are related to blood flow, about 2% of the plasma passing through the capillaries is filtered. In contrast, the diffusion of water is 40 times greater than the rate by which it is brought to the capillaries by blood flow. The transcapillary exchange of solutes is also primarily governed by diffusion. Thus, diffusion is the key factor in providing exchange of gases, substrates, and waste products between the capillaries and the tissue cells.

The process of diffusion is described by Fick's law:

$$J = -DA\frac{dc}{dx} \qquad (20\text{-}3)$$

where

J = quantity of a substance moved per unit time (t)
D = free diffusion coefficient for a particular molecule (the value is inversely related to the square root of the molecular weight)
A = cross-sectional area of the diffusion pathway
dc/dx = concentration gradient of the solute

Fick's law is also expressed as

$$J = -PS(C_o - C_i) \qquad (20\text{-}4)$$

where

P = capillary permeability to the substance
S = capillary surface area
C_i = concentration of the substance inside the capillary
C_o = concentration of the substance outside the capillary

Hence, the PS product provides a convenient expression of available capillary surface, because permeability is rarely altered much under physiological conditions.

In the capillaries, diffusion of lipid-insoluble molecules is restricted to the pores. The mean size of the pores can be calculated by measurement of the diffusion rate of an uncharged molecule whose free diffusion coefficient is known. Movement of solutes across the capillary endothelium is complex and involves corrections for attractions between solute and solvent molecules, interactions between solute molecules, pore configuration, and charge on the molecules relative to charge on the endothelial cells. Such solute motion is not simply a matter of random thermal movements of molecules down a concentration gradient.

For small molecules, such as water, NaCl, urea, and glucose, the capillary pores offer little restriction to diffusion (in other words, they have a low **reflection coefficient**). Diffusion of these substances is so rapid that the mean concentration gradient across the capillary endothelium is extremely small. The greater the size of the lipid-insoluble molecules, the more restricted is the diffusion through capillaries. Diffusion eventually becomes minimal when the mo-

lecular weight of the molecules exceeds about 60,000. With small molecules, the only limitation to net movement across the capillary wall is the rate at which blood flow transports the molecules to the capillary. The transport of these molecules is said to be **flow limited.**

With flow-limited small molecules, the concentration of the molecule in the blood reaches equilibrium with its concentration in the interstitial fluid at a location near the origin of the capillary from its parent arteriole. Its concentration falls to negligible levels near the arterial end of the capillary (Fig. 20-5, *A*). If the flow is large, the small molecule can still be present at a distant locus downstream in the capillary. A somewhat larger molecule will move farther along the capillary before it reaches an insignificant concentration in the blood. Furthermore, the number of still larger molecules that enter the arterial end of the capillary but that cannot pass through the capillary pores equals the number that leaves the venous end of the capillary (Fig. 20-5, *A*).

With large molecules, diffusion across the capillaries becomes the limiting factor (**diffusion limited).** In other words, capillary permeability to a large solute molecule limits its transport across the capillary wall (Fig. 20-5, *A*). The diffusion of small lipid-insoluble molecules is so rapid that diffusion limits the blood-tissue exchange only when the distances between capillaries and parenchymal cells are great (e.g., tissue edema or very low capillary density) (Fig. 20-5, *B*).

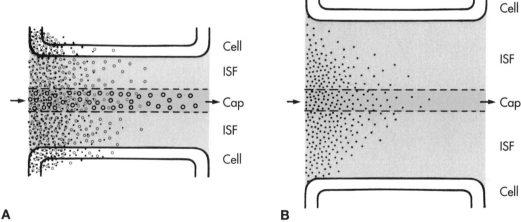

A   **B**

■ **Fig. 20-5** Flow- and diffusion-limited transport from capillaries *(Cap)* to tissue. **A,** Flow-limited transport. The smallest water-soluble inert tracer particles *(black dots)* reach negligible concentrations after passing only a short distance down the capillary. Larger particles *(colored circles)* with similar properties travel farther along the capillary before reaching insignificant intracapillary concentration. Both substances cross the interstitial fluid *(ISF)* and reach the parenchymal tissue *(Cell).* Because of their size, more of the smaller particles are taken up by the tissue cells. The largest particles *(black circles)* cannot penetrate the capillary pores and hence do not escape from the capillary lumen except by pinocytotic vesicle transport. An increase in the volume of blood flow or an increase in capillary density increases tissue supply for the diffusible solutes. Note that capillary permeability is greater at the venous end of the capillary (also in the venule, not shown) because of the larger number of pores in this region. **B,** Diffusion-limited transport. When the distance between the capillaries and the parenchymal tissue is large, as a result of edema or low capillary density, diffusion becomes a limiting factor in the transport of solutes from capillary to tissue even at high rates of capillary blood flow.

Movement of lipid-soluble molecules across the capillary wall is not limited to capillary pores (only about 0.02% of the capillary surface), because these molecules can pass directly through the lipid membranes of the entire capillary endothelium. Consequently, *lipid-soluble molecules move rapidly between blood and tissue. The degree of lipid solubility (oil-to-water partition coefficient) provides a good index of the ease of transfer of lipid molecules through the capillary endothelium.*

Oxygen and carbon dioxide are both lipid soluble, and they readily pass through the endothelial cells. Calculations based on (1) the diffusion coefficient for O_2, (2) the capillary density and diffusion distances, (3) the blood flow, and (4) the tissue O_2 consumption indicate that the O_2 supply of normal tissue at rest and during activity is not limited by diffusion or by the number of open capillaries.

Measurements of Po_2 and of the O_2 saturation of blood in the microvessels indicate that in many tissues, the O_2 saturation at the entrance of the capillaries has decreased to a saturation of about 80% as the result of diffusion of O_2 from arterioles and small arteries. Also, CO_2 loading and the resulting intravascular shifts in the oxyhemoglobin dissociation curve occur in the precapillary vessels. Hence, in addition to gas exchange at the level of the capillaries, O_2 and CO_2 pass directly between adjacent arterioles and venules, and possibly between arteries and veins (**countercurrent exchange**). This countercurrent exchange represents a diffusional shunt of gas away from the capillaries, and, at low blood flow rates, this shunt may limit the supply of O_2 to the tissue.

Capillary filtration. The permeability of the capillary endothelial membrane is not uniform throughout all body tissues. For example, the liver capillaries are quite permeable, and albumin escapes from them at a rate several times greater than that from the less permeable muscle capillaries. Also, permeability is not uniform along the length of the capillary. The venous ends are more permeable than the arterial ends, and permeability is greatest in the venules. The greater permeability at the venous end of the capillaries and in the venules is attributed to the greater number of pores in these regions of the microvessels.

The sites where filtration occurs have been controversial. Some water passes through the capillary endothelial cell membranes, but most flows through apertures (**pores**) in the endothelial walls of the capillaries (Figs. 20-6 and 20-7). The pores in skeletal and cardiac muscle capillaries have diameters of about 4 nm. Electron microscopy has revealed clefts between adjacent endothelial cells in mouse cardiac muscle, and the gap at the narrowest point is about 4 nm (Figs. 20-6 and 20-7). The clefts (pores) are sparse and represent only about 0.02% of the capillary surface area. In cerebral capillaries, where the blood-brain barrier blocks the entry of many small molecules, pores are absent.

In addition to clefts, some of the more porous capillaries (e.g., in kidney, intestine) contain **fenestrations** (Fig. 20-7) 20 to 100 nm wide, whereas other capillaries (e.g., in liver) have a **discontinuous endothelium** (Fig. 20-7). Fenestrations and discontinuous endothelium permit passage of molecules that are too large to pass through the intercellular clefts of the endothelium. *The direction and magnitude of the movement of water across the capillary wall can be estimated as the algebraic sum of the hydrostatic and osmotic pressures that exist across the membrane.* An increase in intracapillary hydrostatic pressure favors movement of fluid from the vessel interior to the interstitial space, whereas an increase in the concentration of osmotically active particles within the vessels favors movement of fluid into the vessels from the interstitial space.

Hydrostatic forces. The hydrostatic pressure (blood pressure) within the capillaries is not constant. Instead, it depends on the arterial pressure and the venous pressure, and on the precapillary (arterioles) and postcapillary (venules and small veins) resistances. An increase in arterial or venous pressure elevates capillary hydrostatic pressure, whereas a reduction in the arterial or venous pressure has the opposite effect. An increase in arteriolar resistance or closure of arteries reduces capillary pressure, whereas a greater resistance to flow in the venules and veins increases capillary pressure.

Hydrostatic pressure is the principal force in capillary filtration. However, changes in the venous resistance affect capillary hydrostatic pressure more than do changes in arteriolar resistance. A given change in venous pressure produces a greater effect on capillary hydrostatic pressure than does the same change in arterial pressure. About 80% of an increase in venous pressure is transmitted back to the capillaries.

Capillary hydrostatic pressure (P_c) varies from tissue to tissue. Average values, obtained from direct measurements in human skin, are about 32 mm Hg at the arterial end of the capillaries and about 15 mm Hg at the venous end of the capillaries at the level of the heart (Fig. 20-8). When a person stands, the hydrostatic pressure increases in the legs and decreases in the head (see Chapter 23).

Tissue pressure, or more specifically interstitial fluid pressure (P_i) outside the capillaries, opposes capillary filtration. $P_c - P_i$ constitutes the driving force for filtration. Normally, P_i is close to zero, so that P_c essentially represents the hydrostatic driving force.

Osmotic forces. The key factor that restrains fluid loss from the capillaries is the osmotic pressure of the plasma proteins (such as albumin). This osmotic pressure is called the **colloid osmotic pressure** or **oncotic pressure** (π_p). The total osmotic pressure of plasma is about 6000 mm Hg, whereas the oncotic pressure is only about 25 mm Hg. Nevertheless, this small oncotic pressure is an important factor in fluid exchange across the capillary wall. The reason the oncotic pressure is important is that the plasma proteins are essentially confined to the intravascular space, whereas the electrolytes are virtually of equal concentration on both sides of the capillary endothelium. The relative permeability of solute to water influences the actual magnitude of the osmotic pressure. The **reflection coefficient** (σ) is the relative impediment to the passage of a substance through the capillary membrane. The reflection coefficient of water is zero and that of albumin (to which the endothelium is essentially impermeable) is 1. Filterable solutes have reflection

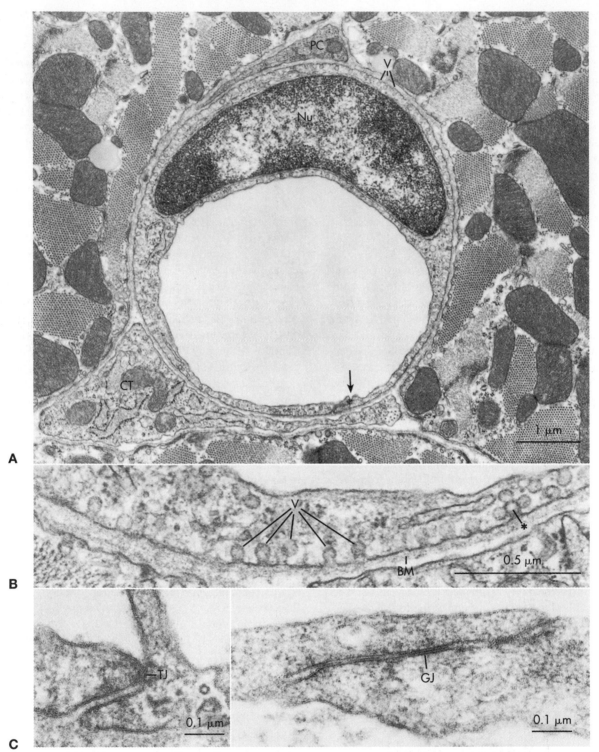

■ **Fig. 20-6** **A,** Cross-sectioned capillary in a mouse ventricular wall. The luminal diameter is approximately 4 μm. In this thin section, the capillary wall is formed by a single endothelial cell (*Nu,* endothelial nucleus), which forms a functional complex *(arrow)* with itself. The thin pericapillary space is occupied by a pericyte *(PC)* and a connective tissue *(CT)* cell ("fibroblast"). Note the numerous endothelial vesicles *(V).* **B,** Detail of the endothelial cell in **A,** showing plasmalemmal vesicles *(V),* attached to the endothelial cell surface. These vesicles are especially prominent in vascular endothelium and are involved in transport of substances across the blood vessel wall. Note the complex alveolar vesicle (*). *BM,* Basement membrane. **C,** Junctional complex in a capillary of mouse heart. "Tight" junctions *(TJ)* typically form in these small blood vessels and appear to consist of fusions between apposed endothelial cell surface membranes. **D,** Interendothelial junction in a muscular artery of monkey papillary muscle. Although tight junctions similar to those of capillaries are found in these large blood vessels, extensive junctions that resemble gap junctions in the intercalated disks between myocardial cells often appear in arterial endothelium (example shown at *GJ*).

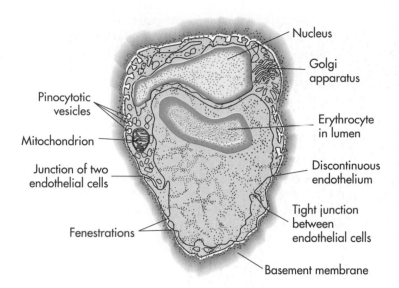

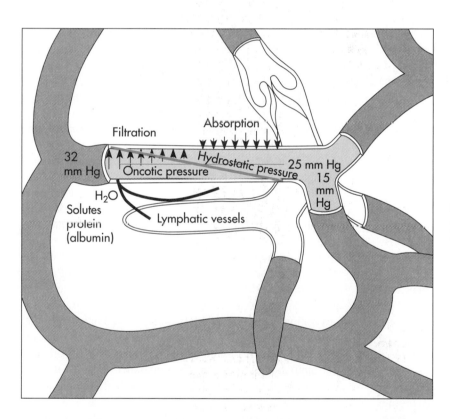

■ **Fig. 20-7**   Diagrammatic sketch of an electron micrograph of a composite capillary in cross section.

■ **Fig. 20-8**   Schematic representation of the factors responsible for filtration and absorption across the capillary wall and the formation of lymph.

coefficients between 0 and 1. Also, different tissues have different reflection coefficients for the same molecule. Hence, movement of a given solute across the endothelial wall varies with the tissue. The true oncotic pressure (π) is defined by the equation

$$\pi = \sigma RT (C_i - C_o) \qquad (20\text{-}5)$$

where

σ	= reflection coefficient
R	= gas constant
T	= absolute temperature
C_i and C_o	= solute (albumin) concentration, inside and outside the capillary respectively.

Of the plasma proteins, albumin is the most important in determining oncotic pressure. The average albumin molecule (molecular weight 69,000) is approximately half the size of the average globulin molecule (molecular weight 150,000), and it is present in almost twice the concentration as that of the globulins (4.5 vs. 2.5 g/dl of plasma). Albumin also exerts a greater osmotic force than can be accounted for solely on the basis of the number of molecules dissolved in a unit volume of plasma. Therefore, it cannot be completely replaced by inert substances of appropriate molecular size, such as dextran. This additional osmotic force becomes disproportionately great at high concentrations of albumin (as in plasma), and this force is weak to absent in dilute solutions of albumin (as in interstitial fluid).

The reason for this behavior of albumin is its negative charge when the blood pH is normal. Albumin binds a small number of chloride ions, which increases the negative charge, and hence the ability to retain more sodium ions inside the capillaries (see Chapter 2). This small increase in electrolyte concentration of the plasma over that of the interstitial fluid produced by the negatively charged albumin enhances its osmotic force to that of an ideal solution that contains a solute of molecular weight 37,000. If albumin did indeed have a molecular weight of 37,000, it would not be retained by the capillary endothelium because of albumin's small size. Hence, albumin could not function as a counterforce to capillary hydrostatic pressure. If, however, albumin did not exert this enhanced osmotic force, a concentration of about 12 g of albumin/per deciliter of plasma would be required to achieve a plasma oncotic pressure of 25 mm Hg. Such a high albumin concentration would greatly increase blood viscosity and hence would increase the resistance to blood flow through the vascular system.

Small amounts of albumin escape from the capillaries and enter the interstitial fluid, where they exert a very small osmotic force (0.1 to 5 mm Hg). This force, πi, is small because of the low concentration of albumin in the interstitial fluid, and because at low concentrations albumin cannot enhance the osmotic force as much as it does at high concentrations.

With prolonged standing, particularly when associated with some elevation of venous pressure in the legs (such as that caused by pregnancy) or with sustained increases in venous pressure (as seen in congestive heart failure), filtration is greatly enhanced, and it exceeds the capacity of the lymphatic system to remove the capillary filtrate from the interstitial space.

The concentration of the plasma proteins may also change in different pathological states and thus alter the osmotic force and movement of fluid across the capillary membrane. The plasma protein concentration is increased in **dehydration** (e.g., water deprivation, prolonged sweating, severe vomiting, diarrhea). In this condition, water moves by osmotic forces from the tissues to the vascular compartment. In contrast, the plasma protein concentration is reduced in **nephrosis** (a renal disease characterized by protein loss, which appears in the urine), and edema may occur.

When capillary injury is extensive, as in severe burns, intravascular fluid and plasma protein leak into the interstitial space in the damaged tissues. The protein that escapes from the vessel lumen increases the oncotic pressure of the interstitial fluid. This greater osmotic force outside the capillaries leads to additional fluid loss and possibly to a severe dehydration of the patient.

Balance of hydrostatic and osmotic forces. The relationship between hydrostatic pressure and oncotic pressure, and the role of these forces in regulating fluid passage across

the capillary endothelium, were expounded by Starling in 1896. This relationship constitutes the **Starling hypothesis.** It can be expressed by the equation

$$Q_f = k[(P_c + \pi_i) - (P_i + \pi_p)] \qquad (20\text{-}6)$$

where

Q_f = fluid movement
P_c = capillary hydrostatic pressure
P_i = interstitial fluid hydrostatic pressure
π_p = plasma oncotic pressure
π_i = interstitial fluid oncotic pressure
k = filtration constant for the capillary membrane

Filtration occurs when the algebraic sum is positive; absorption occurs when it is negative.

Traditionally, filtration was considered to occur at the arterial end of the capillary and absorption was considered to occur at its venous end, because of the gradient of hydrostatic pressure along the capillary. This scheme is true for the idealized capillary, as depicted in Fig. 20-8. However, direct observations have revealed that many capillaries only filter, whereas others only absorb. In some vascular beds (e.g., the renal glomerulus), hydrostatic pressure in the capillary is high enough to cause filtration along the entire length of the capillary. In other vascular beds (e.g., the intestinal mucosa), the hydrostatic and oncotic forces are such that absorption occurs along the whole capillary.

As discussed above, capillary pressure depends on several factors, the principal one being the contractile state of the precapillary vessel. Normally, arterial pressure, venous pressure, postcapillary resistance, interstitial fluid hydrostatic and oncotic pressures, and plasma oncotic pressure are relatively constant. A change in precapillary resistance influences fluid movement across the capillary wall. Because water moves so quickly across the capillary endothelium, the hydrostatic and osmotic forces equilibrate along the entire capillary. Hence, in the normal state, filtration and absorption across the capillary wall are well balanced. Only a small percentage (2%) of the plasma that flows through the vascular system is filtered. Of this, about 85% is absorbed in the capillaries and venules. The remainder returns to the vascular system as lymph fluid, along with the albumin that escapes from the capillaries.

In the lungs, the mean capillary hydrostatic pressure is only about 8 mm Hg (see Chapter 27). Because the plasma oncotic pressure is 25 mm Hg and the lung interstitial fluid pressure is approximately 15 mm Hg, the net force slightly favors reabsorption. Despite the predominance of reabsorption, pulmonary lymph is formed. This lymph consists of fluid that is withdrawn from the capillaries osmotically by the small amount of plasma protein that escapes through the capillary endothelium.

In pathological conditions, such as left ventricular failure or stenosis of the mitral valve, pulmonary capillary hydrostatic pressure may exceed plasma oncotic pressure. When this occurs, it may cause **pulmonary edema,** a condition in which excessive fluid accumulates in the pulmonary interstitium. This fluid accumulation seriously interferes with gas exchange in the lungs.

Capillary filtration coefficient. The rate of fluid movement (Q_f) across the capillary membrane depends not only on the algebraic sum of the hydrostatic and osmotic forces across the endothelium (ΔP), but also on the area (A_m) of the capillary wall available for filtration, the distance (Δx) across the capillary wall, the viscosity (η) of the filtrate, and the filtration constant (k) of the membrane. These factors may be expressed by the equation

$$Q_r = \frac{kA_m\Delta P}{\eta\Delta x} \qquad (20\text{-}7)$$

The dimensions of Q_r are units of flow per unit of pressure gradient across the capillary wall per unit of capillary surface area. This expression, which describes the flow of fluid through the membrane pores, is essentially Poiseuille's law for flow through tubes (see Chapter 18).

Because the thickness of the capillary wall and the viscosity of the filtrate are relatively constant, they can be included in the filtration constant, k. If the area of the capillary membrane is not known, the rate of filtration can be expressed per unit weight of tissue. Hence, the equation can be simplified to

$$Q_f = k_t\Delta P \qquad (20\text{-}8)$$

where k_t is the capillary filtration coefficient for a given tissue, and the units for Q_f are milliliters per minute per 100 g of tissue per mm Hg pressure.

In any given tissue, the filtration coefficient per unit area of capillary surface, and hence the capillary permeability, is not changed by various physiological conditions, such as arteriolar dilation and capillary distention, or by such adverse conditions as hypoxia, hypercapnia, or reduced pH. When capillaries are injured (as by toxins or severe burns) significant amounts of fluid and protein leak out of the capillaries into the interstitial space. This increase in capillary permeability is reflected by an increase in the filtration coefficient.

Because capillary permeability is constant under normal conditions, the filtration coefficient can be used to determine the relative number of open capillaries (that is, the capillary surface area available for filtration in tissue). For example, increased metabolic activity of contracting skeletal muscle relaxes the precapillary resistance vessels and hence opens more capillaries. This process, called **capillary recruitment,** increases the filtering surface area.

Disturbances in hydrostatic-osmotic balance. Relatively small changes in arterial pressure may have little effect on filtration. The change in pressure may be countered by adjustments of the precapillary resistance vessels (autoregulation, see Chapter 21), so that hydrostatic pressure in the open capillaries remains constant. However, a severe reduction in arterial pressure usually evokes arteriolar constriction. This constriction is mediated by the sympathetic nervous system. This response may occur in hemorrhage,

and it is often accompanied by a fall in venous pressure. These changes lead to a decrease in capillary hydrostatic pressure. However, the low blood pressure in hemorrhage causes a decrease in blood flow (and hence in O_2 supply) to the tissue, with the result that vasodilator metabolites accumulate and relax the arterioles. Precapillary vessel relaxation also occurs because of the reduced transmural pressure (autoregulation, see Chapter 21). Consequently, absorption predominates over filtration. These responses to hemorrhage constitute one of the compensatory mechanisms employed by the body to restore blood volume (see Chapter 24).

An increase in venous pressure alone, as occurs in the feet when a person stands up, would elevate capillary pressure and enhance filtration. However, the increase in transmural pressure closes precapillary vessels (myogenic mechanism, see Chapter 21), and hence the capillary filtration coefficient actually decreases. This reduction in capillary surface available for filtration prevents large amounts of fluid from leaving the capillaries and entering the interstitial space.

A large amount of fluid can move rapidly across the capillary wall. In a normal individual, the filtration coefficient (k_t) for the whole body is about 0.006 ml/min/100 g of tissue/mm Hg. For a 70-kg man, an elevation of venous pressure of 10 mm Hg for 10 minutes would increase filtration from capillaries by 342 ml. Edema does not usually occur, because the fluid is returned to the vascular compartment by the lymphatic vessels. When edema does develop, it usually appears in the dependent parts of the body, where the hydrostatic pressure is greatest, but its location and magnitude are also determined by the type of tissue. Loose tissues, such as the subcutaneous tissue around the eyes or in the scrotum, are more prone to collect larger quantities of interstitial fluid than are firm tissues, such as in a muscle, or encapsulated structures, such as in a kidney.

Pinocytosis. Some transfer (pinocytosis) of substances across the capillary wall can occur in tiny pinocytotic vesicles. These vesicles (Figs. 20-6 and 20-7), formed by a pinching off of the endothelial cell membrane, can take up substances on one side of the capillary wall, move them by kinetic energy across the cell, and deposit their contents on the other side. The amount of material that can be transported in this way is very small relative to that moved by diffusion. However, pinocytosis may be responsible for the movement of large (30 nm) lipid-insoluble molecules between the blood and interstitial fluid. The number of pinocytotic vesicles in endothelium varies with the tissue (muscle > lung > brain) and the number increases from the arterial to the venous end of the capillary.

LYMPHATICS

The terminal vessels of the lymphatic system consist of a widely distributed, closed-end network of highly permeable lymph capillaries. These lymph capillaries resemble blood capillaries, with two important differences: tight junctions are not present between endothelial cells, and fine filaments anchor lymph vessels to the surrounding connective tissue. With muscular contraction, these fine strands pull on the lymphatic vessels to open spaces between the endothelial cells. These spaces permit the entrance of protein and large particles into the lymphatic vessels. The lymph capillaries drain into larger vessels that finally enter the right and left subclavian veins, where they connect with the respective internal jugular veins.

Only cartilage, bone, epithelium, and tissues of the central nervous system are devoid of lymphatic vessels. The function of lymphatic vessels is to return the plasma capillary filtrate to the circulation. This task is accomplished by virtue of tissue pressure, and it is facilitated by intermittent skeletal muscle activity, contractions of the lymphatic vessels, and an extensive system of one-way valves. In this respect, lymphatic vessels resemble the veins, although the larger lymphatic vessels do have thinner walls than the corresponding veins, and they contain only a small amount of elastic tissue and smooth muscle.

The volume of fluid transported through the lymphatics in 24 hours is about equal to an animal's total plasma volume. The amount of protein returned by the lymphatics to the blood in a day is about one fourth to one half of the circulating plasma proteins. The lymphatic vessels are the only means whereby the protein that leaves the vascular compartment can be returned to the blood. Net back diffusion of protein into the capillaries cannot occur against the large protein concentration gradient. If the protein were not removed by the lymph vessels, it would accumulate in the interstitial fluid and act as an oncotic force to draw fluid from the blood capillaries to produce edema.

In addition to returning fluid and protein to the vascular bed, the lymphatic system filters the lymph at the **lymph nodes** and removes foreign particles, such as bacteria. The largest lymphatic vessel, the **thoracic duct,** not only drains the lower extremities, but it also returns the protein lost through the permeable liver capillaries. The thoracic duct also carries substances absorbed from the gastrointestinal tract. The principal substance is fat, in the form of chylomicrons.

Lymph flow varies considerably. The flow is almost nil from resting skeletal muscle, and it increases during exercise in proportion to the degree of muscular activity. It is increased by any mechanism that enhances the rate of blood capillary filtration: such mechanisms include, for example, increased capillary pressure or permeability, or decreased plasma oncotic pressure. When either the volume of interstitial fluid exceeds the drainage capacity of the lymphatics or the lymphatic vessels become blocked, interstitial fluid accumulates. Such accumulation occurs chiefly in the more compliant tissues (e.g., subcutaneous tissue), and it gives rise to clinical edema.

SUMMARY

1. Blood flow through the capillaries is chiefly regulated by contraction of the arterioles (resistance vessels).

2. The capillaries, which consist of a single layer of endothelial cells, can withstand high transmural pressure by virtue of their small diameter. According to the law of Laplace, T (wall tension) = P (transmural pressure) × r (radius of the capillary).

3. The endothelium is the source of nitric oxide and prostacyclin, which relax vascular smooth muscles.

4. Water and small solutes move between the vascular and interstitial fluid compartments through capillary pores mainly by diffusion, but also by filtration and absorption.

5. Because the rate of transcapillary diffusion is about 40 times greater than the blood flow in the tissues, exchange of small lipid-insoluble molecules is flow limited. The larger the molecules, the slower is their diffusion. Large lipid-insoluble molecules are diffusion limited. Molecules larger than about 60,000 kDa are essentially confined to the vascular compartment.

6. Lipid-soluble substances, such as CO_2 and O_2, pass directly through the lipid membranes of the capillary, and the rate of transfer is directly proportional to the lipid solubility of the substance.

7. Capillary filtration and absorption are described by the Starling equation: Fluid movement = $k[(P_c + \pi_i) - (P_i + \pi_p)]$, where P_c = capillary hydrostatic pressure, P_i = interstitial fluid hydrostatic pressure, π_i = interstitial fluid oncotic pressure, and π_p = plasma oncotic pressure. Filtration occurs when the algebraic sum of these terms is positive; absorption occurs when it is negative.

8. Large molecules can move across the capillary wall in vesicles by a process called pinocytosis. The vesicles are formed from the lipid membrane of the capillaries.

9. Fluid and protein that have escaped from the blood capillaries enter the lymphatic capillaries and are transported via the lymphatic system back to the blood vascular compartment.

BIBLIOGRAPHY

Journal articles

Aukland K: Why don't our feet swell in the upright position? *News Physiol Sci* 9:214, 1994.

Aukland K, Reed RK: Interstitial-lymphatic mechanisms in the control of extracellular fluid volume, *Physiol Rev* 73:1, 1993.

Bates DO, Lodwick D, Williams B: Vascular endothelial growth factor and microvascular permeability, *Microcirculation* 6:83, 1999.

Curry FRE: Regulation of water and solute exchange in microvessel endothelium: studies in single perfused capillaries, *Microcirculation* 1:11, 1994.

Davies PF: Flow-mediated endothelial mechanotransduction, *Physiol Rev* 75:519, 1995.

Feng Q, Hedner T: Endothelium-derived relaxing factor (EDRF) and nitric oxide. II. Physiology, pharmacology, and pathophysiological implications, *Clin Physiol* 10:503, 1990.

Levick JR, Mortimer PS: Fluid "balance" between microcirculation and interstitium in skin and other tissues: revision of the classical filtration-reabsorption scheme, *Prog Appl Microcirc* 23:42, 1999.

Michel CC: One hundred years of Starling's hypothesis, *News Physiol Sci* 11:229, 1996.

Michel CC, Neal CR: Openings through endothelial cells associated with increased permeability, Microcirculation 6:45, 1999.

Pries AR et al: Resistance to blood flow in microvessels in vivo, *Circ Res* 75:904, 1994.

Rippe B, Haraldsson B: Transport of macromolecules across microvascular walls: the two-pore theory, *Physiol Rev* 74:163, 1994.

Welsch DG, Segal SS: Endothelial and smooth muscle cell conduction in arterioles controlling blood flow, *Am J Physiol* 274:H178, 1998.

Xia J, Duling BR: Patterns of excitation-contraction coupling in arterioles: dependence on time and concentration, *Am J Physiol* 274:H323, 1998.

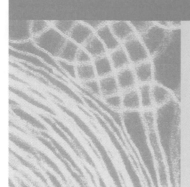

chapter twenty-one

The Peripheral Circulation and Its Control

The peripheral circulation is essentially under dual control: centrally through the nervous system, and locally by the conditions in the tissues surrounding the blood vessels. The relative importance of these two control mechanisms varies in the different tissues. In some areas of the body, such as the skin and splanchnic regions, neural regulation of blood flow predominates, whereas in other regions, such as the heart and brain, this mechanism plays only a minor role.

The vessels chiefly involved in regulating the rate of blood flow throughout the body are called the **resistance vessels** (arterioles). As their name implies, these vessels offer the greatest resistance to the flow of blood pumped to the tissues by the heart, and thus these vessels are important in the maintenance of the arterial blood pressure. The walls of these resistance vessels are composed in large part of smooth muscle fibers (see Fig. 14-1). The presence of smooth muscle in these vessels allows the vessel lumen to vary. When this smooth muscle contracts strongly, the endothelial lining folds inward and completely obliterates the vessel lumen. When the smooth muscle is completely relaxed, the vessel lumen is maximally dilated. Some resistance vessels are closed at any given time. In addition, the smooth muscle in these vessels is partially contracted (which accounts for the tone of these vessels). Were all the resistance vessels in the body to dilate simultaneously, the arterial blood pressure would fall precipitously.

VASCULAR SMOOTH MUSCLE

Vascular smooth muscle is responsible for the control of total peripheral resistance, arterial and venous tone, and the distribution of blood flow throughout the body. The smooth muscle cells are small, mononucleate, and spindle shaped. They are generally arranged in helical or circular layers around the larger blood vessels and in a single circular layer around arterioles (Fig. 21-l, A and B). Parts of endothelial cells project into the vascular smooth muscle layer at various points (**myoendothelial junctions**) along the arterioles (Fig. 21-1, C). These projections suggest a functional inter-

action between endothelium and adjacent vascular smooth muscle. In general, the close association between action potentials and contraction in skeletal and cardiac muscle cells cannot be demonstrated in vascular smooth muscle. Vascular smooth muscle also lacks transverse tubules.

Graded changes in the membrane potential of smooth muscle cells are often associated with variations in force. Contractile activity of these cells is generally elicited by neural or humoral stimuli. However, smooth muscle behavior varies in different vessels. For example, some vessels in the portal or mesenteric circulation contain longitudinally oriented smooth muscle that is spontaneously active. The smooth muscle cells of these vessels generate action potentials that correlate with the contractions and the electrical coupling between cells.

The vascular smooth muscle cells contain many thin (actin) filaments and comparatively few thick (myosin) filaments. These filaments are aligned in the long axis of the cell, but they do not form visible striated sarcomeres. Nevertheless, the sliding filament mechanism appears to operate in this tissue, and phosphorylation of cross-bridges regulates their rate of cycling. Compared with skeletal muscle, smooth muscle contracts more slowly and develops high forces. Such force can be maintained for long periods with low adenosine triphosphate (ATP) utilization. Futhermore, smooth muscle operates over a considerable range of lengths under physiological conditions (see Chapter 13). Cell-to-cell conduction occurs via gap junctions, just as in cardiac muscle (see Chapter 16).

The interaction between myosin and actin leads to contraction in smooth muscle cells, as it does in skeletal muscle cells. This interaction, again as in skeletal muscle, is controlled by the myoplasmic Ca^{2+} concentration. However, the molecular mechanism whereby Ca^{2+} regulates contraction of smooth and skeletal muscle differs. For example, smooth muscle lacks troponin and fast sodium channels. The increased myoplasmic concentration of Ca^{2+} that elicits contraction can be achieved through voltage-gated calcium channels (**electromechanical coupling**) and through receptor-mediated

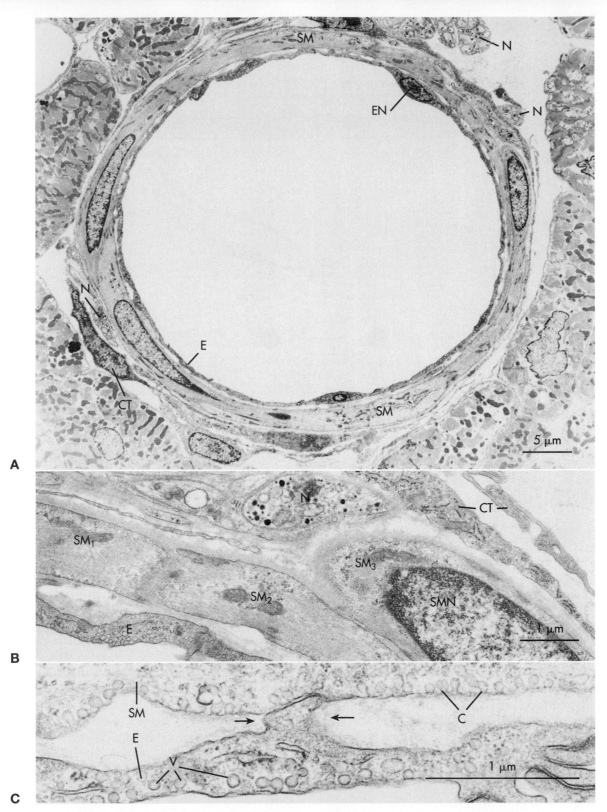

■ **Fig. 21-1** **A,** Low-magnification electron micrograph of an arteriole in cross section (inner diameter of approximately 40 μm) in cat ventricle. The wall of the blood vessel is composed largely of vascular smooth muscle cells *(SM)* whose long axes are directed approximately circularly around the vessel. A single layer of endothelial cells *(E)* forms the innermost portion of the blood vessel. Connective tissue elements *(CT)* such as fibroblasts and collagen make up the adventitial layer at the periphery of the vessel; nerve bundles also appear in this layer *(N)*. *EN,* Endothelial cell nucleus. **B,** Detail of the wall of the blood vessel in **A.** This field contains a single endothelial layer *(E)*, the medial smooth muscle layer (three smooth muscle cell profiles: *SM₁, SM₂, SM₃)*, and the adventitial layer [containing nerves *(N)* and connective tissue *(CT)*]. *SMN,* Smooth muscle nucleus. **C,** Another region of the arteriole, showing the area in which the endothelial *(E)* and smooth muscle *(SM)* layers are apposed. A projection of an endothelial cell *(between arrows)* is closely applied to the surface of the overlying smooth muscle, forming a "myoendothelial junction." Plasmalemmal vesicles are prominent in both the endothelium *(V)* and the smooth muscle cell (where such vesicles are known as "caveolae," *C*).

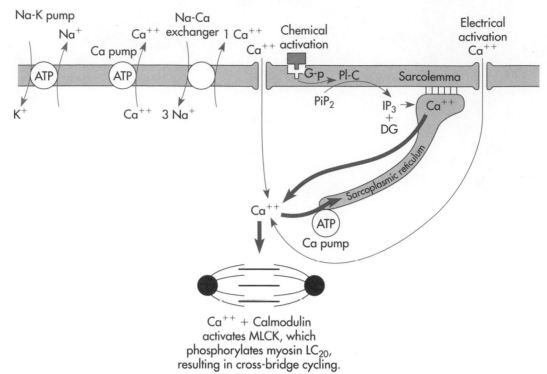

Fig. 21-2 Excitation-contraction coupling in vascular smooth muscle. Calcium can enter the cell via electrically activated channels (*electromechanical coupling*) or via receptor-operated channels (chemical activation, termed *pharmacomechanical coupling*) in the sarcolemma. Calcium is also released from the sarcoplasmic reticulum in response to inositol trisphosphate *(IP₃)* stimulation and is taken back into the sarcoplasmic reticulum by a calcium pump. Calcium is extruded from the cell by a calcium pump and by the Na-Ca exchanger. *G-p,* Guanine nucleotide binding protein; *Pl-C,* phospholipase C; *PiP₂,* phosphatidylinositol bisphosphate; *DG,* diacyglycerol; *MLCK,* myosin light chain kinase; *LC,* light chain kinase, molecular weight 20,000.

calcium channels (**pharmacomechanical coupling**) in the sarcolemma, as well as through the release of Ca^{2+} from the sarcoplasmic reticulum (Fig. 21-2). The cells relax when intracellular free Ca^{2+} is (1) pumped back into the sarcoplasmic reticulum, (2) pumped out of the cell by the calcium pump in the cell membrane, and (3) removed by the Na-Ca exchanger (see Chapter 13).

Pharmacomechanical coupling is the predominant mechanism for eliciting contraction of vascular smooth muscle. Agents that evoke such contraction or relaxation include catecholamines, histamine, acetylcholine, serotonin, angiotensin, adenosine, nitric oxide, CO_2, K^+, H^+, and prostaglandins (see Fig. 20-4). Such substances activate receptors in the vascular smooth muscle membrane. These receptors in turn activate phospholipase C in a reaction coupled to guanine nucleotide binding proteins (G proteins). The phospholipase C hydrolyzes phosphatidylinositol bisphosphate in the membrane to yield diacylglycerol and inositol trisphosphate; the latter releases Ca^{2+} from the sarcoplasmic reticulum. The Ca^{2+} binds to calmodulin, which in turn binds to myosin light chain kinase. This activated Ca^{2+}-calmodulin-myosin kinase complex phosphorylates the light chains (20,000 d) of myosin. The phosphorylated myosin ATPase is

then activated by actin, and the resulting cross-bridge cycling initiates contraction.

Finally, the sensitivity of the contractile regulatory apparatus to Ca^{2+} is increased by agonists. Although the mechanism for this enhanced sensitivity is still unclear, it appears to involve G proteins. Relaxation occurs when the myosin light chain kinase is inactivated by dephosphorylation, and the cytosolic Ca^{2+} is lowered by sarcoplasmic reticulum uptake and by extrusion by the Ca pump and the Na-Ca exchanger. Local humoral changes alter the contractile state of vascular smooth muscle, and factors such as increased temperature or increased carbon dioxide levels relax this tissue.

Most of the arteries and veins of the body are supplied solely by fibers of the sympathetic nervous system. These nerve fibers exert a tonic contractile effect on the blood vessels. This effect has been demonstrated by cutting or freezing the sympathetic nerves to a vascular bed (such as muscle), which results in an increase in blood flow (the blood vessels relax). Activation of the sympathetic nerves, either directly or through a reflex, enhances vascular resistance. In contrast to the sympathetic nerves, the parasympathetic nerves tend to decrease vascular resistance, but they innervate only a

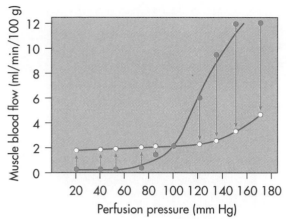

■ **Fig. 21-3**   Pressure-flow relationship in the skeletal muscle vascular bed of the dog. *Closed circles* represent the flows obtained immediately after abrupt changes in perfusion pressure from the control level *(point where lines cross).* *Open circles* represent the steady-state flows obtained at the new perfusion pressure. (Redrawn from Jones RD, Berne RM: *Circ Res* 14:126, 1964.)

small fraction of the blood vessels in the body, mainly in certain viscera.

INTRINSIC OR LOCAL CONTROL OF PERIPHERAL BLOOD FLOW

Autoregulation and Myogenic Regulation

In certain tissues, the blood flow is adjusted to the existing metabolic activity of the tissue. Furthermore, when tissue metabolism is steady, changes in perfusion pressure (arterial blood pressure) evoke vascular resistance changes that tend to maintain a constant blood flow. This mechanism, which is illustrated graphically in Fig. 21-3, is commonly referred to as **autoregulation** of blood flow.

In the skeletal muscle preparation from which the data in Fig. 21-3 were gathered, the muscle was completely isolated from the rest of the animal and was in a resting state. From a control pressure of 100 mm Hg, the pressure was abruptly increased or decreased. The blood flows observed immediately after changing the perfusion pressure are represented by the closed circles. Maintenance of the altered pressure at each new level was followed within 30 to 60 seconds by a return of flow toward the control levels; the open circles represent these steady-state flows. Over the pressure range of 20 to 120 mm Hg, the steady-state flow was relatively constant. Calculation of the hydraulic resistance (pressure/flow) across the vascular bed during steady-state conditions shows that the resistance vessels constricted with elevation of the perfusion pressure but dilated with reduction of perfusion pressure.

Why blood flow remains constant in the presence of an altered perfusion pressure may be explained by the **myogenic mechanism.** *According to this mechanism, the vascular smooth muscle contracts in response to an increase in pressure difference across the wall of a blood vessel (the transmural pressure) and it relaxes in response to a decrease in transmural pressure.*

An example of a myogenic response is shown in Fig. 21-4. Arterioles isolated from the hearts of young pigs were cannulated at each end (Fig. 21-4, *A*), and the transmural pressure (intravascular pressure minus extravascular pressure) and flow through the arteriole could be adjusted to desired levels. With no flow through the arteriole, successive increase of transmural pressure elicited progressive decreases in the vessel diameter (Fig. 21-4, *B*). This response was independent of the endothelium because it was identical in intact vessels and in vessels that had been stripped of endothelium (Fig. 21-4, *C*). Arterioles that were relaxed by direct action of nitroprusside on the vascular smooth muscle showed only a passive increase in diameter when transmural pressure was increased. The mechanism that allows vessel distention to elicit contraction is still unknown. However, because stretch of vascular smooth muscle has been shown to raise the intracellular concentration of Ca^{2+}, an increase in transmural pressure is believed to activate membrane calcium channels.

In normal subjects, blood pressure is maintained at a fairly constant level via the baroreceptor reflex. Hence, the myogenic mechanism might be ineffectual under normal conditions. However, when a person changes from a lying to a standing position, the transmural pressure rises in the lower extremities, and the precapillary vessels constrict in response to this imposed stretch. This constriction, coupled with the hydrostatic pressure imposed by the vertical column of blood from the heart to the feet, results in cessation of flow in most capillaries. After flow stops, capillary filtration diminishes progressively. This change in filtration continues until the increases in plasma oncotic pressure and in interstitial fluid pressure balance the elevated capillary hydrostatic pressure produced by the change to a vertical position.

Endothelium-Mediated Regulation

As discussed in Chapter 20, stimulation of the endothelium can elicit a vasoactive response of the vascular smooth muscle. To demonstrate this response experimentally, transmural pressure is kept constant in an isolated arteriole (as in Fig. 21-4, *A*). The flow is then increased progressively by raising the perfusion fluid reservoir connected to one end of the arteriole, while the reservoir connected to the other end of the arteriole is simultaneously lowered by an equal distance. This maneuver increases the longitudinal pressure gradient along the vessel, and vasodilation occurs (Fig. 21-5, *A*). The vasodilation is presumably caused by the release of nitric oxide from the endothelium in response to the shear stress caused by the increase in flow. If the arteriole is stripped of endothelium, the vessel does not dilate in response to the increased flow (Fig. 21-5, *B*).

If arteriolar resistance did not increase when a subject stands, the hydrostatic pressure in the lower parts of the legs would reach such high levels that large volumes of fluid would pass from the capillaries into the interstitial fluid compartment and produce edema.

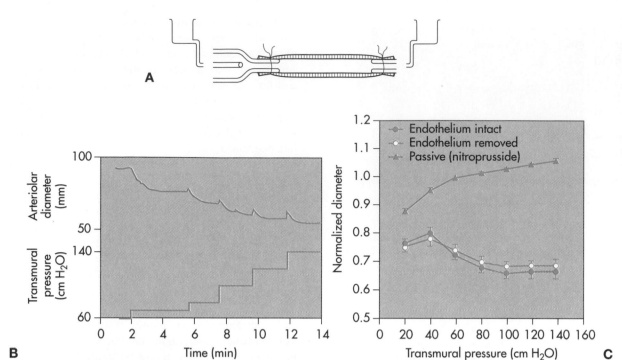

Fig. 21-4 **A,** Constrictor response of the arteriole to an increase in transmural pressure is unaffected by removal of its endothelium. **B,** Diagram of cannulated arteriole. When the smooth muscle is relaxed by nitroprusside, the arteriole is passively distended by the increase in transmural pressure. **C,** Constriction of an isolated cardiac arteriole in response to increases in transmural pressure without flow through the blood vessel. (Redrawn from Kuo L, Davis MJ, Chilian WM: *Am J Physiol* 259:H1063, 1990.)

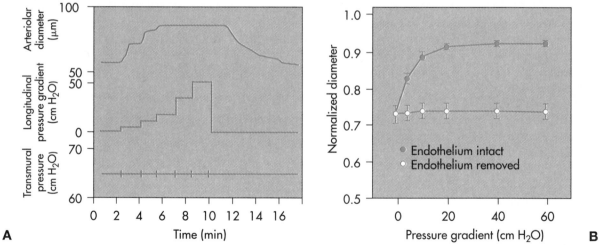

Fig. 21-5 **A,** Flow-induced vasodilation in an isolated cardiac arteriole at constant transmural pressure. Flow was increased progressively by increasing the pressure gradient in the long axis of the arteriole (longitudinal pressure gradient). **B,** Flow-induced vasodilation is abolished by removal of the endothelium of the arteriole. (Redrawn from Kuo L, Davis MJ, Chilian WM: *Am J Physiol* 259:H1063, 1990.)

Metabolic Regulation

Blood flow in a given tissue is governed by the metabolic activity of the tissue. Any intervention that results in an inadequate O_2 supply prompts the formation of vasodilator metabolites. These metabolites are released from the tissue and act locally to dilate the resistance vessels. When the

metabolic rate of the tissue increases or the O_2 delivery to the tissue decreases, more vasodilator substance is released.

Candidate vasodilator substances. Many substances have been proposed as mediators of metabolic vasodilation. Some of the earliest vasodilators suggested were lactic acid, CO_2, and hydrogen ions. However, the decrease in vascular resistance induced by supernormal concentrations of these dilator agents is substantially less than the dilation observed when metabolic activity is increased physiologically.

Changes in O_2 tension can change the contractile state of vascular smooth muscle. An increase in Po_2 elicits contraction; a decrease elicits relaxation. However, measurements of Po_2 in the resistance vessels indicate that over a wide range of Po_2 (11 to 343 mm Hg), the O_2 tension and arteriolar diameter are not well correlated. Hence the observed changes in arteriolar diameter are more compatible with the release of a vasodilator metabolite from the tissue than with a direct effect of Po_2 on the vascular smooth muscle.

Potassium ions, inorganic phosphate ions, and interstitial fluid osmolarity can also induce vasodilation. Both K^+ and phosphate are released and osmolarity is increased during skeletal muscle contraction. Therefore, these factors may contribute to **active hyperemia** (increased blood flow caused by enhanced tissue activity). However, significant increases of phosphate concentration and in osmolarity are not consistently observed during muscle contraction, and they may increase blood flow only transiently. Therefore, they probably do not mediate the vasodilation observed during muscular activity. Potassium is released with the onset of skeletal muscle contraction or with an increase in cardiac muscle activity. Hence, potassium release could be responsible for the initial decrease in vascular resistance observed in response to physical exercise or to increased cardiac work. However, K^+ release is not sustained, despite continued arteriolar dilation throughout the period of enhanced muscle activity. Furthermore, reoxygenated venous blood obtained from active cardiac and skeletal muscles does not elicit vasodilation when the blood is infused into a test vascular bed. It is difficult to see how oxygenation of the venous blood could alter its K^+ or phosphate content or its osmolarity and thereby neutralize its vasodilator effect. Therefore, some agent other than potassium must mediate the vasodilation associated with the metabolic activity of the tissue.

Adenosine, which contributes to the regulation of coronary blood flow, may also participate in the control of the resistance vessels in skeletal muscle. Also, some of the prostaglandins may be important vasodilator mediators in certain vascular beds. Thus, many candidates have been proposed as mediators of metabolic vasodilation, and the relative contribution of each remains a subject for future investigation.

Basal vessel tone. Metabolic control of vascular resistance by the release of a vasodilator substance is predicated on the existence of a **basal vessel tone.** This tonic activity in vascular smooth muscle is readily demonstrable, but, in contrast to tone in skeletal muscle, the tone in vascular smooth muscle is independent of the nervous system. Thus, some metabolic factor must be responsible for maintaining this tone. The following factors may be involved: (1) the myogenic response to the stretch imposed by the blood pressure, (2) the high O_2 tension of arterial blood, or (3) the presence of calcium ions.

Reactive hyperemia. Experiments that test the duration of reactive hyperemia after a vessel is occluded provide evidence for the existence of a local metabolic factor that reg-

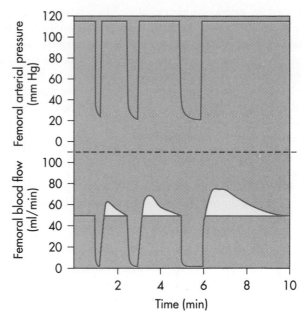

■ **Fig. 21-6**   Reactive hyperemia in the hind limb of the dog after 15-, 30-, and 60-second occlusions of the femoral artery. (Berne RM: Unpublished observations.)

ulates tissue blood flow. If arterial inflow to a vascular bed is stopped temporarily, the blood flow, on release of the occlusion, immediately exceeds the flow that prevailed before occlusion, and the flow gradually returns to the control level. This increase in blood flow is called **reactive hyperemia.**

In the experiment depicted in Fig. 21-6, blood flow to the leg was stopped by clamping the femoral artery for 15, 30, and 60 seconds. Release of the 60-second occlusion resulted in a peak blood flow that was 70% greater than the control flow, and the flow returned to the control level within 110 seconds.

When this same experiment is performed in humans by inflating a blood pressure cuff on the upper arm, dilation of the resistance vessels of the hand and forearm, immediately after release of the cuff, is evident from the bright red color of the skin and the fullness of the veins. Within limits, the peak flow and particularly the duration of the reactive hyperemia are proportional to the duration of the occlusion (Fig. 21-6). If the extremity is exercised during the occlusion period, reactive hyperemia is increased. These observations, and the close relationship that exists between metabolic activity and blood flow in the unoccluded limb, are consistent with a metabolic mechanism in the local regulation of tissue blood flow.

Coordination of arterial and arteriolar dilation. When the vascular smooth muscle of the arterioles relaxes in response to vasodilator metabolites whose release is caused by a decrease in the ratio of the oxygen supply to the oxygen demand of the tissue, resistance may diminish concomitantly in the small upstream arteries that feed these arterioles. The result is a blood flow greater than that produced by arteriolar dilation alone. Two possible mechanisms can account for this coordination of arterial and arteriolar dilation. First, the process of vasodilation in the microvessels is a propagated one, and when dilation is initiated in the arterioles, it can propagate along the vessels from the arterioles back to the small arteries. Second, the metabolite-mediated dilation of the arterioles accelerates blood flow in the feeder arteries. This greater velocity of blood flow increases the shear stress on the arterial endothelium, which can in turn induce vasodilation by release of nitric oxide (Fig. 21-5).

Disease of the arterial walls can lead to obstruction of the arteries, and symptoms, called **intermittent claudication,** appear when the arterial disease occurs in the legs. The symptoms consist of leg pain when the subject walks or climbs stairs, and the pain is relieved by rest. The disease is called **thromboangiitis obliterans,** and it appears most frequently in men who are smokers. With minimal walking, the resistance vessels become maximally dilated by local metabolite release; when the oxygen demand of the muscles increases with more rapid walking, blood flow cannot increase sufficiently to meet the muscle needs for oxygen, and pain caused by muscle ischemia results.

EXTRINSIC CONTROL OF PERIPHERAL BLOOD FLOW

Sympathetic Neural Vasoconstriction

A number of regions in the cerebral medulla influence cardiovascular activity. Stimulation of the dorsal lateral medulla (**pressor** region) evokes vasoconstriction, cardiac acceleration, and enhanced myocardial contractility. Stimulation of cerebral centers caudal and ventromedial to the pressor region decreases the arterial blood pressure. This **depressor** area exerts its effect by direct inhibition of spinal regions and by inhibition of the medullary pressor region. These areas are not true anatomic centers, in which a discrete group of cells is discernible, but they constitute "physiological" centers.

From the vasoconstrictor regions, fibers descend in the spinal cord and synapse at different levels of the thoracolumbar region (T1 to L3). Fibers from the intermediolateral gray matter of the cord emerge with the ventral roots, and they join the paravertebral sympathetic chains through the white communicating branches (see Chapter 11). These preganglionic myelinated fibers may pass up or down the sympathetic chains to synapse in the ganglia within the chains or in outlying ganglia. Postganglionic unmyelinated branches then join the corresponding segmental spinal nerves to innervate the peripheral arteries and veins. Postganglionic sympathetic fibers from the various ganglia join the larger arteries and accompany them as an investing network of fibers to the resistance and capacitance vessels.

The cerebrospinal vasoconstrictor regions are tonically active. Reflexes or humoral stimuli that enhance this activity increase the frequency of impulses that reach the terminal neural branches to the vessels. A constrictor neurohumor (**norepinephrine**) is then released at the terminals and it elicits constriction (α-adrenergic effect) of the resistance vessels. Inhibition of the vasoconstrictor areas diminishes the frequency of impulses in the efferent nerve fibers, and vasodilation results. In this way, neural regulation of the peripheral circulation is accomplished mainly by altering the frequency of impulses in the sympathetic nerves to the blood vessels.

Surgical section of the sympathetic nerves to an extremity abolishes sympathetic vascular tone and thereby increases blood flow to that limb. With time, vascular tone is regained by an increase in basal (intrinsic) tone.

Both the pressor and depressor regions may undergo rhythmic changes in tonic activity, and these changes are manifested as oscillations of arterial pressure. Some rhythmic changes (**Traube-Hering waves**) occur at the frequency of respiration and are caused by a cyclic fluctuation in sympathetic impulses to the resistance vessels. Other fluctuations in sympathetic activity (**Mayer waves**) occur at a frequency lower than that of respiration.

Sympathetic Constrictor Influence on Resistance and Capacitance Vessels

The vasoconstrictor fibers of the sympathetic nervous system supply the arteries, arterioles, and veins, but the neural influence on the larger vessels is much less than it is on the arterioles and small arteries. Capacitance vessels (veins) are more responsive to sympathetic nerve stimulation than are resistance vessels; the capacitance vessels reach maximal constriction at a lower frequency of stimulation than do the resistance vessels. However, capacitance vessels lack β-adrenergic receptors, and they do not respond to vasodilator metabolites. Norepinephrine is the neurotransmitter released at the sympathetic nerve terminals in the blood vessel. Many factors, such as circulating hormones and particularly locally released substances, modify the release of norepinephrine from the vesicles in the nerve terminals.

The response of the resistance and capacitance vessels of the cat to stimulation of the sympathetic fibers is illustrated in Fig. 21-7. When the arterial pressure is held constant, sympathetic fiber stimulation reduces the blood flow (constriction of the resistance vessels) and decreases the blood volume of the tissue (constriction of the capacitance vessels). The abrupt decrease in tissue volume in this experiment was caused by movement of blood out of the capacitance vessels and out of the hindquarters of the cat, whereas the late, slow progressive decline in volume *(to the right of the arrow)* was caused by movement of extravascular fluid into the capillaries and hence away from the tissue. The loss of tissue fluid is a consequence of the lowered capillary hydrostatic pressure brought about by constriction of the resistance vessels. With constriction of the resistance vessels, a new equilibrium of the forces responsible for filtration and absorption across the capillary wall (see Chapter 20) is established.

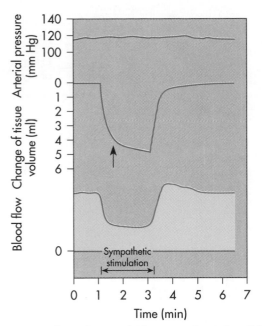

■ **Fig. 21-7**   Effect of sympathetic nerve stimulation (2 Hz) on blood flow and tissue volume in the hindquarters of the cat. The *arrow* denotes the change in slope of the tissue volume curve where the volume decrease caused by emptying of capacitance vessels ceases and loss of extravascular fluid becomes evident. (From Mellander S: *Acta Physiol Scand* 50 [suppl 176]:1, 1960.)

In addition to active changes (contraction and relaxation of the vascular smooth muscle) in vessel caliber, passive changes are also caused by alteration of the intraluminal pressure. An increase in intraluminal pressure distends the vessels, and a decrease reduces the caliber of the vessels as a consequence of the elastic recoil of the vessel walls.

When the vascular tone is basal, approximately one third of the blood volume of a tissue can be mobilized when the sympathetic nerves are stimulated at physiological frequencies. The basal tone is very low in capacitance vessels; if these vessels are denervated experimentally, the increases in volume evoked by maximal doses of acetylcholine are small. Therefore, when the vascular tone is basal, the blood volume is close to the maximal blood volume of the tissue. More blood can be mobilized from the capacitance vessels in the skin than from those in the muscle. This disparity depends in part on the greater sensitivity of the skin vessels to sympathetic stimulation, but also in part because the basal tone is lower in skin vessels than in muscle vessels. Therefore, in the absence of neural influence, the skin capacitance vessels contain more blood than do the muscle capacitance vessels.

Blood is mobilized from capacitance vessels in response to physiological stimuli. For example, during physical exercise, activation of the sympathetic nerve fibers constricts the peripheral veins and hence augments the cardiac filling pressure. In arterial hypotension (as in hemorrhage), the capacitance vessels constrict and thereby correct the decreased central venous pressure associated with blood loss.

In hemorrhagic shock, the resistance vessels constrict and thereby assist in the maintenance of a normal arterial blood pressure. With arterial hypotension, the enhanced arteriolar constriction also leads to a small mobilization of blood from the tissue by virtue of recoil of the postarteriolar vessels when the intraluminal pressure is reduced. Furthermore, extravascular fluid is mobilized because of greater fluid absorption into the capillaries in response to the lowered capillary hydrostatic pressure (see also Chapter 24).

Parasympathetic Neural Influence

The efferent fibers of the cranial division of the parasympathetic nervous system innervate the blood vessels of the head and of some of the viscera, whereas fibers of the sacral division supply blood vessels of the genitalia, bladder, and large bowel. Skeletal muscle and skin do not receive parasympathetic innervation. Because only a small proportion of the resistance vessels of the body receives parasympathetic fibers, the effect of these cholinergic fibers on total vascular resistance is small.

Stimulation of the parasympathetic fibers to the salivary glands induces marked vasodilation. A vasodilator polypeptide, **bradykinin,** formed locally from the action of an enzyme on a plasma protein substrate in the glandular lymphatics mediates the vasodilation. Bradykinin is formed in other exocrine glands, such as the lacrimal and sweat glands. Its presence in sweat may be partly responsible for the dilation of cutaneous blood vessels.

Humoral Factors

Epinephrine and norepinephrine exert a powerful effect on the peripheral blood vessels. In skeletal muscle, epinephrine in low concentrations dilates resistance vessels (β-**adrenergic effect**) but in high concentrations it produces constriction (α-**adrenergic effect.**) In all vascular beds the primary effect of norepinephrine is vasoconstriction. When stimulated, the adrenal gland can release epinephrine and norepinephrine into the systemic circulation. However, under physiological conditions, the effect of catecholamine release from the adrenal medulla is less important than is norepinephrine release from sympathetic nerve endings.

Vascular Reflexes

Areas of the cerebral medulla that mediate sympathetic and vagal effects are under the influence of neural impulses that originate in the baroreceptors, chemoreceptors, hypothalamus, cerebral cortex, and skin. These areas of the medulla are also affected by changes in the blood concentrations of CO_2 and O_2.

Arterial baroreceptors. The **baroreceptors** (or **pressoreceptors**) are stretch receptors located in the carotid sinuses. The carotid sinuses are the slightly widened areas at the origins of the internal carotid arteries. Baroreceptors are also located in the aortic arch (Figs. 21-8 and 21-9). Impulses that arise in the carotid sinus travel up the carotid

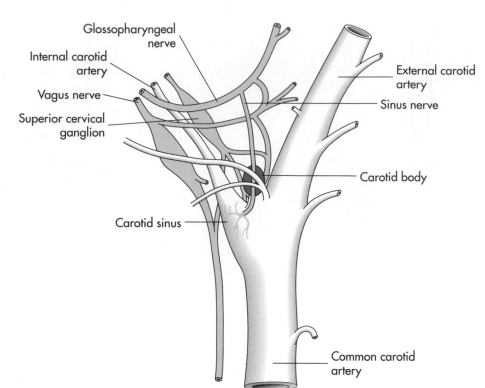

Glossopharyngeal nerve

Internal carotid artery

Vagus nerve

Superior cervical ganglion

External carotid artery

Sinus nerve

Carotid body

Carotid sinus

Common carotid artery

■ **Fig. 21-8** Diagrammatic representation of the carotid sinus and carotid body and their innervation in the dog. (Redrawn from Adams WE: *The comparative morphology of the carotid body and carotid sinus*, Springfield, Ill, 1958, Charles C Thomas.)

sinus nerve (nerve of Hering) to the glossopharyngeal nerve and, via the latter, to the **nucleus of the tractus solitarius (NTS)** in the medulla. The NTS is the site of the central projections of the chemoreceptors and baroreceptors.

Stimulation of the NTS inhibits sympathetic nerve impulses to the peripheral blood vessels (depressor effect), whereas lesions of the NTS produce vasoconstriction (pressor effect). Impulses that arise in the baroreceptors of the aortic arch reach the NTS via afferent fibers in the vagus nerves.

The baroreceptor nerve terminals in the walls of the carotid sinus and aortic arch respond to the vascular stretch and deformation induced by changes in the arterial blood pressure. The frequency of firing of these nerve terminals is enhanced by an increase in arterial blood pressure and diminished by a reduction in arterial blood pressure. An increase in impulse frequency, as occurs with a rise in arterial pressure, inhibits the cerebral vasoconstrictor regions, and it results in peripheral vasodilation and a lowering of the arterial blood pressure. Contributing to this lowering of the blood pressure is a bradycardia brought about by activation of the cardiac branches of the vagus nerves.

The carotid sinus and aortic baroreceptors do not cause equally powerful effects on peripheral resistance. The carotid sinus baroreceptors are more sensitive than are those in the aortic arch. Changes in carotid sinus pressure evoke greater alterations in systemic arterial pressure than do equivalent changes in aortic arch pressure.

The carotid sinus with its sinus nerve can be isolated from the rest of the circulation and perfused by either a donor animal or an artificial perfusion system. Under these conditions, changes in the pressure within the carotid sinus are associated with reciprocal changes in the blood pressure

of the donor animal. The receptors in the walls of the carotid sinus are more responsive to pulsatile pressures than to constant pressures. This is illustrated in Fig. 21-10, which shows that at normal levels of mean arterial blood pressure (about 100 mm Hg) a barrage of impulses from a single fiber of the sinus nerve is initiated in early systole by the pressure rise, and only a few spikes are observed during late systole and early diastole. At lower arterial pressures, these phasic changes are even more evident, but the overall frequency of discharge is reduced. The blood pressure threshold for eliciting sinus nerve impulses is about 50 mm Hg, and a maximal sustained firing is reached at around 200 mm Hg. Because the baroreceptors do adapt, their response at any mean arterial pressure level is greater to a large than to a small pulse pressure.

This response is illustrated in Fig. 21-11, which shows the effects of damping the pulsations in the carotid sinus on the firing frequency in a fiber of the sinus nerve and on the systemic arterial pressure. When the pulse pressure in the carotid sinuses is reduced by adding an air chamber to the system, but mean pressure remains constant, the rate of neural impulses recorded from a sinus nerve fiber decreases and the systemic arterial pressure increases. Restoration of the pulse pressure in the carotid sinus restores the frequency of sinus nerve discharge and the systemic arterial pressure to control levels (Fig. 21-11).

The resistance increases that occur in response to reduced pressure in the carotid sinus vary from one peripheral vascular bed to another. These variations allow blood flow to be redistributed. In the anesthetized dog, for example, the resistance changes elicited by altering carotid sinus pressure are greatest in the femoral vessels, less in the renal vessels, and least in the mesenteric and celiac vessels.

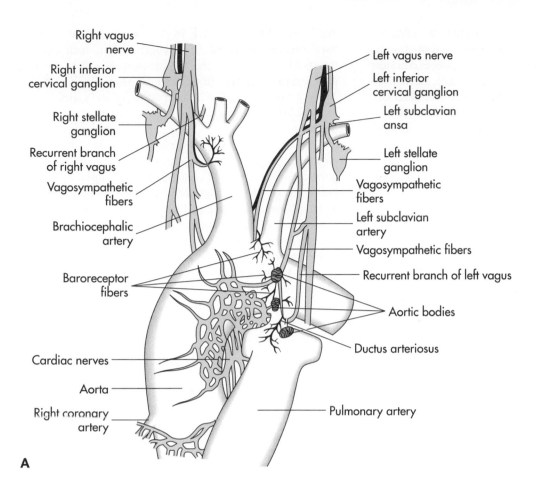

Right vagus nerve

Right inferior cervical ganglion

Right stellate ganglion

Recurrent branch of right vagus

Vagosympathetic fibers

Brachiocephalic artery

Baroreceptor fibers

Cardiac nerves

Aorta

Right coronary artery

Left vagus nerve

Left inferior cervical ganglion

Left subclavian ansa

Left stellate ganglion

Vagosympathetic fibers

Left subclavian artery

Vagosympathetic fibers

Recurrent branch of left vagus

Aortic bodies

Ductus arteriosus

Pulmonary artery

A

■ Fig. 21-9 **A,** Anterior view and **B,** posterior view of the aortic arch showing the innervation of the aortic bodies and pressoreceptors in the dog. (Modified from Nonidez JF: *Anat Rec* 69:299, 1937.)

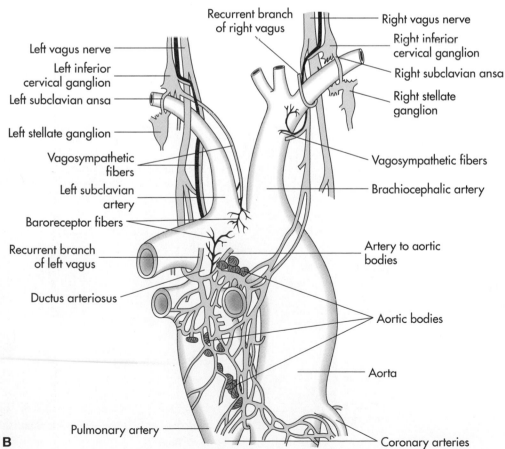

Recurrent branch of right vagus

Left vagus nerve

Left inferior cervical ganglion

Left subclavian ansa

Left stellate ganglion

Vagosympathetic fibers

Left subclavian artery

Baroreceptor fibers

Recurrent branch of left vagus

Ductus arteriosus

Pulmonary artery

Right vagus nerve

Right inferior cervical ganglion

Right subclavian ansa

Right stellate ganglion

Vagosympathetic fibers

Brachiocephalic artery

Artery to aortic bodies

Aortic bodies

Aorta

Coronary arteries

B

Furthermore, the sensitivity of the carotid sinus reflex can be altered. Local application of norepinephrine or stimulation of sympathetic nerve fibers to the carotid sinuses enhances the sensitivity of the receptors in the sinus, such that a given increase in intrasinus pressure produces a greater depressor response. Baroreceptor sensitivity decreases in hypertension, because the carotid sinuses become stiffer as a result of the high intraarterial pressure. Under these conditions, a given increase in carotid sinus pressure elicits a smaller decrease in systemic arterial pressure than it does at a nor-

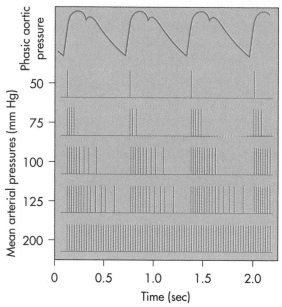

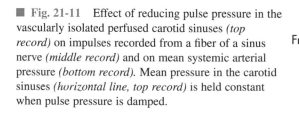

■ **Fig. 21-10**   Relationship of phasic aortic blood pressure in the firing of a single afferent nerve fiber from the carotid sinus at different levels of mean arterial pressure.

mal level of blood pressure. In other words, the set point of the baroreceptors is raised in hypertension, such that the threshold is increased and the pressure receptors are less sensitive to changes in transmural pressure.

As would be expected, denervation of the carotid sinus can produce temporary and, in some instances, prolonged hypertension.

The arterial baroreceptors play a key role in short-term adjustments of blood pressure in response to relatively abrupt changes in blood volume, cardiac output, or peripheral resistance (as in exercise). However, long-term control of blood pressure—that is, over days or weeks—is determined by the fluid balance of the individual, namely, the balance between fluid intake and fluid output. By far the single most important organ in the control of body fluid volume, and hence of blood pressure, is the kidney (see also Chapter 36).

> In some individuals, the carotid sinus is abnormally sensitive to external pressure. Hence, tight collars or other forms of external pressure over the region of the carotid sinus may elicit marked hypotension and fainting. Such hypersensitivity is known as the **carotid sinus syndrome.**

Cardiopulmonary baroreceptors. Cardiopulmonary receptors are located in the atria, ventricles, and pulmonary vessels. These baroreceptors are innervated by vagal and sympathetic afferent nerves. Cardiopulmonary reflexes are tonically active and can alter peripheral resistance in response to changes in intracardiac, venous, or pulmonary vascular pressure.

The atria contain two types of cardiopulmonary baroreceptors: those activated by the tension developed during atrial contraction (**A receptors**) and those activated by the stretch

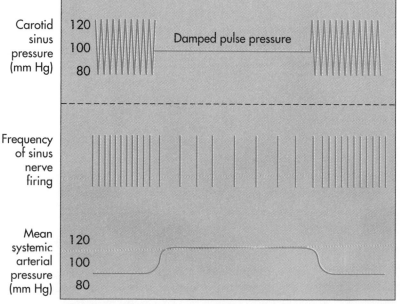

■ **Fig. 21-11**   Effect of reducing pulse pressure in the vascularly isolated perfused carotid sinuses *(top record)* on impulses recorded from a fiber of a sinus nerve *(middle record)* and on mean systemic arterial pressure *(bottom record)*. Mean pressure in the carotid sinuses *(horizontal line, top record)* is held constant when pulse pressure is damped.

of the atria during atrial filling (**B receptors**). Stimulation of these atrial receptors sends impulses up vagal fibers to the vagal center in the medulla. Consequently, the sympathetic activity is decreased to the kidney and increased to the sinus node. These changes in sympathetic activity increase renal blood flow, urine flow, and heart rate (see also Chapter 17).

Activation of the cardiopulmonary receptors can also initiate a reflex that lowers arterial blood pressure by inhibiting the vasoconstrictor center in the cerebral medulla. Stimulation of the cardiopulmonary receptors inhibits angiotensin, aldosterone, and vasopressin (antidiuretic hormone) release; interruption of the reflex pathway has the opposite effects.

The role that activation of these baroreceptors plays in the regulation of blood volume is apparent in the body's responses to hemorrhage. The reduction in blood volume (hypovolemia) enhances sympathetic vasoconstriction in the kidney and increases the secretion of renin, angiotensin, aldosterone, and antidiuretic hormone (see also Chapter 24). The renal vasoconstriction (primarily afferent arterioles) reduces glomerular filtration and increases renin release from the kidney. Renin acts on a plasma substrate to yield angiotensin, which releases aldosterone from the adrenal cortex. The enhanced release of antidiuretic hormone increases water reabsorption and the release of aldosterone increases sodium and water reabsorption. The results are retention of salt and water by the kidney, and hence the blood volume increases. Angiotensin II (formed from antiotensin I by the converting enzyme) also raises systemic arteriolar tone.

Peripheral chemoreceptors. These chemoreceptors consist of small, highly vascular bodies in the region of the aortic arch (**aortic bodies,** Fig. 21-9) and just medial to the carotid sinuses (**carotid bodies,** Fig. 21-8). These vascular bodies are sensitive to changes in the Po_2, Pco_2, and pH of the blood. Although they are primarily involved in the regulation of respiration, they also influence the vasomotor regions. A reduction in arterial blood O_2 tension (Pao_2) stimulates the chemoreceptors. The increased activity in the afferent nerve fibers from the carotid and aortic bodies stimulates the vasoconstrictor regions, and and thereby increases the tone of the resistance and capacitance vessels.

The chemoreceptors are also stimulated by increased arterial blood CO_2 tension ($Paco_2$) and by reduced pH. However, the reflex effect is small compared with the direct effects of hypercapnia (high $Paco_2$) and of acidosis on the vasomotor regions in the medulla. When hypoxia and hypercapnia occur simultaneously, the effects of the chemoreceptors are greater than the sum of the effects of each of the two stimuli when they act alone. The effects of hypoxia plus hypercapnia on blood pressure, heart rate, and respiration are shown in Fig. 21-12 (see also Chapters 17 and 29).

Chemoreceptors are also located in the heart. These cardiac chemoreceptors are activated by ischemia of the cardiac muscle, and they transmit the precordial pain (**angina pectoris**) associated with an inadequate blood supply to the myocardium.

Hypothalamus. Optimal function of the cardiovascular reflexes requires the integrity of the pontine and hypothalamic structures. Furthermore, these structures are responsible for behavioral and emotional control of the cardiovascular system (see also Chapter 11). Stimulation of the anterior hypothalamus produces a drop in blood pressure and bradycardia, whereas stimulation of the posterolateral region of the hypothalamus increases blood pressure and heart rate. The hypothalamus also contains a temperature-regulating center that affects the blood vessels in the skin. Stimulation by cold applications to the skin or by cooling of the blood perfusing the hypothalamus results in constriction of the skin vessels and in heat conservation, whereas warm stimuli

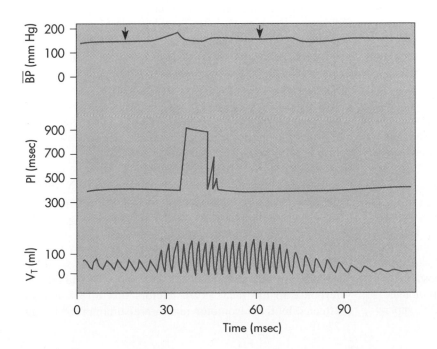

■ **Fig. 21-12**   Effects of stimulation of the isolated perfused carotid body chemoreceptors at constant carotid sinus perfusion pressure, by substituting hypoxic blood (Po_2, 31.1 mm Hg; Pco_2, 84.9 mm Hg; pH, 7.242) for arterial blood (Po_2, 140.4 mm Hg; Pco_2, 42.1 mm Hg; pH, 7.33) between arrows. Note that the bradycardia was transient. The enhanced respiratory response abolishes bradycardia and can produce tachycardia, especially with sustained stimulation of the carotid body receptors (see Figs. 17-14 and 17-15). The increase in pulse interval *(PI)* indicates a decrease in heart rate. $\overline{BP}$, Mean arterial blood pressure; V_T, tidal volume. (Redrawn from Daly MdeB, Kouner PI, Angell-James JE, Oliver JA: *Clin Exp Pharmacol Physiol* 5:511, 1978.)

to the skin result in cutaneous vasodilation and enhanced heat loss.

When subjects are exposed to high altitudes, the low Pa_{O_2} stimulates the peripheral chemoreceptors to increase the rate and depth of respiration. This is the main mechanism involved in an attempt to restore the oxygen supply to the body (see also Chapter 29).

Cerebrum. The cerebral cortex can also affect the blood flow distribution in the body. Stimulation of the motor and premotor areas can affect blood pressure; usually a pressor response is obtained. However, vasodilation and depressor responses may be evoked, as in blushing or fainting, in response to an emotional stimulus.

Skin and viscera. Painful stimuli can elicit either pressor or depressor responses, depending on the magnitude and location of the stimulus. Distention of the viscera often evokes a depressor response, whereas painful stimuli on the body surface usually evoke a pressor response.

Pulmonary reflexes. Inflation of the lungs initiates a reflex that induces systemic vasodilation and a decrease in arterial blood pressure. Conversely, collapse of the lungs evokes systemic vasoconstriction. Afferent fibers that mediate this reflex run in the vagus nerves and possibly also in the sympathetic nerves. Their stimulation by stretch of the lungs inhibits the vasomotor areas. The magnitude of the depressor response to lung inflation is directly related to the degree of inflation and to the existing level of vasoconstrictor tone (see also Chapter 17).

Central chemoreceptors. Increases in Pa_{CO_2} stimulate chemosensitive regions of the medulla (the central chemoreceptors), and they elicit vasoconstriction and increased peripheral resistance. Reduction in Pa_{CO_2} below normal levels (in response to hyperventilation) decreases the tonic activity in these areas in the medulla and thereby decreases peripheral resistance. The chemosensitive regions are also affected by changes in pH. A lowering of blood pH stimulates, and a rise in blood pH inhibits, these cerebral areas. These effects of changes in Pa_{CO_2} and in blood pH may operate through changes in cerebrospinal fluid pH, as may also the respiratory center.

Oxygen tension has little direct effect on the medullary vasomotor region. The primary effect of hypoxia is mediated by reflexes via the carotid and aortic chemoreceptors. Moderate reduction of Pa_{O_2} stimulates the vasomotor region, but severe reduction depresses vasomotor activity in the same manner by which other areas of the brain are depressed by very low O_2 tensions.

Cerebral ischemia, which may occur because of excessive pressure exerted by an expanding intracranial tumor, results in a marked increase in peripheral vasoconstriction. The stimulation is probably caused by a local accumulation of CO_2 and a reduction of O_2, and possibly by excitation of intracranial baroreceptors. With prolonged, severe ischemia, central depression eventually supervenes, and blood pressure falls.

BALANCE BETWEEN EXTRINSIC AND INTRINSIC FACTORS IN REGULATION OF PERIPHERAL BLOOD FLOW

Dual control of the peripheral vessels by intrinsic and extrinsic mechanisms evokes a number of important vascular adjustments. Such regulatory mechanisms enable the body to direct blood flow to the areas where it is most needed and away from the areas that have fewer requirements. In some tissues, the effects of the extrinsic and intrinsic mechanisms are fixed; in other tissues, the ratio is changeable, and it depends on the state of activity of that tissue.

In the brain and heart, which are vital structures with a limited tolerance for a reduced blood supply, intrinsic flow-regulating mechanisms are dominant. For instance, massive discharge of the vasoconstrictor region via the sympathetic nerves, which might occur in severe, acute hemorrhage, has negligible effects on the cerebral and cardiac resistance vessels, whereas the cutaneous, renal, and splanchnic blood vessels become greatly constricted (see also Chapter 17).

In the skin, the extrinsic vascular control is dominant. Not only do the cutaneous vessels participate strongly in a general vasoconstrictor discharge, but they also respond selectively through hypothalamic pathways to subserve the heat loss and heat conservation functions required in body temperature regulation. However, intrinsic control can be demonstrated by local temperature changes that can modify or override the central influence on resistance and capacitance vessels (see also Chapter 16).

In skeletal muscle, the extrinsic and intrinsic mechanisms interact. In resting skeletal muscle, neural control (vasoconstrictor tone) is dominant, as can be demonstrated by the large increase in blood flow that occurs immediately after section of the sympathetic nerves to the tissue. At the start of physical exercise, such as running, blood flow increases in the leg muscles. After the onset of exercise, the intrinsic flow-regulating mechanism assumes control, and vasodilation occurs in the active muscles because of the local increase in metabolites. Vasoconstriction occurs in the inactive tissues, as a manifestation of the general sympathetic discharge. However, constrictor impulses that reach the resistance vessels of the active muscles are overridden by the local metabolic effect. Operation of this dual control mechanism thus provides increased blood flow where it is required and shunts it away from relatively inactive areas (see also Chapter 16). Similar effects may be achieved in response to an increase in Pa_{CO_2}. Normally, the hyperventilation associated with exercise keeps Pa_{CO_2} at normal levels. However, were Pa_{CO_2} to increase, a generalized vasoconstriction would occur, because of stimulation of the medullary vasoconstrictor region by CO_2. In the active muscles, where the CO_2 concentration would be highest, the smooth muscle of the arterioles would relax in response to the local P_{CO_2}. Factors that affect and are affected by the vasomotor region are summarized in Fig. 21-13.

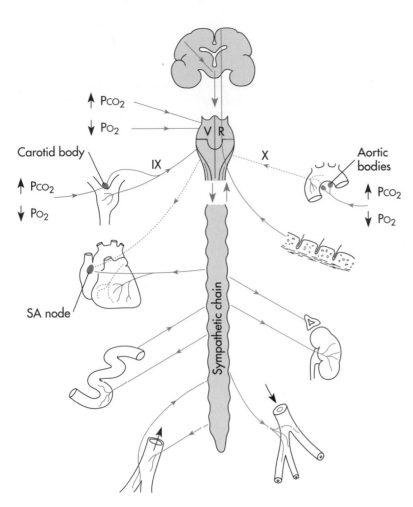

■ **Fig. 21-13** Schematic diagram illustrating the neural input and output of the vasomotor region *(SR)*. *IX,* Glossopharyngeal nerve; *X,* vagus nerve.

SUMMARY

1. The arterioles (resistance vessels) mainly regulate blood flow through their downstream capillaries. The smooth muscle, which makes up most of the walls of the arterioles, contracts and relaxes in response to neural and humoral stimuli.

2. Autoregulation of blood flow occurs in most tissues. This process is characterized by a constant blood flow in the face of a change in perfusion pressure. A logical explanation of autoregulation is the myogenic mechanism, whereby an increase in transmural pressure elicits a contraction of the vascular smooth muscle and a decrease in transmural pressure elicits a relaxation.

3. The striking parallelism between tissue blood flow and tissue oxygen consumption indicates that blood flow is regulated largely by a metabolic mechanism. A decrease in the oxygen supply to oxygen demand ratio of a tissue releases a vasodilator metabolite that dilates arterioles and thereby enhances the oxygen supply.

4. Neural regulation of blood flow is almost completely accomplished by the sympathetic nervous system. Sympathetic nerves to blood vessels are tonically active; inhibition of the vasoconstrictor center in the medulla reduces peripheral vascular resistance. Stimulation of the sympathetic nerves constricts the resistance and capacitance (veins) vessels.

5. Parasympathetic fibers innervate the head, viscera, and genitalia; they do not innervate the skin and muscle.

6. The baroreceptors in the internal carotid arteries and aorta are tonically active and regulate blood pressure on a moment-to-moment basis. Stretch of these receptors by an increase in arterial pressure initiates a reflex that inhibits the vasoconstrictor center in the medulla and induces vasodilation. Conversely, a decrease in arterial pressure disinhibits the vasoconstrictor center and induces vasoconstriction.

7. The baroreceptors in the internal carotid arteries predominate over those in the aorta, and they respond more vigorously to changes in pressure (stretch) than they do to elevated or reduced nonpulsatile pressures. In other words, they adapt to an imposed constant pressure.

8. Cardiopulmonary baroreceptors are also present in the cardiac chambers and large pulmonary vessels. They have less influence on blood pressure but participate in blood volume regulation.

9. Peripheral chemoreceptors (carotid and aortic bodies) and central chemoreceptors in the medulla oblongata are stimulated by a decrease in blood oxygen tension (Pa_{O_2}) and by an increase in blood carbon dioxide tension (Pa_{CO_2}). Stimulation of these chemoreceptors increases the rate and depth of respiration, but it also produces peripheral vasoconstriction.

10. Peripheral resistance, and hence blood pressure, are affected by stimuli that arise in the skin, viscera, lungs, and brain.

11. The combined effect of neural and local metabolic factors distributes blood to active tissues and diverts it from inactive tissues. In vital structures, such as in the heart and brain and in contracting skeletal muscle, the metabolic factors predominate.

BIBLIOGRAPHY

Journal articles

Berg BR, Cohen JD, Sarelius IH: Direct coupling between blood flow and metabolism at the capillary level in striated muscle, *Am J Physiol* 272:H2693, 1997.

Cowley AW Jr: Long-term control of blood pressure, *Physiol Rev* 72:231, 1992.

Ellsworth ML et al: The erythrocyte as a regulator of vascular tone, *Am J Physiol* 269:H2155, 1995.

Hainsworth R: Reflexes from the heart, *Physiol Rev* 71:617, 1991.

Hickner RC et al: Role of nitric oxide in skeletal muscle blood flow at rest and during dynamic exercise in humans, *Am J Physiol* 273:H405, 1997.

Hirst GDS, Edwards FR: Sympathetic neuroeffector transmission in arteries and arterioles, *Physiol Rev* 69:546, 1989.

Kuo L, Davis JJ, Chilian WM: Endothelium-dependent flow-induced dilation of isolated coronary arterioles, *Am J Physiol* 259:H1063, 1990.

Marshall JM: Peripheral chemoreceptors and cardiovascular regulation, *Physiol Rev* 74:543, 1994.

Monos E, Berczi V, Nadasy G: Local control of veins: biomechanical, metabolic, and humoral aspects, *Physiol Rev* 75:611, 1995.

Persson PB: Modulation of cardiovascular control mechanisms and their interaction, *Physiol Rev* 76:193, 1996.

Shen Y-T et al: Relative roles of cardiac receptors and arterial baroreceptors during hemorrhage in conscious dogs, *Circ Res* 66:397, 1990.

Sun D et al: Enhanced release of prostaglandins to flow-induced arteriolar dilation in eNOS knockout mice, *Circ Res* 85:288, 1999.

chapter twenty-two

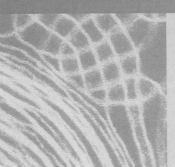

Control of Cardiac Output: Coupling of Heart and Blood Vessels

Four factors control cardiac output: heart rate, myocardial contractility, preload, and afterload (Fig. 22-1). Heart rate and myocardial contractility are strictly **cardiac factors;** that is, these factors originate in the cardiac tissues, although they are controlled by various neural and humoral mechanisms. Preload and afterload, however, are factors that are mutually dependent on the behavior of the heart and the vasculature. On the one hand, preload and afterload are important *determinants of* cardiac output. On the other hand, preload and afterload are themselves *determined by* the cardiac output and by certain vascular characteristics. Because these factors constitute a functional coupling between the heart and blood vessels, preload and afterload will be called **coupling factors.**

To understand the regulation of cardiac output, therefore, the nature of the coupling between the heart and the vascular system must be appreciated. In this chapter, we use two kinds of graphs to analyze the interactions between the cardiac and vascular components of the circulatory system. These graphs represent two important functional relationships between **cardiac output** and **central venous pressure** (i.e., the pressure in the right atrium and thoracic venae cavae).

The curve that defines one of these relationships is called the **cardiac function curve.** It is an expression of the well-known **Frank-Starling relationship** and it illustrates the dependence of cardiac output on preload (i.e., the central venous, or right atrial, pressure). The cardiac function curve is a characteristic of the heart itself; in fact, it is usually studied in hearts completely isolated from the rest of the circulatory system. This curve has already been discussed in detail in Chapters 16 and 17. We use this curve later in this chapter in association with the other characteristic curve in order to analyze the interactions between the heart and the vasculature.

The second curve, called the **vascular function curve,** defines the dependence of central venous pressure on cardiac output. This relationship depends only on certain vascular system characteristics, namely, the peripheral vascular resistance, the arterial and venous compliances, and the blood volume. The vascular function curve is entirely independent of the characteristics of the heart. Because of this independence, it can be derived experimentally even if the heart is replaced by a mechanical pump.

VASCULAR FUNCTION CURVE

The vascular function curve defines the changes in central venous pressure that are caused by changes in cardiac output. In this curve, the central venous pressure is the **dependent variable** (or **response**), and cardiac output is the **independent variable** (or **stimulus**). These variables are opposite to those of the cardiac function curve, in which the central venous pressure (or preload) is the **independent variable** and the cardiac output is the **dependent variable.**

The simplified model of the circulation illustrated in Fig. 22-2 helps explain how the cardiac output determines the level of central venous pressure. In this simplified model, all the essential components of the cardiovascular system have been lumped into four basic elements. The right and left sides of the heart, as well as the pulmonary vascular bed, constitute a **pump-oxygenator,** much like the artificial heart-lung machine that is used to perfuse the body during open heart surgery. The high-resistance microcirculation is designated the **peripheral resistance.** Finally, the compliance of the system is subdivided into two components, the **arterial compliance, C_a,** and the **venous compliance, C_v.** As defined in Chapter 19, the compliance (C) of a blood vessel is the increase in volume (ΔV) that is accommodated in that vessel per unit change of transmural pressure (ΔP); that is,

$$C \equiv \Delta V/\Delta P \qquad (22\text{-}1)$$

The venous compliance is about 20 times greater than the arterial compliance. In the example that follows, the ratio of C_v to C_a is set at 19:1 to simplify the calculations. Thus, if it were necessary to add x ml of blood to the arterial system to produce a 1 mm Hg increase in arterial pressure, then $19x$ ml

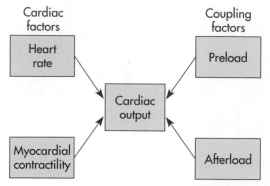

Fig. 22-1 The four factors that determine cardiac output.

of blood would need to be added to the venous system to raise the venous pressure by the same amount.

To show why a change in cardiac output causes an inverse change in central venous pressure, let us first endow our hypothetical model with certain characteristics that mimic those of an average adult person (Fig. 22-2, *A*). Therefore, the flow (Q_h) generated by the heart (i.e., the cardiac output) will be 5 L/min; the mean arterial pressure, P_a, will be 102 mm Hg; and the central venous pressure, P_v, will be 2 mm Hg. The peripheral resistance, R, is the ratio of arteriovenous pressure difference ($P_a - P_v$) to flow (Q_r) through the resistance vessels; this ratio will equal 20 mm Hg/L/min.

An arteriovenous pressure difference of 100 mm Hg is sufficient to force a flow (Q_r) of 5 L/min through a peripheral resistance of 20 mm Hg/L/min (Fig. 22-2, *A*). Under equilibrium conditions, this flow (Q_r) is precisely equal to the flow (Q_h) pumped by the heart. From heartbeat to heartbeat the volume (V_a) of blood in the arteries and the volume (V_v) of blood in the veins remain constant, because the volume of blood transferred from the veins to the arteries by the heart equals the volume of blood that flows from the arteries through the resistance vessels and into the veins.

Effects of Cardiac Arrest on Arterial and Venous Pressures

Figure 22-2, *B*, illustrates the status of the circulation at the very beginning of an episode of cardiac arrest; that is, $Q_h = 0$. In the instant immediately after the arrest of the heart, the volumes of blood in the arteries (V_a) and veins (V_v) have not had time to change appreciably. Because the arterial and venous pressures depend on V_a and V_v, respectively, these pressures are identical to the respective pressures in Fig. 22-2, *A* (i.e., $P_a = 102$ and $P_v = 2$). This arteriovenous pressure gradient of 100 mm Hg forces a flow (Q_r) of 5 L/min through the peripheral resistance of 20 mm Hg/L/min. Thus, although cardiac output (Q_h) now equals 0 L/min, the flow through the microcirculation equals 5 L/min. In other words, the potential energy stored in the arteries by the preceding pumping action of the heart causes blood to be transferred from arteries to veins. This transfer occurs initially at the control rate, even though the heart can no longer transfer blood from the veins into the arteries.

As time passes and the heart continues in arrest, the blood flow through the resistance vessels causes the blood volume in the arteries to decrease progressively and the blood volume in the veins to increase progressively at the same absolute rate. Because the arteries and veins are elastic structures, the arterial pressure falls gradually and the venous pressure rises gradually. This process continues until the arterial and venous pressures become equal (Fig. 22-2, *C*). Once this condition is reached, the flow (Q_r) from the arteries to the veins through the resistance vessels is zero, as is the cardiac output (Q_h).

When the effects of cardiac arrest reach this state of equilibrium (Fig. 22-2, *C*), the pressure attained in the arteries and veins depends on the relative compliances of these vessels. If the arterial (C_a) and venous (C_v) compliances are equal, the decline in P_a would equal the rise in P_v, because the decrease in arterial volume would equal the increase in venous volume (principle of conservation of mass). Both P_a and P_v would attain the average of their combined values in Fig. 22-2, *A*; that is, $P_a = P_v = (102 + 2)/2 = 52$ mm Hg.

However, C_a and C_v in a living subject are *not* equal. The veins are much more compliant than are the arteries; the compliance ratio ($C_v:C_a$) is approximately 19, which is the ratio that we have assumed for the model. Consequently, when the effects of cardiac arrest reach equilibrium in an intact subject, the pressure in the arteries and veins is much less than the average value of 52 mm Hg that occurs when C_a and C_v compliances are equal. Hence, the transfer of blood from arteries to veins at equilibrium induces a fall in arterial pressure 19 times greater than the concomitant rise in venous pressure. As Fig. 22-2, *C*, shows, P_v would increase by 5 mm Hg (to 7 mm Hg), whereas P_a would fall by $19 \times 5 = 95$ mm Hg (to 7 mm Hg). This equilibrium pressure, which prevails in the circulatory system in the absence of flow, is referred to as either the **mean circulatory pressure** or the **static pressure.** The pressure in the static system reflects the total volume of blood in the system and the overall compliance of the system.

We have used the example of cardiac arrest to facilitate an understanding of the vascular function curve. We can now begin to assemble a vascular function curve (Fig. 22-3). As stated previously, the independent variable (plotted along the abscissa) is the cardiac output, and the dependent variable (plotted along the ordinate) is the central venous pressure. Two important points on this curve can be derived from the example illustrated in Fig. 22-2. One point (*A* in Fig. 22-3) represents the control state; that is, when cardiac output is 5 L/min, P_v is 2 mm Hg (as depicted in Fig. 22-2, *A*). Then, when the heart is arrested (cardiac output = 0), P_v becomes 7 mm Hg at equilibrium (Fig. 22- 2, *C*); this pressure is the mean circulatory pressure (P_{mc} in Fig. 22-3).

The inverse relation between P_v and cardiac output simply denotes that when cardiac output is suddenly decreased, the rate at which blood flows from arteries to veins through the capillaries is temporarily greater than the rate at which the heart pumps the blood from the veins back into the arteries. During that transient period, a net volume of

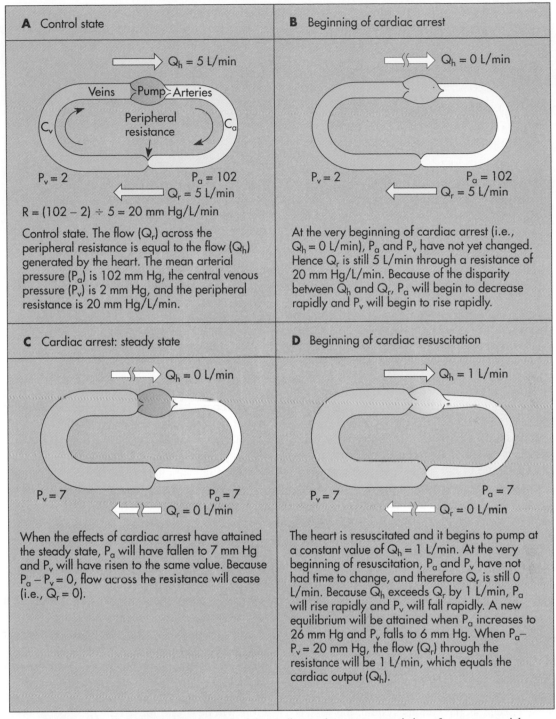

A   Control state

$Q_h = 5$ L/min

Veins — Pump — Arteries

Peripheral resistance

C_v C_a

$P_v = 2$ $P_a = 102$

$Q_r = 5$ L/min

$R = (102 - 2) \div 5 = 20$ mm Hg/L/min

Control state. The flow (Q_r) across the peripheral resistance is equal to the flow (Q_h) generated by the heart. The mean arterial pressure (P_a) is 102 mm Hg, the central venous pressure (P_v) is 2 mm Hg, and the peripheral resistance is 20 mm Hg/L/min.

B   Beginning of cardiac arrest

$Q_h = 0$ L/min

$P_v = 2$ $P_a = 102$

$Q_r = 5$ L/min

At the very beginning of cardiac arrest (i.e., $Q_h = 0$ L/min), P_a and P_v have not yet changed. Hence Q_r is still 5 L/min through a resistance of 20 mm Hg/L/min. Because of the disparity between Q_h and Q_r, P_a will begin to decrease rapidly and P_v will begin to rise rapidly.

C   Cardiac arrest: steady state

$Q_h = 0$ L/min

$P_v = 7$ $P_a = 7$

$Q_r = 0$ L/min

When the effects of cardiac arrest have attained the steady state, P_a will have fallen to 7 mm Hg and P_v will have risen to the same value. Because $P_a - P_v = 0$, flow across the resistance will cease (i.e., $Q_r = 0$).

D   Beginning of cardiac resuscitation

$Q_h = 1$ L/min

$P_v = 7$ $P_a = 7$

$Q_r = 0$ L/min

The heart is resuscitated and it begins to pump at a constant value of $Q_h = 1$ L/min. At the very beginning of resuscitation, P_a and P_v have not had time to change, and therefore Q_r is still 0 L/min. Because Q_h exceeds Q_r by 1 L/min, P_a will rise rapidly and P_v will fall rapidly. A new equilibrium will be attained when P_a increases to 26 mm Hg and P_v falls to 6 mm Hg. When $P_a - P_v = 20$ mm Hg, the flow (Q_r) through the resistance will be 1 L/min, which equals the cardiac output (Q_h).

■ **Fig. 22-2**   **A** to **D**, Simplified model of the cardiovascular system, consisting of a pump, arterial compliance (C_a), peripheral resistance, and venous compliance (C_v).

blood is transferred from arteries to veins; hence, P_a falls and P_v rises.

Now, let us see what happens when cardiac output is suddenly increased. This example will illustrate how a third point (*B* in Fig. 22-3) on the vascular function curve is derived. Consider that the arrested heart is suddenly restarted and immediately begins pumping blood from the veins into the arteries at a rate of 1 L/min (Fig. 22-2, *D*). When the heart

first begins to beat, the arteriovenous pressure gradient is zero, and hence no blood is transferred from the arteries through the capillaries and into the veins. Thus, when beating resumes, blood is depleted from the veins at the rate of 1 L/min, and the arterial blood volume is repleted from the venous blood volume at that same absolute rate. Hence, P_v begins to fall and P_a begins to rise. Because of the difference in arterial and venous compliances, P_a

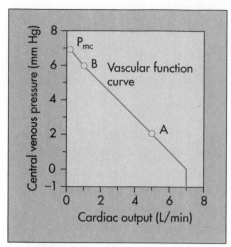

■ **Fig. 22-3** Changes in central venous pressure produced by changes in cardiac output. The mean circulatory pressure (or static pressure), P_{mc}, is the equilibrium pressure throughout the cardiovascular system when cardiac output is 0. Points *B* and *A* represent the values of venous pressure at cardiac outputs of 1 and 5 L/min, respectively.

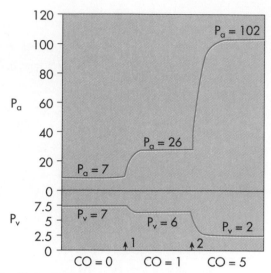

■ **Fig. 22-4** The changes in arterial *(P_a)* and venous *(P_v)* pressures in the circulatory model shown in Fig. 22-3. The total peripheral resistance is 20 mm Hg/L/min, and the ratio of C_v to C_a is 19:1. The cardiac output (CO) is 0 to the left of arrow *1*. It is increased to 1 L/min at arrow *1* and to 5 L/min at arrow *2*.

will rise at a rate 19 times greater than the rate at which Pv will fall.

The resultant arteriovenous pressure gradient causes blood to flow through the peripheral resistance. If the heart maintains a constant output of 1 L/min, P_a will continue to rise and P_v will continue to fall until the pressure gradient becomes 20 mm Hg. This gradient will force a flow of 1 L/min through a resistance of 20 mm Hg/L/min. This gradient will be achieved by a 19 mm Hg rise (to 26 mm Hg) in P_a and a 1 mm Hg fall (to 6 mm Hg) in P_v. This equilibrium value of $P_v = 6$ mm Hg for a cardiac output of 1 L/min also appears on the vascular function curve of Fig. 22-3 (point *B*). The 1 mm Hg reduction in P_v reflects a net transfer of blood from the venous to the arterial side of the circuit.

The reduction of P_v that can be evoked by a sudden increase in cardiac output is limited. At some critical maximal value of cardiac output, sufficient fluid will be transferred from the venous to the arterial side of the circuit for P_v to fall below the ambient pressure. In a system of very distensible vessels, such as the venous system, the vessels will be collapsed by the greater external pressure. This venous collapse acts as an impediment to venous return to the heart. Hence, it limits the maximal value of cardiac output to 7 L/min in this example (Fig. 22-3), regardless of the capabilities of the pump. For readers interested in the mathematical derivation of these results, the basic equations are presented here.

Mathematical Analysis of the Vascular Function Curve
The definition of peripheral resistance is

$$R \equiv (P_a - P_v)/Q_r, \qquad (22\text{-}2)$$

where R is peripheral resistance, P_a is arterial pressure, P_v is venous pressure, and Q_r is blood flow through the resistance vessels (see page 360). At equilibrium, Q_r equals cardiac output, Q_h. Assume that R = 20, and that Q_r had been increased from 0 to a constant value of 1 L/min (Fig. 22-4, arrow *1*). If we solve equation 22-2 for the value of P_a when the system has reached equilibrium (i.e., $Q_r = Q_h$):

$$P_a = P_v + Q_r R = P_v + (1 \times 20) \qquad (22\text{-}3)$$

Thus, P_a will increase to a value 20 mm Hg greater than P_v. It will continue to be 20 mm Hg above P_v as long as the pump output is maintained at 1 L/min and the peripheral resistance remains at 20 mm Hg/L/min.

We can calculate what the actual changes in P_a and P_v will be when Q_h attains a constant value of 1 L/min. The arterial volume increase needed to achieve the required level of P_a depends entirely on the arterial compliance C_a. For a rigid arterial system (low compliance), this volume will be small; for a very distensible system (like the human vascular system), the volume will be large. Whatever the magnitude, however, the change in volume represents the transfer of some quantity of blood from the venous to the arterial side of the circuit.

For a given total blood volume, any increase in arterial volume (ΔV_a) must equal the decrease in venous volume (ΔV_v); that is,

$$\Delta V_a = -\Delta V_v \qquad (22\text{-}4)$$

From the general definition of compliance,

$$C_a = \Delta V_a/\Delta P_a, \text{ and } C_v = \Delta V_v/\Delta P_v \qquad (22\text{-}5)$$

By solving equation 22-5 for ΔV_a and ΔV_v, and substituting the results into equation 22-4:

$$\Delta P_v / \Delta P_a = -C_a / C_v \qquad (22\text{-}6)$$

Given that C_v is 19 times greater than C_a, then the increment in P_a will be 19 times greater than the decrement in P_v; that is,

$$\Delta P_a = -19\ \Delta P_v \qquad (22\text{-}7)$$

To calculate the absolute values of P_a and P_v, let ΔP_a represent the difference between the prevailing P_a and the mean circulatory pressure (P_{mc}); that is, let

$$\Delta P_a = P_a - P_{mc} \qquad (22\text{-}8)$$

and let ΔP_v represent the difference between the prevailing P_v and the mean circulatory pressure:

$$\Delta P_v = P_v - P_{mc} \qquad (22\text{-}9)$$

Substituting these values for ΔP_a and ΔP_v into equation 22-7,

$$P_a - P_{mc} = -19(P_v - P_{mc}) \qquad (22\text{-}10)$$

By solving equations 22-3 and 22-10 simultaneously:

$$P_a = P_{mc} + 19, \text{ and } P_v = P_{mc} - 1 \qquad (22\text{-}11)$$

Hence, if the mean circulatory pressure equals 7 mm Hg, P_a increases to 26 mm Hg and P_v decreases to 6 mm Hg when Q_h increases from 0 to 1 L/min (Fig. 22-4). These pressure changes provide the required arteriovenous pressure gradient of 20 mm Hg.

If the pump output is abruptly increased to a constant level of 5 L/min (Fig. 22-4, arrow *2*) and peripheral resistance remains constant at 20 mm Hg/L/min, an additional volume of blood again will be transferred from the venous to the arterial side of the circuit. It will progressively accumulate in the arteries until P_a reaches a level of 100 mm Hg above P_v, as shown by substitution into equation 22-3:

$$P_a = P_v + Q_r R = P_v + (5 \times 20) \qquad (22\text{-}12)$$

By solving equations 22-10 and 22-12 simultaneously, we find that when the pump output is increased to 5 L/min, P_a rises to a value of 95 mm Hg above P_{mc}, and P_v falls to a value 5 mm Hg below P_{mc}. In Fig. 22-4, therefore, P_v declines to 2 mm Hg and P_a rises to 102 mm Hg. The resultant pressure gradient of 100 mm Hg will force a cardiac output of 5 L/min through a constant peripheral resistance of 20 mm Hg/L/min.

The following equation for the vascular function curve (P_v as a function of Q_r) in the model is derived from equations 22-2, 22-6, 22-8, and 22-9:

$$P_v = -[RC_a / (C_a + C_v)]\ Q_r + P_{mc} \qquad (22\text{-}13)$$

Note that the slope of the vascular function curve depends only on R, C_a, and C_v. Note also that when $Q_r = 0$, $P_v = P_{mc}$; that is, when flow is zero, P_v (and P_a) equal the mean circulatory pressure.

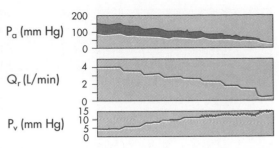

■ **Fig. 22-5** The changes in arterial *(P_a)* and central venous *(P_v)* pressures produced by changes in systemic blood flow *(Q_r)* in a canine right-heart bypass preparation. Stepwise changes in Q_r were produced by altering the rate of a mechanical pump. (From Levy MN: *Circ Res* 44:739, 1979.)

Factors That Influence the Vascular Function Curve

Venous pressure dependence on cardiac output. Experimental and clinical observations have shown that changes in cardiac output do indeed evoke the alterations in P_a and P_v that have been predicted by our simplified model. In an experiment on an anesthetized dog, a mechanical pump was substituted for the right ventricle (Fig. 22-5). As the pump output, Q, was decreased gradually in a series of small steps, P_a fell and P_v rose progressively. The changes in P_a and P_v evoked by the alterations in blood flow in this experiment resemble those derived from our simplified model (Fig. 22-4).

Similarly, cardiac output may decrease abruptly when a major coronary artery suddenly becomes occluded in a human patient. The **acute heart failure** that occurs as a result of **myocardial infarction** (death of myocardial tissue) is usually accompanied by a fall in arterial blood pressure and a rise in central venous pressure.

Blood volume. The vascular function curve is affected by variations in total blood volume. During circulatory standstill (zero cardiac output, such as occurs during cardiac arrest), the mean circulatory pressure depends only on total vascular compliance and blood volume, as stated previously. Thus, for a given vascular compliance, the mean circulatory pressure is increased when blood volume is expanded **(hypervolemia)** and is decreased when blood volume is diminished **(hypovolemia).** This relationship is illustrated by the Y-axis intercepts in Fig. 22-6, where the mean circulatory pressure is 5 mm Hg after hemorrhage and 9 mm Hg after transfusion, as compared with the value of 7 mm Hg at normal blood volume **(normovolemia).**

Furthermore, the differences in P_v during hypervolemia, normovolemia, and hypovolemia in the static system are preserved at each level of cardiac output. As a result, the vascular function curves parallel each other (Fig. 22-6). To illustrate, consider the example of hypervolemia, in which the mean circulatory pressure is 9 mm Hg. In Fig.

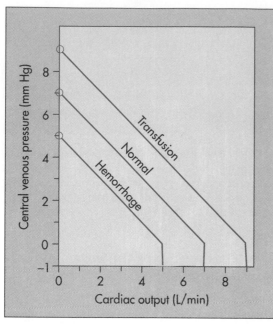

■ **Fig. 22-6** Effects of increased blood volume *(transfusion curve)* and of decreased blood volume *(hemorrhage curve)* on the vascular function curve. Similar shifts in the vascular function curve can be produced by increases and decreases, respectively, in venomotor tone.

22-6, both P_a and P_v would be 9 mm Hg, instead of 7 mm Hg, when the cardiac output is zero. If the peripheral resistance is 20 mm Hg/L/min, and if cardiac output is suddenly increased to 1 L/min (e.g., at arrow 1 in Fig. 22-4), an arteriovenous pressure gradient of 20 mm Hg is still necessary for 1 L/min to flow through the resistance vessels. This condition does not differ from the example for normovolemia. If we assume the same ratio of C_v to C_a (19:1), the pressure gradient would be achieved by a 1 mm Hg decline in Pv and a 19 mm Hg rise in P_a. Hence, a change in cardiac output from 0 to 1 L/min would evoke the same 1 mm Hg reduction in P_v irrespective of the blood volume, as long as C_a, C_v, and peripheral resistance were independent of blood volume. Equation 22-13 also shows that the slope of the vascular function curve remains constant as long as C_a, C_v, and R do not change.

From Fig. 22-6, it is also apparent that the cardiac output at which $P_v = 0$ varies directly with the blood volume. Therefore, the maximal value of cardiac output becomes progressively more limited as the total blood volume is reduced. However, the central venous pressure at which the veins collapse (illustrated by the sharp change in slope of the vascular function curve) is not significantly altered by changes in blood volume. This pressure depends only on the ambient pressure surrounding the central veins. The ambient pressure is the pleural pressure in the thorax (see Chapter 26).

Venomotor tone. The effects of changes in venomotor tone on the vascular function curve closely resemble those for changes in blood volume. In Fig. 22-6, for example, the

transfusion curve could just as well represent increased venomotor tone, whereas the hemorrhage curve could represent decreased tone. During circulatory standstill, for a given blood volume, the pressure within the vascular system will rise as the tension exerted by the smooth muscle within the vascular walls increases (these contractile changes in the arteriolar and venous smooth muscle are under nervous and humoral control). The fraction of the blood volume located within the arterioles is very small, whereas the blood volume in the veins is large (see Fig. 14-2). Therefore, changes in peripheral resistance (arteriolar tone) will have no significant effect on the mean circulatory pressure, but changes in venous tone can alter the mean circulatory pressure appreciably. Hence, mean circulatory pressure rises with increased venomotor tone and falls with diminished venomotor tone.

Experimentally, the mean circulatory pressure attained about 1 minute after abrupt circulatory standstill is usually substantially above 7 mm Hg, even when blood volume is normal. This high pressure level is attributable to the generalized venoconstriction that is caused by cerebral ischemia, activation of the chemoreceptors, and reduced excitation of the baroreceptors. If resuscitation is not successful, this reflex response subsides as central nervous activity ceases, and the mean circulatory pressure usually falls to a value close to 7 mm Hg.

Blood reservoirs. Venoconstriction is considerably greater in certain regions of the body than in others. In effect, *vascular beds that undergo significant venoconstriction constitute blood reservoirs.* The vascular bed of the skin is one of the major blood reservoirs in humans. Blood loss evokes profound subcutaneous venoconstriction, which gives rise to the characteristically pale appearance of the skin in response to hemorrhage. The resultant diversion of blood away from the skin frees up several hundred milliliters of blood that can be perfused through more vital regions of the body. The vascular beds of the liver, lungs, and spleen are also important blood reservoirs. In the dog, the spleen is packed with red blood cells, and the spleen can constrict to a small fraction of its normal size. During hemorrhage, this mechanism autotransfuses blood of high erythrocyte content into the general circulation. In humans, however, the volume changes of the spleen are considerably less extensive (see also Chapter 24).

Peripheral resistance. The changes in the vascular function curve induced by changes in arteriolar tone are shown in Fig. 22-7. As noted, the amount of blood in the arterioles is small—they contain only about 3% of total blood volume (see Chapter 14). Hence, changes in the contractile state of these vessels do not significantly alter the mean circulatory pressure. Thus, vascular function curves that represent different peripheral resistances converge at a common point on the abscissa.

Equation 22-13 above indicates that P_v varies inversely with the total peripheral resistance (TPR) when all other factors remain constant. Physiologically, the relationship between P_v and TPR can be explained as follows: if cardiac output is held constant, a sudden increase in TPR causes a progressively greater volume of blood to be retained in the arterial system. Blood volume in the arterial system continues to increase until P_a rises sufficiently to force a flow of blood equal to the cardiac output through the resistance vessels. In the absence of any change in total blood volume, this increase in arterial blood volume is accompanied by an equivalent decrease in venous blood volume. Hence, an increase in TPR diminishes P_v. Furthermore, the reduction in P_v will be proportionate to the increment in TPR. This relationship between TPR and P_v, together with the inability of peripheral resistance to affect the mean circulatory pressure, accounts for the clockwise rotation of the vascular function curves in response to increased arteriolar constriction (Fig. 22-7). Similarly, arteriolar dilation produces a counterclockwise rotation from the same vertical axis intercept. A higher maximal level of cardiac output is attainable when the arterioles are dilated than when they are constricted (Fig. 22-7).

Interrelationships between cardiac output and venous return. Cardiac output and venous return are tightly linked. Except for small, transient disparities, the heart cannot pump any more blood than is delivered to it through the venous system. Similarly, because the circulatory system is a closed circuit, the venous return to the heart must equal the cardiac output over any appreciable time interval. The flow around the entire closed circuit depends on the capability of the pump, the characteristics of the circuit, and the total volume of fluid in the system.

Thus, we can assert that cardiac output and venous return are simply two terms for the flow around this closed circuit. Cardiac output is the volume of blood being pumped by the heart per unit time. Venous return is the volume of blood returning to the heart per unit time. At equilibrium, these two flows are equal. In the following section, we apply certain techniques of circuit analysis to gain some insight into the control of flow around the circuit.

RELATING THE CARDIAC FUNCTION CURVE TO THE VASCULAR FUNCTION CURVE
Coupling between the Heart and the Vasculature

In accordance with Starling's law of the heart, cardiac output depends closely on right atrial (or central venous) pressure. Furthermore, right atrial pressure is approximately equal to right ventricular end-diastolic pressure, because the normal tricuspid valve acts as a low-resistance junction between the right atrium and ventricle. In the discussion that follows, graphs of cardiac output as a function of central venous pressure (P_v) are called **cardiac function curves.** Extrinsic regulatory influences may be expressed as shifts in such curves, as indicated in Chapter 17.

A typical cardiac function curve is plotted on the same coordinates as a normal vascular function curve in Fig. 22-8. The cardiac function curve is plotted according to the usual convention; that is, the independent variable (P_v) is plotted along the abscissa, and the dependent variable (cardiac output) is plotted along the ordinate. In accordance with the

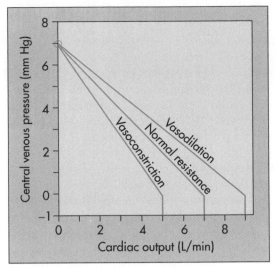

■ Fig. 22-7   Effects of arteriolar dilation and constriction on the vascular function curve.

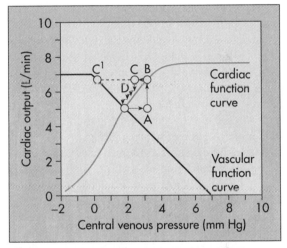

■ Fig. 22-8   Typical vascular and cardiac function curves plotted on the same coordinate axes. Note that to plot both curves on the same graph, the X and Y axes for the vascular function curves had to be reversed; compare the assignment of axes with that in Figs. 22-3, 22-6, and 22-7. The coordinates of the equilibrium point, at the intersection of the cardiac and vascular function curves, represent the stable values of cardiac output and central venous pressure at which the system tends to operate. Any perturbation (e.g., a sudden increase in venous pressure to point *A*) institutes a sequence of changes in cardiac output and venous pressure that restore these variables to their equilibrium values.

Frank-Starling mechanism, the cardiac function curve reveals that a rise in P_v increases the cardiac output.

Conversely, the vascular function curve describes an inverse relationship between cardiac output and P_v; that is, a rise in cardiac output diminishes P_v. P_v is the dependent variable (or response) and cardiac output is the independent variable (or stimulus) for the vascular function curve. Therefore, to plot a vascular function curve in the conventional manner, P_v should be scaled along the Y axis and cardiac output should be scaled along the X axis. Note that this convention is honored for the vascular function curves displayed in Figs. 22-3, 22-6, and 22-7.

To plot the cardiac and vascular function curves on the same set of axes requires a modification of the plotting convention for one of these curves. We have arbitrarily chosen to violate the convention for the vascular function curve. Note that the vascular function curve in Fig. 22-8 is intended to reflect how P_v (scaled along the X axis) varies in response to a change of cardiac output (scaled along the Y axis).

When the cardiovascular system is represented by a given pair of cardiac and vascular function curves, the intersection of these two curves defines the **equilibrium point** of that system. The coordinates of this equilibrium point represent the values of cardiac output and P_v at which the system tends to operate. Only transient deviations from such values of cardiac output and P_v are possible, as long as the given cardiac and vascular function curves accurately describe the system.

The tendency of the cardiovascular system to operate about this equilibrium point may best be illustrated by examining its response to a sudden perturbation. Consider the changes caused by a sudden rise in P_v from the equilibrium point to point A in Fig. 22-8. Such a change in P_v might be induced by the rapid injection, during ventricular diastole, of a given volume of blood on the venous side of the circuit, and the simultaneous withdrawal of an equal volume from the arterial side of the circuit. Thus, although P_v rises, the total blood volume remains constant.

As defined by the cardiac function curve, this elevated P_v would increase cardiac output (from A to B) during the next ventricular systole. The increased cardiac output in turn would transfer a net quantity of blood from the venous to the arterial side of the circuit, with a consequent reduction in P_v. In one heartbeat the reduction in P_v would be small (from B to C) because the heart would transfer only a tiny fraction of the total venous blood volume over to the arterial side. Because of this reduction in P_v, the cardiac output during the very next beat diminishes (from C to D) by an amount dictated by the cardiac function curve. Because D is still above the intersection point, the heart will pump blood from the veins to the arteries at a rate greater than that at which the blood will flow across the peripheral resistance from arteries to veins. Hence, P_v will continue to fall. This process will continue in diminishing steps until the point of intersection is reached. Only one specific combination of cardiac output and venous pressure—the equilibrium point, denoted by the coordinates of the point of the curves' intersection—will satisfy simultaneously the requirements of the cardiac and vascular function curves. The stable operation of the system at the equilibrium point (A, in Fig. 22-8) indicates that cardiac output equals venous return.

Myocardial Contractility

Combinations of cardiac and vascular function curves may also help explain the effects of alterations in ventricular contractility on cardiac output and P_v. In Fig. 22-9, the lower

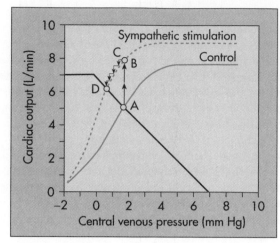

■ **Fig. 22-9**   An enhancement of myocardial contractility, as by cardiac sympathetic nerve stimulation, causes the equilibrium values of cardiac output and central venous pressure *(P_v)* to shift from the intersection *(point A)* of the control vascular and cardiac function curves *(continuous curve)* to the intersection *(point D)* of the same vascular function curve with the cardiac function curve *(dashed curve)* that represents the response to sympathetic stimulation.

cardiac function curve represents the control state, whereas the upper curve reflects the influence of improved myocardial contractility. This pair of curves is analogous to the "family" of ventricular function curves shown in Fig. 17-19. The enhancement of ventricular contractility represented by the upper curve in Fig. 22-9 might be achieved experimentally by electrical stimulation of the cardiac sympathetic nerves. When the effects of such neural stimulation are restricted to the heart, the vascular function curve is unaffected. Therefore, only one vascular function curve is needed for this hypothetical intervention, as shown in Fig. 22-9.

During the control state of our hypothetical model, the equilibrium values for cardiac output and P_v are designated by point A in Fig. 22-9. Cardiac sympathetic nerve stimulation abruptly raises cardiac output to point B, because of the enhanced myocardial contractility. However, this high cardiac output increases the net transfer of blood from the venous to the arterial side of the circuit, and consequently P_v then begins to fall (to point C). The reduction in P_v then leads to a small decrease in cardiac output. However, the cardiac output is still sufficiently high to effect the net transfer of blood from the venous to the arterial side of the circuit. Thus, P_v and cardiac output both continue to fall gradually until a new equilibrium point *(D)* is reached. This equilibrium point is located at the intersection of the vascular function curve with the new cardiac function curve. Point D lies above and to the left of the control equilibrium point *(A)*, and indicates that sympathetic stimulation can evoke a greater cardiac output despite the lower level of P_v.

The actual biological response of an experimental animal to an enhancement of myocardial contractility is mimicked by the hypothetical change predicted by our model. In the

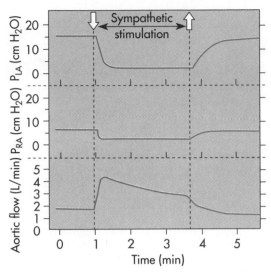

■ **Fig. 22-10**   During electrical stimulation of the left stellate ganglion (which contains cardiac sympathetic nerve fibers), the aortic blood flow (cardiac output) increased while pressures in the left atrium (P_{LA}) and right atrium (P_{RA}) diminished. These data conform with the conclusions derived from Fig. 22-9, in which the equilibrium values of cardiac output and venous pressure are observed to shift from point A to point D (i.e., cardiac output increased, but central venous pressure decreased) during cardiac sympathetic nerve stimulation. (Redrawn from Sarnoff SJ et al: *Circ Res* 8:1108, 1960.)

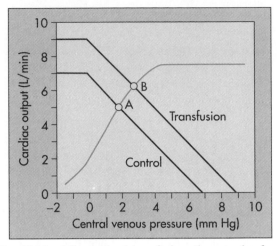

■ **Fig. 22-11**   After a blood transfusion, the vascular function curve is shifted to the right. Therefore, cardiac output and venous pressure are both increased, as denoted by the translocation of the equilibrium point from *A* to *B*.

experiment depicted in Fig. 22-10, the left stellate ganglion of an anesthetized dog was stimulated during the time denoted by the two arrows. During neural stimulation, the cardiac output (aortic flow) rose quickly to a peak value and then fell gradually to a steady-state value significantly greater than the control level. The increased aortic flow was accompanied by reductions in right and left atrial pressures $(P_{RA}$ and $P_{LA})$.

Blood Volume

Changes in blood volume do not directly affect myocardial contractility, but they do influence the vascular function curve in the manner shown in Fig. 22-6. Therefore, to understand how changes in blood volume affect cardiac output and P_v, the appropriate cardiac function curve is plotted along with the vascular function curves that represent the control and experimental states.

Figure 22-11 illustrates the response to a blood transfusion. Equilibrium point *B,* which denotes the values for cardiac output and P_v after transfusion, lies above and to the right of the control equilibrium point *A.* Thus, transfusion increases both cardiac output and P_v. Hemorrhage causes the opposite effect. Mechanistically, the change in ventricular filling pressure (central venous pressure) evoked by a given change in blood volume alters cardiac output by changing the sensitivity of the contractile proteins to the prevailing concentration of intracellular Ca^{2+}, as explained in Chapters 16 and 17. For reasons explained earlier in this chapter, pure increases or decreases in venomotor tone elicit responses

that are analogous to those evoked by increases or decreases, respectively, of total blood volume.

Heart failure is a general term that applies to conditions in which the pumping capability of the heart is impaired to the extent that the tissues of the body are not adequately perfused. In heart failure, myocardial contractility is impaired. Heart failure may be acute or chronic. Consequently, in a graph of cardiac and vascular function curves, the cardiac function curve is shifted downward and to the right, as depicted in Fig. 22-12.

Acute heart failure may be caused by **toxic quantities of drugs or anesthetics** or by certain pathological conditions, such as **coronary artery occlusion.** In acute heart failure, blood volume does not change immediately. In Fig. 22-12, therefore, the equilibrium point shifts from the intersection *(A)* of the normal curves to the intersection *(B* or *C)* of the normal vascular function curve with one of the curves that depict depressed cardiac function.

Chronic heart failure may occur in such conditions as **essential hypertension** or **ischemic heart disease.** In chronic heart failure, both the cardiac function and the vascular function curves shift. The vascular function curve shifts because of an increase in blood volume caused in part by fluid retention by the kidneys. The fluid retention is related to the concomitant reduction in glomerular filtration rate and to the increased secretion of aldosterone by the adrenal cortex (see also Chapters 36 and 45). The resultant hypervolemia is reflected by a rightward shift of the vascular function curve, as shown in Fig. 22-12. Hence, with moderate degrees of heart failure, P_v is elevated, but cardiac output may be normal *(D)*. With more severe degrees of heart failure, P_v is still greater, but cardiac output is subnormal *(E)*.

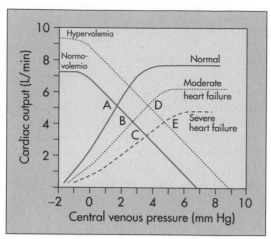

■ Fig. 22-12 Moderate or severe heart failure shifts the cardiac function curves downward and to the right. Before blood volume changes, the cardiac output decreases and central venous pressure rises (from control equilibrium point *A* to point *B* or point *C*). After the increase in blood volume that usually occurs in heart failure, the vascular function curve is shifted to the right. Hence, central venous pressure may be elevated with no reduction in cardiac output (point *D*) or (in severe heart failure) with some reduction in cardiac output (point *E*).

Peripheral Resistance

Analysis of the effects of changes in peripheral resistance on cardiac output and P_v is also complex, because both the cardiac and vascular function curves shift. When peripheral resistance increases (Fig. 22-13), the vascular function curve is rotated counterclockwise, but it converges on the same P_v axis intercept as the control curve (Fig. 22-7). Note that vasoconstriction causes a counterclockwise rotation of the vascular function curve in Fig. 22-13, but a clockwise rotation in Fig. 22-7. The direction of rotation differs, because the axes for the vascular function curves were reversed in these two figures, for reasons explained earlier in this chapter. The cardiac function curve in Fig. 22-13 is also shifted downward, because at any given P_v the heart is able to pump less blood against the greater cardiac afterload imposed by the increased peripheral resistance. Because both curves in Fig. 22-13 are displaced downward, the new equilibrium point, *B*, falls below the control point, *A;* that is, an increase in peripheral resistance diminishes the cardiac output.

Whether point *B* falls directly below point *A* or lies slightly to the right or left of it depends on the magnitude of the shift in each curve. For example, if a given increase in peripheral resistance shifts the vascular function curve more than it does the cardiac function curve, equilibrium point *B* will fall below and to the left of *A;* that is, both cardiac output and P_v will diminish. Conversely, if the cardiac function curve is displaced more than the vascular function curve, point *B* falls below and to the right of point *A;* that is, cardiac output decreases, but P_v rises.

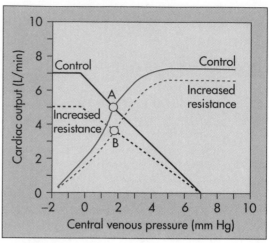

■ Fig. 22-13 An increase in peripheral resistance shifts the cardiac and the vascular function curves downward. At equilibrium, the cardiac output is less *(B)* when the peripheral resistance is high than when it is normal *(A).*

A MORE COMPLETE THEORETICAL MODEL: THE TWO PUMP SYSTEM

The preceding discussion shows that the interrelations between cardiac output and central venous pressure are complicated and perplexing, even in an oversimplified circulation model that includes only one pump and only the systemic circulation. However, in reality, the cardiovascular system includes the systemic and pulmonary circulations and two pumps: the left and right ventricles. The interrelations between ventricular outputs, arterial pressures, and atrial pressures are therefore much more complex.

Fig. 22-14 shows a more complete, but still oversimplified, cardiovascular system model that contains two pumps in series (the left and right ventricles) and two vascular beds in series (the systemic and pulmonary vasculature). The series arrangement requires that the flows pumped by the two ventricles be virtually equal to each other over any substantial period; otherwise, all the blood would ultimately accumulate in one or the other of the vascular systems. Because the cardiac function curves for the two ventricles differ substantially, the filling (atrial) pressures for the two ventricles must differ appropriately in order to ensure equal stroke volumes (see Fig. 17-18).

Any contractility change that affects the two ventricles differently alters the distribution of blood volume in the two vascular systems. For example, if a coronary artery to the left ventricle becomes suddenly occluded, left ventricular contractility will be impaired, and **acute left ventricular failure** will ensue. In the instant after occlusion, left atrial pressure will not change and the left ventricle will begin to pump a diminished flow. If the right ventricle is not affected by the acute coronary artery occlusion, the right ventricle will initially continue to pump the normal flow. The disparate right and left ventricular outputs will result in a progressive increase in left atrial pressure

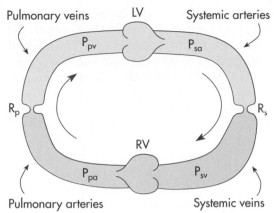

Fig. 22-14 A simplified cardiovascular system model that consists of left *(LV)* and right *(RV)* ventricles, systemic *(R_s)* and pulmonary *(R_p)* vascular resistances, systemic arterial and venous compliances, and pulmonary arterial and venous compliances. P_{sa} and P_{sv} are the pressures in the systemic arteries and veins, respectively; P_{pa} and P_{pv} are the pressures in the pulmonary arteries and veins, respectively.

and a progressive decrease in right atrial pressure. Therefore, left ventricular output will increase toward the normal value and right ventricular output will fall below the normal value. This process will continue until the outputs of the two ventricles again become equal. At this new equilibrium, the outputs of the two ventricles will be subnormal. The elevated left atrial pressure will be accompanied by an equally elevated pulmonary venous pressure, which can have serious clinical consequences. The high pulmonary venous pressure can increase lung stiffness and lead to respiratory distress by increasing the mechanical work of pulmonary ventilation (see Chapter 26). Furthermore, the high pulmonary venous pressure will elevate the hydrostatic pressure in the pulmonary capillaries and may therefore lead to the transudation of fluid from the pulmonary capillaries to the pulmonary interstitium or into the alveoli themselves (**pulmonary edema**) (see Chapter 27). The last of these consequences may be lethal.

Two basic principles to keep in mind about ventricular function are that (1) the left ventricle pumps blood through the systemic vasculature, and (2) the right ventricle pumps blood through the pulmonary vasculature. However, these principles do not necessarily imply that both ventricles are essential for the systemic and pulmonary vascular beds to be perfused adequately. To understand better the relationships between the two ventricles and the two vascular beds, let us examine right ventricular function in more detail.

In the circulatory system model shown in Fig. 22-14, consider the hemodynamic consequences that would prevail if the right ventricle suddenly ceased to function as a pump but instead served merely as a passive, low-resistance conduit between the systemic veins and the pulmonary arteries.

Under these conditions, the only remaining functional pump would be the left ventricle. The left ventricle would then be required to pump blood through both the systemic and pulmonary resistances (for our purposes, consider the resistance to the flow of blood through the inactive right ventricle to be negligible).

Normally, the pulmonary vascular resistance is about 10% as great as the systemic vascular resistance. Because the two resistances are in series with one another, the total resistance would be 10% greater than the systemic resistance alone (see Chapter 18). In a normal cardiovascular system, a 10% increase in systemic vascular resistance would increase mean arterial pressure (and hence left ventricular afterload) by approximately 10%. This increase would not drastically affect left ventricular function. However, under certain conditions, this increase in mean arterial pressure could significantly alter the function of the cardiovascular system. *If the 10% increase in total resistance is achieved by adding a small resistance (i.e., the pulmonary vascular resistance) to that of the much larger systemic resistance, and if the pulmonary vascular resistance is separated from the systemic resistance by a large compliance (the combined systemic venous and pulmonary arterial compliance), the 10% increase in total resistance could drastically impair the operation of the cardiovascular system.*

The simulated effects of inactivating the pumping action of the right ventricle in a hydraulic analog of the circulatory system are shown in Fig. 22-15. In the model, the right and left ventricles generate cardiac outputs that vary directly with their respective filling pressures. Under control conditions (when the right ventricle is functioning normally), the outputs of the left and right ventricles are equal (5 L/min). The right ventricular pumping action causes the pressure in the pulmonary artery (not shown) to exceed the pressure in the pulmonary veins (P_{pv}) by an amount that will force fluid through the pulmonary vascular resistance at a rate of 5 L/min.

When the right ventricle ceases pumping (arrow *1*), the systemic venous and pulmonary arterial systems, along with the right ventricle itself, become a common passive conduit with a large compliance (Fig. 22-14). When the right ventricle ceases to transfer blood actively from the pulmonary veins to the pulmonary arteries, the pulmonary arterial pressure (P_{pa}) decreases rapidly (not shown), and systemic venous pressure (P_{sv}) rises rapidly to a common value (about 5 mm Hg in Fig. 22-15). At this low pressure, however, fluid flows from the pulmonary arteries to the pulmonary veins at a greatly reduced rate. At the start of right ventricular arrest, the left ventricle is pumping fluid from the pulmonary veins to the systemic arteries at the control rate of 5 L/min, which greatly exceeds the rate at which blood returns to the pulmonary veins once the right ventricle ceases to operate. Hence, the pulmonary venous pressure (P_{pv}) drops sharply. Because the pulmonary venous pressure is the preload for the left ventricle, the left ventricular (cardiac) output drops abruptly as well, to attain a steady-state value of about 2.5 L/min. This effect in turn leads to a rapid reduction

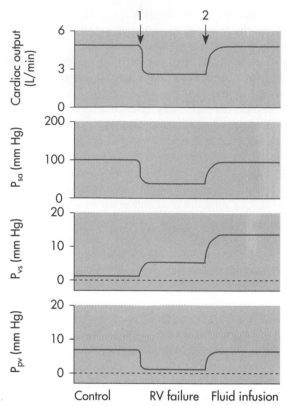

■ **Fig. 22-15** The changes in cardiac output, systemic arterial pressure *(P_{sa})*, systemic venous pressure *(P_{sv})*, and pulmonary venous pressure *(P_{pv})* evoked by simulated right ventricular failure and by simulated fluid infusion in the circulatory model shown in Fig. 22-14. At arrow *1*, the pumping action of the right ventricle was discontinued (simulated right ventricular failure), and the right ventricle served only as a low-resistance conduit. At arrow *2*, the fluid volume in the system was expanded, and the right ventricle continued to serve only as a conduit. (Modified from Furey SA, Zieske HA, Levy MN: *Am Heart J* 107:404, 1984.)

in systemic arterial pressure (P_{sa}). In short, *stoppage of right ventricular pumping markedly curtails cardiac output, systemic arterial pressure, and pulmonary venous pressure and raises systemic venous pressure moderately* (Fig. 22-15).

Most of the hemodynamic problems induced by inactivation of the right ventricle can be reversed by increasing the fluid (blood) volume of the system (arrow *2*, Fig. 22-15). If fluid is added until the pulmonary venous pressure (left ventricular preload) is raised to its control value, the cardiac output and systemic arterial pressure are restored almost to normal, but systemic venous pressure is abnormally elevated. If left ventricular function is normal, adding a normal left ventricular preload will evoke a normal left ventricular output; the 10% increase in peripheral resistance caused by adding the pulmonary vascular resistance to that of the systemic vascular resistance does not impose a serious burden on the left ventricular pumping capacity.

When the right ventricle is inoperative, however, the pulmonary blood flow will not be normal unless the usual pulmonary arteriovenous pressure gradient (about 10 to 15 mm Hg) prevails. Hence, the systemic venous pressure (P_{sv})

must exceed the pulmonary venous pressure (P_{pv}) by this amount. Maintenance of high systemic venous pressures may lead to the accumulation of tissue fluid (**edema**) in the dependent regions of the body. Such edema is a characteristic finding in patients with **right ventricular heart failure.**

With these findings in mind, we may characterize the principal function of the right ventricle as follows. From the viewpoint of providing sufficient flow of blood to all the tissues in the body, the left ventricle alone can carry out this function. The operation of two ventricles in series is not essential to provide adequate blood flow to the tissues. *The crucial function of the right ventricle is to prevent the rise in systemic venous (and pulmonary arterial) pressure that would be required to force the normal cardiac output through the pulmonary vascular resistance.* A normal right ventricle, by preventing an abnormal rise in systemic venous pressure, prevents the occurrence of extensive edema in the dependent regions of the body.

Clinically, **right ventricular heart failure** may be caused by occlusive disease predominantly of the coronary vessels to the right ventricle. These vessels are affected much less commonly than are the vessels to the left ventricle. The major hemodynamic effects of acute right heart failure are pronounced reductions in cardiac output and in arterial blood pressure, and the principal treatment is the infusion of blood or plasma. Bypass of the right ventricle (by anastomosing the right atrium to the pulmonary artery) may be performed surgically for patients with certain **congenital cardiac defects,** such as severe narrowing of the tricuspid valve or maldevelopment of the right ventricle. The effects of acute right heart failure or of right ventricular bypass are directionally similar to those predicted above by the analysis of the model shown in Fig. 22-15.

ROLE OF HEART RATE IN CONTROL OF CARDIAC OUTPUT

Cardiac output is the product of stroke volume and heart rate. The above analysis of the control of cardiac output has been restricted to the control of stroke volume, and the role of the heart rate has been ignored. We now consider the effects of changes in heart rate on cardiac output. The analysis is complex, because a change in heart rate alters the other three factors (preload, afterload, and contractility) that determine stroke volume (Fig. 22-1). An increase in heart rate, for example, shortens the duration of diastole. Hence, ventricular filling is diminished; that is, preload is reduced. If an increase in heart rate did alter cardiac output, the arterial pressure would change; that is, afterload would be altered. Finally, a rise in heart rate would increase the net influx of Ca^{2+} per minute into the myocardial cells (see also Chapter 17), and this influx would enhance myocardial contractility.

The effects of changes in heart rate on cardiac output have been studied extensively in human subjects and in

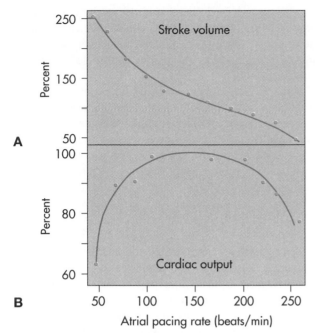

Fig. 22-16   The changes in stroke volume (**A**) and cardiac output (**B**) induced by changing the rate of atrial pacing in an anesthetized dog. (Redrawn from Kumada M, Azuma T, Matsuda K: *Jpn J Physiol* 17:538, 1967.)

experimental animals, and the results are similar to those shown in Fig. 22-16. As the atrial pacing frequency was gradually increased in an anesthetized dog, the stroke volume (SV) progressively diminished (Fig. 22-16, *A*). Presumably, the decrease in SV was caused by the reduced time for ventricular filling. The changes in SV were evidently not inversely proportional to the changes in heart rate (HR), because the direction of the change in cardiac output (Q_h) was influenced markedly by the actual level of HR (Fig. 22-16, *B*). For example, as the pacing frequency was increased from 50 to 100 beats/min, an increase in HR augmented Q_h. Because $Q_h = SV \times HR$, the decrease in SV over this frequency range must have been proportionately less than the increase in HR.

Over the frequency range from about 100 to 200 beats/min, however, Q_h was not affected significantly by changes in pacing frequency (Fig. 22-16, *B*). Hence, as the pacing frequency was increased, the decrease in SV must have been approximately equal to the increase in HR. Also, generalized vascular autoregulation tends to keep tissue blood flow constant (see also Chapter 21). This adaptation leads to changes in preload and afterload that keep Q_h nearly constant.

Finally, at excessively high pacing frequencies (above 200 beats/min in Fig. 22-16), further increases in HR decreased Q_h. Therefore, the induced decrease in SV must have exceeded the increase in HR over this high range of pacing frequencies. Evidently, at such high pacing frequencies, the ventricular filling time was so severely restricted that compensation was inadequate and cardiac output decreased sharply. Although the relationship of Q_h to HR is character-

istically that of an inverted U in the general population, the relationship varies quantitatively among subjects and among physiological states.

The characteristic relationship between cardiac output and heart rate explains the urgent need for treatment of patients who have excessively slow or excessively fast heart rates. Profound **bradycardias** (slow rates) may occur as a result of a very slow sinus rhythm in patients with **sick sinus syndrome** or as a result of a slow idioventricular rhythm in patients with **complete atrioventricular block.** In either rhythm disturbance, the capacity of the ventricles to fill during a prolonged diastole is limited (often by the noncompliant pericardium). Hence, cardiac output usually decreases substantially, because the very slow heart rate cannot be counterbalanced by a sufficiently large stroke volume. Consequently, these bradycardias often require the installation of an artificial pacemaker.

Excessively high heart rates in patients with **supraventricular** or **ventricular tachycardias** often require emergency treatment, because these patients have cardiac outputs that may be critically low. In such patients, the filling time is so restricted at very high heart rates that even small additional reductions in filling time cause disproportionately severe reductions in filling volume. Slowing the tachycardia to a more normal rhythm can usually be accomplished pharmacologically, but **cardioversion,** by delivering a strong electric current across the thorax or directly to the heart through an implanted device, may be required in emergencies (see Chapter 15).

Strong correlations between heart rate and cardiac output must be interpreted cautiously, as must all correlations between important factors. In exercising subjects, for example, cardiac output and heart rate usually increase proportionately, and the stroke volume may remain constant or increase only slightly (see also Chapter 24). The temptation is great to conclude that the increase in cardiac output must be caused by the observed increase in heart rate. However, Fig. 22-16 emphasizes that over a wide range of heart rates, a change in heart rate may have little influence on cardiac output, and several studies on exercising subjects have confirmed these findings.

The principal increase in cardiac output during exercise must therefore be attributed to other factors (see also Chapter 24). Such ancillary factors include the pronounced reduction in peripheral vascular resistance because of the vasodilation in the active skeletal muscles, and the increased contractility of the cardiac muscle associated with the generalized increase in sympathetic neural activity. Nevertheless, the increase in heart rate is still an important factor, even if it cannot be assigned a key causative role. Abundant data show that if the heart rate cannot increase normally during exercise, the augmentation of cardiac output and the capacity for exercise are severely limited. Stroke volume changes only slightly during exercise. Therefore, *the increase in heart rate may play an important permissive role in augmenting cardiac output during physical exercise.*

ANCILLARY FACTORS THAT AFFECT THE VENOUS SYSTEM AND CARDIAC OUTPUT

In earlier sections of this chapter, we oversimplified the interrelationships between central venous pressure and cardiac output by restricting our discussion to the effects evoked by individual variables. However, because the cardiovascular system is regulated by so many feedback control loops, its responses are rarely simple. A change in blood volume, for example, not only affects cardiac output directly by the Frank-Starling mechanism, but it also triggers reflexes that alter other aspects of cardiac function (such as heart rate, atrioventricular conduction, and myocardial contractility) and other characteristics of the vascular system (such as peripheral resistance and venomotor tone). Several other factors, especially gravity and respiration, also regulate cardiac output.

Gravity

Gravitational forces may profoundly affect cardiac output. For example, soldiers standing at attention for a long time may faint because gravity causes blood to pool in the dependent blood vessels, and thereby reduces cardiac output. Warm ambient temperatures interfere with the compensatory vasomotor reactions, and the absence of muscular activity exaggerates these effects. Gravitational effects are amplified in airplane pilots during pullouts from dives. The centrifugal

force in the footward direction may be several times greater than the force of gravity. Pilots characteristically black out momentarily during the pullout maneuver, as blood is drained from the cephalic regions and pooled in the lower parts of the body.

Some of the explanations that have been advanced to explain the gravitationally induced reduction in cardiac output have not been accurate. It has been argued that when an individual is standing, the forces of gravity impede venous return to the heart from the dependent regions of the body. This statement is incomplete, however, because it ignores the gravitational counterforce on the arterial side of the same vascular circuit, and this counterforce facilitates venous return.

In this sense, the vascular system resembles a U tube. To understand the effects of gravity on flow through this U-shaped hydraulic system, let us examine the U tube models depicted in Figs. 22-17 and 22-18. In Fig. 22-17, all the U tubes represent rigid cylinders of constant diameter. With both limbs of the U tube oriented horizontally *(A)*, the flow depends only on the pressures at the inflow and outflow ends of the tube (P_i and P_o, respectively), the viscosity of the fluid, and the length and radius of the tube, in accordance with Poiseuille's equation (see Chapter 18). When the cross-sectional area of the tube is constant, the pressure gradient is uniform; hence, the pressure midway down the tube (P_m) equals the average of the inflow and outflow pressures.

However, when the U tube is oriented vertically (tube *B* to *D*), hydrostatic forces must now be considered. In tube *B*,

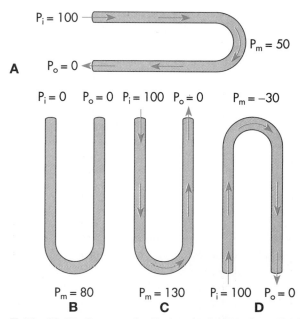

■ **Fig. 22-17** Pressure distributions in rigid U tubes, all with the same dimensions. For a given inflow pressure ($P_i = 100$) and outflow pressure ($P_o = 0$), the pressure at the midpoint (P_m) depends on the orientation of the U tube, but the flow through the tube is independent of the orientation.

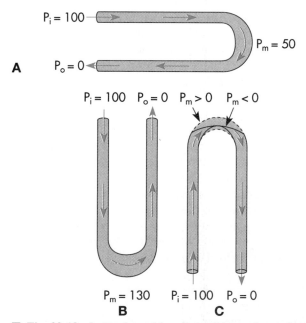

■ **Fig. 22-18** In U tubes with a distensible section at the bend, even when inflow pressures (P_i) are the same for each tube and the outflow pressures (P_o) are the same for each tube, the resistance to flow and the fluid volume contained within each tube vary with the orientation of the tube. P_m is the pressure at the midpoint of each tube.

both limbs are open to atmospheric pressure and both ends are located at the same hydrostatic level; hence, there is no flow. The pressure, P_m, at the midpoint of the tube equals ρhg, where ρ is the density of the fluid, h is the height of the U tube, and g is the acceleration of gravity. In this example, the midpoint pressure of tube *B* is 80 mm Hg.

Now consider tube *C*. This tube is oriented in the same direction as is tube *B,* but a 100 mm Hg pressure difference is applied across the two ends. The flow in tube *C* precisely equals that in *A,* because the pressure gradient, tube dimensions, and fluid viscosity are all the same in tubes *A* and *C.* Gravitational forces are precisely equal in magnitude but opposite in direction in the two limbs of tube *C.* Because the flow in tube *C* will be the same as that in *A,* the pressure drop will be 50 mm Hg at the midpoint, because of the viscous losses that result from flow. Furthermore, gravity will tend to increase pressure by 80 mm Hg at the midpoint, just as in tube *B.* The actual pressure at the midpoint of tube *C* will be the algebraic sum of the viscous loss and hydrostatic gain, or 130 mm Hg in this example.

In tube *D,* a pressure gradient of 100 mm Hg is applied to the same U tube (i.e., *C*), but the tube is oriented in the opposite direction ("upside down"). Gravitational forces will be so directed that the pressure at the midpoint will tend to be 80 mm Hg less than that at the end of the U tube. However, viscous losses will still produce a 50 mm Hg pressure drop at the midpoint relative to P_i. Hence, when the tube is oriented as in tube D, pressure at the midpoint of the U tube will be 30 mm Hg (i.e., 30 mm Hg below the ambient pressure). Flow will of course be the same as in tubes *A* and *C,* for the reasons stated for tube C.

As we can see from Fig. 22-17, in a system of rigid U tubes, gravitational effects do not alter the rate of fluid flow. However, experience does show that gravity affects the cardiovascular system, sometimes dramatically. The reason is that the vessels are *distensible,* not rigid. These gravitational effects can be explained by analyzing the pressures in a set of U tubes with distensible components (at the bends in the tubes of Fig. 22-18). In tubes *A* and *B,* the pressure distributions will resemble those in tubes *A* and *C,* respectively, of Fig. 22-17. Because the pressure is higher at the bend of tube *B* than at the bend of tube *A* in Fig. 22-18 and because the segments are distensible in this region, the distention at the bend in tube *B* will exceed that at the bend in tube *A.* The extent of the distention will depend on the compliance of these tube segments. Because flow varies directly with the tube diameter, the flow through tube *B* in Fig. 22-18 will exceed the flow through tube *A* for a given pressure difference applied at the ends.

Because orienting a U tube with its bend downward actually increases rather than diminishes flow, how then is the observed impairment of cardiovascular function explained when the orientation of the body is similarly changed? The reason is that the cardiovascular system is a closed circuit of constant fluid (blood) volume, whereas the U tube is an open conduit supplied by a fluid source of unlimited volume. In the dependent regions of the cardiovascular system, the dis-

tention occurs more on the venous than on the arterial side of the circuit, because the venous compliance is so much greater than the arterial compliance. Such venous distention is readily observed on the back of the hands when the arms are allowed to hang down below the level of the right atrium.

The hemodynamic effects of such venous distention **(venous pooling)** resemble those caused by the hemorrhage of an equivalent volume of blood from the body. When an adult person shifts from a supine position to a relaxed standing position, 300 to 800 ml of blood pools in the legs. This pooling may reduce cardiac output by about 2 L/min. The compensatory adjustments to assumption of a standing position are similar to the adjustments to blood loss (see also Chapter 24). For example, the diminished baroreceptor excitation triggers a reflex that speeds the heart rate, strengthens the cardiac contraction, and constricts the arterioles and veins. The baroreceptor reflex has a greater effect on the resistance than on the capacitance vessels.

Many of the drugs used to treat chronic **hypertension** interfere with the reflex adaptation to standing. Similarly, astronauts exposed to weightlessness lose their adaptations after a few days in space, and they experience pronounced difficulties when they first return to earth. When such astronauts and other individuals with impaired reflex adaptations stand, their blood pressures may drop substantially. This response is called **orthostatic hypotension,** which may cause lightheadedness or fainting.

When a U tube is rotated so that the bend is directed upward (Fig. 22-18, tube C), the effects are opposite to those that take place in tube *B.* The pressure at the bend of tube *C* would tend to be −30 mm Hg, just as in tube *D* of Fig. 22-17. However, because the ambient pressure exceeds the internal pressure, the distensible segment of tube *C* will collapse. Flow will then cease, and therefore the decline of pressure associated with viscous flow will disappear. When flow stops in U tube *C,* the pressure at the top of each limb will be 80 mm Hg less than at the bottom (the hydrostatic pressure difference). Hence, in the left (or inflow) limb, the pressure will approach 20 mm Hg. As soon as this pressure exceeds ambient pressure (0 mm Hg), the collapsed tubing will be forced open and flow will begin. With the initiation of flow, however, pressure at the bend will again drop below the ambient pressure. Thus, the tubing at the bend will flutter; that is, it will fluctuate between the open and closed states.

When a subject raises an arm above the level of his or her heart, the cutaneous veins in the hand and forearm collapse, for the reasons already described. Fluttering does not occur here, because the deeper veins are protected from collapse by being tethered to surrounding structures. This protection allows the deep veins to accommodate the flow that is ordinarily carried by the collapsed superficial veins. In our hydraulic model, this protection can be simulated by adding a rigid tube (representing the deeper veins) in parallel with the collapsible tube (representing the superficial veins) at the bend of tube *C* in Fig. 22-18. The collapsible tube would no longer flutter but would remain closed. All flow would occur through the rigid tube, just as in tube *D* in Fig. 22-17.

> The superficial veins in the neck are ordinarily partially collapsed when a normal individual is sitting or standing. Venous return from the head is conducted largely through the deeper cervical veins, which are protected from collapse, as stated above. When central venous pressure is abnormally elevated, the superficial neck veins are distended, and they do not collapse even when the subject sits or stands. Such cervical venous distension is an important clinical sign of **congestive heart failure.**

Muscular Activity and Venous Valves

When a recumbent person stands but remains at rest, the pressure rises in the veins in the dependent regions of the body (Fig. 22-19). The venous pressure in the legs increases gradually and does not reach an equilibrium value until almost 1 minute after standing. The slowness of this rise in P_v is attributable to the venous valves, which permit flow only toward the heart. When a person stands, the valves prevent blood in the veins from falling toward the feet. Hence, the column of venous blood is supported at numerous levels by these valves. Because of these valves, the venous column can be thought of as consisting of many discontinuous segments. However, blood continues to enter the column from many venules and small tributary veins, and the pressure continues to rise. As soon as the pressure in one segment exceeds that in the segment just above it, the intervening valve is forced open. Ultimately all the valves are open and the column is continuous, similar to the status in the outflow limbs of the U tubes shown in Figs. 22-17 and 22-18.

Precise measurement reveals that the final level of P_v in the feet during quiet standing is only slightly greater than that in a static column of blood extending from the right atrium to the feet. This finding indicates that the pressure drop caused by blood flow from the foot veins to the right atrium is very small. This very low resistance justifies considering all the veins as a common venous compliance in the circulatory system model illustrated in Fig. 22-2.

When an individual who has been standing quietly begins to walk, the venous pressure in the legs decreases appreciably (Fig. 22-19). Because of the intermittent venous compression exerted by the contracting leg muscles and because of the operation of the venous valves, blood is forced from the veins toward the heart (see Fig. 23-11). Hence, muscular contraction lowers the mean venous pressure in the legs and serves as an **auxiliary pump.** Furthermore, muscular contraction prevents venous pooling and lowers capillary hydrostatic pressure. In this way, muscular contraction reduces the tendency for edema fluid to collect in the feet during standing.

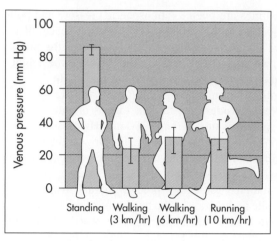

■ **Fig. 22-19**   Mean pressures (±95% confidence intervals) in the foot veins of 18 human subjects during quiet standing, walking, and running. (From Stick C, Jaeger H, Wizleb E: *J Appl Physiol* 72:2063, 1992.)

> This auxiliary pumping mechanism generated by skeletal muscle contractions is much less effective in people with **varicose veins** in their legs. The valves in these defective veins do not function properly, and therefore when the leg muscles contract, the blood in the leg veins is forced in the retrograde as well as in the antegrade direction. Thus, when an individual with varicose veins stands or walks, the venous pressure in the ankles and feet is excessively high. The consequent high capillary pressure leads to the accumulation of edema fluid in the ankles and feet.

Circulatory Effects of Respiratory Activity

The normal, periodic activity of the respiratory muscles causes rhythmic variations in vena caval flow (Fig. 22-20). During respiration, the reduction in intrathoracic pressure is transmitted to the lumina of the thoracic blood vessels. The reduction in central venous pressure during inspiration increases the pressure gradient between extrathoracic and intrathoracic veins. The consequent acceleration of venous return to the right atrium is shown in Fig. 22-20 as an increase in superior vena caval blood flow from 5.2 ml/sec during expiration to 11 ml/sec during inspiration.

The exaggerated reduction in intrathoracic pressure achieved by a strong inspiratory effort against a closed glottis (called **Müller's maneuver**) does not increase venous return proportionately. The extrathoracic veins collapse near their entry into the chest when their internal pressures fall below the ambient level. As the veins collapse, flow into the chest momentarily stops. The cessation of flow raises pressure upstream, forcing the collapsed segment to open again. The process is repetitive; the venous segments adjacent to the chest alternately open and close.

During normal expiration, flow into the central veins decelerates. However, the mean rate of venous return during normal respiration exceeds the flow during a brief period of **apnea** (cessation of respiration). Hence, normal inspiration apparently facilitates venous return more than normal expiration impedes it. In part, this facilitation of venous return is implemented by the valves in the veins of the extremities and neck. These valves prevent any reversal of flow during expiration. Thus, the respiratory muscles and venous valves constitute an **auxiliary pump** for venous return.

Sustained expiratory efforts increase intrathoracic pressure and thereby impede venous return. Straining against a closed glottis (termed Valsalva's maneuver) regularly occurs during coughing, defecation, and heavy lifting. Intrathoracic pressures in excess of 100 mm Hg have been recorded in trumpet players, and pressures over 400 mm Hg have been observed during paroxysms of coughing. Such pressure

increases are transmitted directly to the lumina of the intrathoracic arteries. After coughing stops, the arterial blood pressure may fall precipitously because of the preceding impediment to venous return.

The dramatic increase in intrathoracic pressure induced by coughing constitutes an **auxiliary pumping mechanism** for the blood, despite its concurrent tendency to impede venous return. Patients undergoing certain diagnostic procedures, such as coronary angiography or electrophysiological testing of cardiac function, are at increased risk for ventricular fibrillation. Such patients are trained to cough rhythmically on command during such procedures. If ventricular fibrillation does occur, each cough can generate substantial arterial blood pressure increases, and enough cerebral blood flow may be promoted to sustain consciousness. The cough raises the intravascular pressure equally in intrathoracic arteries and veins. Blood is propelled through the extrathoracic tissues, however, because the increased pressure is transmitted to the extrathoracic arteries, but not to the extrathoracic veins, because the venous valves prevent backflow from the intrathoracic to the extrathoracic veins.

Artificial Respiration

In most forms of artificial respiration (mouth-to-mouth resuscitation, mechanical respiration), lung inflation is achieved by applying endotracheal pressures above atmospheric pressure, and expiration occurs by passive recoil of the thoracic cage (see Chapter 26). Thus, lung inflation is accompanied by an appreciable rise in intrathoracic pressure. Vena caval flow decreases sharply during the phase of positive-pressure lung inflation (indicated by the progressive rise in endotracheal pressure in the central portion of Fig. 22-21). When

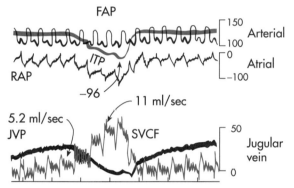

■ **Fig. 22-20** During a normal inspiration intrathoracic *(ITP)*, right atrial *(RAP)*, and jugular venous *(JVP)* pressures decrease, and flow in the superior vena cava *(SVCF)* increases (from 5.2 to 11 ml/sec). All pressures are in mm H₂O, except for femoral arterial pressure *(FAP)*, which is in mm Hg. (Modified from Brecher GA: *Venous return,* New York, 1956, Grune & Stratton.)

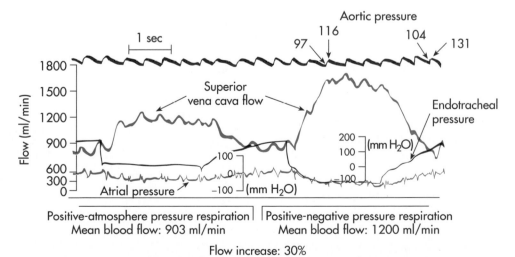

■ **Fig. 22-21** During intermittent positive-pressure respiration, the flow in the superior vena cava is approximately 30% greater when the lungs are deflated actively by applying negative endotracheal pressure *(right side)* than when they are allowed to deflate passively against atmospheric pressure *(left side).* (Modified from Brecher GA: *Venous return,* New York, 1956, Grune & Stratton.)

negative endotracheal pressure (indicated by the abrupt decrease in endotracheal pressure in the right half of Fig. 22-21) is used to facilitate deflation, vena caval flow accelerates more than when the lungs are allowed to deflate passively (near the left border of Fig. 22-21).

SUMMARY

1. Two important relationships between cardiac output (Q_h) and central venous pressure (P_v) prevail in the cardiovascular system: one relationshipo applies to the heart and the other relationship applies to the vascular system.

2. With respect to the heart, Q_h varies directly with P_v (or preload) over a very wide range of P_v. This relationship is represented by the cardiac function curve, and it expresses the Frank-Starling mechanism.

3. With respect to the vascular system, P_v varies inversely with Q_h. This relationship is represented by the vascular function curve, and it reflects the fact that as Q_h increases, a greater fraction of the total blood volume resides in the arteries and a smaller volume resides in the veins.

4. The principal cardiac mechanisms that govern the cardiac output are the changes in numbers of myocardial crossbridges that interact and in the affinity of the contractile proteins for calcium.

5. The principal factors that govern the vascular function curve are the arterial and venous compliances, the peripheral vascular resistance, and the total blood volume.

6. The equilibrium values of Q_h and P_v that prevail under a given set of conditions are determined by the intersection of the cardiac and vascular function curves.

7. At very low and very high heart rates, the heart is unable to pump an adequate Q_h. At very low heart rates, the increase in filling during diastole cannot compensate for the small number of cardiac contractions per minute. At very high heart rates, the large number of contractions per minute cannot compensate for the inadequate filling time.

8. Gravity influences Q_h because the veins are so compliant, and substantial quantities of blood tend to pool in the veins of the dependent portions of the body.

9. Respiration changes the pressure gradient between the intrathoracic and extrathoracic veins. Hence, respiration serves as an auxiliary pump, which may affect the mean level of Q_h and may induce rhythmic changes in stroke volume during the various phases of the respiratory cycle.

BIBLIOGRAPHY

Journal articles

Aukland K: Why don't our feet swell in the upright position? *News Physiol Soc* 9:214, 1994.

Geddes LA, Wessale JL: Cardiac output, stroke volume, and pacing rate, *J Cardiovasc Electrophysiol* 2:408, 1991.

Herron TJ, Korte FS, McDonald KS: Power output is increased after phosphorylation of myofibrillar proteins in rat skinned cardiac myocytes, *Circ Res* 89:1184, 2001.

Konhilas JP, Irving TC, de Tombe PP: Myofilament calcium sensitivity in skinned rat cardiac trabeculae: role of interfilament spacing, *Circ Res* 90:59, 2002.

Lacolley PJ et al: Microgravity and orthostatic intolerance: carotid hemodynamics and peripheral responses, *Am J Physiol* 264:H588, 1993.

Laks H et al: Modification of the Fontan procedure, *Circulation*, 92:2943, 1995.

Lurie KG, Benditt D: Syncope and the autonomic nervous system, *J Cardiovasc Electrophys* 7:760, 1996.

Monos E, Bérczi V, Nadasy G: Local control of veins: biomechanical, metabolic, and humoral aspects, *Physiol Rev* 75:611, 1995.

Risöe C, Tan W, Smiseth OA: Effect of carotid sinus baroreceptor reflex on hepatic and splenic vascular capacitance in vagotomized dogs, *Am J Physiol* 266:H1528, 1994.

Rothe CF: Mean circulatory filling pressure: its meaning and measurement, *J Appl Physiol* 74:499, 1993.

Seymour RS, Hargens AR, Pedley TJ: The heart works against gravity, *Am J Physiol* 265:R715, 1993.

Sheriff DD et al: Dependence of cardiac filling pressure on cardiac output during rest and dynamic exercise in dogs, *Am J Physiol* 265:H316, 1993.

Shoukas AA: Overall systems analysis of the carotid sinus baroreceptor reflex control of the circulation, *Anesthesiology* 79:1402, 1993.

Stick C, Jaeger H, Witzleb E: Measurement of volume changes and venous pressure in the human lower leg during walking and running, *J Appl Physiol* 72:2063, 1992.

Tyberg JV et al: Ventricular interaction and venous capacitance modulate left ventricular preload, *Can J Cardiol* 12:1058, 1996.

Ursino M, Antonucci M, Belardinelli E: Role of active changes in venous capacity by the carotid baroreflex: analysis with a mathematical model, *Am J Physiol* 267:H2531, 1994.

Young ME et al: Intrinsic diurnal variations in cardiac metabolism and contractile function, *Circ Res* 89:1199, 2001.

chapter twenty-three

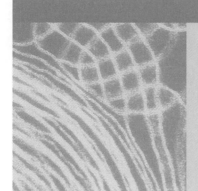

Special Circulations

CORONARY CIRCULATION
Functional Anatomy of Coronary Vessels

The right and left coronary arteries arise at the root of the aorta behind the right and left cusps of the aortic valve, respectively. These arteries provide the entire blood supply to the myocardium. The right coronary artery principally supplies the right ventricle and atrium. The left coronary artery, which divides near its origin into the anterior descending and the circumflex branches, mainly supplies the left ventricle and atrium. However, some overlap exists between the regions supplied by the left and right arteries. In humans, the right coronary artery is dominant (supplying most of the myocardium) in about 50% of individuals. The left coronary artery is dominant in another 20%, and the flow delivered by each main artery is about equal in the remaining 30%. The epicardial distribution of the coronary arteries and veins is illustrated in Fig. 23-1.

After the coronary arterial blood has passed through the capillary beds, most of it returns to the right atrium through the coronary sinus, but some of the coronary venous blood reaches the right atrium by way of the anterior coronary veins. In addition, vascular communications directly link the vessels of the myocardium and the cardiac chambers; these communications are the **arteriosinusoidal, arterioluminal,** and **thebesian vessels.** The arteriosinusoidal channels consist of small arteries or arterioles that lose their arterial structure as they penetrate the chamber walls, where they divide into irregular, endothelium-lined sinuses. These sinuses anastomose with other sinuses and with capillaries, and they communicate with the cardiac chambers. The arterioluminal vessels are small arteries or arterioles that open directly into the atria and ventricles. The thebesian vessels are small veins that connect capillary beds directly with the cardiac chambers and that also communicate with cardiac veins. All the minute vessels of the myocardium communicate in the form of an extensive plexus of subendocardial vessels. However, the myocardium does not receive significant nutritional blood flow directly from the cardiac chambers.

Measurement of Coronary Blood Flow

Coronary blood flow is most commonly measured in humans by a technique called **thermodilution.** Thermodilution is the same procedure used to measure cardiac output (see Chapter 16) except that the indicator (cold saline) is ejected at the tip of a catheter inserted into the coronary sinus via a peripheral vein. The thermal sensor (thermistor) is located on the catheter a few centimeters from the catheter tip. The greater the coronary sinus outflow, the less is the temperature decrease produced by the cold saline injection. This method does not measure total coronary blood flow, because only about two thirds of coronary arterial inflow returns to the venous circulation through the coronary sinus. However, almost all the blood flow that does empty into the coronary sinus comes from the left ventricle. Hence, the thermodilution method provides a good estimate of left ventricular coronary blood flow.

Right and left coronary artery flow, as well as flow in the major branches of the left coronary artery, can be measured by injection of a radioactive tracer (e.g., ^{133}Xe) through a catheter threaded into one of the coronary arteries via a peripheral artery. Myocardial clearance of the isotope is monitored with a detector appropriately placed over the precordium.

In the major coronary arteries, blood flow can also be measured by the **pulsed Doppler technique.** An ultrasound signal is emitted from a crystal at the tip of a cardiac catheter inserted, via a peripheral (e.g., femoral) artery, into the origin of the coronary artery to be studied. The sound is reflected by the flowing blood, and the frequency shift of the reflected sound is proportional to the blood flow.

Coronary blood flow can also be estimated by video densitometry, in which the movement of a bolus of a radiopaque substance injected into the coronary artery is monitored by rapid sequential radiographs. Similarly, intracoronary injection of microbubbles and tracking of their movement by echocardiography are used to measure coronary blood flow. Cine computed tomography and magnetic resonance imaging

413

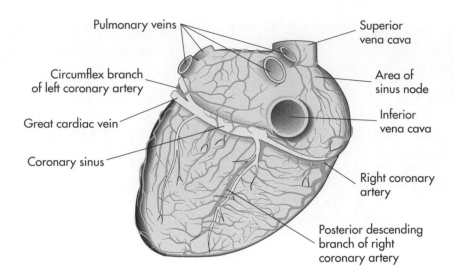

POSTERIOR VIEW

■ **Fig. 23-1** Anterior and posterior surfaces of the heart, illustrating the location and distribution of the principal coronary vessels.

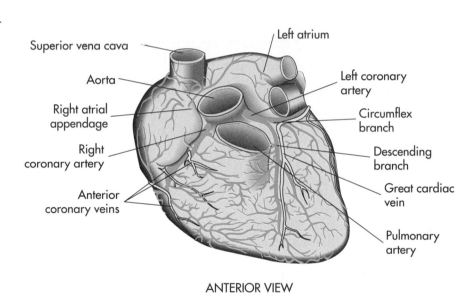

ANTERIOR VIEW

are also used to determine total and regional myocardial blood flow.

Factors That Influence Coronary Blood Flow

Physical factors. *The primary factor responsible for perfusion of the myocardium is the aortic pressure, which is, of course, generated by the heart itself.* Changes in aortic pressure generally evoke parallel directional changes in coronary blood flow. This is caused in part by changes in coronary perfusion pressure. However, the major factor in the regulation of coronary blood flow is a change in arteriolar resistance engendered by changes in the metabolic activity of the heart. When the metabolic activity of the heart increases, coronary resistance decreases; when cardiac metabolism decreases, coronary resistance increases (see Chapter 21).

If a cannulated coronary artery is perfused by blood from a pressure-controlled reservoir, perfusion pressure can be altered without changing aortic pressure and cardiac work. Under these conditions, abrupt variations in perfusion pres-

sure produce equally abrupt changes in coronary blood flow. However, maintenance of the perfusion pressure at the new level is associated with a return of blood flow toward the initial level (Fig. 23-2). This phenomenon is an example of autoregulation of blood flow and is discussed in Chapter 21. Ordinarily, blood pressure is kept within narrow limits by the baroreceptor reflex mechanisms. Hence, changes in coronary blood flow are mainly caused by changes in the diameter of the coronary resistance vessels in response to the metabolic demands of the heart.

In addition to providing the pressure to drive blood through the coronary vessels, the heart also influences its blood supply by the squeezing effect (**extravascular compression**) of the contracting myocardium on the blood vessels that course through it. This force is so great during early ventricular systole that blood flow in the large coronary arteries that supply the left ventricle is briefly reversed. Maximal left coronary inflow occurs in early diastole, when the ventricles have relaxed and extravascular compression of the coronary vessels

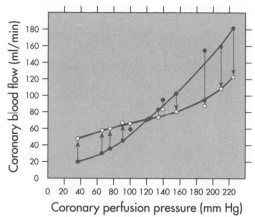

■ **Fig. 23-2** Pressure-flow relationships in the coronary vascular bed. At constant aortic pressure, cardiac output, and heart rate, coronary artery perfusion pressure was abruptly increased or decreased from the control level indicated by the point where the two lines cross. The closed circles represent the flows that were obtained immediately after the change in perfusion pressure; the open circles represent the steady-state flows at the new pressures. There is a tendency for flow to return toward the control level (autoregulation of blood flow), and this is most prominent over the intermediate pressure range (about 60 to 180 mm Hg). (From Berne RM, Rubio R: Coronary circulation. In *Handbook of physiology*, sect 2, *The cardiovascular system: the heart*, vol I, Bethesda, Md, 1979, American Physiological Society.)

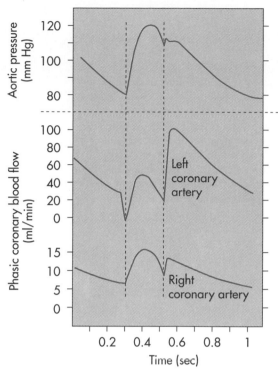

■ **Fig. 23-3** Comparison of phasic coronary blood flow in the left and right coronary arteries.

is virtually absent. This pattern is seen in the phasic coronary flow curve for the left coronary artery (Fig. 23-3). After an initial reversal in early systole, left coronary blood flow follows the aortic pressure until early diastole, when it rises abruptly and then declines slowly as aortic pressure falls during the remainder of diastole.

> The minimal extravascular resistance and absence of left ventricular work during diastole can be used to improve myocardial perfusion in patients with damaged myocardium and low blood pressure. In a method called **counterpulsation,** an inflatable balloon is inserted into the thoracic aorta through a femoral artery. The balloon is inflated during each ventricular diastole and deflated during each systole. This procedure enhances coronary blood flow during diastole by raising diastolic pressure at a time when coronary extravascular resistance is lowest. Furthermore, it reduces cardiac energy requirements by lowering aortic pressure (afterload) during ventricular ejection.

Left ventricular myocardial pressure (pressure within the wall of the left ventricle) is greatest near the endocardium and least near the epicardium. However, under normal conditions, this pressure gradient does not impair endocardial blood flow, because a greater blood flow to the endocardium during diastole compensates for the greater blood flow to the epicardium during systole. In fact, when minute radioactive spheres are injected into the coronary arteries, their distribu-

tion indicates that the blood flow to the epicardial and endocardial halves of the left ventricle is approximately equal under normal conditions. Because extravascular compression is greatest at the endocardial surface of the ventricle, an explanation for the equality of epicardial and endocardial blood flow is that the tone of the endocardial resistance vessels is less than the tone of the epicardial vessels.

The flow pattern in the right coronary artery is similar to that in the left coronary artery (Fig. 23-3). However, because of the lower pressure developed during systole by the thin right ventricle, reversal of blood flow does not occur in the right ventricle in early systole. Hence, systolic blood flow constitutes a much greater proportion of total coronary inflow than it does in the left coronary artery.

The extent to which extravascular compression restricts coronary inflow can be readily seen when the heart is suddenly arrested in diastole, or with the induction of ventricular fibrillation. Figure 23-4 depicts mean left coronary flow when the vessel was perfused with blood at a constant pressure from a reservoir. At the arrow in Fig. 23-4, *A,* ventricular fibrillation was electrically induced and an immediate and substantial increase in blood flow occurred. Subsequent increase in coronary resistance over a period of many minutes reduced myocardial blood flow to below the level that existed before induction of ventricular fibrillation (Fig. 23-4, *B,* before stellate ganglion stimulation).

Under abnormal conditions, when diastolic pressure in the coronary arteries is low (such as in severe hypotension, in partial **coronary artery occlusion,** or in severe **aortic**

■ **Fig. 23-4**   **A,** Unmasking of the restricting effect of ventricular systole on mean coronary blood flow by induction of ventricular fibrillation during constant pressure perfusion of the left coronary artery. **B,** Effect of cardiac sympathetic nerve stimulation on coronary blood flow and coronary sinus blood O_2 tension in the fibrillating heart during constant pressure perfusion of the left coronary artery. (Berne RM: Unpublished observations.)

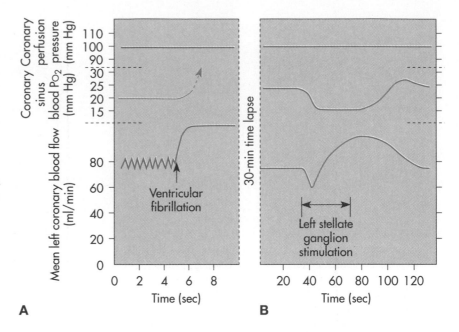

stenosis), the ratio of endocardial to epicardial blood flow falls below a value of l. This ratio indicates that the blood flow to the endocardial regions is more severely impaired than that to the epicardial regions of the ventricle. The redistribution of coronary blood flow is also reflected in an increase in the gradient of myocardial lactic acid and of myocardial adenosine concentrations from epicardium to endocardium. For this reason, the myocardial damage observed in **arteriosclerotic heart disease** (e.g., after coronary occlusion) is greatest in the inner wall of the left ventricle.

Tachycardia and bradycardia have dual effects on coronary blood flow. A change in heart rate is accomplished chiefly by the shortening or lengthening of diastole. In tachycardia the proportion of time spent in systole, and consequently the period of restricted inflow, increases. However, this mechanical reduction in mean coronary flow is overridden by the dilation of the coronary resistance vessels associated with the increased metabolic activity of the more rapidly beating heart. With bradycardia the opposite is true; restriction of coronary inflow is less (more time in diastole), but so are the metabolic (O_2) requirements of the myocardium.

Neural and neurohumoral factors. Stimulation of the sympathetic nerves to the heart elicits a marked increase in coronary blood flow. However, the increase in flow is associated with an increased heart rate and a more forceful systole. The stronger myocardial contraction and the tachycardia (with the consequence that a greater proportion of time is spent in systole) tend to restrict coronary flow. The increase in myocardial metabolic activity, however, tends to dilate the coronary resistance vessels. The increase in coronary blood flow elicited by cardiac sympathetic nerve stimulation reflects the sum of these factors. In perfused hearts in which the mechanical effect of extravascular compression is eliminated by cardiac arrest or by ventricular fibrillation, an initial coronary vasoconstriction is often observed. After this initial vasoconstriction, the metabolic effect evokes vasodilation (Fig. 23-4, *B*).

Furthermore, if the β-adrenergic receptors are blocked to eliminate the chronotropic effects (those that affect the heart rate) and inotropic effects (those that affect contractility), direct reflex activation of the sympathetic nerves to the heart increases coronary resistance. These observations indicate that the *primary action of the sympathetic nerve fibers on the coronary resistance vessels is vasoconstriction.*

α- and β-Adrenergic agonists, as well as α- and β-adrenergic antagonists, reveal the presence of α-adrenergic receptors (constrictors) and β-adrenergic receptors (dilators) on the coronary vessels. Coronary resistance vessels also participate in the baroreceptor and chemoreceptor reflexes, and the sympathetic constrictor tone of the coronary arterioles can be modulated by such reflexes. Nevertheless, coronary resistance is predominantly under local nonneural control.

Vagus nerve stimulation slightly dilates the coronary resistance vessels, and activation of the carotid and aortic chemoreceptors can decrease slightly the coronary resistance via the vagus nerves to the heart. The failure of strong vagal stimulation to increase coronary blood flow is not due to insensitivity of the coronary resistance vessels to acetylcholine; intracoronary administration of this agent elicits marked vasodilation.

Metabolic factors. A striking characteristics of the coronary circulation is the close relationship between the level of myocardial metabolic activity and the magnitude of the coronary blood flow (Fig. 23-5). This relationship is also found in the denervated heart and in the completely isolated heart, whether in the beating or in the fibrillating state. The fibrillating ventricles continue to fibrillate for many hours when the coronary arteries are perfused with arterial blood from some external source. With the onset of ventricular fibrillation, an abrupt increase in coronary blood flow occurs because of the removal of extravascular compression (Fig. 23-4). Flow then gradually returns toward, and often falls below, the prefibrillation level. The increase in coronary resistance that occurs despite the elimination of extravascular

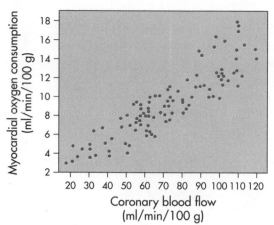

■ Fig. 23-5 Relationship between myocardial oxygen consumption and coronary blood flow during a variety of interventions that increased or decreased myocardial metabolic rate. (From Berne RM, Rubio R: Coronary circulation. In *Handbook of physiology,* sect 2, *The cardiovascular system: the heart,* vol I, Bethesda, Md, 1979, American Physiological Society.)

compression demonstrates the heart's ability to adjust its blood flow to meet its energy requirements. The fibrillating heart uses less O_2 than does the pumping heart, and blood flow to the myocardium is reduced accordingly.

The mechanism that links cardiac metabolic rate and coronary blood flow remains unsettled. However, it appears that *a decrease in the ratio of oxygen supply to oxygen demand releases a vasodilator substance from the myocardial cells into the interstitial fluid, where it relaxes the coronary resistance vessels.* As diagrammed in Fig. 23-6, a decrease in arterial blood oxygen content or in coronary blood flow, or an increase in metabolic rate, all decrease the oxygen supply/demand ratio. In response to the decrease in the oxygen supply/demand ratio, a vasodilator substance, such as adenosine, is released. This substance dilates the arterioles and thereby adjusts the oxygen supply to the oxygen demand. A decrease in oxygen demand diminishes the vasodilator release and permits a greater expression of basal tone.

Numerous agents, generally referred to as **metabolites,** mediate the vasodilation that accompanies increased cardiac

work. Accumulation of vasoactive metabolites may also be responsible for **reactive hyperemia** (see Chapter 21), because the duration of the enhanced coronary flow after release of the briefly occluded vessel is, within certain limits, proportional to the duration of the period of occlusion. Among the factors implicated in reactive hyperemia are CO_2, hydrogen ions, potassium ions, hypoxia, and adenosine.

Among these agents, adenosine is an important physiological mediator of reactive hyperemia. According to the adenosine hypothesis, a reduction in myocardial O_2 tension produced by inadequate coronary blood flow, hypoxemia, or increased metabolic activity of the heart, leads to the myocardial release of adenosine. This nucleoside enters the interstitial fluid space to reach the coronary resistance vessels, and induces vasodilation by activating adenosine receptors.

Potassium release from the myocardium accounts for about half of the initial decrease in coronary resistance. However, it cannot be responsible for the increased coronary flow observed during prolonged enhancement of cardiac metabolic activity, because the release of adenosine from the cardiac muscle is transitory. Little evidence exists that CO_2 hydrogen ions or O_2 play a significant *direct* role in the regulation of coronary blood flow. Factors that alter coronary vascular resistance are illustrated in Fig. 23-7.

Effects of Diminished Coronary Blood Flow

Most of the oxygen in the coronary arterial blood is extracted during one passage through the myocardial capillaries. Thus, the supply of oxygen to the myocardial cells is **flow limited:** any substantial reduction in coronary blood flow will curtail the delivery of oxygen to the myocardium, because the extraction of oxygen from each unit volume of blood is nearly maximal even when blood flow is normal.

A reduction of coronary flow that is neither too prolonged nor too severe to cause myocardial **necrosis** (cell death) can still cause substantial (but temporary) dysfunction of the heart. For example, a relatively brief period of severe ischemia followed by reperfusion can cause a pronounced mechanical dysfunction (called **myocardial stunning**). The heart eventually fully recovers from the dysfunction.

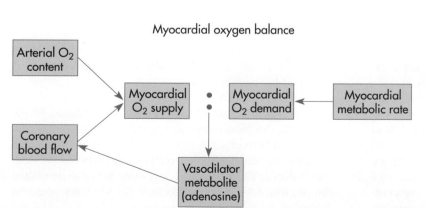

■ Fig. 23-6 Imbalance in the oxygen supply/oxygen demand ratio alters coronary blood flow by the rate of release of a vasodilator metabolite from the cardiomyocytes. A decrease in the ratio elicits an increase in vasodilator release, whereas an increase in the ratio has the opposite effect.

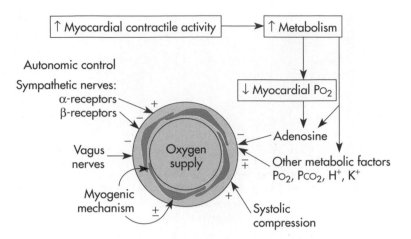

■ **Fig. 23-7**   Schematic representation of factors that increase (+) or decrease (−) coronary vascular resistance. The intravascular pressure (arterial blood pressure) stretches the vessel wall.

The pathophysiological basis for myocardial stunning appears to be a combination of intracellular calcium overload, initiated during the period of ischemia, combined with the generation of hydroxyl and superoxide free radicals early in the period of reperfusion. These changes impair the responsiveness of the myofilaments to calcium.

Myocardial stunning may be evident in patients who have had an **acute coronary artery occlusion** (a so-called heart attack). If the patient is treated sufficiently early by **coronary bypass surgery** or **balloon angioplasty** and if adequate blood flow is restored to the ischemic region, the myocardial cells in this region may recover fully. However, for many days or even weeks, the contractility of the myocardium in the affected region may be grossly subnormal.

Prolonged reductions in coronary blood flow (**myocardial ischemia**) may critically and permanently impair the mechanical and electrical behavior of the heart. Diminished coronary blood flow as a consequence of coronary artery disease (usually **coronary atherosclerosis**) is one of the most common causes of serious cardiac disease. The ischemia may be global (it affects an entire ventricle) or regional (it affects some fraction of the ventricle). The impairment of the mechanical contraction of the affected myocardium is produced not only by the diminished delivery of oxygen and metabolic substrates, but also by the accumulation of potentially harmful substances (e.g., K^+, lactic acid, H^+) in the cardiac tissues. If the reduction of coronary flow to any region of the heart is sufficiently severe and prolonged, necrosis of the affected cardiac cells will result.

The relationships between coronary perfusion pressure, cardiac behavior, and myocardial metabolic activity in an experimental model of **myocardial hibernation** are shown in Fig. 23-8. When the perfusion pressure in isolated hearts was diminished over the range from 160 to about 70 mm Hg, the intraventricular pressure developed by those hearts progressively diminished. However, the intracellular pH and inorganic phosphate concentrations and the efflux of lactic acid remained essentially unaffected. The process is called hibernation because the

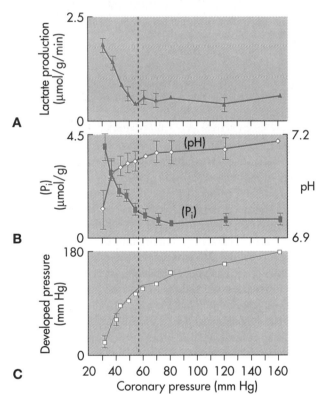

■ **Fig. 23-8**   Effects of changes in coronary perfusion pressure on myocardial lactate production (**A**), on inorganic phosphate levels *(p_i)* and intracellular pH (**B**), and on the pressure developed during left ventricular contraction (**C**) in a group of five ferret hearts. (Modified from Kitikaze M, Marban E: *J Physiol [Lond]* 414:455, 1989.)

down-regulation of metabolism tends to preserve the viability of the cardiac tissues.

Only when the perfusion pressure was reduced below 60 mm Hg did these metabolic variables change substantially (Fig. 23-8). The changes in developed force and in cardiac metabolism were readily reversible when perfusion pressure was restored. The changes in developed pressure correlated directly with the transient intracellular Ca^{2+} currents measured during each ventricular contraction.

Cusps of aortic valve   Cardiac catheter

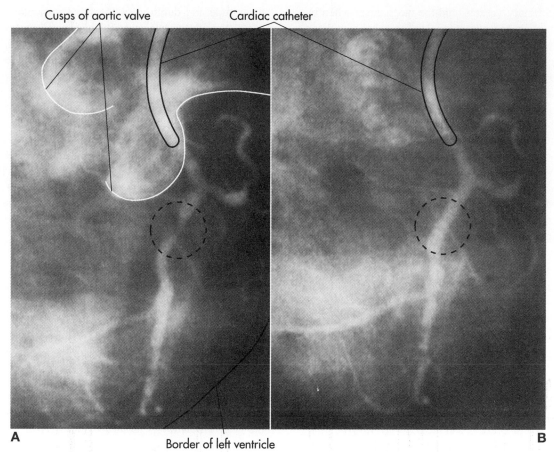

A

B

Border of left ventricle

■ **Fig. 23-9** **A,** Angiogram (intracoronary radiopaque dye) of a person with marked narrowing of the circumflex branch of the left coronary artery *(encircled).* Reflux of dye into the root of the aorta outlines two of the aortic valve cusps. **B,** The same segment of the coronary artery after angioplasty. (Courtesy Dr. Eric R. Powers.)

Myocardial hibernation occurs mainly in patients with coronary artery disease, just as does myocardial stunning. The coronary blood flow in these patients is diminished persistently and significantly, and the mechanical function of the heart is impaired. If coronary blood flow is restored to normal by bypass surgery or angioplasty, mechanical function returns to normal.

Coronary Collateral Circulation and Vasodilators

In the normal human heart, there are virtually no functional intercoronary channels. Abrupt occlusion of a coronary artery or one of its branches leads to ischemic necrosis and eventual fibrosis of the areas of myocardium supplied by the occluded vessel. However, if a coronary artery narrows slowly and progressively over a period of days or weeks, collateral vessels develop and may furnish sufficient blood to the ischemic myocardium to prevent or reduce the extent of necrosis. Collateral vessels may develop between branches of occluded and nonoccluded arteries. They originate from preexisting small vessels that undergo proliferative changes

of the endothelium and smooth muscle. These changes may occur in response to wall stress and to chemical agents released by the ischemic tissue.

Numerous surgical attempts have been made to enhance the development of coronary collateral vessels. However, the techniques used do not increase the collateral circulation over and above that produced by coronary artery narrowing alone. When discrete occlusions or severe narrowing occur in coronary arteries, as in **coronary atherosclerosis,** the lesions can be bypassed with an artery or a vein graft. In many cases the narrow segment can be dilated by inserting a balloon-tipped catheter into the diseased vessel via a peripheral artery and then inflating the balloon. Distension of the vessel by balloon inflation **(angioplasty)** can produce a lasting dilation of a narrowed coronary artery (Fig. 23-9).

A variety of drugs that induce coronary vasodilation are available and are used in patients with coronary artery disease to relieve **angina pectoris,** the chest pain associated with myocardial ischemia. Many of these compounds are organic nitrates and nitrites. They do not selectively dilate the coronary vessels, and the mechanism whereby they accomplish their beneficial effects has not been established. The arterioles that would dilate in response to the drugs are undoubtedly already maximally dilated by the ischemia responsible for the symptoms.

In fact, in a patient with marked narrowing of a coronary artery, administration of a vasodilator can fully dilate normal vessel branches that are parallel to the narrowed segment, and thereby reduce the head of pressure to the partially occluded vessel. The reduced pressure to the narrowed vessel will further compromise blood flow to the ischemic myocardium. This phenomenon is known as **coronary steal,** and it can occur in response to a vasodilator drug, such as dipyridamole, which acts by blocking cellular uptake and metabolism of endogenous adenosine. Nitrites and nitrates alleviate angina pectoris, at least partly, by reducing cardiac work and myocardial oxygen requirements. This is accomplished by relaxing the great veins, which reduces cardiac preload, and by decreasing arterial blood pressure, which reduces afterload.

Cardiac Oxygen Consumption and Work

The volume of O_2 consumed by the heart depends on the amount and type of activity that the heart performs. Under basal conditions, myocardial O_2 consumption is about 8 to 10 ml/min/100 g of heart. It can increase several-fold during exercise and decrease moderately under such conditions as hypotension and hypothermia. The O_2 content of cardiac venous blood is normally low (about 5 ml/dl), and the myocardium can receive little additional O_2 by further O_2 extraction from the coronary blood. Therefore, increased O_2 demands of the heart must be met mainly by an increase in coronary blood flow. In experiments in which the heartbeat is arrested but coronary perfusion is maintained, O_2 consumption falls to 2 ml/min/100 g or less, which is still six to seven times greater than the O_2 consumption for resting skeletal muscle.

Left ventricular work per beat (**stroke work**) is approximately equal to the product of the stroke volume and the mean aortic pressure against which the blood is ejected by the left ventricle (see Chapter 19). At resting levels of cardiac output, the kinetic energy component is negligible (see Chapter 18). However, at high cardiac outputs, as in strenuous exercise, the kinetic energy component can account for up to 50% of total cardiac work. Simultaneously halving the aortic pressure and doubling the cardiac output, or vice versa, will result in the same value for cardiac work. However, *the O_2 requirements are greater for any given amount of cardiac work when a major proportion of the work is pressure work, as opposed to volume work.* An increase in cardiac output at a constant aortic pressure (volume work) is accomplished with only a small increase in left ventricular O_2 consumption, whereas increased arterial pressure at constant cardiac output (pressure work) is accompanied by a large increase in myocardial O_2 consumption. Thus, myocardial O_2 consumption may not correlate well with overall cardiac work. The magnitude and duration of the left ventricular pressure do correlate with the left ventricular O_2 consumption.

The work of the right ventricle is one seventh that of the left ventricle, because pulmonary vascular resistance is much less than systemic vascular resistance.

The greater energy demand of pressure work than of volume work is clinically important, especially in **aortic stenosis.** In this condition, left ventricular O_2 consumption is increased mainly because of the high intraventricular pressures developed during systole. However, coronary perfusion pressure, and hence oxygen supply, is either normal or reduced because of the pressure drop across the narrowed orifice of the diseased aortic valve (see also Chapter 18).

Cardiac Efficiency

As with a mechanical engine, the efficiency of the heart can be calculated as the ratio of the work accomplished to the total energy utilized. If the average O_2 consumption is assumed to be 9 ml/min/100 g for the two ventricles, a 300-g heart will consume 27 ml O_2/min. This value is equivalent to 130 small calories when the respiratory quotient is 0.82. Together, the two ventricles do about 8 kg-m of work per minute, which is equivalent to 18.7 small calories. Therefore, the gross efficiency of the heart is about 14%.

$$18.7/130 \times 100 = 14\% \qquad (23\text{-}1)$$

The net efficiency of the heart is slightly higher (18%) and is determined by subtracting the O_2 consumption of the nonbeating (asystolic) heart (about 2 ml/min/100 g) from the total cardiac O_2 consumption in the calculation of efficiency. Therefore, the efficiency of the heart as a pump is relatively low, and it is comparable to the efficiency of many common mechanical devices. During physical exercise, efficiency improves, because mean blood pressure shows little change, whereas cardiac output and work increase considerably, without a proportional increase in myocardial O_2 consumption. The energy expended in cardiac metabolism that does not contribute to the propulsion of blood through the body is dissipated in the form of heat. The energy of the flowing blood is also dissipated as heat, chiefly in its passage through the arterioles.

Substrate Utilization

The heart is versatile in its use of substrates, and within certain limits, the uptake of a particular substrate is directly proportional to its arterial concentration. The use of one substrate by the heart is also influenced by the presence or absence of other substrates. For example, the addition of lactate to the blood that perfuses a heart metabolizing glucose leads to a reduction in glucose uptake, and vice versa. At normal blood concentrations, glucose and lactate are consumed at about equal rates.

In contrast, pyruvate uptake is very low, as is its arterial concentration. For glucose, the threshold concentration is about 4 mM. Below this blood level, no glucose is taken up by the myocardium. Insulin reduces the glucose threshold and increases the rate of glucose uptake by the heart. A very low threshold exists for the cardiac utilization of lactate; insulin does not affect its uptake by the myocardium. Under hypoxic conditions, glucose utilization is facilitated by an increase in the rate of transport across the myocardial cell wall. However, lactate cannot be metabolized by the hypoxic heart and it is in fact produced by the heart under anaerobic conditions. Associated with lactate production by the hypoxic heart is the breakdown of cardiac glycogen.

Of the total cardiac O_2 consumption, only 35% to 40% can be accounted for by the oxidation of carbohydrate. Thus, the heart derives the major part of its energy from oxidation of noncarbohydrate sources. The chief noncarbohydrate fuels used by the heart are esterified and nonesterified fatty acid, which account for about 60% of the myocardial O_2 consumption in subjects in the postabsorptive state. The various fatty acids have different thresholds for myocardial uptake, but these acids are generally used in direct proportion to their arterial concentration. Ketone bodies, especially acetoacetate, are readily oxidized by the heart, and they contribute a major source of energy in diabetic acidosis. As is true of carbohydrate substrates, utilization of a specific noncarbohydrate is influenced by the presence of other substrates, whether noncarbohydrate or carbohydrate. Therefore, within certain limits, the heart preferentially uses the substrate that is available in the largest concentration. The contribution to myocardial energy expenditure provided by the oxidation of amino acids is small.

Normally the heart derives its energy by oxidative phosphorylation, in which each mole of glucose yields 36 mol of adenosine triphosphate (ATP). However, during hypoxia, glycolysis takes over, and 2 mol of ATP is provided by each mole of glucose; β-oxidation of fatty acids is also curtailed. If hypoxia is prolonged, cellular creatine phosphate and eventually adenosine triphosphate (ATP) are depleted.

In ischemia, lactic acid accumulates and decreases the intracellular pH. This condition inhibits glycolysis, fatty acid use, and protein synthesis, and therefore it results in cellular damage and eventually in necrosis of myocardial cells.

CUTANEOUS CIRCULATION

The oxygen and nutrient requirements of the skin are relatively small. In contrast to most other body tissues, the supply of oxygen and nutrients is not the chief factor in the regulation of cutaneous blood flow. The primary function of the cutaneous circulation is the maintenance of a constant body temperature. Consequently, the skin undergoes wide fluctuations in blood flow, depending on whether the body needs to lose or conserve heat. Mechanisms responsible for alterations in skin blood flow are mainly activated by changes in ambient and internal body temperatures.

Regulation of Skin Blood Flow

Neural factors. The skin contains essentially two types of resistance vessels: **arterioles** and **arteriovenous (AV)** anastomoses. The arterioles are similar to those found elsewhere in the body. AV anastomoses shunt blood from the arterioles to the venules and venous plexuses; hence, they bypass the capillary bed. The anastomoses are found in the fingertips, palms of the hands, toes, soles of the feet, ears, nose, and lips. AV anastomoses differ morphologically from the arterioles; the anastomoses are either short, straight, or long coiled vessels, about 20 to 40 µm in luminal diameter, with thick muscular walls richly supplied with nerve fibers (Fig. 23-10). These vessels are almost exclusively under sympathetic neural control, and they dilate maximally when their nerve supply is interrupted. Conversely, reflex stimulation of the sympathetic fibers to these vessels may produce constriction to the point of complete obliteration of the vascular lumen. Although AV anastomoses do not exhibit **basal tone** (tonic activity of the vascular smooth muscle independent of innervation), they are highly sensitive to vasoconstrictor agents, such as epinephrine and norepinephrine. Furthermore, AV anastomoses are not under metabolic control, and they do not show reactive hyperemia or autoregulation of blood flow. *Thus, the regulation of blood flow through these anastomotic channels is governed principally by the nervous system in response to reflex activation by temperature receptors or from higher centers of the central nervous system.*

Most of the resistance vessels in the skin exhibit some basal tone and are under the dual control of the sympathetic nervous system and local regulatory factors. Neural control is more important than local control in the skin vessels. Stimulation of sympathetic nerve fibers to blood vessels in the skin induces vasoconstriction, and cutting the sympathetic nerves induces vasodilation. After chronic denervation of the cutaneous blood vessels, the degree of tone that existed before denervation is gradually regained over a period of several weeks. This restoration of tone is accomplished by an enhancement of basal tone. Denervation of the skin vessels results in enhanced sensitivity to circulation catecholamines (**denervation hypersensitivity**). As noted above, epinephrine and norepinephrine elicit only vasoconstriction in cutaneous vessels.

Parasympathetic vasodilator nerve fibers do not innervate the cutaneous blood vessels. However, stimulation of the sweat glands, which are innervated by cholinergic fibers of the sympathetic nervous system, dilates the skin resistance vessels. Sweat contains an enzyme that acts on a protein moiety in the tissue fluid to produce **bradykinin,** a polypeptide with potent vasodilator properties. Bradykinin, formed locally, dilates the arterioles and increases blood flow to the skin.

Certain skin vessels, particularly those in the head, neck, shoulders, and upper chest, are regulated by the higher centers in the brain. Blushing, in response to embarrassment or anger, and blanching, in response to fear or anxiety, are examples of cerebral inhibition and stimulation, respectively, of the sympathetic nerve fibers to the affected cutaneous regions.

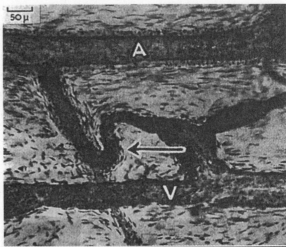

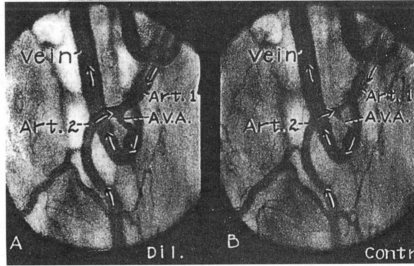

■ **Fig. 23-10** *Top,* Arteriovenous anastomosis in the human ear injected with Berlin blue. *A,* Artery; *V,* vein; arrow points to AV anastomosis. The walls of the AV anastomosis in the fingertips are thicker and more cellular. (From Pritchard MML, Daniel PM: *J Anat* 90:309, 1956.) *Bottom,* Two frames from a motion picture record of the same relatively large artiovenous anastomosis *(A.V.A.)* in a stable rabbit ear chamber installed 3 ½ months previously. *Frame A,* A.V.A. dilated; *Frame B,* contracted. On this day the lumen of the A.V.A. measured 51 μm dilated and 5 μm contracted at its narrowest point. (From Clark ER, Clark EL: *Am J Anat* 54:229, 1934.)

In contrast to AV anastomoses in the skin, the resistance vessels display autoregulation of blood flow and reactive hyperemia. If the arterial inflow to a limb is stopped by inflating a blood pressure cuff briefly, the skin becomes bright red below the point of vascular occlusion when the cuff is subsequently deflated. This increased cutaneous blood flow (reactive hyperemia) is also manifested by distention of the superficial veins in the affected extremity. Autoregulation of blood flow in the skin is best explained by a myogenic mechanism (see Chapter 21).

The fingers and toes of some individuals are very sensitive to cold. Upon exposure to cold, the arterioles to the fingers and toes constrict. The consequent ischemia is characterized by a localized blanching of the skin associated with tingling, numbness, and pain. The blanching is followed by cyanosis (a dark blue color of the skin) and later by redness, as the arterial spasm subsides. The cause of this scondition, called **Raynaud's disease,** is unknown, and it occurs most frequently in young women.

The role of temperature in the regulation of skin blood flow. *The primary function of the skin is to maintain a constant internal environment and protect the body from adverse changes. Ambient (outside) temperature is one of the most important external variables with which the body must contend. Thus, it is not surprising that the vasculature of the skin is chiefly influenced by environmental temperature.* Exposure to cold elicits a generalized cutaneous vasoconstriction that is most pronounced in the hands and feet. This response is chiefly mediated by the nervous system. Arrest of the circulation to a hand by a pressure cuff and immersion of that hand in cold water induce vasoconstriction in the skin of the other extremities that are exposed to room temperature. When the circulation to the chilled hand is not occluded, the reflex generalized vasoconstriction is caused in part by the cooled blood that returns to the general circulation. This returned blood then stimulates the temperature-regulating center in the anterior hypothalamus. Direct application of cold to this region of the brain evokes cutaneous vasoconstriction.

The skin vessels of the cooled hand also respond directly to cold. Moderate cooling or a brief exposure to severe cold (0° to 15° C) constricts the resistance and capacitance vessels, including the AV anastomoses. However, prolonged exposure to severe cold evokes a secondary vasodilator response. Prompt vasoconstriction and severe pain are elicited by immersion of the hand in ice water. However, this response is soon followed by dilation of the skin vessels, with reddening of the immersed part and alleviation of the pain. With continued immersion of the hand, alternating periods of constriction and dilation occur, but the skin temperature rarely drops as much as it did in response to the initial vasoconstriction. Prolonged severe cold, of course, damages tissue. The rosy faces of people exposed to a cold environment are examples of **cold vasodilation.** However, the blood flow through the skin of the face may be greatly reduced, despite the flushed appearance. The red color of the slowly flowing blood is mainly caused by the reduced oxygen uptake by the cold skin and the cold-induced shift to the left of the oxyhemoglobin dissociation curve (see Chapter 28).

Direct application of heat to the skin not only dilates the local resistance and capacitance vessels and AV anastomoses, but it also dilates reflexly blood vessels in other parts of the body. The local effect is independent of the vascular nerve supply, whereas the reflex vasodilation is a combined response to stimulation of the anterior hypothalamus by the returning warmed blood and to stimulation of cutaneous heat receptors in the heated regions of the skin.

The close proximity of the major arteries and veins permits considerable heat exchange (**countercurrent**) *between them.* Cold blood that flows in veins from a cooled hand toward the heart takes up heat from adjacent arteries; this warms the venous blood and cools the arterial blood. Heat exchange, of course, takes place in the opposite direction when the extremity is exposed to heat. Thus, heat conservation is enhanced during exposure of extremities to cold environments, and heat conservation is minimized during exposure of the extremities to warm environments.

Skin Color: Relationship to Skin Blood Volume, Oxyhemoglobin, and Blood Flow

The color of the skin is determined mainly by the pigment content. However, the degree of pallor or ruddiness is mainly a function of the amount of blood in the skin, except when the skin is very dark. With little blood in the venous plexus, the skin appears pale, whereas with moderate to large quantities of blood in the venous plexus, the skin displays a color. This color may be red, blue, or some shade between, depending on the degree of oxygenation of the blood in the subcutaneous vessels. For example, a combination of vasoconstriction and reduced hemoglobin can impart an ashen gray color to the skin. A combination of venous engorgement and reduced hemoglobin content can impart a dark purple hue.

Skin color provides little information about the rate of cutaneous blood flow. Rapid blood flow may be accompanied by pale skin when the AV anastomoses are open, slow blood flow may be associated with red skin when the skin is exposed to cold.

SKELETAL MUSCLE CIRCULATION

The rate of blood flow in skeletal muscle varies directly with the contractile activity of the tissue and the type of muscle. Blood flow and capillary density in red muscle (slow-twitch, high-oxidative) are greater than in white muscle (fast-twitch, low-oxidative). In resting muscle, the precapillary arterioles contract and relax intermittently. Thus, at any given moment most of the capillary bed is not perfused. Consequently, total blood flow through quiescent skeletal muscle is low (1.4 to 4.5 ml/min/100 g). During exercise, the resistance vessels relax and the muscle blood flow may increase to 15 to 20 times the resting level. The magnitude of this increase depends on the intensity of the exercise.

Regulation of Skeletal Muscle Blood Flow

Muscle circulation is regulated by neural and local factors. As with all tissues, physical factors such as arterial pressure, tissue pressure, and blood viscosity influence muscle blood flow. However, another physical factor, the squeezing effect of the active skeletal muscle, affects blood flow in the vessels. With intermittent contractions, inflow is restricted and venous outflow is enhanced during each contraction (Fig. 23-11). The venous valves prevent backflow of blood in the veins between contractions, and the valves thereby aid in the forward propulsion of the blood. With strong sustained contractions, such as those that occur during exercise, the vascular bed can be compressed to the point at which blood flow actually ceases temporarily.

When the valves of the superficial leg veins are incompetent, as may occur during pregnancy, thrombophlebitis, or obesity, the veins become dilated and tortuous. Such **varicose veins** can be treated by surgical removal, intravenous injection of sclerosing solutions, or the use of elastic stockings.

Neural factors. Although the resistance vessels of muscle possess a high degree of basal tone, they also display tone in response to continuous low-frequency activity in the sympathetic vasoconstrictor nerve fibers. The basal frequency of firing in the sympathetic vasoconstrictor fibers is only about 1 to 2 per second, and maximal vasoconstriction occurs at frequencies of about 10 per second.

The vasoconstriction evoked by sympathetic nerve activity is caused by the release of norepinephrine from nerve fiber endings. Intraarterial injection of norepinephrine in skeletal muscle elicits only vasoconstriction, whereas the responses to epinephrine is dose dependent. Low doses of epinephrine produce vasodilation whereas large doses cause vasoconstriction.

The tonic activity of the sympathetic nerves is greatly influenced by reflexes from the baroreceptors. An increase in carotid sinus pressure dilates the vascular bed of muscle,

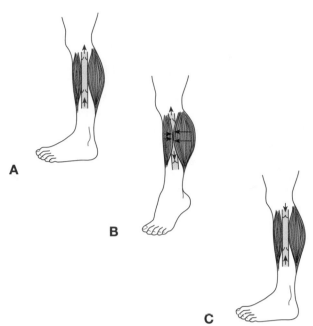

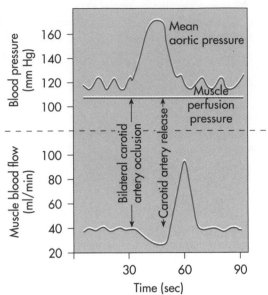

■ **Fig. 23-11**   Action of the muscle pump in venous return from the legs. **A,** Standing at rest, the venous valves are open and blood flows upward toward the heart by virtue of the pressure generated by the heart and transmitted through the capillaries to the veins from the arterial side of the vascular system (vis a tergo). **B,** Contraction of the muscle compresses the vein so that the increased pressure in the vein drives blood toward the thorax through the upper valve and closes the lower valve in the uncompressed segment of the vein just below the point of muscular compression. **C,** Immediately after muscle relaxation, the pressure in the previously compressed venous segment falls and the reversed pressure gradient causes the upper valve to close. The valve below the previously compressed segment opens because pressure below it exceeds that above it. The segment then fills with blood from the foot. As blood flow continues from the foot, the pressure in the previously compressed segment rises. When it exceeds the pressure above the upper valve, this valve opens and continuous flow occurs as in **A.**

■ **Fig. 23-12**   Evidence for participation of the muscle vascular bed in vasoconstriction and vasodilation mediated by the carotid sinus baroreceptors after common carotid artery occlusion and release. In this preparation, the sciatic and femoral nerves constituted the only direct connection between the hind leg muscle mass and the rest of the dog. The muscle was perfused by blood at a constant pressure that was completely independent of the animal's arterial pressure. (Redrawn from Jones RD, Berne RM: *Am J Physiol* 204:461, 1963.)

whereas a decrease in carotid sinus pressure elicits vasoconstriction (Fig. 23-12). When the existing sympathetic constrictor tone is high, as in the experiment illustrated in Fig. 23-12, the decrease in blood flow evoked by common carotid artery occlusion is small, but the increase in flow after the release of occlusion is large. The vasodilation produced by baroreceptor stimulation is caused by inhibition of sympathetic vasoconstrictor activity.

The resistance vessels in skeletal muscle contribute significantly to maintenance of the arterial blood pressure, because skeletal muscle constitutes a large fraction of the body's mass, and hence the muscle vasculature constitutes the largest vascular bed. Therefore, participation of the skeletal muscle vessels in vascular reflexes is important in maintaining a normal arterial blood pressure.

A comparison of the sympathetic neural effects on the blood vessels of the muscle and skin is summarized in Fig. 23-13. Note that the lower the basal tone of the skin vessels, the greater their constrictor response; and note also the absence of active cutaneous vasodilation.

Local factors. In active skeletal muscle, blood flow is regulated by metabolic factors (see Chapter 21). In resting muscle, neural factors predominate, and they superimpose neurogenic tone on the basal tone (Fig. 23-13). Cutting the sympathetic nerves to muscle abolishes the neural component of vascular tone, and it unmasks the intrinsic basal tone of the blood vessels. *The neural and local mechanisms that regulate blood flow oppose each other, and during muscle contraction the local vasodilator mechanism supervenes.* However, during exercise, strong sympathetic nerve stimulation attenuates slightly the vasodilation induced by locally released metabolites.

CEREBRAL CIRCULATION

Blood reaches the brain through the internal carotid and vertebral arteries. The vertebral arteries join to form the basilar artery, which, in conjunction with branches of the internal carotid arteries, forms the **circle of Willis.**

A unique feature of the cerebral circulation is that it lies within a rigid structure, the cranium. Because intracranial contents are incompressible, any increase in arterial inflow, as induced by arteriolar dilation, must be associated with a comparable increase in venous outflow. The volume of blood and of extravascular fluid can vary considerably in most body tissues. In the brain, however, the volume of blood and

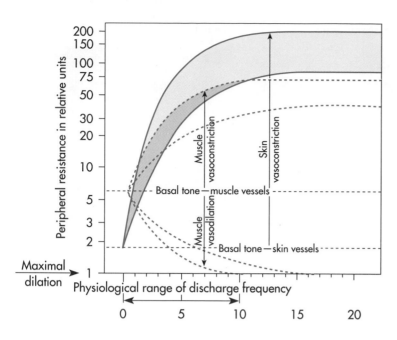

■ **Fig. 23-13** Basal tone and the range of response of the resistance vessels in muscle *(dashed lines)* and skin *(shaded area)* to stimulation and section of the sympathetic nerves. Peripheral resistance is plotted on a logarithmic scale. (Redrawn from Celander O, Folkow B: *Acta Physiol Scand* 29:241, 1953.)

extravascular fluid is relatively constant; a change in one of these fluid volumes must be accompanied by a reciprocal change in the other. In contrast to most other organs, the rate of total cerebral blood flow is maintained within a narrow range; in humans, it averages 55 ml/min/100 g of brain.

Estimation of Cerebral Blood Flow

Total cerebral blood flow can be measured in humans by the nitrous oxide (N₂O) method, which is based on the Fick principle (see Chapter 16). The subject breathes a gas mixture of 15% N_2O, 21% O_2, and 64% N_2 for 10 minutes, which is sufficient time to permit equilibration of the N_2O between the brain tissue and the blood leaving the brain. Simultaneous samples of arterial blood (which can be taken from any artery) and mixed cerebral venous blood (taken from the internal jugular vein) are taken at the start of N_2O administration. Similar techniques, involving radioactive gases, have been developed more recently.

Regulation of Cerebral Blood Flow

Of all the body tissues, the brain is the least tolerant of ischemia. Interruption of cerebral blood flow for as little as 5 seconds results in loss of consciousness, and ischemia lasting just a few minutes results in irreversible tissue damage. Fortunately, regulation of the cerebral circulation is mainly under direction of the brain itself. Local regulatory mechanisms and reflexes originating in the brain maintain cerebral circulation at a relatively constant level.

Neural factors. The cerebral vessels are innervated by the cervical sympathetic nerve fibers that accompany the internal carotid and vertebral arteries into the cranial cavity. The importance of neural regulation of the cerebral circulation is controversial. The sympathetic control of the cerebral vessels appears to be weaker than in other vascular beds, and the contractile state of the cerebrovascular smooth muscle appears to depend mainly on local metabolic factors.

Elevation of intracranial pressure, as caused by a brain tumor, results in an increase in systemic blood pressure. This response, called **Cushing's phenomenon,** is apparently evoked by ischemic stimulation of vasomotor regions in the medulla. Cushing's phenomenon helps maintain cerebral blood flow in such conditions as expanding intracranial tumors.

Local factors. *Generally, total cerebral blood flow is relatively constant. However, regional blood flow in the brain is associated with regional neural activity.* For example, movement of one hand results in increased blood flow only in the hand area of the contralateral sensorimotor and premotor cortex. Also, talking, reading, and other stimuli to the cerebral cortex are associated with increased blood flow in the appropriate regions of the contralateral cortex (Fig. 23-14). Glucose uptake also corresponds with regional cortical neuronal activity. For example when the retina is stimulated by light, uptake of ¹⁴C-2-deoxyglucose is enhanced in the visual cortex.

The cerebral vessels are very sensitive to carbon dioxide tension. Increases in arterial blood CO_2 tension (Pa_{CO_2}) elicit marked cerebral vasodilation; inhalation of 7% CO_2 increases cerebral blood flow twofold. Conversely, decreases in Pa_{CO_2}, which can be caused by hyperventilation, diminish cerebral blood flow. CO_2 causes these changes by altering perivascular (and probably intracellular vascular smooth muscle) pH, which in turn alters arterial resistance to flow. By independently changing P_{CO_2} and bicarbonate concentration, pial vessel diameter and blood flow have been shown to be inversely related to the pH, regardless of the level of the P_{CO_2}.

Carbon dioxide can diffuse to the vascular smooth muscle from the brain tissue or from the lumen of the vessels, whereas hydrogen ions in the blood are prevented from reaching the arteriolar smooth muscle by the **blood-brain**

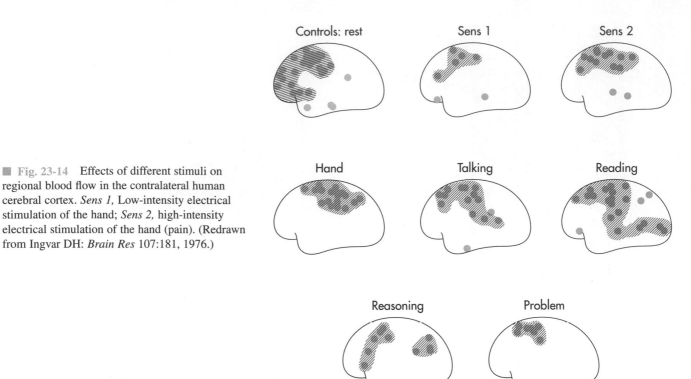

■ Fig. 23-14   Effects of different stimuli on regional blood flow in the contralateral human cerebral cortex. *Sens 1,* Low-intensity electrical stimulation of the hand; *Sens 2,* high-intensity electrical stimulation of the hand (pain). (Redrawn from Ingvar DH: *Brain Res* 107:181, 1976.)

barrier. Hence, the cerebral vessels dilate when the hydrogen ion concentration of the cerebrospinal fluid is increased, but these vessels dilate only minimally in response to an increase in the hydrogen ion concentration of the arterial blood.

The K^+ concentration also affects cerebral blood flow. Stimuli such as hypoxia, electrical stimulation of the brain, and seizures elicit rapid increases in cerebral blood flow and in the perivascular K^+ concentration. The increases in K^+ concentration are similar in magnitude to those that produce pial arteriolar dilation when K^+ is applied topically to these vessels. However, the increase in K^+ is not sustained throughout the period of cerebral stimulation. Hence, only the initial increase in cerebral blood flow can be attributed to the release of K^+.

Adenosine also affects cerebral blood flow. Adenosine levels of the brain increase in response to ischemia, hypoxemia, hypotension, hypocapnia, electrical stimulation of the brain, and induced seizures. When applied topically, adenosine is a potent dilator of the pial arterioles. In fact, any intervention that either reduces the O_2 supply to the brain or increases the O_2 requirements of the brain results in rapid (within 5 seconds) formation of adenosine in the cerebral tissue. Unlike the channges in pH or K^+, the adenosine concentration of the brain increases with initiation of the change in O_2 supply, and it remains elevated throughout the period of O_2 imbalance. The adenosine that is released into the cerebrospinal fluid when the brain O_2 supply is diminished becomes incorporated into the adenine nucleotides in the cerebral tissues. These local factors—pH, K^+, and adenosine—may all act in concert to adjust the cerebral blood flow to the metabolic activity of the brain.

The cerebral circulation displays reactive hyperemia and excellent autoregulation when the arterial blood pressure is between 60 and 160 mm Hg. Mean arterial pressures below 60 mm Hg result in reduced cerebral blood flow and subsequently in syncope, whereas mean pressures above 160 may lead to increased permeability of the blood-brain barrier and consequently to cerebral edema. Autoregulation of cerebral blood flow is abolished by hypercapnia or by any other potent vasodilator. None of the candidates for metabolic regulation of cerebral blood flow accounts for this phenomenon. Hence, autoregulation of cerebral blood flow is probably mediated by a myogenic mechanism, although experimental proof is still lacking.

INTESTINAL CIRCULATION

Anatomy

The gastrointestinal tract is supplied by the celiac, superior mesenteric, and inferior mesenteric arteries. The superior mesenteric artery is the largest aortic branch, and it carries over 10% of the cardiac output. Small mesenteric arteries form an extensive vascular network in the submucosa of the gastrointestinal tract (Fig. 23-15). The arterial branches penetrate the longitudinal and circular muscle layers of the tract, and they give rise to third- and fourth-order arterioles. Some third-order arterioles in the submucosa supply the tips of the villi.

The direction of the blood flow in the capillaries and venules in a villus is opposite to that in the main arteriole (Fig. 23-16). This arrangement is a **countercurrent exchange system** (see Chapter 36). An effective countercurrent exchange also permits diffusion of O_2 from arterioles to venules. At low blood flow rates, a substantial portion of the O₂ of the blood may be shunted from arterioles to venules near the base of the villus. Thus, the supply of O₂ to the mucosal cells at the tip of the villus is reduced. When intestinal blood flow is very low, the shunting of O₂ is

exaggerated, and it may cause extensive necrosis of the intestinal villi.

Neural Regulation

The neural control of the mesenteric circulation is almost exclusively sympathetic. Increased sympathetic activity constricts the mesenteric arterioles and capacitance vessels. These responses are mediated by α-adrenergic receptors, which are prepotent in the mesenteric circulation; however, β-adrenergic receptors are also present. Infusion of a β-receptor agonist, such as isoproterenol, causes vasodilation.

In response to aggressive behavior or to artificial stimulation of the hypothalamic "defense" area, pronounced vasoconstriction occurs in the mesenteric vascular bed. This vasoconstriction shifts blood flow from the less important intestinal circulation to the more crucial skeletal muscles, heart, and brain.

Autoregulation

Autoregulation of blood flow in the intestinal circulation is not as well developed as in certain other vascular beds, such as those in the brain and kidney. The principal mechanism responsible for autoregulation is metabolic, although a myogenic mechanism probably also participates (see Chapter 21). The adenosine concentration in the mesenteric venous blood rises fourfold after brief arterial occlusion. It also rises during enhanced metabolic activity of the intestinal mucosa, such as during absorption of food. Adenosine is a potent vasodilator in the mesenteric vascular bed, and it may be the principal metabolic mediator of autoregulation. However, potassium and altered osmolality may also contribute to autoregulation.

The O₂ consumption of the small intestine is more rigorously controlled than is the blood flow. Experiments have shown that the O₂ uptake of the small intestine remained constant when arterial perfusion pressure was varied between 30 and 125 mm Hg.

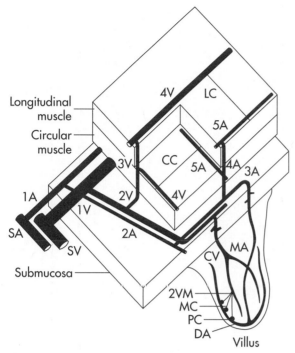

■ **Fig. 23-15** Distribution of small blood vessels to the rat intestinal wall. *Sa,* Small artery; *SV,* small vein; *1A* to *5A,* first- to fifth-order arterioles; *1V* to *4V,* first- to fourth-order venules; *CC* and *LC,* capillaries in circular and longitudinal muscle layers; *MA* and *CV,* main arteriole and collecting venule of a villus; *DA,* distribution arteriole; *2VM,* second-order mucosal venule; *PC,* precapillary sphincter; *MC,* mucosal capillary. (From Gore RW, Bohlen HG: *Am J Physiol* 233:H685, 1977.)

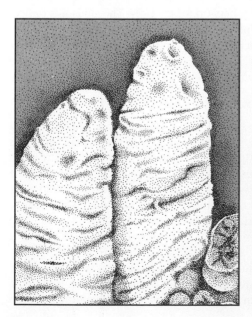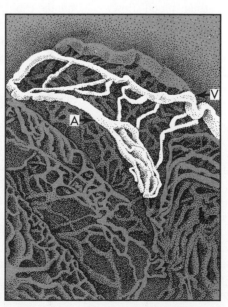

■ **Fig. 23-16** Scanning electron micrographs of rabbit intestinal villi *(left panel)* and corrosion cast of the microcirculation in the villus *(right panel)*. *A,* Arteriole; *V,* venule. (From Gannon BJ, Gore RW, Rogers PAW: *Biomed Res* 2[suppl]:235, 1981.)

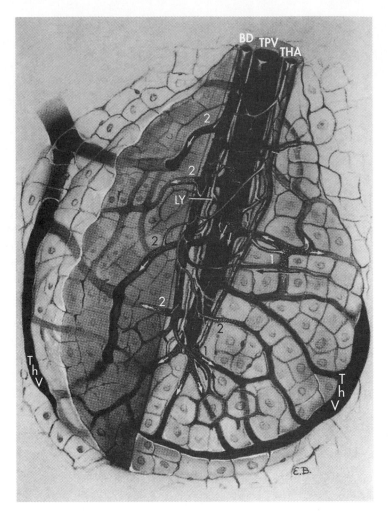

■ **Fig. 23-17**   Microcirculation to a hepatic acinus. *THA,* Terminal hepatic arteriole; *TPV,* terminal portal venule; *BD,* bile ductule; *ThV,* terminal hepatic venule; *LY,* lymphatic. The hepatic arterioles empty either directly *(1)* or through the peribiliary plexus *(2)* into the sinusoids that run from the terminal portal venule to the terminal hepatic venules. (From Rappaport SM: *Microvasc Res* 6:212, 1973.)

Functional Hyperemia

Food ingestion increases intestinal blood flow. The secretion of certain gastrointestinal hormones contributes to this hyperemia. **Gastrin** and **cholecystokinin** augment intestinal blood flow, and they are secreted when food is ingested. The absorption of food also affects intestinal blood flow. Undigested food has no vasoactive influence, whereas several products of digestion are potent vasodilators. Among the various constituents of chyme, the principal mediators of mesenteric hyperemia are glucose and fatty acids.

HEPATIC CIRCULATION
Anatomy

The blood flow to the liver is normally about 25% of cardiac output. *The hepatic blood flow is derived from two sources: the portal vein and the hepatic artery.* Ordinarily, the portal vein provides about three fourths of the blood flow. Because the portal venous blood has already passed through the gastrointestinal capillary bed, much of the O_2 of the portal vein blood flow has already been extracted. The hepatic artery delivers the remaining one fourth of the blood, which is fully saturated with O_2. *Hence, about three fourths of the O_2 used by the liver is derived from the hepatic arterial blood.*

The small branches of the portal vein and hepatic artery give rise to terminal portal venules and hepatic arterioles (Fig. 23-17). These terminal vessels enter the hepatic acinus (the functional unit of the liver) at its center. Blood flows from these terminal vessels into the sinusoids, which constitute the capillary network of the liver. The sinusoids radiate toward the periphery of the acinus, where they connect with the terminal hepatic venules. Blood from these terminal venules drains into progressively larger branches of the hepatic veins, which are tributaries of the inferior vena cava.

Hemodynamics

The mean blood pressure in the portal vein is about 10 mm Hg, and the mean blood pressure in the hepatic artery is about 90 mm Hg. The resistance of the vessels upstream to the hepatic sinusoids is considerably greater than that of the downstream vessels. Consequently, the pressure in the sinusoids is only 2 or 3 mm Hg greater than that in the hepatic veins and inferior vena cava. The ratio of presinusoidal to postsinusoidal resistance in the liver is much greater than is that in almost any other vascular bed. Hence, drugs and other interventions that alter the presinusoidal resistance usually affect the pressure in the sinusoids only slightly. Such changes in presinusoidal resistance have little effect on the fluid exchange across the sinusoidal wall. However, *changes in hepatic and in central venous pressure are transmitted almost quantitatively to the hepatic sinusoids, and they profoundly affect the transsinusoidal exchange of fluids.*

Regulation of Flow

Blood flow in the portal venous and hepatic arterial systems varies reciprocally. When blood flow is curtailed in one system, the flow increases in the other system. However, the ensuing increase in flow in one system usually does not fully compensate for the reduction in flow in the other system.

The portal venous system does not autoregulate. As portal venous pressure and flow are raised, resistance either remains constant or it decreases. The hepatic arterial system does autoregulate, however, and adenosine may be involved in this adjustment of blood flow.

When central venous pressure is elevated, as in **congestive heart failure,** large quantities of plasma water transude from the liver into the peritoneal cavity; such a fluid accumulation in the abdomen is known as **ascites.** Extensive fibrosis of the liver, as in the various types of **hepatic cirrhosis,** leads to a pronounced increase in hepatic vascular resistance, and thereby raises the pressure substantially in the portal venous system. The consequent increase in capillary hydrostatic pressure through the splanchnic circulation also leads to extensive fluid transudation into the abdominal cavity. Furthermore, the pressure may rise substantially in other veins that anastomose with the portal vein. For example, the esophageal veins may enlarge considerably to form **esophageal varices.** These varices may rupture and lead to severe, frequently fatal, internal bleeding. To prevent these grave problems associated with elevated portal venous pressure in cirrhosis of the liver, an anastomosis **(portacaval shunt)** is often created surgically between the portal vein and inferior vena cava to lower the portal venous pressure.

The liver tends to maintain a constant O_2 consumption, because the extraction of O_2 from the hepatic blood is very efficient. The rate of O_2 delivery to the liver varies; the liver compensates by an appropriate change in the fraction of O_2 extracted from the blood. This extraction is facilitated by the distance between the presinusoidal vessels at the acinar center and the postsinusoidal vessels at the periphery of the acinus (Fig. 23-17). The substantial distance between these types of vessels prevents a countercurrent exchange of O_2, contrary to the countercurrent exchange that occurs in an intestinal villus (Fig. 23-16).

The sympathetic nerves constrict the presinusoidal resistance vessels in the portal venous and hepatic arterial systems. Neural effects on the capacitance vessels are more important, however. The liver contains about 15% of the total blood volume of the body. Under appropriate conditions, such as in response to hemorrhage, about half of the hepatic blood volume can be rapidly expelled by constriction of the capacitance vessels (see also Chapter 24). *Hence, the liver*

constitutes an important blood reservoir in humans. In certain other species, such as the dog, the spleen is a more important blood reservoir.

FETAL CIRCULATION

In Utero

Before birth, the circulation of the fetus differs from that of the postnatal infant. The most important difference is that the fetal lungs are functionally inactive, and the fetus depends completely on the placenta for O_2 and nutrient supply. Oxygenated fetal blood from the placenta passes through the umbilical vein to the liver. Approximately half of the flow from the placenta passes though the liver, and the remainder bypasses the liver and reaches the inferior vena cava through the **ductus venosus** (Fig. 23-18). In the inferior vena cava, blood from the ductus venosus joins the blood returning from the lower trunk and extremities. This combined stream in turn merges with the blood from the liver through the hepatic veins.

The streams of blood tend to maintain their identities in the inferior vena cava and are divided into two streams of unequal size by the edge of the interatrial septum **(crista dividens).** The larger stream, which contains mainly blood from the umbilical vein, is shunted from the inferior vena cava to the left atrium through the **foramen ovale** (Fig. 23-18). The other stream passes into the right atrium, where it merges with blood returning from the upper parts of the body through the superior vena cava and with blood from the myocardium.

In contrast to the adult, in whom the right and left ventricles pump in series, the ventricles in the fetus operate essentially in parallel. Because the pulmonary vascular resistance of the fetus is large, only one tenth of right ventricular output passes through the lungs. The remainder passes from the pulmonary artery through the ductus arteriosus to the aorta at a point distal to the origins of the arteries to the head and upper extremities. Blood flows from the pulmonary artery to the aorta, because the pulmonary vascular resistance is high and the diameter of the ductus arteriosus is as large as that of the descending aorta.

The large volume of blood that passes through the foramen ovale into the left atrium is joined by blood returning from the lungs, and it is pumped out by the left ventricle into the aorta. Most of the blood in the ascending aorta goes to the head, upper thorax, and arms; the remainder joins blood from the ductus arteriosus and supplies the rest of the body. The amount of blood pumped by the left ventricle is about half that pumped by the right ventricle. The major fraction of the blood that passes down the descending aorta comes from the ductus arteriosus and right ventricle and flows by way of the two umbilical arteries to the placenta.

Fig. 23-18 indicates the O_2 saturations of the blood at various points of the fetal circulation. Fetal blood that leaves the placenta is 80% saturated, but the saturation of the blood that passes through the foramen ovale is reduced to 67%. This reduction in O_2 saturation is caused by mixing with

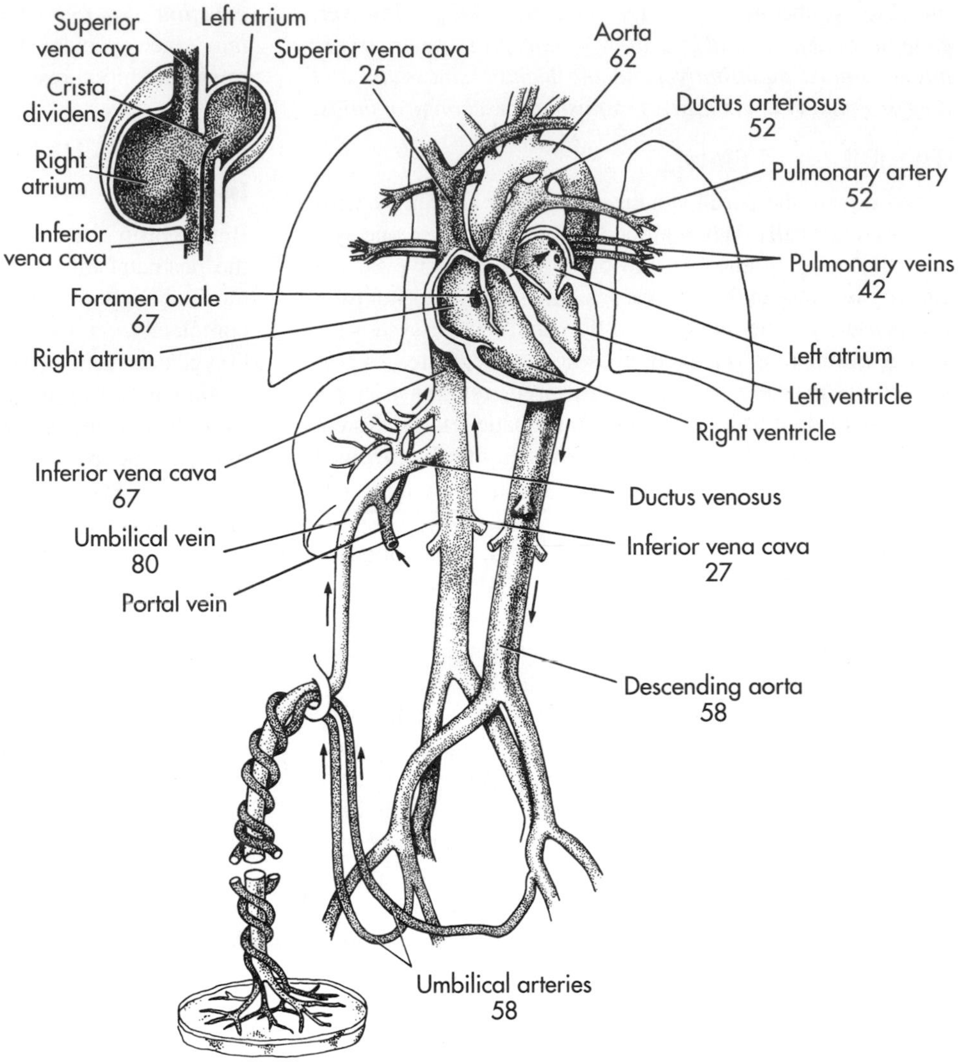

■ **Fig. 23-18** Schematic diagram of the fetal circulation. The numbers represent the percentage of O_2 saturation of the blood flowing in the indicated blood vessel. The inset at upper left illustrates the direction of flow of a major portion of the inferior vena caval blood through the foramen ovale to the left atrium. (Data from Dawes GS, Mott JC, Widdicombe JG: *J Physiol* 126:563, 1954.)

desaturated blood returning from the lower part of the body and the liver. Addition of the desaturated blood from the lungs reduces the O_2 saturation of left ventricular blood to 62%, which is the level of saturation of the blood reaching the head and upper extremities.

The blood in the right ventricle, which is a mixture of desaturated superior vena caval blood, coronary venous blood, and inferior vena caval blood, is only 52% saturated with O_2. When the major portion of this blood traverses the ductus arteriosus and joins that pumped out by the left ventricle, the resulting O_2 saturation of the blood traveling to the lower part of the body and back to the placenta is 58%. Thus, the tissues that receive the most highly saturated blood are the liver, heart, and upper parts of the body, including the head.

At the placenta, the chorionic villi dip into the maternal sinuses, and O_2, CO_2, nutrients, and metabolic waste products are exchanged across the membranes. The barrier to exchange prevents equilibration of PO_2 between the two circulations at normal rates of blood flow. Therefore, the O_2 tension of the fetal blood that leaves the placenta is very low. Were it not for the fact that fetal hemoglobin has a greater affinity for O_2 than does adult hemoglobin, the fetus would not receive an adequate O_2 supply. The fetal oxyhemoglobin dissociation curve is shifted to the left. Therefore, at equal pressures of O_2, fetal blood carries significantly more O_2 than does maternal blood.

In early fetal life, the high glycogen levels that prevail in the cardiac myocytes may protect the heart from acute periods of hypoxia. The glycogen levels decrease in late fetal life, and they reach adult levels by term.

If a pregnant woman is subjected to hypoxia, the reduced blood O_2 tension in the fetus evokes tachycardia and an increase in blood flow through the umbilical vessels. If the hypoxia persists or if flow through the umbilical vessels is impaired, fetal distress occurs and is manifested initially as bradycardia.

Circulatory Changes That Occur at Birth

The umbilical vessels have thick muscular walls that react to trauma, tension, sympathomimetic amines, bradykinin, angiotensin, and changes in PO_2. In animals in which the umbilical cord is not tied, hemorrhage of the newborn is minimized by constriction of these large umbilical vessels in response to the stimuli cited above.

Closure of the umbilical vessels increases the total peripheral resistance and the arterial blood pressure. When blood flow through the umbilical vein ceases, the ductus venosus, a thick-walled vessel with a muscular sphincter, closes. The factor that initiates closure of the ductus venosus is unknown.

Immediately after birth, the asphyxia caused by constriction or clamping of the umbilical vessels, together with the cooling of the body, activates the respiratory center of the newborn infant. As the lungs fill with air, pulmonary vascular resistance decreases to about one tenth of the value that existed before lung expansion. This vascular resistance change is not caused by the presence of O_2 in the lungs, because the change is just as great if the lungs are filled with nitrogen. However, filling the lungs with liquid does not reduce pulmonary vascular resistance.

After birth, the left atrial pressure is raised above that in the inferior vena cava and right atrium by (1) the decrease in pulmonary resistance, with the consequent large flow of blood through the lungs to the left atrium; (2) the reduction of flow to the right atrium, caused by occlusion of the umbilical vein; and (3) the increased resistance to left ventricular output produced by occlusion of the umbilical arteries. The reversal of the pressure gradient across the atria abruptly closes the valve over the foramen ovale, and the septal leaflets fuse over several days.

The decrease in pulmonary vascular resistance causes the pressure in the pulmonary artery to fall to about one-half its previous level (to about 35 mm Hg). This change in pressure, coupled with a slight increase in aortic pressure, reverses the flow of blood through the ductus arteriosus. However, within several minutes, the large ductus arteriosus begins to constrict. This constriction produces turbulent flow, which is manifested as a murmur in the newborn infant. Constriction of the ductus arteriosus is progressive and is usually complete within 1 to 2 days after birth. Closure of the ductus arteriosus appears to be initiated by the high O_2 tension of the arterial blood passing through it; pulmonary ventilation with O_2 closes the ductus, whereas ventilation with air low in O_2 opens this shunt vessel. Whether O_2 acts directly on the ductus or through the release of a vasoconstrictor substance is not known.

The ductus arteriosus occasionally fails to close after birth. This congenital cardiovascular abnormality, called **patent ductus arteriosus,** can be corrected surgically.

At the time of birth, the walls of the two ventricles are about equal in thickness. In addition, the muscle layer of the pulmonary arterioles is thick; this thickness is partly responsible for the high pulmonary vascular resistance of the fetus. After birth, the thickness of the walls of the right ventricle diminishes, as does the muscle layer of the pulmonary arterioles. The left ventricular walls also become thicker. These changes progress over a period of weeks after birth.

SUMMARY

Coronary Circulation

1. The physical factors that influence coronary blood flow are the viscosity of the blood, the frictional resistance of the vessel walls, the aortic pressure, and the extravascular compression of the vessels within the walls of the left ventricle.

2. Left coronary blood flow is restricted during ventricular systole by extravascular compression, and the flow is greatest during diastole when the intramyocardial vessels are not compressed.

3. Neural regulation of coronary blood flow is much less important than metabolic regulation. Activation of the cardiac sympathetic nerves constricts the coronary resistance vessels. However, the enhanced myocardial metabolism caused by the associated increase in heart rate and contractile force produces vasodilation, which overrides the direct constrictor effect of sympathetic nerve stimulation. Stimulation of the cardiac branches of the vagus nerves slightly dilates the coronary arterioles.

4. A striking parallelism exists between metabolic activity of the heart and coronary blood flow. A decrease in oxygen supply or an increase in oxygen demand apparently releases a vasodilator substance that decreases coronary resistance. Of the known factors (CO_2, O_2, H^+, K^+, adenosine) that can mediate this response, adenosine appears to be the most likely candidate.

5. Prolonged, severe reduction in coronary blood flow leads to myocardial cell necrosis and thereby impairs cardiac contraction.

6. Moderate, sustained reductions in coronary blood flow may evoke myocardial hibernation, which is a reversible impairment of mechanical performance associated with a down-regulation of cardiac metabolism.

7. Transient periods of severe ischemia followed by reperfusion may induce myocardial stunning, a temporary stage of impaired mechanical performance by the heart.

8. In response to gradual occlusion of a coronary artery, collateral vessels from adjacent unoccluded arteries develop and supply blood to the compromised myocardium distal to the point of occlusion.

9. The myocardium functions only aerobically, and in general it uses substrates in proportion to their arterial concentration.

Skin Circulation

1. Most of the resistance vessels in the skin are under dual control of the sympathetic nervous system and local vasodilator metabolites. The arteriovenous anastomoses found in the hands, feet, and face, however, are solely under neural control.

2. The main function of skin blood vessels is to aid in the regulation of body temperature by constricting to conserve heat and by dilating to lose heat.

3. Skin blood vessels dilate directly and reflexly in response to heat, and they constrict directly and reflexly in response to cold.

Skeletal Muscle Circulation

1. Skeletal muscle blood flow is regulated centrally by the sympathetic nerves and locally by the release of vasodilator metabolites.

2. In subjects at rest, neural regulation of blood flow is paramount, but it yields to metabolic regulation during muscle contractions (such as during exercise).

Cerebral Circulation

1. Cerebral blood flow is predominantly regulated by metabolic factors, especially CO_2, K^+, and adenosine.

2. Increased regional cerebral activity produced by stimuli such as touch, pain, hand motion, talking, reading, reasoning, and problem solving are associated with enhanced blood flow in the activated area of the contralateral cerebral cortex.

Intestinal Circulation

1. The microcirculation in the intestinal villi constitutes a countercurrent exchange system for O_2. The presence of this countercurrent exchange system places the villi in jeopardy in states of low blood flow.

2. The splanchnic resistance and capacitance vessels are very responsive to changes in sympathetic neural activity.

Hepatic Circulation

1. The liver receives about 25% of cardiac output; about three fourths of this output is from the portal vein and about one fourth from the hepatic artery.

2. When flow is diminished in either the portal or hepatic system, flow in the other system usually increases, but not proportionately.

3. The liver tends to maintain a constant O_2 consumption, in part because its mechanism for extracting O_2 from the blood is so efficient.

4, The liver normally contains about 15% of the total blood volume. It serves as an important blood reservoir for the body.

Fetal Circulation

1. In the fetus, a large percentage of right atrial blood passes through the foramen ovale to the left atrium, and a large percentage of pulmonary arterial blood passes through the ductus arteriosus to the aorta.

2. At birth, the umbilical vessels, ductus venosus, and ductus arteriosus close by contraction of their muscle layers.

3. The reduction in pulmonary vascular resistance caused by lung inflation is the main factor that reverses the pressure gradient between the atria, and thereby closes the foramen ovale.

BIBLIOGRAPHY

Journal articles

Bolli R: Myocardial "stunning" in man, *Circulation* 86:1671, 1992.

Chrissobolis S, Sobey CG: Evidence that rho-kinase activity contributes to cerebral vascular tone in vivo and is enhanced during chronic hypertension: comparison with protein kinase C, *Circ Res* 88:774: 2001.

Escourrou P et al: Cardiopulmonary and carotid baroflex control of splanchnic and forearm circulation, *Am J Physiol* 264:H777, 1993.

Faraci FM, Heistad DD: Regulation of the cerebral circulation: role of endothelium and potassium channels, *Physiol Rev* 78:53, 1998.

Gjuissani DA et al: Dynamics of cardiovascular responses to repeated partial umbilical cord compression in late-gestation sheep fetus, *Am J Physiol* 273:H2351, 1997.

Goto M, VanBavel E, Giezeman MJMM: Vasodilatory effect of pulsatile pressure on coronary resistance vessels, *Circ Res* 79:1039, 1996.

Hoffman JIE, Spaan JAE: Pressure-flow relations in coronary circulation, *Physiol Rev* 70:331, 1990.

Ito S: Role of nitric oxide in glomerular arterioles and macula densa, *News Physiol Sci* 9:115, 1994.

Kusuoka H, Marban E: Cellular mechanisms of myocardial stunning, *Annu Rev Physiol* 54:243, 1992.

Lautt WW, Legare DJ: Passive autoregulation of portal venous pressure: distensible hepatic resistance, *Am J Physiol* 263:G702, 1992.

Lautt WW, Schafer J, Legare DJ: Hepatic blood flow distribution: consideration of gravity, liver surface, and norepinephrine on regional heterogeneity, *Can J Physiol* 71:128, 1993.

Maass-Moreno R, Rothe CF: Contribution of large hepatic veins to postsinusoidal vascular resistance, *Am J Physiol* 262:G14, 1992.

Marshall JM: Skeletal muscle vasculature and systemic hypoxia, *News Physiol Sci* 10:274, 1995.

Olsson RA, Pearson JD: Cardiovascular purinoceptors, *Physiol Rev* 70:761, 1990.

Schaper W: Molecular mechanisms of coronary collateral vessel growth, *Circ Res* 79:911, 1996.

Symons JD, Firoozmand E, Longhurst JC: Repeated dipyridamole administration enhances collateral-dependent flow and regional function during exercise: a role for adenosine, *Circ Res* 73:503, 1993.

Tysebnko VA, Yanchuk PI: Central nervous control of hepatic circulation, *J Auton Nerv Syst* 33:255, 1991.

Zellers TM, McCormick J, Wu Y: Interaction among ET-1, endothelium-derived nitric oxide, and prostacyclin in pulmonary arteries and veins, *Am J Physiol* 267:H139, 1994.

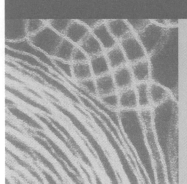

chapter twenty-four

Interplay of Central and Peripheral Factors in the Control of the Circulation

The primary function of the circulatory system is to deliver the supplies needed for tissue metabolism and growth and to remove the products of metabolism. In previous chapters, we have discussed the contributions of the component parts of the cardiovascular system to maintain adequate tissue perfusion under different physiological conditions.

In this chapter, we explore the interrelationships among the various components of the circulatory system. The autonomic nervous system and the baroreceptors and chemoreceptors play key roles in regulating the cardiovascular system. However, the control of fluid balance by the kidney, adrenal cortex, and central nervous system, with maintenance of a constant blood volume, is also very important.

In any well-regulated system, one way to evaluate the extent and sensitivity of its regulatory mechanisms is to disturb the system and to observe how it restores the preexisting steady state. Disturbances in the form of physical exercise and hemorrhage are used in the following sections to illustrate the operation of the various regulatory factors.

EXERCISE

The cardiovascular adjustments that take place during exercise consist of a combination of neural and local (chemical) factors. The neural factors include (1) **central command,** (2) reflexes that originate in the contracting muscle, and (3) the baroreceptor reflex.

Central command is the cerebrocortical activation of the sympathetic nervous system that produces cardiac acceleration, increased myocardial contractile force, and peripheral vasoconstriction. Reflexes are activated intramuscularly by stimulation of mechanoreceptors (by stretch, tension) and chemoreceptors (by products of metabolism) in response to muscle contraction. Impulses from these receptors travel centrally via small myelinated (group III) and unmyelinated (group IV) afferent nerve fibers. The group IV unmyelinated fibers may represent the muscle chemoreceptors, as no morphological chemoreceptor has been identified. The central connections of this reflex are unknown, but the efferent limb

consists of sympathetic nerve fibers to the heart and peripheral blood vessels. The baroreceptor reflex is described in Chapter 21, and the local factors that influence skeletal muscle blood flow (metabolic vasodilators) are described in Chapter 23. Vascular chemoreceptors are important in the regulation of the cardiovascular system during exercise. Evidence for this assertion comes from the observations that the pH, Pco_2, and Po_2 of arterial blood remain normal during exercise, and that the vascular chemoreceptors are located on the arterial side of the circulatory system.

Mild to Moderate Exercise

In humans or trained animals, anticipation of physical activity inhibits the vagal nerve impulses to the heart and increases sympathetic discharge. The simultaneous inhibition of parasympathetic areas and activation of sympathetic areas of the medulla increase heart rate and myocardial contractility. The tachycardia and enhanced contractility increase cardiac output.

Peripheral resistance. When cardiac stimulation occurs, the sympathetic nervous system also changes vascular resistance in the periphery. In skin, kidneys, splanchnic regions, and inactive muscle, sympathetic-mediated vasoconstriction increases vascular resistance, and thereby diverts blood away from these areas (Fig. 24-1). This increased vascular resistance persists throughout the period of exercise.

As cardiac output and blood flow to active muscles increase with progressive increases in the intensity of exercise, visceral blood flow (i.e., to the splanchnic and renal vasculatures) decreases. Blood flow to the myocardium increases, whereas flow to the brain is unchanged. Skin blood flow initially decreases during exercise, and then it increases as body temperature rises with increments in the duration and intensity of exercise. Skin blood flow finally decreases when the skin vessels constrict as total body O_2 consumption nears its maximal value (Fig. 24-1).

The major circulatory adjustment to prolonged exercise occurs in the vasculature of the active muscles. Local formation of vasoactive metabolites dilates the resistance vessels

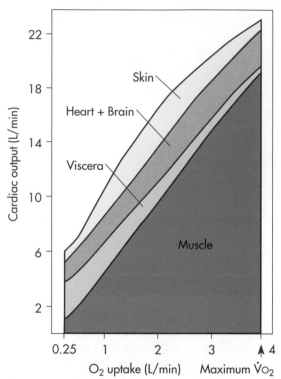

■ Fig. 24-1 Approximate distribution of cardiac output at rest and at different levels of exercise up to the maximal O_2 consumption ($\dot{V}O_{2max}$) in a normal young man. (Redrawn from Ruch HP, Patton TC: *Physiology and biophysics,* ed 12, Philadelphia, 1974, WB Saunders.)

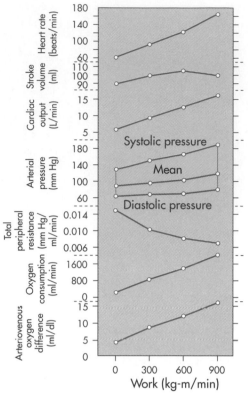

■ Fig. 24-2 Effect of different levels of exercise on several cardiovascular variables. (Data from Carlsten A, Grimby G: *The circulatory response to muscular exercise in man,* Springfield, Ill, 1966, Charles C Thomas.)

markedly. This dilation progresses with increases in the intensity of exercise. Potassium is one of the vasodilator substances released by the contracting muscle, and this ion may be partly responsible for the initial decrease in vascular resistance in the active muscles. Other contributing factors may be the release of adenosine and a decrease in tissue pH during sustained exercise. The local accumulation of metabolites relaxes the terminal arterioles. As a result, blood flow through the muscle may increase 15-fold to 20-fold above the resting level. This metabolic vasodilation of the precapillary vessels in active muscles occurs very soon after the onset of exercise. The decrease in total peripheral resistance (TPR) enables the heart to pump more blood at a lesser load and it pumps more efficiently than if TPR were unchanged (see Chapters 22 and 23).

Marked changes in the capillary circulation also occur during exercise. Only a small percentage of the capillaries are perfused at rest, whereas in actively contracting muscle, all or nearly all of the capillaries contain flowing blood **(capillary recruitment).** The surface area available for exchange of gases, water, and solutes is increased many times. Furthermore, the hydrostatic pressure in the capillaries is increased because of the relaxation of the resistance vessels. Hence, water and solutes move into the muscle tissue. Tissue pressure rises and remains elevated during exercise as fluid continues to move out of the capillaries; this

tissue fluid is carried away by the lymphatics. Lymph flow is increased as a result of the rise in capillary hydrostatic pressure and of the massaging effect of the contracting muscles on the valve-containing lymphatic vessels (see Fig. 23-11).

Contracting muscle avidly extracts O_2 from the perfusing blood and thereby increases arteriovenous O_2 difference (Fig. 24-2). This release of O_2 from the blood is facilitated by the shift in the oxyhemoglobin dissociation curve during exercise. During exercise, the high concentration of CO_2 and the formation of lactic acid reduce the tissue pH. This decrease in pH plus the increase in temperature in the contracting muscle shifts the oxyhemoglobin dissociation curve to the right (see Chapter 28). Therefore, at any given partial pressure of O_2, less O_2 is held by the hemoglobin in the red cells, and consequently more O_2 is available for the tissues. Oxygen consumption may increase as much as sixtyfold, with only a fifteenfold increase in muscle blood flow. Muscle myoglobin may serve as a limited O_2 store during exercise, and it can release the attached O_2 at very low partial pressures. However, the myoglobin can also facilitate O_2 transport from capillaries to mitochondria by serving as an O_2 carrier.

Cardiac output. Because the enhanced sympathetic drive and the reduced parasympathetic inhibition of the sinoatrial node continue during exercise, tachycardia persists. If the workload is moderate and constant, the heart rate will reach a certain level and remain there throughout the period of exercise. However, if the workload increases, the heart rate increases concomitantly until a plateau of about 180 beats/min is reached during strenuous exercise. In contrast to the large increase in heart rate, the increase in stroke volume is only about 10% to 35%, the larger values occurring in trained individuals (Fig. 24-2). In well-trained distance runners, whose cardiac outputs can reach six to seven times the resting level, stroke volume reaches about twice the resting value.

Thus, the increase in cardiac output observed during exercise is correlated principally with an increase in heart rate. If the baroreceptors are denervated, the cardiac output and heart rate responses to exercise are small compared with those in animals with normally innervated baroreceptors. However, in dogs with total cardiac denervation, exercise still increases cardiac output as much as it does in normal animals. This increase in cardiac output is achieved chiefly by means of an elevated stroke volume. However, if a β-adrenergic receptor antagonist is given to the dogs with denervated hearts, exercise performance is impaired. The β-adrenergic receptor blocker apparently prevents the cardiac acceleration and enhanced contractility caused by increased amounts of circulating catecholamines. Therefore, the increase in cardiac output necessary for maximal exercise performance is limited.

Venous return. In addition to the contribution made by sympathetically mediated constriction of the capacitance vessels in both exercising and nonexercising parts of the body, venous return is aided by the auxillary pumping action of the working skeletal muscles and the muscles of respiration (see also Chapter 22). The intermittently contracting muscles compress the veins that course through them. Because the venous valves are oriented toward the heart, the contracting muscle pumps blood back toward the right atrium (see Chapter 23). In exercise, the flow of venous blood to the heart is also aided by the deeper and more frequent respirations that increase the pressure gradient between the abdominal and thoracic veins (intrathoracic pressure becomes more negative during exercise).

In humans, blood reservoirs do not contribute much to the circulating blood volume. In fact, blood volume is usually reduced slightly during exercise, as evidenced by a rise in the hematocrit ratio. This decrease in blood volume is caused by water loss externally through sweating and enhanced ventilation, and by fluid movement into the contracting muscle.

However, fluid loss is counteracted in several ways. The fluid loss from the vascular compartment into the contracting muscles eventually reaches a plateau as the interstitial fluid pressure rises and opposes the increased hydrostatic pressure in the capillaries of the active muscle. Fluid loss is partially offset by movement of fluid from the splanchnic regions and inactive muscle into the bloodstream. This influx of fluid results (1) from the decrease of hydrostatic pressure in the capillaries of these tissues, and (2) from an increase in the plasma osmolarity, because of movement of osmotically active molecules into the blood from the contracting muscle. In addition, reduced urine formation by the kidneys helps to conserve body water.

The large volume of venous blood returning to the heart is so effectively pumped through the lungs and out into the aorta that central venous pressure remains essentially constant. Thus, the Frank-Starling mechanism of a greater initial fiber length does not account for the greater stroke volume in moderate exercise. X-ray films of individuals at rest and during exercise reveal a decrease in heart size during exercise. However, during maximal or near-maximal exercise, right atrial pressure and end-diastolic ventricular volume do increase. Thus, the Frank-Starling mechanism contributes to the enhanced stroke volume in very vigorous exercise.

Arterial pressure. If the exercise involves a large proportion of the body musculature, such as in running or swimming, the reduction in total vascular resistance can be considerable. Nevertheless, arterial pressure starts to rise with the onset of exercise, and the increase in blood pressure roughly parallels the severity of the exercise performed (Fig. 24-2). Therefore, the increase in cardiac output is proportionally greater than the decrease in TPR. The vasoconstriction produced in the inactive tissues by the sympathetic nervous system (and to some extent by the release of catecholamines from the adrenal medulla) is important for maintenance of normal or increased blood pressure. Sympathectomy or drug-induced block of the adrenergic sympathetic nerve fibers decreases the arterial pressure (hypotension) during exercise.

Sympathetic neural activity also elicits vasoconstriction in active skeletal muscle when additional muscles are recruited. In experiments in which one leg is working at maximal levels and then the other leg starts to work, blood flow decreases in the first working leg. Furthermore, blood levels of norepinephrine rise significantly during exercise, and most of the norepinephrine is released from the sympathetic nerves to the active muscles.

As body temperature rises during exercise, the skin vessels dilate in response to thermal stimulation of the heat-regulating center in the hypothalamus, and the TPR decreases further. This reduction in TPR would reduce blood pressure were it not for the increased cardiac output and the constriction of arterioles in the renal, splanchnic, and other tissues.

In general, the mean arterial pressure rises during exercise as a result of the increase in cardiac output. However, the effect of enhanced cardiac output is offset by an overall decrease in TPR, and therefore the mean blood pressure increases only slightly. Vasoconstriction in the inactive vascular beds helps to maintain a normal arterial blood pressure for adequate perfusion of the active tissues. The actual mean arterial pressure attained during exercise thus represents a balance between cardiac output and TPR (see Chapter 19). Systolic pressure usually increases more than diastolic pressure, which results in an increase in pulse pressure (Fig. 24-2). The larger pulse pressure is primarily attributable to a greater stroke volume, but also to a more rapid ejection of blood by the left ventricle and a diminished peripheral runoff during the brief ventricular ejection period (see also Chapters 16 and 19).

Severe Exercise

During exhaustive exercise, the compensatory mechanisms begin to fail. Heart rate attains a maximal level of about 180 beats/min, and stroke volume reaches a plateau. The heart rate may then decrease, resulting in a fall in blood pressure. The subject also frequently becomes dehydrated. Sympathetic vasoconstrictor activity supersedes the vasodilator influence on the vessels of the skin. However, vasoconstriction of skin vessels also decreases the rate of heat loss. Body temperature is normally elevated in exercise. Reduction in heat loss through cutaneous vasoconstriction can lead to very high body temperatures and to acute distress during severe exercise. The tissue and blood pH decrease as a result of increased lactic acid and CO_2 production. The reduced pH is probably the key factor that determines the maximal amount of exercise a given individual can tolerate. Muscle pain, a subjective feeling of exhaustion, and a loss of will to continue determine the exercise tolerance. A summary of the neural and local effects of exercise on the cardiovascular system is diagrammed in Fig. 24-3.

Postexercise Recovery

When exercise stops, heart rate and cardiac output abruptly decrease—the sympathetic drive to the heart is essentially removed. In contrast, TPR remains low for some time after the exercise is stopped, presumably because of the accumulation of vasodilator metabolites in the muscles during the exercise period. As a result of the reduced cardiac output and persistence of vasodilation in the muscles, arterial pressure falls, often below preexercise levels, for brief periods. Blood pressure is then stabilized at normal levels by the baroreceptor reflexes.

Limits of Exercise Performance

The two main factors that limit skeletal muscle performance in the human body are the rate of O_2 utilization by the muscles and the O_2 supply to the muscles. O_2 usage by muscle is probably not a critical factor. During exercise, maximal O_2 consumption ($\dot{V}O_{2max}$) by a large percentage of the body muscle mass is unchanged or increases only slightly when additional muscles are activated. In fact, during exercise of a large muscle mass, as in vigorous bicycling, the addition of bilateral arm exercise without change in the cycling efforts produces only a small increase in cardiac output and $\dot{V}O_{2max}$ However, the additional arm exercise decreases blood flow to the legs. This centrally mediated (baroreceptor reflex) vasoconstriction during maximal cardiac output prevents the fall in blood pressure that would otherwise be caused by metabolically induced vasodilation in the active muscle. If muscle O_2 usage were a significant limiting factor, recruitment of more contracting muscles would use much more O_2 to meet the enhanced O_2 requirements.

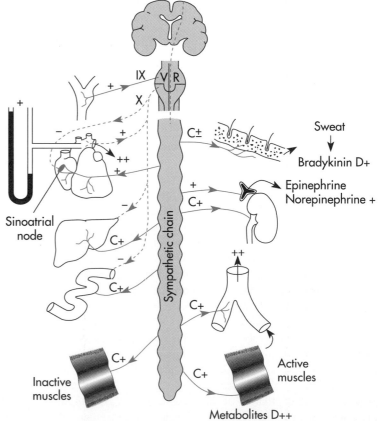

■ **Fig. 24-3**   Cardiovascular adjustments in exercise. *VR,* Vasomotor region; *C,* vasoconstrictor activity; *D,* vasodilator activity; *IX,* glossopharyngeal nerve; *X,* vagus nerve, +, increased activity, –, decreased activity.

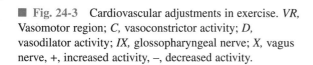

Limitation of O_2 supply could be caused by inadequate oxygenation of blood in the lungs or limitation of the supply of O_2-laden blood to the muscles. Failure to fully oxygenate blood by the lungs can be excluded, because even with the most strenuous exercise at sea level, arterial blood is fully saturated with O_2. Therefore, O_2 delivery to the active muscles (or blood flow, because arterial blood O_2 content is normal) appears to be the limiting factor in muscle performance. This limitation could be caused by the inability to increase cardiac output beyond a critical level. In turn, this inability is caused by a limitation of stroke volume, because heart rate reaches maximal levels before $\dot{V}O_{2max}$ is reached. *Hence, the major factor that limits muscle performance is the pumping capacity of the heart.*

During exercise of a small group of muscles, such as those found in the hand, the limiting factor is unknown, but it appears to lie within the muscle.

Physical Training and Conditioning

The response of the cardiovascular system to regular exercise is to increase its capacity to deliver O_2 to the active muscles and to improve the ability of the muscle to utilize O_2. The $\dot{V}O_{2max}$ varies with the level of physical conditioning. Training progressively increases the $\dot{V}O_{2max}$, which reaches a plateau at the highest level of conditioning. Highly trained athletes have a lower resting heart rate, a greater stroke volume, and a lower peripheral resistance than they had before training or after deconditioning. The low resting heart rate is caused by a higher vagal tone and a lower sympathetic tone. During exercise, the maximal heart rate of the trained individual is the same as that in the untrained, but it is attained at a higher level of exercise.

The trained person also exhibits a low vascular resistance in the muscles. For example, if an individual exercises one leg regularly over an extended time and does not exercise the other leg, the vascular resistance is lower and the $\dot{V}O_{2max}$ is higher in the "trained" leg than in the "untrained" leg. Physical conditioning is also associated with greater extraction of O_2 from the blood (greater arteriovenous O_2 difference) by the muscles. With long-term training, capillary density in skeletal muscle increases. Also, an increase in the number of arterioles may account for the decrease in muscle vascular resistance. The numbers of mitochondria increase, as do the oxidative enzymes in the mitochondria. In addition, the levels of ATPase activity, myoglobin, and enzymes involved in lipid metabolism increase in response to physical conditioning.

Endurance training, such as running or swimming, increases left ventricular volume without increasing left ventricular wall thickness. In contrast, strength exercises, such as weight lifting, increase left ventricular wall thickness (hypertrophy) with little effect on ventricular volume. However, this increase in wall thickness is small relative to that observed in chronic hypertension, in which afterload is persistently elevated because of high peripheral resistance.

HEMORRHAGE

In an individual who has lost a large quantity of blood, the principal system affected is the cardiovascular system. The arterial systolic, diastolic, and pulse pressures decrease and the arterial pulse is rapid and feeble. The cutaneous veins collapse, and they fill slowly when compressed centrally. The skin is pale, moist, and slightly cyanotic. Respiration is rapid, but the depth of respiration may be shallow or deep.

Course of Arterial Blood Pressure Changes

Cardiac output decreases as a result of blood loss (see Chapter 22). The changes in mean arterial pressure evoked by an acute hemorrhage in experimental animals are illustrated in Fig. 24-4. If sufficient blood is rapidly withdrawn to decrease the mean arterial pressure to 50 mm Hg, the pressure then tends to rise spontaneously toward the control level over the next 20 or 30 minutes. In some animals (curve *A*, Fig. 24-4), this trend continues and normal pressures are regained within a few hours. In other animals (curve *B*, Fig. 24-4), the pressure rises initially after the cessation of hemorrhage. The pressure then begins to decline, and it continues to fall at an accelerating rate until death ensues. This progressive deterioration of cardiovascular function is termed **hemorrhagic shock.** *At some time after the hemorrhage, the deterioration of the cardiovascular system becomes irreversible. A lethal outcome can be prevented only temporarily by any known therapy, including massive transfusions of donor blood.*

Compensatory Mechanisms

The changes in arterial pressure immediately after an acute blood loss (Fig. 24-4) indicate that certain compensatory mechanisms must operate. Any mechanism that raises the

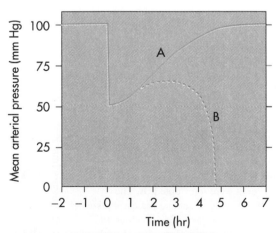

■ Fig. 24-4   Changes in mean arterial pressure after a rapid hemorrhage. At time zero, the animal is bled rapidly to a mean arterial pressure of 50 mm Hg. After a period in which the pressure returns toward the control level, some animals continue to improve until the control pressure is attained (curve *A*). However, in other animals, the pressure will begin to decline until death ensues (curve *B*).

arterial blood pressure toward normal in response to the reduction in pressure may be designated a **negative feedback mechanism.** This mechanism is termed *negative* because the direction of the secondary change in pressure is opposite to the direction of the initiating change after the acute blood loss. The following negative feedback responses are evoked: (1) the baroreceptor reflexes, (2) the chemoreceptor reflexes, (3) cerebral ischemia responses, (4) reabsorption of tissue fluids, (5) release of endogenous vasoconstrictor substances, and (6) renal conservation of salt and water.

Baroreceptor reflexes. The reduction in mean arterial pressure and in pulse pressure during hemorrhage decreases the stimulation of the baroreceptors in the carotid sinuses and aortic arch (see Chapter 21). Several cardiovascular responses are thus evoked, all of which tend to restore the normal level of arterial pressure. Reduction of vagal tone and enhancement of sympathetic tone increase heart rate and enhance myocardial contractility.

The increased sympathetic tone also produces generalized venoconstriction, which has the same hemodynamic consequences as a transfusion of blood (see Chapters 21 and 22). Sympathetic activation constricts certain blood reservoirs. In effect, this vasoconstriction acts as an autotransfusion of blood into the circulating bloodstream. In the dog, considerable quantities of blood are mobilized by the contraction of the spleen. In humans, the cutaneous, pulmonary, and hepatic vasculatures constitute the principal blood reservoirs.

Generalized arteriolar constriction is a prominent response to the diminished baroreceptor stimulation during hemorrhage. The reflex increase in peripheral resistance minimizes the fall in arterial pressure caused by the reduction of cardiac output. Fig. 24-5 shows the effect of an 8% blood loss on mean aortic pressure in a group of dogs. When both vagi were cut to eliminate the influence of the aortic arch baroreceptors, and only the carotid sinus baroreceptors were operative (Fig. 24-5, *A*), this hemorrhage decreased mean aortic pressure by 14%. This pressure change did not differ significantly from the pressure decline (12%) evoked by the same

hemorrhage before vagotomy (not shown). When the carotid sinuses were denervated and the aortic baroreceptor reflexes were intact, the 8% blood loss decreased mean aortic pressure by 38% (Fig. 24-5, *B*). Hence, the carotid sinus baroreceptors were more effective than the aortic baroreceptors in attenuating the fall in pressure. The aortic baroreceptor reflex must also have been operative, however, because when both sets of afferent baroreceptor pathways were interrupted (Fig. 24-5, *C*), an 8% blood loss reduced arterial pressure by 48%.

Although arteriolar constriction is widespread during hemorrhage, it is by no means uniform. Vasoconstriction is most pronounced in the cutaneous, skeletal muscle and splanchnic vascular beds, and it is slight or absent in the cerebral and coronary circulations in response to hemorrhage. In many instances, the cerebral and coronary vascular resistances are diminished. *Thus, the reduced cardiac output is redistributed to favor flow through the brain and the heart.*

In the early stages of mild to moderate hemorrhage, the changes in renal resistance are usually slight. The tendency for increased sympathetic activity to constrict the renal vessels is counteracted by autoregulatory mechanisms (see Chapters 21 and 34). With more prolonged and severe hemorrhages, however, renal vasoconstriction becomes intense. The reductions in renal circulation are most severe in the outer layers of the renal cortex. The inner zones of the cortex and outer zones of the medulla are spared.

The severe renal and splanchnic vasoconstriction during hemorrhage favors the heart and brain. However, if such constriction persists too long, it may be detrimental. Frequently, patients survive the acute hypotensive period of a prolonged, severe hemorrhage, only to die several days later from kidney failure that results from renal ischemia. Intestinal ischemia may also have dire effects. In the dog, for example, intestinal bleeding and extensive sloughing of the mucosa occur after only a few hours of hemorrhagic hypotension. Furthermore, the diminished splanchnic flow swells the centrilobular cells in the liver. The resulting obstruction of the hepatic sinusoids raises portal venous pressure, and this response intensifies intestinal blood loss. Fortunately, the

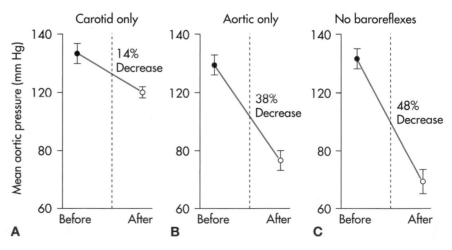

■ Fig. 24-5 Changes in mean aortic pressure in response to an 8% blood loss in three groups of dogs. **A,** The carotid sinus baroreceptors were intact and the aortic reflexes were interrupted. **B,** The aortic reflexes were intact and the carotid sinus reflexes were interrupted. **C,** All sinoaortic reflexes were abrogated. (Data from Shepherd JT: *Circulation* 50:418, 1974; derived from the data of Edis AJ: *Am J Physiol* 221:1352, 1971.)

pathological changes in the liver and intestine are usually much less severe in humans than in dogs.

Chemoreceptor reflexes. Reductions in arterial pressure below about 60 mm Hg do not evoke any additional responses through the baroreceptor reflexes, because this pressure level constitutes the threshold for stimulation (see Chapter 21). However, low arterial pressure may stimulate peripheral chemoreceptors because hypoxia develops in the chemoreceptor tissue as a consequence of inadequate local blood flow. Chemoreceptor excitation may then enhance the already existent peripheral vasoconstriction evoked by the baroreceptor reflexes. Also, respiratory stimulation assists venous return by the auxiliary pumping mechanism described in Chapter 22.

Cerebral ischemia. When the arterial pressure falls below about 40 mm Hg as a consequence of blood loss, the resulting cerebral ischemia activates the sympathoadrenal system. The sympathetic nervous discharge is several times greater than the maximal neural activity that occurs when the baroreceptors cease to be stimulated. Therefore, the vasoconstriction and facilitation of myocardial contractility may be pronounced. With more severe degrees of cerebral ischemia, however, the vagal centers also become activated. The resulting bradycardia may aggravate the hypotension that initiated the cerebral ischemia

Reabsorption of tissue fluids. The arterial hypotension, arteriolar constriction, and reduced venous pressure during hemorrhagic hypotension lower the hydrostatic pressure in the capillaries. The balance of these forces promotes the net reabsorption of interstitial fluid into the vascular compartment (see Chapter 20). The rapidity of this response is displayed in Fig. 24-6. In a group of cats, 45% of the estimated blood volume was removed over a 30-minute period. The mean arterial blood pressure declined rapidly to about 45 mm Hg. The pressure then returned rapidly, but only temporarily, to near the control level. The plasma colloid osmotic pressure declined markedly during the bleeding and contin-

ued to decrease more gradually for several hours. The reduction in colloid osmotic pressure reflects the dilution of the blood by tissue fluids that contain little protein.

Considerable quantities of fluid may thus be drawn into the circulation during hemorrhage. About 0.25 ml of fluid per minute per kilogram of body weight may be reabsorbed. Approximately 1 L of fluid per hour might be autoinfused from the interstitial spaces into the circulatory system of the average individual after an acute blood loss.

Substantial quantities of fluid may also be slowly shifted from intracellular to extracellular spaces. This fluid exchange is probably mediated by secretion of cortisol from the adrenal cortex in response to hemorrhage. Cortisol appears to be essential for the full restoration of plasma volume after hemorrhage.

Endogenous vasoconstrictors. The **catecholamines** epinephrine and norepinephrine are released from the adrenal medulla in response to the same stimuli that evoke widespread sympathetic nervous discharge (see Chapter 45). Blood levels of catecholamines are high during and after hemorrhage. When animals are bled to an arterial pressure level of 40 mm Hg, the level of catecholamines increases as much as 50 times.

Epinephrine comes almost exclusively from the adrenal medulla, whereas norepinephrine is derived from both the adrenal medulla and the peripheral sympathetic nerve endings. These humoral substances reinforce the effects of sympathetic nervous activity listed previously.

Vasopressin (antidiuretic hormone), a potent vasoconstrictor, is actively secreted by the posterior pituitary gland in response to hemorrhage (see Chapter 43). The plasma concentration of vasopressin rises progressively as the arterial blood pressure diminishes (Fig. 24-7). The receptors responsible for the augmented release of vasopressin are the sinoaortic baroreceptors and stretch receptors in the left atrium.

The diminished renal perfusion during hemorrhagic hypotension leads to the secretion of **renin** from the

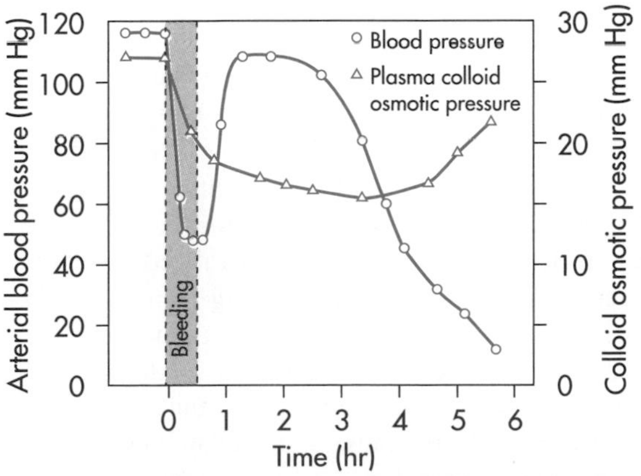

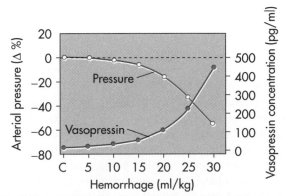

■ **Fig. 24-6** Changes in arterial blood pressure and plasma colloid osmotic pressure in response to withdrawal of 45% of the estimated blood volume over a 30-minute period, beginning at time zero. The data are the average values for 23 cats. (Redrawn from Zweifach BW: *Anesthesiology* 41:157, 1974.)

■ **Fig. 24-7** Mean percentage changes in arterial blood pressure and in plasma vasopressin concentration in response to blood loss (0.5 mg/kg/min) in a group of 12 dogs; the maximal volume of blood withdrawn was 30 ml/kg. (Redrawn from Shen YT, Cowley AW Jr, Vatner SF: *Circ Res* 68:1422, 1991.)

juxtaglomerular apparatus (see Chapter 36). This enzyme acts on a plasma protein, **angiotensinogen,** to form the decapeptide **angiotensin I,** which in turn is cleaved to the active octapeptide, angiotensin II, by the angiotensin converting enzyme; angiotensin II is a very powerful vasoconstrictor.

Renal conservation of salt and water. Fluid and electrolytes are conserved by the kidneys during hemorrhage in response to various stimuli, including the increased secretion of vasopressin noted previously (Fig. 24-7). The lower arterial pressure decreases the glomerular filtration rate and thus curtails the excretion of water and electrolytes. Also, the diminished renal blood flow raises the blood levels of angiotensin II, as described above. This polypeptide accelerates the release of **aldosterone** from the adrenal cortex. Aldosterone in turn stimulates sodium reabsorption by the renal tubules. Sodium is actively reabsorbed, and water accompanies the sodium passively (see also Chapter 36).

Decompensatory Mechanisms

In contrast to the negative feedback mechanisms just described, latent **positive feedback mechanisms** are also evoked by hemorrhage. These mechanisms exaggerate any primary change initiated by the blood loss. Specifically, positive feedback mechanisms aggravate the hypotension induced by blood loss and tend to initiate "vicious" cycles, which may lead to death.

Whether a positive feedback mechanism will lead to a vicious cycle depends on the gain of that mechanism. Gain is defined as the ratio of the secondary change evoked by a given mechanism to the initiating change itself. A gain greater than 1 induces a vicious cycle; a gain less than 1 does not. For example, consider a positive feedback mechanism with a gain of 2. If mean arterial pressure were to decrease by 10 mm Hg, a positive feedback mechanism with a gain of 2 would then evoke a secondary pressure reduction of 20 mm Hg, which in turn would cause a further decrease of 40 mm Hg. In other words, each change would induce a subsequent change that is twice as great. Hence, mean arterial pressure would decline at an ever-increasing rate until death occurred. This process is depicted in curve *B* in Fig. 24-4.

Conversely, a positive feedback mechanism with a gain of 0.5 would also exaggerate any change in mean arterial pressure, but the change would not necessarily lead to death. For example, if arterial pressure suddenly decreased by 10 mm Hg, the positive feedback mechanism would initiate a secondary, additional fall of 5 mm Hg. This decrease in turn would provoke a further decrease of 2.5 mm Hg. The process would continue in ever-diminishing steps until the arterial pressure approached an equilibrium value.

Some of the more important positive feedback mechanisms that are evident during hemorrhage include (1) cardiac failure, (2) acidosis, (3) central nervous system depression, (4) aberrations of blood clotting, and (5) depression of the reticuloendothelial system.

Cardiac failure. The role of cardiac failure in the progression of shock during hemorrhage is controversial. All

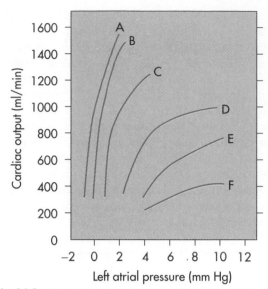

■ **Fig. 24-8** Ventricular function curve for the left ventricle during the course of hemorrhagic shock. Curve *A* represents the control function curve; curve *B*, 117 min; curve *C*, 247 min; curve *D*, 280 min; curve *E*, 295 min; and curve *F*, 310 min after the initial hemorrhage. (Redrawn from Crowell JW, Guyton AC: *Am J Physiol* 203:248, 1962.)

investigators agree that the heart fails terminally, but opinions differ about the importance of cardiac failure during earlier stages of hemorrhagic hypotension. Shifts to the right in ventricular function curves (Fig. 24-8) constitute experimental evidence of a progressive depression of myocardial contractility during hemorrhage.

The hypotension induced by hemorrhage reduces the coronary blood flow and therefore depresses ventricular function. The consequent reduction in cardiac output leads to a further decline in arterial pressure, a classic example of a positive feedback mechanism. Furthermore, the reduced blood flow to the peripheral tissues leads to an accumulation of vasodilator metabolites. The accumulation of these substances decreases peripheral resistance and therefore aggravates the fall in arterial pressure.

Acidosis. The inadequate blood flow during hemorrhage affects the metabolism of all cells in the body. The decreased oxygen delivery to the cells accelerates the production of lactic acid and other acid metabolites by the tissues. Furthermore, impaired kidney function prevents adequate excretion of the excess H^+, and generalized metabolic acidosis ensues (Fig. 24-9). The resulting depressant effect of acidosis on the heart further reduces tissue perfusion and thus aggravates the metabolic acidosis. Acidosis also diminishes the reactivity of the heart and resistance vessels to neurally released and circulating catecholamines, and thereby intensifies the hypotension.

Central nervous system depression. The hypotension in shock reduces cerebral blood flow. Moderate degrees of cerebral ischemia induce a pronounced sympathetic nervous stimulation of the heart, arterioles, and veins, as noted above.

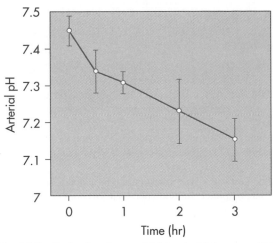

■ **Fig. 24-9**   Reduction in arterial blood pH (mean ± SD) in a group of 11 dogs whose blood pressure had been held at a level of 35 mm Hg by bleeding into a reservoir, beginning at time zero. (Modified from Markov AK et al: *Circ Shock* 8:9, 1981.)

In severe hypotension, however, the cardiovascular centers in the brainstem eventually become depressed because of inadequate cerebral blood flow. The resulting loss of sympathetic tone then reduces cardiac output and peripheral resistance. The consequent reduction in mean arterial pressure intensifies the inadequate cerebral perfusion.

Various endogenous **opioids,** such as **enkephalins** and **β-endorphin,** may be released into the brain substance or into the circulation in response to the same stresses that provoke circulatory shock. Opioids are contained, along with catecholamines, in secretory granules in the adrenal medulla and in sympathetic nerve terminals, and they are released together in response to stress. Similar stimuli release β-endorphin and adrenocorticotropic hormone (ACTH) from the anterior pituitary gland. Opioids depress the brainstem centers that mediate some of the compensatory autonomic adaptations to blood loss, endotoxemia, and other shock-provoking stresses. Conversely, the opioid antagonist **naloxone** improves cardiovascular function and survival in various forms of shock.

Aberrations of blood clotting. *The alterations of blood clotting after hemorrhage are typically biphasic. An initial phase of hypercoagulability is followed by a secondary phase of hypocoagulability and fibrinolysis.* In the initial phase, platelets and leukocytes adhere to the vascular endothelium, and intravascular clots, or **thrombi,** develop within a few minutes of the onset of severe hemorrhage. Coagulation may be extensive throughout the small blood vessels.

The initial phase is further enhanced by the release of thromboxane A_2 from various ischemic tissues. Thromboxane A_2 aggregates platelets. As more platelets aggregate, more thromboxane A_2 is released and more platelets are trapped. This form of positive feedback intensifies and prolongs the clotting tendency. The mortality from certain standard shock-provoking procedures has been reduced considerably

by the administration of anticoagulants such as heparin (see Chapter 14).

Reticuloendothelial system. During the course of hemorrhagic hypotension, reticuloendothelial system (RES) function becomes depressed. The phagocytic activity of the RES is modulated by an **opsonic protein.** The opsonic activity in plasma diminishes during shock, and this change may account in part for the depression of RES function. As a result, the antibacterial and antitoxin defense mechanisms are impaired. Endotoxins from the normal bacterial flora of the intestine constantly enter the circulation. Ordinarily, they are inactivated by the RES, principally in the liver. When the RES is depressed, these endotoxins invade the general circulation. *Endotoxins produce profound, generalized vasodilation, mainly by inducing the abundant synthesis of an isoform of nitric oxide synthase in the smooth muscle of blood vessels throughout the body.* The profound vasodilation aggravates the hemodynamic changes caused by blood loss.

In addition to their role in inactivating endotoxin, the macrophages release many of the mediators associated with shock. These mediators include acid hydrolases, neutral proteases, oxygen free radicals, certain coagulation factors, and the following arachidonic acid derivatives: prostaglandins, thromboxanes, and leukotrienes. Macrophages also release certain **monokines** that modulate temperature regulation, intermediary metabolism, hormone secretion, and the immune system.

Interactions of Positive and Negative Feedback Mechanisms

Hemorrhage provokes a multitude of circulatory and metabolic derangements. As we have seen, some of these changes are compensatory and others are decompensatory. Some of these feedback mechanisms possess a high gain and others possess a low gain. Furthermore, the gain of any specific mechanism varies with the severity of the hemorrhage. For example, with only a slight loss of blood, mean arterial pressure is within the normal range and the gain of the baroreceptor reflexes is high. With greater losses of blood, when mean arterial pressure is below 60 mm Hg (i.e., below the threshold for the baroreceptors), further reductions of pressure have no additional influence through the baroreceptor reflexes. Hence, below this critical pressure, the baroreceptor reflex gain is zero or near zero.

As a general rule, with minor degrees of blood loss, the gains of the negative feedback mechanisms are high, whereas those of the positive feedback mechanisms are low. The opposite is true with more severe hemorrhages. The gains of the various mechanisms are additive algebraically. Therefore, whether a vicious cycle develops depends on whether the sum of the positive and negative gains exceeds 1. Total gains in excess of 1 are of course more likely with severe losses of blood. Therefore, to avert a vicious cycle, serious hemorrhages must be treated quickly and intensively, preferably by whole blood transfusions, before the process becomes irreversible.

SUMMARY

Exercise

1. In anticipation of exercise, the vagus nerve impulses to the heart are inhibited and the sympathetic nervous system is activated by central command. The result is an increase in heart rate, myocardial contractile force, and regional vascular resistance.

2. With exercise, vascular resistance increases in the skin, kidneys, splanchnic regions, and inactive muscles and decreases markedly in the active muscles. The overall effect is a pronounced reduction in total peripheral resistance. This change in resistance, along with the auxiliary pumping action of the contracting skeletal muscles, leads to a large increase in venous return.

3. The increase in heart rate and the enhanced myocardial contractility, both induced by activation of the cardiac sympathetic nerves, enable the heart to transfer the blood to the pulmonary and systemic circulations, thereby increasing cardiac output. Stroke volume increases only slightly. Oxygen consumption and blood oxygen extraction increase, and systolic and mean blood pressure increase slightly.

4. As body temperature rises during exercise, the skin blood vessels dilate. However, when heart rate becomes maximal during severe exercise, the skin vessels constrict. This increases the effective blood volume but causes greater increases in body temperature and a feeling of exhaustion.

5. The limiting factor in exercise performance is the delivery of blood to the active muscles.

Hemorrhage

1. Acute blood loss induces the following hemodynamic changes: tachycardia, hypotension, generalized arteriolar constriction, and generalized venoconstriction.

2. Acute blood loss invokes a number of negative feedback (compensatory) mechanisms, such as baroreceptor and chemoreceptor reflexes, responses to moderate cerebral ischemia, reabsorption of tissue fluids, release of endogenous vasoconstrictors, and renal conservation of water and electrolytes.

3. Acute blood loss also induces a number of positive feedback (decompensatory) mechanisms, such as cardiac failure, acidosis, central nervous system depression, aberrations of blood coagulation, and depression of the reticuloendothelial system.

4. The outcome of acute blood loss depends on the sum of gains of the positive and negative feedback mechanisms and on the interactions between these mechanisms.

BIBLIOGRAPHY

Journal articles

Astiz ME, Rackow EC, Weil MH: Pathophysiology and treatment of circulatory shock, *Crit Care Clin* 9:183, 1993.

Baker CH, Sutton ET: Arteriolar endothelium-dependent vasodilation occurs during endotoxin shock, *Am J Physiol* 264:H1118, 1993.

Buckwalter JB, Clifford PS: Autonomic control of skeletal muscle blood flow at the onset of exercise, *Am J Physiol* 277:H1872, 1999.

Cameron JD, Dart AM: Exercise training increases total systemic arterial compliance in humans, *Am J Physiol* 266:H693, 1994.

Fitts RH: Cellular mechanisms of muscle fatigue, *Physiol Rev* 74:49, 1994.

Gryglewski RJ et al: Protective role of pulmonary nitric oxide in the acute phase of endotoxemia in rats, *Circ Res* 82:819, 1998.

Herbertson MJ, Werner HA, Walley KR: Nitric oxide synthase inhibition partially prevents decreased LV contractility during endotoxemia, *Am J Physiol* 270:H1979, 1996.

Herd JA: Cardiovascular response to stress, *Physiol Rev* 71:305, 1991.

Iellamo F et al: Baroreflex control of sinus node during dynamic exercise in humans: effects of central command and muscle reflexes, *Am J Physiol* 272:H1157, 1997.

Kulics JM, Collins HL, Dicarlo SE: Postexercise hypertension is mediated by reductions in sympathetic nerve activity, *Am J Physiol* 276:H27, 1999.

Lefer AM, Lefer DJ: Pharmacology of the endothelium in ischemia-reperfusion and circulatory shock, *Annu Rev Pharmacol Toxicol* 33:71, 1993.

O'Leary DS et al: Is active skeletal muscle functionally vasoconstricted during dynamic exercise in conscious dogs? *Am J Physiol* 272:R386, 1997.

Share L: Control of vasopressin release: an old but continuing story, *News Physiol Sci* 11:7, 1996.

Sheriff DD et al: Dependence of cardiac filling pressure on cardiac output during rest and dynamic exercise in dogs, *Am J Physiol* 265:H316, 1993.

Szabo C: Alterations in nitric oxide production in various forms of circulatory shock, *New Horizons* 3:2, 1995.

Thiemermann C: Role of l-arginine: nitric oxide pathway in circulatory shock, *Adv Pharmacol* 28:45, 1994.

Tschakorsky ME, Hughson RL: Ischemic muscle chemoreflex response elevates blood flow in nonischemic exercising human forearm muscle, *Am J Physiol* 277:H635, 1999.

Yao Y-M et al: Significance of NO in hemorrhage-induced hemodynamic alterations, organ injury, and mortality in rats, *Am J Physiol* 270:J1615, 1996.

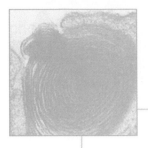

The Respiratory System

M. M. Cloutier
R. S. Thrall

chapter twenty-five

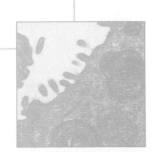

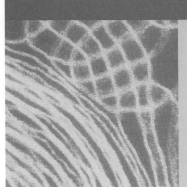

Structure and Function of the Respiratory System

When you can't breathe, nothing else matters.

Slogan of the American Lung Association

INTRODUCTION

The lung has three major functions: gas exchange, host defense, and metabolism. The primary function of the lung is gas exchange, which consists of the movement of oxygen into the body and the removal of carbon dioxide. In addition to gas exchange, the lung also functions as a barrier between the world outside and the inside of the body. And finally, the lung is a metabolic organ that synthesizes and metabolizes different compounds.

Breathing is automatic and under the control of the central nervous system. Gas exchange, or the process of respiration, begins with the act of inspiration, which is initiated by the contraction of the diaphragm, the major muscle of respiration. Upon contraction, the diaphragm protrudes into the abdominal cavity moving the abdomen outward. The descent of the diaphragm creates a negative pressure inside the chest. The upper airway (glottis) opens, creating a portal that connects the outside world to the respiratory system. Because gases flow from higher to lower pressure, air moves into the lungs from the outside, much like the way a vacuum cleaner sucks air into the canister. Lung volume increases, oxygen (O_2) is taken up, and carbon dioxide (CO_2) is eliminated at the level of the alveolus. During exhalation, the diaphragm (and other respiratory muscles) relaxes, the pressure inside the chest increases, and gas flows passively out of the lungs.

The important respiratory components of gas exchange are the gas(es) being inhaled, the characteristics of the conducting airways, the gas-exchanging unit (alveolar capillary network), the pulmonary circulation that regulates blood flow through the gas-exchanging unit, and the muscles that move the gas in and out of the lung. In addition to the respiratory system, a systemic circulatory system brings oxygen to the tissues and cells throughout the body and removes CO_2 from these sites. Thus, both the respiratory system and

the systemic circulatory system are essential for health and well-being.

The lungs are a remarkable feat of engineering. They receive the entire right ventricular cardiac output and they are called upon at birth to function without cessation. The lungs are contained in a space with a volume of approximately 4 L, but they have a surface area for gas exchange that is the size of a tennis court (~85 m^2). This large surface area is comprised of myriads of independently functioning respiratory units. Unlike the heart, but similar to the kidneys, the lungs demonstrate functional unity; that is, each unit is structurally identical and functions just like every other unit. Because the divisions of the lung and the sites of disease are designated by their anatomic locations (right upper lobe, left lower lobe, etc.), students must fully understand pulmonary anatomy in order to clinically relate respiratory physiology and pathophysiology.

GROSS ANATOMY

The respiratory tract (or system) begins at the nose and ends in the most distal alveolus. Thus, the nasal cavity, the posterior pharynx, the glottis and vocal cords, the trachea, and all the divisions of the tracheobronchial tree are included in the respiratory system. The **upper airway** consists of all structures from the nose to the vocal cords, including sinuses and the larynx, whereas the **lower airway** consists of the trachea, airways, and alveoli.

UPPER AIRWAYS

The major function of the upper airways is to "condition" inspired air, so that by the time it reaches the trachea, it is at body temperature and fully humidified. The nose also functions to filter, entrap, and clear particles greater than 10 μm in size. Finally, the nose provides the sense of smell. Neuronal endings in the roof of the nose above the superior turbinate carry impulses through the cribriform plate to the olfactory bulb. The volume of the nose in an adult is approximately

445

20 ml, but the cross-sectional area is greatly increased by the nasal turbinates, which are a series of three continuous ribbons of tissue that protrude into the nasal cavity (Fig. 25-1). In humans, the volume of air entering the nares each day is in the order of 10,000 to 15,000 L.

Resistance to air flow in the nose during quiet breathing accounts for ~50% of the total respiratory system resistance, which is ~8 cm $H_2O/L/sec$. Nasal resistance increases with viral infections and with increased airflow, such as during exercise. When nasal resistance becomes too high, mouth breathing begins.

The interior of the nose is lined by the respiratory epithelium, which is interspersed with surface secretory cells. The flow of mucus clears the main nasal passages approximately every 15 minutes. Nasal secretions contain important immunoglobulins, inflammatory cells, and interferons, which are the first step in host defense.

The paranasal sinuses are lined by ciliated epithelium, and they nearly surround the nasal passages. The fluid covering their surface is continually being propelled into the nose along the principal line of inspiratory flow. In some sinuses (e.g., the maxillary sinus) the opening (ostium) of the sinus is at the upper edge of the sinus, which makes them particularly susceptible to mucus retention (Fig. 25-1). The ostia are readily obstructed in the presence of nasal edema, resulting in retention of secretions and secondary infection (sinusitis). The sinuses have two major functions—they lighten the skull, which makes upright posture easier, and they offer resonance to the voice. They may also protect the brain during frontal trauma.

The major structures of the larynx include the epiglottis, arytenoids, and vocal cords. With some infections, these structures can become edematous (swollen) and can contribute significantly to airflow resistance. The epiglottis and arytenoids "hood" or cover the vocal cords during swallowing. Thus, under normal circumstances, they function to inhibit aspiration into the lower respiratory tract. The act of swallowing food after mastication (chewing) usually occurs within 2 seconds, and it is synchronized closely with muscle reflexes that coordinate the opening and closing of the airway. Hence, air is allowed to enter and food and liquids are kept out. Patients with neuromuscular diseases have altered muscle reflexes and they can lose this coordinated swallowing mechanism. Thus, they may become susceptible to aspiration of food and liquid, with the risk of pneumonia.

LOWER AIRWAYS

The trachea bifurcates (branches) into two mainstem bronchi, which enter the lungs, which are subdivided by fissures that form incomplete divisions (Fig. 25-2). The right lung, located in the right hemithorax, has three lobes (the right upper lobe, the right middle lobe, and the right lower lobe). The left lung is divided into the left upper lobe, which includes the lingula, the homologous lobe of the right middle lobe, and the left lower lobe. Both the right and left lung are covered by the visceral pleura and are encased by the parietal pleura over p5 of the last version. The interface of these two pleuras allows for the smooth gliding of the lung as it expands in the chest and produces a potential space. Air can enter between the visceral and parietal pleuras either because of trauma, surgery, or rupture of a group of alveoli creating a pneumothorax. Because the right and left lungs and their pleuras are separate, a pneumothorax will involve only the right or left hemithorax.

The tracheobronchial system (also called the tracheobronchial "tree") consists of all of the airways, beginning with the trachea. Air flows into the lung through the trachea and airways. As the airways divide and penetrate deeper into the lung, they become narrower, shorter, and more numerous (using a tree analogy, the branches become smaller as they approach the leaves). The trachea divides at the carina (named because it has the appearance of the "keel" of a boat) into the right and left mainstem bronchi, which in turn divide into the lobar bronchi and then the segmental bronchi (Fig. 25-3). The airways continue to divide in what is called a dichotomous or asymmetric branching pattern, until they form terminal bronchioles that are distinguished by being the smallest airways without alveoli.

The bronchopulmonary segment, the region of the lung supplied by a segmental bronchus, is the **functional anatomical unit** of the lung. Disease usually involves a segment at a time and surgical resection follows along segments. The airways can be further divided into two types: cartilaginous airways, or bronchi, and noncartilaginous airways, or bronchioles (Table 25-1).

Bronchi are the conductors of air between the external environment and the distal sites of gas exchange (i.e., the alveoli). The amount of cartilage decreases as the airways become smaller and smaller, and the cartilage disappears completely in airways that are approximately 1 mm in diameter. Airways from the trachea to the terminal bronchioles contain no alveoli, and thus they do not participate in gas exchange. These airways form the anatomic dead space,

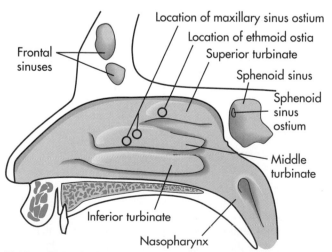

■ Fig. 25-1 Nasal passage structure demonstrating superior, middle, and inferior turbinates. Approximate locations of some sinus ostia are shown.

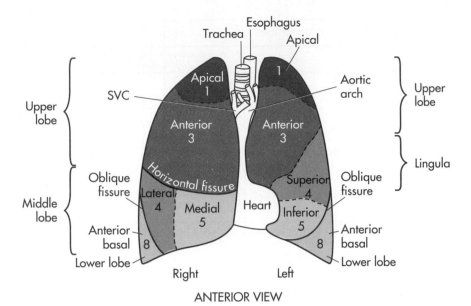

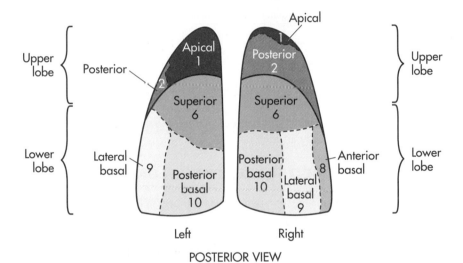

Fig. 25-2 Topography of the lung demonstrating the lobes, segments, and fissures. Numbers refer to specific bronchopulmonary segments that are also shown in Fig. 25-3.

Fig. 25-3 Segments: *1,* Apical; *2,* posterior; *3,* anterior; *4,* lateral (superior); *5,* medial (inferior); *6,* superior; *7,* medial basal; *8,* anterior basal; *9,* lateral basal; *10,* posterior basal. Bronchopulmonary segments, anterior view. Segment numbers same as in Fig. 25-2.

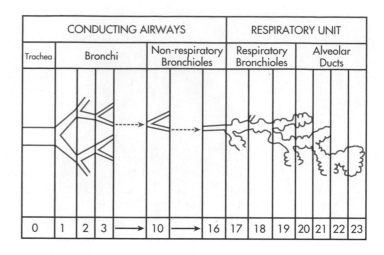

■ **Fig. 25-4**   Conducting airways and terminal respiratory units of the lung. The relative size of the respiratory unit is greatly enlarged. Figures at the bottom indicate the approximate number of generations from trachea to alveoli, which may vary from as few as 10 to as many as 27. (From Weibel ER: *Morphometry of the human lung,* Heidelberg, Germany, 1963, Springer-Verlag.)

■ **Table 25-1**   Anatomical characteristics of bronchi and bronchioles

	Cartilage present	Size	Epithelium	Blood supply	Alveoli	Volume
Bronchi	Yes	>1 mm	Pseudostratified Columnar	Bronchial	No	
Terminal bronchioles	No	<1 mm	Cuboidal	Bronchial	No	>150 ml
Respiratory bronchioles	No	<1 mm	Cuboidal	Pulmonary	Yes	2500 ml

which has a volume in adults of approximately 150 ml. The number of different branches from the trachea to the terminal bronchioles can vary from as few as 10 to as many as 25 (Fig. 25-4).

Bronchioles are smaller than 1 mm in diameter, they lack cartilage, and they have a simple cuboidal epithelium. Bronchioles are embedded into the connective tissue framework of the lung, and thus their diameter increases and decreases with lung volume. Bronchioles are further subdivided, depending upon their function. Nonrespiratory bronchioles include terminal bronchioles, which serve as conductors of the gas stream, whereas respiratory bronchioles contain alveoli that function as sites of gas exchange. The area from the terminal bronchiole to the alveolus is occasionally called the secondary lobule or acinus (Fig. 25-5). The amazing anatomic feature of this area is that it is only ~5 mm in length, but the total volume of the acini comprises the single largest volume of the lung, at approximately 2500 ml!

The respiratory (gas-exchanging) unit consists of the respiratory bronchioles, the alveolar ducts, and the alveoli, and it is the **basic physiological unit** of the lung. The respiratory bronchioles, as previously mentioned, are the first bronchioles that have alveoli. Each branching of the respiratory bronchioles results in an increased number and size of the alveoli, until the respiratory bronchiole terminates in an opening to a group of alveoli (Fig. 25-6). This terminal opening is called an alveolar duct. In addition to the difference in function between the conducting airways and the terminal respiratory unit, the conducting airways receive their blood supply from the bronchial circulation, whereas the terminal

respiratory units receive their blood supply from the pulmonary arteries.

BLOOD SUPPLY TO THE LUNG

The lung has two separate blood supplies. The first is the pulmonary circulation, which brings deoxygenated blood from the right ventricle to the gas-exchanging units. At the gas-exchanging units, oxygen is picked up and carbon dioxide is removed from the blood before it is returned to the left atrium for distribution to the rest of the body. The second blood supply is the bronchial circulation, which arises from the aorta and provides nourishment to the lung parenchyma. The circulation to the lung is unique in its dual circulation and in its ability to accommodate large volumes of blood at low pressure.

The pulmonary capillary bed is the largest vascular bed in the body. It covers a surface area of 70 to 80 m², which is nearly as large as the alveolar surface area. The network of capillaries is so dense that it might be considered to be a sheet of blood interrupted by small vertical supporting posts (Fig. 25-7). The capillary volume in the lung at rest is approximately 70 ml. During exercise, this volume increases and approaches ~200 ml. This increase occurs, in part, through the recruitment of closed or compressed capillary segments as an increased cardiac output raises the pulmonary vascular pressure. In addition, open capillaries can enlarge as their internal pressure rises. This occurs when the lungs fill with blood, as it does in left heart failure, which is associated with an elevated left atrial pressure (see Chapter 16). The pulmonary veins return blood to the left atrium

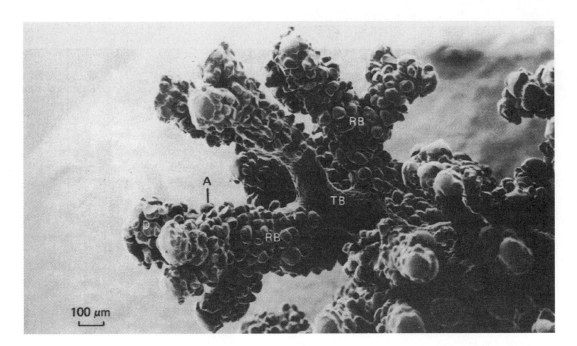

■ **Fig. 25-5**
Transition of terminal bronchiole. Scanning electron micrographs of airway branches peripheral to terminal bronchiole in silicon-rubber cast of cat lung. *A,* Alveolus; *RB,* respiratory bronchiole; *TB,* terminal bronchiole. Note absence of alveoli in terminal bronchiole.

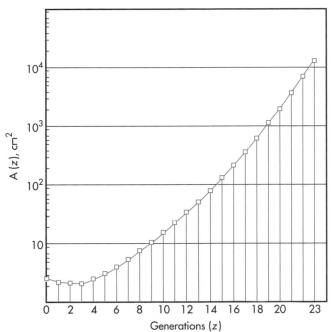

■ **Fig. 25-6**   Increase in surface area. Total cross section of the airways in the human lung by generation. Although each generation of airway is smaller than its parent, the *total* cross-sectional area of each generation is greater than the *total* area of the previous generation. (From Weibel ER: *Morphometry of the human lung,* Heidelberg, Germany, 1963, Springer-Verlag.)

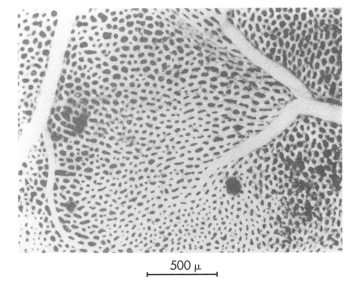

■ **Fig. 25-7**   Sheet of blood. View of an alveolar wall (in the frog) showing the dense network of capillaries. A small artery *(left)* and vein *(right)* can also be seen. The individual capillary segments are so short that the blood forms an almost continuous sheet. (From Maloney JE, Castle BL: *Respirat Physiol* 7:150, 1969.)

through conventional and supernumerary branches. Because of their larger numbers and thinner walls, the pulmonary veins provide a large reservoir for blood, and these veins can either increase or decrease their capacitance to provide a constant left ventricular output in the face of a variable pulmonary arterial flow.

Pulmonary arteries and veins with diameters larger than 50 μm contain smooth muscle. These vessels actively regulate their diameter and thus alter resistance to blood flow.

The bronchial arteries, usually three in number, provide a source of well-oxygenated systemic blood to the lungs. These arteries accompany the bronchial tree and divide with it (Fig. 25-8). They nourish the walls of the bronchi, bronchioles, blood vessels, and nerves, and they perfuse the lymph nodes and most of the visceral pleura. Approximately one third of the blood returns to the right atrium through the bronchial veins, whereas the remainder drains into the left atrium via pulmonary veins. This deoxygenated blood, which mixes with oxygen-enriched blood in the pulmonary veins, contributes to the small alveolar-arterial oxygen difference in normal individuals. In the presence of diseases such as cystic fibrosis, the bronchial arteries, which normally receive only 1% to 2% of the cardiac output, increase in size (hypertrophy), and they could receive as much as 10% to 20% of the cardiac output. Erosion into these vessels secondary to infection is responsible for the hemoptysis (coughing up blood) that occurs in this disease.

MUSCLES OF RESPIRATION

The muscles of respiration are skeletal muscles. Their structure and function are identical to those of other skeletal muscles; that is, their force of contraction increases when they are stretched, and it decreases when the muscles are shorter. Thus, the force of contraction of respiratory muscles increases with increasing lung volume.

The lungs are located within the thoracic cavity, and they are in intimate contact with the chest wall. Dividing the thoracic cavity from the abdominal cavity is the diaphragm, the major muscle of respiration. The diaphragm is a thin, musculotendinous, dome-shaped sheet of muscle that is inserted into the lower ribs, and it separates the thoracic from the abdominal cavity (Fig. 25-9). The zone of opposition is the region where the diaphragm is in direct contact with the lower ribs. This zone of opposition enhances the transmission of the abdominal pressure across the diaphragm directly

to the rib cage. The diaphragm is innervated by the right and left phrenic nerves, which have their origins at the third to fifth cervical segments of the spinal cord (C3 to C5). The arterial blood supply to the diaphragm originates from branches of the intercostal arteries, and the veins drain into the inferior vena cava. Contraction of the diaphragm forces the abdominal contents downward and forward. This increases the vertical dimension of the chest cavity, and creates a pressure difference between the thorax and abdomen. In addition, the rib margins are lifted and moved out, which increases the transverse diameter of the thorax. The 12 ribs on either side articulate with the thoracic vertebrae. The ribs can rotate only upward, which increases the transverse diameter of the thorax. The curvature of the diaphragm, when it is contracted, results in a substantial increase in thoracic volume.

In adults, the diaphragm can generate airway pressures up to 150 to 200 cm H_2O during a maximal inspiratory effort. During quiet breathing (tidal breathing), the diaphragm moves approximately 1 cm. However, during vital capacity (deep breath) maneuvers, the diaphragm can move as much as 10 cm. If the diaphragm is paralyzed, it moves higher up in the thoracic cavity during inspiration, because of the fall in intrathoracic pressure. This paradoxical movement of the diaphragm can be demonstrated by fluoroscopy.

The other significant muscles of inspiration are the external intercostal muscles, which pull the ribs upward and forward during inspiration. This causes an increase in both the lateral and the anteroposterior diameters of the thorax (Fig. 25-10). Innervation of these muscles originates from the intercostal nerves that arise from the same level of the spinal cord. Paralysis of these muscles has no significant effect on respiration, because of the importance of the diaphragm.

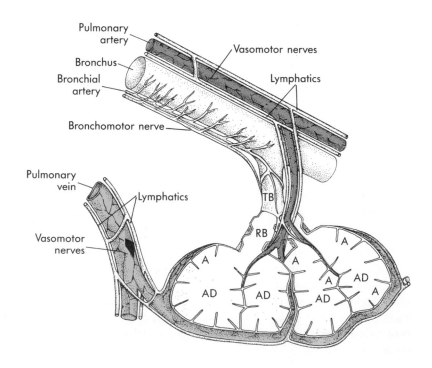

■ **Fig. 25-8**   The anatomic relation between the pulmonary artery, the bronchial artery, the airways, and the lymphatics. *TB,* Terminal bronchioles; *RB,* respiratory bronchioles; *A,* alveoli; *AD,* alveolar ducts.

This is why individuals with high spinal cord injuries can breathe on their own. It is only when the injury is above C3 that individuals are completely ventilator dependent.

Accessory muscles of inspiration (the scalene muscles that elevate the sternocleidomastoid, the alae nasi that cause nasal flaring, and the small muscles in the neck and head) do not contract during normal breathing. However, they do contract vigorously during exercise and when airway obstruction is significant, and they actively pull up on the rib cage. During normal breathing, they anchor the sternum and upper ribs. All of the rib cage muscles are voluntary muscles that

are supplied by intercostal arteries and veins and that are innervated by motor and sensory intercostal nerves.

The upper airway must remain patent during inspiration. Therefore, the pharyngeal wall muscles (the genioglossus and arytenoid muscles) are also considered to be muscles of inspiration.

Exhalation during normal breathing is passive, but it becomes active during exercise and hyperventilation. The most important muscles of exhalation are those of the abdominal wall (rectus abdominus, internal and external oblique, and transversus abdominus) and the internal intercostal muscles that oppose the external intercostal muscles (i.e., they pull the ribs downward and inward). Maximal lengthening of the respiratory muscles at high lung volumes and maximal shortening of the respiratory muscles at low lung volumes limit maximal inspiratory and maximal expiratory volume, respectively.

The inspiratory muscles do the work of breathing. During normal breathing, work is low and the inspiratory muscles have significant reserve. Respiratory muscles can be trained to do more work, but there is a finite limit to the work they can perform. Respiratory muscle fatigue is a major factor in the development of respiratory failure.

Because respiratory muscles provide the driving force for ventilation, diseases that affect the mechanical properties of the lung affect the muscles of respiration. For example, in chronic obstructive pulmonary disease, the work of breathing secondary to airflow obstruction is increased. Exhalation is no longer passive, but it requires active, expiratory muscle contraction. In addition, the total lung capacity (TLC) is increased. The greater TLC forces the diaphragm downward, shortens the muscle fibers, and decreases the radius of curvature. As a result, the function and efficiency of the diaphragm are decreased. In addition,

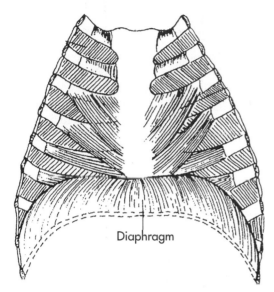

■ **Fig. 25-9** The diaphragm. Diagram illustrating the position of the diaphragm in the thorax. View from the inside of the thorax. (From Fishman AP: *Pulmonary diseases and disorders*, ed 2, vol 1, New York, 1988, Mc Graw-Hill, p. 68.)

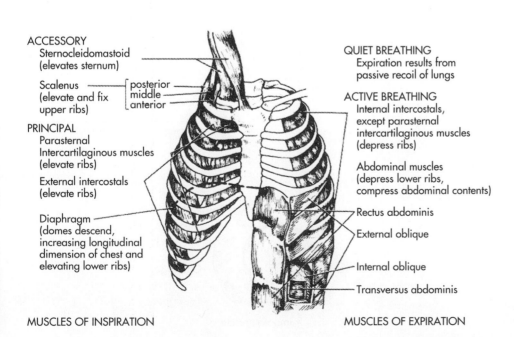

ACCESSORY
Sternocleidomastoid (elevates sternum)

Scalenus (elevate and fix upper ribs) — posterior, middle, anterior

PRINCIPAL
Parasternal Intercartilaginous muscles (elevate ribs)

External intercostals (elevate ribs)

Diaphragm (domes descend, increasing longitudinal dimension of chest and elevating lower ribs)

QUIET BREATHING
Expiration results from passive recoil of lungs

ACTIVE BREATHING
Internal intercostals, except parasternal intercartilaginous muscles (depress ribs)

Abdominal muscles (depress lower ribs, compress abdominal contents)

Rectus abdominis

External oblique

Internal oblique

Transversus abdominis

MUSCLES OF INSPIRATION

MUSCLES OF EXPIRATION

■ **Fig. 25-10** Muscles of respiration. Diagram of the anatomy of the major respiratory muscles. *Left side,* inspiratory muscles; *right side,* expiratory muscles. (From Garrity ER, Sharp JT. In *Pulmonary and critical care update,* vol 2, Park Ridge, Ill, 1986, American College of Chest Physicians.)

the respiratory muscles can fatigue just as other skeletal muscles do when the workload increases.

Respiratory muscle can also weaken in patients with the neuromuscular diseases Guillain-Barré syndrome and myasthenia gravis. In these diseases, sufficient respiratory muscle weakness can impair movement of the chest wall. Respiratory failure can occur even though the mechanical properties of the lung and chest wall are normal.

CELLS OF THE AIRWAYS

Ciliated Cells

The respiratory tract to the level of the bronchioles is lined by a pseudostratified, ciliated columnar epithelium (Fig. 25-11). These cells maintain the level of the periciliary fluid, a 5 μm layer of water and electrolytes in which cilia and the mucociliary transport system function. The depth of the periciliary fluid is maintained by the movement of various ions across the epithelium (Fig. 25-12). Active (i.e., energy-dependent) chloride secretion into the airway lumen occurs through chloride (Cl⁻) channels in the apical membrane. These chloride channels are regulated by intracellular cyclic

AMP (cAMP) and calcium. Sodium (Na^+) is absorbed through sodium channels in the apical membrane. Both chloride secretion and sodium absorption translocate water secondarily (osmotic equilibrium) and the balance between Cl^- secretion and Na^+ absorption regulates the depth of the periciliary fluid. A sodium-potassium adenosine triphosphate (ATP) pump in the basolateral membrane maintains the gradient for sodium absorption. An Na-Cl cotransporter in the basolateral membrane links sodium and chloride flux, which raises chloride above its electrochemical equilibrium and chloride then diffuses across the apical membrane into the airway lumen. The sodium that accompanies chloride is then transported back across the basolateral membrane by the Na,K-ATPase pump.

Mucus Production

Three types of cellular structures are responsible for mucus production in the airways: surface secretory cells (SSC), submucosal glands, and Clara cells. Surface secretory cells, also known as *goblet cells*, are interspersed among the epithelial cells. In general, there is one goblet cell to five or six ciliated cells. Goblet cells decrease in number between the fifth and twelfth lung division and they disappear beyond the

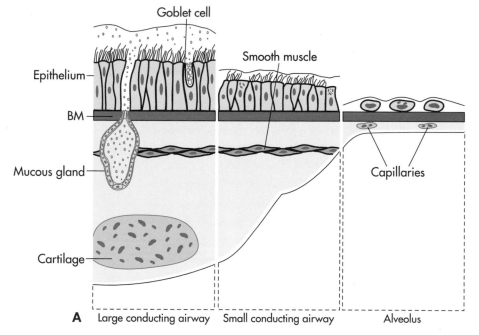

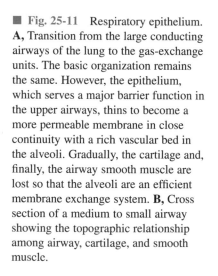

■ **Fig. 25-11** Respiratory epithelium. **A,** Transition from the large conducting airways of the lung to the gas-exchange units. The basic organization remains the same. However, the epithelium, which serves a major barrier function in the upper airways, thins to become a more permeable membrane in close continuity with a rich vascular bed in the alveoli. Gradually, the cartilage and, finally, the airway smooth muscle are lost so that the alveoli are an efficient membrane exchange system. **B,** Cross section of a medium to small airway showing the topographic relationship among airway, cartilage, and smooth muscle.

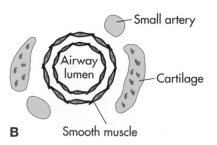

twelfth tracheobronchial division in normal individuals. Goblet cells increase in number and propagate into bronchioles in response to chronic cigarette smoke and other pollutants. Thus, they contribute to the airway obstruction that occurs in smokers.

Submucosal tracheobronchial glands are present wherever there is cartilage in the tracheobronchial tree. These glands empty to the surface epithelium through a ciliated duct, and they are lined by mucous and serous cells (Fig. 25-13). Submucosal tracheobronchial glands increase in number and size in chronic bronchitis, and they extend down to the level of the bronchioles in pulmonary disease.

In normal individuals, Clara cells are found at the level of the bronchioles, where the goblet cells and submucosal glands have disappeared. These Clara cells contain granules and they may have a secretory function, or they may play a role in epithelial regeneration after injury.

Mucus and inhaled particles are removed from the airways by the rhythmic beating of the cilia on the top of the

pseudostratified, columnar epithelium (Fig. 25-14). Each epithelial cell contains about 200 cilia. Each cilium consists of a central dynein doublet surrounded peripherally by nine single tubules. The central doublet contains an ATPase enzyme, and it is probably responsible for the contractile beat of the cilia. Mucociliary transport is described in Chapter 30.

Cells of the Alveoli

The alveoli are polygonal in shape and are ~250 μm in diameter. An adult has on average 300,000 alveoli (Figs. 25-15 and 25-16). Three different cell types (Type I, II, and III cells) line the alveoli (Fig. 25-17). The most important cells are the Type I and Type II epithelial cells in the epithelium of the alveolus. The Type I epithelial cell is the primary cell responsible for gas exchange.

The **Type I cell** is a very flat, elongated cell with extremely thin cytoplasm and a flattened nucleus; it occupies ~95% of the surface area of the alveolus, and it is the primary site for gas exchange. The thin cytoplasm of the Type I cell is ideal for optimal gas diffusion. In addition, the basement membranes of the Type I cells and the capillary endothelium are fused. This arrangement minimizes the thickness and aids gas exchange.

The **Type II epithelial cell** is a small, cuboidal cell that is usually found in the "corners" of the alveolus; it occupies ~2% of the surface area. The Type II cell synthesizes pulmonary surfactant, and it is also responsible for regeneration of the normal alveolar structure subsequent to injury.

The Type I cell is prone to cytotoxic agents. When the Type I cell dies, the epithelial layer is denuded. In response to this type of injury, the Type II cell is stimulated to replicate, and it eventually differentiates into a Type I cell. This alteration restores normal alveolar structure. Under normal conditions the Type I and Type II cells exist in approximately a 1:1 ratio. However, in an injured lung (especially with

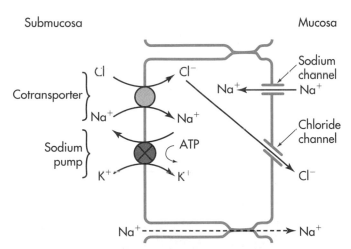

■ **Fig. 25-12** Ion transport. Chloride secretion and sodium absorption in airway epithelial cells. A cotransporter in the basolateral membrane links sodium and chloride flux leading to a build-up in chloride above its electrochemical equilibrium. A sodium pump in the same membrane maintains a sodium gradient. A sodium channel and a chloride channel in the apical membrane provide for sodium influx and chloride efflux out of the cell. Osmotic equilibrium is maintained by the diffusion of water accompanying net solute flux.

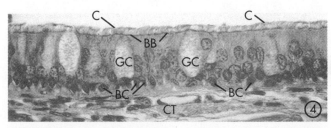

■ **Fig. 25-13** Scanning electron micrograph of airway. The ciliated, pseudostratified, columnar epithelium of a bronchus. Each cilium is connected to a basal body *(BB)*, which collectively appear at the base of the cilia *(C)* as a dark band. Goblet cells *(GC)* and basal cells *(BC)*, the potential precursors of the ciliated cells, are shown. *CT*, Connective tissue.

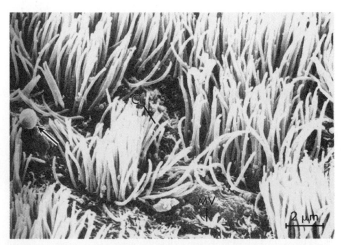

■ **Fig. 25-14** Scanning electron micrograph of cilia blanket. Surface view of bronchiolar epithelium shows tufts of cilia *(Ci)* forming on individual ciliated cells and microvilli *(MV)* on other cells. Note secretion droplet in process of release from goblet cell *(arrow)*.

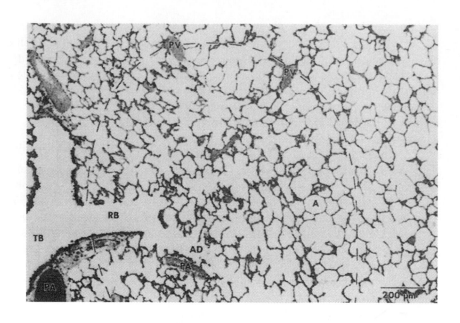

■ **Fig. 25-15** Alveoli. The terminal respiratory unit consists of the alveoli *(A)* and the alveolar ducts *(AD)* arising from a respiratory bronchiole *(RB).* Each unit is roughly spherical, as suggested by the dashed outline. Pulmonary venous vessels *(PV)* are peripherally located. *TB* identifies a terminal bronchiole. *PA* identifies a pulmonary artery. (Normal sheep lung, somewhat underinflated, 1-μm-thick glycol methacrylate section, light microscopy.)

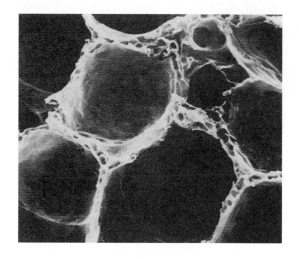

■ **Fig. 25-16** Alveoli. Scanning electron micrograph of air-filled lung fixed by vascular perfusion at 80% of lung capacity *(TLC).* Note smooth surface of the lung at 80% TLC. (From Gil J et al: *J Appl Physiol* 47:990, 1979.)

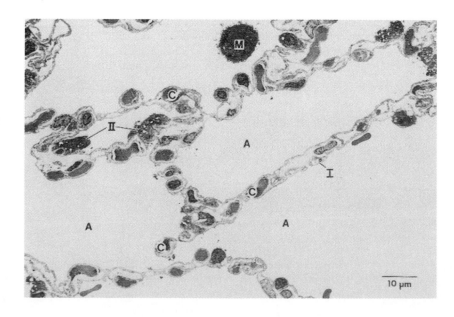

■ **Fig. 25-17** Types I and II thick-thin section. A large fraction of the alveolar wall consists of capillaries and their contents *(C).* The alveolar walls are folded and the alveoli *(A)* are collapsed because this section is from a human lung surgical specimen that was excised and immediately immersed in fixative. This procedure probably also accounts for the three red blood cells in the alveolar air spaces. *M,* Alveolar macrophage; *I,* Type I pneumonocyte; *II,* Type II pneumonocyte (transmission electron microscopy).

pulmonary fibrosis), the alveolar epithelium is lined entirely with Type II cells. This condition is not conducive to optimal gas exchange. The repair system is an example of phylogeny recapitulating ontogeny, because the epithelium of the alveolus is entirely comprised of Type II cells until very late into gestation.

Type III pneumocytes are also known as **brush cells,** because of their characteristic appearance by electron microscopy. These brush cells can be found throughout the lung, and thus they are not unique to the alveolus. They are closely associated with nerves, and they may function as a chemoreceptor.

SURFACTANT

The lungs have a unique substance, called **surfactant,** which compensates for the harsh environment established by the air-to-liquid interface in which it must function. Surface tension forces at the air-liquid interfaces are high, and they influence function. This is illustrated clearly by comparing the volume pressure curves of the saline-filled and air-filled lungs. Higher pressure is required to fully inflate the lung with air than with saline, due to the different surface tension forces in the air-filled and saline-filled lungs (Fig. 25-18).

Surfactants are generally considered to be soaps or detergents, and they act to decrease surface tension. Pulmonary surfactant is a complex mixture of phospholipids, neutral lipids, fatty acids, and proteins. This substance constitutes a thin film that lines the surface of the alveoli. It has "anti-stick" and surface tension-lowering properties, and it acts as a barrier at the air-liquid interface.

As shown in Table 25-2, surfactant contains 85% to 90% lipids (of which 85% are phospholipids and 5% are neutral lipids) and 10% to 15% protein. The major phospholipid in surfactant is phosphatidylcholine, of which approximately

75% is present as dipalmitoyl phosphatidylcholine (DPPC). DPPC is the major surface-active component in surfactant, and it readily decreases surface tension. The second most abundant phospholipid is phosphatidylglycerol (PG), which comprises 1% to 10% of total surfactant. These lipids are important in the formation of the monolayer on the alveolar-air interface, and PG is important in the spreading of surfactant over a large surface area. The surfactant is secreted from the small cuboidal-shaped Type II cells, which occupy only ~2% of the surface area of the alveoli. The surfactant must spread over the remaining surface area. This is accomplished with the aid of surfactant components, such as PG, which have spreading properties. Cholesterol and cholesterol esters account for the majority of the neutral lipids; their precise functional role is not yet determined, but they may aid in stabilizing the lipid structure.

Four specific surfactant proteins comprise 2% to 5% of the weight of surfactant. The most studied surfactant protein is SP-A, which is expressed in alveolar Type II epithelial cells and in Clara cells in the lung. SP-A is involved in the regulation of surfactant turnover, in the immune regulation within the lung, and in the formation of tubular myelin. Tubular myelin is the term used to describe a precursor stage of surfactant as it is initially secreted from the Type II cell and has not yet spread.

Two hydrophobic surfactant specific proteins are SP-B and SP-C. SP-B may be involved in the formation of tubular myelin. Recent studies have shown that SP-B is involved in the surface activity of surfactant, and that this protein may increase the intermolecular and intramolecular order of the phospholipid bilayer. These findings support the concept that SP-B resists surface tension by increasing the lateral stability of the phospholipid layer. Another recent study confirmed that the 25 amino-terminal peptides of SP-B stabilize the phospholipid layer by increasing the collapse pressure of surfactant phospholipids. This action may prevent the squeezing out of the phospholipids from the monolayers at the alveolar air-liquid interface. A specific charge interaction between the cationic peptide and an anionic lipid, such as PG, may be responsible for this stabilization. SP-C may be

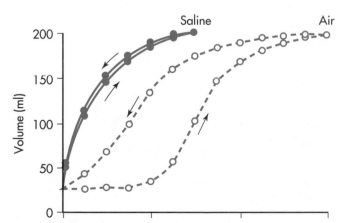

■ **Fig. 25-18** Volume-pressure curves of lungs filled with saline and with air. The arrows indicate whether the lung is being inflated or deflated; note that when using saline, hysteresis (i.e., the difference between inflation and deflation limbs of the curve) is virtually eliminated. (From Clements JA, Tierney DF. In Feen WO, Rahn H, editors: *Handbook of physiology,* Section 3, *Respiration,* vol II, Washington, DC, 1964, American Physiological Society, p. 1565.)

■ **Table 25-2** Composition of mature surfactant

	Percentage of total weight
Lipid	85-90
Protein	10-15

	Percentage of lipids
Phospholipids	85-90
Neutral lipids	5
Glycolipids	5-10

	Percentage of total phospholipids
Phosphatidylcholine	70-80
Dipalmitoyl phosphatidylcholine	45-50
Phosphatidylglycerol	7-10
Phosphatidylethanolamine	3-5

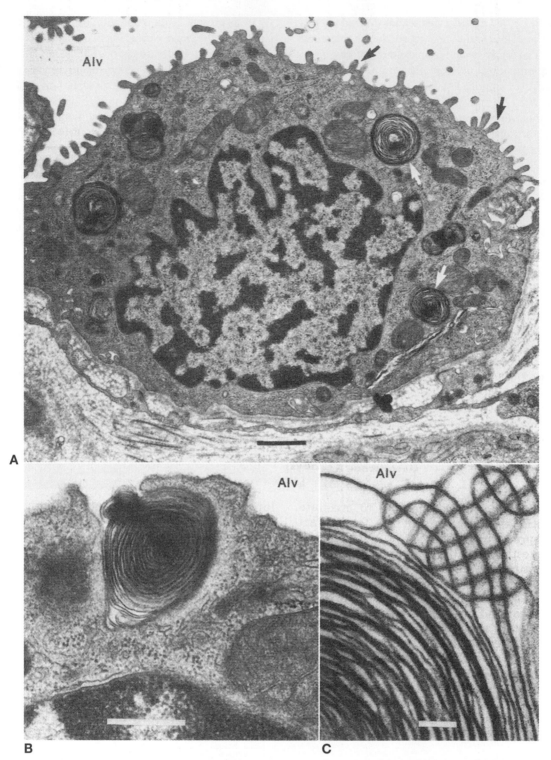

■ **Fig. 25-19   A,** Type II epithelial cell from a human lung showing characteristic lamellar inclusion bodies *(white arrows)* within cell and microvilli *(black arrows)* projecting into alveolus *(Alv).* Bar = 0.5 μm. **B,** Early exocytosis of lamellar body into alveolar space of a human lung. **C,** Secreted lamellar body and newly formed tubular myelin in alveolar liquid in a fetal rat lung. Membrane continuities between outer lamellae and adjacent tubular myelin provide evidence of intraalveolar tubular myelin formation. Bar = 0.1 μm. (Courtesy Dr. Mary C. Williams.)

involved in the spreading ability and in the surface activity of surfactant. Another recently discovered surfactant specific protein, SP-D, is a glycoprotein with an apparent molecular weight of 43 kDa. This substance contains an N-terminal collagenous domain and a carboxy-terminal glycosylated domain similar to SP-A. The function of SP-D is unknown at this time.

Pulmonary surfactant is synthesized in the alveolar Type II epithelial cell, and it is stored as preformed units in lamellar bodies in the cytoplasm. These preformed lamellar bodies have distinctive swirling patterns that are readily observed by electron microscopy, and they are uniquely characteristic of Type II epithelial cells (Fig. 25-19). Secretion of surfactant into the airway occurs via exocytosis of the lamellar body by both constitutive and regulated mechanisms. Numerous agents, including β-adrenergic agonists, activators of protein kinase C, leukotrienes, and purinergic agonists have been shown to stimulate the secretion of surfactant. The major route of clearance of pulmonary surfactant within the lung is through reuptake by Type II cells. Minor contributions to surfactant clearance occur through absorption into lymphatics and clearance by alveolar macrophages. After being taken up by the Type II cell, the phospholipids are either recycled for resecretion or they are degraded and reutilized in the synthesis of new phospholipids. These processes have recently been shown to be regulated developmentally in the fetal lung.

Pulmonary surfactant offers several physiological advantages, such as (1) reducing the work of breathing by reducing surface tension forces, (2) preventing collapse and sticking of alveoli upon expiration with antistick properties, and (3) stabilizing alveoli, especially those that tend to deflate at low surface tension.

SURFACTANT AND SURFACE TENSION

Surface tension is a measure of the attractive force of the surface molecules per unit length of the material to which they are attached. The units of surface tension are those of a force applied per unit length. For a sphere (such as an alveolus), the relationship between the pressure within the sphere (P_s) and the tension in the wall is described by the law of LaPlace:

$$P_s = \frac{2T}{r}$$

where T is the wall tension (dynes/cm) and r is the radius of the sphere.

In the absence of surfactant, the surface tension at the air-liquid interface would remain constant and the transmural (transalveolar) pressure needed to keep it at that volume would be greater at lower lung (alveolar) volumes (Fig. 25-20, *A*). Thus, it would require a greater transmural pressure to produce a given increase in alveolar volume at lower lung volumes that at higher lung volumes. Stated another way, the transmural pressure necessary to keep an alveolus inflated would decrease as the transpulmonary pressure (i.e., lung volume) increases, and, conversely, the transmural pressure necessary to keep an alveolus inflated would increase as the transpulmonary pressure (i.e., lung volume) decreases. This would create instability of alveolar inflation and alveolar collapse.

Surfactant stabilizes the inflation of alveoli because it allows the surface tension to decrease as the alveoli become larger (Fig. 25-20, *B*). As a result, the transmural pressure required to keep an alveolus inflated increases as lung volume (and transpulmonary pressure) increases, and it decreases as lung volume decreases.

In addition to surfactant, another mechanism, namely interdependence, contributes to the stability of the alveoli (Fig. 25-21). Alveoli, except for those on the pleural surface, are surrounded by other alveoli. The tendency of one alveolus to collapse is opposed by the traction exerted by the surrounding alveoli. Thus, the collapse of a single alveolus stretches and distorts the surrounding alveoli, which in turn are connected to other alveoli. Small openings (pores of Kohn) in alveolar walls connect adjacent alveoli, whereas the canals of Lambert connect terminal airways to adjacent alveoli. The pores of Kohn and the canals of Lambert provide collateral ventilation and prevent alveolar collapse (atelectasis).

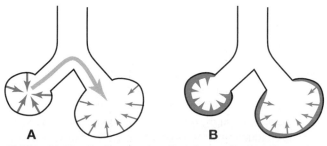

■ **Fig. 25-20** Surface tension in spheres. Surface forces in a sphere attempt to reduce the area of the surface and generate a pressure within the sphere. By LaPlace's law, the pressure generated is inversely proportional to the radius of the sphere. **A,** Surface forces in a smaller sphere generate a higher pressure (P_S; *heavier arrows*) than those in the larger sphere (P_L; *lighter arrows*). As a result, air moves from the small sphere (higher pressure) to the larger sphere (lower pressure; *shaded line*). This causes the small sphere to collapse and the large sphere to become overdistended. **B,** Surfactant *(shaded layer)* lowers surface tension, and lowers it more in the smaller sphere than in the larger sphere. The net result is that P_S is approximately equal to P_L, and the spheres are stabilized.

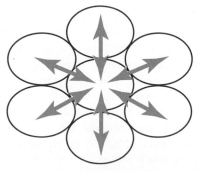

■ **Fig. 25-21** Interdependence. The tendency of one alveolus to collapse *(shaded area)* is countered by opposing traction from the surrounding alveoli.

In 1959, Avery and Mead discovered that the lungs of premature infants who died of hyaline membrane disease (HMD) were deficient in surfactant. HMD, also known as respiratory distress syndrome (RDS), is characterized by progressive atelectasis and respiratory failure in premature infants. It is a major cause of morbidity and mortality in the neonatal period. The major surfactant deficiency in premature infants is the lack of PG. In general, as the level of PG increases in amniotic fluid, the mortality rate decreases. Recently, this research has culminated in successful attempts to treat HMD in premature infants with surfactant replacement therapy. Today, surfactant replacement therapy is the standard care for premature infants.

LYMPHOID TISSUE AND THE LYMPHATIC SYSTEM

The lymphatic network in the lung has two major functions: (1) fluid filtration and (2) host defense. The lymphatic capillaries are the terminal vessels of the lymphatic system, and they are highly specialized to filter fluid from the interstitial spaces and return it to the circulation. Although the lymphatic capillaries are somewhat similar to blood capillaries, they have several distinct features that aid in fluid filtration and clearance: (1) no tight junctions between endothelial cells, (2) fine filaments that anchor lymph vessels to adjacent connective tissue (such that with each muscle contraction, the endothelial junctions open for fluid transport), and (3) a valvular structure to enhance lymph flow in one direction. Interstitial fluid enters the lymphatic vessels via lymphatic capillaries. The fluid drains to the larger lymphatic vessels, and it eventually returns to the blood by way of large veins. The main right lymphatic ducts follow the right side of the trachea, and they enter the venous system at the right jugular and subclavian veins. The left lymphatic ducts follow a similar pattern on the left side, and they enter the venous system in the left subclavian vein. Changes in tissue pressure and contractions of the lymphatic vessels drive the interstitial fluid into the lymphatic capillaries. Lung lymphatic flow is very active. The fluid volume moved through the lymphatics in 24 hours is equal to an animal's total plasma volume. One fourth to one half of the total plasma proteins can move through the lymphatics in 24 hours.

The lymphatic system filters fluid and particulates in the lung through various organized lymphoid structures: lymph nodes, lymph nodules, lymph aggregates, and a diffuse submucosal network of scattered lymphocytes and dendritic cells. The lungs have an extensive lymphatic system, and they have been referred to as a lymphoid organ. The lungs are considered part of the mucosal immune system that communicates with the gastrointestinal tract and mammary glands. The anatomical structures of the lymphoid tissue in the lung become less organized as one transcends the lung from the uppermost airways (hilum) to the periphery (alveoli). Lymph nodes and nodules predominate in the upper airway, and diffuse interstitial lymphocytes predominate at the

alveoli. There are no organized lymphoid structures in the alveolar spaces. Mature lymph nodes with germinal centers are common in the hilar area of the mainstem bronchi. Lymph nodules, often referred to as bronchus-associated lymphoid tissue (BALT), are the next level of organization. Although they are not true lymph nodes (they lack a germinal center), they are still considered a major processing center for antigens. They reside in the upper airways around major airway branches and blood vessels. The epithelium associated with areas of BALT is specialized, and it is referred to as a lymphoepithelium. It is comprised of a mix of epithelial cells and lymphocytes. This lymphoepithelium lacks ciliated epithelial cells. Hence, there is a break in the mucociliary clearance system, and therefore fluid flow into this BALT area is enhanced. BALT appears to be very similar to the Peyer's patches (GALT) in the gastrointestinal tract, and a communication network exists within the mucosal immune system.

Scattered lymphocytes and plasma cells can readily be found throughout the tracheobronchial tree. In most lymphoid tissue, T lymphocytes are comprised predominantly of cells with $\alpha\beta$ T cell receptors (TCR$\alpha\beta$). However, in the respiratory and gastrointestinal systems, scattered submucosal T lymphocytes have a disproportionately high number of lymphocytes with $\gamma\delta$ T cell receptors (TCR$\gamma\delta$) cells. These TCR$\gamma\delta$ cells may be a first line of defense in these environmentally exposed organs. Dendritic cells also line the respiratory and gastrointestinal tracts in a pattern similar to scattered lymphocytes. The dendritic cells are of macrophage lineage, and their phagocytic ability may also play a major role as antigen-presenting cells. This may be a necessary step to optimizing the immune response and to enable antibody class switching (IgM>IgG>IgE). The innate and adaptive immune functions of the lung, including alveolar macrophages and natural killer (NK) cells, are discussed in Chapter 30.

SMOOTH MUSCLE, CONNECTIVE TISSUE, AND OTHER CELLS

Fibroblasts are the cells of the interstitium. They synthesize and secrete collagen and elastin, which are the extracellular proteins that play a major role in matrix formation and in the physiology of the lung. Collagen is the major component of lung structure that limits lung distensibility. Elastin is the major contributor to elastic recoil of the lung.

Cartilage is a tough, resilient connective tissue that supports the conducting airways of the lung. The cartilage in the trachea forms rings that encircle about 80% of the trachea. The amount of cartilage decreases further down the respiratory system and disappears at the level of the bronchioles.

In addition to the cartilage, the airway epithelium rests on spiral bands of smooth muscle, which can dilate or constrict in response to chemical, irritant, or mechanical stimulation.

Kulchitsky cells are neuroendocrine cells that are derived from neural crest cells. They secrete biogenic amines, including dopamine and 5-hydroxytryptamine (serotonin). These cells are more numerous in the fetus than in adults, and they appear to be the cells of origin for a rare bronchial tumor called a **bronchial carcinoid tumor.** They are frequently found in clumps throughout the tracheobronchial tree. Their functional significance in the respiratory tract is not known. They appear, however, to be related to the argentaffin cells of the gastrointestinal tract.

INNERVATION

The main function of the nervous system is to enable the organism or a specific organ to communicate with both the internal and external environments. The nervous system contains sensory, integrative, and motor components that detect stimuli, integrate responses, and ultimately generate functional activities, such as movement or glandular secretion (Fig. 25-22). The central nervous system (CNS) is the main control center for respiration. The peripheral nervous system (PNS) includes both sensory and motor components, and it acts as the integrator between the CNS and the environment. Sensory and motor neurons of the PNS transmit peripheral signals to the CNS. Somatic motor neurons innervate skeletal muscles, and the autonomic neurons innervate smooth muscle, cardiac muscle, and glands (see Chapter 11).

The lung is innervated by the autonomic nervous system of the PNS, which is under CNS control. There are four distinct components of the autonomic nervous system: parasympathetic (constriction), sympathetic (relaxation), nonadrenergic noncholinergic inhibitory (relaxation), and nonadrenergic noncholinergic stimulatory (constriction).

Stimulation of the **parasympathetic** system leads to airway constriction, blood vessel dilatation, and increased glandular secretion. Stimulation of the **sympathetic** system causes airway relaxation, blood vessel constriction, and inhibition of glandular secretion (Fig. 25-23). The functional unit of the autonomic nervous system is comprised of pre- and postganglionic neurons that are located in the CNS and postganglionic neurons that are located in the ganglia of the specific organ. As with most organ systems, the CNS and PNS work in cohort to maintain homeostasis. There is no voluntary motor innervation in the lung, nor are there pain fibers. Pain fibers are found only in the pleura.

The parasympathetic innervation of the lung originates from the medulla in the brainstem (cranial nerve X). Preganglionic fibers from the vagal nuclei descend in the vagus nerve to ganglia adjacent to airways and blood vessels in the lung.

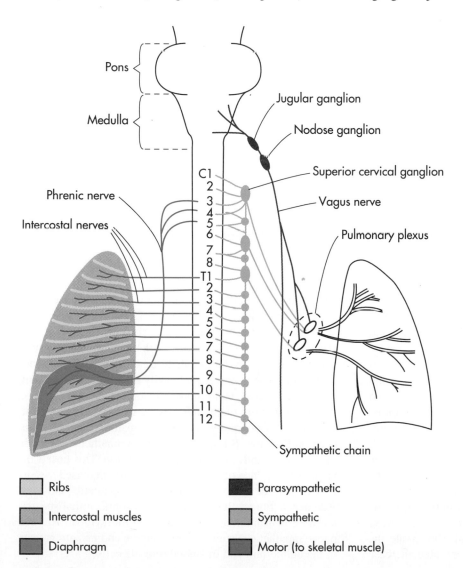

■ **Fig. 25-22** Innervation of the lungs. Schematic depiction of the autonomic innervation (motor and sensory) of the lung and the somatic (motor) nerve supply to the intercostals muscles and diaphragm.

Pons

Medulla

Phrenic nerve

Intercostal nerves

Jugular ganglion

Nodose ganglion

Superior cervical ganglion

Vagus nerve

Pulmonary plexus

C1
2
3
4
5
6
7
8
T1
2
3
4
5
6
7
8
9
10
11
12

Sympathetic chain

□ Ribs

□ Intercostal muscles

■ Diaphragm

■ Parasympathetic

□ Sympathetic

■ Motor (to skeletal muscle)

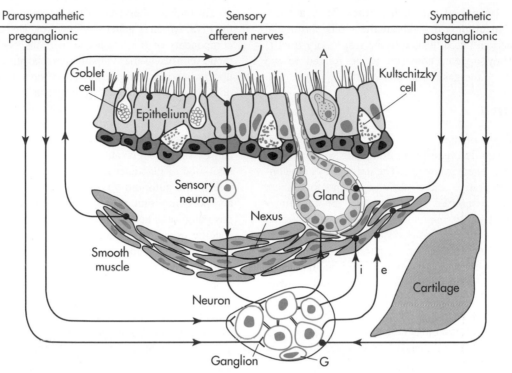

■ **Fig. 25-23**   Innervation. Schematic summary of the innervation of the airways. In the human lung, parasympathetic, preganglionic fibers descend into the vagus and terminate in the ganglia. The ganglia contain excitatory neurons that are cholingeric and inhibitory neurons that are nonadrenergic. Other neurons with an integrative function are probably also present. Glial cells *(G)* are present in the ganglia. Blood vessels and collagen are excluded from the neuropil. Postganglionic fibers to the smooth muscle are excitatory *(e)* or inhibitory *(i)*. Excitatory fibers may also terminate in the glands. Sensory afferent endings are present in the epithelium and the smooth muscle. The neurons associated with these endings may be in the vagus or the vagal nuclei. Sensory neurons may also be present in the mucosa, and fibers from these neurons may terminate in the ganglia, as in the gastrointestinal tract. Sympathetic postganglionic fibers terminate on the ganglia in humans and in other species, but adrenergic fibers to the glands or smooth muscle, although found in some mammals, have not been demonstrated in humans. In the epithelium, there are cells, such as Kultchitsky-type cell and the granular cell *(A),* found only in the chicken, whose functions are unknown. Nerves may be related to these cells. The human airway smooth muscle cells are connected by low resistance junctions and these connections may permit muscle mass to act as a syncytium. (From Richardson JB: *Am Rev Respir Dis* 119:785, 1978.)

Postganglionic fibers from the ganglia then complete the network by innervating smooth muscle cells, blood vessels, and bronchial epithelial cells (including goblet cells and submucosal glands). The anatomic locations of the parasympathetic nervous system enhance specific organ responses without influencing other organs. Both the preganglionic and postganglionic fibers contain excitatory (cholinergic) and inhibitory (nonadrenergic) motor neurons. Acetylcholine and substance P are neurotransmitters of excitatory motor neurons; dynorphin and vasoactive intestinal peptide are neurotransmitters of inhibitory motor neurons. Parasympathetic stimulation through the vagus nerve is responsible for the slightly constricted smooth muscle tone in the normal resting lung. Parasympathetic innervation is greater in the larger airways, and it diminishes toward the smaller conducting airways in the periphery. Parasympathetic fibers also innervate the bronchial glands, and these fibers, when stimulated, increase the synthesis of mucus glycoprotein, which raises the viscosity of the mucus.

Whereas the response of the parasympathetic nervous system is very specific and local, the response of the sympathetic nervous system tends to be more general. Mucous glands and blood vessels are heavily innervated by the sympathetic nervous system; however, smooth muscles are not. Neurotransmitters of the adrenergic nerves include norepinephrine and dopamine, although dopamine has no influence on the lung. Stimulation of the sympathetic nerves in the mucous glands increases water secretion. This upsets the balanced response of increased water and increased viscosity between the sympathetic and parasympathetic pathways. Adrenergic fibers, although present in some animal species, are absent in humans. In addition to the sympathetic and parasympathetic systems, afferent nerve endings are present in the epithelium and in smooth muscle cells.

CENTRAL CONTROL OF RESPIRATION

Breathing is an automatic, rhythmic, and centrally regulated process with voluntary control. The central nervous system, and, in particular, the brainstem, functions as the main control center for respiration (Fig. 25-24). Despite widely varying demands for oxygen uptake and carbon dioxide removal, arterial levels of O_2 and CO_2 are normally kept within close limits. Regulation of respiration requires (1) the generation and maintenance of a respiratory rhythm; (2) the modulation of this rhythm by sensory feedback loops and reflexes that allow adaptation to various conditions and minimize energy costs; and (3) the recruitment of respiratory muscles that can contract appropriately for gas exchange. Unlike the heart, which begins beating at approximately 6 weeks of gestation, rhythmic respirations do not begin until birth.

The central pattern generator (CPG) is most likely composed of several groups of cells in the brainstem that have the property of a pacemaker. The CPG integrates peripheral input from stretch receptors in the lung, from oxygen receptors in the carotid body, and from central input from the hypothalamus and amygdala. This input may be excitatory or inhibitory. In addition, because phrenic nerve output is absent between inspiratory efforts, an inspiratory on-off switch appears to operate in the system, and this switch inhibits the CPG during exhalation. The control of respiration is described in greater detail in Chapter 29.

GROWTH AND DEVELOPMENT: CONGENITAL LUNG DISEASE

The epithelial portion of the lung arises as a pouch from the primitive foregut at approximately 22 to 26 days after fertilization of the ovum. This single lung bud branches into primitive right and left lungs. Over the next 2–3 weeks, further branching occurs to create the irregular dichotomous branching pattern (Fig. 25-25). Reid has described "three Laws of Lung Development": (1) the bronchial tree is devel-

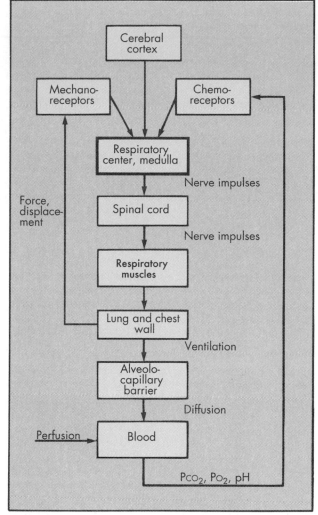

■ **Fig. 25-24** Central control. Block diagram of the respiratory control system. Ventilation and perfusion come together near the bottom, and their output sets arterial and alveolar carbon dioxide and oxygen partial pressures, and in part arterial hydrogen ion concentration, pH. These outputs feed back to the controllers via chemoreceptors located in strategic places.

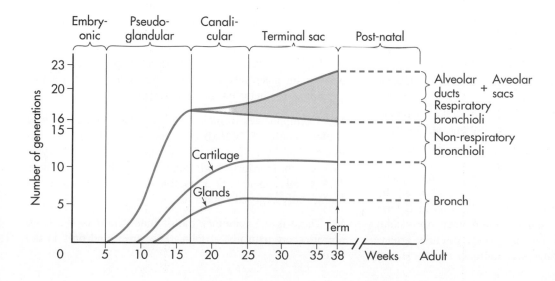

■ **Fig. 25-25** Lung growth. Chronology in lung development. (From Burn PH. In Fishman AP, Fisher AB, Geiger SR, editors: *Handbook of physiology,* Section 3, The respiratory system, vol I, Bethesda, Md, 1985, American Physiological Society.)

■ Table 25-3   Pulmonary congenital diseases

Congenital anomaly	Description
Congenital lobar emphysema	Overdistention of a lobe of unclear etiology but probably secondary to partial bronchial airway obstruction
Congenital lymphangiectasis	Congenital dilatation and over-growth of the pulmonary lymphatic system
Congenital cystic adenomatoid malformation	Developmental overgrowth of pulmonary tissue in the region of the end bronchioles with suppression of alveolar growth
Pulmonary agenesis, aplasia, hypoplasia	Diminished or absent pulmonary tissue, due to failure of development of the respiratory system from the foregut
Congenital bronchial stenosis	Stricture of the mainstem or middle lobe bronchus
Tracheal and esophageal deformities: vascular ring	A host of vascular anomalies that result in tracheal or bronchial compression and/or collapse
Tracheoesophageal fistula	Communication between the esophagus and the trachea resulting in aspiration
Thoracic wall deformities: pectus carinatum, pectus excavatum	Sternal protrusion or depression

oped by week 16 of intrauterine life; (2) alveoli develop after birth, and the number increases until the age of 8 years, and the size increases until growth of the chest wall finishes with adulthood; (3) preacinar vessels (arteries and veins) parallel the development of the airways, whereas the intraacinar vessels parallel that of the alveoli.

Thus, intrauterine events that occur prior to 16 weeks of gestation will affect the number of airways. For example, failure of the pleuroperitoneal canal to close and to separate the chest and abdominal cavities results in displacement of the intestines into the involved hemithorax. This condition, called congenital diaphragmatic hernia, occurs at 6 to 8 weeks of gestation; it occurs most often on the left, and it involves the foramen of Bochdalek. The lung on the affected side is smaller than usual, because it has been compressed by the presence of intestine. Also, the number of airways is decreased, because the failure of the pleuroperitoneal canal to close occurred very early in gestation. Even after the intestine has been surgically placed back into the abdomen, the small, hypoplastic (underdeveloped) lung will develop new alveoli, but the number of airways will remain decreased.

Another congenital anomaly is called pulmonary sequestration. This normally represents a malformation of the primitive respiratory and vascular systems, in which fetal lung tissue is segregated from the main tracheobronchial apparatus and ultimately has its own systemic artery. Although timing of this congenital anomaly is not clear, it probably appears early as an accessory bronchopulmonary bud that arises from the foregut.

Other important pulmonary congenital diseases are listed in Table 25-3.

SUMMARY

1. The lung has three functions: gas exchange, host defense, and metabolism.

2. The lung demonstrates anatomical and physiological unity; that is, each unit is structurally identical and it functions just like every other unit.

3. The bronchopulmonary segment is the **functional anatomical unit** of the lung. The segment of the lung supplied by a segmental bronchus is called the bronchopulmonary segment.

4. The terminal respiratory (gas-exchanging) unit, which consists of the respiratory bronchiole, alveolar ducts, and alveoli, is the **basic physiological unit** of the lung.

5. The lung has two separate blood supplies. The first is the pulmonary circulation, which brings deoxygenated blood from the right ventricle to the gas-exchanging units. In these units, oxygen is picked up and carbon dioxide is removed before the blood returns to the left atrium, for distribution to the rest of the body.

6. The second blood supply is the bronchial circulation, which arises from the aorta and provides nourishment to the lung parenchyma.

7. The circulation to the lung is unique in its dual circulation and in its ability to accommodate large volumes of blood (high capacitance, e.g., during exercise) at low pressure.

8. As a result of surfactant, the transmural pressure required to keep an alveolus inflated increases as lung volume (and transpulmonary pressure) increases and decreases as lung volume decreases.

9. The fluid volume moved through the lymphatics in 24 hours is equal to an animal's total plasma volume, and 25% to 50% of the total plasma proteins can move through the lymphatics in 24 hours.

10. BALT is similar to the Peyer's patches (GALT) that occur in the gastrointestinal tract, and a network of communication exists between the two systems.

11. T lymphocytes in most lymphoid tissue are comprised predominantly of TCRαβ cells, but in the lung and gastrointestinal system, scattered submucosal T lymphocytes have a disproportional high number of TCRγδ cells. These TCRγδ cells appear to be a first line of defense in these environmentally exposed organs.

12. There is no voluntary motor innervation in the lung, nor are there pain fibers. Pain fibers are found only in the pleura.

13. Stimulation of the parasympathetic system leads to airway constriction, blood vessel dilatation, and increased glandular secretion.

14. Stimulation of the sympathetic system causes airway relaxation, blood vessel constriction, and inhibition of glandular secretion.

BIBLIOGRAPHY

Journal articles

Baile EM: The anatomy and physiology of the bronchial circulation, *J Aerosol Med* 9(1):1, 1996.

Boggs DS, Kinasewitz GT: Review: pathophysiology of the pleural space, *Am J Med Sci* 309(1):53, 1995.

Creuwels LA, van Golde LM, Haagsman HP: The pulmonary surfactant system: biochemical and clinical aspects, *Lung* 175(1):1, 1997.

Factor P: Role and regulation of lung Na, K-ATPase, *Cell Mol Biol* 47(2):347, 2001.

Fehrenbach H: Alveolar epithelial type II cell: defender of the alveolus revisited. *Respir Res* 2(1):33, 2001.

Gandevia SC et al: Human respiratory muscles: sensations, reflexes and fatiguability, *Clin Exp Pharmacol Physiol* 25(10):757, 1998.

Hallman M, Glumoff V, Ramet M: Surfactant in respiratory distress syndrome and lung injury, *Comp Biochem Physiol A Mol Integr Physiol* 129(1):287, 2001.

Horsfield K, Cumming G: Morphology of the bronchial tree in man, *J Appl Physiol* 24:373, 1968.

Jeffrey PK: The development of large and small airways, *Am J Respir Crit Care Med* 157(5 Pt 2):S174, 1998.

Jobe AH, Ikegami M: Lung development and function in preterm infants in the surfactant treatment era, *Annu Rev Physiol* 62:825, 2000.

Khubchandani KR, Snyder JM: Surfactant protein A (SP-A): the alveolus and beyond, *FASEB J* 15(1):59, 2001.

Kravitz RM: Congenital malformations of the lung, *Pediatr Clin North Am* 41(3):453, 1994.

Massaro D, Massaro GD: Invited review: pulmonary alveoli: formation, the "call for oxygen," and other regulators, *Am J Physiol Lung Cell Mol Physiol* 282(3):L345, 2002.

Muratore CS, Wilson JM: Congenital diaphragmatic hernia: where are we and where do we go from here? *Semin Perinatol* 24(6):418, 2000.

Nettesheim P, Koo JS, Gray T: Regulation of differentiation of the tracheobronchial epithelium, *J Aerosol Med* 13(3):207, 2000.

Pison U et al: Host defence capacities of pulmonary surfactant: evidence for "non-surfactant" functions of the surfactant system, *Eur J Clin Invest* 24(9):586, 1994.

Poole DC et al: Diaphragm structure and function in health and disease, *Med Sci Sports Exerc* 29(6):738, 1997.

Rogers DE: Airway goblet cells: responsive and adaptable front-line defenders, *Eur Respir J* 7(9):1690, 1994.

Witte CL, Witte MH: Disorder of lymph flow, *Acad Radiol* 2(4):324, 1995.

Books and monographs

Avery ME, Fletcher BD, Williams R: *The lung and its disorders in the newborn infant*, ed 4, Philadelphia, 1981, WB Saunders Co.

Chernick V: *Kendig's disorders of the respiratory tract in children*, ed 5, Philadelphia, 1990, WB Saunders Co.

Fishman AP, editor: *Pulmonary diseases and disorders*, ed 2, vol 1, New York, 1988, McGraw-Hill.

Fishman AP, editor: *Pulmonary diseases and disorders*, ed 3, New York, 1998, McGraw-Hill.

George RB et al, editors: *Chest medicine: essentials of pulmonary and critical care medicine*, ed 3, Baltimore, Williams & Wilkins, 1995.

Leff AR, Schumacker PT: *Respiratory physiology: basics and applications*, Philadelphia, 1993, WB Saunders Co.

Murray JF: *The normal lung*, ed 2, Philadelphia, 1986, WB Saunders Co.

Murray JF, Nadel JA, editors: *Textbook of respiratory medicine*, ed 3, Philadelphia, 2000, WB Saunders Co.

Reith EJ, Ross MH: *Atlas of descriptive histology*, ed 2, New York, 1970, Harper & Row.

Weibel ER: *The pathway for oxygen: structure and function of the mammalian respiratory system*, Cambridge, Mass, 1984, Harvard University Press.

West JB: *Respiratory physiology: the essentials*, ed 1, Baltimore, 1974, Williams & Wilkins.

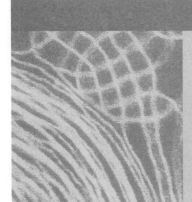

chapter twenty-six

Mechanical Properties of the Lung and Chest Wall: Static and Dynamic

STATIC LUNG MECHANICS

Lung Volumes

Before examining how air moves in and out of the lung, it is important to describe the various volumes of the lung and how they are measured. *Lung mechanics* is the study of the mechanical properties of the lung and chest wall. *Chest wall* is a term commonly used in lung mechanics to describe the properties of all of the structures that are outside of the lungs and that move during breathing. These structures include the rib cage, diaphragm, abdominal cavity, and anterior abdominal muscles. *Static mechanics* are the mechanical properties of a lung whose volume is not changing with time. The interaction between the lung and the chest wall determines the lung volume, and it is the lung volume that plays a major role in gas exchange and in the work of breathing. The static volumes of the lungs are shown in Fig. 26-1.

All lung volumes are subdivisions of the total lung capacity (TLC), and they are measured in liters. They are reported either as volumes or capacities. A *capacity* is composed of two or more volumes. Many of the lung volumes are measured by having the patient breathe through a mouthpiece and tubing that are connected to a spirometer (Fig. 26-2). The subject is asked first to breathe normally, and the volume of air (the tidal volume) that is moved with each quiet breath is recorded. The subject is then asked to inhale maximally, and then to exhale fully and completely.

The total volume of exhaled air, from a maximal inspiration to a maximal exhalation, is the **vital capacity (VC).** The **residual volume (RV)** is the air remaining in the lung after a complete exhalation. This volume is established during the first several breaths after birth. The **total lung capacity (TLC)** is the sum of the VC and the RV; it is the total volume of air contained in the lungs and it includes the volume of air that can be moved (VC) and the volume of air that is always present in the lung (RV).

The **functional residual capacity (FRC)** is the volume of air in the lung at the end of exhalation during quiet breathing. The FRC is also called the resting volume of the lung.

The FRC is composed of the RV and the *expiratory reserve volume,* or ERV (the volume of air that can be exhaled from FRC to RV).

The **RV/TLC** ratio is used to distinguish different types of pulmonary disease. In normal individuals, the ratio is usually less than 0.25. An elevated RV/TLC ratio, induced by an increase in RV out of proportion to an increase in TLC, is due to air trapping secondary to airway obstruction. This abnormal ratio occurs in a group of pulmonary diseases known as *obstructive pulmonary diseases.* An elevated RV/TLC ratio caused by a decrease in TLC occurs in individuals with restrictive types of lung disease. The measurement of these lung volumes is described later.

Determinants of Lung Volume

Why can't we inspire to levels above the TLC or exhale beyond the levels of RV? The answers lie in the properties of the lung parenchyma, and in the interactions between the lungs and the chest wall. The lungs are elastic; they expand when stresses are applied, and they recoil passively when stresses are released. The lungs are enclosed by the chest wall, which expands during inspiration. The lungs and chest wall always move together in healthy individuals.

Lung volumes are determined by the balance between the lung's elastic recoil properties and the properties of the muscles of the chest wall. TLC occurs when the forces of inspiration decrease because of muscle lengthening. The forces are insufficient to overcome the increasing force required to distend the lung and chest wall. RV occurs when the expiratory muscle force is insufficient to further reduce the chest wall volume. As the chest wall is squeezed by the expiratory muscles, the recoil pressure of the chest wall increases. The expiratory muscles shorten and their capacity to generate force decreases; the point at which the force generated by the expiratory muscles cannot overcome the outward recoil of the chest wall determines the RV.

The FRC is the volume of the lung at the end of a normal exhalation. It is determined by the balance between the elastic recoil pressure generated by the lung parenchyma to

464

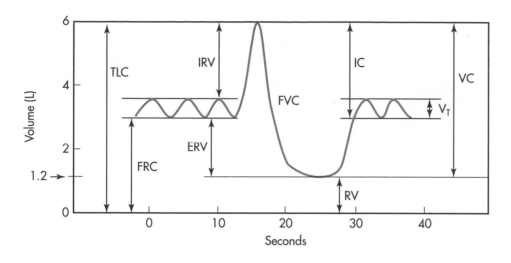

■ **Fig. 26-1** The various lung volumes and capacities. *TLC,* Total lung capacity; *FRC,* functional residual capacity; *IRV,* inspiratory reserve volume; *ERV,* expiratory reserve volume; *RV,* residual volume; *IC,* inspiratory capacity; V_T, tidal volume; *VC,* vital capacity; *FVC,* forced vital capacity.

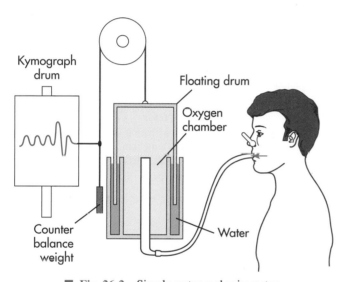

■ **Fig. 26-2** Simple water-seal spirometer.

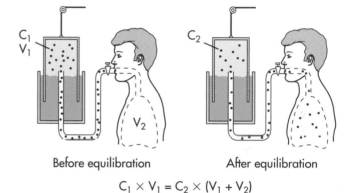

$$C_1 \times V_1 = C_2 \times (V_1 + V_2)$$

■ **Fig. 26-3** Measurement of lung volume by helium dilution.

become smaller and the pressure generated by the chest wall to become larger. When the chest wall is weak, the FRC decreases (lung elastic recoil > chest wall muscle force). In the presence of airway obstruction, the FRC increases because of premature airway closure, which traps air in the lung.

Measurement of Lung Volumes

RV and TLC can be measured in two ways: by helium dilution and by body plethysmography. In the helium dilution technique, a known concentration of an inert gas (such as helium) is added to a box of known volume. The box is then connected to a volume that is unknown (the lung volume to be measured). After adequate time for distribution of the inert gas, the new concentration of the inert gas is measured. The change in the concentration of the inert gas is then used to determine the new volume in which the inert gas has been distributed (Fig. 26-3). Specifically,

$$C_1 \times V_1 = C_2(V_1 + V_2)$$

where C_1 is the concentration of helium in the closed box of known volume (V_1), and C_2 is the concentration of helium after it has equilibrated in the new volume ($V_1 + V_2$). If the measurement is recorded when the individual has exhaled fully, V_2 is the residual volume. If it is measured at the end of a normal tidal volume breath, V_2 is the functional residual capacity.

Measuring Lung Volumes by Helium Dilution: An Example

The volume of the spirometer is 2 L, and to it a volume of helium is added to yield a concentration of 10%. The subject breathes in and out of the box. After 2 to 3 minutes of breathing quietly, the concentration of helium at the end of a normal exhalation (FRC) is 6.3%. The FRC is

$$C_1 \times V_1 = C_2(V_1 + V_2)$$
$$0.10 \times 2\ L = 0.063(2\ L + FRC)$$
$$FRC = 1.17\ L$$

Now the subject exhales to residual volume and th concentration is 7.1%. The residual volume is

$$C_1 \times V_1 = C_2(V_1 + V_2)$$
$$0.10 \times 2\ L = 0.071(2\ L + RV)$$
$$RV = 0.82\ L$$

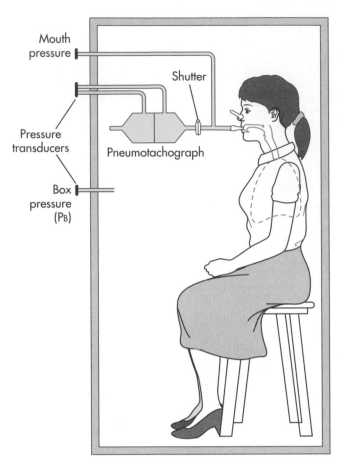

■ Fig. 26-4   The body plethysmograph.

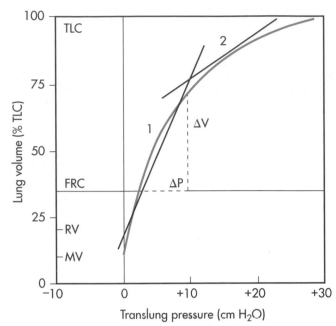

■ **Fig. 26-5**   Deflation pressure volume curve (PV). Because of hysteresis caused by surfactant, the deflation PV curve is used for measurements. Compliance at any point along this curve is the change in volume per change in pressure. From the curve it can be seen that lung compliance varies with lung volume. Compare compliance at 1 vs. 2. By convention, lung compliance is the change in pressure in going from FRC to FRC + 1 L.

Another way of measuring lung volumes is with a body plethysmograph (body box). This method uses Boyle's gas law, which states that pressure × volume is constant (at a constant temperature). The subject sits in an airtight box (Fig. 26-4) and breathes through a mouthpiece that is connected to a flow sensor (pneumotach). The subject then makes panting respiratory efforts against a closed mouthpiece. During the expiratory phase of the maneuver, the gas in the lung becomes compressed, the lung volume decreases, and the pressure inside the box falls, because the gas volume in the box increases. Knowing the volume of the box and measuring the change in pressure of the box at the mouth, the change in volume of the lung can be calculated. Thus,

$$P_1 \times V = P_2(V - \Delta V)$$

where P_1 and P_2 are the mouth pressures and V is the FRC.

In normal individuals the FRC measured by helium dilution and the FRC measured by plethysmography are essentially the same. This is not true in individuals with lung disease. The FRC measured by helium dilution measures the resting volume in the lung that communicates with the airways, whereas the FRC measured by plethysmography measures the total volume in the lung at the end of a normal exhalation. If a significant amount of gas is trapped in the lung (because of premature airway closure), the FRC determined by plethysmography will be considerably greater than the FRC measured by helium dilution.

Lung Compliance

Lung compliance (C_L) is a measure of the elastic properties of the lung, and it is a reflection of lung distensibility. Compliance of the lungs is defined as the change in lung volume evoked by a 1 cm H_2O change in the distending pressure of the lung. The units of compliance are ml (or L)/cm H_2O. A large lung compliance refers to a lung that is readily distended. A small lung compliance or "stiff" lung is a lung that is not easily distended. The compliance of the lung (C_L) is thus

$$C_L = \frac{\Delta V}{\Delta P}$$

where ΔV is the change in volume and ΔP is the change in pressure. The lung compliance is the slope of the line between any two points on the deflation limb of the pressure-volume loop (Fig. 26-5). The compliance of the normal human lung is about 0.2 L/cm H_2O, but it varies with lung volume. For this reason, the compliance per unit volume, or the **specific compliance,** is measured (Fig. 26-6).

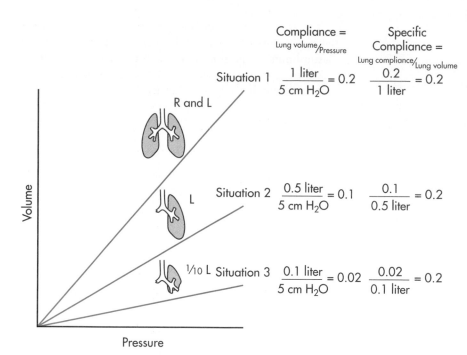

Compliance =
Lung volume/Pressure

Specific
Compliance =
Lung compliance/Lung volume

Situation 1 $\dfrac{1 \text{ liter}}{5 \text{ cm H}_2\text{O}} = 0.2$ $\dfrac{0.2}{1 \text{ liter}} = 0.2$

R and L

Situation 2 $\dfrac{0.5 \text{ liter}}{5 \text{ cm H}_2\text{O}} = 0.1$ $\dfrac{0.1}{0.5 \text{ liter}} = 0.2$

L

¹⁄₁₀ L   Situation 3 $\dfrac{0.1 \text{ liter}}{5 \text{ cm H}_2\text{O}} = 0.02$ $\dfrac{0.02}{0.1 \text{ liter}} = 0.2$

Volume

Pressure

■ **Fig. 26-6**   Relationship between compliance and lung volume. Imagine a lung in which a 5 cm H_2O change in pressure results in a 1 L change in volume. If half of the lung is removed, the compliance will decrease but when corrected for the volume of the lung there is no change (specific compliance). Even when the lung is reduced by 90%, the specific compliance is unchanged.

Measurement of Compliance

Compliance can be measured with an esophageal balloon that is connected to a pressure transducer and a spirometer. Esophageal balloon pressure is a measure of pleural pressure (P_{pl}). When the lung is not moving (that is, airflow is zero), the pleural pressure is subatmospheric or negative. This is because the lungs are elastic and they always tend to collapse. This tendency of the lung to collapse is resisted by the chest wall. Hence the P_{pl}, when the volume is constant, reflects the elastic pressure or recoil of the lung at that volume. If lung volume is increased by a known amount (ΔV) and volume is then held constant, the new P_{pl} is more negative (lung recoil is greater). The ΔV divided by the change in P_{pl} is the lung compliance.

Lung Compliance: An Example

A patient inhales 2 L of air and holds his breath with his glottis open. At the beginning of inspiration his esophageal pressure is –5 cm H_2O. During breath holding his esophageal pressure is –7.5 cm H_2O. What is his lung compliance?

$$C_L = \frac{\Delta V}{\Delta P} = \frac{2.0 \text{ L}}{-5(-7.5) \text{ cm H}_2\text{O}} = 0.8 \text{ L/cm H}_2\text{O}$$

This lung has a high compliance compatible with loss of elastic recoil as is seen in individuals with emphysema.

The compliance of the lung is affected by several respiratory disorders. In emphysema, the lung is more compliant; that is, for every 1 cm H_2O increase in pressure the increase in volume is greater than in the normal lung (see example) (Fig. 26-7). In contrast, in pulmonary fibrosis, the lung is noncompliant; that is, for every 1 cm change in water pressure, the change in volume is less.

Lung-Chest Wall Interactions

The lung and chest wall move together in healthy people. Separating these structures is the pleural space, which is best thought of as a potential space, because of its small volume. Because the lung and chest wall move together, changes in their respective volumes are equal. The pressure changes across the lung and across the chest wall are defined as the *transmural pressures*. For the lung, this transmural pressure is called the *transpulmonary (or translung) pressure* (P_L), and it is defined as the pressure difference between the airspaces (alveolar pressure, P_A) and the pressure surrounding the lung (pleural pressure, P_{pl}). That is,

$$P_L = P_A - P_{pl}$$

The lung requires a positive transpulmonary pressure in order to increase its volume; the lung volume increases with increasing transpulmonary pressure. The lung assumes its smallest size when the transpulmonary pressure is zero. The lung, however, is not devoid of air when the transpulmonary pressure is zero because of the surface tension lowering properties of surfactant.

The *transmural pressure (P_w) across the chest wall* is the difference between the pleural pressure and the pressure surrounding the chest wall (P_b), which is the barometric pressure or body surface pressure. That is,

$$P_w = P_{pl} - P_b$$

During the inspiratory phase of quiet breathing, the chest wall expands to a larger volume. Because the pleural pressure is negative relative to atmospheric pressure during quiet breathing, the transmural pressure across the chest wall is negative.

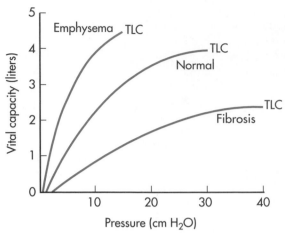

■ **Fig. 26-7** Fibrosis/emphysema pressure/volume curve.

The pressure across the respiratory system (P_{rs}) is the sum of the pressure across the lung and the pressure across the chest wall. That is,

$$P_{rs} = P_L + P_w$$
$$= (P_A - P_{pl}) + (P_{pl} - P_b)$$
$$= P_A - P_b$$

The pressure-volume relationships for the lung alone, for the chest wall alone, and for the intact respiratory system are shown in Fig. 26-8. A number of important observations can be made by examining the pressure-volume curves of the lung, chest wall, and respiratory system. Note that the transmural pressure across the respiratory system at FRC is zero. At TLC, both the lung and chest wall pressures are positive, and they both require positive transmural distending pressures. The resting volume of the *chest wall* is the volume at which the transmural pressure for the chest wall is zero, and it is approximately 60% of the TLC. At volumes greater than 60% of TLC the chest wall is recoiling inward, whereas at volumes below 60% of TLC, the chest wall tends to recoil outward (see Fig. 26-8).

The transmural distending pressure for the *lung alone* flattens at pressures greater than 20 cm H_2O, because the elastic limits of the lung have been reached. Thus, further increases in transmural pressure produce no change in volume and compliance is low. Further distension is limited by the connective tissue (collagen, elastin) of the lung. If further pressure is applied, the alveoli near the lung surface can rupture and air can escape into the pleural space. This is called a pneumothorax.

The relationship between pleural, alveolar, and elastic recoil pressure is shown in Fig. 26-9. The alveolar pressure is the sum of the pleural pressure and the elastic recoil pressure of the lung.

$$P_A = P_{el} + P_{pl}$$

Because $P_L = P_A - P_{pl}$,

$$P_L = (P_{el} + P_{pl}) - P_{pl}$$

Thus,

$$P_L = P_{el}$$

In general, P_L is the pressure distending the lung, whereas P_{el} is the pressure tending to collapse the lung.

Pressure-Volume Relationships

As previously mentioned, gas flows from an area of higher pressure to an area of lower pressure. This applies to both bulk flow of air into the airways, as well as to the movement of oxygen and carbon dioxide across the alveolar surface. Blood flow through the lung and breathing bring fresh sources of blood and air to the alveolar surface. Both pulmonary blood flow and alveolar ventilation can change significantly depending upon the metabolic needs of the individual. Such needs vary from quiet sleep to maximal activity. Minute ventilation is the volume of gas that is moved per unit of time. It is equal to the volume of gas moved with each breath (tidal volume) times the number of breaths per minute.

■ **Fig. 26-8** The relaxation pressure-volume curve of the lung, chest wall, and respiratory system. The curve for the respiratory system is the sum of the individual curves. The curve for the lung is the same as Fig. 26-5.

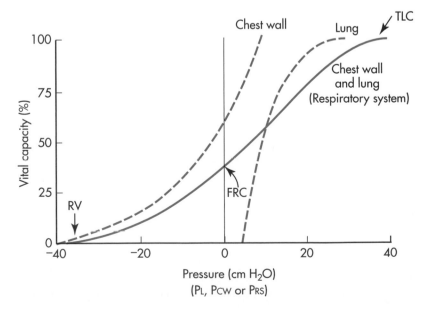

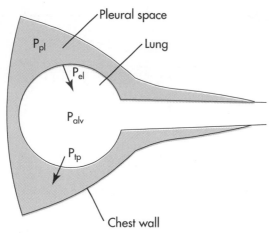

■ **Fig. 26-9** The relationship between the transpulmonary pressure (P_L), the pleural, alveolar, and elastic recoil pressures of the lung. The alveolar pressure is the sum of the pleural pressure and the elastic recoil pressure.

$$\dot{V}_E = V_T \times f$$

where $\dot{V}_E$ is minute ventilation in ml or L/min, V_T is tidal volume, in ml or L, and f is frequency or the number of breaths per minute.

Before inspiration begins, the pressure inside the pleura (pleural pressure) in normal individuals is approximately –5 cm H_2O. That is, the pressure in the pleural space is negative relative to atmospheric pressure. This negative pressure is created by the elastic recoil of the lung, and it acts to pull the lung away from the chest wall. At this point, the alveolar pressure is zero, because with no gas flow there is no pressure drop along the airways. With the onset of inspiration, the diaphragm and chest wall muscles shorten, which causes a downward movement of the diaphragm and outward and upward movements of the rib cage. Alveolar pressure falls below zero, and when the glottis is open, gas moves into the airways.

To understand the relationship between changes in pressure and changes in volume, it is helpful to examine the pressure changes during inspiration and expiration. In normal individuals during a tidal volume maneuver, alveolar pressure decreases at the start of inspiration. This decrease in alveolar pressure is usually small (1-3 cm H_2O) in normal individuals. In individuals with airway obstruction, the decrease is much greater, because in order for a pressure drop to occur across obstructed airways, a larger negative inspiratory force must be generated.

Intrapleural pressure also falls during inspiration. This decrease equals the sum of the lung elastic recoil, which increases as the lung inflates, and the pressure drops along the airways as gas flows from atmospheric pressure (zero) to the pressure in the alveolus (negative, relative to atmospheric pressure). Airflow stops when the alveolar pressure and the atmospheric pressure become equal.

On exhalation, the diaphragm moves higher into the chest, intrapleural pressure increases (i.e. becomes less negative),

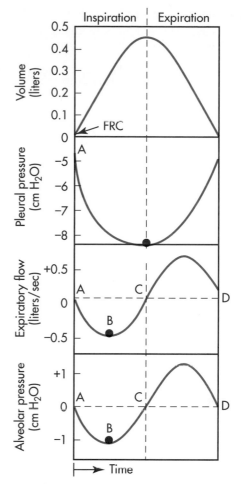

■ **Fig. 26-10** Changes in alveolar and pleural pressure during a tidal volume breath. Inspiration is to the left of the vertical dotted line and exhalation is to the right. Positive (relative to atmosphere) pressures are above the horizontal dotted line and negative pressures are below. See text for details. At points of no airflow, alveolar pressure is zero.

alveolar pressure becomes positive, the glottis opens and gas again flows from a higher (alveolus) to a lower (atmospheric) pressure. In the alveolus, the driving force for exhalation is the sum of the elastic recoil of the lung and the intrapleural pressure. The pressure events during inspiration and exhalation are shown in Fig. 26-10.

A few calculations may clarify these points. At the end of exhalation, the lung is at its resting volume (functional residual capacity). The pleural pressure is negative (–5 cm H_2O in normal individuals) because of the pressure generated by the elastic recoil of the lungs. Just before inspiration begins, P_A is zero and there is no gas flow. At this point, the transpulmonary pressure (i.e., the transmural pressure for the lung), as previously defined is

$$P_L = P_A - P_{pl}$$
$$P_L = 0 - (-5 \text{ cm } H_2O)$$
$$= 5 \text{ cm } H_2O$$

At this same time, the transmural pressure for the chest wall, defined as the pleural pressure minus the pressure outside of the chest wall, is

$$P_W = P_{pl} - P_b$$
$$= -5 \text{ cm H}_2\text{O} - (0)$$
$$= -5 \text{ cm H}_2\text{O}$$

Thus, the pressure across the respiratory system (transpulmonary + trans–chest wall pressures) is

$$P_{rs} = P_L + P_w$$
$$= 5 \text{ cm H}_2\text{O} + (-5 \text{ cm H}_2\text{O})$$
$$= 0$$

In the absence of airflow, the pressure across the respiratory system is zero.

Note that at the resting volume of the lung (the FRC), the elastic recoil of the lung acts to decrease lung volume, but it is balanced by the recoil of the chest wall that acts to increase the lung volume. At FRC, the forces are equal and opposite, and the muscles are relaxed.

At end inspiration, similar events occur, and alveolar pressure is zero. At this time, pleural pressure is approximately –8 cm H_2O, and hence the transpulmonary pressure is

$$P_L = P_A - P_{pl} = 0 - (-8 \text{ cm H}_2\text{O})$$
$$= 8 \text{ cm H}_2\text{O}$$

The trans–chest wall pressure at end inspiration is

$$P_w = P_{pl} - P_b = -8 \text{ cm H}_2\text{O} - (0)$$
$$= -8 \text{ cm H}_2\text{O}$$

The pressures now are different, but again the pressure across the respiratory system is zero and there is no airflow. This is different than the FRC because this volume is being maintained by the active contraction of the muscles of respiration.

When the chest is opened, as during thoracic surgery, the lung recoils until the transpulmonary pressure is zero and the chest wall increases in size. The lungs do not, however, become airless, but they retain approximately 10% of their total lung capacity.

DYNAMIC LUNG MECHANICS

In this section we examine the principles that control air movement in and out of the lung. *Dynamic lung mechanics* is that aspect of mechanics that studies the lung in motion.

Dynamic Compliance

Previously, we examined compliance in terms of static changes, that is, we have determined compliance at discrete times. Breathing and temporal components create a set of dynamic mechanical properties that affect the pressure in the lung and chest wall.

A dynamic pressure-volume curve can be created by having an individual breathe over a normal lung volume range (usually from FRC to FRC + 1 L). The mean dynamic compliance of the lung (dyn C_L) is calculated as the slope of the

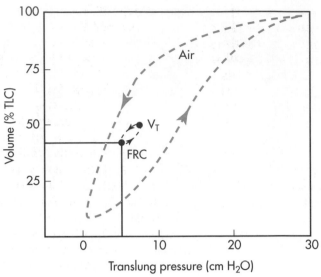

■ Fig. 26-11 Inflation : deflation pressure-volume curve. The direction of inspiration and exhalation is shown by the arrows. The difference between the inflation and deflation pressure volume curves is due to surface tension variation with changes in lung volume.

line that joins the end-inspiratory and end-expiratory points of no flow (Fig. 26-11).

Dynamic compliance is always less than static compliance, and it increases during exercise. This is because during tidal volume breathing, a small change in alveolar surface area is insufficient to bring additional surfactant molecules to the surface and so the lung is less compliant. During exercise, the opposite occurs; there are large changes in tidal volume and more surfactant material is incorporated into the air-liquid interface. Therefore, the lung is more compliant.

Sighing and yawning increase dynamic compliance by increasing the tidal volume by restoring the normal surfactant layer. Both of these respiratory activities are important to maintaining normal lung compliance. In contrast to the lung, the *dynamic compliance of the chest wall* is not significantly different from its static compliance.

Airflow in Airways

Air flows through a tube when there is a pressure difference at the two ends of the tube. Specifically, during inspiration evoked by the contraction of the diaphragm, the pleural pressure becomes more negative. As a result, gas flows into the lung (from the higher to the lower pressure), assuming that the glottis is open and that there is no obstruction to gas flow.

At low flow rates, in a cylindrical tube, the stream of gas is parallel to the walls of the tube and laminar flow occurs (see Chapter 18). As the flow rate increases and particularly as the airways divide, the flow stream becomes unsteady and small eddies occur. At higher flow rates, the flow stream is disorganized and *turbulence* occurs (see Chapter 18).

In laminar flow, the gas traveling in the center of the tube moves most rapidly, whereas the gas in direct contact with the walls of the tube remains stationary. In fact, when laminar flow is fully developed, the gas in the center of the tube moves twice as fast as the average velocity. This changing velocity across the diameter of the tube is known as the *velocity profile*. The pressure flow characteristics of laminar flow were first described by the French physician, Poiseuille (see Chapter 18). In straight circular tubes, the flow rate ($\dot{V}$), is defined by the following equation:

$$\dot{V} = \frac{P\pi r^4}{8nl}$$

where P is the driving pressure, r is the radius of the tube, n is the viscosity of the fluid, and l is the length of the tube. It can be seen that the driving pressure (P) is proportional to the flow rate ($\dot{V}$). The flow resistance, R, across a set of tubes is the change in driving pressure (ΔP) divided by flow rate, or

$$R = \frac{\Delta P}{\dot{V}} = \frac{8nl}{\pi r^4}$$

The units of resistance are cm $H_2O/L \cdot$ sec. There are a number of important conclusions that can be derived from this equation. The first is the importance of radius in determining resistance. If the radius of the tube is reduced in half, the resistance will increase 16-fold. If, however, the tube length is increased 2-fold, the resistance will increase only 2-fold. Thus, the radius of the tube is the principal determinant of the resistance. Stated in another way, resistance is inversely proportional to the fourth power of the radius, and it is directly proportional to the length of the tube and to the viscosity.

In turbulent flow, gas movement occurs both parallel and perpendicular to the axis of the tube. Pressure is proportional to the flow rate squared. Viscosity of the gas increases with the gas density, and therefore the pressure drop increases for a given flow. The gas along the wall of the tube remains stationary, but there is less variation in gas velocity as a function of the position of a gas particle in the tube. Overall, gas velocity is blunted, because energy is consumed in the process of generating the eddies and chaotic movement. As a consequence, a higher driving pressure is needed to support a given turbulent flow than to support a given laminar flow.

Whether flow through a tube is laminar or turbulent depends upon the Reynold's number (see Chapter 18). Reynold's number (R_e) is a dimensionless value that expresses the ratio of two dimensionally equivalent terms (kinematic/viscosity).

$$R_e = \frac{2rvd}{\eta}$$

where d is the fluid density, v is the average velocity, r is the radius, and η is the viscosity. In straight tubes, turbulence occurs when the Reynold's number is greater than 2000. From this relationship, it can be seen that turbulence is most likely to occur when the average velocity of gas flow is high and the radius is large. In contrast, a low-density gas, such as helium, is less likely to cause turbulent flow.

In marginally laminar or disturbed flow, the characteristics of both laminar and turbulent flow are seen. Flow through

much of the tube may be laminar, but it becomes more turbulent at sites where the tubes narrow or branch or where the walls of the tube become irregular.

Although the above relationships apply well to smooth cylindrical tubes, the application of the above principles to a complicated system of tubes, such as the conducting airways, is difficult. During quiet breathing, gas flow at the mouth is approximately 1 L/sec. Gas velocities of 150 cm/sec will occur in an adult with a tracheal diameter of 3 cm. Because air has a density of 0.0012 g/ml and a viscosity of 1.83×10^{-4} g/(cm/sec), the Reynolds number is greater than 2000. Hence, turbulent flow occurs in the trachea, even during quiet breathing.

> **Gas Flow in the Trachea During Quiet Breathing: An Example**
>
> $$R_e = \frac{2rvd}{\eta}$$
>
> $$R_e = \frac{2 \cdot 1.5 \text{ cm} \cdot 150 \text{ cm/sec} \cdot 0.0012 \text{ g/ml}}{1.83 \times 10^{-4} \text{ g/sec} \cdot \text{cm}}$$
>
> $$R_e = \frac{0.54}{0.000183}$$
>
> $$= 2951$$
>
> that is, turbulent flow is present

Turbulence is also promoted by the glottis and vocal cords, which produce some irregularity and obstruction in the tubes. As gas flows distally, the increase in total cross-sectional area increases dramatically, and gas velocities decrease significantly. As a result, gas flow becomes more laminar in the smaller airways, even during maximal ventilation. Overall, the gas flow in the larger airways (nose, mouth, glottis, and bronchi) is turbulent, whereas the gas flow in the smaller airways is laminar. Breath sounds heard with a stethoscope reflect the turbulent airflow. Laminar flow is silent.

Lung Resistance

Airflow resistance in the airways (R_{aw}) differs in the large airways (>2 mm diameter: first eight airway generations), the medium size airways (subsegmental bronchi; ~2 mm), and the small airways (<2 mm; bronchioles). Therefore, R_{aw} is equal to the sum of these resistances (i.e., $R_{aw} = R_{large} + R_{medium} + R_{small}$). From Poiseuille's equation, one might conclude that the major site of airways resistance is in the smallest airways. In fact, however, the major site of resistance along the bronchial tree is the large bronchi. The smallest airways contribute very little to the overall total resistance of the bronchial tree (Fig. 26-12). The reason for this is 2-fold. First, airflow velocity decreases substantially as the effective cross-sectional area increases. Second and most importantly, the airways exist mainly in parallel, rather than in series. Because the resistance of this area, composed of many airways in parallel, is the inverse of the sum of the individual resistances, the overall resistance of the small airways is very small. As an example, assume that each of three tubes

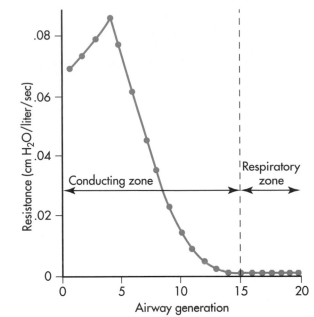

■ **Fig. 26-12**   Airways resistance as a function of the airway generation. In the normal lung, most of the resistance to airflow occurs in the first eight airway generations.

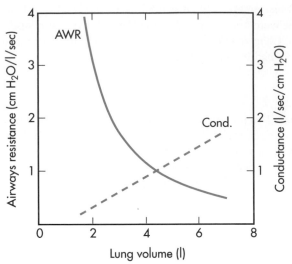

■ **Fig. 26-13**   Airway resistance *(AWR)* and conductance *(Cond.)* as a function of lung volume.

has a resistance of 3 cm H_2O. If the tubes are in series, the total resistance (R_{tot}) is the sum of the individual resistances:

$$R_{tot} = R_1 + R_2 + R_3 = 3 + 3 + 3 = 9 \text{ cm } H_2O$$

If the tubes are in parallel (as they are in small airways) the total resistance is the sum of the inverse of the individual resistances:

$$R_{tot} = 1/R_1 + 1/R_2 + 1/R_3 = 1/3 + 1/3 + 1/3 = 1 \text{ cm } H_2O$$

This relationship is in marked contrast to the pulmonary blood vessels in which most of the resistance is located in the small vessels.

Resistance: An Example

If the resistance of the entire respiratory system (R_{aw}) is 2 cm H_2O/L • sec and the trachea to segmental bronchi ("large") airways contribute 80% to the total resistance, the subsegmental (~2 mm, "medium") airways contribute 15% and the "small" (<2 mm) airways the remainder, what are the individual resistances of the small, medium, and large airways?

Large airways = 0.80×2 cm H_2O/L • sec = 1.6 cm H_2O/L/sec
Medium airways = 0.15×2 cm H_2O/L • sec =
                                              0.30 cm H_2O/L/sec
Small airways = 0.05×2 cm H_2O/L • sec = 0.10 cm H_2O/L/sec

In this example, tripling the resistance in the small airways by an obstruction would increase Raw by only 2.2 cm H_2O/L/sec, a 10% change. Thus, significant small airway disease can exist without a substantial change in Raw.

In the lungs, the trachea divides into the mainstem bronchi, which in turn divide into the lobar, then the segmental, and finally the subsegmental bronchi. In comparing the airways from the trachea to the respiratory bronchioles, the number of airway branches increases as the size of each branch decreases. As the airway diameter decreases, the resistance offered by each airway increases, but the large increase in the number of parallel pathways reduces the resistance at each generation of branching (Fig. 25-6). During normal breathing, approximately 80% of the resistance to airflow at FRC occurs in the airways with diameters greater than 2 mm. Because the small airways contribute so little to total lung resistance, the measurement of airway resistance is a poor test for detecting small airway obstruction.

Factors That Contribute to Resistance

In healthy individuals, lung resistance is approximately 1 cm H_2O/liter • sec. One of the most important factors affecting resistance is lung volume, because the caliber of the airways increases with increasing lung volume. As a result, resistance to airflow decreases with increasing lung volume, and it increases with decreasing lung volume. If the reciprocal of resistance (i.e., conductance) is plotted against lung volume, the relationship is linear (Fig. 26-13). In the presence of increased airway resistance, breathing at a higher lung volume will reduce airway resistance. Patients with increased airway resistance frequently have high lung volumes. Other factors that increase resistance include airway mucus, edema, and contraction of bronchial smooth muscle, all of which decrease the caliber of the airways.

The density and viscosity of the inspired gas also affect airway resistance. When gas density increases, such as during a dive, the airway resistance increases. When an oxygen-helium mixture is breathed, the decrease in gas density decreases the airway resistance. This decrease has been exploited in the treatment of **status asthmaticus,** a condition associated with increased airway resistance due to a combination of bronchospasm, edema, and mucus. In patients with this condition, breathing in an oxygen-helium mixture decreases the airway resistance.

Measurement of Airways Resistance

To calculate total airway resistance, alveolar pressure, airflow, and velocity must be measured. Airflow at the mouth can be measured with a flowmeter. Alveolar pressure can be measured either with an esophageal balloon attached to a pressure transducer to measure pleural pressure, or with a body plethysmograph.

Measuring R_{aw} with an Esophageal Balloon: An Example

At an expiratory flow rate of 0.5 L/min, the esophageal balloon pressure is 7.5 cm H_2O and the pressure at the mouth is 7.0 cm H_2O. What is the pulmonary resistance?

$$R_{aw} = \frac{\Delta P}{\dot{V}} = \frac{P_{pl} - P_{mouth}}{\dot{V}}$$

$$= \frac{7.5 \text{ cm } H_2O - 7.0 \text{ cm } H_2O}{0.5 \text{ L/sec}}$$

$$= 1.0 \text{ cm } H_2O/\text{L/sec}$$

Although this method actually measures the *pulmonary* resistance (which is equal to the airway resistance, plus a small component due to lung tissue resistance), it is also a good approximation of airway resistance. Airway resistance can also be measured with a body plethysmograph.

In normal adults, *airway* resistance with the lungs at FRC is 1 to 3 cm H_2O/L/sec. Resistance is greater in young children, because their airways are smaller. As explained below, a strong negative correlation exists between resistance and maximal expiratory flow. A high resistance is associated with decreased expiratory flow.

Neurohumoral Regulation of Airway Resistance

In addition to the effects of disease, airway resistance can be affected or regulated by various neural and humoral agents. Stimulation of efferent vagal fibers, either directly or reflexly, increases airway resistance and decreases anatomical and dead space secondary to airway constriction (recall that the vagus nerve innervates airway smooth muscle). In contrast, stimulation of the sympathetic nerves and release of the postganglionic neurotransmitter norepinephrine inhibit airway constriction.

Reflex stimulation of the vagus nerve by smoke inhalation, dust, cold air, or other irritants can result in airway constriction and coughing. Agents such as histamine, acetylcholine, thromboxane A_2, prostaglandin F_2, and leukotrienes (LTB$_4$, C$_4$, and

D_4) are released by various resident and recruited airway cells in response to various triggers. These agents act directly on airway smooth muscle to cause constriction and an increase in airway resistance. Methacholine, a histamine-like compound, is inhaled by patients who have asthma to provoke airway constriction. Although everyone is capable of responding to methacholine, patients with asthma develop airway obstruction at much lower concentrations of methacholine.

Measurements of Expiratory Flow

Expiratory flows can be measured by spirometry, an important clinical tool for diagnosing and monitoring the course of many respiratory diseases. In addition to measuring lung volumes (Fig. 26-2), spirometry assesses the rate at which the lung changes volume during a forced breathing maneuver. When spirometry is performed from total lung capacity (TLC), spirometry measures the **forced vital capacity (FVC),** the single most important pulmonary function test. In this maneuver, the subject inhales maximally and then exhales as rapidly and completely as possible.

Spirometry. The FVC maneuver can be displayed in two different ways, namely by the spirogram and by the flow-volume loop. In the spirogram method, the volume of gas exhaled is plotted against time, as shown in Fig. 26-14. The spirogram provides four major test results: (1) the FVC, (2) the forced expiratory volume in 1 second (FEV$_1$), (3) the ratio of the FEV$_1$ to the FVC (FEV$_1$/FVC), and (4) the average mid-maximal expiratory flow (FEF$_{25-75}$).

The total volume of air that is exhaled during a forced exhalation is called the FVC, and it is reported in liters. The volume of air that is exhaled in the first second during the maneuver is called the forced expiratory volume in 1 second (or FEV$_1$), and it too is reported in liters. In normal individuals, at least 72% of the vital capacity can be exhaled in the first second. Thus, the FEV$_1$/FVC ratio is greater than 72% in normal individuals. If this ratio is less than 72%, the results suggest difficulty in exhaling due to obstruction, and it is a hallmark of obstructive pulmonary disease. The third measure made by the spirogram is the average flow rate over the middle section of the vital capacity. This test has several names, including the **MMEF (mid-maximal expiratory flow)** and the **FEF$_{25-75}$ (forced expiratory flow from 25 to 75% of the vital capacity).** It can be calculated from the spirogram by dividing the vital capacity into quarters, dropping a line from the first (25%) and third (75%) quartiles, and then connecting the lines and measuring the slope. Volume/time is a flow rate and thus the slope is a flow rate (the only real flow rate that can easily be obtained from the spirogram). The maximum or peak expiratory flow rate (PEFR) can also be obtained from the spirogram by measuring the maximum slope. However, this is rarely done, because there are easier measurement techniques.

Lung Volumes by Spirometry: An Example

What are
1. FVC = 5.0 L
2. FEV$_1$ = 3.8 L

■ **Fig. 26-14** The clinical spirogram (**A**) and expiratory flow volume curve (**B**). The subject takes a maximal inspiration and then exhales as rapidly, as forcibly, and as maximally as possible. The volume exhaled is plotted as a function of time. In the spirogram that is reported in clinical settings, exhaled volume increases from the bottom of the trace to the top (**A**). This is in contrast to the physiologist's view of the same maneuver (Fig. 26-1) in which the exhaled volume increases from the top to the bottom of the trace. Note the locations of TLC and RV on both tracings.

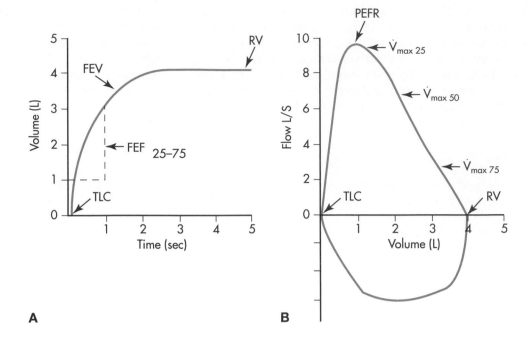

A   **B**

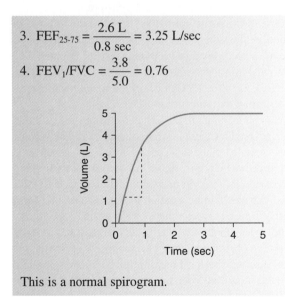

3. $FEF_{25-75} = \dfrac{2.6\ L}{0.8\ sec} = 3.25\ L/sec$

4. $FEV_1/FVC = \dfrac{3.8}{5.0} = 0.76$

This is a normal spirogram.

Flow-volume loop. The second way that the FVC maneuver can be displayed is by recording the instantaneous flow rate versus volume. This is called the *flow-volume loop*. The flow-volume loop can record instantaneous flow both during exhalation (expiratory flow-volume loop) and during inspiration (inspiratory flow-volume loop) (Fig. 26-14, *B*). The flow-volume loop is created in much the same way as the spirogram. The subject puts a mouthpiece in his mouth and breathes normally (tidal volume). He is then asked to take a maximal inspiration to total lung capacity, and then to breathe out as fast and as rapidly as he can, until he can exhale no further (a maximal exhalation to RV); he then takes a rapid and maximal inspiration. Flow rates above the horizontal line are expiratory, whereas flow rates below the horizontal line are inspiratory. The point at which inspiration is maximal is the total lung capacity, whereas the point at which exhalation is maximal is the residual volume.

The flow-volume loop yields data for four main pulmonary function tests. Again, the total amount of air that can be exhaled is called the FVC. The greatest flow rate achieved during the maneuver is called the **peak expiratory flow rate (PEFR)**. The flow-volume loop can be divided into quarters. The instantaneous flow rate, at which 50% of the VC remains to be exhaled, is called the **FEF_{50}** (also known as the **$\dot{V}max_{50}$**). The flow rate at which 75% of the VC has been exhaled is called the $\dot{V}max$ 75% (**$\dot{V}max_{75}$**), and the flow rate at which 25% of the VC has been exhaled is called the $\dot{V}max$ 25% (**$\dot{V}max_{25}$**).

Pulmonary Function and the Expiratory Flow-Volume Curve: An Example

1. FVC = 5.0
2. PEFR = 10 L/sec
3. $\dot{V}max_{50}$ = 7.5 L/sec
4. $\dot{V}max_{75}$ = 3.8 L/sec

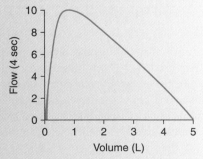

This is a normal expiratory flow-volume curve.

Determinants of Maximal Flow

Inspection of the flow-volume loop reveals that the maximum inspiratory flow is the same or slightly greater than the

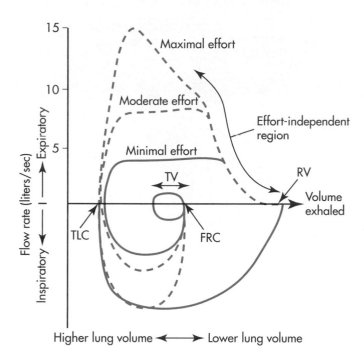

■ **Fig. 26-15** Isovolume curves. Three superimposed expiratory flow maneuvers are made with increasing effort. Note that peak inspiratory and expiratory flow rates are *effort dependent*, whereas expiratory flow rates later in expiration are *effort independent*.

maximal expiratory flow. Three major factors are responsible for the maximum inspiratory flow. First is the force generated by the inspiratory muscles that decreases as lung volume increases above RV. Second, the static recoil pressure of the lung increases as the lung volume increases above RV. This opposes the force generated by the inspiratory muscles, and it tends to reduce maximum inspiratory flows. However, airway resistance decreases with increasing lung volume as the airway caliber increases. The combination of the inspiratory muscle force, the static recoil of the lung, and the changes in airway resistance causes maximal inspiratory flow to occur about halfway between TLC and RV.

During exhalation, maximal flow occurs early (in the first 20%) in the maneuver, and it decreases progressively toward the RV. Even with increasing effort, maximal flows will decrease as RV is approached ("expiratory flow limitation"; see below for an explanation). Expiratory flow limitation can be demonstrated by asking an individual to perform three forced expiratory maneuvers with increasing effort. Figure 26-15 shows the results of these three maneuvers. As effort increases, peak expiratory flow increases. However, the flow rates at lower lung volumes converge; this indicates that with modest effort, a maximal expiratory flow is achieved. No amount of effort will increase these flow rates when lung volumes are diminished. For this reason, expiratory flow rates at lower lung volumes are said to be *effort independent*, because maximal flow is achieved with modest effort. In this range, the expiratory flow rate is flow limited by the lung, and no amount of additional effort can increase the flow rate beyond this limit. In contrast, events early in the expiratory maneuver are said to be *effort dependent,* that is, increasing effort generates increasing flow rates. In general, the first 20% of flow in the expiratory flow-volume loop is effort dependent.

Flow Limitation and the Equal Pressure Point

What is the mechanism for expiratory flow limitation? Flow limitation occurs when the airways, which are intrinsically floppy, distensible tubes, become compressed. The airways become compressed when the pressure outside of the airway exceeds the pressure inside the airway.

Figure 26-16 shows the events that occur during expiratory flow limitation at two different lung volumes. The collective airways and alveoli are surrounded by the pleural space and the chest wall. The airways are shown as tapered tubes, because the total or collective airway cross-sectional area decreases from the alveoli to the trachea. At the start of exhalation, but before any gas flow occurs, the pressure inside the alveolus (P_A) is zero (no airflow), and the pleural pressure (in this example) is −30 cm H_2O. The transpulmonary pressure is thus +30 cm H_2O ($P_L = P_A − P_{pl}$). Because there is no flow, the pressure inside the airways is zero and the pressure across the airways (P_{ta}, transairway pressure) is +30 cm H_2O [$P_{ta} = P_{airway} − P_{pl} = 0 − (−30$ cm $H_2O)$]. This positive transpulmonary and transairway pressure holds the alveoli and the airways open.

When exhalation begins and the diaphragm relaxes, the pleural pressure rises to +60 cm H_2O. Alveolar pressure also rises; this is due in part to the increase in pleural pressure (60 cm H_2O), and in part to the elastic recoil pressure of the lung at that lung volume. Alveolar pressure is thus the sum of the pleural pressure and the elastic recoil pressure (which in this case is 30 cm H_2O). This is the driving pressure for expiratory gas flow. Because the alveolar pressure ($P_A = P_{el} + P_{pl} = 30$ cm $H_2O + 60$ cm $H_2O = 90$ cm H_2O in this example) exceeds the atmospheric pressure, gas begins to flow from the alveolus to the mouth when the glottis opens. As

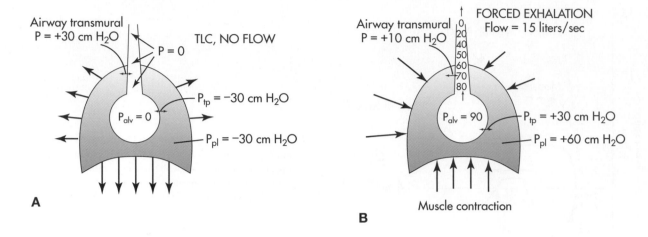

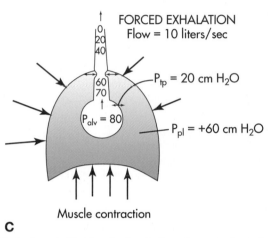

■ **Fig. 26-16**   Flow limitation. **A,** End inspiration, before the start of exhalation. **B,** At the start of a forced exhalation. **C,** Expiratory flow limitation later in a forced exhalation. Expiratory flow limitation occurs at locations where airway diameter is narrowed as a result of a negative transmural pressure. See text for further explanation.

gas flows out of the alveoli, the transmural pressure across the airways decreases (i.e., the pressure head for expiratory gas flow dissipates). This occurs for two reasons: first, there is a resistive pressure drop caused by the frictional pressure loss associated with flow (expiratory airflow resistance), and second, as the cross-sectional area of the airways decreases toward the trachea, the gas velocity increases. This acceleration of gas flow further decreases the pressure (see Chapter 18).

Thus, as air moves out of the lung, the driving pressure for expiratory gas flow decreases. In addition, the mechanical tethering that holds the airways open at high lung volumes diminishes as lung volume decreases. There is a point between the alveoli and the mouth at which the pressure inside the airways equals the pressure that surrounds the airways. This point is called the *equal pressure point*. Airways toward the mouth become compressed, because the pressure outside is greater than the pressure inside *(dynamic airway compression)*. As a consequence, the transairway pressure now becomes negative [$P_{ta} = P_{airway} - P_{pl} = 58 - (+60) = -2$ cm

H_2O just beyond the equal pressure point]. No amount of effort will increase the flow further, because the higher pleural pressure tends to collapse the airway at the equal pressure point, just as it also tends to increase the gradient for expiratory gas flow. Under these conditions, airflow is independent of the total driving pressure. Hence, the independent expiratory effort flow is limited. It is also why airway resistance is greater during exhalation than during inspiration.

In the absence of lung disease, the equal pressure point occurs in the airways that contain cartilage, and thus they resist deformation. The equal pressure point, however, is not static. As lung volume decreases, and as the elastic recoil pressure decreases, the equal pressure point moves closer to the alveoli. What happens in individuals with lung disease? Imagine, an individual with airway obstruction secondary to a combination of mucus accumulation and airway inflammation. At the start of exhalation, the driving pressure for expiratory gas flow is the same as in the normal individual, that is, the driving pressure is the sum of the elastic recoil pressure and the pleural pressure.

■ **Table 26-1**   Normal values

Lung volumes	
Functional residual capacity	2.4 L
Total lung capacity	6 L
Tidal volume	0.5 L
Breathing frequency	12/min

Mechanics	
Pleural pressure, mean	–5 cm H_2O
Chest wall compliance (at FRC)	0.2 L/cm H_2O
Lung compliance (at FRC)	0.2 L/cm H_2O
Airway resistance	2.0 cm H_2O/L/sec

As exhalation proceeds, however, the resistive drop in pressure increases due to the decrease in airway radius secondary to the mucus accumulation and the inflammation. As a result, the locus at which the pressure inside of the airway is equal to the pressure outside now occurs in the smaller airways that are devoid of cartilage. These airways become compressed, and they readily collapse as the equal pressure point becomes closer to the alveolus. Premature airway closure occurs, and this results in air trapping and an increase in lung volume. The increase in lung volume initially helps to offset the increase in airway resistance due to the mucus accumulation and inflammation by increasing the airway caliber and the elastic recoil. As inflammation progresses or as mucus accumulates, flow is limited and maximal expiratory flow rates decrease. Premature airway closure is responsible for the appearance of crackles on auscultation in individuals with lung disease. The crackles can be due to mucus accumulation, airway inflammation, fluid in the airways, or any mechanism responsible for airway narrowing or compression, and it can also be due to loss of elastic recoil (emphysema). In fact, acute and chronic lung diseases can change the expiratory flow-volume relationship by changes in (1) static lung recoil pressures, (2) airways resistance and the distribution of resistance along the airways, (3) loss of mechanical tethering of intraparenchymal airways, (4) changes in the stiffness or mechanical properties of the airways, and (5) differences in the severity of the above changes in various lung regions.

Uses of Spirometry and Body Plethysmography

Spirometry and lung volume measurements can provide important clinical information. Predicted values vary with age, gender, ethnicity, and height, and, to a lesser extent, with weight. Normal ranges are larger for flow rates than for volumes (Table 26-1). Abnormalities in values indicate abnormal pulmonary function, and they can be used to predict abnormalities in gas exchange. These values can detect the presence of abnormal lung function long before respiratory symptoms develop, and they determine disease severity and the response to therapy. For example, an improved response of >12% in FEV_1 after administration of a bronchodilator is considered a clinically significant improvement.

WORK OF BREATHING

Breathing requires the use of respiratory muscles (diaphragm, intercostals, etc.), which expend energy. Therefore, work is involved in the inspiration and exhalation of each breath. Work is required to overcome the inherent mechanical properties of the lung (i.e., elastic and flow-resistive forces) to move both the lungs and the chest wall. In the respiratory system the work of breathing is calculated by multiplying the change in volume times the pressure exerted across the respiratory system. That is,

Work of breathing (W) = Pressure (P) × Change in volume (ΔV)

Although methods are not available to measure the total amount of work involved in breathing, one can estimate the mechanical work by measuring the volume and pressure changes during a respiratory cycle. Analysis of pressure-volume curves can be used to illustrate these points (Fig. 26-17). In Figure 26-17, *A* represents a respiratory cycle of a normal lung. The static inflation-deflation curve is represented by line ABC. The total mechanical workload is represented by the trapezoidal area OAECD. *A* breakdown of the trapezoidal areas of Fig. 26-17, *A,* enables one to appreciate the individual aspects of the mechanical work load, which include the following:

OABCD: work necessary to overcome elastic resistance
AECF:　work necessary to overcome nonelastic resistance
AECB:　work necessary to overcome nonelastic resistance during inspiration
ABCF:　work necessary to overcome nonelastic resistance during expiration

(represents stored elastic energy from inspiration)

In restrictive lung diseases, such as pulmonary fibrosis, in which lung compliance is decreased, the pressure-volume curve is shifted to the right. Hence, the work of breathing has increased significantly (Fig. 26-17, *B*), as indicated by the increase in the trapezoidal area of OAECD. In obstructive lung diseases, such as asthma or chronic bronchitis, in which airway resistance is elevated (Fig. 26-17, *C*), greater negative pleural pressures are needed to maintain proper inspiratory flow rates. In addition to the increase in total inspiratory work (OAECD), individuals with obstructive lung diseases have an increase in positive pleural pressure during exhalation due to the increase in resistance and also to the increased expiratory workload, which is visualized as area DFO. The stored elastic energy, represented by area ABCF of Fig. 26-17, *A*, is not sufficient, and additional energy is needed for exhalation. Respiratory muscles can perform increased work over long periods of time. But like other skeletal muscles, they can fatigue and respiratory failure may ensue.

In addition to the diseases mentioned above, the work of breathing is influenced by breathing patterns. The work of breathing is increased when deeper breaths are taken (increase in tidal volume requires more elastic work to overcome), or

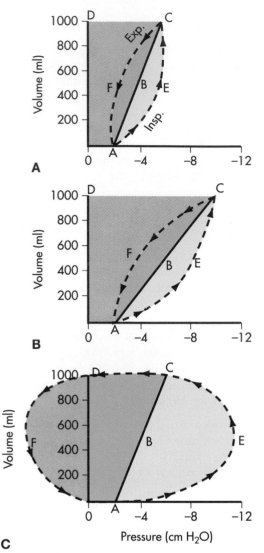

Fig. 26-17 The mechanical work done during a respiratory cycle on a normal lung **(A),** a lung with reduced compliance **(B),** and a lung with increased airway resistance **(C).**

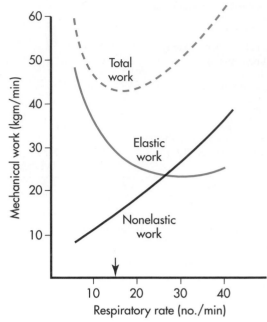

Fig. 26-18 The effect of respiratory rate on the elastic, nonelastic, and total mechanical work of breathing at a given level of alveolar ventilation. Subjects tend to adopt the respiratory rate at which the total work of breathing is minimal *(arrow).*

when the respiratory rate increases (increase in minute ventilation requires more flow resistance forces to overcome) (Fig. 26-18). As would be anticipated, normal individuals and individuals with lung disease adopt respiratory patterns such that the work of breathing is minimal. Patients with pulmonary fibrosis (elastic work) breathe more shallowly and rapidly and those with obstructive lung disease (no elastic work) breathe more slowly and deeply.

CLINICAL IMPLICATIONS

In emphysema, a chronic obstructive pulmonary disease (COPD), the alveolar and capillary walls are progressively destroyed. This results in larger than normal changes in lung volume for small changes in transpulmonary pressure, which results in increased lung compliance. The decrease in elastic recoil also results in movement of the equal pressure point toward the alveolus and toward premature airway closure.

This produces air trapping and increases in RV, FRC, and TLC. Airway resistance is also increased. These changes in lung volume increase the work of breathing by stretching the respiratory muscles and by decreasing their efficiency.

In chronic bronchitis, the other large category of COPD, mucus accumulation and airway inflammation cause the equal pressure point to move toward the alveolus, which leads to increases in RV, FRC, and TLC. Compliance, however, is normal.

In restrictive lung diseases, such as pulmonary fibrosis, lung compliance is decreased and changes in transpulmonary pressure elicit smaller than normal changes in lung volume. The changes in pulmonary function values in obstructive and restrictive pulmonary diseases are shown in Table 26-2.

In the third trimester of pregnancy, the enlarged uterus increases intraabdominal pressure and restricts the movement of the diaphragm. The FRC, as a result, decreases. This

Table 26-2 Patterns of abnormalities in pulmonary function tests

Pulmonary function measurement	Obstructive pulmonary disease	Restrictive pulmonary disease
FVC (L)	↓	↓
FEV_1 (L)	↓	↓
FEV_1/FVC	↓	N
FEF_{25-75} (L/sec)	↓	N
PEFR (L/sec)	↓	N
FEF_{50} (L/sec)	↓	N
FEF_{75} (L/sec)	↓	N
Slope of FV curve	↓	N to ↑

N, Normal; ↑, increased; ↓, decreased.

change in lung volume results in decreased lung compliance and increased airway resistance in otherwise healthy women.

SUMMARY

1. Lung volumes play a major role in gas exchange and in the work of breathing.

2. Lung volumes are determined by the balance between the lung's elastic recoil properties and the properties of the muscles of the chest wall.

3. The vital capacity is the single most important pulmonary function measurement; it is the maximal amount of air that an individual can either inspire or exhale.

4. The functional residual capacity (FRC) is the resting volume of the lung. It is determined by the balance between the lung elastic recoil pressure, which operates to decrease the lung volume, and the pressure generated by the chest wall to become larger. At FRC, the pressure difference across the respiratory system is zero.

5. Lung compliance is a measure of the elastic properties of the lung. A loss of elastic recoil, as seen in patients with emphysema, is associated with an increase in lung compliance.

6. In diseases associated with pulmonary fibrosis, lung compliance is decreased.

7. A positive transpulmonary pressure is needed to increase lung volume. The pressure across the respiratory system is zero at points of no air flow (end inspiration and end exhalation).

8. Resistance to airflow is the change in pressure per unit of flow. Airway resistance is determined by airway caliber and length, as well as by gas velocity and density.

9. Airway resistance is highly sensitive to changes in airway radius and varies with the inverse of the fourth power of the radius. Resistance to airflow is higher in turbulent than in laminar flow.

10. The first eight airway generations are the major site of airway resistance.

11. Airway resistance decreases with increases in lung volume and with decreases in gas density.

12. The equal pressure point is the point at which the pressures inside and surrounding the airway are the same.

13. As lung volume and elastic recoil decrease, the equal pressure point moves toward the alveolus in normal individuals. In individuals with chronic obstructive pulmonary disease (COPD), at any lung volume, the equal pressure point is closer to the alveolus.

14. Predicted values for lung volumes and expiratory flow rates vary by age, gender, ethnicity, and height, and, to a lesser extent, by weight.

15. Pulmonary function tests (spirometry, flow-volume loop, body plethysmography) can detect abnormalities in lung function before individuals become symptomatic.

16. COPD is characterized by increases in lung volume and in airway resistance, and by decreases in expiratory flow rates.

17. Emphysema, a specific type of COPD, is further characterized by increased lung compliance.

18. Restrictive lung diseases are characterized by decreases in lung volume, normal expiratory flow rates, and resistance, and a marked decrease in lung compliance.

REFERENCES

Journal articles

Brown RH, Mitzner W: Effects of lung inflation and airway muscle tone on airway diameter in vivo, *J Appl Physiol* 80:1581, 1996.

Cheung D et al: Relationship between loss in parenchymal recoil pressure and maximal airway narrowing in subjects with alpha-1-antitrypsin deficient, *Am J Respir Crit Care Med* 155:135, 1997.

Contreras G et al: Ventilatory drive and respiratory muscle function in pregnancy, *Am Rev Respir Dis* 144:837, 1991.

D'Angelo E et al: Pulmonary and chest wall mechanics in anesthetized paralyzed humans, *J Appl Physiol* 70:2602, 1991.

Lai-Fook SJ, Rodarte JR: Pleural pressure distribution and its relationship to lung volume and interstitial pressure, *J Appl Physiol* 70:967, 1991.

Zapletal A et al: Lung recoil and the determination of airflow limitation in cystic fibrosis and asthma, *Pediatr Pulmonol* 15:13, 1993.

Books and monographs

George RB et al, editors: *Chest medicine: essentials of pulmonary and critical care medicine*, ed 3, Baltimore, Md., 1995, Williams & Wilkins.

Hyatt RE, Scanlon PD, Nakamura M, editors: *Interpretation of pulmonary function tests. A practical guide*, Philadelphia, 1997, Lippincott Williams & Wilkins.

Leff AR, Schumacker PT: *Respiratory physiology: basics and applications*, Philadelphia, 1993, WB Saunders.

Murray JF: *The normal lung*, ed 2, Philadelphia, 1986, WB Saunders.

West JB: *Respiratory physiology—the essentials*, Baltimore, Md., 1974, Williams & Wilkins.

chapter twenty-seven

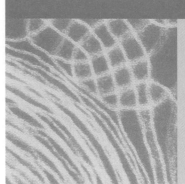

Ventilation (V̇), Perfusion (Q̇), and V̇/Q̇ Relationships

Although ventilation and pulmonary blood flow (perfusion) are important individual components in the primary function of the lung, the relationship between ventilation and perfusion (determined by the $\dot{V}/\dot{Q}$ ratio) is the major determinant of normal gas exchange. To fully understand the $\dot{V}/\dot{Q}$ ratio, however, we must first examine ventilation and pulmonary blood flow individually.

VENTILATION

Ventilation is the process by which fresh gas moves in and out of the lung. As previously described, minute (or total) ventilation ($\dot{V}_E$) is the volume of air that enters or leaves the lung per minute, and it is described by

$$\dot{V}_E = f \times TV$$

where f is the frequency, or number of breaths/minute, and TV, also known as V_T, is the tidal volume or volume of air inspired (or exhaled) per breath. Tidal volume varies with age, gender, body position, and metabolic activity. In an average-sized adult, TV is 500 ml. In children, the tidal volume is 3 to 5 ml/kg.

ALVEOLAR VENTILATION

Composition of a Gas Mixture

The process of respiration brings oxygen from the ambient air to the alveoli, where oxygen is taken up and carbon dioxide is excreted. Alveolar ventilation thus begins with ambient air. Ambient air is a gas mixture composed mainly of nitrogen and oxygen, with minute quantities of carbon dioxide, argon, and other inert gases. The composition of a gas mixture can be described in terms of either the gas fractions or the corresponding partial pressure. Because ambient air is a gas, it obeys the gas laws. The two most important gas laws governing ambient air and alveolar ventilation are Boyle's law and Dalton's law. Boyle's law states that when temperature is

constant, pressure (P) and volume (V) are directly related, that is

$$P_1V_1 = P_2V_2$$

Dalton's law states that the partial pressure of a gas in a gas mixture is the pressure that the gas would exert if it occupied the total volume of the mixture in the absence of the other components.

When these gas laws are applied to ambient air, two important principles arise. The first is that when the components are viewed in terms of gas fractions (F), the sum of the individual gas fractions must equal one.

$$1.0 = F_N + F_{O_2} + F_{argon\ and\ other\ gases}$$

When Boyle's gas law is applied, the sum of the **partial pressures** (in mm Hg) or of the **tensions** (in torr) of a gas must be equal to the total pressure. Thus, at sea level, where the partial pressure is 760 mm Hg, the partial pressures of the gases in the atmospheric air [also known as the barometric partial pressure (P_b)] are

$$P_b = P_{O_2} + P_{N_2} + P_{argon\ and\ other\ gases}$$
$$760\ mm\ Hg = P_{O_2} + P_{N_2} + P_{argon\ and\ other\ gases}$$

The second important principle is that the partial pressure of a gas (P_{gas}) is equal to the fraction of gas in the gas mixture (F_{gas}) times the total or ambient (barometric) pressure.

$$P_{gas} = F_{gas} \times P_b$$

Ambient air is composed of approximately 21% oxygen and 79% nitrogen. Therefore, the partial pressure of oxygen in ambient air (P_{O_2}) is

$$P_{O_2} = F_{O_2} + P_b$$
$$P_{O_2} = 0.21 \times 760\ mm\ Hg$$
$$= 159\ mm\ Hg\ or\ 159\ torr$$

This is the oxygen tension (i.e., the partial pressure of oxygen) at the mouth at the start of inspiration. It is evident that the oxygen tension at the mouth can be altered in one of two ways—by changing the fraction of oxygen or by changing the barometric (atmospheric) pressure. For example, if the fraction of oxygen is increased through the administration of supplemental oxygen, the partial pressure of atmospheric oxygen will be increased. On the other hand, if the atmospheric (barometric) pressure is decreased, for example, by high altitude, the partial pressure of ambient oxygen will decrease.

As inspiration begins, the ambient gases are brought into the airways, where they become warmed to body temperature and are humidified. Inspired gases become saturated with water vapor, which exerts a partial pressure. Because the total pressure remains constant at the barometric pressure, water vapor dilutes the total pressure of the other gases. **Water vapor pressure** at body temperature is 47 mm Hg. To calculate the partial pressure of a gas in a *humidified* mixture, the water vapor partial pressure must be subtracted from the total barometric pressure. Thus, in the conducting airways the partial pressure of oxygen is

$$P_{trachea O_2} = (P_b - P_{H_2O}) \times F_{O_2}$$
$$P_{trachea O_2} = (760 - 47 \text{ mm Hg}) \times 0.21$$
$$= 150 \text{ mm Hg}$$

and the partial pressure of nitrogen is

$$P_{trachea N_2} = (760 - 47 \text{ mm Hg}) \times 0.79$$
$$= 563 \text{ mm Hg}$$

Note that the total pressure has remained 760 mm Hg (150 + 563 + 47 mm Hg). Water vapor pressure, however, has reduced the partial pressures of oxygen and nitrogen. The conducting airways do not participate in gas exchange. Therefore, the partial pressures of oxygen, nitrogen, and water vapor remain unchanged in the airways until the gas reaches the alveolus.

ALVEOLAR GAS COMPOSITION

When the inspired gas reaches the alveolus, oxygen is transported across the alveolar membrane, and carbon dioxide moves from the capillary bed into the alveolus. The process by which this occurs is described in Chapter 28. At the end of inspiration and with the glottis open, the total pressure in the alveolus is atmospheric; the same gas laws apply, namely the partial pressures of the gases in the alveolus must equal the total pressure, that in this case is atmospheric. The

composition of the gas mixture, however, is changed, and it can be described as

$$1.0 = F_{O_2} + F_{N_2} + F_{H_2O} + F_{CO_2} + F_{argon \text{ and other gases}}$$

Nitrogen and argon are inert gases, and therefore the fraction of these gases in the alveolus does not change. The fraction of water vapor also does not change, because the gas is already fully saturated, and it is at body temperature by the time the gas reaches the trachea. As a consequence of gas exchange, the fraction of oxygen in the alveolus decreases and the fraction of carbon dioxide in the alveolus increases. Because of the changes in the fractions of oxygen and carbon dioxide, the partial pressures exerted by these gases also change. The partial pressure of oxygen in the alveolus (P_{AO_2}) is given by the *alveolar gas equation*, which is also called the *ideal alveolar oxygen equation:*

$$P_{AO_2} = P_{IO_2} - \frac{P_{ACO_2}}{R}$$

$$= (P_b - P_{H_2O}) \bullet F_{IO_2} - \frac{P_{ACO_2}}{R}$$

P_{IO_2} is the inspired partial pressure of oxygen, which is equal to the fraction (F) of the inspired oxygen (F_{IO_2}) times the difference between the barometric pressure (P_b) and the water vapor pressure (P_{H_2O}). P_{ACO_2} is the carbon dioxide tension of the alveolar gas, and R is the respiratory exchange ratio or respiratory quotient. The **respiratory quotient** is the ratio of carbon dioxide excreted ($\dot{V}_{CO_2}$) to the oxygen taken up ($\dot{V}_{O_2}$) by the lungs. This quotient is the number of carbon dioxide molecules produced relative to the number of oxygen molecules consumed by metabolism and is dependent upon intake. The respiratory quotient varies between 0.7 and 1.0. In states of exclusive fatty acid metabolism, R is 0.7, whereas in states of exclusive carbohydrate metabolism, R is 1.0. Because the respiratory quotient is rarely measured, it is considered to be 0.8 under usual circumstances. Hence, the quantity of oxygen taken up exceeds the quantity of carbon dioxide that is released in the alveoli. The alveolar air equation is a very important equation in respiratory medicine.

The partial pressures of oxygen, carbon dioxide, nitrogen, and H_2O from ambient air to the alveolus are shown in Table 27-1.

The fraction of carbon dioxide in the alveolus is a function of the rate of carbon dioxide production by the cells during

■ **Table 27-1** Total and partial pressures of respiratory gases in ideal alveolar gas and blood at sea level barometric pressure (760 mm Hg)

	Ambient air (dry)	Moist tracheal air	Alveolar gas (R = 0.80)	Systemic arterial blood	Mixed venous blood
P_{O_2}	159	150	102	90	40
P_{CO_2}	0	0	40	40	46
P_{H_2O}, 37°C	0	47	47	47	47
P_{N_2}	601	563	571*	571	571
P_{TOTAL}	760	760	760	760	704†

*P_{N_2} is increased in alveolar gas by 1% because R is <1 normally.

†P_{TOTAL} is less in venous than in arterial blood because P_{O_2} has decreased more than P_{CO_2} has increased.

metabolism and the rate at which the carbon dioxide is eliminated from the alveolus. This process is known as *alveolar ventilation.* Even though ventilation is episodic, that is, it occurs only during inspiration, alveolar ventilation is described as a *continuous* gas flow through the alveoli that exchange gas with the pulmonary capillary blood. The relationship between carbon dioxide production and alveolar ventilation is defined by the *alveolar carbon dioxide equation,*

$$\dot{V}_{CO_2} = \dot{V}_A \times F_{ACO_2}$$

where $\dot{V}_{CO_2}$ is the rate of carbon dioxide production by the body, $\dot{V}_A$ is the alveolar ventilation, and F_{ACO_2} is the fraction of carbon dioxide in dry alveolar gas. This relationship demonstrates that the rate of elimination of CO_2 from the alveolus is related to the alveolar ventilation and to the fraction of CO_2 in the alveolus. The alveolar P_{ACO_2} is defined by the following:

$$P_{ACO_2} = F_{ACO_2} \times (P_b - P_{H_2O})$$

Hence, we can substitute in the previous equation and demonstrate the following relationship:

$$P_{ACO_2} = \frac{\dot{V}_{CO_2} \times (P_b - P_{H_2O})}{\dot{V}_A}$$

This equation demonstrates a number of interesting and important relationships. First, there is an inverse relationship between the partial pressure of carbon dioxide in the alveolus (P_{ACO_2}) and the alveolar ventilation ($\dot{V}_A$), irrespective of the exhaled CO_2. Specifically, if ventilation is doubled, the P_{ACO_2} will be decreased by 50%. Conversely, if ventilation is decreased by one-half, the partial pressure of CO_2 in the alveolus will be doubled. Second, if a constant alveolar ventilation ($\dot{V}_A$) is maintained, but the metabolic production of carbon dioxide ($\dot{V}_{CO_2}$) is doubled, the partial pressure of carbon dioxide in the alveolus (P_{ACO_2}) will be increased by 100%.

Clinically, this principle is applied in patients who are being mechanically ventilated and who cannot self-regulate their breathing. An increase in the partial pressure of carbon dioxide in the blood indicates that the partial pressure of carbon dioxide in the alveoli has increased. If the same patient develops a fever and cannot increase his alveolar ventilation, his arterial P_{CO_2} will rise as a result of the greater CO_2 production. The relationship between alveolar ventilation and alveolar P_{CO_2} is shown in Fig. 27-1.

In normal individuals, the alveolar P_{CO_2} is regulated to remain constant at about 40 mm Hg. Specialized chemoreceptors monitor the P_{CO_2} in the arterial blood and in the brainstem, and the minute ventilation varies in accordance with the level of P_{CO_2}. Increases or decreases in arterial P_{CO_2}, particularly when they are associated with changes in the arterial pH, have profound effects upon cell behavior, including enzyme and transport functions. Hence, the arterial P_{CO_2} is tightly regulated.

An increase in arterial P_{CO_2} results in an (respiratory) acidosis (pH < 7.35) whereas a decrease in arterial P_{CO_2} results in an (respiratory) alkalosis (pH > 7.45). Hypercapnia is an elevation in arterial P_{CO_2}, and it is secondary to inadequate alveolar sentilation (hypoventilation) relative to CO_2 production. Conversely, hyperventilation occurs when alveolar

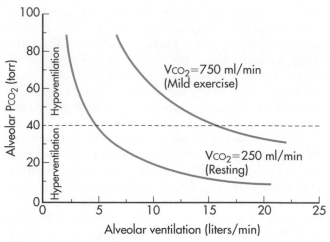

■ **Fig. 27-1**   Alveolar P_{CO_2} as a function of alveolar ventilation in the lung. Each line corresponds to a given metabolic rate associated with a constant production of carbon dioxide (V_{CO_2} isometabolic line). Normally, alveolar ventilation is controlled to maintain an alveolar P_{CO_2} of about 40 torr. During *hypoventilation* the alveolar ventilation is low relative to V_{CO_2}, and alveolar P_{CO_2} rises. During *hyperventilation* the alveolar ventilation is excessive relative to V_{CO_2} so the alveolar P_{CO_2} falls.

ventilation exceeds CO_2 production, and it decreases arterial P_{CO_2} (hypocapnia).

Distribution of Ventilation

Ventilation is not uniformly distributed in the lung, due in large part to the effects of gravity. If the chest is oriented in the upright position, the alveoli near the apex of the lung are more expanded than are alveoli at the base. This is because the pleural pressure is less at the apex than at the base, because the weight of the lung tends to pull it downward away from the chest wall. If the pleural pressure is decreased, the static translung pressure ($P_L = P_A - P_{pl}$) must be increased, and the alveolar volume increases in this area.

As inspiration begins, the alveoli at the apex and at the base of the lung have different volumes (see Fig. 27-2). Alveoli at the lung base are located along the steeper portion of the pressure:volume curve, and they receive more of the ventilation (i.e., they have a greater compliance). In contrast, the expanded alveoli at the apex are closer to the top of the pressure:volume curve. They have a lower compliance, and thus they receive proportionately less of the tidal volume.

In the absence of gravity, such as experienced by the astronauts in space, this type of nonuniformity disappears. The effect is also less pronounced when one is supine rather than upright, and it is less when one is supine rather than prone. This behavior occurs because the diaphragm is pushed cephalad when one is supine, and it affects the size of all of the alveoli.

In addition to gravitational effects on the distribution of ventilation, the ventilation in the terminal respiratory units is not uniform. This is caused by variable airway resistance (R) or compliance (C), and it may be described quantitatively by the time constant (τ):

$$\tau = R \times C$$

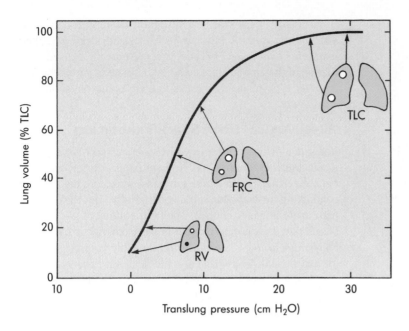

■ **Fig. 27-2**   Regional distribution of lung volume. Because of suspension of the lung from top to bottom, pleural pressure (P_{pl}) and translung pressure, P_L, of units at the top will be greater than those at the bottom. The effect is greatest at residual volume *(RV)*, is less at *FRC*, and disappears at total lung capacity *(TLC)*.

Alveolar units with long time constants fill and empty slowly. Thus, a unit with increased airway resistance or with increased compliance will take longer to fill and longer to empty. In normal adults, the respiratory rate is about 12 breaths/minute, the inspiratory time is about 2 seconds, and the expiratory time is about 3 seconds. In normal individuals this time is sufficient to approach equilibrium (Fig. 27-3). In the presence of an increased resistance or an increased compliance, however, equilibrium is not reached.

Single Breath Nitrogen Test

The single breath nitrogen test can be used to assess the uniformity of ventilation. The subject takes a single maximal inspiration of 100% O_2. During the subsequent exhalation, the nitrogen concentration of the exhaled air is measured. Air (100% O_2, 0% nitrogen) initially exits from the conducting airways; then the nitrogen concentration begins to rise as alveolar emptying occurs. Finally, there is a plateau concentration of nitrogen as only the alveoli that contain nitrogen empty (Fig. 27-4).

DEAD SPACE

Air within the conducting airways does not participate in gas exchange. This volume of air in the conducting airways is called the **anatomical dead space (V_D).** The volume of air in the anatomical dead space is determined by the anatomy (size and number) of the conducting airways. When V is used to denote volume, the subscripts T, D, and A are used to denote tidal, dead space, and alveolar, respectively. A "dot" above V denotes a volume per unit of time (n). Thus,

$$V_T = V_D + V_A$$

Therefore,

$$V_T \times n = V_D \times n + V_A \times n$$

or

$$\dot{V}_E = \dot{V}_D + \dot{V}_A$$

$\dot{V}_E$ is the exhaled minute volume and $\dot{V}_D$ and $\dot{V}_A$ are the dead space and alveolar ventilation per minute, respectively.

In the normal adult, the volume of gas at functional residual capacity (FRC) contained in the conducting airways is approximately 100 to 200 ml compared to the 3 L of gas in the entire lung. With each tidal breath (approximately 500 ml), fresh gas moves first into the conducting airways and then into the alveoli. The ratio of the volume of the conducting airways (dead space) to the tidal volume describes the fraction of each breath that is wasted in "ventilating" the conducting airways. This volume is related to the tidal volume (V_T) and to the minute ventilation ($\dot{V}_E$) in the following way:

$$\dot{V}_D = \frac{V_D}{V_T} \times \dot{V}_E$$

The equation above indicates that the dead space ventilation (V_D) varies inversely with the tidal volume (V_T). The larger the tidal volume the smaller the dead space ventilation.

Dead Space: An Example

If the dead space is 150 ml, and the tidal volume increases from 500 to 600 ml, for the same minute ventilation, what is the effect on dead space ventilation?

$V_T = 500$ ml

$$V_D = \frac{150 \text{ ml}}{500 \text{ ml}} \cdot \dot{V}_E \qquad\qquad V_D = \frac{150 \text{ ml}}{600 \text{ ml}} \cdot \dot{V}_E$$
$$= 0.30 \qquad\qquad\qquad\qquad = 0.25$$

As tidal volume increases, the dead space ventilation decreases for the same minute ventilation.

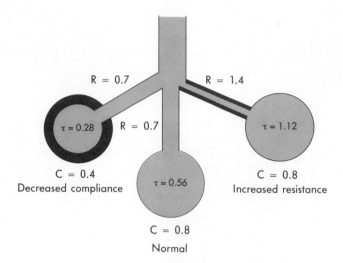

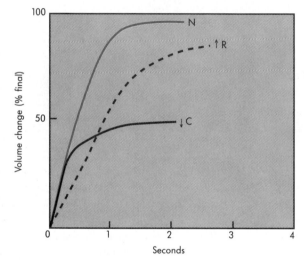

Fig. 27-3 Examples of local regulation of ventilation due to variation of resistance (R) or compliance (C) of individual lung units. In the upper schema, the normal lung has a time constant, τ, of 0.56 second. This unit reaches 97% of final equilibrium in 2 seconds, the normal inspiratory time, as shown in the lower graph. The unit at the right has a 2-fold increase in resistance; hence, its time constant is doubled. That unit fills more slowly and reaches only 80% equilibrium during a normal breath. The unit is underventilated. The unit on the left has reduced compliance (stiff), which acts to reduce its time constant. This unit fills faster than the normal unit but receives only half the ventilation of a normal unit.

Fig. 27-4 The single-breath nitrogen washout curve is a simple useful pulmonary function test of regional ventilation distribution. It clearly shows that not all lung units have equal $\dot{V}/\dot{Q}$. The well-ventilated units (short time constant) empty faster than less well-ventilated units (long time constant). The portion of the curve up to the vertical dashed line represents the washout of dead space air mixed with alveolar gas. The long alveolar plateau rises slowly (<2%) if ventilation distribution is relatively uniform, as shown here. The final phase, after the second vertical line, shows very late, slowly emptying alveoli. This phase is accentuated with age.

Normally, dead space ventilation represents 20% to 30% of the minute ventilation. This dead space is called *anatomic dead space*, because it represents the wasted ventilation of the airways that do not participate in gas exchange. Another type of dead space is known as the physiological dead space.

Physiological Dead Space Ventilation

Imagine a diseased lung in which some alveoli are not perfused, but they continue to be ventilated. These ventilated but not perfused areas of the lung, in a sense, are just like the conducting airways that are also ventilated, but they do not participate in gas exchange. The total volume of gas in each breath that does not participate in gas exchange is called the *physiological dead space ventilation*. This volume includes the anatomical dead space and the dead space secondary to the ventilated, but not perfused, alveoli, or to the alveoli that are overventilated relative to the amount of perfusion. Thus, the physiological dead space is always as great as the anatomical dead space, and in the presence of disease, it may be considerably greater than the anatomical dead space. In healthy individuals, the physiological dead space normally represents 25% to 30% of the minute ventilation.

Measurements of Dead Space

Dead space in the lungs is usually not measured clinically. There are, however, two different ways that dead space can be determined. The first is by measuring the P_{CO_2} in alveolar gas and in mixed expired gas. The dilution of carbon dioxide in mixed expired gas relative to that in the alveolar gas is measured, and it is a function of the amount of wasted ventilation relative to the minute ventilation. This is because the conducting airways are ventilated, but not perfused, and the alveoli do not contribute to the CO_2 in expired gas. Exhaled gas is collected in a bag over a period of time, and the P_{CO_2} in the arterial blood (which is the same as the P_{ACO_2} in the alveolus) and in the collection bag (P_{ECO_2}) are measured. The dead

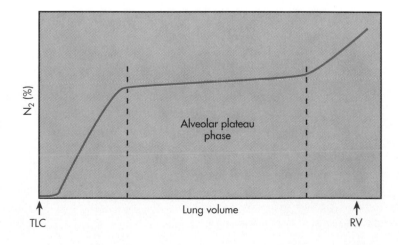

space ventilation as a function of the tidal volume (V_D/V_T) is described by the following equation:

$$\frac{V_D}{V_T} = 1 - \frac{P_{ECO_2}}{P_{ACO_2}}$$

This is called the **Bohr dead space equation**, because it was originally described by the physiologist Christian Bohr at the turn of the twentieth century.

Dead space ventilat ion can also be measured by **Fowler's method.** The patient takes a single breath of 100% oxygen, and then exhales into a tube that continuously measures the N_2 concentration in the exhaled gas. As the subject exhales, the anatomical dead space empties first. This volume contains 100% oxygen and 0% nitrogen, because it has not participated in any gas exchange. As the alveoli begin to empty, the oxygen falls and the nitrogen begins to rise. Finally, the concentration of nitrogen is almost uniform, and it represents alveolar gas almost entirely. This phase of expired air exhalation is called the alveolar plateau. The volume with initially 0% nitrogen plus half of the rising nitrogen volume is equal to the anatomical dead space.

Fowler's and Bohr's methods do not measure exactly the same thing. Fowler's method measures the volume of the conducting airways down to the level at which the inspired gas is rapidly diluted with gas already in the lung. Thus, Fowler's method measures anatomical dead space. In contrast, Bohr's method measures the volume of the lung that does not eliminate CO_2. Thus, Bohr's method measures physiologic dead space. In normal individuals, the anatomical and physiological dead spaces differ only slightly. In people with lung disease, however, the difference can be very large.

Measurement of Dead Space: An Example

Consider that a patient is breathing into a spirometer at a tidal volume of 500 ml and at a respiratory frequency of 12 breaths/minute. The inspired gas is switched to 100% at the end of a full exhalation, and the nitrogen concentration is monitored at the lips during the following exhalation. The nitrogen concentration is zero for the first 130 ml, and then it increases to a constant level of 50% when the exhaled gas is 170 ml and it remains at this level for the duration of exhalation. What is the dead space?

$$V_D = 130 + \frac{1}{2}(170 - 130)$$
$$= 150 \text{ ml}$$

PERFUSION

Perfusion is the process by which deoxygenated blood passes through the lung and becomes reoxygenated.

THE PULMONARY CIRCULATION

Consider that the pulmonary circulation begins with the right atrium. Deoxygenated blood from the right atrium enters the right ventricle via the tricuspid valve, and it is then pumped *under low pressure* (9-24 mm Hg) into the pulmonary artery through the pulmonic valve. The pulmonary artery (pulmonary trunk), which is about 3 cm in diameter, branches quickly (5 cm from the right ventricle) into the right and left main pulmonary arteries, which supply blood to the right and left lungs, respectively. The arteries of the pulmonary circulation are the only arteries that carry deoxygenated blood. The deoxygenated blood in the pulmonary arteries passes through a progressively smaller series of branching vessels (vessel diameters: arteries >500 μm, arterioles 10-200 μm, capillaries <10 μm), and they end in a complex mesh-like network of capillaries (see Chapter 25, Fig. 25-7). The sequential branching pattern of the pulmonary arteries follows a pattern similar to the airway branching, such that there are supporting vascular structures for each airway. The functions of the pulmonary circulatory system are (1) to reoxygenate the blood and to dispense of CO_2, (2) to aid in fluid balance in the lung, and (3) to distribute metabolic products of the lung. Oxygenation of red blood cells occurs in the capillaries that surround the alveolus, where the pulmonary capillary bed and the alveoli come together in the alveolar wall in a unique configuration for optimal gas exchange (Fig. 27-5). Gas exchange occurs through this alveolar-capillary network.

The total blood volume of the pulmonary circulation is about 500 ml, which is about 10% of the circulating blood volume. It is estimated that 75 ml of blood is present in the alveolar-capillary network of normal adults at any one time. During exercise this blood volume can be increased by over 50% to 150 to 200 ml, due to the recruitment of new capillaries secondary to an increase in pressure and flow. This recruitment of new capillaries is a unique feature of the lung, and it allows for compensation and adjustments to stress, as in the case of exercise. The oxygenated blood leaves the alveolus through a network of small pulmonary venules (15 to 500 μm in diameter) and veins. These small vessels quickly coalesce to form larger pulmonary veins (>500 μm in diameter), through which the oxygenated blood returns to the left atrium of the heart. In contrast to arteries, arterioles, and capillaries, which closely follow the branching patterns of the airways, venules and veins run quite distant from the airways.

STRUCTURAL FEATURES OF THE PULMONARY AND BRONCHIAL CIRCULATION

Structure of the Pulmonary Circulation

The arteries of the pulmonary circulation are thin walled, with minimal smooth muscle. They are seven times more compliant than systemic vessels, and they are easily distensible. This highly compliant state of the pulmonary arterial vessels requires much less work (lower pressures throughout the pulmonary circulation) for blood flow through the pulmonary circulation than do the more muscular, noncompliant arterial walls of the systemic circulation (Table 27-2).

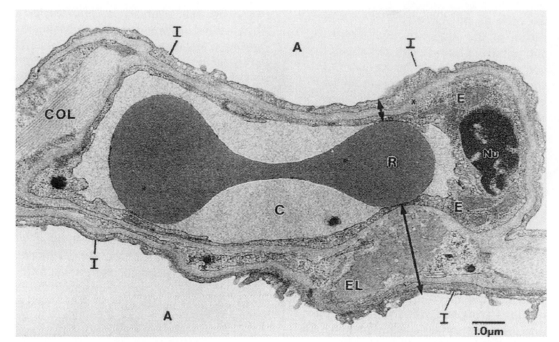

■ **Fig. 27-5** Cross section of an alveolar wall showing the path for oxygen and carbon dioxide diffusion. The thin side of the alveolar wall barrier *(short double arrow)* consists of type I epithelium *(I)*, interstitium (*) formed by the fused basal laminae of the epithelial and endothelial cells, capillary endothelium *(E)*, plasma in the alveolar capillary *(C)*, and finally the cytoplasm of the red blood cell *(R)*. The thick side of the gas exchange barrier *(long double arrow)* has an accumulation of elastin *(EL)*, collagen *(COL)*, and matrix that jointly separate the alveolar epithelium from the alveolar capillary endothelium. As long as the red blood cells are flowing, oxygen and carbon dioxide diffusion probably occurs across both sides of the air:blood barrier. *A,* Alveolus; *Nu,* nucleus of the capillary endothelial cell. (Human lung speciman, transmission electron microscopy.)

■ **Table 27-2** Pressures in the pulmonary circulation of normal, resting, supine adult humans

	mm Hg	*cm H$_2$O*
Pulmonary artery*		
Systolic/diastolic	24/9	33/11
Mean	14	19
Arterioles		
Mean	12	16
Capillaries		
Mean	10.5	14
Venules		
Mean	9	12
Left atrium		
Mean	8	11

*The pulmonary arterial and left atrial pressures are measured at cardiac catheterization; the former directly, the latter by wedging the arterial catheter in a branch of the pulmonary artery.

The vessels in the pulmonary circulation, under normal circumstances, are in a dilated state and have larger diameters than do similar arteries in the systemic system. All of these factors contribute to a very compliant, low-resistance circulatory system, which aids in the flow of blood through the pulmonary circulation via the relatively weak pumping action of the right ventricle. This low-resistance, low-work system also explains why the right ventricle is less muscular than the left ventricle. The pressure gradient differential for the pulmonary circulation from the pulmonary artery to the left atrium is only 6 mm Hg (14 mm Hg pulmonary artery minus 8 mm Hg left atrium) (Fig. 27-6). It is almost 15 times less than the pressure gradient differential of 87 mm Hg present in the systemic circulation (90 mm Hg in the aorta, minus 3 mm Hg in the right atrium).

Structures of the Extraalveolar and Alveolar Vessels and the Pulmonary Microcirculation

Although anatomically not well defined, vessels in the pulmonary circulation can be divided into three categories (extraalveolar, alveolar, and microcirculation) based on differences in their physiological properties. These properties may change during conditions such as stress and exercise. The extraalveolar vessels (arteries, arterioles, veins, and venules) are generally larger. They are not influenced by alveolar pressure changes, but they are affected by intrapleural and interstitial pressure changes. Alterations in either the intrapleural pressure or the interstitial pressure, which are affected by lung volume and the retractive force generated by elastin, can vastly influence vessel caliber. At high lung volumes, a decrease in pleural pressure increases the caliber

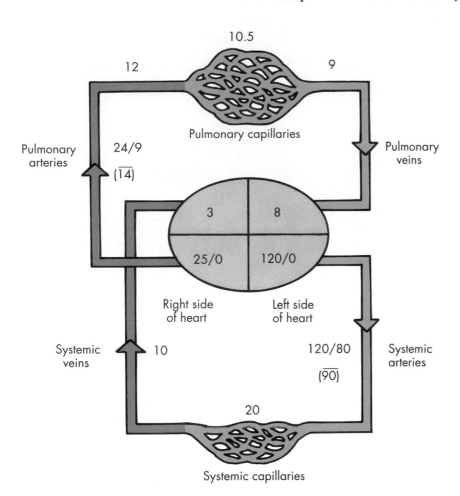

■ **Fig. 27-6** Schematic representation of the phasic and mean pressures within the systemic and pulmonary circulations in a normal, resting human adult lying supine (dorsal recumbency). The units are millimeters of mercury (mm Hg) for easy comparison. The driving pressure in the systemic circuit ($P_{ao} - P_{ra}$) = 90 – 3 = 87 mm Hg, whereas the driving pressure in the pulmonary circuit ($P_{pa} - P_{la}$) = 14 – 8 = 6 mm Hg. As cardiac output must be the same in both circuits in the steady state because they are in series, the resistance to flow through the lungs is less than 10% that of the rest of the body. Note also that the pressures in the left heart chambers are higher than those in the right heart. Any congenital openings between the right and left sides of the heart favor left-to-right flow.

of extraalveolar vessels. In contrast, at low lung volumes, an increase in pleural pressure has a constrictive effect.

Alveolar vessels are the capillaries within the interalveolar septa, and they are very sensitive to shifts in alveolar pressure but not to changes in pleural or interstitial pressure. An increase in alveolar pressure, which occurs when positive-pressure ventilation is applied, can compress the capillaries and block blood flow. This effect is discussed later in this chapter in reference to blood flow in the zone 1 region. Finally, the term pulmonary microcirculation is used to describe small vessels, which participate in liquid and solute exchange in the maintenance of fluid balance in the lung.

Structure of the Alveolar-Capillary Network

The sequential branching pattern of the pulmonary arteries culminates with the branching of the small arterioles into the alveolar wall. This unique pattern establishes a dense mesh-like network of capillaries and alveoli that has little structure other than the thin epithelial lining cells of the alveolus, the endothelial cells of the vessels, and their supportive matrix. This alveolar-capillary network has an alveolar surface area of about 70 m^2 (about the size of a tennis court). The structural matrix and the tissue components of this alveolar-capillary network provide the only barrier between gas in the airway and blood in the capillary. This barrier comprises the type I alveolar epithelial cell, the capillary endothelial

cell, and their respective basement membranes. The basement membranes are back to back. The distance for gas exchange through the basement membrane barrier is only about 1 to 2 μm thick. Surrounded mostly by air, this alveolar-capillary network creates an ideal environment for gas exchange. Red blood cells pass through this network in less than 1 second, which is sufficient time for CO_2 and O_2 gas exchange. In addition to gas exchange, this network also functions in fluid regulation within the lung. At the pulmonary capillary level, the balance between hydrostatic pressure and oncotic pressure results in a small net movement of fluid out of the vessels and into the interstitial space.

The fluid is then removed from the lung interstitium by the lymphatic system, and it then enters the circulation via the vena cava in the area of the hilus. In normal adults it is estimated that an average of 30 ml of fluid/hour is returned to the circulation via this route.

The Starling equation (see also Chapter 20) is used to calculate fluid flux within this capillary network:

$$\text{Flux (flow in ml/min)} = K_{fc}[\,(P_w - P_{is}) - \sigma_d(\pi_{jv} - \pi_{is})\,]$$

Where

K_{fc} = capillary filtration coefficient on the total number of perfused capillaries

P_{jv} = intravascular hydrostatic pressure

P_{is} = interstitial hydrostatic pressure

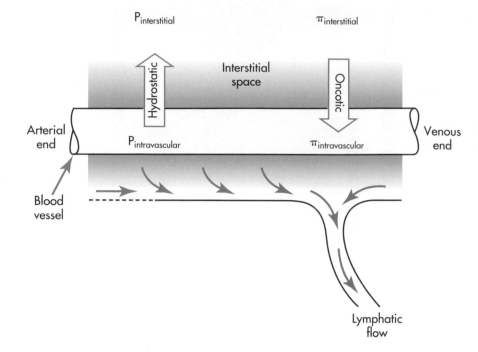

Pulmonary Capillary Fluid Balance

■ **Fig. 27-7** Factors influencing lung fluid balance. The Starling equation summarizes the balance of forces favoring fluid flux into or out of the pulmonary vessels. Normally there is a net flux of fluid out of the vessels, which is drained from the interstitial space by the lymphatic system.

σ_d = reflection coefficient (reflects the permeability of the membrane to protein)

π_{jv} = intravascular colloid osmotic pressure

π_{is} = interstitial colloid osmotic pressure

In principle, the Starling equation illustrates the forces that create the net flux of fluid out of the pulmonary capillaries (Fig. 27-7). However, in practice it is not possible to calculate this flux. Many of the parameters needed cannot be measured. For instance, the K_{fc} is dependent on the number of capillaries actually being perfused, which cannot be determined.

The alveolar epithelium (type I and type II epithelial cells) establishes a tight restrictive barrier that inhibits fluids from entering the airspace. This barrier is highly advantageous, because any fluid in the airspace will interfere with gas diffusion. This alveolar-capillary network is also very fragile and susceptible to various injurious agents and events. The type I cell is the site of gas diffusion from the air into the capillaries, but it is quite susceptible to injury, perhaps due to its thin, elongated shape and large surface area. In certain disease states, such as interstitial lung diseases, the type I cell dies, leaving a denuded alveolar epithelium that is associated with increased permeability. The cuboidal shaped type II epithelial cell then proliferates and differentiates into type I cells and thereby tends to restore the normal lung architecture.

Structure of the Bronchial Circulation

The existence of a second, separate circulatory system in the lung with oxygenated blood from the systemic circulation was first observed by Frederich Ruysch in the latter half of the seventeenth century. This second circulatory system is the **bronchial circulation,** and it provides systemic arterial perfusion to the trachea, upper airways, surface secretory cells, glands, nerves, visceral pleural surface, lymph nodes, pulmonary arteries, and pulmonary veins. The bronchial circulation perfuses the upper respiratory tract; it does not reach the terminal or respiratory bronchioles or the alveolus. The return of venous blood from the capillaries of the bronchial circulation to the heart occurs either through true bronchial veins or through bronchopulmonary veins. True bronchial veins are present in the region of the hilus and blood flows into either the azygos, hemiazygos, or intercostal veins prior to entering the right atrium. The bronchopulmonary veins are formed through a network of tributaries that comprises the bronchial and pulmonary circulatory vessels, which anastomose and form vessels with an admixture of blood from both circulatory systems. Blood from these anastomosed vessels returns to the left atrium through pulmonary veins. About two thirds of the total bronchial circulation is returned to the heart via the pulmonary veins and this anastomosis route.

The bronchial circulation receives only about 1% of the total cardiac output, compared to almost 100% for the pulmonary circulation. In contrast to the pulmonary circulation, the bronchial circulation has angiogenesis capabilities. Such capabilities are particularly important for repair when tissues are damaged. However, this property can also be detrimental, as in the case of tumor angiogenesis. The major pathway for tumor angiogenesis in the lung is via the bronchial circulation. The physiological function of the bronchial circulation remains an enigma, because lung transplant studies have shown that adult lungs can function normally in the absence of a bronchial circulatory system. The bronchial circulation is more prominent in neonates and young children, and it may play a greater role in bringing nutrients to the developing lung.

PULMONARY VASCULAR RESISTANCE

Factors that influence blood flow include pulmonary vascular resistance (PVR), gravity, alveolar pressure, and the arterial to venous pressure gradient. Blood flows through the pulmonary circulation in a pulsatile manner and parallels the pressure gradient in this low-resistance system. PVR is the change in pressure from the pulmonary artery (P_{PA}) to the left atrium (P_{LA}) divided by the flow (Q_T), which is the cardiac output.

$$PVR = \frac{P_{PA} - P_{LA}}{Q_T}$$

Under normal circumstances,

$$PVR = \frac{14 \text{ mm Hg} - 8 \text{ mm Hg}}{6 \text{ L/min}} = 1.0 \text{ mm Hg/L/min}$$

This resistance is about 10 times less than that in the systemic circulation. The low resistance in the pulmonary circulation has two unique features that allow for increased blood flow upon demand. All of the available vessels are not used under normal resting conditions. This allows for compensation and recruitment of new vessels upon increased demand, such as during exertion or exercise, and with little or no increase in pulmonary artery pressure. In addition, the distensibility of the blood vessels in the pulmonary circulation enables the vessels to increase their diameter with only a minimal increase in pulmonary arterial pressure.

Lung volume can affect PVR through its influence on alveolar vessels, mainly the capillaries (Fig. 27-8). At end inspiration, the fully distended air-filled alveoli compress the alveolar capillaries and increase PVR. In contrast to the capillary beds in the systemic circulation, the capillary bed in the lung has a major influence on PVR, and it accounts for about 40% of the resistance. This stretching effect during inspiration has an opposite effect on the larger extraalveolar vessels, which increase in diameter due to radial traction and elastic recoil. During exhalation, the deflated alveoli apply the least resistance and PVR is diminished. Thus, at high lung volume, PVR is greatest, and at low lung volume, PVR is least.

DISTRIBUTION OF PULMONARY BLOOD FLOW

Because the pulmonary circulation is a low-pressure/low-resistance system, it is influenced by gravity much more dramatically than is the systemic circulation. This gravitational effect and other factors contribute to an uneven distribution

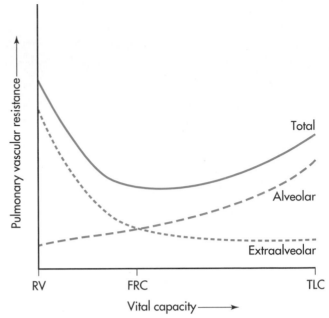

■ **Fig. 27-8** Schematic representation of the effects of changes in vital capacity on total pulmonary vascular resistance and the contributions to the total afforded by alveolar and extraalveolar vessels. During inflation from residual volume *(RV)* to total lung capacity *(TLC)*, resistance to blood flow through alveolar vessels increases, whereas resistance through extraalveolar vessels decreases. Thus changes in total pulmonary vascular resistance form a U-shaped curve during lung inflation, with the nadir at functional residual capacity *(FRC)*.

of blood flow in the lung. In upright subjects, under normal resting conditions, blood flow increases from the apex of the lung (lowest flow) to the base of the lung, where it is greatest. Similarly, in a supine individual, blood flow is less in the uppermost (anterior) regions and greater in the lower (posterior) regions. In the supine subject, blood flow becomes equal in both the apical and basal regions of the lung. Under conditions of stress, such as exercise, the difference in the blood flow in the apical and basal regions in upright subjects becomes less, due mainly to the increase in demand and the increase in arterial pressure.

Upon leaving the pulmonary artery, blood must travel up to the apex of the lung, against gravity in upright subjects. One can estimate that for every 1 cm increase in height above the heart, there is a corresponding decrease in hydrostatic pressure. A change of 1 cm in height is equivalent to a change in hydrostatic pressure of 0.74 mm Hg. Thus, the pressure in a segment of pulmonary artery that is 10 cm above the heart will be 7.4 mm Hg less than the pressure in a segment of pulmonary artery that is at the level of the heart. At this point the arterial pressure would be 6.6 mm Hg (arterial pressure at level of the heart 14 mm Hg minus 7.4 mm Hg). Conversely a segment of lung 5 cm below the heart will experience an increase in pulmonary arterial pressure of 3.7 mm Hg and thus have a pulmonary arterial pressure of 17.7 mm Hg. The effect of gravity on blood flow equally affects arteries and veins. It is obvious that there are wide variations in arterial

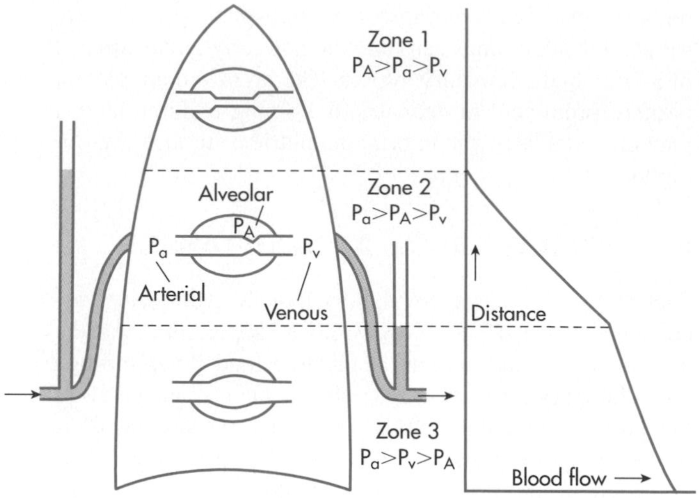

■ **Fig. 27-9** Model to explain the uneven distribution of blood flow in the lung based on the pressures affecting the capillaries. (From West JB, Dollery CT, Naimark J: *J Appl Physiol* 19:713, 1964.)

and venous pressures from the apex to the base of the lung. These variations will not only influence the flow but also the ventilation/perfusion relationships. In addition to the pulmonary arterial pressure (P_a) to pulmonary venous pressure (P_v) gradients, differences in the pulmonary alveolar pressure (P_A) also influence blood flow in the lung.

In referring to blood flow, the lung has been classically divided into three zones based on different physiological aspects of function in each zone or region (Fig. 27-9). Zone 1 represents the lung apex, where it is possible to have no blood flow. This could occur at the very top of the lung, where the P_a is so low that it can be exceeded by P_A. The capillaries collapse because of the greater external P_A, thereby preventing blood flow. Under normal conditions, this zone does not exist; however, this state could be reached during positive-pressure mechanical ventilation or if a physiological alteration sufficiently decreases P_a. Under conditions of decreased arterial pressure, the blood flow rises only to the level at which the arterial and alveolar pressures are equal; above this, there is no flow. Under normal circumstances and in an upright subject, most of the lung functions in what is referred to as zones 2 and 3. In zone 2, which comprises the upper one third of the lung, the P_a is greater than the P_A, which also is greater than P_v. Because P_A is greater than P_v, the greater external P_A partially collapses the capillaries and causes a "damming" effect. This phenomenon is often referred to as the "waterfall" effect. In zone 3, P_a is greater than P_v, which is greater than P_A, and blood flows in this area in accordance with the pressure gradients. Because the effect of gravity is equal in both arteries and veins, the pressure differential between the base and the apex of the lung does not change. Flow is increased in the basal area due to an increase in transmural pressure, which distends the vessels and thus lowers the resistance.

ACTIVE REGULATION OF BLOOD FLOW

Although the passive mechanisms of blood flow regulation discussed earlier in this chapter represent the major factors

that influence blood flow in the lung, several active mechanisms also regulate blood flow in the lung. The smooth muscle around the pulmonary vessels is much thinner than that around the systemic vessels, but it is sufficient to affect vessel caliber, and thus PVR. Low and high oxygen levels also have a major impact on blood flow. Hypoxic vasoconstriction occurs in small arterial vessels in response to decreased arterial P_{O_2}. The response is local, and it may be a protective response by shifting the blood flow from the hypoxic areas to normal areas in an effort to enhance gas exchange. Isolated, local hypoxia does not alter PVR; approximately 20% of the vessels need to be hypoxic before a change in PVR can be measured. Low inspired oxygen levels due to exposure to high altitude will have a greater effect on PVR. High concentrations of inspired oxygen can dilate pulmonary vessels and decrease PVR.

In addition to alterations in oxygen, a wide range of other factors and mediators can influence vessel caliber (Table 27-3). Under normal conditions, these factors play a very minor role; however, in pathological conditions their influence can be dramatic. Most of these factors can be released by local cells or by inflammatory cells. These factors have a short half-life and their effects are usually local.

VENTILATION-PERFUSION RELATIONSHIPS

We have already examined ventilation ($\dot{V}$) and lung perfusion ($\dot{Q}$) in isolation. Both are essential elements in the normal functioning of the lung, but they are insufficient to ensure normal *gas exchange*. For example, consider the situation in which blood is perfusing an area of the lung that is not ventilated. Overall ventilation and perfusion in the lung may be normal, but in this specific area of the lung, normal gas exchange cannot occur because ventilation is absent. Thus, without ventilation the blood entering and leaving the area would be unchanged and would remain deoxygenated. Similarly, imagine an area of the lung with normal ventilation but no perfusion. Gas entering and leaving the alveoli in this area would be unchanged; that is, these alveoli would not participate in gas exchange because blood flow is absent.

■ **Table 27-3** Compounds with active regulatory properties on pulmonary blood flow

Pulmonary vasoconstrictors

Low P_{AO_2}
Thromboxane A_2
α-Adrenergic catecholamines
Angiotensin
Leukotrienes
Neuropeptides
Serotonin
Endothelin
Histamine
Prostaglandins
High CO_2

Pulmonary vasodilators

High P_{AO_2}
Prostacyclin
Nitric oxide
Acetylcholine
Bradykinin
Dopamine
β-Adrenergic catecholamines

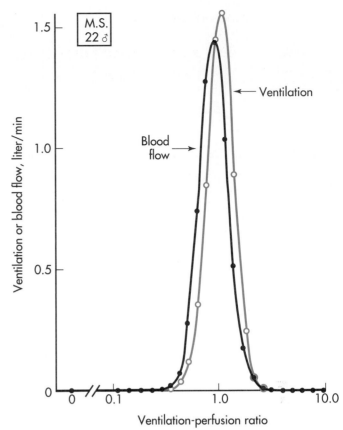

■ **Fig. 27-10** The distribution of ventilation and blood flow in a normal 22-year-old man. Both distributions are positioned about a ventilation:perfusion ratio close to 1.0; the curves are symmetrical on a log scale with no areas of high or low ventilation:perfusion ratios, and there is no shunt (ventilation:perfusion ratio = zero). (From Wagner PD et al: *J Clin Invest* 54.54, 1974.)

The ventilation:perfusion ratio (also referred to as the $\dot{V}/\dot{Q}$ ratio) is defined as the ratio of ventilation to blood flow. This ratio can be defined for a single alveolus, for a group of alveoli, or for the entire lung. At the level of a single alveolus, the ratio is defined as the alveolar ventilation ($\dot{V}_A$) divided by the capillary flow. At the level of the lung, the ratio is defined as the total alveolar ventilation divided by the cardiac output.

In normal individuals, alveolar ventilation and blood flow are each distributed uniformly to the gas-exchanging units, and the alveolar ventilation is slightly less than the pulmonary blood flow. In normal resting individuals, alveolar ventilation is about 4.0 L/min and pulmonary blood flow is about 5.0 L/min. Thus, in the normal lung, the overall ventilation:perfusion ratio is about 0.8, but the range of $\dot{V}/\dot{Q}$ ratios varies widely in different lung units (Fig. 27-10). If ventilation and blood flow are mismatched, both O_2 and CO_2 transfer are impaired. When ventilation exceeds perfusion, the ventilation:perfusion ratio is greater than one ($\dot{V}/\dot{Q} > 1$) and when perfusion exceeds ventilation the ventilation:perfusion ratio is less than 1 ($\dot{V}/\dot{Q} < 1$). In individuals with cardiopulmonary disease, mismatching of pulmonary blood flow and alveolar ventilation is the most frequent cause of systemic arterial hypoxemia.

A normal ventilation:perfusion ratio does not mean that ventilation and perfusion to that lung unit are normal; it simply means that the relationship between ventilation and perfusion is normal. For example, in lobar pneumonia, ventilation to the affected lobe is decreased. If perfusion to this area remains unchanged, perfusion would exceed ventilation; that is, the ventilation:perfusion ratio would be less than 1 ($\dot{V}/\dot{Q} < 1$). However, the decreased ventilation to this area evokes hypoxic vasoconstriction in the pulmonary capillary bed supplying this lobe. The result is a decrease in per-

fusion to the affected area and a more "normal" ventilation:perfusion ratio. However, neither the ventilation nor the perfusion to this area is normal (both are decreased) but the relationship between the two is in the normal range.

Regional Differences in Ratios

Because gravity evokes regional differences in ventilation and perfusion, even in the normal lung, the ventilation:perfusion ratio in different areas of the lung is greater than or less than the normal value of about 0.8. In an upright subject, as ventilation and blood flow are measured sequentially from the top of the lung to the bottom, ventilation increases more slowly than does blood flow. Hence, the $\dot{V}/\dot{Q}$ ratio at the top of the lung is high, whereas the $\dot{V}/\dot{Q}$ ratio at the bottom of the lung is abnormally low. The relationship between ventilation and perfusion from the top to the bottom of the lung is shown in Fig. 27-11. Note that although the overall ventilation:perfusion ratio in the normal lung is about 0.8, the local values constitute a wide range of $\dot{V}/\dot{Q}$ ratios.

Alveolar : Arterial Difference

Before we examine ventilation:perfusion ratios in greater depth, we must examine the relationship between the alveolar

Ventilation-Perfusion Relationships

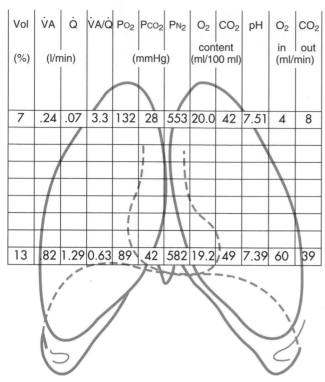

Vol	V̇A	Q̇	V̇A/Q̇	PO₂	PCO₂	PN₂	O₂	CO₂	pH	O₂	CO₂
(%)	(l/min)			(mmHg)			content (ml/100 ml)			in | out (ml/min)	
7	.24	.07	3.3	132	28	553	20.0	42	7.51	4	8
13	82	1.29	0.63	89	42	582	19.2	49	7.39	60	39

■ **Fig. 27-11** Regional differences in gas exchange down the normal lung. Only the apical and basal values are shown for clarity.

O_2 and the arterial O_2. Under ideal conditions, alveolar and arterial O_2 would be equal. Even in normal individuals, alveolar and arterial O_2 differ slightly. The difference between the alveolar O_2 (P_{AO_2}) and the arterial P_{O_2} (P_{aO_2}) is called the AaD_{O_2}. An increased difference in the AaD_{O_2} is a hallmark of abnormal O_2 exchange. This small difference is not caused by "imperfect" gas exchange, but by the small number of veins that bypass the lung and empty directly into the arterial circulation. The thebesian vessels of the left ventricular myocardium drain directly into the left ventricle (rather than into the coronary sinus in the right atrium), and some bronchial veins and mediastinal veins drain into pulmonary veins. This results in venous admixture and a decrease in arterial P_{O_2} (this is an example of an anatomic shunt, see below). Approximately 2% to 3% of the cardiac output is shunted in this way.

Clinically, the effectiveness of gas exchange is determined by measuring the oxygen and carbon dioxide in the arterial blood. This can be done by inserting a needle into a peripheral artery and measuring the P_{aO_2} and P_{aCO_2}. By measuring the barometric pressure, the fraction of oxygen in the inspired air, the water vapor pressure, the alveolar CO_2 (which is equal to the arterial CO_2), and the respiratory quotient (usually considered to be 0.8), we can calculate the alveolar P_{AO_2} from the alveolar air equation. The difference then between the alveolar P_{AO_2} and the arterial P_{aO_2} is the AaD_{O_2}. In normal individuals breathing room air, the AaD_{O_2} is less than 15 mm Hg. The mean value rises approximately 3 mm Hg per decade of life. Hence, an AaD_{O_2} less than 25 mm Hg is considered to be the upper limit of normal.

Using the AaD_{O_2}: An Example

An individual with pneumonia is receiving 30% supplemental O_2 by a facemask. An *arterial* blood gas reveals a pH 7.40, a P_{aCO_2} 44 mm Hg, and a P_{aO_2} 70 mm Hg. What is his AaD_{O_2}? (Assume he is at sea level and his respiratory quotient is 0.8.) Using the alveolar air equation:

$$P_{AO_2} = F_{IO_2}(P_h - P_{H_2O}) - P_{ACO_2}/R$$
$$P_{AO_2} = 0.3(760 - 47) - 40/0.8$$
$$= 164 \text{ mm Hg}$$
$$AaD_{O_2} = P_{AO_2} - P_{aO_2}$$
$$= 164 - 70 = 94 \text{ mm Hg}$$

This elevated AaD_{O_2} suggests that this patient has a lung disease (in this case, pneumonia).

As shown below, abnormalities in arterial P_{aO_2} can occur in the presence or absence of an abnormal AaD_{O_2}. Hence, the relationship between P_{aO_2} and the AaD_{O_2} is useful in determining the cause of an abnormal P_{aO_2} and in predicting the response to therapy (particularly to supplemental oxygen administration). Causes of a reduction in arterial P_{O_2} (arterial hypoxemia) and their effect on the AaD_{O_2} are shown in Table 27-4. Each of these causes is discussed in greater detail later.

Diffusion abnormalities are an uncommon cause of decreased arterial P_{aO_2} in resting subjects, but they assume greater significance during exercise, when the P_{aO_2} is decreased and the AaD_{O_2} is increased.

ARTERIAL BLOOD GAS ABNORMALITIES

Arterial hypoxemia is said to be present when the arterial P_{aO_2} is below the normal range. In general, an arterial P_{aO_2} less than 80 mm Hg is abnormal in an adult who is breathing room air at sea level. *Hypoxia* occurs when there is

■ **Table 27-4**   Causes of hypoxemia

Cause	Arterial P_{O_2}	AaD_{O_2}	Arterial P_{O_2} response to 100% O_2
Anatomical shunt	Decreased	Increased	No change in P_{O_2}
Decreased F_{IO_2}	Decreased	Normal	Increased P_{aO_2}
Physiological shunt	Decreased	Increased	Increased P_{aO_2}
Low ventilation:perfusion ratio	Decreased	Increased	Increased P_{aO_2}
Hypoventilation	Decreased	Normal	Increased P_{aO_2}

insufficient oxygen to carry out normal metabolic functions. Thus, hypoxia and hypoxemia are frequently used interchangeably. Hypercapnia is defined as an increase in arterial P_{aCO_2} above the normal range (40 ± 2 mm Hg) and hypocapnia as an abnormally low arterial P_{aCO_2} (usually less than 35 mm Hg).

VENTILATION : PERFUSION IN A SINGLE ALVEOLUS

A useful way to examine the interaction and relationship between ventilation and perfusion is the two-lung unit model (Fig. 27-12). Two alveoli are ventilated, each of which is supplied by a part of the cardiac output. When ventilation is uniform, half of the inspired gas goes to each alveolus, and when perfusion is uniform, half of the cardiac output goes to each alveoli. In this normal unit, the ventilation:perfusion ratios in each of the alveoli are the same and are equal to 1. The alveoli are perfused by mixed venous blood that is deoxygenated and contains increased P_{aCO_2}. Alveolar O_2 is higher than mixed venous O_2 and this provides a gradient for the movement of oxygen into the blood. In contrast, mixed venous CO_2 is greater than the alveolar CO_2. This provides a gradient for the movement of CO_2 into the alveolus. Note that in this ideal model, alveolar-arterial O_2 values do not differ.

ANATOMICAL SHUNT

Now imagine that a certain amount of mixed venous blood bypasses the gas exchange unit and goes directly into the arterial blood (Fig. 27-13). In this example, let the alveolar ventilation, the distribution of alveolar gas, and the composition of alveolar gas be normal. The distribution of the cardiac output is changed, however. Some of it goes through the pulmonary capillary bed that supplies the two gas exchange units, whereas the rest of it bypasses the gas exchange units and goes directly into the arterial blood. The blood that bypasses the gas exchange unit is said to be "shunted," and because the blood is deoxygenated, the model is said to be a right-to-left shunt. Most often these anatomical shunts occur within the heart, and they occur when deoxygenated blood from the right atrium or ventricle crosses the septum and mixes with blood from the left atrium or ventricle. The effect of this right-to-left shunt is to mix deoxygenated blood with oxygenated blood, and it results in varying degrees of arterial hypoxemia.

An important feature of an anatomical shunt is that the hypoxemia cannot be abolished by giving the individual 100% oxygen to breathe. This condition prevails because the blood that bypasses the ventilation is never exposed to the enriched oxygen, and thus it continues to be deoxygenated. Because the blood that is not being shunted is exposed to the enriched oxygen and it does increase its arterial P_{O_2}, the

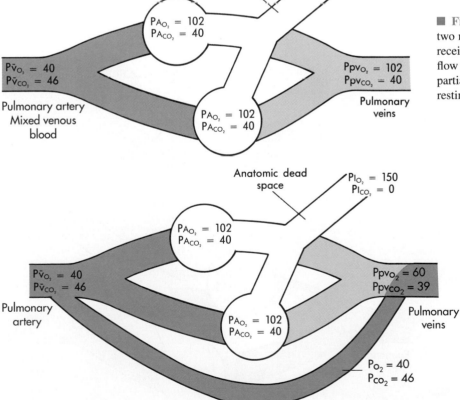

■ **Fig. 27-12** Simplified lung model showing two normal parallel lung units. Both units receive equal quantities of fresh air and blood flow for their size. The blood and alveolar gas partial pressures, *P*, are normal values in a resting person.

■ **Fig. 27-13** Right-to-left shunt. Alveolar ventilation is normal but a portion of the cardiac output bypasses the lung and mixes with oxygenated blood. The P_{aO_2} will vary depending on the size of the shunt.

arterial P_{O_2} does increase in the presence of an anatomical shunt. Normally, the hemoglobin in the blood that perfuses the ventilated alveoli is almost fully saturated. Therefore, most of the added O_2 is in the form of dissolved O_2 that is not well utilized (see Chapter 28).

An anatomical shunt does not usually increase the arterial P_{CO_2}, even though the shunted blood has an elevated level of CO_2. This condition prevails because the central chemoreceptors respond to any elevation in CO_2 with an increase in ventilation. This reduces the arterial P_{CO_2} to the normal range. Sometimes, the level of P_{aCO_2} is below the normal range. This prevails because if the hypoxemia is severe, the increased respiratory drive secondary to the hypoxemia increases the ventilation and further decreases the P_{aCO_2}.

PHYSIOLOGICAL SHUNT

Next let us analyze the response to discontinuing the ventilation to one of the lung units (Fig. 27-14). All of the ventilation now goes to the other lung unit, while the perfusion is equally distributed between both of the lung units. The lung unit without ventilation but with perfusion has a $\dot{V}/\dot{Q}$ ratio = 0. The blood perfusing this unit is mixed venous blood; because there is no ventilation, no gas is exchanged in the unit, and the blood leaving this unit continues to be mixed venous blood. This condition is called a physiological shunt (or venous admixture), but it is similar in its effect to an anatomical shunt; that is, deoxygenated blood

bypasses a gas-exchanging unit and admixes with arterial blood. Clinically, atelectasis (which is obstruction to ventilation of a gas-exchanging unit with subsequent loss of volume) is an example of a lung region with a $\dot{V}/\dot{Q} = 0$. Examples of the obstruction to ventilation include mucus plugs, airway edema, foreign bodies, and tumors in the airway.

VENTILATION : PERFUSION MISMATCHING

Mismatching between ventilation and perfusion is the most common cause of arterial hypoxemia in patients with respiratory disorders. In the most common example, the composition of mixed venous blood, total blood flow (cardiac output), and the distribution of blood flow are all normal. However, in Fig. 27-15, the same total alveolar ventilation is distributed unevenly between the two gas exchange units. Because blood flow is equally distributed, the unit with the decreased ventilation has a $\dot{V}/\dot{Q}$ ratio <1, whereas the unit with the increased ventilation has a $\dot{V}/\dot{Q} > 1$. This causes the alveolar and end-capillary gas compositions to vary. Both the arterial O_2 and the arterial CO_2 contents will be abnormal in the blood that has come from the unit with the decreased ventilation ($\dot{V}/\dot{Q}$ is much less than 1). The unit with the increased ventilation ($\dot{V}/\dot{Q} > 1$) will have a lower CO_2 and a higher O_2 content, because it is being overventilated. The actual arterial P_{O_2} and P_{CO_2} will vary, depending upon the relative contribution of each of these units to the

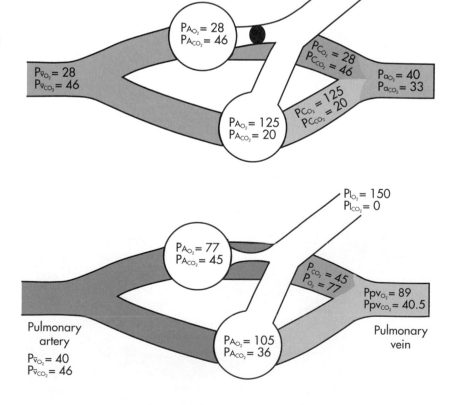

■ **Fig. 27-14** Schema of a physiological shunt (venous admixture). Notice the marked decrease in arterial P_{O_2} compared with P_{CO_2}. The AaD_{O_2} is 85 mm Hg.

$P_{I_{O_2}} = 150$
$P_{I_{CO_2}} = 0$

$P_{A_{O_2}} = 28$
$P_{A_{CO_2}} = 46$

$P_{\bar{v}_{O_2}} = 28$
$P_{\bar{v}_{CO_2}} = 46$

$P_{C_{O_2}} = 28$
$P_{C_{CO_2}} = 46$

$P_{a_{O_2}} = 40$
$P_{a_{CO_2}} = 33$

$P_{A_{O_2}} = 125$
$P_{A_{CO_2}} = 20$

$P_{C_{O_2}} = 125$
$P_{C_{CO_2}} = 20$

■ **Fig. 27-15** Effects of ventilation:perfusion mismatching on gas exchange. The decrease in ventilation to the one lung unit could be due to mucous obstruction airway edema, bronchospasm, a foreign body, or a tumor.

$P_{I_{O_2}} = 150$
$P_{I_{CO_2}} = 0$

$P_{A_{O_2}} = 77$
$P_{A_{CO_2}} = 45$

$P_{C_{O_2}} = 45$
$P_{O_2} = 77$

$Ppv_{O_2} = 89$
$Ppv_{CO_2} = 40.5$

Pulmonary artery
$P_{\bar{v}_{O_2}} = 40$
$P_{\bar{v}_{CO_2}} = 46$

$P_{A_{O_2}} = 105$
$P_{A_{CO_2}} = 36$

Pulmonary vein

arterial blood. In this instance, the alveolar-arterial oxygen gradient (AaD_{O_2}) will be different. This disparity occurs because the relative overventilation of one unit does not fully compensate (either by adding extra oxygen or removing extra carbon dioxide) for the disturbances created by underventilating the other unit. The failure to compensate is greater in the case of oxygen than in that of CO_2. This failure is predictable by the flatness of the upper part of the oxyhemoglobin dissociation curve, in comparison with the slope of the CO_2 dissociation curve (see Chapter 28). In other words, an increased ventilation raises the alveolar P_{O_2}, but it adds little extra O_2 content to the blood. However, the steeper slope of the CO_2 curve indicates that more CO_2 would be eliminated when the ventilation increases. This response occurs because hemoglobin is close to being 100% saturated in these overventilated areas, whereas CO_2 moves by diffusion. Hence, as long as a CO_2 gradient is maintained, CO_2 diffusion will occur.

HYPOVENTILATION

Alveolar O_2 is determined by a balance between the rate of O_2 removal and the rate of O_2 replenishment by ventilation. The rate of O_2 removal is determined by the blood flow through the lung and the metabolic demands of the tissues. If ventilation decreases, alveolar P_{O_2} will decrease, and the arterial P_{O_2} will subsequently decrease. In addition, alveolar ventilation and alveolar CO_2 are directly related. When ventilation is halved, the alveolar CO_2 content and thus the arterial CO_2 content doubles (see the alveolar gas equation on page 481). This process of decreased ventilation is called **hypoventilation.** Hypoventilation always decreases the P_{aO_2} level and increases the P_{aCO_2} level, except when the subject breathes an enriched source of oxygen.

One of the hallmarks of hypoventilation is a normal AaD_{O_2}. This will occur when the gas exchange and the perfusion to the alveolus are normal; that is, the lung is functioning normally. The problem is that the rate of ventilation to the unit is decreased. There are few instances of "pure" hypoventilation, because as ventilation decreases, areas of atelectasis develop ($\dot{V}/\dot{Q} = 0$); atelectasis creates regions with $\dot{V}/\dot{Q}$ ratios = 0 and an increase in the AaD_{O_2}.

DIFFUSION ABNORMALITY

Abnormalities in the diffusion of O_2 across the alveolar-capillary barrier could also result in arterial hypoxia. Equilibration between the alveolar and capillary O_2 and CO_2 contents occurs rapidly and in a fraction of the time that it takes for red blood cells to go through the pulmonary capillary network. Hence, diffusion equilibrium almost always occurs in normal subjects even during exercise when the transit time of red blood cells through the lung increases significantly. An alveolar-arterial P_{O_2} difference, attributable to incomplete diffusion (diffusion disequilibrium), has been observed in normal individuals only during exercise at high altitude (10,000 ft or greater). Even in indi-

viduals with abnormal diffusion capacities, diffusion disequilibrium at rest is unusual. In contrast, abnormalities of diffusion are much more likely to affect arterial blood gas composition during exercise and the effects are accentuated at altitude.

Alveolar capillary block, or thickening of the air-blood barrier, is less common as a cause of decreased diffusing capacity than is a reduction in pulmonary capillary blood volume. The mechanism of hypoxemia is also different. As capillaries are progressively destroyed or obstructed, previously unperfused capillaries are progressively recruited until the velocity of blood flow through the remaining vessels finally increases. Recall that the lung "accepts" the entire cardiac output; flow remains normal even with destruction of capillaries until all capillaries have been recruited. Flow through the remaining capillaries then increases. When this process is severe, the time available for gas exchange in patients at rest may resemble what is observed in normal individuals during exercise. During exercise, the transit time in these individuals may be too short to permit equilibration.

DISEASES ASSOCIATED WITH HYPOXIA

Several types of congenital heart disease may cause cyanosis. The most common of the cyanotic congenital heart diseases is the tetralogy of Fallot. This disease is characterized by pulmonary valve stenosis and a ventricular septal defect (a hole in the septum between the right and left ventricles). As a result, the pressure in the right ventricle increases, and deoxygenated blood is shunted from the right to the left ventricle (an anatomical shunt), bypassing the lung.

The Guillain-Barré syndrome is an acute neuromuscular disease associated with ascending muscle weakness. When respiratory muscles are involved, particularly the diaphragm, minute ventilation (tidal volume × frequency) decreases, P_{aO_2} decreases, and P_{aCO_2} increases.

Asthma is a chronic inflammatory lung disease that is characterized by periodic exacerbations. When the patient is well, pulmonary function tests and arterial blood gases are normal. During an exacerbation, airway inflammation, bronchospasm, and airway edema are evident. This results in airflow obstruction and areas of poor ventilation ($\dot{V}/\dot{Q}$ mismatch).

MECHANISMS OF HYPERCARBIA

Two major mechanisms account for the development of hypercarbia: hypoventilation and wasted ventilation. As previously noted, alveolar ventilation and alveolar CO_2 are directly related. When ventilation is halved, alveolar CO_2 and thus P_{aCO_2} doubles. Hypoventilation always decreases the P_{aO_2} and increases the P_{aCO_2}, except when the subject breathes an enriched source of oxygen.

Wasted ventilation occurs when pulmonary blood flow decreases markedly in the presence of normal ventilation ($\dot{V}/\dot{Q} > 1 \rightarrow \infty$). This occurs most often because of a pulmonary embolus that obstructs blood flow. The embolus halts blood flow to pulmonary areas with normal ventilation ($\dot{V}/\dot{Q} = \infty$). In this situation, the ventilation is wasted, because it fails to oxygenate any of the mixed venous blood. The ventilation to the perfused regions of the lung is less than ideal (i.e., there is relative "hypoventilation" to this area, because this area now receives all of the pulmonary blood flow with a "normal" ventilation). If compensation does not occur, the P_{aCO_2} would increase and the P_{aO_2} would decrease. Compensation after a pulmonary embolus, however, begins almost immediately; the distribution of ventilation shifts to the areas being perfused. As a result, changes in the arterial CO_2 and O_2 contents are minimized.

EFFECT OF 100% O$_2$ ON ARTERIAL BLOOD GAS ABNORMALITIES

One of the ways that a right-to-left shunt can be distinguished from other causes of hypoxemia is by having the individual breathe 100% oxygen through a nonrebreathing facemask for approximately 15 minutes. When the subject breathes 100% oxygen, all of the nitrogen in the alveolus is replaced by oxygen. Thus, alveolar O_2, from the alveolar air equation, is

$$P_{AO_2} = 1.0 \, (P_b - P_{H_2O}) - P_{aCO_2}/0.8$$
$$= 1.0 \, (760 - 47) - 40/0.8$$
$$= 663 \text{ mm Hg}$$

In the normal lung, the alveolar oxygen content rapidly increases, and it provides the gradient for oxygen transfer into the capillary blood. This is associated with a marked increase in the arterial oxygen content (Table 27-4). Similarly, over the 15 to 20-minute period of breathing enriched oxygen, even areas with very low $\dot{V}/\dot{Q}$ ratios will develop a high alveolar oxygen pressure as the nitrogen is replaced by oxygen. In the presence of normal perfusion to these areas, there is a gradient for gas exchange and the end-capillary blood is highly enriched in oxygen. In contrast, in the presence of a right-to-left shunt, oxygenation is not corrected, because mixed venous blood continues to flow through the shunt and to mix with blood that has perfused normal units. The poorly oxygenated blood from the shunt lowers the arterial oxygen content and maintains (and even augments) the AaD_{O_2}. An elevated alveolar-arterial O_2 difference during a properly conducted study with 100% O_2 signifies the presence of a right-to-left shunt; the magnitude of the difference can be used to quantify the proportion of the cardiac output that is shunted.

EFFECT OF CHANGING CARDIAC OUTPUT

Changes in cardiac output are the only nonrespiratory factor that affects gas exchange. Decreasing cardiac output diminishes the O_2 content, and it increases the CO_2 content in the mixed venous blood. Increasing the cardiac output has the opposite effect. This change in O_2 and CO_2 content will have little effect on the arterial O_2 and CO_2 levels in individuals with normal lungs, unless cardiac output is extremely low. In the presence of lung disease secondary to ventilation:per-

fusion mismatching or in the presence of an anatomical shunt, the composition of mixed venous blood will have a significant effect upon the arterial levels of O_2 and CO_2. For any level of $\dot{V}/\dot{Q}$ abnormality, a decrease in cardiac output is associated with an increasingly abnormal P_{aO_2}.

REGIONAL DIFFERENCES

We have already examined regional differences in ventilation and in perfusion, and in the relationship between ventilation and perfusion. We have also examined the effects of various physiological abnormalities (e.g., shunt, $\dot{V}/\dot{Q}$ mismatch, and hypoventilation) on arterial oxygen and carbon dioxide levels. Before leaving this topic, however, it should be noted that because the $\dot{V}/\dot{Q}$ ratio varies in different regions of the lung, the end-capillary blood coming from these regions will have different oxygen and carbon dioxide levels. These disparities are shown in Fig. 27-11, and they demonstrate the complexity of the lung. First recall that the volume of the lung at the apex is less than the volume at the bases. As previously described, ventilation and perfusion are less at the apex than at the base, but the differences in perfusion are greater than the differences in ventilation. Thus, the $\dot{V}/\dot{Q}$ ratio is abnormally high at the apex and abnormally low at the base, and the $\dot{V}/\dot{Q}$ ratio decreases from the apex to the base of the lung. This difference in ventilation:perfusion ratios is associated with a difference in alveolar O_2 and CO_2 contents between the apex and the base. The alveolar O_2 content is higher and the alveolar CO_2 content is lower in the apex than in the base. This results in differences in end-capillary contents for these gases. The P_{O_2} is lower, and consequently the oxygen content is lower for end-capillary blood at the lung base than at the apex. In addition, there is significant variation in the blood pH in the end capillaries in these regions, because of the variation in CO_2 content in the presence of a constant base excess.

Because of the decreased blood flow at the apex, the oxygen consumed and the CO_2 produced are also decreased in this region. Because the CO_2 produced is more closely linked to ventilation, whereas the oxygen consumed is more closely linked to perfusion, the CO_2 produced is higher because ventilation exceeds perfusion. As a result, the respiratory quotient (CO_2 produced/O_2 consumed) is higher at the apex than at the base. During exercise, when blood flow to the apex increases and becomes more uniform in the lung, the differences between contents of gases in the apex and in the base of the lung diminish.

SUMMARY

1. The sum of the partial pressures of a gas must equal the total pressure. The partial pressure of a gas (P_{gas}) is equal to the fraction of gas in the gas mixture (F_{gas}) times the total pressure (P_{tot}).

2. The conducting airways do not participate in gas exchange. Therefore, the partial pressures of oxygen, nitro-

gen, and water vapor remain unchanged in the airways until the gas reaches the alveolus.

3. The partial pressure of oxygen in the alveolus is given by the *alveolar air equation*. This equation is used to calculate the AaD_{O_2}, the most useful measurement of abnormal arterial O_2.

4. The relationship between carbon dioxide production and alveolar ventilation is defined by the *alveolar carbon dioxide equation*. There is an inverse relationship between the partial pressure of carbon dioxide in the alveolus (P_{ACO_2}) and the alveolar ventilation (V_A), irrespective of the exhaled quantity of CO_2. In normal individuals, the alveolar P_{ACO_2} is tightly regulated to remain constant around 40 mm Hg.

5. There are regional differences in ventilation and perfusion, due in large part to the effects of gravity.

6. The volume of air in the conducting airways is called the anatomical dead space. Deadspace ventilation (V_D) varies inversely with tidal volume (V_T).

7. The total volume of gas in each breath that does not participate in gas exchange is called the physiological dead space ventilation. It includes the anatomical dead space and the dead space secondary to ventilated, but not perfused, alveoli or alveoli overventilated relative to the amount of perfusion.

8. The pulmonary circulation is a low-pressure, low-resistance system with a driving pressure that is almost one-sixteenth that of the systemic circulation.

9. The recruitment of new capillaries is a unique feature of the lung, and allows for stress adjustments as in the case of exercise. The arteries of the pulmonary circulation are thin walled, and they have minimal smooth muscle. The pulmonary vessels are seven times more compliant than the systemic vessels.

10. The extraalveolar vessels are generally large vessels (arteries, arterioles, veins, and venules) that are not influenced by alveolar pressure changes, but they are affected by intrapleural and interstitial pressure changes.

11. *Pulmonary vascular resistance* is the change in pressure from the pulmonary artery (P_{PA}) to the left atrium (P_{LA}) divided by the cardiac output (Q_T). This resistance is about 10 times less than in the systemic circulation.

12. In upright, resting subjects, blood flow increases linearly from the apex of the lung to the base of the lung, where the flow is the greatest.

13. The lung has been classically divided into three zones. Zone 1 represents the apex region, where blood does not flow under certain conditions. In zone 2, which comprises the upper one-third of the lung, the P_a is greater than the P_A, which is greater than P_v. In zone 3, P_a is greater than P_v, which is greater than P_A, and blood flow in this area parallels the pressure gradients.

14. Hypoxic vasoconstriction occurs in small arterial vessels in response to a decreased P_{O_2}. Local hypoxia does not alter PVR.

15. The ventilation:perfusion ratio (also referred to as the $V̇/Q̇$ ratio) is defined as the ratio of ventilation to blood flow. In the normal lung, the overall ventilation:perfusion ratio is about 0.8. When ventilation exceeds perfusion, the ventilation:perfusion ratio is greater than 1 ($V̇/Q̇ > 1$), and when perfusion exceeds ventilation, the ventilation:perfusion ratio is less than 1 ($V̇/Q̇ < 1$).

16. The $V̇/Q̇$ ratio at the top of the lung is high (increased ventilation relative to very little blood flow), whereas the $V̇/Q̇$ ratio at the bottom of the lung is very low. In normal individuals on room air the AaD_{O_2} is less than 15 mm Hg.

17. There are four mechanisms of hypoxemia: anatomical shunt, physiological shunt, $V̇/Q̇$ mismatching, and hypoventilation.

18. There are two mechanisms of hypercarbia: increase in dead space and hypoventilation.

19. A change in cardiac output is the only nonrespiratory factor that affects gas exchange.

REFERENCES

Journal articles

Bongartz G et al: Pulmonary circulation, *Eur Radiol* 8(5):698, 1998.

Glenny RW: Blood flow distribution in the lung, *Chest* 114:8S, 1998.

Henig NR, Pierson DJ: Mechanisms of hypoxemia, *Respir Care Clin North Am* 6(4):501, 2000.

Weir K, Archer SL: The mechanism of acute hypoxic pulmonary vasoconstriction: the tale of two channels, *FASEB J* 9:183, 1995.

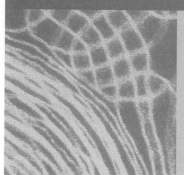

chapter twenty-eight

Oxygen and Carbon Dioxide Transport

The intracellular metabolism of oxygen (O_2) provides the cell with its major source of energy, which enables the cell to carry out active cellular processes. Oxygen metabolism occurs within the mitochondrial electron transport system, and it results in the generation of adenosine triphosphate (ATP). Energy is produced by the subsequent hydrolysis of ATP to adenosine diphosphate (ADP) and inorganic phosphate.

O_2 delivery to the tissue drives the intracellular metabolism of O_2. The respiratory and circulatory systems function together to transport sufficient O_2 from the lungs to the tissues to sustain normal cellular activity. As O_2 is transported to the tissue, a product of active cellular metabolism, namely carbon dioxide (CO_2), is transported from the tissues to the blood, and it is eventually exhaled through the lungs. Unique transport mechanisms not only enable these two processes (O_2 uptake and CO_2 exhalation) to occur simultaneously, but they also facilitate each other. That is, the uptake of O_2 into the tissues enhances the elimination of CO_2, and vice versa (Fig. 28-1). To gain an understanding of the mechanisms involved in the transport of these gases, one must consider gas diffusion properties, as well as transport and delivery processes.

GAS DIFFUSION

Gas Diffusion and Diffusing Capacity of the Lung for CO (D_{LCO})

Diffusion is the major mechanism of gas movement throughout the respiratory system. Diffusion is important both for gas movement from the smaller airways to the alveoli (air → air), and for gas movement across the alveoli into the blood (air → liquid) and from the blood into the tissue (liquid → tissue). The velocity of inspired air for gas distribution decreases as the air approaches the alveoli, because of the multiple bifurcations of the respiratory tract and the increasing cross-sectional area. Once in the alveolus, gas diffusion is aided by the **pores of Kohn**, which function as interalveolar canals. Diffusion through the pores of Kohn occurs

under normal conditions, but it becomes even more significant in the ventilation of alveoli whose airways are obstructed. The obstruction is caused by increased mucus production in disease states such as cystic fibrosis, acute asthma, and chronic bronchitis. The process of gas diffusion is passive, non–energy dependent, and similar whether in a gas or liquid state. Gases for the most part will maintain their molecular characteristics when they are in the liquid state and the gases establish what is referred to as a **partial pressure (P).** As previously described (Chapter 27), the sum of the partial pressures of the various gases in inspired air equals the *total pressure;* thus, if the partial pressure of one gas decreases, the partial pressure of another gas must rise. This concept is particularly important when evaluating the partial pressures of oxygen (P_{O_2}) and carbon dioxide (P_{CO_2}) in blood; theoretically, when one partial pressure increases, the other must decrease, if the total pressure remains constant. Gas diffusion follows the partial pressure gradient from higher pressure to lower pressure.

The rates of O_2 transport from the lungs into the blood and from the blood into the tissue, and vice versa for CO_2, are predicted by the gas diffusion laws. **Fick's law** states that the diffusion ($\dot{V}$) of a gas across a sheet of tissue is *directly* related to the surface area (A) of the tissue, the diffusion constant (D) of the specific gas, and the partial pressure difference ($P_1 - P_2$) of the gas on each side of the tissue, and it is *inversely* related to tissue thickness (T) (Fig. 28-2). That is,

$$\dot{V}_{gas} = \frac{A \cdot D(P_1 - P_2)}{T}$$

The two key anatomical locations for O_2 diffusion are at the alveolar-capillary membrane (air → liquid) and at the blood capillary-tissue barrier (liquid → tissue). Fick's equation demonstrates that the major rate-limiting step for diffusion is at the liquid to tissue (t) interface. At this step, T is the tissue thickness from the capillaries to the mitochondria in the tissue cells. A is the capillary surface area, and the pressure gradient is $P_1 - P_2$, whereas in the alveolus, the pressure gradient is $P_{AO_2} - P_{CO_2}$.

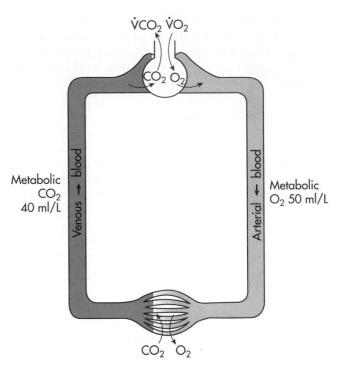

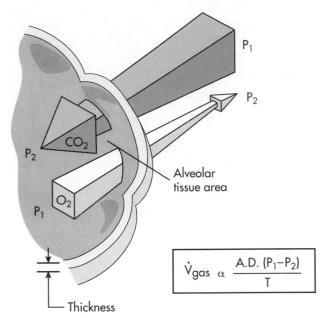

■ Fig. 28-1 Oxygen and carbon dioxide transport occur in both arterial and venous blood. However, the extracted or utilized oxygen is present in arterial blood where it is transferred from arterial capillaries to the tissue. Only ~25% of transported oxygen is actually taken up by the tissue. The source of exhaled carbon dioxide is venous blood; it is expired via the pulmonary capillaries. The flow rates for oxygen ($\dot{V}O_2$) and carbon dioxide ($\dot{V}CO_2$) shown are for 1 liter of blood. The ratio of CO_2 production to O_2 consumption is the respiratory exchange ratio, R, which at rest is ~0.80.

■ Fig. 28-2 Fick's law states that the diffusion of a gas across a sheet of tissue is *directly* related to the surface area of the tissue, the diffusion constant of the specific gas, and the partial pressure difference of the gas on each side of the tissue, and is *inversely* related to the tissue thickness.

The ratio of AD/T represents the conductance (1/resistance) of a gas from the alveolus to the blood. The diffusing capacity of the lung (D_L) is its conductance (AD/T) when considered for the entire lung; thus, applying Fick's equation, the D_L can be calculated as follows:

$$\dot{V} = \frac{A \cdot D(P_1 - P_2)}{T}$$
$$\dot{V} = D_L(P_1 - P_2)$$
$$D_L = \frac{\dot{V}}{(P_1 - P_2)}$$

Fick's law of diffusion could be used to assess the diffusion properties of O_2 in the lung, except that ΔP (alveolar − capillary P_{O_2}) cannot be determined, because the capillary P_{O_2} cannot be measured. This limitation can be overcome by using carbon monoxide (CO) rather than O_2. Because carbon monoxide has a *low* solubility in the capillary membrane, the rate of CO equilibrium across the capillary is slow and the partial pressure of CO in the capillary blood remains close to zero. This is in contrast to the *high* solubility of CO in blood. Thus, the only limitation for CO diffusion is the alveolar-capillary membrane, which makes CO a useful gas

for calculating D_L. The capillary partial pressure (P_2 above) is essentially zero for CO, and, therefore, D_L can be measured from the $\dot{V}_{CO}$ and the average partial pressure of CO in the alveolus. That is,

$$D_L = \frac{\dot{V}_{CO}}{P_{ACO}}$$

The Measurement of D_{LCO}: An Example

A patient with interstitial pulmonary fibrosis (a restrictive process) inhales a single breath of 0.3% CO from the residual volume to the total lung capacity. He holds his breath for 10 seconds and then exhales. After the exhaled gas is discarded from the dead space, a representative sample of alveolar gas is obtained near the end of exhalation. The average alveolar CO is 0.1 torr, and 0.25 ml of CO has been taken up. The diffusion capacity for CO in this patient is

$$D_{LCO} = \frac{\dot{V}_{CO}}{P_{ACO}} = \frac{0.25 \text{ ml}/10 \text{ sec} \times 60 \text{ sec/min}}{0.1 \text{ torr}}$$
$$= 15 \text{ ml/min/torr}$$

The normal range for D_{LCO} is 20 to 30 ml/min/torr. In patients with interstitial pulmonary fibrosis, there is an initial alveolar inflammatory response and subsequent scar formation (connective tissue deposition) within the interstitial space. The inflammation and scar tissue thicken the interstitial space and make it more difficult for gas to diffuse. Hence, D_{LCO} decreases. This is a classic characteristic of a restrictive lung disease process; gas readily

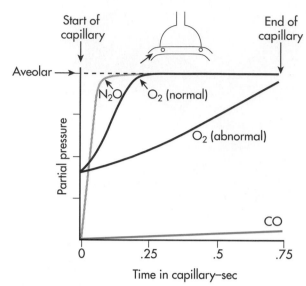

■ **Fig. 28-3** Uptake of nitrous oxide, carbon monoxide, and oxygen in blood relative to their partial pressures and the transit time of the red blood cell in the capillary. For gases which are perfusion limited (nitrous oxide and oxygen), their partial pressures have equilibrated with alveolar pressure prior to exiting the capillary. In contrast, for carbon monoxide, a gas which is diffusion limited, its partial pressure does not reach equilibrium with alveolar pressure. Oxygen uptake in various disease conditions can become diffusion limited.

enters the alveolus, but its ability to diffuse into the blood is restricted.

Perfusion and diffusion limitation. Different gases have different solubility factors, which result in varying diffusion coefficients. For gases such as nitrous oxide (N_2O), ether, and, helium, which are insoluble in blood and do not combine chemically with blood, equilibration between alveolar gas and blood occurs rapidly (significantly less than the 0.75 second that the red blood cell spends in the capillary bed), and it is driven by the difference in partial pressure (Fig. 28-3). This type of gas exchange is **perfusion limited,** because blood leaving the capillary has reached equilibrium with alveolar gas. As illustrated in Fig. 28-3, the partial pressure of N_2O peaks quickly and is maximal by 0.25 second, at which point no further N_2O is transferred.

In contrast, for a gas such as carbon monoxide (CO), which has a low solubility in the alveolar-capillary membrane but a high solubility in blood, equilibration between alveolar gas and blood occurs very slowly (significantly greater than the 0.75 second transit time of the red blood cells in the capillary). CO is highly soluble in blood at partial pressures below 1 to 2 torr. At partial pressures greater than 2 torr, CO solubility is slight, as the CO content increases only by adding dissolved CO. Equilibration is not reached during the transit time, and therefore the partial pressure increases only slightly (Fig. 28-3). Because of the high avidity of CO for hemoglobin, large amounts of CO can be taken up in blood with little increase in its partial pressure. Exchange of CO

still occurs as the red blood cell leaves the end of the capillary, because its equilibration is slow relative to the time spent in the capillary. This type of gas transfer is **diffusion limited.** This occurs for CO because its solubility in the membrane is slight, but its solubility in blood is great. In the absence of red blood cells, CO uptake would be perfusion limited, because the blood plasma has a low solubility for CO.

Like CO, both CO_2 and O_2 have a low solubility in the membrane of the blood gas barrier, but they have a high solubility in blood because they combine with hemoglobin. However, their rate of equilibration is sufficiently rapid for complete equilibration to occur during the transit time of the red blood cells within the capillary. Equilibration for O_2 and CO_2 usually occurs within 0.25 second (Fig. 28-3). Thus, O_2 and CO_2 transfers are normally perfusion limited. Note that CO_2 has a greater overall rate of diffusion (about 20 times) in blood than does oxygen but a lower membrane to blood solubility ratio. As a consequence, O_2 and CO_2 reach equilibrium in approximately the same amount of time.

Diffusion limitation for O_2 and CO_2 could occur if the red blood cell spent less than 0.25 second in the capillary bed. Occasionally, this occurs in very fit athletes during vigorous exercise and in healthy subjects who exercise at high altitude.

OXYGEN TRANSPORT

Oxygen is carried in the blood in both the dissolved gaseous state in plasma, and it is bound to hemoglobin (Hgb) as oxyhemoglobin ($HgbO_2$) within red blood cells. O_2 transport occurs primarily in the $HgbO_2$ form; the contribution of dissolved O_2 is minimal. The Hgb not bound to O_2 is referred to as deoxyhemoglobin or reduced hemoglobin. At a P_{aO_2} of 100 mm Hg, only 3 ml of O_2 is dissolved in 1 L of plasma. The contribution of hemoglobin within the red blood cell enhances the O_2-carrying capacity of blood by about 65-fold.

Hemoglobin as a Transport Molecule

Structure. Hemoglobin has a molecular weight of 66,500, and it consists of four nonprotein O_2-binding *heme* groups and four polypeptide chains. These components make up the *globin* protein portion of the Hgb molecule (Fig. 28-4). Iron is present in each heme group in the reduced ferrous (Fe^{2+}) form, and it is the site of O_2 binding. The binding of O_2 to hemoglobin alters the absorption of hemoglobin, which is responsible for the change in color between oxygenated arterial blood ($HgbO_2$) and deoxygenated venous blood (Hgb). The readily reversible binding of O_2 to hemoglobin facilitates the delivery of O_2 to the tissue from the blood. The binding and dissociation of O_2 with Hgb occur in milliseconds, which accounts for the transit time of 0.75 second for the red blood cells in the capillaries. The four polypeptide chains in adult Hgb (hemoglobin type A, HgbA) have two α chains and two β chains whereas the polypeptide chains of fetal Hgb (HgbF) have two α chains and two γ chains. This change in the structure of HgbF increases its affinity for O_2, and it aids in the transport of O_2 across the placenta. As will be discussed later in this chapter, HgbF is

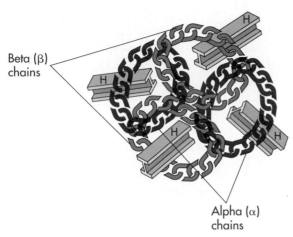

Beta (β) chains

Alpha (α) chains

■ **Fig. 28-4** Schematic illustration of a hemoglobin molecule showing the globin (protein) component with two alpha and beta chains and the four iron containing heme groups (oxygen binding) positioned in the center of each globin portion. Each hemoglobin molecule can bind four oxygen molecules.

not affected or inhibited by the glycolysis product, 2,3-diphosphoglycerate, in red blood cells, and thus O_2 uptake is enhanced. During the first year of life, HgbF is replaced by HgbA.

There are about 280 million Hgb molecules per red blood cell, and this profusion of Hgb provides a unique and efficient mechanism for the transport of O_2. Because the amount of hemoglobin present in each red blood cell is relatively constant, the amount of hemoglobin in blood is directly proportional to the percent of the blood volume that is occupied by red blood cells (this fraction is called the hematocrit). It should be noted that **myoglobin**, the O_2-carrying and storage protein of muscle tissue, is similar to hemoglobin in structure and function, except that myoglobin has only one subunit of the hemoglobin molecule; thus its molecular weight is about 25% that of hemoglobin. Myoglobin aids in the transfer of O_2 from the blood to the muscle cells, and in the storage of O_2, which is especially critical when the O_2 supply is inadequate.

Abnormal hemoglobin. Abnormalities of the hemoglobin molecule occur when the sequence or spatial arrangements of the globin polypeptide chains are altered, and they result in abnormal hemoglobin function.

Sickle Cell Anemia

In an inherited, homozygous condition known as *sickle cell anemia,* individuals have an amino acid substitution (valine for glutamic acid) on the β chain of the hemoglobin molecule. This creates a sickle cell hemoglobin (HgbS), which when unbound to O_2 (deoxyhemoglobin) forms a gel that distorts the normal biconcave shape of the red blood cell to a crescent or "sickle" form. This change in shape increases the tendency of the red blood cell to form thrombi or clots that obstruct small vessels,

and it creates a clinical condition known as a "sickle cell crisis." The symptoms of such a crisis vary depending on the site of the obstruction. If it occurs in the central nervous system, the patient suffers a stroke. If it occurs in the lung, the patient can develop a pulmonary infarction (tissue death) of the lung tissue. If the molecule is in the homozygous form, the clinical condition is life-shortening. However, if the molecule is in the heterozygous form, the condition is not life-threatening, and the subjects are resistant to malaria. Thus, there is a survival advantage to the heterozygous individual in regions in the world in which malaria is prevalent.

When oxygen combines with hemoglobin, the iron usually remains in the ferrous state. In a condition known as **methemoglobinemia,** compounds such as nitrites and various cyanides (which may be released in the environment during the burning of plastics, or in electroplating or mining) can oxidize the iron molecule in the heme group, and thereby change it from the reduced ferrous state to the oxidized ferric state (Fe^{3+}). Hemoglobin with iron in the ferric state is brown instead of red. Methemoglobin blocks the release of O_2 from hemoglobin, and thereby inhibits the delivery of O_2 to the tissues. This is a critical aspect of reversible O_2 transport. Under normal conditions, about 1% to 2% of hemoglobin binding sites are in the ferric state. Intracellular enzymes, such as glutathione reductase, can reduce the methemoglobin back to the functioning ferrous state. Patients with methemoglobinemia have an absence of glutathione reductase.

Dissolved Oxygen

Oxygen diffuses passively from the alveolus and dissolves in the plasma. In its dissolved form, O_2 maintains its molecular structure and gaseous state. It is this form that is measured clinically as the P_{aO_2} in an arterial blood gas sample. The quantity of oxygen that dissolves in a fluid, such as blood, is predicted by the gas laws (Henry's law and Graham's law), and it depends on the partial pressure of the gas and on the temperature. **Henry's law** states that the amount of gas that dissolves in a liquid at a given temperature is proportional to the partial pressure of the gas. The rate of diffusion of a gas through a liquid is best described by **Graham's law,** which states that the diffusion rate is directly proportional to the solubility coefficient of the gas and inversely proportional to the square root of its gram molecular weight (GMW). The solubility coefficient for oxygen at 37° C and at 760 mm Hg is 0.0244 ml/mm Hg/ml H_2O and for CO_2, it is 0.592 ml/mm Hg/ml H_2O. Thus, CO_2 is about 24 times more soluble than is oxygen in blood. However, because the GMW of oxygen (GMW-32) is smaller than that of CO_2 (GMW-44) the oxygen will have a faster diffusion rate. The overall result is that CO_2 has an overall greater rate of diffusion (about 20 times) than does oxygen in blood.

In a healthy normal adult, approximately 0.3 ml of O_2 is dissolved in 100 ml of blood. This is commonly expressed as 0.3 volumes percent (vol%), where the vol% is equal to the ml O_2 per 100 ml of blood. Only a small percentage of O_2 is carried in this dissolved form, and its contribution to total O_2 transport is small. When the O_2 content in blood is calculated, the dissolved O_2 is frequently ignored, although ideally it should be considered. The small amount of additional dissolved O_2 can, however, be significant in individuals with severe hypoxemia. The dissolved O_2 content is the product of the oxygen solubility (0.00304 ml O_2/dl • torr) times the oxygen tension (torr).

Oxygen Bound to Hemoglobin, and the Oxyhemoglobin Dissociation Curve

The majority of O_2 in plasma quickly diffuses into the red blood cells, where it chemically binds to the heme groups of the hemoglobin molecule and forms oxyhemoglobin ($HgbO_2$). The chemical binding of O_2 to hemoglobin occurs in the lung and this $HgbO_2$ complex is the major transport mechanism for oxygen. O_2 binding is also reversible at the tissue level, where hemoglobin gives up its oxygen to the tissue. The number of O_2 molecules bound to hemoglobin is dependent on the partial pressure of O_2 in the blood. The oxyhemoglobin dissociation curve illustrates the relationship between the oxygen partial pressure (P_{O_2}) in the blood and the percentage of O_2 binding sites occupied by oxygen molecules (Fig. 28-5). As the partial pressure of O_2 rises, hemoglobin saturation increases. The curve, however, is S-shaped, not linear, and this raises a number of interesting observations. The curve begins to plateau at a P_{O_2} of around 50 mm Hg, and it flattens at a P_{O_2} of about 70 mm Hg. At partial pressures below 60 mm Hg, oxygen readily binds to hemoglobin as the P_{O_2} increases. At a P_{O_2} of 60 mm Hg, hemoglobin is 90% saturated; increases in P_{O_2} above this level will influence hemoglobin saturation only slightly. Specifically, increasing the P_{O_2} from 60 to 100 mm Hg will increase the hemoglobin saturation by only 7%. The clinical significance of the flat portion of the oxyhemoglobin dissociation curve is that a drop in P_{O_2} from about 100 mm Hg to about 60 mm Hg still results in a hemoglobin saturation of more than 90%, which virtually ensures adequate O_2 transport. Also, increasing the P_{O_2} above 100 mm Hg has little effect on the oxygen content in the blood, because hemoglobin is already fully saturated. In the steep portion of the curve, blood oxygen content and thus oxygen delivery to the tissue are significantly compromised when the P_{O_2} falls below 60 mm Hg. The clinical significance of this portion of the curve is that a large amount of O_2 is released from hemoglobin with only a small change in P_{O_2}. This response facilitates the diffusion of O_2 to the tissue. The point on the curve at which 50% of the hemoglobin is saturated with O_2 (two oxygen molecules on one Hgb molecule) is called the P_{50} (Fig. 28-6). In adults at sea level, this condition occurs at a P_{O_2} of 27 mm Hg.

The oxyhemoglobin dissociation curve can be shifted either to the right or left in various clinical conditions. The curve is shifted to the right when the affinity of hemoglobin for O_2 decreases. This decreases the binding of O_2 to hemoglobin at a given P_{O_2}; thus, the P_{50} will be increased. The

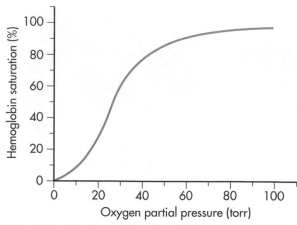

■ Fig. 28-5 Oxyhemoglobin dissociation curve showing the relationship between the partial pressure of oxygen in blood and the percentage of the hemoglobin binding sites that are occupied by oxygen molecules (percent saturation). Adult hemoglobin (HgbA) is about 60% saturated at a P_{O_2} of 30 torr, 90% saturated at 60 torr, and about 75% saturated at 40 torr.

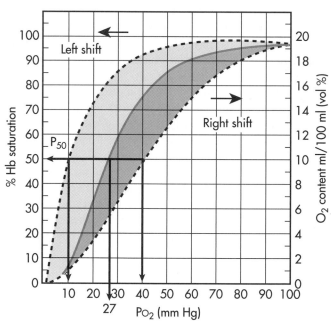

■ Fig. 28-6 The P_{50} represents the partial pressure at which hemoglobin is 50% saturated with oxygen. When the oxygen dissociation curve shifts to the right, the P_{50} increases. When the curve shifts to the left, the P_{50} decreases.

curve is shifted to the left when the affinity of hemoglobin for O_2 increases. This results in a lower P_{50}. Processes that shift the oxyhemoglobin dissociation curve are listed in Fig. 28-7.

Factors That Shift the Oxyhemoglobin Dissociation Curve

pH and CO_2: the Bohr effect. Changes in blood pH will shift the oxyhemoglobin dissociation curve. A decrease in pH shifts the curve to the right (enhancing O_2 dissocia-

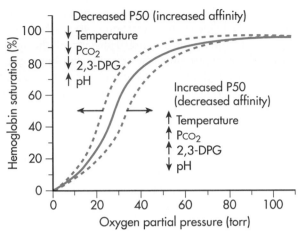

■ **Fig. 28-7** Factors which shift the oxyhemoglobin dissociation curve. The affinity of hemoglobin for oxygen is expressed as the P_{50}. Increases in P_{CO_2} temperature, or 2,3-diphosphoglycerate (2,3-DPG) or decreases in pH shift the oxyhemoglobin dissociation curve to the right (increased P_{50} = decreased affinity), while opposite changes shift the curve to the left (decreased P_{50} = increased affinity) relative to the standard value of 27 torr.

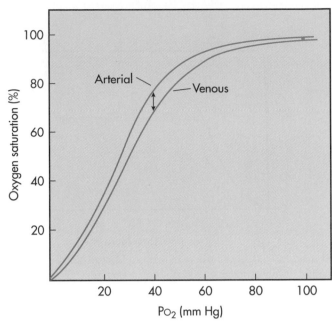

■ **Fig. 28-8** Normal arterial and venous $HgbO_2$ equilibrium curves. In the lung, the effect of the shift to the left caused by a decrease in hydrogen ion concentration enhances oxygen uptake. In the systemic capillaries, significant O_2 unloading begins at about P_{O_2} = 70 mm Hg. The rising hydrogen ion concentration caused by the entry of CO_2 shifts the curve to the right, enhancing oxygen dissociation. The P_{50} of the arterial curve is 26 mm Hg; the P_{50} of the venous curve is 29 mm Hg.

tion) whereas an increase in pH shifts the curve to the left (increasing O_2 affinity). During cellular metabolism, CO_2 is released into the blood, and therefore the generation of hydrogen ions increases and pH decreases. This results in a shift of the dissociation curve to the right, which indicates that the effect is beneficial by aiding in the release of O_2 from Hgb and the diffusion of O_2 into the tissues and cells. The shift to the right is probably due not only to the decrease in pH, but also to a direct effect of CO_2 on hemoglobin. Conversely, as blood passes through the lungs, CO_2 is exhaled, which results in a decrease in hydrogen ions and an increase in pH; these changes result in a shift to the left in the dissociation curve. The higher hemoglobin affinity for O_2 enhances the binding of O_2 to hemoglobin. This effect of CO_2 on the affinity of hemoglobin for oxygen is known as the **Bohr effect** (after the Danish physiologist, Christian Bohr). The Bohr effect is caused in part by the change in pH that occurs as CO_2 increases, and in part to the direct effects of CO_2 on hemoglobin. The Bohr effect enhances O_2 delivery to the tissues and the O_2 uptake in the lungs (Fig. 28-8).

Temperature. The body temperature increases during muscular exercise. This effect shifts the dissociation curve to the right and it enables more O_2 to be released in the tissues, where it is needed because the demand increases. During cold weather, a decrease in body temperature, especially in the extremities (lips, fingers, toes, and ears), shifts the O_2 dissociation curve to the left (higher Hgb affinity). In this instance, the P_{aO_2} concentration may be normal, but the release of O_2 in these extremities is not facilitated. That is why these anatomical areas display a bluish coloration with exposure to cold.

2,3-Diphosphoglycerate. Mature red blood cells do not have mitochondria, and therefore they respire via anaerobic glycolysis. Large quantities of a metabolic intermediary,

2,3-diphosphoglycerate (2,3-DPG), are formed within the red blood cell during glycolysis. The affinity of Hgb for O_2 decreases proportionately as 2,3-DPG levels increase in the red blood cell. Thus, the oxyhemoglobin dissociation curve is shifted to the right. The affinity of 2,3-DPG for Hgb is greater than that of O_2 for Hgb; as a result, 2,3-DPG directly competes with O_2 for Hgb binding sites. Conditions that increase 2,3-DPG include hypoxia, decreased Hgb concentration, and increased pH. Red blood cells with HgbS (sickle cell trait) have increased levels of 2,3-DPG. Decreased levels of 2,3-DPG are observed in stored blood samples, and thus may present a problem due to the greater Hgb O_2 affinity, which inhibits the unloading of O_2 in tissues.

Fetal hemoglobin. As discussed previously, fetal hemoglobin has a greater affinity for O_2 than does adult hemoglobin. Fetal hemoglobin thus shifts the oxyhemoglobin dissociation curve to the left.

Carbon monoxide. Carbon monoxide (CO) binds to the heme group of the hemoglobin molecule at the same site as O_2 and it forms carboxyhemoglobin, HgbCO. A major difference, however, is illustrated by comparing the oxyhemoglobin and carboxyhemoglobin dissociation curves. The affinity of CO for Hgb is about 200 times greater than it is for O_2 (Fig. 28-9). Thus, small amounts of CO can greatly influence the binding of O_2 to Hgb. In the presence of CO, the affinity of hemoglobin for O_2 is enhanced. This influence shifts the dissociation curve to the left, which further prevents the unloading and delivery of O_2 to tissues. As the P_{CO}

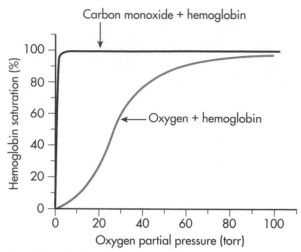

■ **Fig. 28-9** Oxyhemoglobin and carboxyhemoglobin dissociation curves. Carbon monoxide and oxygen compete for the same binding sites on hemoglobin, but CO has an affinity for Hgb that is ~200 times greater than O_2. Thus, above a blood P_{CO} of about 0.5 torr, all of the hemoglobin binding sites are occupied by carbon monoxide.

of blood approaches 1.0 torr, all of the hemoglobin binding sites are occupied by CO, and hemoglobin is unable to bind to O_2. This situation is not compatible with life; it is the mechanism of death in individuals with carbon monoxide poisoning. In healthy individuals, carboxyhemoglobin occupies about 1% to 2% of the Hgb binding sites; however, in cigarette smokers and in individuals who reside in high-density urban traffic areas, occupation of Hgb binding sites can be increased to 10%.

Treatment for individuals with high levels of CO, such as after inhaling car exhaust or inhaling smoke from a burning building, consists of administering high concentrations of O_2 to displace CO from hemoglobin. Increasing the barometric pressure above atmospheric, through the use of a barometric chamber, substantially increases the oxygen tension. This increase in barometric pressure promotes the further dissociation of CO from hemoglobin.

Another gas, nitric oxide (NO), has a great affinity (200,000 times greater than O_2) for Hgb, and it binds irreversibly to Hgb at the same site as does O_2. Endothelial cells can synthesize NO, which has vasodilation properties, and it is used therapeutically as an inhalant in patients with pulmonary hypertension. Although NO poisoning is not common, one should be cautious when administering NO therapy for long periods of time.

Clinical significance of shifts in the oxyhemoglobin dissociation curve. Shifts of the dissociation curve to the right or left have little effect when they occur at oxygen partial pressures within the plateau region (80-100 mm Hg) of the oxyhemoglobin dissociation curve. However, at oxygen partial pressures below 60 mm Hg (the steep part of the curve), shifts in the oxyhemoglobin dissociation curve can dramatically influence O_2 transport. For example, in a patient

who has lung disease and who has an arterial P_{O_2} equal to 60 mm Hg, the hemoglobin saturation is 90%, which is still adequate for normal functioning. However, if the patient experiences a decrease in pH, which will shift the dissociation curve to the right, the hemoglobin saturation could drop to less than 70%, and this would significantly impair O_2 delivery.

Oxygen Saturation

Each hemoglobin molecule can bind up to four oxygen atoms, and each gram of hemoglobin can bind up to 1.34 ml (range of 1.34-1.39 ml depending on methemoglobin levels) of oxygen. The term oxygen saturation (S_{O_2}) refers to the ratio of the amount of O_2 bound to hemoglobin relative to the maximal amount of O_2 (100% oxygen capacity) that can bind hemoglobin. At 100% oxygen capacity, the heme group is fully saturated with oxygen. Correspondingly at 75% S_{O_2}, three of the four heme groups are occupied by O_2. The binding of oxygen to each heme group increases the affinity of the hemoglobin molecule to bind additional O_2. Thus, when three of the heme groups are oxygen bound, the affinity of the fourth heme group to bind oxygen is increased. Because there are about 14 g of Hgb/100 ml of blood, the normal O_2 capacity is 18.76 ml of O_2/100 ml of blood (1 g of Hgb binds 1.34 ml $O_2 \times 14$ g). A mildly anemic individual with an Hgb concentration of 10 g/100 ml of blood and with normal lungs would have an O_2 capacity of only 13.40 ml of O_2/100 ml of blood, and a severely anemic individual with an Hgb concentration of 5 g would have an O_2 capacity of 6.70 ml of O_2/100 ml of blood, which is one-third of normal.

Oxygen Content (Concentration) of Blood

The O_2 content in blood is the volume of O_2 contained per unit volume of blood. The total O_2 content is the sum of the O_2 bound to hemoglobin and the dissolved O_2. The hemoglobin bound O_2 content is determined by the concentration of hemoglobin (in g/dl), the O_2 binding capacity of the hemoglobin (1.34 ml O_2/g Hgb), and the percent saturation of the hemoglobin. The dissolved O_2 content is the product of the O_2 solubility (0.00304 ml O_2/dl • torr) times the O_2 tension (torr). The oxygen content decreases as the CO_2 and CO increase, and it decreases in individuals with anemia (Fig. 28-10).

***

O_2 Content: An Example

An arterial blood gas reveals a P_{aO_2} of 60 torr and an O_2 saturation (Sa_{O_2}) of 90%. The patient's hemoglobin is 14 g/dl. What is the total (Hgb-bound and dissolved) O_2 content?

$$\text{Hgb-bound } O_2 \text{ content} = \frac{1.34 \text{ ml}}{\text{g Hgb}} \cdot \frac{14 \text{ g Hgb}}{\text{dl blood}} \cdot \frac{0.90\% \text{ saturation}}{100}$$

$$= 16.88 \text{ ml/dl blood}$$

$$\text{Dissolved } O_2 \text{ content} = P_{aO_2} \cdot O_2 \text{ solubility}$$

$$= 60 \text{ torr} \cdot 0.00304 \text{ ml } O_2/\text{dl} \cdot \text{torr}$$

$$= 0.18 \text{ ml } O_2/\text{dl}$$

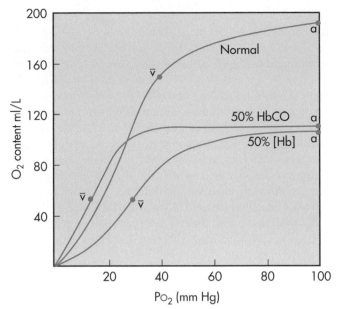

■ Fig. 28-10 Comparison of oxygen content curves under three conditions shows why HbCO is so toxic to the oxygen transport system. Fifty percent [Hb] represents a reduction in circulating hemoglobin by half; 50% HbCO represents binding of half the circulating hemoglobin with CO. The 50% [Hb] and 50% HbCO curves show the same decreased oxygen content in arterial blood. However, CO has a profound effect in lowering venous P_{O_2}. The arterial *(a)* and mixed venous *(v̄)* points of constant cardiac output are indicated.

Total O_2 content	= 16.88 ml/dl + 0.18 ml/dl
	= 17.06 ml/dl blood

The patient is treated with 30% supplemental O_2, and a repeat arterial blood gas reveals a P_{aO_2} of 95 torr, with an O_2 saturation of 97%. What is the total O_2 content now?

Hgb O_2 content = 1.34 ml/dl • 14 g/dl • 0.97
                 = 18.20 ml/dl
Dissolved O_2 content = 95 torr × 0.00304 ml O_2/dl • torr =
                                              0.29 ml/dl
Total O_2 content = 18.20 ml/dl + 0.29 ml/dl = 18.49 ml/dl

Oxygen therapy has significantly increased the total O_2 content. Note again, the very small contribution of dissolved O_2 to the total O_2 content.

Oxygen Delivery

Oxygen delivery from the lungs to the tissue depends on several factors, including cardiac output (Q_t), the hemoglobin content of blood, and the ability of the lung to oxygenate the blood. Thus, the total O_2 delivered (D_{O_2}) to the tissue can be calculated by multiplying the cardiac output (Q_t) times the O_2 content of the arterial blood (C_{aO_2}). That is,

$$D_{O_2} = Q_t × (C_{aO_2}) × 10$$
$$\text{(to change the vol\% from ml } O_2/\text{dl to ml } O_2/\text{L)}$$

Under normal conditions the Q_t is about 5 L/min, and the C_{aO_2} is 20 vol%; thus, the D_{O_2} in a normal individual is approximately

$$D_{O_2} = 5 \text{ L/min} × 20 \text{ vol\%} × 10 = 1000 \text{ ml } O_2/\text{min}$$

Oxygen Consumption

Because not all of the O_2 carried in the blood is unloaded at the tissue level, the principle of conservation of mass (the **Fick** relationship) can be applied to calculate oxygen consumption. The O_2 extracted from the blood by the tissue (that is, the O_2 consumption, or V_{O_2}) is the difference between the arterial O_2 content (C_{aO_2}) and the venous O_2 content (C_{vO_2}), times the cardiac output.

$$V_{O_2} = Q_t[(C_{aO_2} - C_{vO_2}) × 10]$$

Under normal conditions the C_{aO_2} is 20 vol% and the C_{vO_2} is 15 vol%; thus, the amount of O_2 actually extracted is 5 vol% (5 ml of O_2 for each 100/ml of blood or 50 ml of O_2 for each liter of blood). With a cardiac output of 5 L/min, the total amount of O_2 consumed in 1 minute is 250 ml (50 ml O_2/L of blood × 5 L/min).

To gain a greater understanding of the O_2 consumed, consider the **O_2 extraction ratio** (also referred to as the O_2 coefficient ratio), which is the amount of O_2 extracted by the tissue divided by the amount of O_2 delivered:

$$O_2 \text{ extraction ratio} = \frac{C_{aO_2} - C_{vO_2}}{C_{aO_2}}$$
$$\text{Normal } O_2 \text{ extraction ratio} = \frac{20 - 50}{20} = \frac{5}{20} = 0.25$$

This illustrates that Hgb leaves the tissue 75% saturated with O_2 and that under normal conditions, 1000 ml of O_2 is transported in blood/minute, the amount of O_2 delivered to tissue is only 250 ml. Hence, only 25% of the O_2 is actually utilized by the tissue. The O_2 extraction ratio can be dramatically altered, even though the difference in C_{aO_2} and C_{vO_2} remains the same. As shown above, the normal O_2 extraction ratio is 0.25, with a C_{aO_2} and C_{vO_2} difference of 5. In an altered condition, with a C_{aO_2} of 8 and a C_{vO_2} of 3, the O_2 extraction ratio now becomes 0.40, even though the C_{aO_2} and C_{vO_2} difference remains at 5.

$$\text{Altered } O_2 \text{ extraction ratio} = \frac{8 - 3}{8} = \frac{5}{8} = 0.63$$

Hypothermia, relaxation of skeletal muscles, and an increase in cardiac output reduce the O_2 extraction. Conversely, a decrease in cardiac output, anemia, hyperthermia, and exercise increases O_2 extraction (Fig. 28-11).

Tissue Hypoxia

The term, **tissue hypoxia** refers to a condition in which the O_2 available to the cells is insufficient to maintain an aerobic metabolism that is adequate to carry out normal cellular activities. Anaerobic metabolism is then stimulated, which results in the generation of increased levels of lactate and hydrogen ions and the subsequent formation of lactic acid.

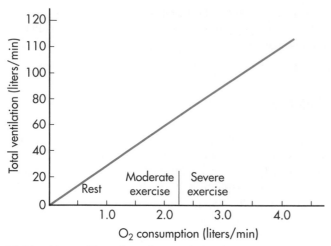

■ **Fig. 28-11** There is a linear relationship between oxygen consumption and alveolar ventilation as the intensity of exercise increases.

The net result can lead to a significant decrease in the blood pH. In cases of severe hypoxia, the extremities, toes, and fingertips, may begin to appear cyanotic (blue-gray coloration) due to the lack of O_2 and the increased amount of deoxyhemoglobin. As shown in Table 28-1, four major types of tissue hypoxia can occur via different mechanisms. **Hypoxic** hypoxia is the most common, and it is due to a variety of lung diseases (chronic obstructive pulmonary disease, pulmonary fibrosis, neuromuscular diseases), which result in decreased P_{AO_2} and/or C_{aO_2}, with subsequent decrease in the O_2 delivery to tissue. **Circulatory** (stagnate) hypoxia is the result of inhibited blood flow to an organ usually due to a vascular disease or an arterial venous shunt. **Anemic** hypoxia is caused by the inability of the blood to carry sufficient O_2, either due to low Hgb (anemia) or to its inability to carry O_2 (as in the case of CO poisoning). **Histological** hypoxia results when a block in the electron transport system in mitochondrial respiration prevents the utilization of O_2 by the cell. Respiratory chain poisons include cyanide, sodium azide, and the pesticide, rotenome.

Tissue oxygenation directly depends upon the hemoglobin concentration, and thus upon the number of red blood cells available in the circulation. Red blood cell production (erythropoiesis) in the bone marrow is controlled by the hormone erythropoietin, which is synthesized in the kidney by cortical interstitial cells. Although Hgb levels are very stable under normal conditions, under conditions of decreased O_2 delivery, low Hgb concentrations, or low P_{aO_2}, the cortical interstitial cells are stimulated to increase erythropoietin secretion. This increases the production of red blood cells. Chronic renal disease can damage the cortical interstitial cells and thereby suppress their ability to synthesize erythropoietin. Anemia ensues, along with decreased Hgb concentrations because of the lack of erythropoietin production. Erythropoietin replacement therapy has been shown to be effective in this condition.

CARBON DIOXIDE TRANSPORT

CO₂ Production, Metabolism, and Diffusion

CO_2 plays a critical role in the maintenance of physiological homeostasis, and it is a major factor in regulating hydrogen ion (H^+) concentrations in blood, cells, and other body tissues. Also, CO_2 is an important chemical stimulus of the chemoreceptors in the peripheral circulation and central nervous system, and hence it plays an important role in the regulation of respiration in normal individuals. The major sources of CO_2 production are in mitochondria during the aerobic cellular metabolism of glucose, and in the conversion of carbohydrates to fats. Carbonic acid, H_2CO_3, is a major product of cellular metabolism, and it is readily metabolized to CO_2 and H_2O. During the metabolism of one glucose molecule, six CO_2 molecules are produced and six O_2 molecules are consumed. In a normal individual under ordinary conditions, CO_2 is produced at a rate of about 200 ml/min, which can be increased 6-fold during conditions of stress or exercise. The body has greater storage capabilities for CO_2 than to O_2. Hence, P_{aO_2} is much more affected by changes in ventilation than is P_{aCO_2}. Whereas P_{aO_2} depends on several factors in addition to alveolar ventilation, arterial P_{aCO_2} depends solely on alveolar ventilation and CO_2

■ **Table 28-1** Tissue hypoxia

		Mechanism			
Type of hypoxia	*Cause*	*P_{aO_2}*	*C_{aO_2}*	*Amount O_2 delivered*	*Amount O_2 utilized*
Hypoxic	Pulmonary disease with ↓P_{aO_2} ↓V/Q ratio	Low	Low	Low	Normal
Circulatory	Vascular disease Arterial-venous shunt (malformation)	Normal	Normal	Low	Normal
Anemic	CO poisoning Anemia	Normal	Low	Low (CO poisoning) Normal (Chronic anemia)	Normal
Histological	Cyanide Sodium azide	Normal	Normal	Normal	Low

production. An inverse relationship exists between alveolar ventilation and P_{aCO_2} (Fig. 27-1, Chapter 27). For example, if a person stops breathing for 1 minute, only a 6 to 10 mm Hg elevation in P_{aCO_2} is observed, whereas a corresponding drop of 40 to 50 mm Hg occurs in P_{aO_2}. The diffusion of CO_2 from the cell to the capillaries occurs through passive diffusion from higher to lower partial pressures of CO_2. When the intracellular concentration of CO_2, or its partial pressure (P_{cCO_2}), exceeds the tissue concentration (P_{tCO_2}), CO_2 moves out of the cell and into the surrounding tissue. Subsequently, the tissue P_{tCO_2} is increased. When it exceeds the arterial P_{cCO_2}, CO_2 diffuses from the tissue into the capillaries just before the blood enters the venous system. The CO_2 is then carried in venous blood to the lungs, where it is excreted via the exhaled gas. CO_2 diffuses readily from the alveolar lumen to the capillaries, and vice versa. Hence, the alveolar P_{ACO_2} and P_{cCO_2} are equal. Under normal conditions the tissue P_{tCO_2} is 50 mm Hg, the venous P_{vCO_2} is 46 mm Hg, and the arterial P_{aCO_2} is 40 mm Hg. The blood level of CO_2 is highest in the veins after the CO_2 has entered the capillaries. Normally the difference in arterial P_{CO_2} and venous P_{CO_2} is about 6 mm Hg. In contrast to the exchange of O_2 from the arterial side of the circulatory system, CO_2 exchange occurs mainly from the venous side.

CO_2 transport

CO_2 is carried and transported through the blood in both plasma and red blood cells in three distinct chemical forms: namely, as bicarbonate (HCO_3^-), dissolved CO_2, and carbamino protein complexes. In plasma, CO_2 binds to various plasma proteins, and in red blood cells, CO_2 binds to hemoglobin. By far the predominant transport mechanism of CO_2 is as HCO_3^- within the red blood cells (Table 28-2).

Once CO_2 diffuses through the tissue and reaches the plasma, it quickly dissolves physically and establishes a partial pressure (P_{aCO_2}). CO_2 readily diffuses from the plasma to the red blood cells, and an equilibrium is established between the red blood cells and the plasma. The major pathway for the generation of HCO_3^- is the reaction of CO_2 with H_2O to form carbonic acid (H_2CO_3), which then dissociates readily to form bicarbonate (HCO_3^-) and free H^+ ions (Fig. 28-12).

$$CO_2 + H_2O \leftrightarrow H_2CO_3 \leftrightarrow H^+ + HCO_3^-$$

This reaction occurs very slowly (seconds) by chemical reaction standards in tissue and plasma, and it is probably not important in those compartments. However, the reaction is catalyzed within the red blood cells by the enzyme carbonic anhydrase, which speeds up the reaction time to a few microseconds, and it is the major source of HCO_3^-. Once formed within the red blood cells, the HCO_3^- diffuses out of the cell in exchange for Cl^-. This Cl^- exchange is referred to as the **chloride shift** (the Hamburger phenomenon or an anionic shift to equilibrium). The Cl^- binds to K^+, which was released by hemoglobin during the transfer of O_2 from hemoglobin to the tissue. The chloride shift maintains the electrostatic homeostasis of the cells. In addition, osmotic equilibrium is maintained in the red blood cell as water also accompanies the Cl^- movement. For this reason, red blood cells are slightly more swollen in the venous system than in the arterial system.

This transformation of CO_2 to carbonic acid to bicarbonate is reversible. These reactions are shifted to the right to generate more bicarbonate when CO_2 enters the blood from the tissue, and they are shifted to the left as more generated CO_2 is exhaled in the lungs.

The free H^+ ions are quickly buffered by binding to plasma proteins, or if the H^+ ions are within the red blood cell, they bind to hemoglobin to form a H • Hgb complex. The H^+ ion buffering is critical to keep the reaction moving toward the synthesis of HCO_3^-; high levels of free H^+ will push the reaction in the opposite direction. Also, this H^+ source is mainly responsible for the slightly more acidic (pH 7.35) venous blood than for the arterial blood (pH 7.40).

$$CO_2 + H_2O \leftrightarrow H^+ + HCO_3^-$$
$$\updownarrow$$
$$H^+ + Hgb \leftrightarrow H \cdot Hgb$$

Although CO_2 is 20 times more soluble in water than is O_2, the dissolved form of CO_2 still constitutes a small fraction of the total transported CO_2. Hence, the dissolved form of CO_2 is much more important in CO_2 transport than is the dissolved form of O_2. Also, one must note that although CO_2 transport and H^+ regulation occur simultaneously, they are independent of each other and are controlled by different factors.

CO_2 Dissociation Curve

In contrast to the behavior of O_2, the dissociation (removal and uptake) of CO_2 from the blood is almost directly related to the P_{CO_2}, and therefore the dissociation curve for CO_2 is linear (Fig. 28-13). The saturation of hemoglobin with O_2

■ Table 28-2   Transport of CO_2 per liter of normal human blood

CO_2	P_{CO_2} (mm Hg)		
	Arterial 40	*Mixed venous 46*	*a-v difference 6*
Dissolved (ml/L)	25	29	4
Carbamino (ml/L)	24	38	14
HCO_3^- (ml/L)	433	455	22
Total (ml/L)	482	522	40

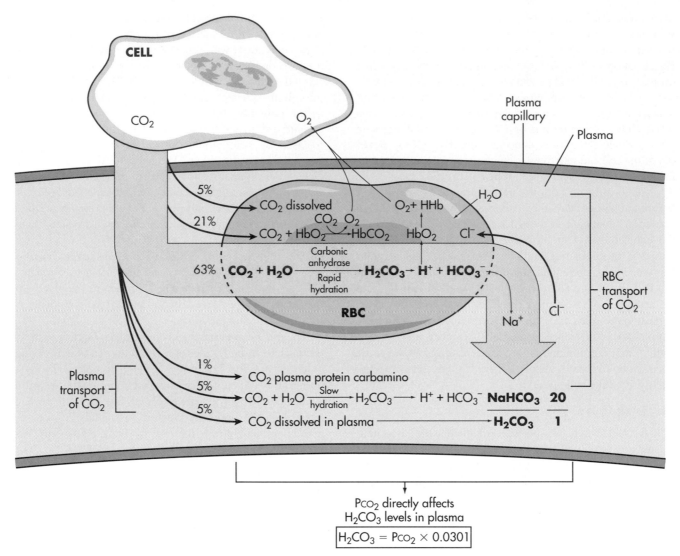

■ **Fig. 28-12** Mechanisms of CO_2 transport. The predominant mechanism by which CO_2 is transported from the tissue cells to lung is in the form of HCO_3^-.

has a major effect on the CO_2 dissociation curve. Although O_2 and CO_2 bind to hemoglobin at different sites, deoxygenated hemoglobin has a greater affinity for CO_2 than does oxygenated hemoglobin. The deoxygenated Hgb more readily forms carbamino compounds, and it also more readily binds the free H^+ ions that are released during the formation of HCO_3^-. Thus, deoxygenated blood (venous blood) freely takes up and transports more CO_2 than does oxygenated arterial blood. The effect of changes in oxyhemoglobin saturation on the relationship of the CO_2 content to P_{CO_2} is referred to as the **Haldane** effect. This effect is reversed in the lung when O_2 is transported from the alveoli to the red blood cells.

In summary, the red blood cell is ideally constructed to transport O_2 and CO_2. Oxygen unloading along the capillary is enhanced by increases in P_{CO_2} and by decreases in pH (Bohr effect), whereas CO_2 loading into the blood is enhanced

by decreases in oxyhemoglobin saturation (Haldane effect). Oxygen is bound to hemoglobin, whereas CO_2 exists in the form of HCO_3^-, which is produced in the red blood cell and transported into the plasma.

Arterial Blood Gas Analysis

The partial pressures of O_2 and CO_2 and blood pH can readily be measured in blood, and they have been shown to be important clinical assessments in the management of patients with lung disease. As stated previously in Chapter 27, the P_{aCO_2} depends directly and inversely on ventilation (Fig. 27-1). Thus, when ventilation is doubled, the P_{aCO_2} will decrease 2-fold, as long as all other factors remain normal. A basic gas law states that the sum of the partial pressures of the gases is equal to the total pressure; if the pressure of one gas decreases, then the pressure of another gas must correspondingly increase.

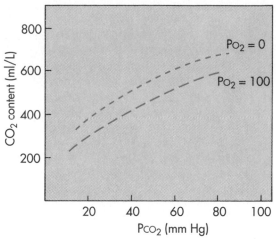

■ **Fig. 28-13**   Blood CO_2 equilibrium curves (arterial and venous). Venous blood can transport more CO_2 than arterial blood at any given P_{CO_2}. Compared with the hemoglobin oxygen equilibrium curve, the CO_2 curves are essentially straight lines between P_{CO_2} of 20 and 80 mm Hg.

Example

A healthy 55-year-old woman is upset because she has just witnessed a bank robbery. She is brought to the emergency room in an agitated, breathless state, and she hyperventilates noticeably. She had a physical examination last week, and her blood gas values were in the normal range; P_{aO_2} = 84 mm Hg (P_{aO_2} levels normally decline with age). One way to estimate an ideal value is P_{aO_2} = 110 – age/2: for this patient 110 – 55/2 = 110 – 28 = 86), P_{CO_2} = 40 mm Hg and pH 7.40. What would you predict her arterial blood gas values to be in her current condition? (For calculation purposes, assume that her ventilation has increased by 50%.)

P_{aCO_2} = 30 mm Hg. If her ventilation rate had doubled (increased by 100%) her P_{aCO_2} would have decreased by half (20 mm Hg). Therefore, a 50% increase would decrease the P_{aCO_2} by 10 mm Hg.

P_{aO_2} = 94 mm Hg. The basic gas laws show that the total pressure must stay constant. Therefore, the decrease alveolar in P_{CO_2} must be accompanied by an equal increase of 10 mm Hg in P_{O_2} using the alveolar air equation (Chapter 27) and a respiratory quotient = 0.8.

pH = 7.48. An acute change in P_{aCO_2} of 10 mm Hg is accompanied by a corresponding inverse change in pH of 0.08 units. The P_{aCO_2} influences the H^+ concentration via the carbonic acid to bicarbonate pathway. A decrease in P_{aCO_2} results in a decrease in H^+ ions and an increase in pH.

SUMMARY

1. The transport of oxygen and carbon dioxide from various anatomical locations and states (air → blood → tissue →

air) is defined by certain basic gas diffusion laws, and the rate of trasnport is dependent upon differential pressure gradients.

2. Gases (N_2O, ether, helium) that have a rapid rate of air to blood equilibration are perfusion limited, and gases (CO) that have a slow air to blood equilibration rate are diffusion limited. Under normal conditions, O_2 transport is perfusion limited, but it can be diffusion limited under certain conditions.

3. D_{LCO} is a classic measurement of the diffusion capability of the alveolar capillary membrane. This factor is especially useful in the diagnosis of restrictive lung diseases, such as interstitial pulmonary fibrosis, and in diseases, such as emphysema, which are associated with destruction of the alveoli.

4. The major transport mechanism of O_2 in the blood is O_2 bound to Hgb within the red blood cell, and for CO_2, it is within red blood cells in the form of HCO_3^-.

5. O_2 binds quickly and reversibly to the heme groups of the Hgb molecule.

6. The ability of CO_2 to alter the affinity of Hgb for O_2 (the Bohr effect) enhances the O_2 delivery to the tissues, and it enhances the O_2 uptake in the lungs.

7. Tissue hypoxia occurs when the amounts of O_2 supplied to the tissues are insufficient to carry out the normal levels of aerobic metabolism.

8. The major source of CO_2 production is in the mitochondria during aerobic cellular metabolism. The reversible reaction of CO_2 with H_2O to form H_2CO_3, and its subsequent dissociation to HCO_3^- and H^+, is catalyzed by the enzyme carbonic anhydrase within red blood cells, and it is the major pathway for HCO_3^- generation.

9. The CO_2 dissociation curve from blood is linear and is directly related to P_{CO_2}.

10. The O_2 dissociation curve is S-shaped not linear. In the plateau area (above 60 mm Hg), increasing the P_{O_2} has only a minimal effect on Hgb saturation. The same response occurs if P_{O_2} decreases from 100 to 60 mm Hg. These changes ensure an adequate saturation of Hgb over a large range of P_{O_2} values. The steep portion of the curve (20-60 mm Hg) illustrates that during O_2 deprivation (low P_{O_2}), O_2 is readily released from Hgb, and the changes in P_{O_2} that facilitate O_2 diffusion to the tissues are slight.

BIBLIOGRAPHY

Journal article

Russell JA, Phang PT: The oxygen delivery-consumption controversy, *Am J Respir Crit Care Med* 149:433, 1994.

Books and monographs

Des Jardins T: *Cardiopulmonary anatomy and physiology: essentials for respiratory care*, ed 3, Albany, NY, 1998, Delmar Publishers.

Leff AR, Schumacker PT: *Respiratory physiology: basics and applications*, Philadelphia, 1993, WB Saunders.

West JB: *Respiratory physiology: the essentials*, Baltimore, 1974, Williams & Wilkins.

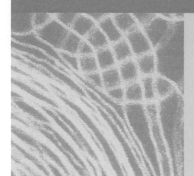

chapter twenty-nine

Control of Respiration

Unlike virtually all other organ systems, respiration demonstrates automaticity as well as self-modulation (voluntary). We breathe without thinking, but we can willingly modify our breathing pattern, and we can hold our breath up to the so-called "breaking point." Our breathing pattern is also modulated by the activities of speech and singing.

Control of ventilation refers to the generation and regulation of rhythmic breathing by the respiratory center in the brainstem, and its modification by the input of information from higher brain centers and from systemic receptors. The goals of breathing, from a mechanical perspective, are to minimize work, and from a physiological perspective, are to maintain blood gases, and, specifically, to regulate arterial P_{CO_2}. A third goal of breathing is to maintain the acid-base environment of the brain through the effects of ventilation on arterial P_{CO_2}.

Respiratory movements have been observed in utero, but regular, automatic respiration begins at birth. The fetus is well suited to its environment, in which the lung is not the gas-exchange unit. The placenta is the organ of gas exchange for the fetus in utero. Its microvilli interdigitate with the maternal uterine circulation, and oxygen transport and carbon dioxide removal from the fetus occur by passive diffusion across the maternal circulation. Blood travels through the umbilical artery to the placenta, and it returns to the fetus through the umbilical vein. The maternal and fetal circulations are separate, and the blood of the fetus and mother does not mix. Compared to the arterial partial pressures in the adult, the partial pressures of oxygen in the blood being delivered to the fetus are low, because the uterus extracts its oxygen from the blood prior to its delivery to the fetus. Thus, the P_{O_2} in the umbilical vein is 30 torr, whereas in the umbilical artery, the P_{O_2} is only 20 torr (see Fig. 23-18). The fetus, however, is able to thrive in this environment because of the presence of fetal hemoglobin, which has a substantially greater affinity for oxygen than does adult hemoglobin. Fetal hemoglobin is discussed on page 503.

VENTILATORY CONTROL: AN OVERVIEW

First, we will describe an overall functional view of ventilatory control, then we will examine its integrated role in maintaining a normal P_{aCO_2}, and finally we will examine each of the major areas in greater detail.

There are four major sites of ventilatory control, namely (1) the respiratory control center, (2) the central chemoreceptors, (3) the peripheral chemoreceptors, and (4) the pulmonary mechanoreceptors (Fig. 25-24). The **respiratory control center** is located in the medulla oblongata of the brainstem. The control center is composed of a number of different nuclei that generate and modify the basic ventilatory rhythm. The center consists of two main parts: (1) a **ventilatory pattern generator,** which sets the rhythmic pattern, and (2) an **integrator,** which processes inputs from higher brain centers and chemoreceptors, and which controls the rate and amplitude of the ventilatory pattern. The integrator controls the pattern generator and determines the appropriate ventilatory drive. Input to the integrator arises from higher brain centers, including the cerebral cortex, hypothalamus, amygdala, limbic system, and cerebellum.

Within the central nervous system, there are **central chemoreceptors,** which are located just below the ventrolateral surface of the medulla. These central chemoreceptors detect changes in the P_{CO_2} and pH of the brainstem interstitial fluid and they modulate ventilation.

Peripheral structures also provide input to the integrator and they control ventilatory drive. Chemosensitive **peripheral chemoreceptors** are located on specialized cells in the aortic arch (**aortic bodies**) and at the bifurcation of the internal and external carotid arteries (**carotid bodies**) in the neck (see Chapter 21). These peripheral chemoreceptors sense the P_{O_2}, P_{CO_2}, and pH of arterial blood, and they feed back information to the integrative nuclei in the medulla through the vagus nerves (aortic bodies) and the carotid sinus nerves, which are branches of the glossopharyngeal nerves (carotid bodies). Finally, the ventilatory pattern can be modulated by pulmonary **mechanoreceptors and irritant**

receptors in the lungs, in response to the degree of lung inflation or the presence of an irritant in the airways (see Fig. 25-24).

The collective output of the respiratory control center to the motor neurons controls the muscles of respiration, and this output determines the automatic, rhythmic pattern of respiration. The responsible motor neurons are located in the anterior horn of the spinal column. The intercostal muscles and the accessory muscles of respiration are controlled by motor neurons that are located in the thoracic region of the spinal column. Diaphragmatic motor neurons are situated in the cervical region of the spine, and they control the activity of the diaphragm through the phrenic nerves.

In contrast to automatic respiration, voluntary respiration bypasses the respiratory control center in the medulla. The neural activity originates in the motor cortex, and information passes directly to the motor neurons in the spine through the corticospinal tracts. The motor neurons to the respiratory muscles thus act as the final site of integration of the voluntary (corticospinal tract) and the automatic (ventrolateral tracts) control of ventilation. Voluntary control of these muscles competes with the automatic influences at the level of the spinal motor neurons, and this competition can be demonstrated by breathholding. At the start of the breathhold, voluntary control dominates the spinal motor neurons. However, as the breathhold continues, the automatic ventilatory control eventually overpowers the voluntary effort and limits the duration of the breathhold.

Motor neurons also innervate the muscles of the upper airway. These neurons are located within the medulla near the respiratory control center. They innervate muscles in the upper airways through the cranial nerves. When activated, they dilate the pharynx and large airways at the initiation of inspiration.

RESPONSE TO CO₂

Ventilation is regulated by the levels of CO_2, O_2, and pH in the arterial blood. Among these regulators, the arterial CO_2 is the most important. Both the rate and depth of breathing are controlled to maintain the P_{aCO_2} close to 40 mm Hg. Even during periods of activity, rest, or sleep, the arterial P_{CO_2} is held to within 2 to 3 mm Hg. The importance of arterial CO_2 in ventilation can be demonstrated by having an individual breathe a low concentration of oxygen, to which CO_2 is added to maintain a constant CO_2. Hypoxemia is sensed by the peripheral chemoreceptors, which increase their rate of firing in response to the decrease in P_{aO_2}. This stimulation in ventilation, however, does not occur until the P_{aO_2} has dropped below 60 mm Hg. Below this level, ventilation is strongly stimulated. However, if arterial P_{aCO_2} is increased by only a small amount (about 5 mm Hg), ventilation is increased even if the level of P_{aO_2} is increased (Fig. 29-1).

The relationship between P_{aCO_2} and ventilation is best shown in a classic experiment that was first performed many years ago. In these experiments, the alveolar P_{O_2} was maintained at a constant level, and the subject rebreathed from a

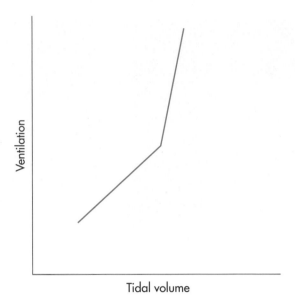

■ **Fig. 29-1**   Relationship between overall ventilation and tidal volume is depicted in awake states when ventilation is increased in response to respiratory stimuli such as hypercapnia. (From Murray JF, Nadel JA, editors: *Textbook of respiratory medicine,* ed 3, vol 1, Philadelphia, 1994, W B Saunders.)

bag so that the inspired P_{CO_2} gradually rose. The effects of alveolar P_{CO_2} on ventilation are shown in Fig. 29-2.

The central and peripheral chemoreceptors detect changes in P_{aCO_2}, and they transmit this information to the medullary respiratory centers. The respiratory control center then regulates minute ventilation and thereby maintains the arterial P_{CO_2} within the normal range. Ventilation increases as P_{CO_2} increases. In the presence of a normal P_{AO_2}, the ventilation increases by about 3 L/min for each millimeter rise in P_{aCO_2}. In the presence of a low P_{AO_2} ventilation is greater for any given P_{ACO_2}, and the increase in ventilation for a given increment in P_{ACO_2} is enhanced (the slope is greater).

The relationship between minute ventilation and the inspired CO_2 concentration is used as a test of CO_2 sensitivity. The slope of the minute ventilation response as a function of the inspired CO_2 is termed the **ventilatory response to CO₂.** It is important to recognize that this relationship is amplified by low oxygen. This change in responsiveness occurs because different mechanisms are responsible for sensing P_{O_2} and P_{CO_2} in the peripheral chemoreceptors. Thus, the presence of both hypercapnia and hypoxemia (often called **asphyxia** when both changes are present) has an additive effect on chemoreceptor output and on the resulting ventilatory stimulation (Fig. 29-3).

Decreasing the arterial P_{CO_2} by hyperventilation reduces the ventilatory drive. Drugs, such as morphine, barbiturates, and anesthetic agents, that depress the respiratory center decrease the ventilatory responses to both CO_2 and O_2. In these instances, the stimulus is inadequate to drive the motor neurons that innervate the muscles of respiration. Hypoventilation causes the arterial P_{CO_2} to increase and the arterial P_{O_2} to decrease.

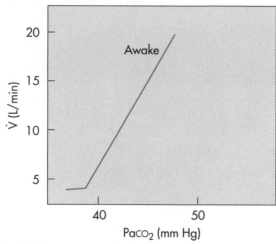

■ **Fig. 29-2** Dose-response curve for ventilation as a function of arterial P_{CO_2}. Sensitivity is defined as the slope of the line and the extrapolated intercept on the abscissa. The normal operating point is at VE = 5 L/min and P_{aCO_2} = 40 mm Hg. The extrapolated intercept of about 35 mm Hg does not occur because other stimuli keep us breathing.

The ventilatory response to CO_2 is also reduced if the work of breathing is increased, such as in individuals with chronic obstructive pulmonary disease. This effect occurs primarily because the neural output of the respiratory center is less effective in promoting ventilation because of the mechanical limitation to ventilation. In addition, the sensitivity of the respiratory control center is reduced in individuals with chronic obstructive pulmonary disease.

CONTROL OF VENTILATION: THE DETAILS

The Respiratory Control Center

Most of the information about the control of ventilation comes from studies in animals in which focal areas of the brain have been destroyed or in which the brainstem has been surgically transected. When the brain is transected between the medulla and the pons, periodic breathing is maintained. These results demonstrate that the inherent rhythmicity of breathing originates in the medulla. Although no single group of neurons in the medulla has been found to be the breathing "pacemaker," two distinct nuclei within the medulla are involved in respiratory pattern generation (Fig. 29-4). One nucleus is the **dorsal respiratory group (DRG),** which is composed of cells in the nucleus tractus solitarius located in the dorsomedial region of the medulla. These cells are primarily responsible for inspiration. The solitary tract is the principal central nervous system (CNS) fiber tract for afferent input from the ninth and tenth cranial nerves that originate from airways and lungs. Hence, the DRG is thought to constitute the initial intracranial processing station for these afferent inputs.

The second group of relevant medullary cells is the **ventral respiratory group** (VRG), which is located in the ventrolateral region of the medulla. This nucleus is composed of three cell groups (the rostral nucleus retrofacialis, the caudal

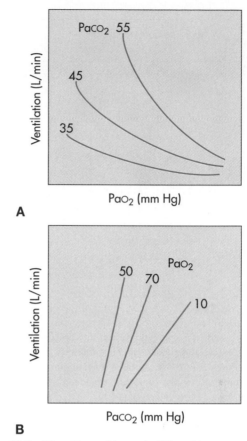

■ **Fig. 29-3** The effects of hypoxia (**A**) and hypercapnia (**B**) on ventilation as the other respiratory gas partial pressure is varied. **A,** At a given P_{aCO_2}, ventilation increases more and more as P_{aO_2} decreases. When P_{aCO_2} is allowed to decrease (the normal condition) during hypoxia, there is a little stimulation of breathing until P_{O_2} falls below 60 mm Hg. The hypoxic response is mediated through the carotid body chemoreceptors. **B,** The sensitivity of the ventilatory response to CO_2 is enhanced by hypoxia.

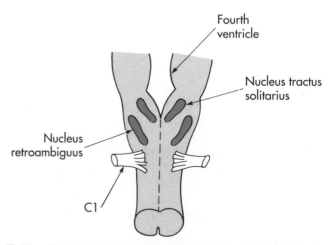

■ **Fig. 29-4** The respiratory control center is located in the medulla (the most primitive portion of the brain). The neurons are mainly in two areas called the *nucleus tractus solitarius* and the *nucleus retroambiguus*.

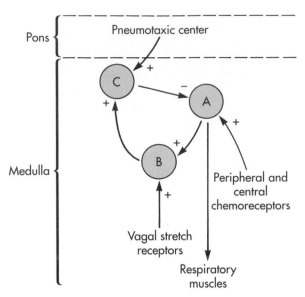

■ **Fig. 29-5**   The basic wiring diagram of the brainstem ventilatory controller. The signs of the main outputs *(arrows)* of the neuron pools indicate whether the outputs are excitatory (+) or inhibitory (−). Pool *A* provides tonic inspiratory stimuli to the muscles of breathing. Pool *B* is stimulated by pool *A* and provides additional stimulation to the muscles of breathing, and pool *B* stimulates pool *C*. Other brain centers feed into pool *C* (inspiratory cutoff switch), which sends inhibitory impulses to pool *A*. Afferent information (feedback) from various sensors acts at different locations: chemoreceptors act on pool *A* and intrapulmonary sensory fibers act via the vagus nerves on pool *B*. A pneumotaxic center in the anterior pons receives input from the cerebral cortex, and it modulates the pool *C* group.

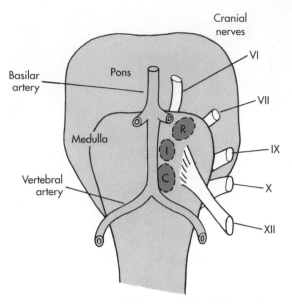

■ **Fig. 29-6**   The locations of the three CO_2 ([H^+])-sensitive areas on the ventrolateral medulla. The receptor cells are not actually at the surface but are close to it. *R*, *I*, and *C* refer to the rostral, intermediate, and caudal receptor areas, respectively.

nucleus retroambiguus, and the nucleus para-ambiguus). The VRG contains both inspiratory and expiratory neurons. The nucleus retrofacialis and the nucleus retroambiguus are active during exhalation, whereas the nucleus paraambiguus is active during inspiration. Discharges from the cells in these areas appear to excite some cells and to inhibit other cells.

Inspiration and exhalation at the level of the respiratory control center involve three phases—one inspiratory and two expiratory (Fig. 29-5). Inspiration begins with an abrupt increase in discharge from cells in the nucleus tractus solitarius, the rostral nucleus retrofacialis, and the nucleus retroambiguus, followed by a steady ramp-like increase in firing rate throughout inspiration. This leads to progressive contraction of the respiratory muscles during automatic breathing. At the end of inspiration, an off-switch event results in a marked decrease in neuron firing, at which point exhalation begins. At the start of exhalation (phase 1), a paradoxical increase in inspiratory neuron firing slows down the expiratory phase by increasing inspiratory muscle tone and expiratory neuron firing. This inspiratory neuron firing decreases and stops during phase II of exhalation. Although many different neurons in the dorsal and ventral respiratory group are involved in ventilation, each cell type appears to have a specific function. For example, the **Hering-Breuer reflex** is an inspiratory-inhibitory reflex that arises from

afferent stretch receptors located in the smooth muscles of the airways. Increasing lung inflation stimulates these stretch receptors and results in early exhalation by stimulating the neurons that are associated with the off-switch phase of inspiratory muscle control.

Thus, rhythmic breathing depends on a continuous (tonic) inspiratory drive from the dorsal respiratory group and on intermittent (phasic) expiratory inputs from the cerebrum, thalamus, cranial nerves, and ascending sensory tracts in the spinal cord.

Central chemoreceptors.   A chemoreceptor is a receptor that responds to a change in the chemical composition of the blood or of other fluid around it. Central chemoreceptors are specialized cells that are located on the ventrolateral surface of the medulla. These chemoreceptors are sensitive to the pH of the surrounding extracellular fluid. Because this extracellular fluid is in contact with the cerebrospinal fluid (CSF), changes in the pH of the CSF affect ventilation by acting on these chemoreceptors (Fig. 29-6).

Cerebrospinal fluid is an ultrafiltrate of plasma that is secreted continuously by the choroid plexus and that is reabsorbed by the arachnoid villi. Because it is in contact with the extracellular fluid in the brain, the cerebrospinal fluid reflects the conditions that surround the cells in the brain. Although the origin of CSF is the plasma, the composition of the CSF is not the same as that of plasma, because a barrier to free ion flow exists between the two sites. This barrier is termed the **blood-brain barrier.** It is composed of endothelial cells, smooth muscle, and the pial and arachnoid membranes, and it regulates ion flow. In addition, the choroid plexus also determines the composition of the CSF. The blood-brain barrier is relatively impermeable to H^+ and HCO_3^- ions, but molecular CO_2 diffuses across it readily. Thus, the P_{CO_2} in the CSF parallels the arterial P_{CO_2} tension.

■ **Table 29-1** Normal values for the composition of cerebrospinal fluid and arterial blood

	CSF	*Arterial*
pH	7.33	7.40
P_{CO_2} (torr)	44	40
HCO_3^- (mEq/L)	22	24

CO_2 is also produced by the cells of the brain as a product of metabolism. As a consequence, the P_{CO_2} in the CSF is usually a few torr higher than that in the arterial blood, and the pH is slightly more acidic (7.33) than in plasma (Table 29-1).

The Henderson-Hasselbach equation relates the pH of the CSF to the bicarbonate ion concentration (HCO_3^-):

$$pH = pK + \log \frac{[HCO_3^-]}{\alpha \cdot P_{CO_2}}$$

where α is the solubility coefficient of 0.03 mmol/L torr, and pK is the negative log of the dissociation constant for carbonic acid. The Henderson-Hasselbach equation demonstrates that increases in P_{CO_2} will be associated with decreases in pH at any given bicarbonate concentration. Likewise, increases in CSF bicarbonate will increase the pH of the CSF at any given P_{CO_2}. As a consequence of this relationship, an increase in arterial P_{CO_2} will increase the P_{CO_2} of the CSF and will decrease the pH of the CSF. The decrease in the pH of the CSF will stimulate the central chemoreceptors and thereby increase the ventilation. Thus, the CO_2 in blood regulates ventilation by its effect on the pH of the CSF. The resulting hyperventilation reduces the P_{CO_2} in the blood, and therefore in the CSF. The cerebral vasodilation that accompanies an increase in arterial P_{CO_2} enhances the diffusion of CO_2 into the CSF.

When the arterial P_{CO_2} changes, homeostatic mechanisms are activated to regulate the change in pH and to bring the system back to normal. The blood-brain barrier regulates the pH of the CSF by adjusting the ionic composition and bicarbonate concentration of the CSF. These changes in CSF bicarbonate concentration, however, occur slowly, over several hours, whereas the changes in P_{CO_2} in the CSF can occur within minutes. Adjustments in ventilation attempt to maintain a normal CSF and arterial pH and P_{CO_2}.

Peripheral chemoreceptors. The carotid and aortic bodies are peripheral chemoreceptors that respond to changes in the arterial P_{O_2} (not the O_2 content), P_{CO_2}, and pH, and they transmit afferent information to the central respiratory control center. The peripheral chemoreceptors are the only chemoreceptors that respond to changes in P_{O_2}, because the central chemoreceptors respond only to changes in P_{CO_2} and pH. Both the central and peripheral chemoreceptors respond to changes in P_{CO_2}, and the peripheral chemoreceptors are responsible for approximately 40% of the ventilatory response to CO_2.

The peripheral chemoreceptors are small, highly vascularized structures. They consist of type 1 (glomus) cells that

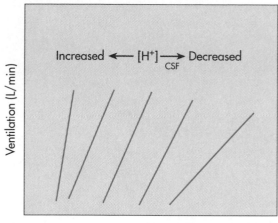

■ **Fig. 29-7** The ventilatory response to P_{CO_2} is affected by the hydrogen ion concentration, [H^+], of the cerebrospinal fluid *(CSF)* and brainstem interstitial liquid. When a subject is in chronic metabolic acidosis (e.g., diabetic acidosis), the [H^+] CSF is increased and the ventilatory response to inspired P_{CO_2} is increased (steeper slope). Conversely, when a subject is in chronic metabolic alkalosis (a relatively uncommon condition), the [H^+] CSF is decreased and the ventilatory response to inspired P_{CO_2} is decreased (reduced slope). The positions of the response lines are also shifted, indicating altered response thresholds.

are rich in mitochondria and endoplasmic reticulum. They also contain several types of cytoplasmic granules (synaptic vesicles) that contain various neurotransmitters including dopamine, acetylcholine, norepinephrine, and neuropeptides. The type I cells are the cells primarily responsible for sensing P_{O_2}, P_{CO_2}, and pH. Small increases in chemoreceptor discharge occur even in response to small decreases in arterial P_{O_2}. However, marked increases in chemoreceptor activity occur when the arterial P_{O_2} decreases below 75 mm Hg. Increases in ventilation result when the P_{O_2} falls below 50 to 60 mm Hg. Afferent nerve fibers synapse with type I cells, and they transmit information to the brainstem through the carotid sinus nerve (carotid body) and vagus nerve (aortic body). How they respond to arterial changes in P_{O_2}, P_{CO_2}, and pH is not known.

It can be seen from the above discussion that ventilation is regulated by changes in arterial and CSF pH, and by their effects on peripheral and central chemoreceptors. Homeostasis, or the return toward normal ventilation, is regulated by changes in HCO_3^- transport in the CSF and by renal compensatory mechanisms (Fig. 29-7). An example will illustrate this relationship.

Imagine flying from New York City to Denver for a weekend of skiing (Fig. 29-8). The barometric pressure in New York is about 760 mm Hg, whereas the barometric pressure in the mountains surrounding Denver, Colorado is 600 mm Hg. At sea level, the P_{O_2} in arterial blood is approximately 95 torr [using the alveolar air equation (Chapter 27), $P_{AO_2} = (760 - 47) \times 0.21 - 40/0.8 = 100$

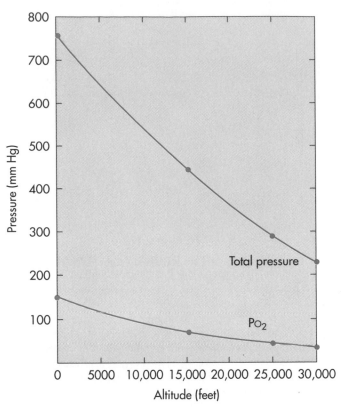

■ Fig. 29-8   Barometric pressure and P_{O_2} fall exponentially as one ascends to high altitude (abscissa). The F_{IO_2} remains constant at 21%.

torr. If the AaD_{O_2} is 5 torr, the $P_{aO_2} = 100 - 5 = 95$ torr]. In the CSF the pH would be about 7.33, the P_{CO_2} would be 44 torr (arterial $P_{CO_2} + CO_2$ produced by metabolism of the brain cells), and the CSF HCO_3^- would be approximately 22 mEq/L.

When you arrive in the mountains, the inspired O_2 abruptly decreases [$P_{IO_2} = (600 - 47) \times 0.21 = 116$ torr] and the alveolar O_2 and arterial O_2 decrease ($P_{AO_2} = 116 - 40/0.8 = 66$ torr $P_{aO_2} = 61$ torr). This decrease in inspired O_2 stimulates the peripheral chemoreceptors, and it increases ventilation. The increase in ventilation decreases the arterial P_{CO_2} and increases the arterial pH. The result of this increase in ventilation is to minimize the hypoxemia by increasing P_{AO_2}. [For example, assume that the P_{ACO_2} decreases to 30 torr. Then, $P_{AO_2} = (600 - 47) \times 0.21 - 30/0.8 = 78$ torr, a 12 torr increase in P_{AO_2}.]

The decrease in arterial P_{CO_2} also decreases the P_{CO_2} of the CSF. Because the bicarbonate concentration is unchanged, the pH of the CSF increases. This increase in the pH of the CSF attenuates the rate of discharge of the central chemoreceptors, and it decreases their contribution to ventilatory drive. Over the next 12 to 36 hours, the bicarbonate concentration in the CSF decreases as ion pumps in the blood-brain barrier are activated. Consequently, the pH of the CSF returns toward normal. Central chemoreceptor discharge increases and minute ventilation is further increased. At the same time that

the bicarbonate concentration in the CSF is decreasing, the bicarbonate ions are gradually excreted from the plasma by the kidneys. This results in a gradual return of the arterial pH toward normal. Peripheral chemoreceptor stimulation increases further as the arterial pH becomes normal (peripheral chemoreceptors are inhibited by the elevated arterial pH). Finally, within 36 hours of arriving at high altitude, minute ventilation increases significantly. This delayed response is greater than the immediate effect of the hypoxemia on ventilation. This further increase in ventilation is due to both central and peripheral chemoreceptor stimulation. Thus, by the end of the weekend, both the arterial pH and the CSF pH are approaching normal; minute ventilation is increased, arterial P_{O_2} is decreased, and arterial P_{CO_2} is decreased.

You now return home. When you land in New York City, the inspired P_{O_2} returns to normal, and the hypoxic stimulus to ventilation is removed. Arterial P_{O_2} returns to normal and the peripheral chemoreceptor stimulation to ventilation decreases. This increases the arterial CO_2 toward normal. The CO_2 in the CSF also increases back toward normal. This increase is associated with a decrease in the pH of the CSF as the bicarbonate concentration in the CSF is now reduced and ventilation is augmented. Over the next 12 to 36 hours, ion pumps in the blood-brain barrier pump HCO_3^- ions back into the CSF, and the pH of the CSF gradually returns toward normal. Similarly, the pH in the blood decreases as the arterial P_{CO_2} rises, because the arterial bicarbonate concentration is also decreased. This stimulates the peripheral chemoreceptors, and minute ventilation remains augmented. Over the next 12 to 36 hours, renal mechanisms increase the blood HCO_3^- concentrations, the arterial pH returns to normal, and the minute ventilation returns to normal.

Chest wall and lung reflexes.   Several reflexes that arise from the chest wall and lungs affect ventilation and ventilatory patterns (Table 29-2). The Hering-Breuer inspiratory-inhibitory reflex is stimulated by increases in lung volume, especially those associated with an increase in **both** ventilatory rate and tidal volume. This stretch reflex is mediated by vagal fibers, and when elicited, this reflex results in the cessation of inspiration by stimulating the off-switch neurons in the medulla. This reflex is inactive during quiet breathing, and it plays a role in **ventilatory** control only when the tidal volumes in adults are greater than 1 L. This reflex may be more important in newborns.

Stimulation of nasal or facial receptors with cold water initiates the **diving reflex.** When this reflex is elicited, apnea or cessation of breathing and bradycardia occur. This reflex protects individuals from aspirating water in the initial stages of drowning. Activation of receptors in the nose is also responsible for the **sneeze reflex.**

Receptors are also present in the nasopharynx and pharynx. Mechanical stimulation of these receptors produces the aspiration, or **sniff, reflex.** This is a strong, short-duration inspiratory effort that brings material from the nasopharynx

■ Table 29-2   Tracheobronchial receptor properties

Receptor type	End-organ location	Stimuli	Reflexes
Myelinated vagal fibers			
Slowly adapting receptor	Among airway smooth muscle cells	Lung inflation	Hering-Breuer inflation reflex Hering-Breuer deflation reflex Inspiratory time-shortening Bronchodilation Tachycardia Hyperpnea
Rapidly adapting receptor (irritant receptor)	Among airway epithelial cells	Lung hyperinflation Exogenous and endogenous agents Histamine Prostaglandins	Hering-Breuer deflation reflex Cough Mucus secretion Bronchoconstriction
Unmyelinated vagal fibers			

C-fiber ending (J receptors)	Pulmonary interstitial space
	Close to pulmonary circulation
	
	Close to bronchial circulation
		Large hyperinflation
		Exogenous and endogenous agents
		  Capsaicin
		  Phenyl diguanide
		  Histamine
		  Bradykinin
		  Serotonin
		  Prostaglandins
			Apnea, followed by rapid shallow breathing
			Bronchoconstriction
			Bradycardia
			Hypotension
			Mucus secretion

to the pharynx where it can be swallowed or expectorated. These receptors are also important in swallowing by inhibiting respiration and by causing laryngeal closure. Only newborn infants can breathe and swallow simultaneously, which allows for more rapid nutrient ingestion.

The larynx contains both superficial and deep receptors. Activation of the superficial receptors results in apnea, cough, and expiratory movements that protect the lower respiratory tract from aspirating foreign materials. The deep receptors are located in the skeletal muscles of the larynx, and they control muscle fiber activation as in other skeletal muscles.

Three major types of receptors are located in the tracheobronchial tree. Inhaled dust, noxious gases, or cigarette smoke stimulate **irritant receptors** in the trachea and in the large airways that transmit information through myelinated vagal afferent fibers. Stimulation of these receptors results in an increase in airway resistance, in reflex apnea, and in cough. These receptors are also known as **rapidly adapting pulmonary stretch receptors. Slowly adapting pulmonary stretch receptors** respond to mechanical stimulation, and they are activated by lung inflation. They also transmit information through myelinated, vagal afferent fibers. The increased lung volume in people with obstructive pulmonary disease stimulates these pulmonary stretch receptors, and it delays the onset of the next inspiratory effort. This explains the long, slow expiratory effort in these individuals, and it is essential to minimize the dynamic, expiratory airway compression. Finally, specialized receptors occur in the lung parenchyma, and they respond to chemical or mechanical stimulation in the lung interstitium. These receptors are called **juxtaalveolar** or **J receptors.** They transmit their afferent input through unmyelinated, vagal C-fibers. They

may be responsible for the sensation of dyspnea (shortness of breath) and the rapid, shallow ventilatory patterns that occur in interstitial lung edema and in some inflammatory lung states.

Somatic receptors are also located in the intercostal muscles, rib joints, accessory muscles of respiration, and tendons that respond to changes in the length and tension of the respiratory muscles. Although they do not directly control respiration, they do provide information about lung volume, and they play a role in terminating inspiration. They are especially important in individuals with increased airway resistance and with decreased pulmonary compliance because they can augment muscle force within the same breath. They also help to minimize the chest wall distortion during inspiration in newborns who have very compliant rib cages.

NONPULMONARY REFLEXES

The ventilatory pattern is also under voluntary control. Purposeful hyperventilation can result in a decrease in the P_{ACO_2} and an increase in the pH of the blood. The alkalosis that accompanies this hyperventilation can cause carpopedal spasm, which is a contraction of the muscles of the hands and feet. An increase in arterial blood pressure stimulates aortic and carotid sinus baroreceptors, and it can cause reflex hypoventilation or apnea.

EXERCISE

Many books and articles have been written about the cardiorespiratory changes that occur during exercise (see Chapter 24). The ability to exercise depends on the capacity

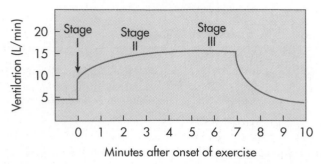

■ **Fig. 29-9** The three stages of exercise: I, onset; II, transient period of adjustment; III, the steady state.

of the cardiac and respiratory systems to increase oxygen delivery to the tissues and to remove carbon dioxide from the body. Ventilation increases immediately when exercise begins, and this increase in minute ventilation closely matches the increase in oxygen consumption and carbon dioxide production that accompanies exercise (Fig. 29-9). Ventilation is linearly related to both CO_2 production and O_2 consumption at low to moderate levels (Fig. 29-10). During maximal exercise, a fit young man can achieve an oxygen consumption of 4 L/min with a minute volume of 120 L/min, which is almost 15 times the resting levels.

Exercise is most remarkable for the lack of significant changes in blood gases. Except at maximal levels, in general, arterial P_{CO_2} decreases slightly and arterial P_{O_2} increases slightly. Arterial pH remains normal at moderate exercise. During heavy exercise, arterial pH begins to fall as lactic acid is liberated during anaerobic metabolism. This decrease in arterial pH stimulates ventilation at a rate that is out of proportion to the level of exercise intensity. The level of exercise at which a sustained metabolic acidosis begins is called the **anaerobic threshhold.** This level is different in fit than in unfit individuals.

The actual cause of the increased ventilation during exercise remains largely unknown. No single mediator or mechanism has been identified to explain why ventilation remains so closely matched to carbon dioxide production. Hypoxic or hypercarbic mechanisms do not play a role, because neither occurs during most exercise. Mechanisms believed to contribute include neural inputs from the motor cortex to the medullary respiratory control center, afferents from muscle and joint mechanoreceptors, or unknown mediators that are released from working muscles.

ABNORMALITIES IN CONTROL OF BREATHING

Changes in ventilatory pattern can occur because of both primary and secondary reasons. During sleep, approximately one third of normal individuals have brief episodes of apnea or hypoventilation, which have no significant effects on arterial P_{O_2} or arterial P_{CO_2}. The apnea usually lasts less than 10 seconds, and it occurs in the lighter stages of slow-wave and rapid eye movement (REM) sleep. In sleep apnea syn-

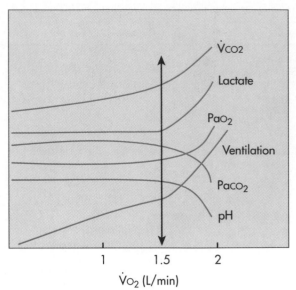

■ **Fig. 29-10** Some important metabolic changes that occur during exercise. The anaerobic threshold *(arrow)* is marked by a sudden change in the measured variables, which is due mainly to the developing lactic acidosis as anaerobic glycolysis takes over more and more of the muscle energy supply caused by the relative failure of the body to supply sufficient oxygen to the muscles at the rate demanded by the level of exercise.

dromes, the duration of apnea is abnormally prolonged, and it changes the arterial P_{O_2} and P_{CO_2}.

There are two major categories of sleep apnea syndromes (Fig. 29-11). The first is **obstructive sleep apnea (OSA).** It is the most common of the sleep apnea syndromes, and it occurs when the upper airway (usually the hypopharynx) closes during inspiration. Although the process is similar to what happens during snoring, it is more severe, it obstructs the airway, and it causes cessation of airflow. The history of individuals with OSA is very similar. A spouse usually reports that the individual snores. The snoring becomes louder and louder and then stops, while the individual continues to make vigorous respiratory efforts. The individual then awakens, falls back to sleep, and continues the same process repetitively throughout the night. The arousal occurs when the arterial hypoxemia and hypercarbia stimulate both peripheral and central chemoreceptors. Respiration is restored briefly before the next apneic event occurs. Individuals with OSA can have hundreds of these events each night. As a consequence, they are sleep deprived even though they do not awaken fully with each episode. Other complications of OSA include polycythemia, right-sided cardiac failure (cor pulmonale), and pulmonary hypertension that is secondary to the recurrent, hypoxic events. The most common cause of OSA is obesity. Other causes include excessive compliance of the hypopharynx, upper airway edema, and structural abnormalities of the upper airway. Treatment includes weight loss, oral appliances to pull the tongue forward, and bilevel positive airway pressure (Bi-PAP) that keeps the upper airway distended during inspiration.

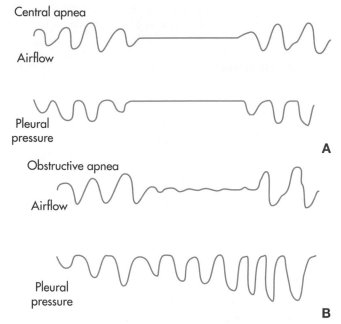

Fig. 29-11 The two main types of sleep apnea. **A,** Central apnea is characterized by no attempt to breathe, as demonstrated by no pleural pressure oscillations. **B,** In obstructive sleep apnea, the pleural pressure oscillations increase as CO_2 rises. This indicates that airflow resistance is very high owing to upper airway obstruction.

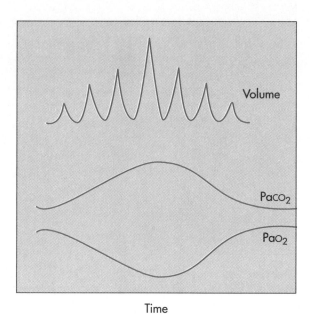

Fig. 29-12 In Cheyne-Stokes breathing, tidal volume and consequently arterial blood gases wax and wane. Generally, Cheyne-Stokes breathing is a sign of vasomotor instability, particularly low cardiac output.

The second sleep apnea syndrome is called **central sleep apnea.** This variant of apnea occurs when the ventilatory drive to the respiratory motor neurons decreases. The individual with central sleep apnea makes no respiratory efforts. The degree of hypercarbia and hypoxemia in individuals with central sleep apnea is less than in individuals with OSA, but the same sequelae (polycythemia, etc.) can occur when central sleep apnea is recurrent and severe.

Central alveolar hypoventilation (CAH), also known as Ondine's curse, is a rare disease in which voluntary breathing is intact, but abnormalities in automaticity exist. It is the most severe of the central sleep apneas. As a result, people with CAH can breathe as long as they don't fall asleep. For these individuals, mechanical ventilation or, more recently, bilateral diaphragmatic pacing (similar to a cardiac pacemaker) can be life-saving.

Sudden infant death syndrome (SIDS) is the most common cause of death in infants in the first year of life, outside of the perinatal period. Although the cause of SIDS is not known, abnormalities in ventilatory control, and particularly in CO_2 responsiveness, have been implicated. Placing infants on their back to sleep (reducing the potential for CO_2 rebreathing) has dramatically decreased (but not eliminated) the death rate from this syndrome.

Cheyne-Stokes ventilation is another abnormality of ventilatory control, and it is characterized by a varying tidal volume and ventilatory frequency (Fig. 29-12). Following a period of apnea, tidal volume and respiratory frequency increase progressively over several breaths, and then they progressively decrease until apnea occurs. This irregular breathing pattern is seen in some individuals with central nervous system diseases, such as head trauma and increases in intracranial pressure. It is also present on occasion in normal individuals during sleep at high altitude. The mechanism for Cheyne-Stokes respiration is not known. In some individuals, it appears to be due to slow blood flow in the brain associated with periods of overshooting and undershooting ventilatory efforts in response to changes in P_{CO_2}.

Apneustic breathing is another abnormal breathing pattern that is characterized by sustained periods of inspiration separated by brief periods of exhalation (Fig. 29-13). The mechanism for this ventilatory pattern appears to be a loss of inspiratory-inhibitory activities that results in the augmented inspiratory drive. The pattern sometimes occurs in individuals with central nervous system injury.

SUMMARY

1. Respiratory control is both automatic and voluntary.

2. Ventilatory control is composed of the respiratory control center, central chemoreceptors, peripheral chemoreceptors, and pulmonary mechanoreceptors.

3. The arterial P_{CO_2} is the major factor that influences ventilation.

4. The respiratory control center is composed of the dorsal respiratory group and the ventral respiratory group. Rhythmic breathing depends on a continuous (tonic) inspiratory drive

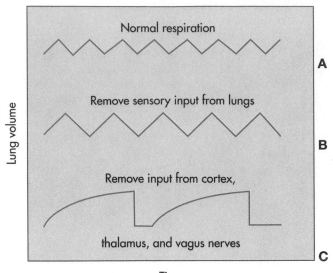

Fig. 29-13 Some patterns of breathing. **A**, Normal breathing at about 15 breaths/min in humans. **B**, The effect of removing sensory input from various lung receptors (mainly stretch) is to lengthen each breathing cycle and to increase tidal volume so that alveolar ventilation is not significantly affected. **C**, When input from the cerebral cortex and thalamus is also eliminated together with vagal blockade, the result is prolonged inspiratory activity broken after several seconds by brief expirations (apneusis).

from the dorsal respiratory group, and on intermittent (phasic) expiratory inputs from the cerebrum, thalamus, cranial nerves, and ascending spinal cord sensory tracts.

5. The peripheral and central chemoreceptors respond to changes in P_{CO_2} and pH. The peripheral chemoreceptors (carotid and aortic bodies) are the only chemoreceptors that respond to changes in P_{O_2}.

6. Acute and chronic hypoxia affect breathing differently because of slow adjustments in cerebrospinal fluid $[H^+]$, which alter CO_2 sensitivity.

7. Irritant receptors protect the lower respiratory tract from particles, chemical vapors, and physical factors, primarily by inducing cough.

8. C-fiber J receptors in the terminal respiratory units are stimulated by distortion of the alveolar walls (by lung congestion or edema).

9. At low to moderate levels of exercise, ventilation is linearly related to both CO_2 production and O_2 consumption.

10. The two most important clinical abnormalities of breathing are obstructive and central sleep apnea.

BIBLIOGRAPHY

Journal articles

Coleridge HM, Coleridge JCG: Pulmonary reflexes: neural mechanisms of pulmonary defense, *Annu Rev Physiol* 56:69, 1994.

de Castro D, Lipski J, Kanjhan R: Electrophysiological study of dorsal respiratory neurons in the medulla oblongata of the rat, *Brain Res* 639:49, 1994.

Ezure K: Synaptic connections between medullary respiratory neurons and considerations on the genesis of respiratory rhythm, *Progr Neurobiol* 35:429, 1990.

Funk GD, Feldman JL: Generation of respiratory rhythm and pattern in mammals: insights from developmental studies, *Curr Opin Neurobiol* 5:778, 1995.

Haddad GG, Jiang C: O_2-Sensing mechanisms in excitable cells: role of plasma membrane K^+ channels, *Annu Rev Physiol* 59:23, 1997.

Lee L-Y et al: Stimulation of vagal pulmonary C-fibers by a single breath of cigarette smoke in dogs, *J Appl Physiol* 66:2032, 1989.

Monteau R, Hilaire G: Spinal respiratory motoneurons, *Progr Neurobiol* 37:83, 1991.

Pisarri TE et al: Rapidly adapting receptors monitor lung compliance in spontaneously breathing dogs, *J Appl Physiol* 68:1997, 1990.

Robin ED et al: Alveolar gas tensions, pulmonary ventilation and blood pH during physiologic sleep in normal subjects, *J Clin Invest* 37:981, 1998.

Sant'Ambrogio G, Tsubone H, Sant'Ambrogio FB: Sensory information from the upper airway: role in the control of breathing, *Respir Physiol* 102:1, 1995.

Voipio J, Ballanyi K: Interstitial P_{CO_2} and pH, and their role as chemostimulants in the isolated respiratory network of neonatal rats, *J Physiol (Lond)* 499:527, 1997.

Books and monographs

Gonzalez C, Dinger B, Fidone SJ: Mechanisms of carotid body chemoreception. In Dempsey JA, Pack AI, editors: *Regulation of breathing,* New York, 1995, Marcel Dekker, pp 391-471.

Jammes Y, Speck DF: Respiratory control by diaphragmatic and respiratory muscle afferents. In Dempsy JA, Pack AI, editors: *Regulation of breathing,* New York, 1995 Marcel Dekker, pp 543-582.

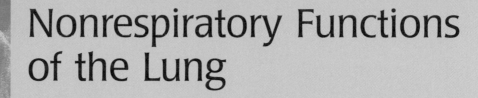

chapter thirty

Nonrespiratory Functions of the Lung

Although gas exchange is the primary function of the lung, the lung also functions as a major defense organ that protects the inside of the body from the outside world. The respiratory system has developed unique systems to bring O_2 and to expel CO_2. It has also developed a series of unique defense systems to cope with environmental exposure and with the constant insult of foreign agents. The respiratory tract is continuously exposed to natural, ubiquitous, foreign substances that vary from inert, nonpathological particles to pathogenic viruses and bacteria. The locations of inhaled dcposed particles vary throughout the respiratory tract, and are based mainly on particle size (Figure 30-1). The distance traveled, the density, and the relative humidity also influence deposition. Because particle deposition varies from one region of the respiratory system to another, the respiratory tract has evolved unique systems to process and dispose of these particles. These systems include (1) a specialized mucosal immune system that involves both innate and adaptive immune responses of unique lymphocytes, macrophages, and dendritic cells; and (2) a mucociliary clearance system in the tracheobronchial region that involves ciliated, epithelial cells that move fluid and trapped particles upward toward the mouth, where they are to be swallowed.

OVERVIEW OF THE IMMUNOLOGICAL DEFENSE SYSTEMS IN THE LUNG

The respiratory, gastrointestinal, and urinary systems have developed specialized defense mechanisms, and together they form the **mucosal immune system.** In these mucosal tissues the immune system must discriminate between what is harmful and what is not. Otherwise, a potent inflammatory response would most certainly occur. Although inflammation is a protective response to injury or to an invading pathogen, its presence is usually harmful. The lung and other mucosal tissues have evolved specific defense mechanisms that are designed to handle the offending agent without inflammation. If this first line fails, then an inflammatory response can be initiated. Present in these mucosal tissues are specialized

immune cells, such as T lymphocytes that possess a selective antigen recognition mechanism, and plasma cells that synthesize IgA, a noncomplement binding antibody (Table 30-1). In addition, specialized mononuclear cells (alveolar macrophages and dendritic cells) are present throughout the respiratory tract, which can process and phagocytize particles without inciting an inflammatory response. These specialized features limit the immunological and inflammatory responses to foreign, nonpathological substances that enter the respiratory system.

THE LUNG AS A SECONDARY LYMPHOID TISSUE

Lymphoid Tissue

Lymphoid tissues are generally classified as either primary (central) or secondary (peripheral). Primary lymphoid tissues are the sites in which stem cells of the lymphoid lineage mature and develop into functioning lymphocytes. In these sites lymphocytes acquire the ability for antigen recognition, tolerance, and the recognition of major histocompatibility molecules (MHC). The thymus (T-lymphocytes), fetal liver (B-lymphocytes), and bone marrow (B-lymphocytes) are **primary** lymphoid tissues in humans. After maturation in the primary lymphoid tissues, the lymphocytes migrate to **secondary** lymphoid tissues, the actual peripheral sites where lymphocytes come in contact with antigens. In these sites, the immune response is initiated with the help of local accessory cells (macrophages, dendritic cells, antigen presenting cells, and epithelial cells). The spleen, lymph nodes, and **mucosa-associated lymphoid tissues (MALT)** make up the major secondary lymphoid tissues. The spleen is the main site that handles blood-borne antigens. Specific regional lymph nodes cover local sites via lymphatic drainage, and MALT covers all mucosal surfaces, such as those in the gastrointestinal (gut-associated lymphoid tissue—GALT), respiratory (bronchus-associated lymphoid tissue—BALT), and urinary systems.

The lymphatic system and the lymphoid tissues in the lungs filter fluids and particulates through such organized

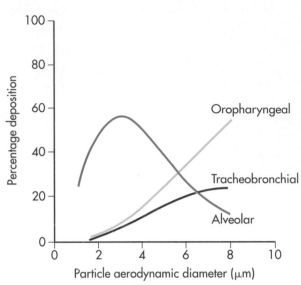

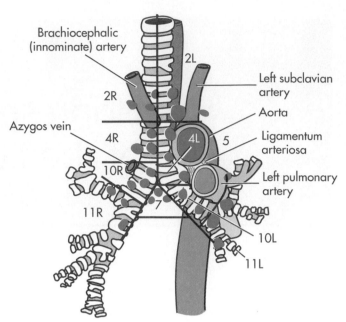

■ **Figure 30-1** Inhaled particles are trapped at different locations in the airways, according to their size. Particles with diameters greater than approximately 5 μm tend to impact into the nasopharynx, oropharynx, or large conducting airways. Smaller particles are more likely to become trapped in the distal airways or in the alveoli. (From Clarke SW, Pavia D: Mucociliary clearance. In Crystal RG, West JB, editors: *The lung: Scientific foundation.* New York, Raven Press, 1991.)

■ **Figure 30-2** American Thoracic Society Map of Regional Pulmonary Nodes. See text. (From Tisi GM, Friedman PJ, Peters RM, et al: *Am Rev Respir Dis* 127: 659, 1983.)

lymphoid structures as lymph nodes, lymph nodules, lymph aggregates (BALT), and a diffuse submucosal network of scattered lymphocytes and dendritic cells. These lymphoid structures are scattered throughout the respiratory tract. Because inhaled particle are dispersed, each lymphoid tissue plays an important unique role in the overall defense of the lung.

Regional Lymph Nodes of the Lung

The lymph nodes that drain the lungs are part of the mediastinal network, which drains the head, neck, lungs, and esophagus.

The regional lymph nodes are not only the sites of antigen presentation via lymph drainage, but they also are the sites that receive cancer cells. Thus, these mediastinal nodes have significant diagnostic importance for the detection of lung cancer (Figure 30-2, Table 30-2).

Mucosa-Associated Lymphoid Tissue (MALT)

The lymphoid tissues of the mucosal areas (gastrointestinal, respiratory, and urinary systems) are organized, and they resemble actual lymph nodes that have a similar repertoire of immune cells. However, they are highly specialized. In contrast to lymph nodes, these tissues are not encapsulated, but they are comprised mainly of aggregates of lymphocytes that reside in submucosa regions. In addition to aggregates of cells, MALT contains a substantial number of solitary B- and T-lymphocytes. These cells are scattered regularly within

■ **Table 30-1** Innate and adaptive immune cells in the respiratory system

Cell type	Location	Function
TCRγδ lymphocytes	Intraepithelial	Selective antigen recognition Immunoregulation (↓ IgE)
TCRαβ lymphocytes	Lamina propria	Specific adaptive immunity Immunoregulation (Th1/Th2 cytokines)
B lymphocytes	Submucosa	IgA antibody synthesis
Dendritic cells	Diffuse in lung interstitium	Antigen presentation Immunoregulation (tolerance)
Alveolar macrophages	Alveoli and alveolar ducts	Phagocytosis Immunoregulation (cytokines)
NK cells	Diffuse in lung interstitium	Targeted cytotoxicity Immunoregulation (tolerance)
NK/T cells	Diffuse in lung interstitium	Immunoregulation (IL-4)

NK, Natural killer.

the connective tissue of the lamina propria (**lamina propria lymphocytes**) and the epithelial layer (**intraepithelial lymphocytes**). The B cells found in MALT can selectively differentiate into IgA-secreting plasma cells when they are stimulated by antigen. MALT provides a first line of defense for these highly exposed mucosal surfaces. In the upper airways of the respiratory tract, they are present in the adenoids and tonsils.

The lymphoid tissue of the lung becomes less organized as one moves from the hilum to the periphery (alveoli). Mature lymph nodes with germinal centers and nodules predominate in the hilar region around the mainstem bronchi, whereas lymph aggregates predominate near the alveoli. Organized lymphoid structures are absent in the alveolar spaces. BALT predominates throughout the conducting airways, whereas aggregates of lymph nodules or solitary lymph nodules are found only sporadically. Although these nodules are not true lymph nodes, they are still a major processing center for antigens. These nodules reside in the upper airways, around the major airway branches and blood vessels.

The epithelium associated with areas of BALT is specialized, and it is referred to as a **lymphoepithelium.** It is comprised of a mix of epithelial cells and lymphocytes. This lymphoepithelium lacks ciliated epithelial cells. The absence of ciliated cells results in a break in the mucociliary clearance system, and thereby enhances fluid and particulate flow into the BALT area (Figure 30-3). Although a highly specialized epithelial cell with many microfolds ("M" cells) has been observed in GALT, it has not yet been observed in BALT. These "M" cells form pockets or invaginations, and antigen processing occurs where clusters of macrophages and lym-

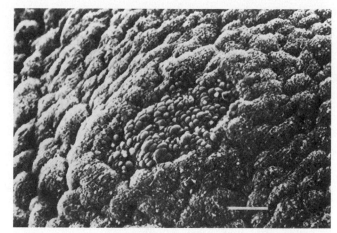

■ **Figure 30-3.** Scanning electron micrograph of rabbit bronchial epithelium showing island of lymphoepithelium surrounded by ciliated epithelium. *Horizontal bar,* 1 mm. (Reprinted by permission from Bienenstock J, Johnston N: A morphologic study of rabbit bronchial lymphoid aggregates and lymphoepithelium. *Lab Invest,* 35:343-348, 1976, Williams & Wilkins, Baltimore.)

phocytes collect (Figure 30-4). BALT is present in humans, but only under pathological conditions, such as during upper respiratory tract infections.

The lung has several unique defense features that limit airway inflammation, which can adversely affect lung function. One of the specialized features of MALT is a unique antibody system, IgA. In submucosal areas, plasma cells synthesize and secrete IgA in a dimer form that is linked by a **J-chain.** The antibody-dimer combination migrates to the

■ Table 30-2   American Thoracic Society definitions of regional nodal stations

X	**Supraclavicular nodes**
2R	**Right upper paratracheal nodes:** nodes to the right of the midline of the trachea, between the intersection of the caudal margin of the innominate artery with the trachea and the apex of the lung
2L	**Left upper paratracheal nodes:** nodes to the left of the midline of the trachea, between the top of the aortic arch and the apex of the lung
4R	**Right lower paratracheal nodes:** nodes to the right of the midline of the trachea, between the cephalic border of the azygos vein and the intersection of the caudal margin of the brachiocephalic artery with the right side of the trachea
4L	**Left lower paratracheal nodes:** nodes to the right of the midline of the trachea, between the top of the aortic arch and the level of the carina, medial to the ligamentum arteriosum
5	**Aortopulmonary nodes:** subaortic and paraaortic nodes, lateral to the ligamentum arteriosum or the aorta or left pulmonary artery, proximal to the first branch of the left pulmonary artery
6	**Anterior mediastinal nodes:** nodes anterior to the ascending aorta or the innominate artery
7	**Subcarinal nodes:** nodes arising caudal to the carina of the trachea but not associated with the lower lobe bronchi or arteries within the lung
8	**Paraesophageal nodes:** nodes dorsal to the posterior wall of the trachea and to the right or left of the midline of the esophagus
9	**Right or left pulmonary ligament nodes:** nodes within the right or left pulmonary artery
10R	**Right tracheobronchial nodes:** nodes to the right of the midline of the trachea, from the level of the cephalic border of the azygos vein to the origin of the right upper lobe bronchus
10L	**Left peribronchial nodes:** nodes to the left of the midline of the trachea, between the carina and the left upper lobe bronchus, medial to the ligamentum arteriosum
11	**Intrapulmonary nodes:** nodes removed in the right or left lung specimen plus those distal to the mainstem bronchi or carina

Modified from Tisis GM, Friedman PJ, Peters RM, et al: *Am Rev Respir Dis* 127:659, 1983.

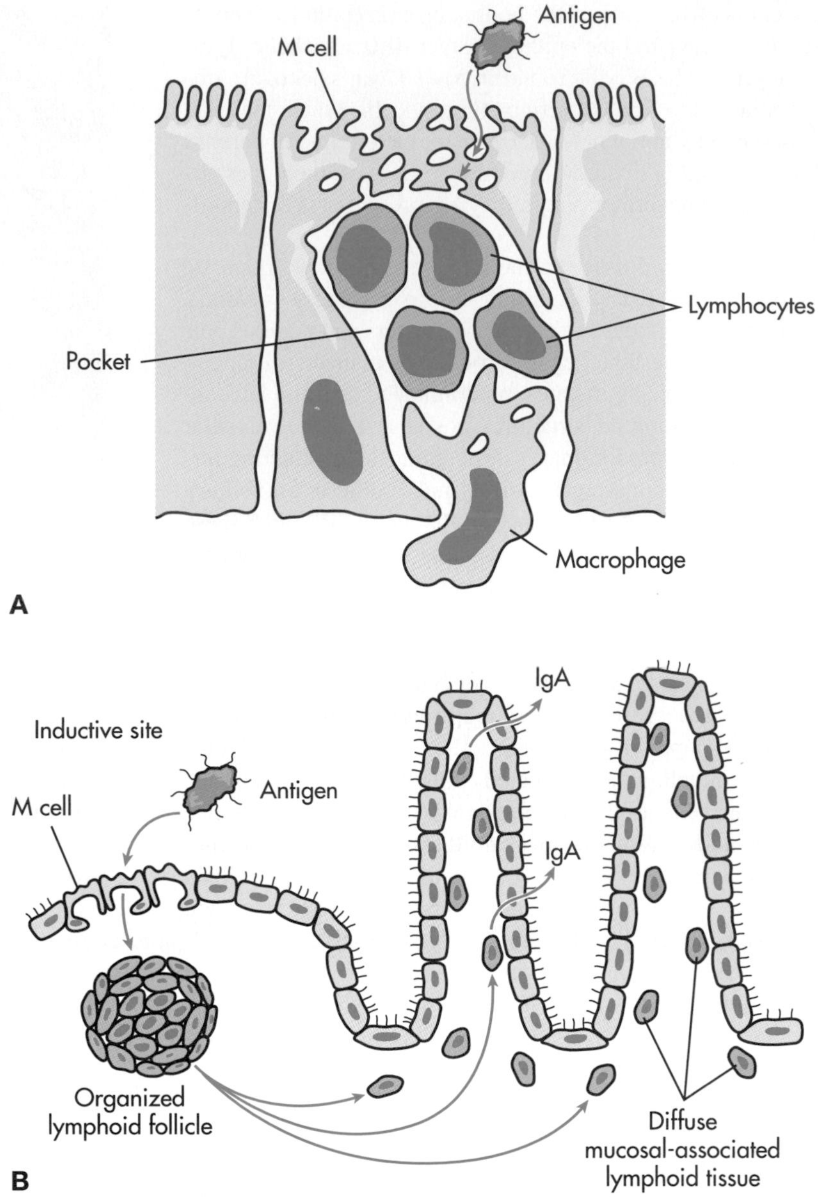

■ **Figure 30-4** Representation of MALT, "M" cells, and IgA synthesis. **A,** "M" cells located in mucosal epithelium endocytose antigen in the lumen and transport it for processing to submucosal pockets of immune cells. **B,** Diagram of mucous membrane showing secretion of IgA antibodies in response to antigen endocytosed by M cells at an inductive site. Activated B cells migrate from the lymphoid follicle to nearby mucosal-associated lymphoid tissue where they differentiate into IgA-producing plasma cells.

submucosal surface of epithelial cells, where it binds to a surface protein receptor, **poly-Ig** (Figure 30-5). The poly-Ig receptor aids in the pinocytosis of the dimer into the epithelial cell and its eventual secretion into the airway lumen. During exocytosis of the IgA complex, the poly-Ig is enzymatically cleaved, and a portion of it (the **secretory piece**) is still associated with the complex. The secretory piece stays attached to the IgA complex in the airway, and it helps to protect it from proteolytic cleavage in the lumen. The IgA•antigen immune complex does not bind complement in the same classical manner as do other immune complexes; this limits its proinflammatory properties. However, the IgA may activate complement via the alternate pathway. The IgA-antibody system is very effective in binding particulates and viruses before they invade epithelial cells, and it aids in the removal of these substances through the mucociliary clearance system.

Another important feature that distinguishes lymph nodes from MALT is that true lymph nodes have an afferent (entering) and efferent (leaving) pattern of lymphatic fluid drainage, whereas this pattern is not present in MALT. Once an antigen is processed through a lymph node, systemic sensitization will soon follow. This does not necessarily occur in MALT. However, direct communication may occur between the organs of MALT, and sensitization via one organ may be transposed to all MALT tissues. The systemic immune system and MALT may work independently of each other, and sensitization of one system may not transpose to the other. These reactions may serve as a defense mechanism that limits sensitization specifically to mucosal tissues.

Immunologic Cells of MALT

TCRγδ Lymphocytes. The vast majority of T lymphocytes are CD3+ cells with T cell receptors (TCR) that are

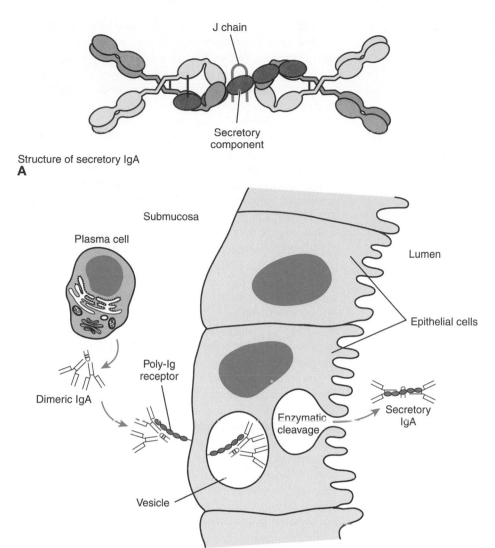

J chain

Secretory
component

Structure of secretory IgA
A

Submucosa

Plasma cell

Lumen

Poly-Ig
receptor

Epithelial cells

Dimeric IgA

Enzymatic
cleavage

Secretory
IgA

Vesicle

Formation of secretory IgA
B

■ **Figure 30-5** Structure and formation of secretory IgA. **A,** Secretory IgA consists of at least two IgA molecules, which are covalently linked via a J chain and covalently associated with the secretory component. The secretory component contains five Ig-like domains and is linked to dimeric (thick black line) between its fifth domain and one of the IgA heavy chains. **B,** Secretory IgA is formed during transport through mucous membrane epithelial cells. Dimeric IgA binds to a poly-Ig receptor on the basolateral membrane of an epithelial cell and is internalized by receptor-mediated endocytosis. After transport of the receptor-IgA complex to the luminal surface, the poly-Ig receptor is enzymatically cleaved, releasing the secretory component bound to the dimeric IgA.

comprised of α and β chains (TCR$\alpha\beta$ cells). A new class of T lymphocytes with the TCR expressing γ and δ chains (TCR$\gamma\delta$ cells) has recently been identified. TCR$\alpha\beta$ and TCR$\gamma\delta$ cells can secrete similar profiles of cytokines, such as interferon γ (IFNγ), IL-2, IL-4, and IL-5. TCR$\gamma\delta$ cells represent a minority of T cells in the peripheral blood of rodents and humans. In mice and humans, these cells are preferentially localized to the epithelial surfaces, including the skin, intestine, and lung. The mechanism by which TCR$\gamma\delta$ cells populate various mucosal areas is not fully understood. However, the mechanism appears to be regulated developmentally, because the population of various mucosal tissues correlates well with the developmental maturation of subpopulations of TCR$\gamma\delta$ cells with different variable region genes (Figure 30-6). These cells are the predominant intraepithelial solitary T cell throughout MALT. This **epitheliotropism** (preferential localization in the epithelium) of TCR$\gamma\delta$ cells suggests that they play a role in immunosurveillance and in the maintenance of normal homeostasis in the airway.

TCR$\gamma\delta$ cells exhibit several unique properties for immunosurveillance. Unlike the TCR$\alpha\beta$ cells, TCR$\gamma\delta$ cells do not depend upon the MHC molecules for antigen presentation and recognition. Instead, TCR$\gamma\delta$ cells may recognize native antigens, such as the heat shock proteins that are expressed by stressed or infected epithelial cells. Accordingly, these cells may be able to eliminate damaged epithelial cells before the adaptive T cell immune system is activated. TCR$\gamma\delta$ cells may, therefore, be the "first line of defense" of epithelial surfaces, and they may prevent the development of inflammation mediated by antigen specific T-cells. Also, TCR$\gamma\delta$ cells may have an immunoregulatory role in allergic respiratory reactions, since they have been shown to suppress selectively the IgE response to inhaled antigen in mice.

The numbers of TCR$\gamma\delta$ cells are increased in the respiratory epithelium and submucosal tissue in biopsies of humans afflicted by asthma and allergic rhinitis. Similarly, patients with immunological pulmonary diseases, such as sarcoidosis and hypersensitivity pneumonitis, have increased numbers of TCR$\gamma\delta$ cells in the peripheral blood and in bronchoalveolar lavage (BAL) fluid.

Natural Killer Cells. Natural killer (NK) cells are derived developmentally from a lymphoid lineage in the bone

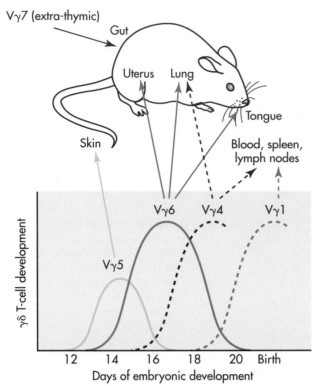

■ Figure 30-6 Mouse γδ T-cell generation is developmentally programmed. γδ T cells bearing T-cell receptors that are encoded by specific Vγ-gene segments are exported from the thymus at defined periods of fetal and neonatal development, and then migrate to and populate different epithelial-rich tissue in adult animals.

marrow, and are a major component of the body's innate immune defense system against invading pathogens such as herpes viruses and various bacterial infections. Although these cells share many functional activities that are similar to lymphocytes, they do not directly fit into the classification of a T- or B- lymphocyte. They usually do not express the T cell marker, CD3, on their cell surface, although a subpopulation of NK cells (NK/T cells) that do express CD3 and secrete high levels of the Th2 cytokine, IL-4 have been described in mice and humans.

NK cells are named for their ability to kill target cells without prior sensitization. The mechanism of killing is through the release of granular enzymes, perforins and serine esterases. These enzymes create holes or pores within the target cell membranes, and these changes lead to cell death. In addition to their cytotoxic activity, they produce cytokines that are similar to those of lymphocytes. These cytokines include IL-4, IL-5, IL-13, IFNγ, and TNFα. The biological activities generated during an innate immune response via NK and NK/T cells can modulate an adaptive immune response. The mechanism of antigen or target cell recognition is not known. However, NK cells have many surface receptors, which display inhibitory activity in response to MHC Class I molecules. Cells that lack or have low expression of MHC Class I molecules are targets for NK cells.

Although they are not abundant, a resident population of functionally active NK cells appears to be present in the lung

interstitium. These resident NK cells have been shown to be the first cells to produce cytokines in an animal model of allergic disease. NK cells have also been observed in BAL fluid, but they are not functionally active.

NK cells also play an important role in the pathogenesis of allergic diseases. NK cell depletion in a murine model of allergic airway disease decreases the content of lung eosinophils and T-cells and decreases the levels of the proinflammatory cytokines, IL-4 and IL-5. Increased numbers of NK cells that produce IL-5 were found in the peritoneal lavage of a model of allergic inflammation. In humans with asthma, the number and activity of NK cells are increased. The NK cells can influence the inflammatory response via several steps in the pathogenesis of allergic diseases. The initial NK cell response may determine whether the response is a full-blown Th2 allergic response or a more quiescent Th1 response. If the NK cell synthesizes IFNγ in response to antigen, a Th1 response is favored; conversely, if the NK/T cell responds with an IL-4 response, a Th2 allergic response is favored. Because IL-4 is required for a plasma cell switchover to IgE synthesis, the NK/T cell could determine whether one develops an allergic response.

Other Resident Cells (Dendritic Cells and Alveolar Macrophages). Whether an inhaled substance stays within the airway lumen or attaches to and penetrates the epithelium determines the fate and type of response generated. Differentiated cells of the myeloid lineage (dendritic cells and alveolar macrophages) are the first nonepithelial cells to contact and respond to a foreign substance. If the foreign material stays within the airspace in the lower respiratory system (alveolar ducts and alveoli), it will be phagocytized by alveolar macrophages. However, if it penetrates and reaches interstitial areas, it will come into contact with dendritic cells. In either case, the macrophage type of mononuclear cells plays a critical role in host defense in the lung.

Dendritic cells (DCs) are derived from the myeloid lineage of monocytes and macrophages, and they have been well documented as a major cell type for antigen presentation to T cells. Although B- and T-lymphocytes are the predominant cells involved in mounting an immune response, they cannot do it maximally without antigen presenting cells, such as the dendritic cell. In 1868, Langerhans cells of the skin were the first dendritic cells to be described. Since then, dendritic cells have been found in the periphery of many tissues. They function mainly as sentinels, not only to capture antigens but also to bring them to lymphocytes to be processed in the various lymphoid tissues. It is estimated that the skin has about 10^9 Langerhans cells located in the epidermal layer. There are two known sources of DCs: the first develops from CD34$^+$ progenitor cells in the bone marrow, and the second is the differentiation of blood monocytes in response to the cytokines GM-CSF and IL-4. The major functions of DCs are to capture, process, and present antigen to T cells, as well as to activate or to suppress the T cell response (Table 30-3).

Most DCs are present in an immature state in peripheral tissues, and they are unable to stimulate the lymphocytes,

■ **Table 30-3** Functions of the dendritic cell

Capture and process antigen

Migrate to lymphoid tissues

Present antigen to lymphocytes via major histocompatibility complex

Activate lymphocytes and enhance stimulatory response

Express lymphocyte co-stimulatory molecules

Secrete cytokines

Induce tolerance

although they are ready to capture and process antigen (Figure 30-7). After contact with antigen, they can mature quite rapidly and migrate to lymphoid tissues to engage lymphocytes.

One major difference between DCs and macrophages is the manner in which they phagocytize and process antigen. Macrophages phagocytize particles and digest them to amino acids in lysosomes with minimal or no binding to the MHC. Immature dendritic cells have nonlysosomal organelle-like endosomal structures that contain high levels of MHC Class II molecules, where endocytosed extracellular particles are processed. During the processing, fragments of antigen plus MHC are extruded to the cell surface for presentation to T cells. In general, DCs present MHC Class II antigens to helper T cells with immune regulatory activity. Intracellular antigens (e.g., viruses, tumor cells, or transplanted cells) are processed and fragmented as typical intracellular proteins within proteasomes. They are then transported from the cytosol to the endoplasmic reticulum, where they complex with MHC Class I molecules and then are carried to the cell surface for expression. DCs present MHC Class I antigens to cytotoxic T cells for direct killing.

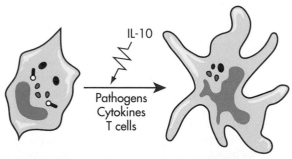

IL-10

Pathogens
Cytokines
T cells

IMMATURE DC	MATURE DC
High intracellular MHCII (MIICs)	High surface MHCII
Endocytosis, including FcR	Low endocytosis and FcR
Low CD54, 58, 80, 86	High CD54, 58, 80, 86
Low CD40, CD25, IL-12	High CD40, CD25, IL-12
Low CD83, p55	High CD83, p55
Low granule antigens	High M342, 2A1,
Actin cables	MIDC-8 antigens
	No actin cables

■ **Figure 30-7** Pheontypic and physiological differences distinguishing immature from mature DCs. The developmental maturation of immature DCs can be regulated by the cytokine IL-10.

DCs are commonly found throughout the respiratory tract in the parenchyma of the lung, and they are usually associated with the epithelium. The upper airways are more densely populated with DCs (Figure 30-8) than are the smaller airways in the more peripheral regions of the lung. The anatomical location of these cells correlates well with particle deposition in the airways. The diversity in staining intensity suggests that subpopulations of DCs or cells differentiate or mature at different stages. DCs with both stimulatory (high co-stimulating molecules and activity) as well as inhibitory (low co-stimulatory molecules and synthesis of high levels of IL-10) properties have been described.

Alveolar macrophages are large, foamy, highly active phagocytic cells that are derived from myeloid progenitor cells in the bone marrow. There appear to be two sources of alveolar macrophages—those that differentiate directly from blood monocytes, and those that arise from cell division of existing alveolar macrophages. The main source in the alveolus seems to be the offspring of existing alveolar macrophages.

Alveolar macrophages are found mostly in the alveolus adjacent to the epithelium and less frequently in the terminal airways and interstitial space (Figure 30-9). They migrate freely throughout the alveolar spaces and serve as a first line of defense in the lower air spaces. They readily and rapidly (usually within 24 hours) phagocytize foreign particles and substances, as well as cellular debris from dead cells. Once a particle is engulfed, the major mechanisms for killing are typical of phagocytic cells. Such mechanisms include oxygen radicals, enzymatic activity, and halogen derivatives within the lysosomes. The ability of the alveolar macrophage to kill foreign material rapidly, and without mounting an inflammatory response, enhances the lung defense system immensely and is a major contributor to the overall defense system. By rapidly phagocytizing particles in the alveolus, the alveolar macrophage inhibits the binding of these substances to the alveolar surface and the possible invasion of them into the interstitial spaces which could cause tissue damage. The alveolar macrophage also has the capability of suppressing an adaptive immune response via T cell mechanisms. It can suppress T cell activity via direct contact with the T cell or via the secretion of soluble factors, such as nitric oxide, prostaglandin E_2, and the immunosuppressive cytokines IL-10 and TGFβ. The proinflammatory cytokines GM-CSF and TNFα inhibit the suppressive activity of the alveolar macrophage. In certain circumstances, such as the inhalation of silica particles, the alveolar macrophage cannot destroy the particulate substance and the cell dies. The result is that the alveolar macrophage now has localized and concentrated silica particles in a region of the lung and this causes tissue destruction.

The fate of the alveolar macrophage varies. It can be taken up into the mucociliary clearance system, it can die within the alveolus and get phagocytized by other alveolar macrophages, or it can migrate into lymphoid tissue or lung interstitium.

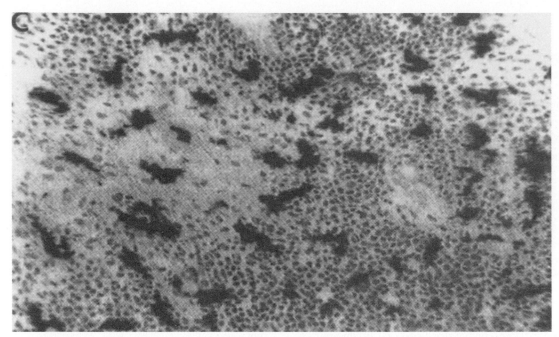

■ **Figure 30-8** The dispersed Ia immunostaining pattern in normal rat tracheal epithelium. Frozen segments of Wistar Furth strain rat trachea were sectioned tangentially and immunostained for Ia.

Normal Adaptive Immune Response

In nonmucosal tissues (i.e., spleen, liver, kidney) the adaptive immune system is the body's primary specific host defense. However, in mucosal tissues, it is a secondary response to a foreign agent. Only after the insulting agent has avoided the unique defense systems established in the respiratory tract is the adaptive immune response summoned. Once triggered, the adaptive immune system in the respiratory tract resembles any systemic organ.

Under normal circumstances, bacteria, such as *Streptococcus pneumoniae,* that commonly come into contact with the upper respiratory system are expelled by the mucociliary clearance system or are handled by MALT via an IgA response. However, if the bacteria elude these first-line defenses, an inflammatory response develops (i.e., bacterial pneumonia), which is followed by a classic adaptive immune response with T-cell activation and antibody synthesis. These responses take a week or two to develop fully before the pneumonia resolves. A typical inflammatory response to a bacterial or viral pneumonia is initially dominated by polymorphonuclear leukocytes. If the response persists, more mononuclear cells infiltrate. As with other organ systems, there is a transient population of blood-borne phagocytic cells (polymorphonuclear leukocytes and macrophages) residing in local vessels ready to immigrate into sites of injury. The first inflammatory cells to respond to the injury via chemotactic mechanisms are the polymorphonuclear leukocytes. The response usually occurs within 4 to 12 hours. If the injury persists, the leukocytes are followed by macrophages within 24 to 72 hours.

If the bacteria or inciting agent persists and is hard to phagocytize, a granulomatous type of response occurs. The body's reaction to *Mycobacterium tuberculosis* is a classic type of granulomatous response; that is, mononuclear cells (lymphocytes and macrophages) form around the agent in an attempt to wall it off and to prevent it from infiltrating into other tissues. This is a T-cell response that is dominated by CD4+ T cells and Th1 cytokines such as IFNγ. A granulomatous response is commonly found in the lung, and it is associated with such diseases as silicosis, sarcoidosis, and the hypersensitivity lung diseases (i.e., Farmer's lung). Although the sequelae to many acute bacterial and viral pneumonias resolve to normal tissue, a common sequela to the chronic granulomatous type of response is scar formation (i.e., pulmonary fibrosis). Extensive injury and cell death (necrosis) occurs during the granulomatous response. The body has no recourse but to lay down collagen to form scar tissue, in essence to sew up the hole left by the necrotic tissue. Scar formation is usually nonreversible. It replaces normal functioning tissue, and therefore imparts a dysfunctional state in affected areas.

Mucociliary Transport. The mucociliary transport system is one of the lungs' primary defense mechanisms. It protects the conducting airways by trapping and removing bacteria, inhaled particles, and cellular debris from the lungs. Ambient air contains many gases in addition to oxygen and nitrogen, as well as particulate material, such as pollen, ash, mineral dust, mold spores, and organic particles. This particulate material must be removed from the lungs. Because new particles and toxic substances are continuously inhaled, even during normal respiration, a continuous system for the clearance of this material is needed. The mucociliary transport system is responsible for this continuous process. Three major components of mucociliary transport are: (a) cilia that beat in a lower layer of nonviscid;

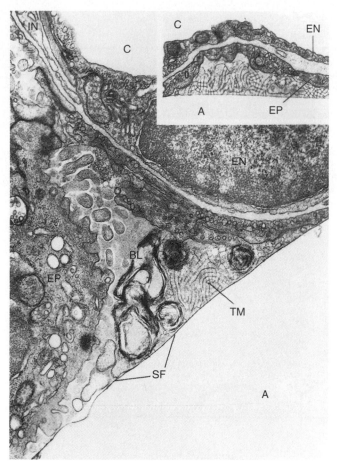

■ **Figure 30-9** Scanning electron micrograph of a normal human lung showing an alveolar macrophage (Ma) attached to the epithelium partly by filopodia (FP) and forming an undulating membrane (U) in the direction of forward movement to the left. Several capillaries (C) are evident, and a type II epithelial cell (EP2) can be seen in the background. (Original magnification × 3700.) (Reprinted by permission from Gehr P et al: The normal human lung: ultrastructure and morphometric estimation of diffusion capacity. *Respir Physiol* 32:121-140, 1978, Williams & Wilkins, Baltimore.)

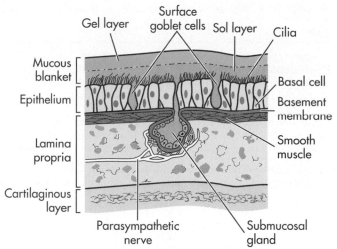

■ **Figure 30-10** Epithelial lining of the tracheobronchial tree. The cilia of the epithelial cell reside in the periciliary fluid layer with the mucus on top. Interspersed between the ciliated epithelial cells are surface secretory (goblet) cells and submucosal glands.

(b) serous fluid (the periciliary fluid); and (c) the mucus layer (Figure 30-10). Effective clearance requires both ciliary activity and respiratory tract fluid (periciliary fluid and mucus). Inhaled material is trapped on the viscoelastic mucus, whereas the watery periciliary fluid allows the cilia to move freely. Only their tips contact the mucus and propel it toward the mouth.

The periciliary fluid layer is produced by active ion transport by the pseudostratified, columnar epithelium that lines the respiratory system and that is joined together by tight junctions. These cells are ciliated, and they line the entire respiratory tract to the level of the bronchioles, where they are replaced by a cuboidal, nonciliated epithelium. As previously described (see Figure 25.12), the serous environment is maintained by the active transport of sodium and chloride across the epithelium. This process is regulated by intracellular cAMP, calcium ions, and ion-specific chloride and sodium channels. Active secretion of Cl⁻ into the airway lumen produces fluid secretion, whereas active Na⁺ absorption accounts for the ability to absorb fluid. The balance between Cl⁻ secretion and Na⁺ absorption regulates the depth of the periciliary fluid at 5-6 μm (Table 30-4). This depth is important for the normal functioning of the cilia. If it is too deep, cilia splash around, and if it is not deep enough, ciliary function is markedly diminished.

Mucus Layer. The mucus, or gel layer lies on top of the periciliary fluid layer, and it is propelled by the cilia. Airway mucus is a complex mixture of macromolecules, such as proteins, glycoproteins, and electrolytes. The mucus layer is 5 to 10 μm thick, and it exists as a discontinuous blanket (i.e., islands of mucus). Three cells produce the mucus layer: surface secretory cells, submucosal tracheobronchial glands, and Clara cells. These cells control both the quantity and composition of the macromolecules in the mucus.

Mucus is composed of glycoproteins, and it consists of groups of oligosaccharides that are attached to a protein backbone, like the bones of a fish are to the vertebral column (Figure 30-11). The mucus has a low viscosity and high elasticity. This elasticity prevents mucus from backsliding during clearance. Mucus is 95% to 97% water.

Surface secretory cells or **goblet cells** are interspersed between every 5 or 6 ciliated cells. They decrease in number between the 5th and 12th lung divisions, and they disappear completely beyond the 12th tracheobronchial division. They secrete neutral and acidic glycoproteins that are rich in sialic acid. In response to a chemical signal, goblet cells discharge their stored material by the process of exocytosis. In this process, membrane-bound storage granules fuse with the plasma membrane and subsequently release their contents into the airway lumen. In the presence of cigarette smoke or in patients with chronic bronchitis, surface secretory cells increase in size and number, and they extend further down the respiratory tract toward the alveolus. Their

■ **Table 30-4** Agents that stimulate chloride secretion in airway epithelia

Agent	Surface	cAMP
β-Adrenergic agonist	Submucosal	↑
Prostaglandin E$_2$	Submucosal	↑
Prostaglandin F$_2$	Submucosal	—
Vasoactive intestinal peptide	Submucosal	↑
Adenosine	Mucosal	↑
Leukotrienes LTC$_4$ and LTD$_4$	Mucosal and submucosal	↑?
Substance P	Mucosal and submucosal	?
Bradykinin	Mucosal and submucosal	↑?

Surface, Side of the epithelium on which the agents act; ↑, increase; ?, uncertainty; —, no measurable change.
From Welsh MJ: Production and control of airway secretions. In Fishman AP: *Pulmonary diseases and disorders,* ed 2, New York, 1988, McGraw-Hill.

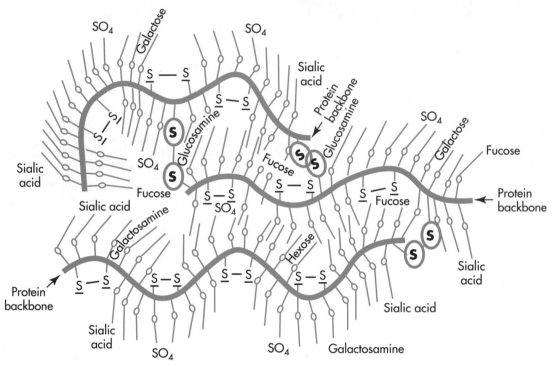

■ **Figure 30-11** Schematic drawing of mucus. Note the protein backbone with glycoprotein side chains and the "O" glycosidic and disulfide bonds.

output also increases, and the chemical composition of their secretions changes.

Submucosal tracheobronchial glands are present normally wherever there is cartilage, and they empty into the airway lumen through a ciliated duct. Glands are increased in number and size, and they can extend to the bronchioles in chronic bronchitis. The secretory component consists of **mucus cells** that are located near the distal end of the tubule, which is lined by "nonspecified" cells and **serous cells** at the distal end of the tubule (Table 30-5). Mucous cells contain large, often confluent, electron-lucent granules, whereas serous cells contain small, discrete electron-dense secretory granules. The mucus cells of the submucosal tracheobronchial glands secrete acid glycoproteins, whereas the serous cells secrete neutral glycoproteins, and they contain lysozyme, lactoferrin, and antileukoprotease. In certain diseases, the chemical composition of the glycoproteins does not change. However, the volume of the secretions increases and the

ratio of neutral glycoproteins to acidic glycoproteins changes. These changes modify the physical properties of the mucus. The associated changes in viscosity and elasticity affect the subsequent clearance of the mucus. Gland secretion is under parasympathetic, adrenergic, and peptidergic (vasoactive intestinal peptide) neural control. Local inflammatory mediators such as histamine and arachidonic acid metabolites stimulate mucus production.

Clara cells are located in the bronchioles, and they contain granules. Although their exact function is not known, they secrete a nonmucinous material that contains carbohydrate and protein. These cells may play a role in bronchial regeneration after injury. Normal individuals produce approximately 100 ml of mucus each day. Although authorities even today refer to the "mucus blanket" in the airways, the mucus layer is actually "spotty," and it varies in thickness from 2 to 5 μm. Most of the volume of the mucus is absorbed by the ciliated, columnar, epithelial lining cells,

■ Table 30-5   Properties of submucosal gland cells

	Serous cells	*Mucous cells*
Granules	Small, electron-dense	Large, electron-lucent
Glycoproteins	Neutral	Acidic
	Lysozyme, lactoferrin	
Hormone	α > β-Adrenergic	β > α-Adrenergic
Receptors	Muscarinic	Muscarinic
Degranulation	α-Adrenergic	β-Adrenergic
	Cholinergic	Cholinergic
	Substance P	

From Welsh MJ: Production and control of airway secretions. In Fishman AP: *Pulmonary diseases and disorders,* ed 2, New York, 1988, McGraw-Hill.

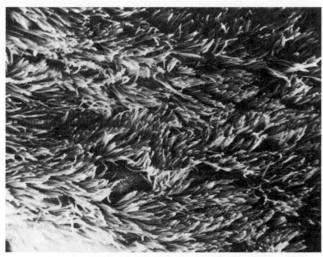

■ **Figure 30-12** Scanning electron micrograph of the luminal surface of a bronchiole from a normal adult man; many cilia are evident surrounding a nonciliated cell (× 2000). Reprinted by permission from Ebert RV, Terracio MJ: *Am Rev Resp Dis,* 111:4, 1975.)

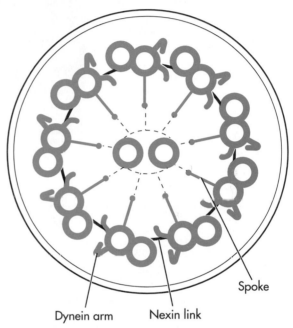

■ **Figure 30-13** Schematic cross-sectional diagram of cilium showing its main structural components. (From Palmbald J et al: Ultrastructural, cellular, and clinical features of the immotile-cilia syndrome. *Ann Rev Med,* 35:481-492, 1984. Reprinted, with permission from Annual Reviews Inc.)

and only 10 ml reaches the glottis each day. This mucus is propelled to the back of the throat, where it is swallowed.

It may be important at this point to distinguish mucus from sputum, which is expectorated mucus. Sputum contains not only serum proteins, but also lipids, electrolytes, calcium and DNA from degenerated white cell nuclei (collectively known as bronchial secretions), and extra bronchial secretions, such as nasal, oral, lingual, pharyngeal, and salivary secretions.

Cilia. Cilia are the microscopic hairlike scrubbers of the respiratory system. There are approximately 200 cilia per cell (Figure 30-12), and they are 2 to 5 μm in length. They have a structure that has been preserved through evolution from protozoa. They are composed of nine microtubular doublets that surround two central microtubules, and they are held together by dynein arms, nexin links, and spokes (Figure 30-13). This structure is ideally suited for their function. The central microtubule doublet contains an ATPase enzyme that is responsible for the contractile beat of the cil-

ium. Coordinated ciliary beating can be detected by the 13th week of gestation.

Cilia beat with a coordinated oscillation in a characteristic, biphasic, wavelike rhythm called metachronism (Figure 30-14). They beat 900 to 1200 strokes/min with a power forward stroke and a slow return or recovery stroke. During their power forward stroke, the tips of the cilia extend upward into the viscous layer, and thereby drag it and the entrapped particles. On the reverse beat, the cilia release the mucus, and they are contained completely in the sol layer. Cilia in the nasopharynx beat in the direction that propels the mucus into the pharynx, whereas cilia in the trachea propel mucus upward toward the pharynx, where it is swallowed. Ciliary beating is powered by ATP. The bending of the cilia occurs by the sliding of dynein arms that interlink each microtubule pair. This causes a bending to one side. Cilia beat in a coordinated fashion; this coordination occurs by cell-to-cell ion flow that results in electrical and metabolic

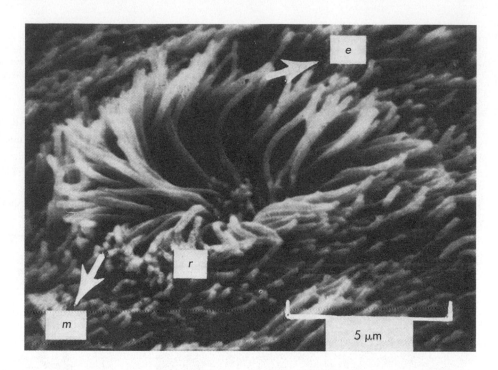

■ **Figure 30-14** Scanning electron micrograph of a metachronal wave on rabbit tracheal epithelium. Cilia that move to the left close to the cell surface in their recovery stroke *(r)* then swing over towards the right in the more erect effective stroke *(e)*. The metachronal wave moves in the direction indicated by the *arrow (m)*. (Micrograph by MJ Sanderson.) (Sanderson MJ, Sleigh MS: Ciliary activity of cultured rabbit tracheal epithelium: beat pattern and metachrony. *J Cell Sci* 47:331-347, 1981.)

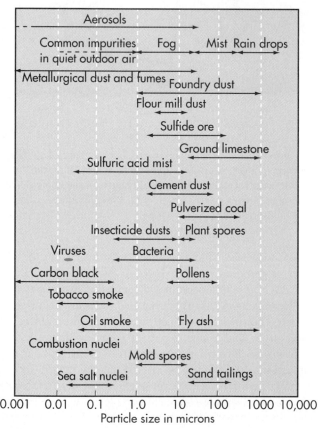

■ **Figure 30-15** Approximate size ranges of common airborne particles. (Modified from Stuart BO: *Arch Intern Med* 131:60, 1973.)

coordination. The mechanism by which cilia and the adjoining cells intercommunicate is unknown.

As previously mentioned, particle deposition in the lung depends on particle size and density, the distance over which the particle travels and the relative humidity of the air (Figure 30-15). Once a particle has deposited itself on the epithelial surface of the airways, it ordinarily is not resuspended in the air stream. Hence, it must by cleared from the airways by some other means. In general, particles larger than 10 µm are deposited by impaction in the nasal passages, and they do not penetrate the lower respiratory tract. In the lower respiratory tract, particles that are 2 to 10 µm in size impact at points where the air stream changes direction (airway birfucations) into the surface, because their inertia prevents them from changing directions rapidly (inertial impaction). This phenomenon usually occurs in areas with turbulent airflow. Such areas include the nasopharynx, trachea, and bronchi to the first 10 to 12 airway generations. In more distal areas, where airflow is slower, smaller particles (0.2-2 µm) deposit on the surface secondary to gravitation (sedimentation). Particles less than 0.2 µm can contact the epithelium as they diffuse in the alveolar gas in the terminal respiratory units. The particles are cleared via endocytosis by the alveolar macrophages, or they are carried away by lymphatics or lymphoid tissue, or they are carried to the beginning of the mucociliary transport system.

The particles deposited along the alveolar walls or in the alveolar ducts are cleared by alveolar macrophages. These macrophages migrate through the alveoli and engulf foreign or effete autologous materials. Phagocytosis requires the presence of both magnesium and calcium ions. Macrophages have potent bactericidal, fungicidal, and virus killing abilities. After they engulf a potentially infectious agent, they undergo a rapid burst in metabolic activity. Unwanted clearance of material by alveolar macrophages is rapid. Within one hour after deposit, approximately 25% of inhaled particles are phagocytized, and within 24 hours, the entire load has been phagocytized.

In the conducting airways, the mucociliary system transports deposited particles from the terminal bronchioles to the major airways, where they are coughed up and either expectorated or swallowed. The transition from the conducting airways and their mucociliary transport system to the terminal respiratory units where alveolar mechanisms become important is the "Achilles heel" in what is otherwise a highly effective system. In individuals with the occupational lung disease called pneumoconiosis (the "black lung" disease of coal miners), the highest concentration of particles is usually seen just beyond the terminal bronchioles. The relatively slow rate of particle clearance in this area may provide an opportunity for particles to leave the airway space and enter the interstitial spaces. The terminal respiratory unit is the most common location of airway damage for all types of occupational lung diseases.

When it functions normally, the mucociliary transport system is highly effective. Deposited particles can be removed in a matter of minutes to hours. In the trachea and main bronchi, the rate of particle clearance is 5 to 20 mm/min, but it is slower in the bronchioles (0.5-1 mm/min). In general, the longer that inhaled material remains in the airways, the greater the probability that lung damage will occur. Once particles in the terminal airways have entered the interstitium, clearance is even slower, and the likelihood of lung damage is even greater.

CLINICAL MANIFESTATIONS OF ALTERED PULMONARY DEFENSE

Diseases Associated with Abnormalities in Innate and Adaptive Immunity

Allergic Diseases. By far the most common pathological conditions associated with mucosal tissues are allergic responses (e.g., allergic asthma, allergic rhinitis, and food and skin allergies). As previously described, the predominant antibody response in MALT is IgA. However, in an allergic response, an antibody switchover response has occurred, and IgE becomes the predominant antibody that is synthesized to the allergen. Sensitized CD4+ T cells and IL-4 are required for this to occur. The IgE binds to the surface of tissue mast cells, and antigen stimulation leads to the degranulation of mast cells (Figure 30-16). The released granules contain many factors, such as eosinophil chemotactic factors and leukotrienes with bronchoconstrictor activity. Symptoms of wheezing, cough, and shortness of breath occur within minutes, and the lesion is associated with an intense eosinophilia and airway edema. Resolution of the inflammatory response can occur spontaneously or in response to therapy (antiinflammatory drugs). Low-grade inflammation may, however, persist, and it can result in permanent changes in airway structure. Such changes are referred to as airway remodeling. The mechanisms for airway remodeling in allergic diseases are not known, but TGFβ may be important.

Hypersensitivity Lung Diseases. An interesting group of difficult to diagnose lung diseases was first described in the 1930s to 1960s (and they continue to be described), and they are caused by nonpathological organisms and dusts. These diseases are referred to as hypersensitivity lung diseases, and they are associated with an altered immune response to the inciting agent. Only a small percentage of equally exposed individuals have contracted the disease, which is caused by an immune response to the agent and not by the agent itself. The allergic response is not typical because the symptoms usually occur 4 to 6 hours post exposure. This contrasts with the immediate type of response to allergens, although some individuals can also have an allergic response. Also, the lesion is not dominated by eosinohils, as it is in an allergic response. The lung pathology can consist either of a polymorphonuclear cell response or of a granulomatous type of response, followed by pulmonary fibrosis.

Autoimmune Diseases. Pulmonary complications are common in chronic systemic diseases with possible autoimmune etiologies, such as rheumatoid arthritis, systemic lupus erythematous, and inflammatory bowel diseases (i.e., Crohn's disease, ulcerative colitis). Why this association exists is not clear, but it may be due to a similar dysregulation of immune responses, which initiate a local pulmonary type of autoimmune disease. **Goodpasture's syndrome** is the classic autoimmune response in the lung. This syndrome is a pulmonary hemorrhagic disease caused by an autoimmune, IgG antibody response to type IV collagen in the basement membrane of the lung. Cell injury and death occur through complement activation via an antibody•antigen complex. This syndrome is associated with an intense glomerulonephritis, in which the disease is thought to be initiated. The type IV collagen antigen in the kidney basement membrane cross reacts with the basement membrane in the lung. Immunofluorescence antibody staining to IgG shows a classic linear pattern of staining.

Genetically Inherited IgA Deficiency. The most common inherited immunoglobulin deficiency is selective IgA deficiency, its prevalence is 1 in 800 births. Although this deficiency is not associated with any particular disease, these patients have a high rate of chronic lung disease, which illustrates the advantages that this antibody has in host defense in the respiratory tract.

Diseases That Affect Mucociliary Clearance

It is important to note that today's urban industrial environment can produce a significant burden even when the mucociliary transport system is normal. In addition, occupations in which airborne particles are inhaled present an even greater challenge to the system. Living or working in environments where large loads of foreign materials are inhaled can lead to the development of chronic lung injury that often develops after many years of exposure. Excessive mucus production can stress the mucociliary system. Excess accumulation of mucus in the airways stimulates the cough reflex, which helps to remove these secretions.

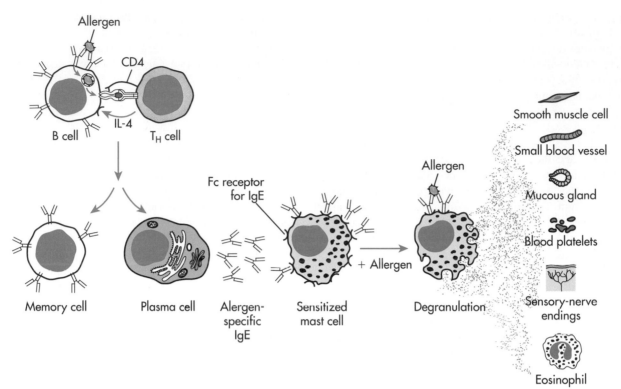

■ **Figure 30-16**   General mechanism underlying an allergic reaction. Exposure to an allergen activates B cells to form IgE-secreting plasma cells. The secreted IgE molecules bind to IgE-specific Fc receptors on mast cells and blood basophils. Upon a second exposure to the allergen, the bound IgE is cross linked, triggering the release of pharmacologically active mediators (green) from mast cells and basophils. The mediators cause smooth-muscle contraction, increased vascular permeability, and vasodilation.

Numerous diseases of the lungs have their origin in abnormalities of lung defense. **Cystic fibrosis** is an autosomal, recessive disease that is characterized by thick, tenacious, dehydrated airway secretions. In this disease, the airway epithelium demonstrates decreased permeability to Cl^-. The Cl^- ion channel in the apical cell membrane fails to open, even under stimulation by cAMP. The result is a thick mucus, with a water content that is less than normal. Furthermore, in cystic fibrosis the goblet cells proliferate and the submucosal glands hypertrophy secondary to irritation or to abnormalities in the surface liquid.

In normal individuals, bronchial secretions owe their viscoelastic properties to the size, length, coiling, and cross-linking of the mucus glycoproteins, which result in flexible elastic fibers. Normal secretions have low viscosity and long relaxation times (they are highly elastic). In **asthma,** a disease associated with bronchospasm, airway inflammation and airway edema, mucus viscosity, instead of elasticity, becomes the major physical property, and a glycoprotein gel is formed. Secretions from individuals with asthma have the highest viscosity of mucus in any disease; on occasion, entire mucus casts of a lobe have been expectorated.

Many processes can result in abnormal ciliary beating, and in abnormal clearance of particles. Ciliary beating is decreased by various factors, such as hypoxia, repeated exposure to the gas phases of tobacco smoke, very dry air,

inflammation, ozone, and pollution. Cilia are also destroyed by infection. Immotile cilia syndrome is associated with abnormal ciliary microstructure, and by cilia throughout the body that consequently do not beat. The triad of situs inversus associated with bronchiectasis, sinusitis, and immotile cilia is termed **Kartagener's syndrome.**

SUMMARY

1. The respiratory system and other mucosal tissues have developed unique immunological and structural features to cope with the constant environmental exposure to foreign substances.

2. The two major components of the lung defense against inhaled particles and other inhaled materials are mucociliary transport in the larger airways and a specialized mucosal immune system.

3. The lung is a secondary lymphoid tissue.

4. BALT is part of the mucosal associated lymphoid tissue (MALT) system, and it is mainly comprised of aggregates of lymph nodules throughout the conducting airways.

5. Atypical immune cells that play important roles in host defense in the lung include NK cells, NK/T cells, dendritic cells, alveolar macrophages, and TCRγδ cells.

6. IgA is the predominant antibody produced by plasma cells in BALT.

7. The epitheliotropism and antigen selectivity of TCRγδ cells make them a likely candidate for "first line" of defense in the lung.

8. NK cells and alveolar macrophages play a major role in the innate immune response in the lung.

9. The three components of mucociliary transport are cilia, periciliary fluid, and mucus.

10. The depth of the periciliary fluid layer is maintained by the balance between Cl^- secretion and Na^+ absorption, and it is essential to normal ciliary beating.

11. Mucus is a complex macromolecule composed of glycoproteins, proteins, electrolytes, and water. The viscoelastic properties of mucus are due to the size, length, coiling, and cross-linking of the mucus glycoproteins. Normal mucus has low viscosity and high elasticity.

12. Three cell types produce mucus: surface secretory cells, tracheobronchial glands and Clara cells.

REFERENCES

1. Christmas SE: Cytokine production by lymphocytes bearing the gamma-delta T-cell antigen receptor. *Chem Immunol* 53:32-46, 1992.
2. Spinozzi F, Agea E, Bistoni O, et al: Increased allergen specific, steroid sensitive γδ T cells in bronchoalveolar lavage fluid from patients with asthma. *Ann Intern Med* 124:223-227, 1996.
3. Holt PG, McMenamin C: IgE and mucosal immunity: studies on the role of intraepithelial Ia+ dendritic cells and γ/δ T-lymphocytes in regulation of T cell activation in the lung. *Clin Exp Allergy* 21:148-152, 1991.
4. Holt PG: Regulation of antigen presenting cell function(s) in lung and airway tissues. *Eur Respir J* 6:120-129, 1993.
5. Bilyk N, Holt PG: Inhibition of the immunosuppressive activity of resident pulmonary alveolar macrophages by granulocyte/macrophage colony stimulating factor. *J Exp Med* 177:1773-1777, 1993.
6. Chakraborty A, Li L, Chakraborty NG, et al: Stimulatory and inhibitory differentiation of human myeloid dendritic cells. *Clin Immunol* 94:88-98, 2000.
7. Stumbles PA, Thomas JA, Pimm CL, et al: Resting respiratory tract dendritic cells preferentially stimulate T helper cell type 2 (Th2) responses and require obligatory cytokine signals for induction of Th1 immunity. *J Exp Med* 188:2019-2031, 1998.
8. Banchereau J, Steinman RM: Dendritic cells and the control of immunity. *Nature* 392:245-252, 1998.
9. Sheehan JK, Thorton DJ, Somerville M, et al: The structure and heterogeneity of respiratory mucus glycoproteins. *Am Rev Respir Dis Suppl* 144:S4, 1991.
10. Verdugo P: Goblet cells secretion and mucogenesis. *Annu Rev Physiol* 52:157, 1990.
11. Daniele RP: Immunoglobulin secretion in the airways. *Annu Rev Physiol* 52:177, 1998.
12. Kerr A: The structure and function of human IgA. *Biochem J* 271:285, 1990.
13. Sommerhoff CP, Finkbeiner WE: Human tracheobronchial submucosal gland cells in culture. *Am J Respir Cell Mol Biol* 2:41, 1990.
14. Smith J, Travis S, Greenberg E, et al: Cystic fibrosis airway epithelia fail to kill bacteria because of abnormal airway surface liquid. *Cell* 85:229-236, 1996.
15. Gashi AA, Nadel JA, Basbaum CB: Tracheal gland mucous cells stimulated in vitro with adrenergic and cholinergic drugs. *Tissue Cell* 21:59, 1989.
16. Welsh MJ: Electrolyte transport by airway epithelia. *Physiol Rev* 67:1143-1184, 1987.
17. Oberdorster G: Lung clearance of inhaled insoluble and soluble particles. *J Aerosol Med* 1:289-330, 1988.
18. Wanner A, Salathe M, O'Riordan TG: Mucociliary clearance in the airways. *Am J Respir Crit Care Med* 154:1868-1902, 1996.
19. Martonen TB: Deposition patterns of cigarette smoke in human airways. *Am Ind Hyg Assoc* 53:6-18, 1992.
20. Salathe M, O'Riordan TG, Wanner A: Treatment of mucociliary dysfunction. *Chest* 110:1048-1057, 1996.

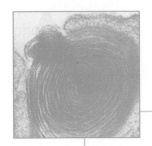

The Gastro-intestinal System

Howard C. Kutchai

chapter thirty-one

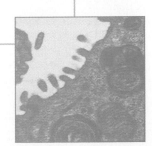

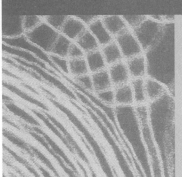

Gastrointestinal Regulation and Motility

The gastrointestinal system consists of the gastrointestinal tract and associated glandular organs that produce secretions. The major structures of the gastrointestinal tract are the mouth, pharynx, esophagus, stomach, duodenum, jejunum, ileum, colon, rectum, and anus. The duodenum, jejunum, and ileum make up the small intestine. Associated glandular organs include the salivary glands, liver, gallbladder, and pancreas.

The major physiological functions of the gastrointestinal system are to digest foodstuffs and absorb nutrient molecules into the bloodstream. The gastrointestinal system carries out these functions by motility, secretion (see Chapter 32), digestion, and absorption (see Chapter 33). **Motility** refers to the movements that mix and circulate the gastrointestinal contents and propel them along the length of the tract. Gastrointestinal contents are usually propelled in the orthograde (forward) direction, that is, away from the mouth and toward the anus. Retrograde (backward) propulsion does occur, however; vomiting is a notable example. **Secretion** refers to the processes by which the glands associated with the gastrointestinal tract release water and substances into the tract. **Digestion** is defined as the processes by which food and large molecules are chemically degraded to produce smaller molecules that can be absorbed across the wall of the gastrointestinal tract. **Absorption** refers to the processes by which nutrient molecules are absorbed by cells that line the gastrointestinal tract and enter the bloodstream.

STRUCTURE OF THE GASTROINTESTINAL TRACT

The structure of the gastrointestinal tract varies greatly from region to region, but common features exist in the overall organization of the tissue. Figure 31-1 depicts the general layered structure of the gastrointestinal tract wall.

The **mucosa** is the innermost layer of the gastrointestinal tract. It consists of an **epithelium,** the **lamina propria,** and the **muscularis mucosae.** The epithelium is a single layer of specialized cells that lines the lumen of the gastrointestinal

tract. The nature of the epithelium varies greatly from one part of the digestive tract to another. The lamina propria consists largely of loose connective tissue that contains collagen and elastin fibrils. The lamina propria is rich in several types of glands and contains lymph nodules and capillaries. The muscularis mucosae is the thin, innermost layer of intestinal smooth muscle. The mucosal folds and ridges are caused by contractions of the muscularis mucosae.

The next layer is the **submucosa.** The submucosa consists largely of loose connective tissue with collagen and elastin fibrils. In some regions of the gastrointestinal tract, glands are present in the submucosa. The larger nerve trunks and blood vessels of the intestinal wall lie in the submucosa.

The next layer, the **muscularis externa,** typically consists of two substantial layers of smooth muscle cells: an inner circular layer and an outer longitudinal layer. In humans and most mammals, the circular layer of the small intestine is subdivided into an **inner dense circular layer,** which consists of smaller, more closely packed cells, and an **outer circular layer.** Contractions of the muscularis externa mix and circulate the contents of the lumen and propel them along the gastrointestinal tract.

The wall of the gastrointestinal tract contains many interconnected neurons. The submucosa contains a dense network of nerve cells in the submucosa called the **submucosal plexus (Meissner's plexus).** The prominent **myenteric plexus (Auerbach's plexus)** is located between the circular and longitudinal smooth muscle layers. These **intramural plexuses,** together with the other neurons of the gastrointestinal tract, constitute the **enteric nervous system.** The enteric nervous system helps to integrate the motor and secretory activities of the gastrointestinal system. If the sympathetic and parasympathetic nerves to the gut are cut, many motor and secretory activities continue, because these processes are directly controlled by the enteric nervous system.

The **serosa,** or **adventitia,** is the outermost layer of the gastrointestinal tract. This layer consists mainly of connective tissue covered with a layer of squamous mesothelial cells.

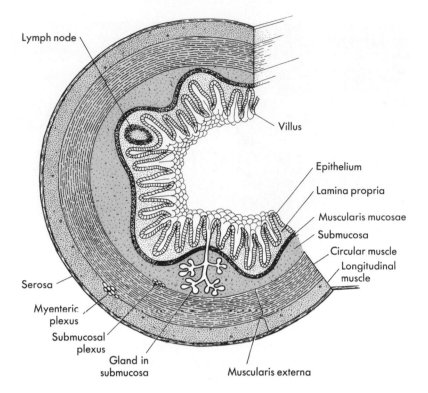

■ **Fig. 31-1** The general organization of the layers of the gastrointestinal tract. (Redrawn from Ham AW: *Histology,* ed 3, Philadelphia, 1957, JB Lippincott.)

REGULATION OF GASTROINTESTINAL TRACT FUNCTIONS

The functions of the gastrointestinal tract are regulated and coordinated by hormones, paracrine agonists, and neurons. Hormones are produced by endocrine cells and are released into the blood to reach their target cells via the circulation. Paracrine agonists are released by cells in the vicinity of the target cells and reach the target cells by diffusion. Regulation may be classified as **endocrine, paracrine,** or **neurocrine,** depending on the cell type that produces the regulatory substance and the route of delivery of the substance to the target cell.

Much of the hormonal and neural regulation of gastrointestinal functions is intrinsic to the gastrointestinal tract. In **intrinsic regulation,** both the cells that regulate and the cells that respond reside in the gastrointestinal tract. However, some hormonal and neural regulation of gastrointestinal functions is **extrinsic.** These extrinsic regulatory mechanisms are mediated by endocrine cells that are located outside the gastrointestinal tract and by neurons whose cell bodies are located in the central nervous system or in prevertebral and paravertebral sympathetic ganglia. These overlapping layers of hormonal and neural control allow for subtle and precise control of gastrointestinal functions.

Gastrointestinal Hormones

Endocrine cells are located in the mucosa or submucosa of the stomach and the intestine, as well as in the pancreas. These endocrine cells produce an array of hormones (Table 31-1). Some of these hormones act on secretory cells located in the wall of the gastrointestinal tract, in the pancreas, or in the liver to alter the rate or the composition of their secre-

■ **Table 31-1** Gastrointestinal hormones

Location of cells that produce the hormone	Hormone	Cells that produce the hormone
Stomach	Gastrin	G
	Somatostatin	D
Duodenum or jejunum	Secretin	S
	Cholecystokinin (CCK)	I
	Motilin	M
	Gastric inhibitory peptide (GIP)	K
	Somatostatin	D
Pancreatic islets	Insulin	b
	Glucagon	a
	Pancreatic polypeptide	PP
	Somatostatin	d
Ileum or Colon	Enteroglucagon	L
	Peptide YY	L
	Neurotensin	N
	Somatostatin	D

GIP is also known as **glucose-dependent insulinotropic peptide** because it stimulates insulin secretion. GIP may be more potent in this action than it is as an inhibitor of gastric motility and secretion.

tions (see Chapter 32). Other hormones act on smooth muscle cells in specific segments of the gastrointestinal tract, on gastrointestinal sphincters, or on the musculature of the gallbladder (see Chapter 32).

Paracrine Mediators in the Gastrointestinal Tract

Paracrine substances regulate the secretory and motor functions of the gastrointestinal tract. For example, histamine is released from cells in the wall of the stomach. The substance is a key physiological agonist of hydrochloric acid (HCl) secretion by gastric parietal cells.

Other paracrine agonists are released by cells of the extensive **gastrointestinal immune system.** The mass of cells with immune function in the gastrointestinal tract is approximately equal to the combined mass of immunocytes (immune cells) in the rest of the body. The gastrointestinal immune system secretes antibodies in response to specific food antigens and mounts an immunological defense against many pathogenic microorganisms.

The components of the gastrointestinal immune system include cells in mesenteric lymph nodes, Peyer's patches in the wall of the intestine, and immunocytes that reside in the mucosa and submucosa (Fig. 31-2). Mucosal and submucosal immunocytes include intraepithelial lymphocytes, B and T lymphocytes, plasma cells, mast cells, macrophages, and eosinophils. These immune cells secrete **inflammatory mediators** such as histamine, prostaglandins, leukotrienes, cytokines, and others. Once released, these mediators diffuse to secretory and smooth muscle cells in the gastrointestinal tract, where they affect their activities and modulate the function of neurons in the gastrointestinal tract. The gastrointestinal immune system is involved in some of the most troublesome gastrointestinal disorders, such as **celiac disease, inflammatory bowel disease,** and **Crohn's disease.**

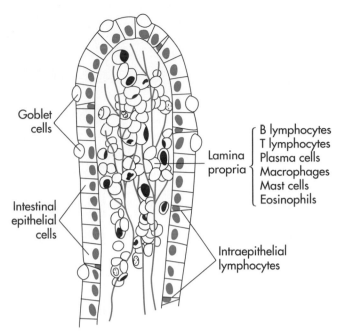

■ **Fig. 31-2** A small intestinal villus showing intraepithelial lymphocytes and various immunocytes in the lamina propria. (Redrawn from Kagnoff MF: Immunology and inflammation of the gastrointestinal tract. In Sleisenger MH, Fordtran JS, editors: *Gastrointestinal disease,* ed 6, Philadelphia, 1997, WB Saunders.)

> Important diseases involve hyperactivity of the gastrointestinal immune system. Patients with **celiac disease,** also known as **celiac sprue** and **gluten enteropathy,** mount an allergic response to gliadin, a component of gluten in wheat flour. As a consequence the villi become shortened and microvilli become much less numerous, so that the absorptive surface of the small intestine is markedly decreased, so that multiple nutrients may be poorly absorbed. Celiac disease is best treated with a diet that excludes gluten. **Inflammatory bowel disease (IBD)** is characterized by an increased population of lymphocytes and macrophages in the lamina propria, where T lymphocytes are involved in causing inflammation. The chronic inflammation of the intestine in most cases results in diarrhea and abdominal pain. The most common IBDs are ulcerative colitis and Crohn's disease. Ulcerative colitis is confined to the colon and can usually be cured by surgical removal of the affected section of colon. Crohn's disease, by contrast, can occur in any part of the small or large intestine and sometimes involves both the small intestine and the colon. In Crohn's disease, if the inflamed segment of bowel is removed, the disease is likely to recur elsewhere.

Innervation of the Gastrointestinal Tract

Sympathetic innervation. *Sympathetic innervation of the gastrointestinal tract is mainly via postganglionic adrenergic fibers whose cell bodies are located in **prevertebral** and **paravertebral** ganglia* (Fig. 31-3). The celiac, superior and inferior mesenteric, and hypogastric plexuses provide sympathetic innervation to various segments of the gastrointestinal tract. Activation of the sympathetic nerves usually inhibits the motor and secretory activities of the gastrointestinal system. *Most of the sympathetic fibers do not directly innervate structures in the gastrointestinal tract but rather terminate on neurons in the intramural plexuses.* Some vasoconstrictor sympathetic fibers directly innervate blood vessels of the gastrointestinal tract. Other sympathetic fibers innervate glandular structures in the wall of the gut.

Although stimulation of the sympathetic input to the gastrointestinal tract inhibits motor activity of the muscularis externa, it induces contraction of the muscularis mucosae and some sphincters. The inhibitory effect of the sympathetic nerves on the muscularis externa does not result from direct action on the smooth muscle cells, because few sympathetic nerve endings lie in the muscularis externa. Rather, the sympathetic nerves influence neural circuits in the enteric nervous system; these circuits provide input to the smooth muscle cells. The sympathetic nerves may reinforce this effect by reducing blood flow to the muscularis externa. Other fibers that travel with the sympathetic nerves may be cholinergic; still others release neurotransmitters that remain to be identified.

Parasympathetic innervation. Parasympathetic innervation of the gastrointestinal tract down to the level of the transverse colon is provided by branches of the vagus nerves (Fig. 31-3). The remainder of the colon, the rectum, and the anus receive parasympathetic fibers from the pelvic nerves

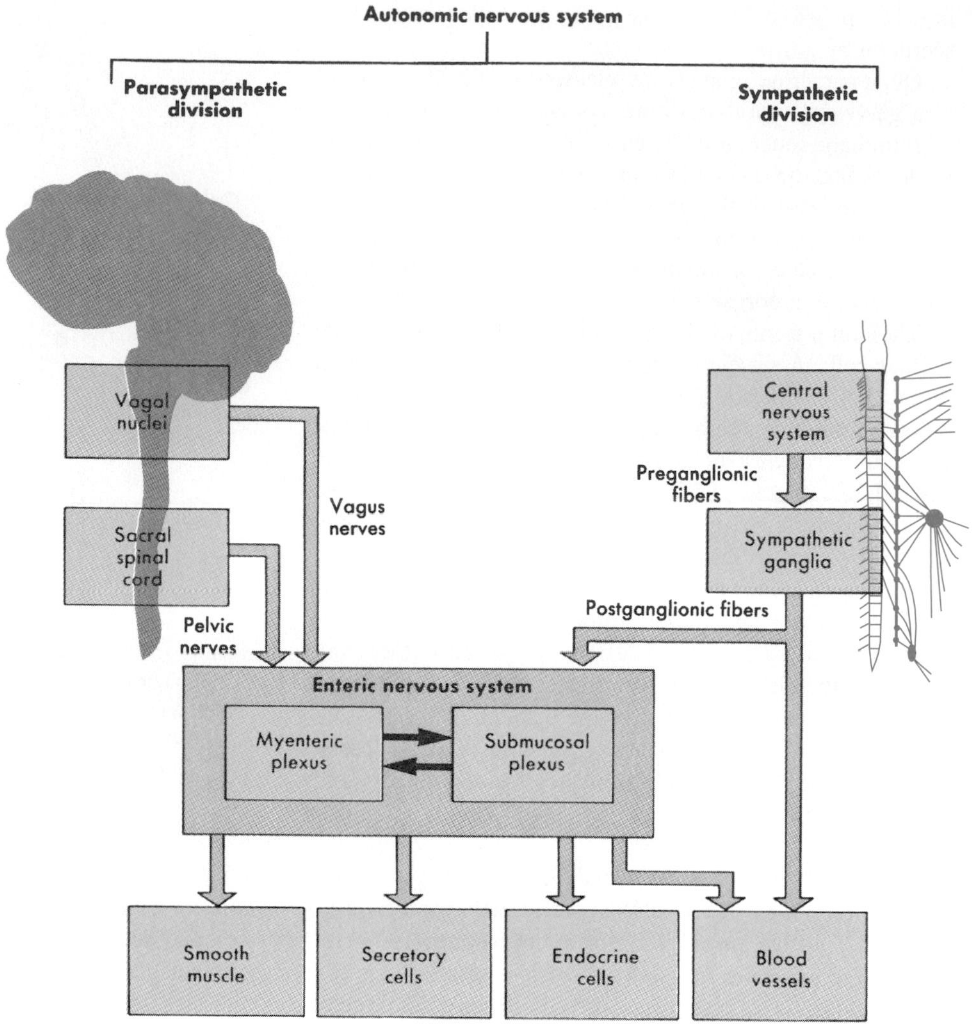

■ **Fig. 31-3**   Major features of the autonomic innervation of the gastrointestinal tract. In most cases the autonomic nerves influence the functions of the gastrointestinal tract by modulating the activities of neurons of the enteric nervous system.

from the sacral spinal cord. Parasympathetic fibers are preganglionic and predominantly cholinergic. Other fibers that travel in the vagus nerve and its branches release other transmitters, some of which have not been identified. The parasympathetic fibers terminate predominantly on the ganglion cells in the intramural plexuses. The ganglion cells then directly innervate the smooth muscle and secretory cells of the gastrointestinal tract. Excitation of parasympathetic nerves usually stimulates the motor and secretory activities of the gastrointestinal tract.

The enteric nervous system. The myenteric and submucosal plexuses are the best defined plexuses in the wall of the gastrointestinal tract (Fig. 31-4). These two plexuses are networks of nerve fibers and ganglion cell bodies. Interneurons in the plexuses connect afferent sensory fibers with efferent neurons to smooth muscle and secretory cells, and thereby form reflex arcs that are located wholly within the gastrointestinal tract wall. Consequently, the myenteric and submucosal plexuses can coordinate activity in the absence of extrinsic innervation of the gastrointestinal tract. Axons of plexus neurons innervate gland cells in the mucosa and submucosa, smooth muscle cells in the muscularis

externa and muscularis mucosae, and intramural endocrine and exocrine cells.

About 10^8 neurons—approximately the same number contained in the spinal cord—reside in the gastrointestinal tract. These gastrointestinal neurons constitute the semiautonomous enteric nervous system. In addition to motor neurons that innervate muscle and secretory cells and blood vessels in the gastrointestinal tract, the enteric nervous system also contains numerous sensory receptors and interneurons. Sensory neurons that respond to mechanical deformation, particular chemical stimuli, pain, and temperature, have been identified. The myenteric and submucosal plexuses give rise to bundles of nerve fibers that form nonganglionated plexuses, such as the **mucosal plexus** and the **deep muscular plexus.**

The extrinsic innervation of the gastrointestinal tract, via sympathetic and parasympathetic nerves, projects primarily onto the neurons of the myenteric and submucosal plexuses to excite or inhibit particular plexus neurons. In this way, the extrinsic innervation influences the motor and secretory functions of the gastrointestinal tract via the enteric nervous system. However, much of the regulation of gastrointestinal

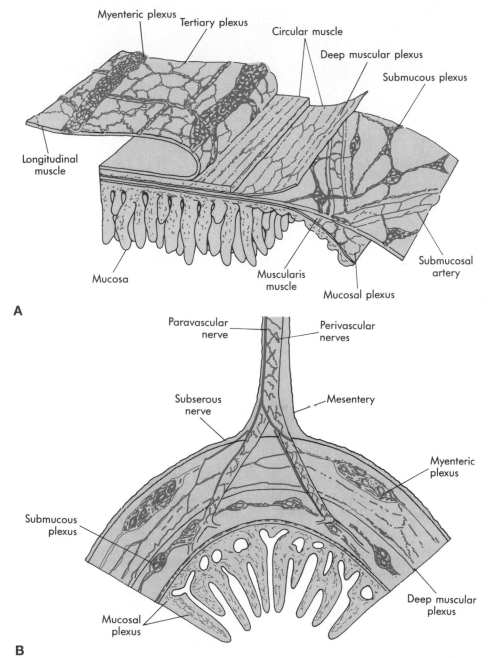

A

B

■ **Fig. 31-4**   Major neural plexuses of the small intestine. (**A,** Seen in whole mounts; **B,** seen in transverse section.) The two ganglionated plexuses are the myenteric and submucosal plexuses. Fibers originating in the myenteric and submucosal plexuses form the nonganglionated plexuses: the tertiary plexus (which innervates the longitudinal layer of muscularis externa), the deep muscular plexus (which supplies the inner dense circular muscle), and the mucosal plexus. Neurons and neuronal processes are shown in color. (Redrawn from Furness JB, Costal M: *Neuroscience* 5:1, 1980.)

activities can be effected by the enteric nervous system, independent of sympathetic or parasympathetic input.

Reflex control. Afferent fibers in the gastrointestinal tract provide the afferent limbs of both **local** and **central reflex arcs** (Fig. 31-5). **Chemoreceptor** and **mechanoreceptor** endings are present in the mucosa and muscularis externa. The cell bodies of many of these sensory receptors are located in the myenteric and submucosal plexuses. The axons of some of these receptor cells synapse with other cells in the plexuses to mediate local reflex activity. Other sensory receptors send signals back to the central nervous system. The complex afferent and efferent innervation of the gastrointestinal tract allows for fine control of secretory and motor activities by intrinsic and extrinsic reflex arcs.

GASTROINTESTINAL SMOOTH MUSCLE

Properties of Gastrointestinal Smooth Muscle Cells

The smooth muscle cells of the gastrointestinal tract are long (about 500 μm in length) and slender (5 to 20 μm across). The cells are arranged in bundles that are separated and defined by connective tissues (see Chapter 13).

Electrophysiology of Gastrointestinal Smooth Muscle

Resting membrane potential. The resting membrane potential of gastrointestinal smooth muscle cells ranges from approximately –40 to –70 mV. The electrogenic Na^+,K^+-ATPase (see Chapter 2) contributes significantly to the

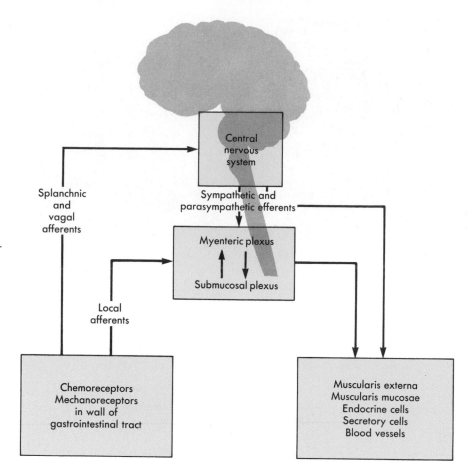

■ **Fig. 31-5** Local and central reflex pathways in the gastrointestinal system.

resting membrane potential in gastrointestinal smooth muscle. In guinea pig taeniae coli, for example, almost one-half of the resting membrane potential results from the electrogenicity of the Na^+,K^+-ATPase.

Slow waves. In most other excitable tissues, the resting membrane potential remains rather constant. In gastrointestinal smooth muscle, the resting membrane potential characteristically varies or oscillates (Fig. 31-6). These oscillations are called **slow waves** (they are also known as the **basic electrical rhythm**). The frequency of slow waves varies from about 3 per minute in the stomach to 12 per minute in the duodenum.

Slow waves are generated by **interstitial cells.** These cells are located in a thin layer between the longitudinal and circular layers of the muscularis externa and in other places in the wall of the gastrointestinal tract. Interstitial cells have properties of both fibroblasts and smooth muscle cells. Their long processes form gap junctions with longitudinal and circular smooth muscle cells. These gap junctions enable the slow waves to be conducted rapidly to both muscle layers. Because gap junctions electrically couple the smooth muscle cells of both longitudinal and circular layers, the slow wave spreads throughout the smooth muscle of each segment of the gastrointestinal tract.

The amplitude and, to a lesser extent, the frequency of the slow waves can be modulated by the activity of intrinsic and extrinsic nerves and by hormones and paracrine sub-

stances. In general, sympathetic nerve activity decreases the amplitude of the slow waves or abolishes them completely, whereas stimulation of parasympathetic nerves increases the amplitude of the slow waves.

If the peak of the slow wave exceeds the cell's threshold to fire action potentials, one or more action potentials may be triggered during the peak of the slow wave (Fig. 31-6). The action potentials enhance contractile force of the smooth muscle.

Action potentials. Action potentials in gastrointestinal smooth muscle are more prolonged (10 to 20 msec) than those of skeletal muscle and have little or no overshoot. The rising phase of the action potential is caused by ion flow through channels that conduct both Ca^{2+} and Na^+ and are relatively slow to open. Ca^{2+} that enters the cell during the action potential helps to initiate contraction (see Chapter 13).

When the membrane potential of gastrointestinal smooth muscle reaches the electrical threshold, typically near the peak of a slow wave, a train of action potentials (1 to 10/sec) is fired (Fig. 31-6). The extent of depolarization of the cells and the frequency of action potentials are enhanced by some hormones and paracrine agonists and by compounds liberated from excitatory nerve endings. Inhibitory hormones and neuroeffector substances hyperpolarize the smooth muscle cells and may diminish or abolish action potential spikes.

Relationship between membrane potential and tension. Slow waves that are not accompanied by action potentials

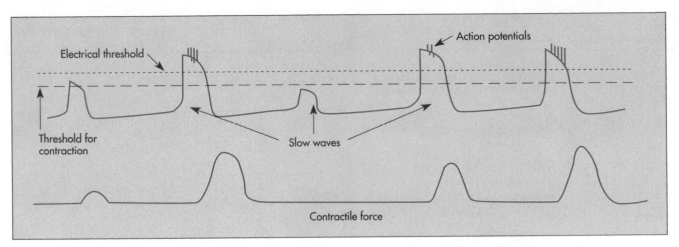

■ **Fig. 31-6** Contraction of small intestinal smooth muscle occurs when the depolarization caused by the slow wave exceeds a threshold for contraction. When depolarization of a slow wave exceeds the electrical threshold, a burst of action potentials occurs. The action potentials elicit a contraction much stronger than occurs in the absence of action potentials. The contractile force increases with increasing number of action potentials. (Modified from Sarna SK: In vivo myoelectric activity: methods, analysis and interpretation. In Wood JD, editor: *Handbook of physiology,* sect 6, *The gastrointestinal system,* vol 1, pt. 2, Bethesda, Md, 1989, American Physiological Society.)

elicit weak contractions of the smooth muscle cells (Fig. 31-6). Much stronger contractions are evoked by the action potentials that are intermittently triggered near the peaks of the slow waves. The greater the number of action potentials that occur at the peak of a slow wave, the more intense is the contraction of the smooth muscle. Because smooth muscle cells contract rather slowly (about one tenth as fast as skeletal muscle cells), the individual contractions caused by each action potential in a train do not cause distinct twitches; rather, they sum temporally to produce a smoothly increasing level of tension (Fig. 31-6).

Between trains of action potentials the tension developed by gastrointestinal smooth muscle falls, but not to zero. This nonzero resting, or baseline, tension of smooth muscle is called **tone.** The tone of gastrointestinal smooth muscle is altered by neuroeffectors, hormones, paracrine substances, and drugs.

Electrical coupling between smooth muscle cells. Neighboring cells are described as "well coupled electrically" if a charge in the membrane potential of one cell spreads rapidly, and with little decrease, to the adjacent cell. The smooth muscle cells of the circular layer are better coupled than are those of the longitudinal layer. The cells of the circular layer are joined by frequent gap junctions that allow the spread of electrical current from one cell to another (see Chapter 4).

NEURAL CONTROL OF GASTROINTESTINAL ACTIVITIES

Control of the contractile and secretory activities of the gastrointestinal tract involves the central nervous system, the enteric nervous system, and hormones and paracrine substances. The autonomic nervous system typically only modulates the patterns of muscular and secretory activity; these activities are controlled more directly by the enteric nervous system.

Neuromuscular Interactions

The neurons of the intramural plexuses send axons to the smooth muscle layers, and each axon may branch extensively to innervate many smooth muscle cells. Neuromuscular interactions in the gastrointestinal tract do not involve true neuromuscular junctions with specialization of the postjunctional membrane, as occurs at neuromuscular junctions in skeletal muscle (see Chapter 4).

The circular smooth muscle layer of the muscularis externa is heavily innervated by excitatory and inhibitory motor nerve terminals that are closely associated with the plasma membranes of the smooth muscle cells of this layer. In contrast, longitudinal smooth muscle cells are much less richly innervated by the neurons of the intrinsic plexuses than are the circular layer cells, and the neuromuscular contacts are not as intimate.

Sympathetic and Parasympathetic Control of Gastrointestinal Function

The major types of sympathetic and parasympathetic input to the gastrointestinal tract are summarized in Table 31-2. Most sympathetic and parasympathetic fibers project not onto muscle or gland cells in the gastrointestinal tract, but rather onto neurons of the enteric nervous system. Exceptions include the direct sympathetic innervation of gastrointestinal blood vessels.

■ **Table 31-2** Extrinsic neurons of the gastrointestinal tract

Neural pathway	Function
In motor pathways	Sympathetic motility-inhibiting neurons
	Sympathetic vasoconstrictor neurons
	Sympathetic secretomotor-inhibiting neurons
	Vagal inputs to enteric inhibitory pathways
	Vagal inputs to enteric excitatory pathways
	Pelvic nerve inputs to enteric excitatory and inhibitory pathways and to enteric vasodilatory pathways
	Vagal inputs promoting gastrin and acid secretion
In sensory pathways	Mechanoreceptor neurons
	Chemoceptive neurons
	Nociceptive neurons

The cell bodies of efferent neurons are in vagal nuclei, sympathetic ganglia, or the sacral spinal cord. The cell bodies of sensory neurons are in vagal nuclei or in dorsal root ganglia. (Adapted from Costa M, Furness JB: In Makhlouf GM, editor: *Handbook of physiology,* sect 6, *The gastrointestinal system,* vol II, *Neural and endocrine biology,* Bethesda, Md, 1989, American Physiological Society.)

■ **Table 31-3** Neurons of the enteric nervous system

Type of neuron	Function
Motor neurons	
Motor neurons to muscle cells	
Excitatory	Promote contraction of smooth muscle
Inhibitory	Inhibit contraction of smooth muscle
Motor neurons to blood vessels	Vasodilator neurons
Moton neurons to epithelial cells	Promote secretion of electrolytes and water
Motor neurons to gland cells	Promote secretion of specific substances
Motor neurons to endocrine cells	Promote secretion of hormones
Sensory neurons	Respond to stretch or to chemical stimuli
Associative neurons	Interneurons in motor, secretomotor, and vasomotor pathways
Intestinofugal neurons	Neurons with cell bodies in enteric ganglia and nerve terminals in sympathetic ganglia

Afferent fibers are abundant in the sympathetic and parasympathetic nerves to the gastrointestinal tract. These fibers carry signals from chemosensitive and mechanosensitive nerve endings in the wall of the gastrointestinal tract. The cell bodies of the afferent fibers in the sympathetic nerves are located primarily in dorsal root ganglia. The cell bodies of the afferent fibers in the branches of the vagus nerves are located in the nodose ganglion and in the solitary nucleus, whereas cell bodies of the afferent fibers in the pelvic nerves are located in sacral dorsal root ganglia. Some central afferent fibers have collaterals that project to enteric neurons or to smooth muscle.

The reflex control of gastrointestinal function effected by autonomic sensory and efferent fibers provides a central level of control that overlies and influences the local reflex control by the enteric nervous system. The central reflex pathways are clearly required for coordination of the activities of gastrointestinal regions that are located far away from one another. An example of this long-range control is the gastrocolic reflex: increased motor and secretory activity in the colon is coordinated with increased contractile and secretory activity in the stomach.

The Enteric Nervous System

As previously stated, the plexuses that make up the enteric nervous system function as a scmiautonomous nervous system that controls the motor and secretory activities of the digestive system. Figure 31-4 depicts the myenteric and submucosal plexuses and their locations in the wall of the intestine. Both plexuses consist of ganglia that are interconnected by tracts of fine, unmyelinated nerve fibers. Some neurons in the ganglia (Table 31-3) are sensory neurons; the sensory endings of these neurons are located in the gastrointestinal tract. Some of the neurons in the enteric ganglia are effector neurons that send axons to smooth muscle cells of the circular or longitudinal layers and muscularis mucosae, to secretory cells of the gastrointestinal tract, or to gastrointestinal blood vessels. Many of the neurons in the enteric ganglia are interneurons; these neurons form part of the neuronal network that integrates the sensory input to the ganglia and formulates the output of the effector neurons.

Neuromodulatory substances. Most of the neurotransmitters and neuromodulatory substances that function in the central nervous system (see Chapter 4) also function in the gastrointestinal tract. Table 31-4 lists some of the neuroactive substances present in the gastrointestinal tract and summarizes current knowledge about the functions of these substances in gastrointestinal control.

Table 31-5 shows the quantitative distribution of neuroactive substances, or biochemical markers of these substances, in neurons of the myenteric and submucosal ganglia of guinea pig small intestine. The distribution of neuroactive substances in myenteric neurons differs from their distribution in submucosal neurons. Enteric neurons often contain more than one putative neurotransmitter or neuromodulator, and these neurons may release more than one neuroactive substance in response to stimulation. The combination of neuroactive substances present in a particular neuron correlates with the morphology and function of the neuron and with its projections.

Functions of enteric neurons. The types of neurons in the enteric nervous system and their major functions are summarized in Table 31-3.

Myenteric neurons. Most neurons in myenteric ganglia are motor neurons. The motor neurons in myenteric ganglia

■ Table 31-4   Substances that may be neurotransmitters or neuromodulators in the enteric nervous system

Substance	Location and function
Established and probable neurotransmitters	
Acetylcholine (ACh)	Excitatory transmitter to smooth muscle, intestinal epithelial cells, parietal cells, certain endocrine cells, and at neuroneuronal synapses
Adenosine triphosphate (ATP)	Inhibitory transmitter to smooth muscle
Calcitonin gene-related peptide (CGRP)	Released by enteric sensory neurons onto interneurons in enteric ganglia and central ganglia
Gastric-releasing peptide	Released by secretomotor neurons onto G cells
Nitric oxide (NO)	Inhibitory transmitter to smooth muscle cells
Substance P (and other tachykinins)	Excitatory transmitter to smooth muscle cells
Vasoactive intestinal peptide (VIP)	Inhibitory transmitter to smooth muscle cells, excitatory secretomotor transmitter to epithelial and gland cells, vasodilatory transmitter
Present in neurons, but transmitter function not established	
Cholecysokinin (CCK)	Present in some secretomotor neurons and interneurons, may contribute to excitation
Dynorphin and related peptides	Present in some secretomotor neurons, interneurons, and motor neurons to muscle
Enkephalins and related peptides	Present in some interneurons and in motor neurons to smooth muscle
Galanin	Present in some secretomotor neurons, interneurons, and inhibitory motor neurons to smooth muscle
Glutamate	May be an excitatory transmitter at synapses between enteric neurons
γ-Aminobutyric acid (GABA)	Present, but transmitter role is not known
Neuropeptide Y	May inhibit secretion of electrolytes and water
Serotonin (5-HT)	May be excitatory transmitter at synapses between enteric neurons
Somatostatin	Present in numerous enteric neurons, but transmitter role is not established

include both excitatory and inhibitory neurons. These neurons project to the smooth muscle cells of the muscularis externa. The myenteric ganglia also contain sensory neurons and interneurons. About one third of neurons in myenteric ganglia are sensory. Other myenteric neurons project to neurons in submucosal ganglia or to mucosal effectors.

Excitatory motor neurons release **acetylcholine** onto **muscarinic receptors** on the smooth muscle cells; they also release **substance P** or other members of the tachykinin family of neuropeptides. Inhibitory motor neurons release **vasoactive intestinal polypeptide (VIP)** and **nitric oxide (NO)**. There is a positive interaction between VIP and NO. NO produced in nerve terminals promotes release of VIP. VIP binds to receptors on smooth muscle cells that are coupled to NO synthase there. NO produced in the smooth muscle cells relaxes them and also diffuses back into nerve terminals to promote more VIP release. ATP is also an inhibitory transmitter in some locations. Quantitatively, NO is the most important mediator of relaxation of gastrointestinal smooth muscles. Most myenteric interneurons release acetylcholine onto **nicotinic receptors** on motor neurons or on other interneurons.

Submucosal neurons. Most neurons in submucosal ganglia regulate glandular, endocrine, and epithelial cell secretion. Stimulatory secretomotor neurons release acetylcholine and VIP onto gland cells or epithelial cells. The submucosal ganglia also have numerous sensory neurons. These neurons are the afferent limbs of the secretomotor reflexes. Traffic in the sensory neurons is evoked by chemical stimuli or by mechanical deformation of the mucosa. Most mucosal sensory neurons do not respond directly to sensory stimuli. Enterochromaffin cells (EC cells) in the mucosa release

■ Table 31-5   Neurochemically identified nerve cell bodies in myenteric ganglia of guinea pig small intestine

Neurochemical	Proportion (%)
Myenteric ganglia about 10,000 neurons/cm length	
Aromatic amine handling	0.5
Acetylcholinesterase	High
Calcium-binding protein	30
Cholecystokinin	6
Calcitonin gene-related peptide	2
Choline acetyltransferase	High
Dynorphin	49
Enkephalin	51
Gastrin-releasing peptide	19
Monoamine oxidase B	10
Neuropeptide Y	28
Nitric oxide (NO)	10
Somatostatin	6
Substance P	37
Vasoactive intestinal peptide	39
Submucosal ganglia about 7000 neurons/cm length	
Dynorphin/galanin/vasoactive intestinal peptide	45
Choline acetyltransferase/cholecystokinin/ calcitonin gene-related peptide/(galanin)/ neuropeptide Y/somatostatin	20
Choline acetyltransferase/substance P	11
Choline acetyltransferase	14
NO synthase	10
Aromatic amine handling	11

Adapted from Costa M, Furness JB: In Makhlouf GM, editor: *Handbook of physiology,* sect 6, *The gastrointestinal system,* vol II, *Neural and endocrine biology,* Bethesda, Md, 1989, American Physiological Society.

serotonin (5-HT) in response to mechanical or chemical stimuli. Sensory neurons are then stimulated by serotonin. Sensory neurons project to enteric ganglia and dorsal root ganglia, where many of them release calcitonin gene-related peptide (CGRP) onto interneurons. Submucosal interneurons release acetylcholine onto other neurons in submucosal ganglia or project to myenteric ganglia. Submucosal ganglia also contain vasodilator neurons that release acetylcholine and/or VIP onto submucosal blood vessels.

Intrinsic reflexes. All of the component cells of an **intrinsic reflex** are located in the wall of the gastrointestinal tract.

Numerous intrinsic reflexes control the motor and secretory activities of each segment of the gastrointestinal tract. A well-characterized intrinsic reflex is shown in Fig. 31-7. *Localized mechanical or chemical stimulation of the intestinal mucosa elicits contraction above (oral to) and relaxation below (anal to) the point of stimulation.*

CHEWING (MASTICATION)

Although chewing is sometimes a voluntary behavior it is more frequently a reflex behavior. Chewing performs several

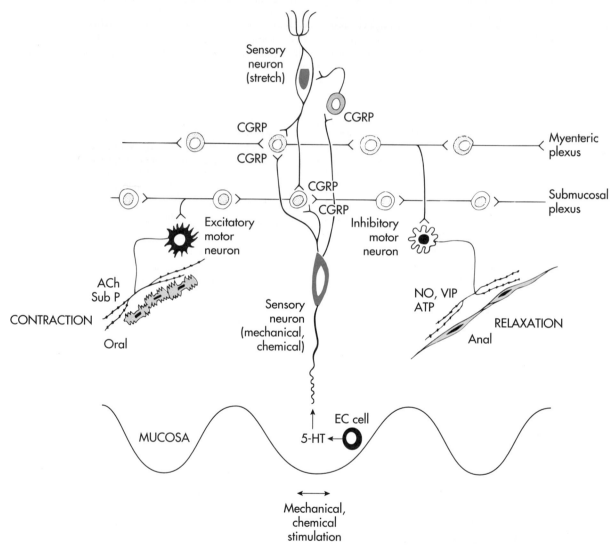

■ **Fig. 31-7**   Localized mechanical or chemical stimulation of the intestinal mucosa or stretch of the muscularis externa typically elicits contraction above and relaxation below the point of stimulation. This figure depicts the neuronal circuitry responsible for this reflex. In the center of the figure are two sensory neurons: a stretch-sensitive neuron with soma in the myenteric plexus (white cytoplasm, colored nucleus) and a chemosensitive or mechanosensitive neuron whose soma is in the submucosal plexus. Stimulation of either of these sensory neurons results in activation of ascending (oral) excitation and descending (anal) inhibition of contraction of the smooth muscle of muscularis externa. Stimuli to the mucosa evoke release of serotonin (5-HT) from enterochromaffin (EC) cells in the mucosa. Sensory neurons are stimulated by 5-HT. The myenteric stretch receptors, by contrast, respond directly to stretch. Sensory neurons release predominantly calcitonin gene-related peptide *(CGRP)* onto interneurons in the enteric plexuses. *ACh,* Acetylcholine; *Sub P,* substance P; *VIP,* vasoactive intestinal peptide; *NO,* nitric oxide. (Courtesy of Dr. Terence K. Smith.)

functions. It lubricates food by mixing it with salivary mucus. If the food contains starch, salivary amylase, an enzyme that breaks down starch, is added to the food during chewing. Finally, chewing mechanically chops food into smaller pieces so that it can be swallowed and propelled more easily, and more readily mixed with the digestive secretions of the stomach and duodenum.

SWALLOWING

Swallowing can be initiated voluntarily, but thereafter it is almost entirely under reflex control. The swallowing reflex is a rigidly ordered sequence of events that propels food from the mouth to the stomach. This reflex also inhibits respiration and prevents the entrance of food into the trachea (Fig. 31-8) during swallowing. *The afferent limb of the swallowing reflex begins when touch receptors, most notably those near the opening of the pharynx, are stimulated.* Sensory impulses from these receptors are transmitted to an area in the medulla and lower pons called the **swallowing center.** Motor impulses travel from the swallowing center to the musculature of the pharynx and upper esophagus via various cranial nerves and to the remainder of the esophagus by vagal motor neurons.

Swallowing can be divided into three phases: oral, pharyngeal, and esophageal.

Oral Phase

The **oral,** or **voluntary, phase,** of swallowing is initiated when the tip of the tongue separates a bolus of food from the mass of food in the mouth. First the tip of the tongue, and later the more posterior portions of the tongue, press against the hard palate. The action of the tongue moves the bolus upward and then backward into the mouth. The bolus is forced into the pharynx, where it stimulates the touch receptors that initiate the swallowing reflex.

Pharyngeal Phase

The **pharyngeal phase** of swallowing involves the following sequence of events, which occurs in less than 1 second:

1. The soft palate is pulled upward and the palatopharyngeal folds move inward toward one another. These movements prevent reflux of food into the nasopharynx and open a narrow passage through which food moves into the pharynx.
2. The vocal cords are pulled together and the larynx is moved forward and upward against the epiglottis. These actions prevent food from entering the trachea and help to open the upper esophageal sphincter.
3. The **upper esophageal sphincter (UES)** relaxes to receive the bolus of food (Fig. 31-9). The superior constrictor muscles of the pharynx then contract strongly to force the bolus deeply into the pharynx.
4. A **peristaltic wave** is initiated with contraction of the pharyngeal superior constrictor muscles, and the wave moves toward the esophagus (Figs. 31-8 and 31-9). This wave forces the bolus of food through the relaxed UES.

During the pharyngeal stage of swallowing, respiration is also reflexly inhibited.

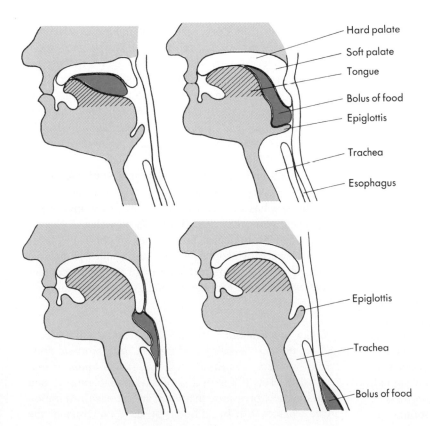

Hard palate
Soft palate
Tongue
Bolus of food
Epiglottis
Trachea
Esophagus

Epiglottis

Trachea

Bolus of food

■ **Fig. 31-8**   Major events involved in the swallowing reflex. (Modified from Johnson LR: *Gastrointestinal physiology,* ed 2, St Louis, 1981, Mosby.)

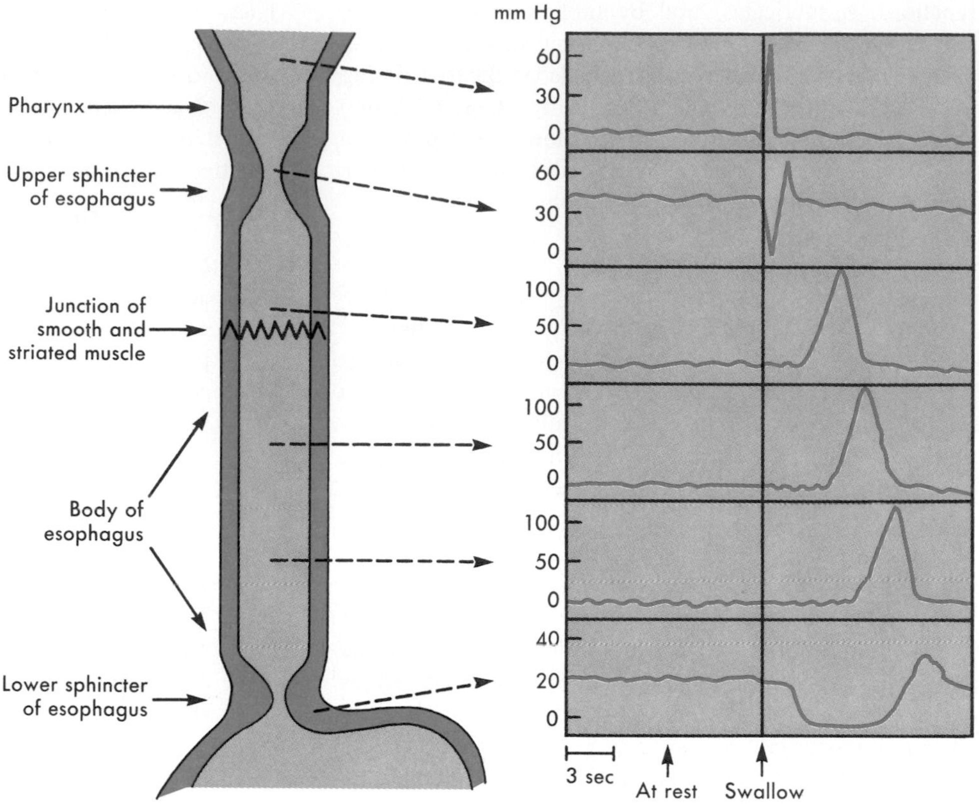

■ **Fig. 31-9** Pressures in the pharynx, esophagus, and esophageal sphincters during swallowing. Note the reflex relaxation of the upper and lower esophageal sphincters and the timing of their relaxation. (Redrawn from Christensen J: In Christensen J, Wingate DL, editors: *A guide to gastrointestinal motility,* Bristol, UK, 1983, John Wright & Sons.)

Esophageal Phase

The **esophageal phase** of swallowing is controlled mainly by the swallowing center. After the bolus of food passes the UES, a reflex action causes the sphincter to constrict. A peristaltic wave, which is called **primary peristalsis,** then begins just below the UES. This wave travels at approximately 3 to 5 cm/sec, and traverses the entire esophagus in less than 10 seconds (Fig. 31-9). Primary peristalsis is controlled by the swallowing center. If the primary peristalsis is insufficient to clear the esophagus of food, distension of the esophagus initiates another peristaltic wave, called **secondary peristalsis.** This peristaltic wave begins above the site of distension and moves downward. Input from esophageal sensory fibers to the central and enteric nervous systems modulates both primary and secondary esophageal peristalsis.

ESOPHAGEAL FUNCTION

Function, Structure, and Innervation of the Esophagus

After food is swallowed, the esophagus functions as a conduit to move the food from the pharynx to the stomach. In the upper third of the esophagus, both the inner circular and the outer longitudinal muscle layers are striated. In the lower third, the muscle layers are composed entirely of smooth muscle cells. The middle third contains both skeletal and smooth muscles. Thus, the esophagus contains a gradient of muscle, from all skeletal at the top to all smooth at the bottom.

The esophageal musculature, both striated and smooth, is mainly innervated by branches of the vagus nerve. Motor fibers of the vagus nerve form motor end plates on the striated muscle fibers. Esophageal striated muscles are dually innervated by excitatory nerves that release acetylcholine and inhibitory nerves that release NO. Esophageal smooth muscle is innervated by visceral motor nerves that are preganglionic parasympathetic fibers that synapse primarily on the nerve cells of the myenteric plexus. *Neurons of the myenteric plexus directly innervate the smooth muscle cells of the esophagus and communicate with one another.* The neural circuits that control esophageal motility are schematized in Fig. 31-10.

The **UES** and the **lower esophageal sphincter (LES)** prevent the entry of air and gastric contents, respectively, into the esophagus. The LES opens with the initiation of esophageal peristalsis (Fig. 31-9). The opening of the LES is mediated by impulses in branches of the vagus nerve. In the absence of esophageal peristalsis, the sphincter remains tightly closed to prevent reflux of the gastric contents, which would cause esophagitis and the sensation known as "heartburn."

Reflux is particularly problematic because the pressure in the thoracic esophagus is close to intrathoracic pressure, which is almost always less than intraabdominal pressure. The difference between intraabdominal and intrathoracic pressures increases during each inspiration (see Chapter 26). In addition, because the crura of the

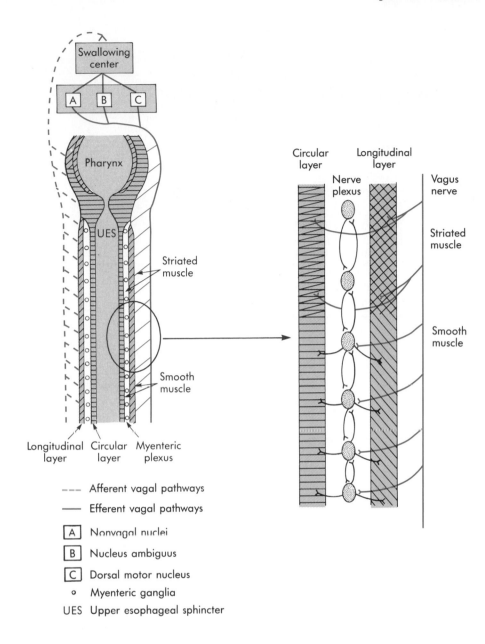

Longitudinal   Circular   Myenteric
layer   layer   plexus

- - - Afferent vagal pathways
⎯⎯ Efferent vagal pathways
[A] Nonvagal nuclei
[B] Nucleus ambiguus
[C] Dorsal motor nucleus
o Myenteric ganglia
UES Upper esophageal sphincter

■ **Fig. 31-10**   Local and central neural circuits involved in the control of esophageal motility. *Left,* Motor neurons reach the esophagus in branches of the vagus nerves, and sensory feedback to the swallowing center is carried by vagal afferent fibers. *Right,* Enlarged view of the circled region of the esophagus to show vagal motor neurons that innervate the striated muscle of the pharynx and upper esophagus, and vagal visceral motor neurons that innervate the smooth muscle of the lower esophagus. Note that the visceral motor neurons terminate predominantly on neurons of the myenteric plexus. Motor neurons to striated and smooth muscle are both excitatory and inhibitory. *UES,* Upper esophageal sphincter. (Adapted from Johnson LR: *Gastrointestinal physiology,* ed 5, St Louis, 1997, Mosby.)

diaphragm wrap around the esophagus at the level of the LES, contraction of the diaphragm helps to increase the pressure in the LES with each inspiration. In individuals with weakness of the diaphragm, and particularly in those with **hiatal hernia,** esophagitis may be caused by increased reflux.

Lower Esophageal Sphincter

Control of LES tone.   The resting pressure in the LES is about 20 mm Hg. The tonic contraction of the circular musculature of the sphincter is regulated by nerves, both intrinsic and extrinsic, and by hormones and neuromodulators. A significant fraction of this basal tone in this sphincter is mediated by vagal cholinergic nerves. Stimulation of sympathetic nerves to the sphincter also causes the LES to contract.

Relaxation of the LES.   The intrinsic and extrinsic innervation of the LES is both excitatory and inhibitory (Fig. 31-11). Vagal excitatory fibers are predominantly cholinergic. The relaxation of the sphincter that occurs in response to primary peristalsis in the esophagus is primarily mediated by vagal fibers that inhibit the circular muscle of the LES. Although the inhibitory neurotransmitter is not known with certainty, it is thought that VIP and NO mediate this relaxation of the LES.

In some individuals, the sphincter fails to relax sufficiently during swallowing to allow food to enter the stomach. This condition is known as **achalasia.** Therapy for achalasia involves either mechanically dilating or surgically weakening the LES or administering drugs that inhibit its tone. In individuals with **diffuse esophageal spasm,** prolonged and painful contraction of the lower

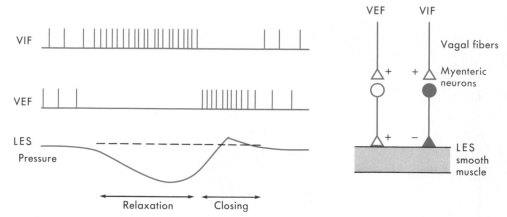

■ **Fig. 31-11**   The lower esophageal sphincter (LES) is innervated by both vagal excitatory fibers (VEF) and vagal inhibitory fibers (VIF). Relaxation of the LES is associated with an increased frequency of action potentials in VIF and decreased frequency of action potentials in VEF. Reciprocal changes occur when the sphincter regains its resting tone. (Adapted from Miolan JP, Roman C: *J Physiol Paris* 74:709, 1978.)

part of the esophagus occurs after swallowing, instead of the normal esophageal peristaltic wave. In individuals with **incompetence of the LES,** gastric juice can move back up into the lower esophagus and erode the esophageal mucosa.

Sensory neurons in the lower esophagus that respond to acid evoke a vagovagal reflux that promotes closure of the LES and relaxation of the stomach.

GASTRIC MOTILITY

The major functions of gastric motility are (1) to allow the stomach to serve as a reservoir for the large volume of food that may be ingested at a single meal, (2) to break food into smaller particles and mix food with gastric secretions so that digestion can begin, and (3) to empty gastric contents into the duodenum at a controlled rate.

Figure 31-12 shows the major anatomic subdivisions of the stomach. *The **fundus** and the **body** of the stomach can accommodate volume increases as large as 1.5 L without a great increase in intragastric pressure;* this phenomenon is called **receptive relaxation.** Distension of the esophagus during swallowing evokes relaxation of the stomach via a vagovagal reflex. Because the contractions of the fundus and body are normally weak, much of the gastric contents remains relatively unmixed for long periods. *The fundus and the body thus serve the reservoir functions of the stomach. In the antrum, however, contractions are vigorous.* These contractions break the food down into smaller pieces and mix the food thoroughly with gastric juice. At this point, the partly digested food is a semisolid mass called *chyme.* The antral contractions "feed" the chyme in small squirts into the duodenal bulb. *Several mechanisms adjust the rate of gastric emptying so that chyme is not*

delivered to the duodenum too rapidly. The physiological mechanisms that underlie gastric motility are discussed below.

Structure and Innervation of the Stomach

The basic structure of the gastric wall follows the general scheme presented in Fig. 31-1. The circular muscle layer of the muscularis externa is more prominent than the longitudinal layer. The muscularis externa of the fundus and the body of the stomach is relatively thin. In contrast, the muscularis externa of the antrum is considerably thicker, and it increases in thickness toward the pylorus. In the antrum and pylorus, the inner layer of obliquely oriented muscle cells is incomplete.

The stomach is richly innervated by extrinsic nerves and by the neurons of the enteric nervous system. Axons from the cells of the intramural plexuses innervate smooth muscle and secretory cells.

Parasympathetic innervation is supplied by the vagus nerves, while sympathetic innervation is provided by the celiac plexus. In general, parasympathetic nerves stimulate gastric smooth muscle motility and gastric secretions, whereas sympathetic activity inhibits these functions. Numerous sensory afferent fibers leave the stomach in the vagus nerves; some of these fibers travel with sympathetic nerves. Other sensory neurons are the afferent links between sensory receptors and the intramural plexuses of the stomach. Some of these afferent fibers relay information about intragastric pressure, gastric distention, intragastric pH, or pain.

Responses to Gastric Filling

When a wave of esophageal peristalsis begins, a reflex causes the LES to relax. This relaxation of the LES is followed by *receptive relaxation of the fundus and body of the stomach.* The stomach will also relax if it is filled directly with gas or

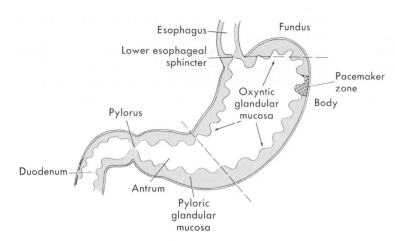

liquid. The nerve fibers in the vagi are a major efferent pathway for reflex relaxation of the stomach. The vagal fibers that mediate this response may release VIP and/or NO as their transmitters.

Mixing and Emptying of Gastric Contents

The muscle layers in the fundus and body are thin; weak contractions characterize these parts of the stomach. As a result, the contents of the fundus and the body settle into layers based on the density of the contents. Gastric contents may remain unmixed for as long as 1 hour after eating. *Fats tend to form an oily layer on top of the other gastric contents. Consequently, fats are emptied later than are the other gastric contents.* Liquids can flow around the mass of food contained in the body of the stomach and are emptied more rapidly into the duodenum (Fig. 31-13). Solid food is emptied more slowly. Large or indigestible particles are retained in the stomach for even longer periods.

When food enters the stomach, gastric contractions begin. These contractions usually begin in the middle of the body of the stomach and travel toward the pylorus. They increase in force and velocity as they approach the gastroduodenal junction. Thus, *the major mixing activity occurs in the antrum of the stomach.* The contents of the antrum are mixed rapidly and thoroughly with gastric secretions as a result of these forceful, rapid contractions. As each peristaltic wave reaches the pylorus, the pyloric sphincter snaps shut, so that the stomach empties in small squirts, one for each peristaltic wave. Food particles larger than 2 mm do not pass through the narrow pyloric opening. The rapid contraction of the terminal antrum propels the chyme back into the antrum; this movement is called retropulsion. Retropulsion is particularly effective at mixing and breaking down gastric contents.

Fed versus Fasted State

After an individual eats, the antrum contracts about three times per minute. As discussed later, the rate of gastric emptying is regulated by feedback mechanisms that diminish the force of antral contractions and enhance contraction of the pyloric sphincter.

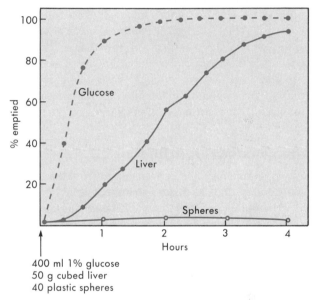

400 ml 1% glucose
50 g cubed liver
40 plastic spheres

■ **Fig. 31-13**   Rates of emptying of different meals from dog stomach. A solution (1% glucose) is emptied faster than a digestible solid (cubed liver). An indigestible solid (7-mm plastic spheres) remains in the stomach until the contractile phase of the migrating myoelectric complex occurs. (Redrawn from Hinder RA, Kelly KA: *Am J Physiol* 233:E335, 1977.)

In a fasted animal, a different pattern of antral contractions occurs. The antrum is quiescent for 75 to 90 minutes, after which a brief period (5 to 10 minutes) of intense electrical and motor activity occurs. *This activity is characterized by strong contractions of the antrum with a relaxed pylorus.* During this period, even large chunks of material that remain from the previous meal are emptied from the stomach. This period of intense contractions is followed by 75 to 90 minutes of quiescence. This cycle of contractions in the stomach is part of a pattern of contractile activity that periodically sweeps from the stomach to the terminal ileum during fasting. This cyclic contractile activity is known as the **migrating myoelectric complex (MMC)** (discussed later).

Electrical Activity and Gastric Contractions

The gastric peristaltic waves occur at about the frequency of the gastric slow waves that are generated by a **pacemaker zone** (Fig. 31-12) located near the middle of the body of the stomach. These waves are conducted toward the pylorus. In humans, the frequency of slow waves is about three per minute.

The gastric slow wave is triphasic (Fig. 31-14), and its shape resembles the action potentials in cardiac muscle. However, the gastric slow wave lasts about 10 times longer than does the cardiac action potential, and it does not overshoot.

Gastric smooth muscle contracts when the depolarization during the slow wave exceeds the threshold for contraction (Fig. 31-14). The greater the extent of depolarization and the longer the muscle cell remains depolarized above the threshold, the greater is the force of contraction. In the gastric antrum, action potential spikes frequently occur during the plateau phase (Fig. 31-15). *The contraction that results from these action potentials is much stronger* than a contraction that occurs in the absence of action potentials. Acetylcholine and the hormone **gastrin** stimulate gastric contractility by increasing the amplitude and duration of the plateau phase of the gastric slow wave. Norepinephrine has the opposite effect.

Gastroduodenal Junction

The pylorus separates the gastric antrum from the first part of the **duodenum,** the **duodenal bulb.** The pylorus functions as a sphincter. The circular smooth muscle of the pylorus forms two ringlike thickenings that are followed by a connective tissue ring that separates the pylorus from the duodenum.

The electrical rhythm of the duodenum is 10 to 12 slow waves per minute, which is much faster than the three per minute of the stomach. The electrical activity of the duodenal bulb is influenced by the basic electrical rhythms of both the stomach and the postbulbar duodenum. The bulb thus contracts somewhat irregularly. However, the contractions of the antrum and duodenum are coordinated; when the antrum contracts, the duodenal bulb is often relaxed.

The essential functions of the gastroduodenal junction are (1) to *allow the carefully regulated emptying of gastric contents* at a rate consistent with the ability of the duodenum to process the chyme and (2) *to prevent regurgitation of duodenal contents* back into the stomach.

> The gastric mucosa is highly resistant to acid, but it may be damaged by bile. The duodenal mucosa has the opposite properties. Thus, if gastric emptying is too rapid, a **duodenal ulcer** may develop. On the other hand, regurgitation of duodenal contents may contribute to **gastric ulcers.** Gastric ulcers may be exacerbated when gastric emptying is slower than normal.

The pylorus is densely innervated by both vagal and sympathetic nerve fibers. Sympathetic fibers increase the constriction of the pyloric sphincter. Vagal fibers are both excitatory and inhibitory to pyloric smooth muscle. Excitatory cholinergic vagal fibers stimulate constriction of the sphincter. Inhibitory vagal fibers release another transmitter, probably **VIP** or **NO,** that relaxes the sphincter. The hormones **cholecystokinin (CCK), gastrin, gastric inhibitory peptide (GIP),** and **secretin** all promote constriction of the pyloric sphincter and thereby slow gastric emptying.

Regulation of Gastric Emptying

The emptying of gastric contents is regulated by both neural and hormonal mechanisms. The duodenal and jejunal mucosa contain receptors that sense acidity, osmotic pressure, certain fats and fat digestion products, and peptides and amino acids (Fig. 31-16). The chyme that leaves the stomach is usually hypertonic, and it becomes even more hypertonic because of the action of the digestive enzymes in the duodenum. *Gastric emptying is slowed by hypertonic solutions in the duodenum, by duodenal pH below 3.5, and by the presence of amino acids and peptides in the duodenum. The presence of fatty acids or monoglycerides (products of fat digestion) in the duodenum also dramatically decreases the rate of gastric emptying.* As a result of these mechanisms:

1. The rate at which fat is emptied into the duodenum does not exceed the rate at which the fat can be emulsified by the bile acids and lecithin of the bile.
2. Acid is not dumped into the duodenum more rapidly than it can be neutralized by pancreatic and duodenal secretions and by other mechanisms.
3. The rates at which the other components of chyme enter the small intestine do not exceed the rate at which the small intestine can process those components.

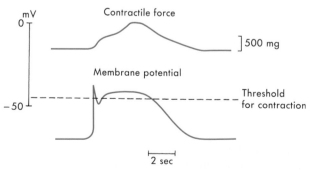

■ **Fig. 31-14**   Relationship between contraction of smooth muscle of dog stomach *(upper tracing)* and intracellularly recorded slow wave *(lower tracing).* Note the triphasic shape of the slow wave in gastric smooth muscle. Contraction occurs when the depolarizing phase of the slow wave exceeds the threshold for contraction, even though there are no action potential spikes on the plateau of the slow wave. When action potentials occur, a much stronger contraction is elicited. (Redrawn from Szurszewski J: *Electrical basis for gastrointestinal motility.* In Johnson LR, editor: *Physiology of the gastrointestinal tract,* New York, 1981, Raven Press.)

The slowing of gastric emptying in response to the different components of the duodenal contents is mediated by neural and hormonal mechanisms:

1. *Acid in the duodenum.* In response to acid in the duodenum, the force of gastric contractions promptly decreases and duodenal motility increases. This response has neural and hormonal components. The presence of acid in the duodenum releases **secretin,** which diminishes the rate of gastric emptying by inhibiting antral contractions and by stimulating contraction of the pyloric sphincter (Fig. 31-17). Neural reflexes evoked by acid in the duedenum also increase contraction of the pyloric sphincter.

2. *Fat-digestion products.* The presence of fat-digestion products in the duodenum and jejunum decreases the rate of gastric emptying. This response results partly from the release of **CCK** from the duodenum and jejunum. CCK decreases the rate of gastric emptying. The presence of fatty acids in the duodenum and jejunum releases another hormone, **GIP,** that also decreases the rate of gastric emptying. In addition to its hormonal effects, CCK also stimulates duodenal neurons that initiate vagovagal reflexes that diminish the rate of gastric emptying.

3. *Osmotic pressure of duodenal contents.* Hyperosmotic solutions in the duodenum and jejunum slow the rate

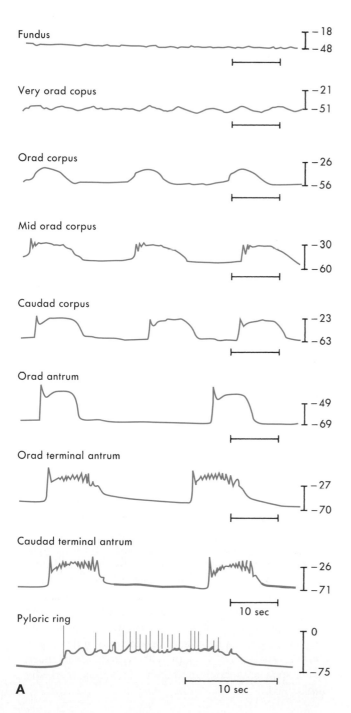

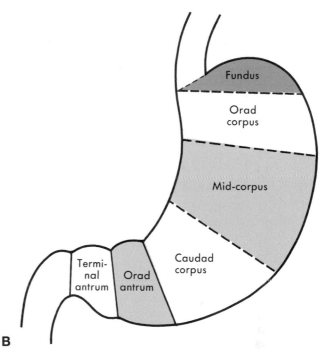

■ **Fig. 31-15**   Intracellular recordings (**A**) of the electrical activity in smooth muscle cells of isolated strips of various regions (**B**) of a dog's stomach. Note that slow waves are absent in the fundus and weak in the orad corpus, and gain in strength and definition toward the antrum. Only in the terminal antrum and pylorus do action potential spikes occur on the plateaus of the slow waves. Action potential spikes are associated with stronger contractions. In the intact stomach, the slow waves in the different parts of the stomach have the same frequency because they are driven by the same pacemaker. In these records, the intrinsic slow wave frequency differs in the isolated strips of muscle. (Redrawn from Szurszewski J: *Electrical basis for gastrointestinal motility.* In Johnson LR, editor: *Physiology of the gastrointestinal tract,* New York, 1981, Raven Press.)

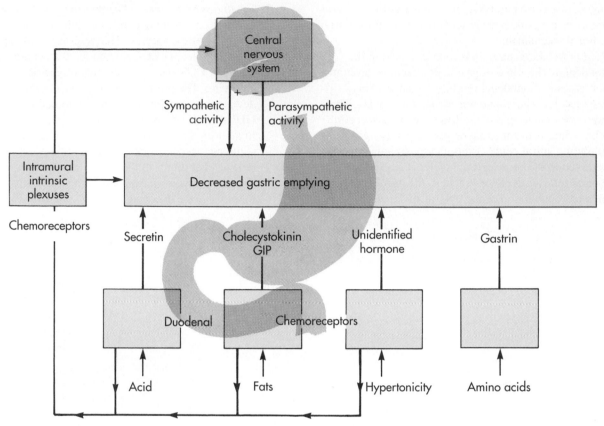

■ **Fig. 31-16** Duodenal stimuli elicit neural and hormonal inhibition of gastric emptying. *GIP,* Gastric inhibitory peptide.

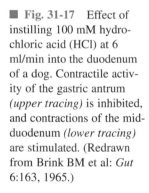
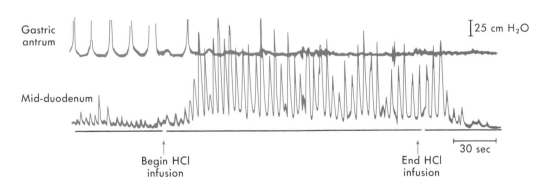

of gastric emptying. This response has both neural and hormonal components. Hypertonic solutions in the duodenum release an unidentified hormone that slows the rate of gastric emptying.

4. *Peptides and amino acids in the duodenum.* Peptides and amino acids release **gastrin** from **G cells** located in the antrum of the stomach and the duodenum. Gastrin increases the strength of antral contractions and increases constriction of the pyloric sphincter; the net effect of these actions usually diminishes the rate of gastric emptying. Release of GIP and CCK is also promoted by the presence of peptides and amino acids in the duodenum; these hormones also

contribute to a decreased rate of gastric emptying in response to amino acids in the duodenum.

In some patients with **duodenal ulcers,** the effectiveness of the mechanisms that release hormones from the duodenum may be diminished. As a result of this malfunction, the rate of gastric emptying or of gastric acid secretion is abnormally high. In normal individuals, instillation of acid into the duodenum via a nasogastric tube dramatically decreases the rate and force of contractions of the gastric antrum. However, in some patients with duodenal ulcer, this response to acid in the duodenum is markedly diminished.

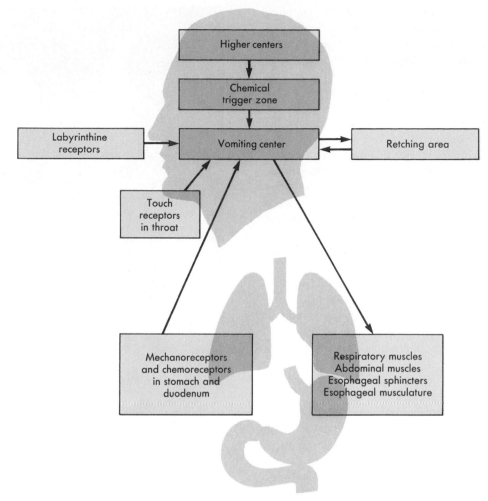

■ Fig. 31-18   Some aspects of control of vomiting.

VOMITING

Vomiting is the expulsion of gastric (and sometimes duodenal) contents from the gastrointestinal tract via the mouth. Vomiting is often preceded by a feeling of nausea, a rapid or irregular heartbeat, dizziness, sweating, pallor, and dilation of the pupils. It is usually preceded by **retching,** in which gastric contents are forced up into the esophagus but do not enter the pharynx.

Vomiting is a reflex behavior controlled and coordinated by a **vomiting center** in the medulla oblongata (Fig. 31-18). Many areas in the body have receptors that provide afferent input to the vomiting center. *Distension of the stomach and duodenum is a strong stimulus that elicits vomiting. Tickling the back of the throat, painful injury to the genitourinary system, dizziness, and certain other stimuli can bring about nausea and vomiting.*

Certain chemicals, called **emetics,** can also elicit vomiting. Some emetics stimulate receptors in the stomach, or more often in the duodenum. **Ipecac,** a commonly used emetic, stimulates duodenal receptors. Other emetics (e.g., **apomorphine**) act on receptors in the floor of the fourth ventricle, in an area known as the **chemoreceptor trigger zone.** The chemorecep-

tor trigger zone lies on the blood side of the blood-brain barrier, and thus it can be reached by most blood-borne substances.

*When the **vomiting reflex** is initiated, the sequence of events is the same regardless of the stimulus that initiates the reflex.* Early events in the vomiting reflex include a wave of **reverse peristalsis** that sweeps from the middle of the small intestine to the duodenum. The pyloric sphincter and the stomach relax to receive intestinal contents. A forced inspiration then occurs against a closed glottis. This inspiration decreases intrathoracic pressure, while a lowering of the diaphragm that also occurs during this inspiration increases intraabdominal pressure. The forced inspiration is followed by a forceful contraction of abdominal muscles, which sharply elevates intraabdominal pressure and drives gastric contents into the esophagus. The LES relaxes reflexly to receive the gastric contents, and the pylorus and antrum contract. *When a person retches, the UES remains closed and prevents vomiting.* When the respiratory and abdominal muscles relax, the esophagus is emptied by secondary peristalsis into the stomach. Often, a series of stronger and stronger retches precedes vomiting.

When a person vomits, the rapid propulsion of gastric contents into the esophagus is accompanied by a reflex relaxation of the UES. **Vomitus** is projected into the pharynx and mouth. Entry of vomitus into the trachea is prevented by movement of the vocal cords closer together, closure of the glottis, and inhibition of respiration.

MOTILITY OF THE SMALL INTESTINE

The small intestine makes up about three fourths of the length of the human gastrointestinal tract. It is about 5 m in length, and chyme typically takes 2 to 4 hours to traverse it.

The first 5% or so of the small intestine is the duodenum, which has no mesentery and has a characteristic histology that distinguishes it from the rest of the small intestine. The remaining small intestine is divided into the **jejunum** and the **ileum.** The jejunum is more proximal and occupies about 40% of the length of the small bowel. The ileum is the remaining distal part of the small intestine.

The small intestine, particularly the duodenum and jejunum, is the site where most digestion and absorption take place. The movements of the small intestine mix chyme with digestive secretions, bring fresh chyme into contact with the absorptive surface of the microvilli, and propel chyme toward the colon.

The most frequent type of movement of the small intestine is called **segmentation.** Segmentation (Fig. 31-19) is characterized by closely spaced contractions of the circular muscle layer. These contractions divide the small intestine into small neighboring segments. In rhythmic segmentation, the sites of the circular contractions alternate, so that an individual segment of gut contracts and then relaxes. *Segmentation effectively mixes chyme with digestive secretions* and brings fresh chyme into contact with the mucosal surface.

In contrast to segmentation, **peristalsis** is the progressive contraction of successive sections of circular smooth muscle. The contractions move along the gastrointestinal tract in an orthograde direction. Peristaltic waves occur in the small intestine but usually involve only a short length of intestine. As in other parts of the digestive tract, the slow waves of the smooth muscle cells determine the timing of intestinal contractions.

Electrical Activity of Small Intestinal Smooth Muscle

Regular slow waves occur all along the small intestine. The frequency is highest (11 to 13 per minute in humans) in the duodenum but declines along the length of the small intestine (to a minimum of 8 or 9 per minute in humans) in the terminal part of the ileum. The slow waves may or may not be accompanied by bursts of action potential spikes (Fig. 31-20). When action potentials occur, they elicit strong smooth muscle contractions that cause the major mixing and propulsive movements of the small intestine. Because action potential bursts are localized to short segments of the intestine, they are responsible for the highly localized contractions of the circular smooth muscle that cause segmentation.

The basic electrical rhythm of the small intestine is

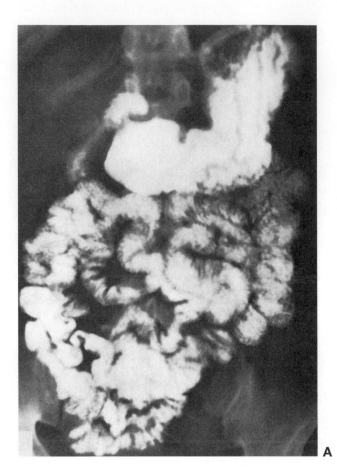

A

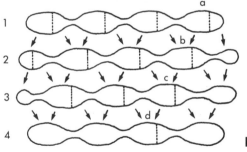

B

■ **Fig. 31-19 A,** X-ray view showing the stomach and small intestine filled with barium contrast medium in a normal individual. Note that segmentation of the small intestine divides its contents into ovoid segments. **B,** The sequence of segmental contractions in a portion of the cat's small intestine. Lines 1 to 4 indicate successive patterns in time. The dotted lines indicate where contractions will occur next. The arrows show the direction of chyme movement. (**A** from Gardner EM et al: *Anatomy: a regional study of human structure,* ed 4, Philadelphia, 1975, WB Saunders. **B** redrawn from Cannon WB: *Am J Physiol* 6:251, 1902.)

entirely intrinsic; that is, it is independent of extrinsic innervation. The frequency of the action potential spike bursts that elicit strong contractions depends on the excitability of the smooth muscle cells of the small intestine. The excitability of the smooth muscle cells is in turn influenced by circulating hormones, the autonomic nervous system, and the enteric neurons. Although direct control of intestinal motility resides in the intramural plexuses, the parasympathetic

Slow

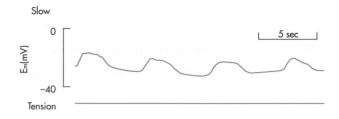

Slow waves and prepotentials that give rise to action

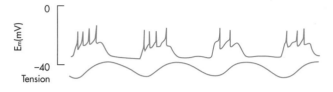

Slow waves and prepotentials that fail to give rise to action

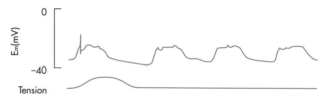

■ **Fig. 31-20** Electrical and contractile activity of isolated longitudinal muscle of rabbit jejunum. The upper tracing in each panel is the transmembrane electrical potential difference (millivolts), and the lower tracing shows contractile tension. Under the conditions shown, the tissue contracts only in response to action potentials. The greater the number of action potentials, the stronger is the contraction. (Redrawn from Bortoff A: *Am J Physiol* 201:203, 1961.)

and sympathetic innervation of the small intestine modulates contractile activity. *Excitability is enhanced by parasympathetic nerves and is inhibited by sympathetic nerves, and both autonomic divisions act via the intramural plexuses.* These modulating extrinsic neural circuits are essential for certain long-range intestinal reflexes (discussed later).

Contractile Behavior of the Small Intestine

Contractions of the duodenal bulb mix the chyme with pancreatic and biliary secretions, and they propel the chyme along the duodenum. Contractions of the duodenal bulb typically occur after contractions of the gastric antrum. This sequence helps prevent regurgitation of duodenal contents back into the stomach.

Segmentation is the most frequent type of movement by the small intestine (Fig. 31-19). The maximal rate of segmental contractions is the same as the frequency of slow waves: 11 or 12 per minute in the duodenum and 8 or 9 per minute in the ileum. In some individuals, the frequency of segmental contractions is fairly constant. In others, periods of segmentation are interrupted by brief periods of relative quiescence.

Short-range peristalsis also occurs in the small intestine, although much less frequently than does segmentation. The relatively low rate of net propulsion of chyme in the small intestine allows time for digestion and absorption.

The importance of the slow rate of propulsion in the small intestine can be demonstrated by treatment of patients with agents that alter small intestinal motility. Administration of **codeine** and other **opiates** markedly reduces the frequency and the volume of stools. This effect results from a decrease in small intestinal motility; this diminished motility in turn increases the transit time of the jejunal contents. The longer transit time allows salts, water, and certain nutrients to be more completely absorbed in the small intestine, so that the volume of contents that enters the colon is less than normal. Treatment with **castor oil,** a potent laxative, causes the opposite effects. Castor oil contains hydroxy fatty acids that stimulate small intestinal motility and decrease small intestinal transit time. Hence, salts and water are delivered to the colon at a rate that overwhelms the ability of the colon to absorb them, and diarrhea results.

Intestinal Reflexes

When a bolus of material is placed in the small intestine, *the intestine typically contracts behind the bolus and relaxes ahead of it* (Fig. 31-7). This response is known as the **law of the intestine.** This action propels the bolus in an orthograde direction, as does a peristaltic wave.

Certain intestinal reflexes can occur along a considerable length of the gastrointestinal tract. These long-range reflexes depend on the function of both intrinsic and extrinsic nerves.

Overdistension of one segment of the intestine relaxes the smooth muscle in the rest of the intestine. This response is known as the **intestinointestinal reflex.**

The stomach and the terminal part of the ileum interact in a reflex called the **gastroileal reflex.** In this response, elevated secretory and motor functions of the stomach increase the motility of the terminal part of the ileum and accelerate the movement of material through the **ileocecal sphincter.** Distension of the ileum evokes neural reflexes and release of peptide YY that diminish the rate of gastric emptying.

Migrating Myoelectric Complex

The contractile behavior of the small intestine previously discussed is characteristic of the period after ingestion of a meal. In a fasted individual or some hours after the processing of a previous meal, the motility of the small intestine follows a different pattern. In this "fasting" pattern, *bursts of intense electrical and contractile activity are separated by longer quiescent periods.* Like the similar pattern that occurs in the stomach during fasting, these bursts of activity in the small intestine and the intervening long periods of quiescence are called the **migrating myoelectric complex (MMC).** An MMC is propagated from the stomach to the terminal ileum.

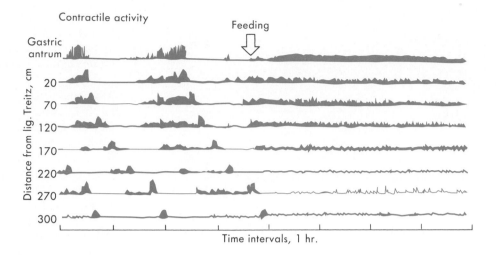

■ **Fig. 31-21** Contractile activity in the stomach and small intestine of a fasting dog, showing the characteristic pattern of the migrating myoelectric complex. The ligament of Treitz marks the border between the duodenum and the jejunum. (From Itoh Z, Sekiguchi T: *Scand J Gastroenterol Suppl* 82:121, 1983.)

In humans, the MMC repeats every 75 to 90 minutes (Fig. 31-21). At about the time that one MMC reaches the distal ileum, a new MMC begins in the stomach. The MMC in the stomach is initiated by vagal impulses that release motilin. Motilin is important in beginning the MMC in the duodenum and small intestine, which does not depend on extrinsic nerves.

Contractions of both stomach and small intestine are more propulsive during the MMC than contractions in a fed individual. In the small intestine, it appears the most propulsive, peristaltic contractions occur just before the period of most intense electrical activity (Fig. 31-21). These peristaltic contractions sweep the contents of the small intestine toward the colon. The MMC has been called the "housekeeper of the small intestine."

The MMC also inhibits the migration of colonic bacteria into the terminal ileum. Individuals with weak or absent MMC contractions may be susceptible to bacterial overgrowth in the ileum. Substances released by the bacteria may stimulate secretion of NaCl and water by the epithelium and increased motility of the ileum and cause diarrhea.

Soon after eating the fed motility pattern returns. Intact vagal innervation is required for this response.

Contractile Activity of the Muscularis Mucosae

Sections of the muscularis mucosae of the small intestine contract irregularly at an average rate of about three contractions per minute. These contractions alter the pattern of ridges and folds of the mucosa, mix the luminal contents, and bring different parts of the mucosal surface into contact with freshly mixed chyme. The villi of the small intestine also contract irregularly, especially in the proximal part of the small intestine. These contractions help to empty the central lacteals of the villi and increase intestinal lymph flow.

Emptying the Ileum

The **ileocecal sphincter,** also known as the **ileocecal valve,** separates the terminal end of the ileum from the **cecum,** the

first part of the colon (Fig. 31-22). Normally, this sphincter is closed. However, short-range peristalsis in the terminal part of the ileum relaxes the sphincter and allows a small amount of chyme to squirt into the cecum. Distension of the distal ileum promotes peristalsis in the ileum and thus the opening of the ileocecal sphincter. Distension of the cecum causes the ileocecal sphincter to close. The ileocecal sphincter normally permits ileal chyme to enter the colon at a rate that allows the colon to absorb most of the salts and water in the chyme. The opening and closing of the ileocecal sphincter are coordinated mainly by the neurons of the intramural plexuses. The extrinsic innervation plays a role in longer-range control of the ileocecal sphincter, such as occurs in the gastroileal reflex.

MOTILITY OF THE COLON

The colon receives 500 to 1500 ml of chyme per day from the ileum. Most of the salts and water that enter the colon are absorbed; the feces normally contain only about 50 to 100 ml of water each day. Colonic contractions mix the chyme and circulate it across the mucosal surface of the colon. As the chyme becomes semisolid, this mixing resembles a kneading process. *Normally, the progress of colonic contents is slow,* about 5 to 10 cm per hour at most.

One to three times daily a wave of contraction, called **mass movement,** occurs in the colon. A mass movement differs from a peristaltic wave because the contracted segments remain contracted for some time. Mass movements push the contents within a significant length of colon in an orthograde direction.

Structure and Innervation of the Colon

The major subdivisions of the colon, or large intestine, are the cecum, the ascending **colon,** the **transverse colon,** the **descending colon,** the **sigmoid colon,** the **rectum,** and the **anal canal** (Fig. 31-22).

The structure of the wall of the large intestine follows the general plan of the gastrointestinal tract presented earlier in this chapter. However, the colon has some characteristic

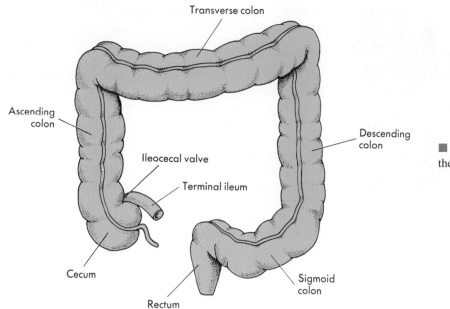

Transverse colon

Ascending colon

Ileocecal valve

Terminal ileum

Cecum

Rectum

Descending colon

Sigmoid colon

■ **Fig. 31-22** Major anatomical subdivisions of the colon.

features. The longitudinal muscle layer of the muscularis externa is concentrated into three bands, called the **taeniae coli.** The longitudinal muscle layer located between the taeniae coli is thin. In contrast, the longitudinal muscle of the rectum and anal canal is substantial and continuous.

Parasympathetic innervation of the cecum and the ascending and transverse colon is via branches of the vagus nerve; that of the descending and sigmoid colon, the rectum, and the anal canal is via the **pelvic nerves** from the sacral spinal cord. The parasympathetic fibers end mainly on neurons of the intramural plexuses. Sympathetic fibers innervate the proximal part of the large intestine via the **superior mesenteric plexus,** the distal part of the large intestine via the **inferior mesenteric** and **superior hypogastric plexuses,** and the rectum and anal canal via the **inferior hypogastric plexus**.

Stimulation of the sympathetic nerves stops colonic movements. Stimulation of the vagal nerves causes segmental contractions of the proximal part of the colon. Stimulation of the pelvic nerves causes expulsive movements of the distal colon and sustained contraction of some segments.

The anal canal is usually kept closed by the internal and external sphincters. The **internal anal sphincter** is a thickening of the *circular smooth muscle* of the anal canal. The **external anal sphincter** is more distal and consists entirely of **striated muscle.** The external anal sphincter is innervated by *somatic motor fibers* via the pudendal nerves. *This innervation allows the anal sphincter to be controlled both by reflexes and voluntarily.*

Motility of the Cecum and Proximal Colon

Most contractions of the cecum and proximal part of the large intestine are segmental, and they are more effective at mixing and circulating the colonic contents than at propelling them. The mixing action facilitates absorption of salts and water by the mucosal epithelium.

Localized segmental contractions divide the colon into neighboring ovoid segments, called **haustra** (Fig. 31-23). Thus, segmentation in the colon is known as **haustration.** The most dramatic difference between haustration and the segmentation that occurs in the small intestine is the regularity of the haustra and the large length of the large intestine involved in haustration at one time. The structural basis for the haustral pattern may be the localized thickenings that occur in the circular muscle of the colon. Haustral contractions, which can increase the local luminal pressure by 10 to 50 mm Hg, result in back-and-forth mixing of luminal contents.

In the proximal colon, "antipropulsive" patterns predominate. Reverse peristalsis and segmental propulsion toward the cecum both take place. Consequently, chyme is retained in the proximal colon, and this retention facilitates the absorption of salts and water.

Motility of the Central and Distal Colon

Normally, a mass movement fills the central and distal parts of the colon with semisolid feces. Segmental haustral contractions knead the feces and thus facilitate the absorption of remaining salts and water. Mass movements then sweep the feces toward the rectum.

Control of Colonic Motility

As in other segments of the gastrointestinal tract, the intramural plexuses directly control the contractile behavior of the colon, while the extrinsic innervation plays a modulating role. Enteric stimulatory motor neurons use acetylcholine and substance P as neurotransmitters; inhibitory enteric motor neurons release VIP and NO onto colonic smooth muscle cells. The extrinsic autonomic nerves to the colon modulate the control of colonic motility by the enteric nervous system. The **defecation reflex** (discussed later) is an exception,

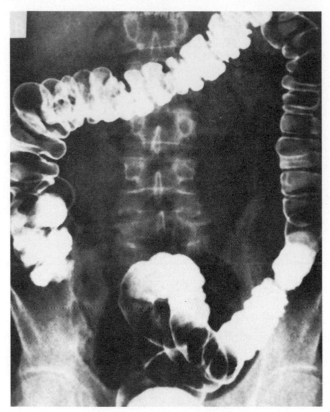

■ **Fig. 31-23**   X-ray image showing a prominent haustral pattern in the colon of a normal individual. (From Keats TE: *An atlas of normal roentgen variants,* ed 2, St Louis, 1979, Mosby.)

because *it requires the function of the spinal cord via the pelvic nerves.*

Electrophysiology of the Colon

Circular muscle. The colon contains two classes of rhythm-generating cells. Interstitial cells near the inner border of the circular muscle produce regular slow waves with a frequency of about six per minute. The slow waves have high amplitude and their shape resembles that of gastric slow waves. Interstitial cells near the outer border of the circular muscle produce **myenteric potential oscillations.** These oscillations are low in amplitude and much higher in frequency than the slow waves.

The circular muscle of the colon does not usually fire action potentials. Contractile agonists, such as acetylcholine released from excitatory enteric motor neurons, enhance contractions by increasing the *duration of some of the slow waves.* These longer slow waves elicit contractions of the circular muscle (Fig. 31-24).

Longitudinal muscle. Longitudinal colonic muscle displays myenteric potential oscillations. In contrast to the circular smooth muscle, however, the longitudinal muscle cells fire occasional action potentials at the peaks of the myenteric potential oscillations. The action potentials elicit contraction of the longitudinal muscle. Contractile agonists increase the frequency of action potentials.

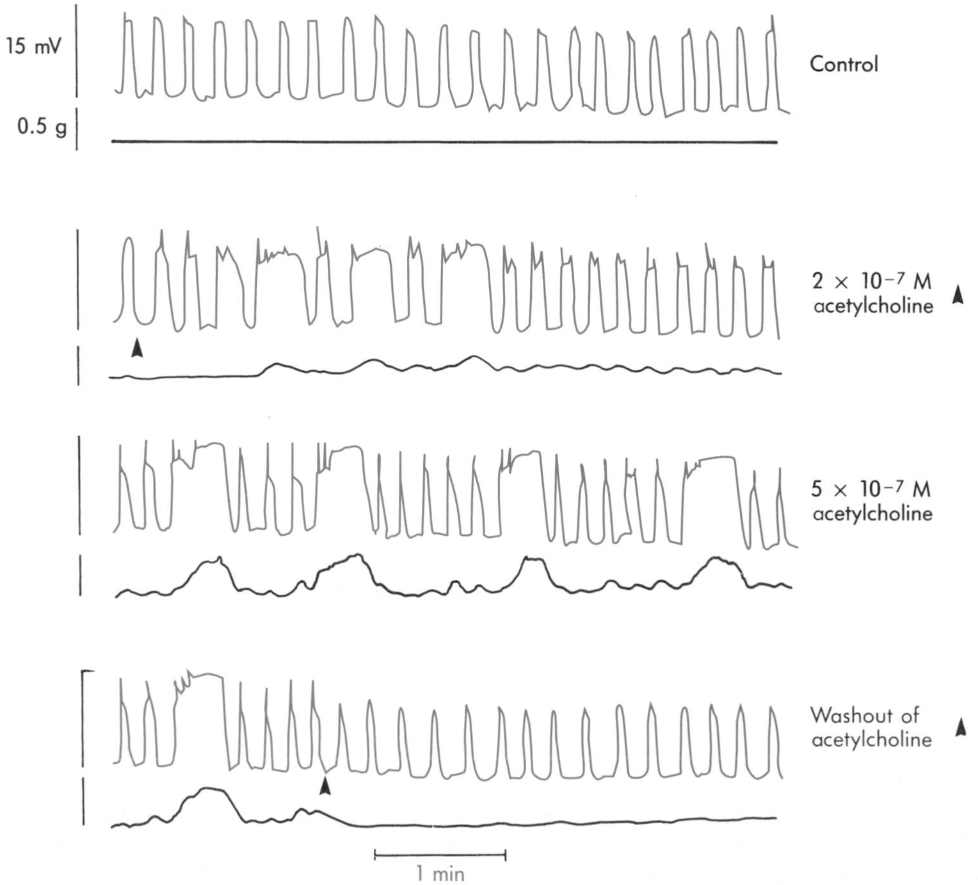

15 mV

0.5 g

Control

■ **Fig. 31-24**   Effects of acetylcholine, a contractile agonist, on electrophysiological and contractile behavior of circular smooth muscle cells of canine colon. In each panel the top trace *(color)* is the membrane potential recording and the bottom trace *(black)* is the contractile response. Superfusion of the preparation with acetylcholine causes somewhat irregular lengthening of the slow waves. The longer slow waves elicit contractions. (Redrawn from Huizenga JD, Chang G, Diamant NE, El-Sharkaway TY: *J Pharmacol Exp Ther* 231:692, 1984.)

2×10^{-7} M acetylcholine

5×10^{-7} M acetylcholine

Washout of acetylcholine

1 min

Reflex Control of Colonic Motility

Distension of one part of the colon causes a relaxation in other parts of the colon. This **colonocolonic reflex** is mediated partly by the sympathetic fibers that supply the colon. Another reflex that functions in the colon is the **gastrocolic reflex**. After a meal enters the stomach, the reflex causes the motility of proximal and distal colon and the frequency of mass movements to increase. The gastrocolic reflex depends on the autonomic innervation to the colon; hormones such as CCK and gastrin may also be involved.

The Rectum and Anal Canal

The rectum is usually empty, or nearly so. The rectum is more active in segmental contractions than is the sigmoid colon, so that the rectal contents tend to move in a retrograde direction into the sigmoid colon. The anal canal is kept tightly closed by the anal sphincters. Just before defecation, a mass movement in the sigmoid colon causes the rectum to fill. *It is the filling of the rectum that brings about reflex relaxation of the internal anal sphincter and reflex constriction of the external anal sphincter* (Fig. 31-25) *and causes the urge to defecate.* Persons who lack functional motor nerves to the external anal sphincter defecate involuntarily when the rectum is filled. The reflex reactions of the sphincters to rectal distention are transient. If defecation is postponed, the sphincters regain their normal tone, and the urge to defecate temporarily subsides.

In **Hirschsprung's disease,** also known as **congenital megacolon,** enteric neurons are congenitally absent from part of the colon. Usually, only the internal anal sphincter and a short length of colon proximal to it lack enteric neurons, but larger segments of the colon may be affected. In a normal person, filling of the rectum by a mass movement leads to reflex relaxation of the distal rectum and the internal anal sphincter. In the absence of enteric neurons, this reflex relaxation does not occur. As a result, functional obstruction of the distal colon and dilation of the colon above the obstruction occur.

Defecation

When the circumstances are appropriate, an individual may voluntarily relax the external anal sphincter to allow defecation to proceed. Highly propulsive contractions of the descending and sigmoid colon are part of the defecation reflex. Defecation is a complex behavior that involves both reflex and voluntary actions. *The integrating center for the reflex action is in the sacral spinal cord, and it is modulated by higher centers.* The principal efferent pathways are cholinergic parasympathetic fibers in the pelvic nerves. The role of the sympathetic nervous system is not significant in normal defecation.

Voluntary actions are also important in defecation. The external anal sphincter is voluntarily held in the relaxed state. Intraabdominal pressure is elevated to aid in expulsion of feces. Evacuation is normally preceded by a deep breath, which moves the diaphragm downward. The glottis then closes, and contractions of the respiratory muscles on full lungs elevate both intrathoracic and intraabdominal pressure. Contractions of the muscles of the abdominal wall further increase intraabdominal pressure, which may be as great as 200 cm H_2O. This increase in pressure helps to force feces through the relaxed sphincters. The muscles of the pelvic floor relax, allowing the floor to drop. This activity helps to straighten out the rectum and prevent rectal prolapse.

SUMMARY

1. The gastrointestinal tract has a characteristic layered structure that consists of mucosa, submucosa, muscularis externa, and serosa; this structure varies somewhat in different parts of the tract.

2. The gastrointestinal tract receives both sympathetic and parasympathetic innervation. Autonomic nerves influence the motor and secretory activities of the gastrointestinal tract and regulate the caliber of blood vessels of the gastrointestinal tract.

3. Contractions of the smooth muscle of the muscularis externa mix and propel the contents of the gastrointestinal tract.

4. Gastrointestinal smooth muscle cells are electrically coupled. Their resting membrane potential oscillates in a rhythm characteristic of each segment of the gastrointestinal tract. The membrane potential oscillations, called slow waves, control the timing and force of contractions of gastrointestinal smooth muscle.

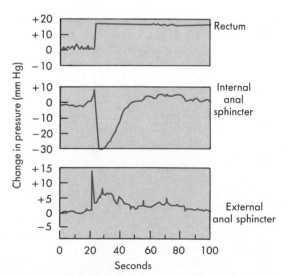

■ **Fig. 31-25** Responses of internal and external anal sphincters to prolonged distension of the rectum. Note that the responses of the sphincters are transient. (Redrawn from Shuster MM et al: *Bull Johns Hopkins Hosp* 116:79, 1965.)

5. The nerve plexuses of the gastrointestinal tract constitute the enteric nervous system. This system contains about the same number of neurons as are present in the spinal cord. The enteric nervous system contains motor neurons, sensory neurons, and interneurons.

6. Enteric sensory neurons function as the afferent arms of enteric reflex arcs by which the enteric nervous system controls most of the motor and secretory activities of the gastrointestinal tract. The autonomic nervous system modulates the activities of the enteric nervous system.

7. Swallowing is a reflex coordinated by a swallowing center in the medulla and pons. The swallowing reflex is initiated by touch receptors in the pharynx. This reflex involves a series of ordered and coordinated motor impulses to the muscles of the pharynx, upper esophageal sphincter, esophageal striated muscle, esophageal smooth muscle, and lower esophageal sphincter.

8. Contractions of the stomach mix food with gastric juice and mechanically break the food down into smaller pieces. Gastric emptying is closely regulated. This regulation ensures that gastric contents are not emptied into the duodenum at a rate faster than the duodenum and jejunum can neutralize gastric acid and process the chyme.

9. Hormonal and neural mechanisms initiated by the presence of acid, fats, peptides, amino acids, and hypertonicity in the duodenum regulate gastric emptying.

10. Segmentation is the major contractile activity of the small intestine. Segmental contractions mix and circulate intestinal contents, but they are not very propulsive. The slow rate of transport of intestinal contents allows adequate time for digestion and absorption.

11. In a fasted individual, a different pattern of motility, called the migrating myoelectric complex (MMC), occurs. The MMC is characterized by 75- to 90-minute periods of quiescence, interrupted by periods of vigorous and intensely propulsive contractions that last 3 to 6 minutes. The MMC sweeps the stomach and the small intestine clear of any debris left from the previous meal.

12. In the proximal colon, antipropulsive contractions predominate, which allows time for absorption of salts and water.

13. In the transverse and descending colon, haustral contractions mix and knead colonic contents to facilitate extraction of salts and water. Mass movements that occur in the colon one to three times daily sweep colonic contents toward the anus.

14. Filling the rectum with feces initiates the defecation reflex. The integrating center for the defecation reflex is in the sacral spinal cord, and the pelvic nerves are the principal motor pathway that regulates the actions of the distal colon, the rectum, the anal canal, and the internal anal sphincter in defecation. Both reflex and voluntary activities are involved in defecation.

BIBLIOGRAPHY

Journal articles

Bolton TB et al: Excitation-contraction coupling in gastrointestinal and other smooth muscles, *Annu Rev Physiol* 61:85, 1999.

Furness JB: Types of neurons in the enteric nervous system, *J Autonom Nerv Syst* 81:87, 2000.

Furness JB et al: Intrinsic primary afferent neurons of the intestine, *Progr Neurobiol* 54:1, 1998.

Goyal RK: Targets of enteric motor neurones: smooth muscle cells, *Gut* 47(Suppl 4):38, 2000.

Goyal RK, Hirnao I: The enteric nervous system, *N Engl J Med* 334:1106, 1999.

Goyal RK, Padmanabhan R, Sang Q: Neural circuits in swallowing and abdominal vagal afferent-mediated lower esophageal sphincter relaxation, *Am J Med* 111(Suppl 8A):95S, 2001.

Horowitz B, Ward SM, Sanders KM: Cellular and molecular basis for electrical rhythmicity in gastrointestinal muscles, *Annu Rev Physiol* 61:19, 1999.

Jourd'heuil D, Grisham MB, Granger DN: Nitric oxide and the gut, *Curr Gastroenterol Rep* 1:384, 1999.

Kunze WA, Furness JB: The entric nervous system and regulation of intestinal motility, *Annu Rev Physiol* 61:117, 1999.

Lammers WJ, Slack JR: Of slow waves and spike patches, *News Physiol Sci* 16:138, 2001.

Makhlouf GM, Murthy KS: Signal transduction in gastrointestinal smooth muscle, *Cell Signal* 9:269, 1997.

Murthy et al: Interplay of VIP and nitric oxide in the regulation of neuromuscular function in the guy, *Ann NY Acad Sci* 805:355, 1996.

Quigley EM: Gastric and small intestinal motility in health and disease, *Gastroenterol Clin North Am* 25:113, 1996.

Tack J, Vanden Berghe P: Neuropeptides and colonic motility: it's all in the little brain, *Gastroenterology* 119:257, 2000.

Thomson AB et al: Small bowel review: normal physiology, *Dig Dis Sci* 46:2588, 2001.

Timmermans JP: Interstitial cells of Cajal: is their role in gastrointestinal function in view of therapeutic perspectives underestimated or exaggerated? *Folia Morphol* 60:1, 2001.

Ward SM, Sanders KM: Physiology and pathophysiology of the interstitial cell of Cajal: from bench to bedside. I. Functional development and plasticity of interstitial cells of Cajal networks, *Am J Physiol* 281(3):G602, 2001.

Wood JD: Enteric nervous control of motility in the upper gastrointestinal tract in defensive states, *Dig Dis Sci* 44 (8 Suppl): 44S, 1999.

Wood JD: Mixing and moving in the gut, *Gut* 45:333, 1999.

Book and monographs

Conklin JL, Christensen J: Motor functions of the pharynx and esophagus. In Johnson RL, editor: *Physiology of the gastrointestinal tract,* ed 3, New York, 1994, Raven Press.

Furness JB, Costa M: *The enteric nervous system,* Edinburgh, 1987, Churchill Livingstone.

Furness JB et al: The enteric nervous system and its extrinsic connections. In Yamada T, editor: *Textbook of gastroenterology,* ed 3, Philadelphia, 1999, Lippincott, Williams & Wilkins.

Gabella G: Structure of muscles and nerves in the gastrointestinal tract. In Johnson RL, editor: *Physiology of the gastrointestinal tract,* ed 3, New York, 1994, Raven Press.

Kamm MA, Lennard-Jones JE, editors: *Gastrointestinal transit,* Petersfield, UK, 1991, Wrightson Biomedical Publishing.

Makhlouf GM: Neuromuscular function of the small intestine. In Johnson RL, editor: *Physiology of the gastrointestinal tract,* ed 3, New York, 1994, Raven Press.

Makhlouf GM: Smooth muscle of the gut. In Yamada T, editor: *Textbook of gastroenterology,* ed 3, Philadelphia, 1999, Lippincott, Williams & Wilkins.

Mayer EM: The physiology of gastric storage and emptying. In Johnson RL, editor: *Physiology of the gastrointestinal tract,* ed 3, New York, 1994, Raven Press.

Miller LJ: Gastrointestinal hormones and receptors. In Yamada T, editor: *Textbook of gastroenterology,* ed 3, Philadelphia, 1999, Lippincott, Williams & Wilkins.

chapter thirty-two

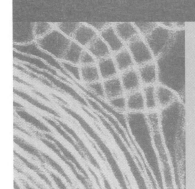

Gastrointestinal Secretions

This chapter deals with the glandular secretion of fluids and compounds that have important functions in the digestive tract. The secretions of the **salivary glands, gastric glands, exocrine pancreas,** and **liver** are considered. The composition and digestive function of each section are discussed, and the regulation of secretory processes is emphasized.

Digestive secretions are released from glands by the action of specific effector substances on the secretory cells. These effector substances may be classified as neurocrine, endocrine, or paracrine (see Chapter 5).

A substance that stimulates a particular cell to secrete is called a **secretagogue.** Although secretagogues are numerous, only a few signal transduction mechanisms (discussed in Chapter 5) mediate secretion.

SECRETION OF SALIVA

In humans, the salivary glands produce about 1 L of saliva each day. Saliva lubricates food to make swallowing easier, and it also facilitates speaking.

> In people who lack functional salivary glands, **xerostomia** (dry mouth), **dental caries,** and infections of the buccal mucosa are prevalent. Saliva contains secretory **immunoglobulins** (antibodies) directed against microorganisms in the mouth, and lysozyme that hydrolyzes a major component of bacterial outer membranes. In the absence of antibodies and lysozyme, organisms that cause buccal infections and dental caries proliferate. The basic pH of saliva also helps prevent dental caries.

Functions of Saliva

Mucins, which are glycoproteins produced by the submaxillary and sublingual glands, lubricate food so that it may be more readily swallowed. The major digestive function of saliva is carried out by the enzyme **salivary amylase,** which breaks down starch. Salivary amylase has the same speci-

ficity as the α-amylase of pancreatic juice (see Chapter 33); it reduces starch to oligosaccharide molecules. The optimal pH for salivary amylase is about 7, but it is active between pH 4 and 11. After mixing with food in the mouth, amylase continues to break down starch in the mass of food in the stomach. Its action is terminated only when the contents of the antrum are mixed with enough gastric acid to lower the pH to less than 4. More than half the starch in a well-chewed meal may be reduced to small oligosaccharides by the action of salivary amylase. However, because of the efficiency with which pancreatic α-amylase digests starch in the small intestine, starch is well absorbed even in the absence of salivary amylase.

Other components of saliva are present in smaller amounts. These components include RNase, DNase, lysozyme, lactoperoxidase, lingual lipase, kallikrein, and secretory immunoglobulin A (IgA).

Structure of Salivary Glands

In humans, the **parotid glands,** the largest salivary glands, are entirely serous. The watery secretion from these glands lacks mucins. The **submandibular** and **sublingual glands** are mixed mucous and serous glands, and they secrete a more viscous saliva that contains mucins. Many smaller salivary glands are present in the oral cavity. The microscopic structure of a mixed salivary gland is depicted in Fig. 32-1. **Serous acinar cells** are located in the **secretory endpieces** (also called **acini**). Serous acinar cells have apical **zymogen granules** that contain salivary amylase and perhaps other salivary proteins also (Fig. 32-2). **Mucous acinar cells** secrete glycoprotein mucins into the saliva. **Intercalated ducts** drain the acinar fluid into larger ducts, the **striated ducts,** which empty into still larger **excretory ducts** (Fig. 32-1). A single large duct brings the secretions of each major gland into the mouth.

The production of saliva by a salivary gland begins in the secretory endpieces, which elaborate a fluid called the **primary secretion.** The cells that line the ducts modify this primary secretion to produce saliva.

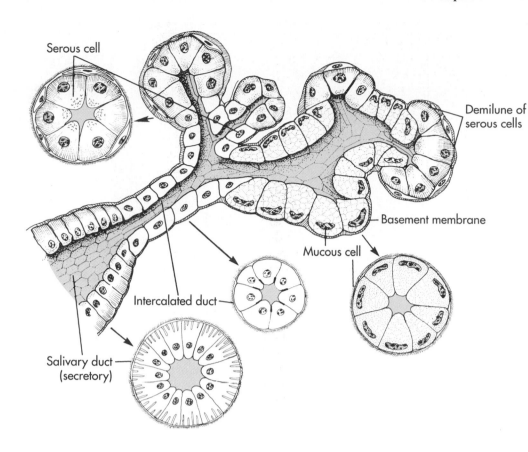

■ **Fig. 32-1** Structure of the human submandibular gland, as seen with the light microscope. (From Braus H: *Anatomie des Menschen,* Berlin, 1934, Julius Springer.)

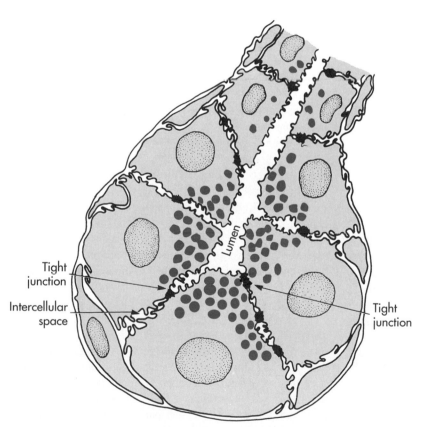

■ **Fig. 32-2** Schematic representation of the cellular morphology of a secretory endpiece of a serous salivary gland. Colored circles represent zymogen granules. Upon stimulation, the contents of zymogen granules are released by exocytosis into the lumen of the acinus. (From Young JA, van Lennep LW: *Morphology of salivary glands,* London, 1978, Academic Press.)

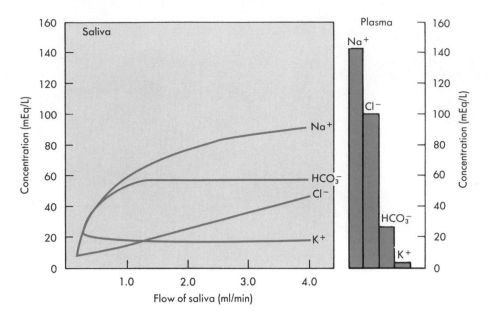

■ **Fig. 32-3** Average composition of parotid saliva as a function of the salivary flow rate. Saliva is hypotonic to plasma at all flow rates, but the tonicity increases with increasing flow rate. The bicarbonate level in saliva exceeds that in plasma, except at very low flow rates. (From Thaysen JH et al: *Am J Physiol* 178:155, 1954.)

Metabolism and Blood Flow of Salivary Glands

The salivary glands produce a prodigious flow of saliva. The maximal rate of saliva production in humans is about 1 ml/min/g of gland; *at this rate, the glands are producing their own weight in saliva each minute!* Salivary glands have a high rate of metabolism and a high blood flow; both are proportional to the rate of saliva formation. *The blood flow to maximally secreting salivary glands is approximately 10 times that of an equal mass of actively contracting skeletal muscle.* Stimulation of the parasympathetic nerves to salivary glands increases blood flow by dilating the vasculature of the glands. **Vasoactive intestinal polypeptide (VIP)** and **acetylcholine** are released from parasympathetic nerve terminals in the salivary glands; both of these compounds contribute to vasodilation during secretory activity.

Secretion of Saliva

Ionic composition of saliva. *In humans, saliva is always hypotonic to plasma.* As shown in Fig. 32-3, salivary concentrations of Na^+ and Cl^- are less than those of plasma. The greater the secretory flow rate, the higher is the tonicity of the saliva; at maximal flow rates, the tonicity of saliva in humans is about 70% of that of plasma. The pH of saliva from resting glands is slightly acidic. During active secretion, however, the saliva becomes basic, and its pH increases to near 8. The increase in pH that accompanies saliva secretion is partly caused by an increase in bicarbonate concentration with increasing flow rate. Except at the lowest salivary flow rates, the concentration of bicarbonate in saliva is greater than the plasma concentration of bicarbonate. The concentration of K^+ in saliva is always much greater than its concentration in plasma. When salivary flow rates are very low, salivary K^+ levels are high.

Secretion of water and electrolytes. A two-stage model of salivary secretion (Fig. 32-4) postulates the following:

1. The secretory endpieces, perhaps with the participation of intercalated ducts, produce a primary secretion that is isotonic to plasma. The amylase concentration of this primary secretion and the rate at which it is secreted vary with the level and type of stimulation. However, the electrolyte composition of the secretion is fairly constant. Levels of Na^+, K^+, HCO_3^-, and Cl^- are close to plasma levels.

2. The excretory ducts, and probably the striated ducts also, modify the primary secretion by extracting Na^+ and Cl^- from, and adding K^+ and HCO_3^- to, the saliva. The ducts only modify the composition of the primary secretion; they do not add to the volume of saliva.

Because the ducts remove more Na^+ and Cl^- ions from saliva than they add K^+ and HCO_3^-, saliva becomes progressively more hypotonic as it flows through the ducts. The faster the flow rate of the saliva through the striated and excretory ducts, the closer to isotonicity it becomes.

Secretion of salivary amylase. As noted previously, serous acinar cells have zymogen granules (Fig. 32-2) that contain salivary amylase. These granules are located in the apical cytoplasm of these cells. When the gland is stimulated to secrete, the zymogen granules fuse with the plasma membrane and release their contents into the lumen of the secretory endpiece by exocytosis.

Neural Control of Salivary Gland Function

The primary physiological control of the salivary glands is by the parasympathetic nervous system. In contrast, the control of most other gastrointestinal secretions is primarily hormonal. Excitation of either sympathetic or parasympathetic nerves to the salivary glands stimulates salivary secretion, but the effects of the parasympathetic nerves are stronger and more long-lasting. Interruption of the sympathetic nerves does not disrupt salivary gland function. If the parasympathetic supply is interrupted, however, salivation is severely impaired and the salivary glands atrophy.

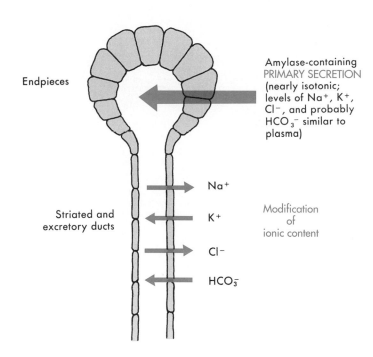

Endpieces

Amylase-containing
PRIMARY SECRETION
(nearly isotonic;
levels of Na⁺, K⁺,
Cl⁻, and probably
HCO₃⁻ similar to
plasma)

Striated and
excretory ducts

Na^+

K^+

Cl^-

HCO_3^-

Modification
of
ionic content

■ **Fig. 32-4** Schematic representation of the two-stage model of salivary secretion. The primary secretion, containing salivary amylase and electrolytes at concentrations similar to those in plasma, is produced by the acinar cells. The striated and excretory ducts modify the composition of saliva by absorbing Na^+ and Cl^- and secreting K^+ and HCO_3^-.

Sympathetic fibers to the salivary glands stem from the superior cervical ganglion. Preganglionic parasympathetic fibers come via branches of the facial and glossopharyngeal nerves (cranial nerves VII and IX, respectively). These fibers form synapses with postganglionic neurons in ganglia in or near the salivary glands. The acinar cells and ducts are supplied with parasympathetic nerve endings.

Parasympathetic stimulation increases the synthesis and secretion of salivary amylase and mucins, enhances the transport activities of the ductular epithelium, greatly increases blood flow to the glands, and stimulates glandular metabolism and growth.

The increase in salivary secretion that results from stimulation of sympathetic nerves is transient. Sympathetic stimulation constricts blood vessels, which causes a decrease in salivary gland blood flow.

Both sympathetic and parasympathetic stimulation cause contraction of myoepithelial cells that surround the acini. This contraction serves to empty the acinar contents into the ducts and thus augments salivary flow.

Ionic Mechanisms of Salivary Secretion

Ion transport in ductular cells. Figure 32-5 shows a simplified model of ion transport processes in the epithelial cells of excretory ducts and probably of striated ducts also. The Na^+,K^+-ATPase located in the basolateral membrane of the epithelial cell maintains the electrochemical potential gradients of Na^+ and K^+ that power most of the other ionic transport processes of the cell. In the apical membrane, the parallel operation of Na^+, H^+, Cl^-, HCO_3^-, and H^+,K^+ exchangers results in the absorption of Na^+ and Cl^- from the luminal fluid and the secretion of K^+ and HCO_3^- into the lumen. The impermeability of the ductular epithelium to water prevents the ducts from absorbing too much water by osmosis.

As noted, both parasympathetic and sympathetic stimulation increase the flow rate of saliva. This increase in flow rate is mediated partly by the inhibition of Na^+ absorption across the luminal membrane of the epithelial cells.

Ion transport in acinar cells. Figure 32-6 shows a simplified view of the mechanisms of ion secretion in serous acinar cells. The basolateral membrane of the cell contains the Na^+,K^+-ATPase and an Na^+, K^+, $2Cl^-$ cotransporter that uses the energy of the Na^+ gradient to power the active uptake of K^+ and Cl^-. Cl^- and bicarbonate leave the acinar cell to enter the luminal fluid via an electrogenic anion channel located in the apical membrane of the acinar cell. Acinar cell fluid secretion is strongly enhanced in response to elevations of intracellular Ca^{2+} concentration.

Cellular Control of Salivary Secretion: Signal Transduction Mechanisms

Control mechanisms in ductular cells. The ducts of salivary glands respond to both cholinergic and adrenergic agonists by increasing the rates of secretion of K^+ and HCO_3^-.

Control mechanisms in serous acinar cells. Acetylcholine, norepinephrine, substance P, and **VIP** are released in salivary glands by specific nerve terminals. Each of these neuroeffectors increases the secretion of salivary amylase and the flow of saliva.

These neuroeffector substances act mainly by elevating the intracellular concentration of cyclic AMP (cAMP) or by increasing the concentration of Ca^{2+} in the cytosol (Fig. 32-7). Acetylcholine, substance P, and norepinephrine acting on α receptors increase the cytosolic concentration of Ca^{2+} in the serous acinar cells. In contrast, norepinephrine acting on β receptors and VIP elevate the cAMP concentration in acinar cells. Agonists that elevate cAMP concentration in serous

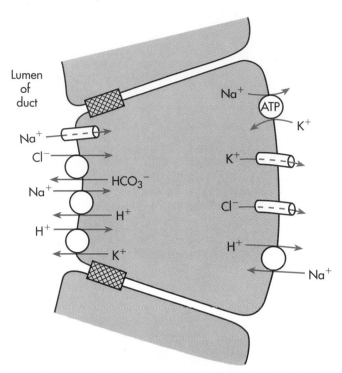

Fig. 32-5 Postulated model of ionic transport mechanisms involved in the absorption of Na^+ and Cl^- and the secretion of K^+ and HCO_3^- by the epithelial cells of the striated and excretory ducts of salivary glands. In the apical membrane, the parallel operation of Na^+, H^+, Cl^-, HCO_3^-, and H^+,K^+ exchangers results in the absorption of Na^+ and Cl^- from the luminal fluid and the secretion of K^+ and HCO_3^- into the lumen. Na^+ is also absorbed from the lumen via an Na^+ channel that is blocked by amiloride. The basolateral membrane contains the Na^+,K^+-ATPase that maintains the gradients of Na^+ and K^+ and Na^+,H^+ exchangers. Basolateral K^+ channels that are activated by increased Ca^{2+} maintain the electronegativity of the cytosol that helps to drive Cl^- absorption across the basolateral membrane via a Cl^- channel. The Cl^- conductance may increase in response to elevated cytosolic levels of Ca^{2+} or cyclic AMP.

acinar cells elicit a secretion that is rich in amylase; agonists that mobilize Ca^{2+} elicit a secretion that is more voluminous but that has a lower concentration of amylase. Ca^{2+} mobilizing agonists may also elevate the concentration of cyclic GMP (cGMP), which may mediate the trophic effects evoked by these agonists.

GASTRIC SECRETION

The stomach serves several functions. It functions as a reservoir that allows the ingestion of a large meal. Later, the stomach empties its contents (now called chyme) into the duodenum at a controlled rate consistent with the ability of the duodenum and small intestine to process the chyme.

The major secretions of the stomach are hydrochloric acid (HCl), pepsins, intrinsic factor, mucus, and bicarbonate. HCl kills most ingested microorganisms. HCl also catalyzes the cleavage of inactive pepsinogens to active **pepsins.** In addition, HCl provides a low pH environment, which is required

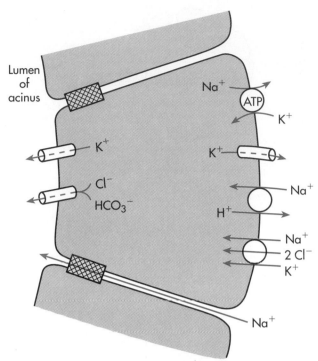

Fig. 32-6 Postulated ionic transport processes involved in secretion of Na^+, Cl^-, and HCO_3^- by serous salivary acinar cells. The basolateral membrane of the cell contains the Na^+,K^+-ATPase and an Na^+, K^+, $2Cl^-$ cotransporter that uses the energy of the Na^+ gradient to power the active uptake of K^+ and Cl^-. As a result, the intracellular electrochemical potential of Cl^- is greater than in the acinar fluid. Cl^- and HCO_3^- leave the acinar cell to enter the luminal fluid via an electrogenic anion channel in the apical membrane of the acinar cell. The electrogenic secretion of anions drives the entry of Na^+ into the acinar lumen, partly via the tight junctions between the acinar cells. Apical and basolateral K^+ channels that are stimulated by elevated cytosolic Ca^{2+} enhance the electronegativity of the cytosol that helps drive Cl^- and HCO_3^- across the luminal membrane, and promote uphill entry of Cl^- across the basolateral membrane by increasing the driving force for Na^+ uptake. The anion conductance of the apical membrane is increased in response to elevation of cytoplasmic Ca^{2+} or cyclic AMP.

for the action of pepsins in digesting proteins and peptides. **Intrinsic factor,** a glycoprotein, binds vitamin B_{12} and allows it to be absorbed in the ileum. The hormone **gastrin,** released by G cells in the gastric antrum, promotes secretion of HCl and pepsinogens. Mucus and bicarbonate secretions protect the stomach from mechanical and chemical damage.

Structure of the Gastric Mucosa

The surface of the gastric mucosa (Fig. 32-8) is covered by columnar **epithelial cells** that secrete mucus and an alkaline fluid that protects the epithelium from mechanical injury and gastric acid. The gastric mucosal surface is studded with **gastric pits;** each pit is the opening of a duct into which one or more **gastric glands** empty (Fig. 32-8, *A*). The gastric pits are so numerous that they account for a significant fraction of the total surface area of the gastric mucosa.

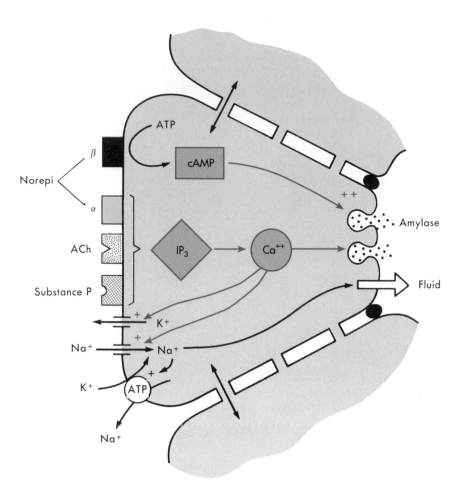

■ **Fig. 32-7**   The cellular mechanisms whereby norepinephrine *(Norepi),* acetylcholine *(ACh),* and substance P evoke salivary secretion. Norepinephrine acting on α-adrenergic receptors, acetylcholine, and substance P increases intracellular Ca^{2+}. Norepinephrine acting on β-adrenergic receptors increases intracellular levels of cyclic AMP *(cAMP).* Effectors that increase cellular cAMP elicit a primary secretion that is richer in amylase than is the secretion evoked by agents that increase intracellular Ca^{2+}. Substances that increase intracellular Ca^{2+} produce a greater volume of acinar cell secretion than do agonists that increase intracellular cAMP. (From Peterson OH. In Johnson RL, editor: *Physiology of the gastrointestinal tract,* New York, 1981, Raven Press.)

The gastric mucosa can be divided into three distinct regions, based on the structures of the glands present. The small **cardiac glandular region,** located just below the lower esophageal sphincter, contains primarily mucus-secreting gland cells. The remainder of the gastric mucosa is divided into the oxyntic (acid-secreting) **glandular region,** located above the gastric notch, and the **pyloric glandular region,** below the notch (see Fig. 31-12).

The structure of a gastric gland from the oxyntic glandular region is illustrated in Fig. 32-8, *B.* The surface epithelial cells extend slightly into the duct opening. **Mucous neck cells,** which secrete mucus, are located in the narrow neck of the gland. **Parietal** or **oxyntic cells,** which secrete HCl and **intrinsic factor,** and **chief** or **peptic cells,** which secrete **pepsinogens,** are located deeper in the gland. Oxyntic glands also contain enterochromaffin-like (ECL) cells that secrete histamine and D cells that secrete somatostatin. Parietal cells are particularly numerous in glands in the fundus, whereas mucus-secreting cells are more numerous in the glands of the pyloric glandular region. Pyloric glands also contain G cells, which secrete the hormone gastrin.

The stomach has the remarkable ability to repair damage to its epithelial surface. Surface epithelial cells are exfoliated into the lumen at a considerable rate during normal gastric function. These cells are replaced by mucous neck cells, which then differentiate into columnar epithelial cells and migrate up out of the necks of the glands.

Gastric Acid Secretion

The fluid secreted into the stomach is called **gastric juice.** Gastric juice is a mixture of the secretions of the surface epithelial cells and the secretions of gastric glands. *Among the important components of gastric juice are HCl, salts, water, pepsins, intrinsic factor, mucus, and bicarbonate.* Secretion of all these components increases after a meal.

Ionic composition of gastric juice. The ionic composition of gastric juice depends on the rate of secretion. Figure 32-9 shows that the higher the secretory rate, the higher is the concentration of hydrogen ions. At lower secretory rates, [H+] decreases and [Na+] increases. [K+] is always higher in gastric juice than in plasma. Consequently, prolonged vomiting may lead to hypokalemia. At all rates of secretion, Cl− is the major anion of gastric juice. At high rates of secretion, gastric juice resembles an isotonic solution of HCl. Gastric HCl converts pepsinogens to active pepsins (see below) and provides an acid pH at which pepsins are active.

The high acidity of gastric juice kills most ingested microorganisms. Individuals who have low rates of gastric acid secretion, either because of disease or because they are taking medications that suppress HCl secretion, are more susceptible to infection by ingested pathogens and may have bacterial overgrowth in the stomach or upper small intestine.

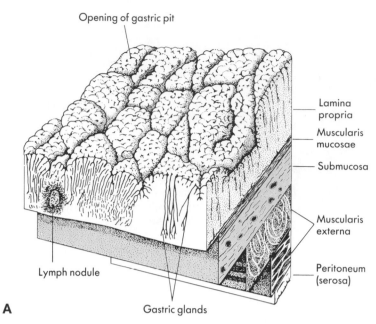

Opening of gastric pit

Lamina
propria

Muscularis
mucosae

Submucosa

Muscularis
externa

Peritoneum
(serosa)

Lymph nodule

Gastric glands

A

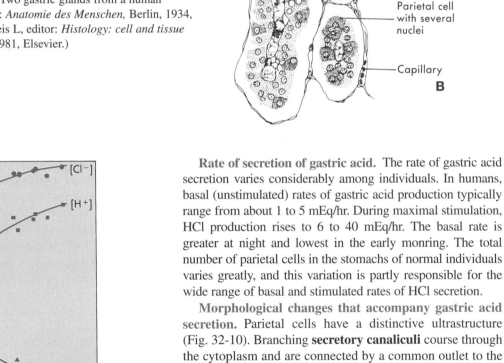

Surface
epithelium

Opening of
gastric pit

Foveolar
cell

Parietal
cell

Neck mucous
cell

Chief cell

Connective
tissue

Parietal cell
with several
nuclei

Capillary

B

■ **Fig. 32-8**   Structure of the gastric mucosa. **A,** Reconstruction of part of the gastric wall. **B,** Two gastric glands from a human stomach. (A from Braus H: *Anatomie des Menschen,* Berlin, 1934, Julius Springer. B from Weis L, editor: *Histology: cell and tissue biology,* ed 5, New York, 1981, Elsevier.)

■ **Fig. 32-9**   Concentrations of ions in gastric juice as a function of the rate of secretion in a normal young person. At low flow rates, gastric juice is hypotonic to plasma. At high flow rates, gastric juice approaches isotonicity and contains predominantly H^+ and Cl^- [From Davenport HW: *Physiology of the digestive tract,* ed 5, Chicago, *Mosby-Year Book;* and adapted from Nordgren B: *Acta Physiol Scand* 58(Suppl 202):1, 1963.]

Rate of secretion of gastric acid. The rate of gastric acid secretion varies considerably among individuals. In humans, basal (unstimulated) rates of gastric acid production typically range from about 1 to 5 mEq/hr. During maximal stimulation, HCl production rises to 6 to 40 mEq/hr. The basal rate is greater at night and lowest in the early monring. The total number of parietal cells in the stomachs of normal individuals varies greatly, and this variation is partly responsible for the wide range of basal and stimulated rates of HCl secretion.

Morphological changes that accompany gastric acid secretion. Parietal cells have a distinctive ultrastructure (Fig. 32-10). Branching **secretory canaliculi** course through the cytoplasm and are connected by a common outlet to the cell's luminal surface. Microvilli line the surfaces of the secretory canaliculi. The cytoplasm of unstimulated parietal cells contains numerous tubules and vesicles, which together are called the **tubulovesicular system.** The membranes of the tubulovesicles contain the transport proteins responsible for secretion of H^+ and Cl^- into the lumen of the gland.

To secrete HCl, parietal cells must undergo a morphological change that is prompted by stimulation. When parietal cells are stimulated to secrete HCl (Fig. 32-10, *B*), tubulovesicular membranes fuse with the plasma membrane of the secretory canaliculi. *This extensive membrane fusion greatly increases the number of HCl-pumping sites available at the surface of the secretory canaliculi.*

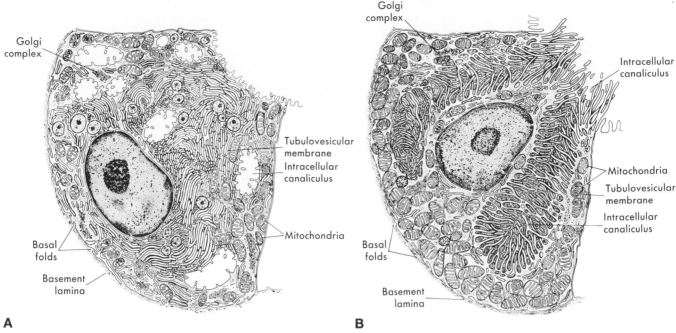

■ **Fig. 32-10** **A,** Drawing of a resting parietal cell with cytoplasm full of tubulovesicles and an internalized intracellular canaliculus. **B,** An acid-secreting parietal cell. Tubulovesicles have fused with the membrane of the intracellular canaliculus, which is now open to the lumen of the gland and lined with abundant, long microvilli. (From Ito S: In Johnson RL, editor: *Physiology of the gastrointestinal tract,* New York, 1981, Raven Press.)

Cellular mechanisms of gastric acid secretion. When parietal cells are secreting gastric acid at the maximal rate, H^+ is pumped against a concentration gradient that is about 1 million-fold: about pH 7 in the parietal cell cytosol to about pH 1 in the lumen of the gastric gland. Also, because the lumen of the stomach is electronegative by 30 to 80 mV relative to the serosa, Cl^- enters the gastric lumen against both chemical and electrical potential differences. Energy is required for transport of both H^+ and Cl^- into gastric juice.

The apical membrane of the parietal cell (the membrane that lines the secretory canaliculus) contains an H^+,K^+-ATPase, which exchanges H^+ for K^+. This ATPase is the primary H^+ pump. Both H^+ and K^+ are pumped against their electrochemical potential gradients. The H^+,K^+-ATPase is closely related to the Na^+,K^+-ATPase of plasma membranes and the Ca^{2+}-ATPase of sarcoplasmic reticulum membranes.

Drugs that specifically inhibit the H^+,K^+-ATPase are available. Substituted benzimidazoles, such as omeprazole, are inactive at neutral pH. At a low pH, however, they are converted to a form that reacts with sulfhydryl groups on the H^+,K^+-ATPase. This reaction inactivates its enzymatic and ion pumping activities. Because the inactivation of H^+,K^+-ATPase by omeprazole is irreversible, the drug is usually administered only once daily.

When H^+ is pumped out of the parietal cell (Fig. 32-11), an excess of HCO_3^- is left behind. HCO_3^- flows down its electrochemical gradient across the basolateral plasma membrane. *The protein that mediates HCO_3^- efflux, called the Cl^-, HCO_3^- countertransporter, also transports Cl^- in the opposite direction. Thus, Cl^- moves against its electrochemical potential gradient into the cell. The energy for this active transport of Cl^- comes from the downhill movement of HCO_3^- across the basolateral membrane.* The basolateral plasma membrane has numerous infoldings that increase the area available for Cl^-/HCO_3^- exchange. As a result of the combined action of the H^+,K^+-ATPase and the Cl^-, HCO_3^- countertransporter, Cl^- is concentrated in the cytoplasm of the parietal cell. The Cl^- leaves the parietal cell at the apical membrane via an electrogenic anion channel.

Stimulation of the parietal cell to secrete H^+ and Cl^-. Histamine, acetylcholine, and gastrin are the three physiological agonists of HCl secretion by parietal cells. Histamine elevates the intracellular concentration of cAMP, while acetylcholine and gastrin elevate the intracellular Ca^{2+} concentration.

The basolateral membranes of parietal cells contain two types of K^+ channels (Fig. 32-11). One type of K^+ channel is activated by cAMP; the other type is activated by Ca^{2+}. Activation of the basolateral K^+ channels hyperpolarizes the cell and thereby increases the driving force for Cl^- to leave the cell. Cl^- leaves the cell through the electrogenic Cl^- channels in the apical membrane on the boundary of the secretory canaliculus. The K^+ channels also mediate the efflux of K^+ that accumulates in the parietal cell via the activity of the H^+,K^+-ATPase.

The conductance of the electrogenic Cl^- channels of the apical membrane is dramatically increased by elevated

■ **Fig. 32-11**   Postulated model of the major ionic transport processes involved in the secretion of H^+ and Cl^- by parietal cells. Cl^- enters the cell across the basolateral membrane against an electrochemical gradient. Cl^- entry is powered by the downhill efflux of HCO_3^-. The high level of HCO_3^- in the cytosol is generated by the extrusion of H^+ across the luminal membrane. H^+ is pumped into the secretory canaliculus by the H^+,K^+-ATPase. Cl^- enters the canalicular fluid by an electrogenic ion channel. The Cl^- conductance of the luminal membrane is increased in response to increased cytosolic Ca^{2+} and cyclic AMP. The conductance of basolateral K^+ channels is also enhanced by the second messengers, and K^+ efflux through these channels increases the electronegativity of the cytosol and increases the driving force for efflux of Cl^- across the apical membrane.

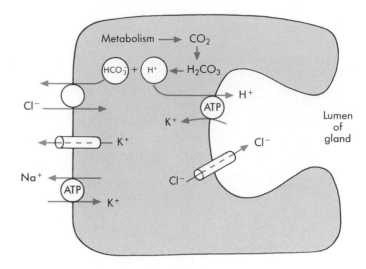

cAMP concentrations and by hyperpolarization of the cell. In addition, cAMP and Ca^{2+} promote the insertion of more Cl^- channels into the luminal membrane and promote the fusion of cytosolic tubovesicles with the membrane of the secretory canaliculi. This latter process increases the number of H^+,K^+-ATPase molecules in the canalicular membrane (Fig. 32-10).

Secretion of Pepsins

Pepsins, often collectively called **pepsin,** are a group of proteases secreted by the chief cells of the gastric glands. **Pepsins are secreted as inactive proenzymes called *pepsinogens.*** Pepsinogens are contained in membrane-bound zymogen granules in the chief cells. Zymogen granules release their contents by exocytosis when the chief cells are stimulated to secrete.

Pepsinogens are converted to active pepsins by the cleavage of acid-labile linkages. The lower the pH, the more rapid is this conversion. Pepsins also act proteolytically on pepsinogens to form more pepsins. Pepsins are most proteolytically active at pH 3 and below. Pepsins may digest as much as 20% of the protein in a typical meal. When the duodenal contents are neutralized, pepsins are inactivated irreversibly by the neutral pH.

Secretion of Intrinsic Factor

Intrinsic factor, a glycoprotein secreted by the parietal cells of the stomach, is required for the normal absorption of vitamin B_{12} (see Chapter 33). Intrinsic factor is released in response to the same stimuli that elicit the secretion of HCl by parietal cells. *Secretion of intrinsic factor is the only gastric function that is essential for human life.*

Secretion of Mucus and Bicarbonate

Mucus and bicarbonate protect the surface of the stomach from the effects of HCl and pepsins.

Secretion of mucus. Secretions that contain glycoprotein mucins are viscous and sticky and are collectively termed **mucus.** Mucins are secreted by mucous neck cells located in the necks of gastric glands and by the surface epithelial cells of the stomach. Mucus is stored in large granules in the apical cytoplasm of mucous neck cells and surface epithelial cells, and is released by exocytosis.

Gastric mucins are about 80% carbohydrate by weight and consist of four similar monomers of about 500,000 daltons each that are linked together by disulfide cross-links (Fig. 32-12). These tetrameric mucins form a sticky gel that adheres to the surface of the stomach. However, this gel is subject to proteolysis by pepsins, which cleave bonds near the center of the tetramers. This process releases fragments that do not form gels, and thus dissolves the protective mucus layer. Maintenance of the protective mucus layer requires continuous synthesis of new tetrameric mucins to replace those mucins that are cleaved by pepsins.

Mucus is secreted at a significant rate in the resting stomach. Secretion of mucus is stimulated by some of the same stimuli that enhance acid and pepsinogen secretion, especially by acetylcholine released from parasympathetic nerve endings near the gastric glands. If the gastric mucosa is mechanically deformed, neural reflexes are evoked that enhance mucus secretion.

Secretion of bicarbonate. The surface epithelial cells also secrete a watery fluid that contains Na^+ and Cl^- concentrations similar to those of plasma, but with higher K^+ and HCO_3^- concentrations than those of plasma. Bicarbonate is entrapped by the viscous mucus that coats the surface of the stomach. *The high HCO_3^- concentration makes the mucus layer alkaline,* and thus the mucus secreted by the resting mucosa lines the stomach with a sticky, viscous, alkaline coat. When food is eaten, the rates of secretion of both mucus and of HCO_3^- increase. The maximal rate of bicarbonate secretion is about 10% of the maximal rate of HCl secretion. Bicarbonate secretion is enhanced by acetylcholine released from nerve endings near the surface epithelial cells.

The gastric mucosal barrier. *The protective mucus gel that forms on the luminal surface of the stomach and alkaline secretions entrapped within it constitute a **gastric mucosal barrier** that prevents damage to the mucosa by*

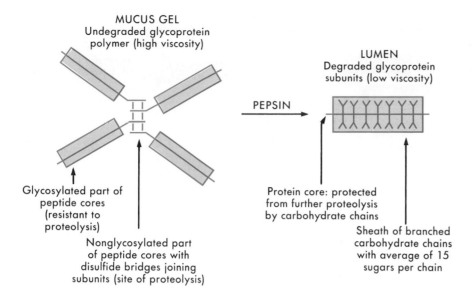

MUCUS GEL
Undegraded glycoprotein
polymer (high viscosity)

LUMEN
Degraded glycoprotein
subunits (low viscosity)

PEPSIN

Glycosylated part of
peptide cores
(resistant to
proteolysis)

Nonglycosylated part
of peptide cores with
disulfide bridges joining
subunits (site of proteolysis)

Protein core: protected
from further proteolysis
by carbohydrate chains

Sheath of branched
carbohydrate chains
with average of 15
sugars per chain

■ **Fig. 32-12** Schematic depiction of the structure of gastric mucins before and after hydrolysis by pepsin. Intact mucins are tetramers of four similar monomers of about 500,000 daltons each that are attached by disulfide cross-links. Each monomer is largely covered by carbohydrate side chains that protect it from proteolytic degradation. The tetrameric mucins form a sticky gel that adheres to the surface of the stomach. The central portion of the mucin tetramer, near the disulfide cross-links, is more susceptible to proteolytic digestion. Pepsins cleave bonds near the center of the tetramers to release fragments about the size of monomers; these fragments do not form gels, so that proteolysis dissolves the gel. (From Allen A: *Br Med Bull* 34:28, 1978.)

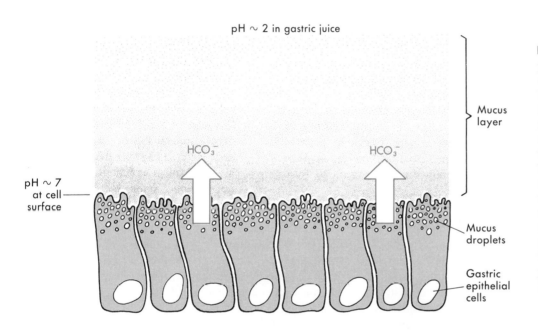

pH ~ 2 in gastric juice

HCO_3^- HCO_3^-

pH ~ 7
at cell
surface

Mucus
layer

Mucus
droplets

Gastric
epithelial
cells

■ **Fig. 32-13** The protection provided to the mucosal surface of the stomach by the bicarbonate-containing mucus layer is known as the gastric mucosal barrier. In man, the mucus layer is about 0.2 mm thick. Buffering by the bicarbonate-rich secretions of the surface epithelial cells and the restraint to convective mixing caused by the high viscosity of the mucus layer allow the pH at the cell surface to remain near 7, whereas the pH in the gastric juice in the lumen is 1 to 2.

gastric contents (Fig. 32-13). The mucus gel layer, which is about 0.2 mm thick, effectively separates the bicarbonate-rich secretions of the surface epithelial cells from the acidic contents of the gastric lumen. The secretions of gastric glands enter the lumen of the stomach via 5- to 7-μm-diameter channels through the mucus layer. The mucus allows the pH of the epithelial cells to be maintained at nearly neutral pH, despite a luminal pH of about 2. Mucus also slows the diffusion of acid and pepsins to the epithelial cell surface. *The protection of the gastric epithelium depends on both mucus and HCO_3^- secretion;* neither mucus alone nor HCO_3^- alone can hold the pH at the epithelial cell surface near neutral.

The gastric mucosal barrier of a normal individual can protect the stomach even when rates of secretion of HCl and pepsins are elevated. If the secretion of either HCO_3^- or mucus is suppressed, however, the gastric mucosal barrier is compromised, and the effects of acid and pepsin on the surface of the stomach may produce **gastric ulcers.**

Aspirin and other nonsteroidal antiinflammatory agents inhibit secretion of both mucus and HCO_3^-; prolonged use of these drugs may damage the mucosal surface and produce gastritis or even gastric ulcers. α-Adrenergic agonists diminish HCO_3^- secretion. This effect may play a role in the pathogenesis of stress ulcers; chronically elevated levels of circulating epinephrine may suppress HCO_3^- secretion sufficiently to decrease protection of the epithelial cell surface.

Control of Gastric Acid Secretion

Control of HCl secretion at the level of the parietal cell. Acetylcholine, histamine, and **gastrin** are the three

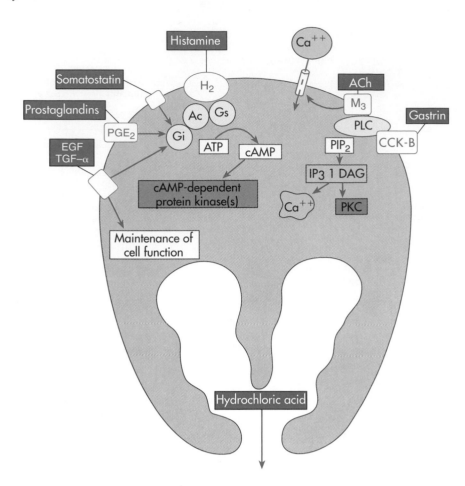

■ **Fig. 32-14** Signal transduction mechanisms of secretagogues and antagonists of acid secretion by parietal cells. Acetylcholine *(ACh)* binds to M_3 muscarinic receptors. Histamine acts via H_2 histamine receptors. Gastrin binds to CCK-B/gastrin receptors. Acetylcholine and gastrin act to open Ca^{2+} channels and to release Ca^{2+} from intracellular stores in order to increase cytosolic free Ca^{2+}. Histamine activates adenylyl cyclase and increases intracellular levels of cyclic AMP *(cAMP)*. The secretagogues activate protein kinase C, cAMP-dependent protein kinase, and Ca^{2+}-calmodulin-dependent kinases. Certain inhibitors of acid secretion, such as somatostatin, prostaglandins of the E class, and epidermal growth factor *(EGF)*, inhibit adenylyl cyclase and lower the cytosolic level of cAMP. *PLC,* Phospholipase C; *PKC,* protein kinase C; *TGF,* transforming growth factor. (From Chew CS: *Curr Opin Gastroenterol* 7:856, 1991.)

physiological agonists of HCl secretion. Each of these secretagogues binds to a distinct class of receptors on the plasma membrane of the parietal cell and directly stimulates the parietal cell to secrete HCl (Fig. 32-14). Acetylcholine is released near parietal cells by cholinergic nerve terminals. Gastrin, a hormone, is produced by G cells in the mucosa of the gastric antrum and the duodenum, and reaches parietal cells via the bloodstream. Histamine, a paracrine agonist, is released from ECL cells in the gastric mucosa and diffuses to the parietal cells. Thus, the control of HCl secretion occurs by all three types of control mechanisms—neurocrine, endocrine, and paracrine—that regulate gastrointestinal secretions.

Cellular mechanisms of parietal cell agonists. The receptors on the parietal cell membrane for acetylcholine, gastrin, and histamine, as well as the intracellular second messengers by which these secretagogues act, are shown in Fig. 32-14. Histamine is the strongest agonist of HCl secretion. Gastrin and acetylcholine are much weaker agonists than histamine. Histamine, acetylcholine, and gastrin potentiate one another's actions on the parietal cell.

Histamine is a major physiological mediator of HCl secretion. Antagonists of H_2 histamine receptors, such as **cimetidine,** block a large portion of the acid secretion elicited by any of the known secretagogues.

Histamine is synthesized and stored in **ECL cells,** which are present in the gastric mucosa. When stimulated by gastrin, the ECL cells release histamine, which diffuses to nearby parietal cells to stimulate HCl secretion. Gastrin is not as potent as histamine in directly stimulating parietal cells to release HCl. Blockers of the H_2 receptors can greatly reduce the physiological response to elevated blood levels of gastrin. Thus, much of the response to gastrin results from gastrin-stimulated release of histamine. Gastrin has important trophic effects: elevation of gastrin levels causes increased size and number of ECL cells.

Histamine binding to H_2 receptors on parietal cell plasma membranes activates adenylyl cyclase and elevates the cytosolic concentration of cAMP. These events stimulate HCl secretion by activating basolateral K^+ channels and apical Cl^- channels; they also cause more H^+,K^+-ATPase molecules and Cl^- channels to be inserted into the apical plasma membrane (Fig. 32-11).

Acetylcholine binds to M_3 muscarinic receptors and opens Ca^{2+} channels in the apical plasma membrane. Acetylcholine also elevates the intracellular Ca^{2+} concentration by promoting release of Ca^{2+} from intracellular stores. An elevated intracellular Ca^{2+} concentration enhances HCl secretion by activating basolateral K^+ channels and by causing more H^+,K^+-ATPase molecules and Cl^- channels to be inserted into the apical plasma membrane.

Gastrin enhances acid secretion by binding to CCK-B receptors to elevate the intracellular Ca^{2+} concentration. **Proglumide** is an antagonist of the binding of gastrin to CCK-B receptors.

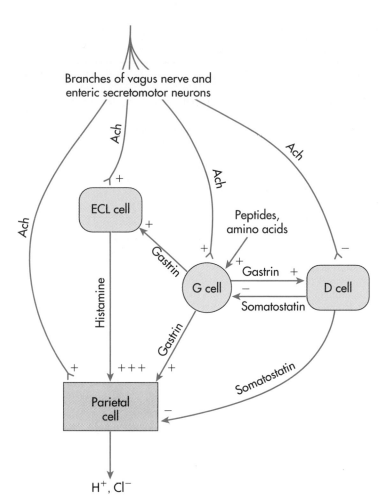

■ Fig. 32-15 Control of gastric secretion of HC1. Histamine (the strongest agonist), acetylcholine *(ACh)*, and gastrin evoke HC1 secretion by parietal cells. Somatostatin from mucosal D cells tonically suppresses HC1 secretion. Vagal impulses stimulate enteric neurons that release ACh to increase secretion of histamine, gastrin, somatostatin, and HC1. Gastrin enhances secretion of histamine by ECL cells. Gastrin increases secretion of somatostatin by D cells and somatostatin acts to inhibit gastrin secretion. The negative effect on HC1 secretion that results from the latter two effects, together with the potent inhibition of parietal cells by somatostatin, helps to prevent the positive feedback loops shown in the figure from evoking uncontrolled high rates of HC1 secretion.

Before the availability of cimetidine and other H_2 receptor blockers, gastric and duodenal ulcers were resistant to drug therapy. Consequently, surgical treatments of ulcers were among the most common surgical operations performed. H_2 receptor blockers revolutionized therapy for gastric and duodenal ulcer disease and for most other disorders related to hypersecretion of gastric acid. More recently drugs that directly inhibit the H^+,K^+-ATPase have been developed. These drugs inhibit HCl secretion even more profoundly than do the H_2 receptor antagonists. Surgical interventions are now rarely necessary. These drugs can dramatically reduce secretion of HCl, and they have few side effects.

Endogenous antagonists of acid secretion. **Somatostatin, prostaglandins** of the E and I series, and **epidermal growth factor (EGF)** act on parietal cells to inhibit HCl secretion by inhibiting adenylyl cyclase and decreasing the cAMP concentration (Fig. 32-14). A prostaglandin analog, called **misoprostol,** suppresses acid secretion in this way.

Somatostatin, released from D cells near the bases of gastric glands, is the most important antagonist of HCl secretion. Somatostatin directly inhibits HCl secretion by parietal cells and also suppresses the release of gastrin from G cells. Somatostatin tonically inhibits HCl secretion, and other inhibitory mechanisms may be mediated largely by somato-

statin. Figure 32-15 summarizes control of HCl secretion by neural, hormonal, and paracrine mechanisms.

In vivo control of acid secretion rate. When the stomach has been empty for several hours, HCl is secreted at a basal rate, which is approximately 10% of the maximal rate. After a meal, the stomach promptly increases the rate of acid secretion. There are three phases of increased acid secretion in response to food: the **cephalic phase,** elicited before food reaches the stomach; the **gastric phase,** elicited by the presence of food in the stomach; and the **intestinal phase,** elicited by mechanisms that originate in the duodenum and upper jejunum (Table 32-1).

The cephalic phase. The cephalic phase of gastric secretion is elicited by the sight, smell, and taste of food. Cephalic phase secretion is entirely mediated by branches of the vagus nerves. Vagal fibers then stimulate enteric neurons that are predominantly cholinergic, and it is these enteric neurons that directly elicit cephalic phase secretion. Acetylcholine released from these neurons directly stimulates parietal cells to secrete HCl. Indirectly, acetylcholine stimulates acid secretion by releasing gastrin from G cells in the antrum and duodenum, and by releasing histamine from ECL cells in the gastric mucosa (Fig. 32-15).

The low pH in the antrum of the stomach inhibits HCl secretion by directly inhibiting parietal cells and by evoking inhibitory neural reflexes. In the absence of food in the

■ **Table 32-1**   Mechanisms for stimulation of gastric acid secretion

Phase	Stimuli	Mechanisms of stimulation of HC1 secretion
Cephalic	Chewing, swallowing, taste, smell of food	Vagal impulses excite enteric secretomotor neurons to parietal, G, and ECL cells
Gastric	Gastric distension	Local and vagovagal reflexes stimulate parietal cells and release of histamine and gastrin
	Peptides and amino acids in lumen	Peptides and amino acids release gastrin from G cells in stomach
Intestinal	Protein digestion products in duodenum	Release of gastrin from G cells in intestine and enterooxyntin
	Distension of duodenum	Enteric and vagovagal reflexes to ECL, G, and parietal cells
	Amino acids and peptides in blood	Release of gastrin from G cells in stomach

■ **Table 32-2**   Mechanisms for inhibition of gastric acid secretion

Phase	Stimuli	Mechanisms of stimulation of HC1 secretion
Cephalic and gastric	Vagovagal and enteric neural impulses	Release of gastrin promotes release of somatostatin by D cells
	Low pH in lumen of stomach	Inhibition of parietal and G cells
Intestinal	Low pH in duodenum	Vagovagal and enteric reflexes that inhibit HC1 secretion
	Digestion products of fats and protein	Secretin and bulbogastrone inhibit parietal cells
		CCK and GIP inhibit parietal cells
	IIypertonicity in duodcnum	Unidentified enterogastrone inhibits HC1 secretion

stomach to buffer the acid secreted, the pH of the antral contents falls rapidly during the cephalic phase. The rate of acid secretion during the cephalic phase may be 40% of the maximal rate, but because of the inhibitory mechanisms evoked by low pH in the antrum, the amount of acid secreted is small.

The brain may also influence gastric acid secretion by other mechanisms, but their physiological importance remains uncertain. Low glucose levels in cerebral blood, which occur, for example, during insulin-induced hypoglycemia, stimulate gastric acid secretion. Certain neuropeptides present in brain neurons, when injected into cerebrospinal fluid, stimulate or inhibit gastric secretion of HCl.

The gastric phase. The gastric phase of gastric secretion is elicited by the presence of food in the stomach. The principal stimuli are distension of the stomach and the presence of amino acids and peptides that result from the actions of pepsins. Most of the acid secreted in response to a meal is secreted during the gastric phase.

Distension of either the body or the antrum of the stomach stimulates mechanoreceptors in the gastric wall. These mechanoreceptors are the afferent arms of local and central reflexes. Both the local and central reflexes are largely cholinergic. The central reflexes have their afferent and efferent fibers in the vagus nerves; thus, they are called **vagovagal reflexes.** Activation of these local and central reflexes causes acetylcholine to be released onto parietal cells, which directly stimulates them to secrete HCl, and onto antral G cells, which are stimulated to release gastrin.

The presence of amino acids, especially tryptophan and phenylalanine, and peptides in the antrum elicits HCl secretion by causing G cells in the antrum to release gastrin. Intact proteins do not have this effect. Other ingested substances that may enhance gastric acid secretion include calcium ions, caffeine, and alcohol. Gastric distention enhances the effects of chemical stimuli of HCl secretion.

Secretion of HCl elicited by any of the mechanisms just described is effectively blocked by bathing the mucosal surface with a solution that has a pH of 2 or less. Once the buffering capacity of the gastric contents is saturated, gastric pH falls rapidly and inhibits further acid release. *In this way, the acidity of gastric contents regulates itself.* Low pH in the lumen of the stomach inhibits HCl secretion by parietal cells by evoking local inhibitory reflexes, by directly inhibiting parietal cell secretion, and by inhibiting the release of gastrin from G cells.

The intestinal phase. The presence of chyme in the duodenum brings about neural and endocrine responses that *first stimulate and later inhibit acid secretion by the stomach.* Early in gastric emptying, when the pH of gastric chyme is greater than 3, stimulation predominates. Later, when the buffer capacity of gastric chyme is exhausted and the pH of chyme emptied into the duodenum falls to less than 3, inhibition prevails. Tables 32-1 and 32-2 summarize the major mechanisms that stimulate and inhibit gastric acid secretion.

Stimulation of secretion. Gastric secretion is enhanced by distension of the duodenum and by the presence of protein digestion products (peptides and amino acids) in the duodenum. Duodenal distension increases gastric acid secretion by means of vagovagal reflexes that stimulate parietal cells and G cells in the gastric antrum. Peptides and amino acids stimulate G cells in the duodenum and proximal jejunum to release gastrin. In addition, amino acids and peptides that are absorbed in the duodenum and jejunum are carried in the blood to the gastric antrum, where they enhance gastrin release by G cells and may also stimulate parietal cells directly.

In addition, protein digestion products prompt the release of the hormone ***entero-oxyntin*** from the duodenum. This poorly characterized hormone also stimulates gastric acid secretion.

Inhibition of secretion. Several different mechanisms that operate during the intestinal phase inhibit gastric secretion (Table 32-2). These mechanisms are evoked by the presence of acid, fat digestion products, and hypertonicity in the duodenum and proximal part of the jejunum.

Acid solutions in the duodenum inhibit gastric acid by parietal cells via enteric and vagovagal reflexes. Acid solutions in the duodenum also release the hormone **secretin** into the bloodstream. Secretin inhibits gastric acid by inhibiting gastrin release by G cells and by decreasing the response of parietal cells to secretagogues. Acid in the duodenal bulb releases another hormone, **bulbogastrone,** which inhibits acid secretion by the parietal cells.

Products of triglyceride digestion in the duodenum and proximal part of the jejunum release two hormones, **gastric inhibitory peptide (GIP)** and **cholecystokinin (CCK),** that inhibit acid secretion by parietal cells.

Hyperosmotic solutions in the duodenum release an unidentified hormone that inhibits gastric acid secretion. Hormones that are released from the intestine and affect gastric secretions are called enterogastrones.

Gastric and Duodenal Ulcers

Ulceration of the gastric or duodenal mucosa occurs in many individuals. The term **peptic ulcer disease** includes both gastric and duodenal ulcers. Among the mechanisms that may contribute to ulcer formation are diminished effectiveness of the gastric mucosal barrier, hypersecretion of acid, and infection by *Helicobacter pylori* bacteria.

Diminished effectiveness of the gastric mucosal barrier, and formation of gastric ulcers, may result from long-term treatment with nonsteroidal antiinflammatory agents. These agents reduce the rates of secretion of mucus and bicarbonate.

Hypersecretion of acid may contribute to formation of duodenal ulcers. In **Zollinger-Ellison syndrome,** a gastrin-secreting tumor results in increased HCl secretion and in the formation of duodenal ulcers.

Helicobacter pylori infection is responsible for nearly all cases of gastric and duodenal ulcers that are not related to medication. *H. pylori* has the highly unusual ability to thrive in an acid environment. The bacteria contain large amounts of urease, an enzyme that catalyzes the conversion of urea to ammonia and CO_2. Ammonia helps to buffer the acid surrounding the bacteria. *H. pylori* colonizes the mucus layer of the stomach and duodenum. It does not actually invade the mucosa; rather, it causes damage by secreting proteins that evoke both cellular and humoral immune responses. The invasion of the mucosa by macrophages and other immunocytes results in **chronic superficial gastritis,** which may lead to ulcer disease.

The stomachs of approximately 40% of all individuals are infected with *H. pylori!* Most of these people have chronic superficial gastritis that causes no intolerable symptoms. In other individuals, *H. pylori* causes more severe

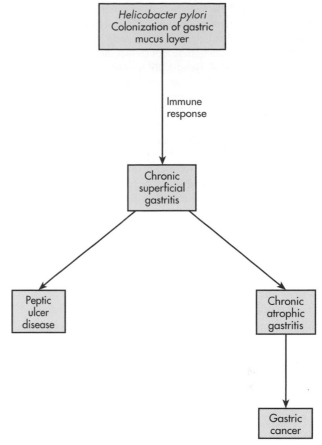

■ **Fig. 32-16** Diseases caused by infection of the gastric mucosal surface by *Helicobacter pylori*. Most individuals whose stomachs are infected with the bacterium have chronic superficial gastritis. It is not known why in certain people this condition progresses to peptic ulcer disease, to more severe gastritis, or to gastric cancer.

gastritis or ulcerations. Chronic severe gastritis caused by *H. pylori* has been implicated in many gastric cancers (Fig. 32-16).

Most duodenal ulcers are also associated with *H. pylori* infection of the stomach. Duodenal ulcer patients are often hypersecretors of HCl; this hypersecretion may be partly attributed to diminished sensitivity to inhibition of HCl secretion by secretin released from the duodenum.

Antibiotic therapy is part of the recommended treatment of gastric or duodenal ulcer disease in *H. pylori*-infected patients. In addition, drugs that suppress HCl secretion are administered, because suppression of HCl secretion renders *H. pylori* more sensitive to antibiotics. Treatment with omeprazole or H_2 receptor antagonists without antibiotics reduces the population of *H. pylori* and promotes healing of ulcers. When administration of blockers of acid secretion is discontinued, however, *H. pylori* again flourishes, and ulcers recur in most cases.

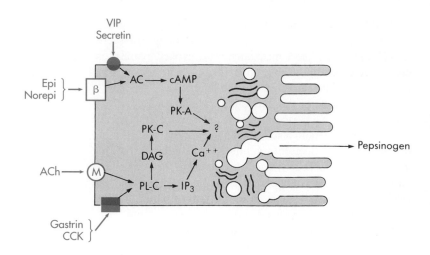

■ **Fig. 32-17** Cellular mechanisms of agonists that elicit pepsinogen secretion by chief cells. Secretin, vasoactive intestinal polypeptide *(VIP)*, and β-adrenergic agonists act via receptors that increase the intracellular level of cyclic AMP *(cAMP)*. Acetylcholine *(ACh)*, gastrin, and cholecystokinin *(CCK)* act by the inositol phosphate pathway to increase intracellular [Ca^{2+}]. The mechanism whereby H^+ ions potentiate secretion of pepsinogens remains to be elucidated. *PK-A*, Protein kinase A; *PK-C*, protein kinase C; *PL-C*, phospholipase C; *DAG*, diacyclglycerol; *IP₃*, inositol trisphosphate. (From Hershey SJ: In *Handbook of physiology*, sect 6, vol III, *The gastrointestinal system*, Bethesda, Md, 1989, American Physiological Society.)

Pepsinogen Secretion

Most of the agents that stimulate parietal cells to secrete acid also release pepsinogens from chief cells (Fig. 32-17). Thus, *the rates of release of acid and pepsinogens from the gastric glands are highly correlated.* Acetylcholine is a potent stimulus for the chief cells to release pepsinogens. Gastrin also directly stimulates chief cells. Acid in contact with the gastric mucosa stimulates pepsinogen release by a local neural reflex. Secretin and CCK, which are released by the duodenal mucosa, also stimulate chief cells to secrete pepsinogens.

PANCREATIC SECRETION

The human pancreas weighs less than 100 g, yet each day it secretes 1 kg (10 times its mass) of pancreatic juice. The pancreas is unusual in that it serves both endocrine and exocrine secretory functions. *The exocrine juice is composed of an* **aqueous component** *and an* **enzyme component.** The aqueous component *is rich in bicarbonate and helps to neutralize duodenal contents. The enzyme component contains enzymes for digesting carbohydrates, proteins, and fats.* Both neural and hormonal signals control pancreatic exocrine secretion. Cholinergic neurons, both vagal neurons and neurons intrinsic to the pancreas, stimulate secretion of the enzyme and the aqueous components of pancreatic juice. **CCK** and **secretin,** hormones released by endocrine cells in the duodenum, stimulate the enzyme and aqueous components, respectively.

Structure and Innervation of the Pancreas

The structure of the exocrine pancreas resembles that of the salivary glands (Figs. 32-1 and 32-2). The pancreas contains microscopic, blind-ended tubules that are surrounded by polygonal acinar cells and are organized into lobules. The primary function of these lobules, or acini, is to secrete the enzyme component of pancreatic juice. The tiny ducts that drain the acini are called **intercalated ducts.** The intercalated ducts empty into somewhat larger **intralobular ducts** (Fig. 32-18). All of the intralobular ducts of a particular lob-

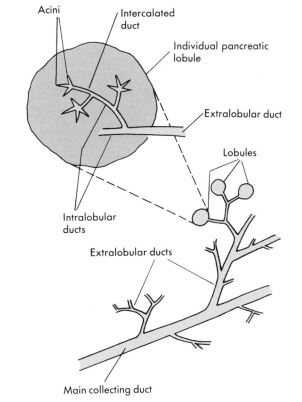

■ **Fig. 32-18** Duct system of the pancreas. (From Swanson CH, Solomon AK: *J Gen Physiol* 62:407, 1973.)

ule then drain into a single **extralobular duct;** this duct in turn empties into still larger ducts. These larger ducts converge into a main duct that enters the duodenum along with the **common bile duct.**

The endocrine portion of the pancreas is composed of cells that reside in the **islets of Langerhans.** Although islet cells account for less than 2% of the volume of the pancreas, their hormones play an essential role in regulating metabolism. **Insulin, glucagon, somatostatin,** and **pancreatic polypeptide** are the hormones that are released from cells of the islets of Langerhans (see Chapter 41). Each of these hormones, when administered intravenously, influences the

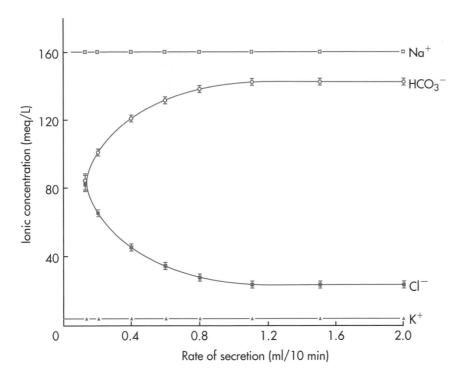

■ **Fig. 32-19** Concentrations of the major ions in the pancreatic juice of anesthetized cats as functions of the secretory flow rate. Secretion was stimulated by intravenous administration of secretin. (From Case RM, Harper AA, Scratcherd T: *J Physiol* 201:335, 1969.)

exocrine secretion of the pancreas, but the exact physiological roles of these effects remain to be established.

The pancreas is supplied by branches of the celiac and superior mesenteric arteries. The portal vein drains the pancreas. The acini and islets are supplied by separate capillary networks. Some of the capillaries that supply the islets converge into venules, which then branch to form a second capillary bed around the acini.

The pancreas is innervated by branches of the vagus nerve. Vagal fibers form synapses with cholinergic neurons that lie within the pancreas; these neurons innervate acinar, duct, and islet cells. Postganglionic sympathetic nerves from the celiac and superior mesenteric plexuses innervate pancreatic blood vessels. Sympathetic activity causes vasoconstriction. *Secretion of pancreatic juice is stimulated by parasympathetic activity and inhibited by sympathetic activity.* Enteric sensory neurons from the stomach and duedenum project onto intrinsic neurons in the pancreas. The enteric neurons evoke **gastropancreatic** and **intestinopancreatic** reflexes that stimulate and also may inhibit secretion by both acinar and duct cells.

Aqueous Component of Pancreatic Juice

The **aqueous component** of pancreatic juice is produced principally by the columnar epithelial cells that line the pancreatic ducts. Pancreatic juice is nearly isotonic to plasma at all rates of flow. The Na^+ and K^+ concentrations of pancreatic juice are similar to those in plasma. HCO_3^- (at levels well above those in plasma) and Cl^- are the major anions contained in pancreatic juice. The HCO_3^- concentration varies from approximately 70 mEq/L at low rates of secretion to more than 130 mEq/L at high secretory rates (Fig. 32-19). Cl^- concentrations vary reciprocally with HCO_3^- concentrations.

The aqueous component secreted by the duct cells is slightly hypertonic to plasma, and its HCO_3^- concentration is high. As the secretion flows through the ducts, water moves into the ducts across the epithelium and makes the pancreatic juice isotonic. In addition, some HCO_3^- is exchanged for Cl^- (Fig. 32-20) as the pancreatic juice makes its way through the ducts.

Under resting conditions, the aqueous component is produced primarily by the intercalated and other intralobular ducts. *When secretion is stimulated by secretin, however, the additional aqueous component is made primarily by the extralobular ducts* (Fig. 32-20). The secretin-stimulated fluid secreted by the extralobular ducts has a higher bicarbonate concentration than does the fluid spontaneously secreted by the intralobular ducts.

A current model of the cellular mechanisms whereby extralobular ducts secrete a bicarbonate-rich fluid is shown in Fig. 32-21. Bicarbonate in the blood that perfuses the pancreas, rather than bicarbonate that is produced by the duct epithelial cell, is the major source of the bicarbonate that is secreted into the lumen of the extralobular duct.

Enzyme Component of Pancreatic Juice

*The secretions of the acinar cells make up the **enzyme component** of pancreatic juice.* The fluid that is secreted by the acinar cells resembles plasma in its tonicity and in the concentrations of various ions; a current view of the ionic transport mechanisms involved is shown in Fig. 32-22. The cells of the intercalated ducts may also contribute to these secretions.

The enzyme component of pancreatic juice contains enzymes that are important for the digestion of all the major classes of foodstuffs (Table 32-3). If pancreatic enzymes are absent, the digestion and absorption of lipids, proteins, and carbohydrates are abnormal.

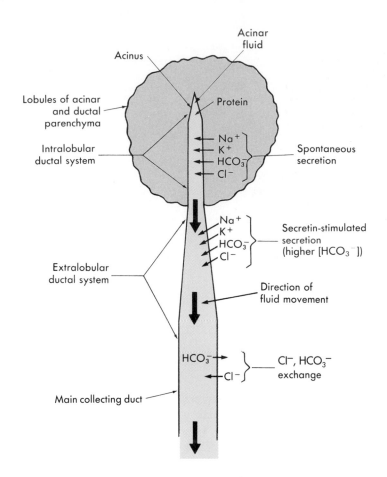

Fig. 32-20 Locations of important transport processes involved in the elaboration of pancreatic juice. Acinar fluid is isotonic and resembles plasma in its concentrations of Na^+, K^+, Cl^-, and HCO_3^-. The secretion of acinar fluid and the proteins it contains is stimulated by cholecystokinin and acetylcholine. A spontaneous secretion that is produced by the intralobular ducts has higher concentrations of K^+ and HCO_3^- than does plasma. The hormone secretin stimulates water and electrolyte secretion by the cells that line the extralobular ducts. The secretin-stimulated secretion is still richer in HCO_3^- than the spontaneous secretion. (From Swanson CH, Solomon AK: *J Gen Physiol* 62:407, 1973.)

Fig. 32-21 Postulated cellular ion transport mechanisms for secretion of bicarbonate-rich fluid by epithelial cells of pancreatic extralobular ducts. Blood is the principal source of the bicarbonate secreted into the duct lumen. Blood perfusing the ducts is acidified by Na^+,H^+ exchangers and H^+,K^+-ATPases in the basolateral membrane, resulting in formation of CO_2 from blood bicarbonate. CO_2 diffuses into the ductular epithelial cell, where its hydration to form H_2CO_3 is catalyzed by carbonic anhydrase *(CA)*. Dissociation of H_2CO_3 to H^+ and HCO_3^-, together with extrusion of H^+ across the basolateral membrane, produces a high intracellular $[HCO_3^-]$. HCO_3^- flows down its electrochemical potential gradient across the luminal membrane via the Cl^-, HCO_3^- exchanger. Cl^- is recycled back into the lumen by the electrogenic Cl^- channels in the luminal membrane. Na^+ enters the luminal fluid by flowing through the tight junctions in response to the negative electrical potential in the lumen that is produced by electrogenic Cl^- transport. Efflux of K^+ through basolateral K^+ channels maintains the intracellular electronegativity that is part of the driving force for the transport of Cl^- and HCO_3^- across the luminal membrane. Secretin, the most important physiological agonist, elevates intracellular cyclic AMP, which dramatically increases the open time of the luminal Cl^- channel. In addition, cAMP probably activates basolateral K^+ channels and promotes the insertion of more H^+,K^+-ATPase molecules into the basolateral membrane. Calcium-mobilizing agonists, such as acetylcholine and CCK, open Ca^{2+}-activated K^+ channels in the basolateral membrane, and in this way mildly enhance secretion when acting alone and markedly potentiate the effects of secretin.

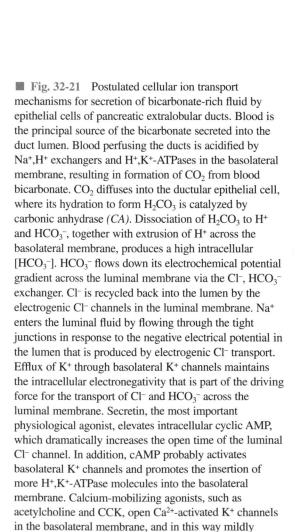

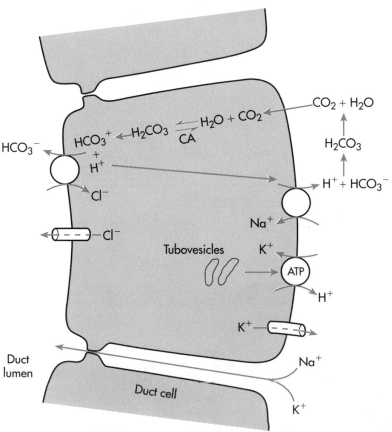

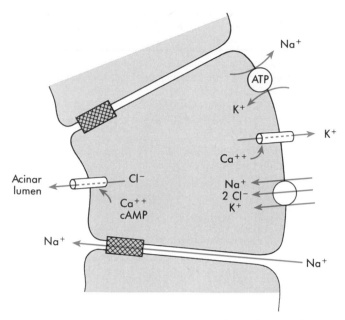

■ **Fig. 32-22** Postulated ionic mechanisms for secretion of NaCl-rich fluid by the pancreatic acinar cells and perhaps by the cells of the intercalated ducts also. The basolateral membrane has an electroneutral transporter that uses the energy of the Na^+ gradient to take up one Na^+ along with one K^+ and two Cl^-; the latter two ions are transported into the cell against their electrochemical potential gradients. Cl^- leaves the cell across the luminal membrane via a Cl^- channel that is activated by cyclic AMP *(cAMP)* and Ca^{2+}. Na^+ enters the lumen via the leaky tight junctions between adjacent acinar cells. The basolateral membrane has Ca^{2+}-activated K^+ channels. Ca^{2+}-mobilizing agonists thus hyperpolarize the cell and thereby increase the force for luminal Cl^- efflux and for basolateral Na^+-driven Cl^- entry.

■ **Table 32-3** Some of the proteins of human pancreatic juice

Protein	Molecular weight	Mass proportion (%)
α-Amylase	54,800	5.3
Triacylglycerol hydrolase	50,500	0.7
Phospholipase A_2	17,500	–
Colipase 1	–	–
Colipase 2	–	–
Procarboxypeptidase A1	46,000	16.8
Procarboxypeptidase A2	47,000	8.1
Procarboxypeptidase B1	47,000	4.4
Procarboxypeptidase B2	47,000	2.9
Trypsinogen 1	28,000	23.1
Trypsinogen 2	26,000	–
Trypsinogen 3	26,700	16.0
Chymotrypsinogen	29,000	1.7
Proelastase 1	30,500	3.1
Proelastase 2	30,500	1.2

Based on data from Scheele G et al: *Gastroenterology* 80:461, 1981.

The proteases contained in pancreatic juice are secreted in an inactive zymogen form. The major pancreatic proteases are **trypsin, chymotrypsin,** and **carboxypeptidase.** The zymogen forms in which they are secreted are **trypsinogen, chymotrypsinogen,** and **procarboxypepti-**

dase, respectively. Trypsinogen is specifically activated by **enteropeptidase** (also called **enterokinase**), which is secreted by the duodenal mucosa. Trypsin then activates trypsinogen, chymotrypsinogen, and procarboxypeptidase. **Trypsin inhibitor,** a protein present in pancreatic juice, prevents the premature activation of proteolytic enzymes within the pancreas.

Pancreatic juice also contains an α-**amylase** that is secreted in active form. Like salivary amylase, **pancreatic amylase** cleaves starch molecules into oligosaccharides. In addition, pancreatic juice contains a number of lipid-digesting enzymes, or **lipases.** Among the major pancreatic lipases are **triacylglycerol hydrolase, cholesterol ester hydrolase,** and **phospholipase A_2.** Pancreatic juice also contains **ribonuclease** and **deoxyribonuclease.** The digestive functions of these pancreatic enzymes are discussed in Chapter 33. A prolonged diet rich in lipids, proteins, or carbohydrates will result in increased concentrations of the appropriate digestive enzymes in pancreatic juice.

The pancreatic enzymes are stored in **zymogen granules** located in the apical cytoplasm of the acinar cells. In response to secretagogues, the contents of the zymogen granule are released by exocytosis into the lumen of the acinus. Acinar cells that have been depleted of zymogen granules can also secrete enzymes; the details of this secretory mechanism remain unclear.

Cl^- enters the acinar lumen via electrogenic Cl^- channels in the apical plasma membranes of the acinar cells (Fig. 32-22) and the ductular epithelial cells (Fig. 32-21). The primary molecular defect in **cystic fibrosis** is a mutation in the gene that encodes this Cl^- channel. As a result of this mutation, the number of Cl^- channels inserted into the plasma membrane is drastically reduced. The decreased transport of Cl^- into the acinar and duct lumens impairs the transport of water and electrolytes. Consequently, in cystic fibrosis, the acini and ducts of the pancreas and the small airways of the lung become clogged with mucus. As a result, the acinar cells and duct system of the pancreas are destroyed, and chronic infections of the lungs can occur. In many infants with cystic fibrosis, pancreatic exocrine function may be irreversibly damaged in utero. Because of the almost complete absence of pancreatic enzymes, infants with cystic fibrosis frequently have severe digestive difficulties, especially in the digestion and absorption of fats.

Regulation of Secretion of Pancreatic Juice

Stimulation of the vagal branches to the pancreas enhances secretion of pancreatic juice, whereas activation of sympathetic fibers inhibits pancreatic secretion, partly by decreasing blood flow to the pancreas. The hormones secretin and CCK, which are released from the duodenal mucosa, stimulate secretion of the aqueous and enzyme components, respectively. Because the production of the

■ **Table 32-4** Control of exocrine pancreatic secretion during the cephalic, gastric, and intestinal phases

Phase	Stimuli of secretion	Mediator or mechanism
Cephalic	Sight, smell, taste of food	Vagal and enteric nerve impulses stimulate acinar and duct cells
Gastric	Distension of stomach	Vagovagal and gastropancreatic reflexes stimulate acinar and duct cells
Intestinal	Acid duodenum (pH <4.5)	Secretin stimulates duct cells
	Amino acids and fatty acids, Ca^{2+}	CCK stimulates afferent arm of vagovagal reflexes to acinar and duct cells
	Distension of duodenum, hypertonicity in duodenum	Enterohepatic reflexes stimulate acinar and duct cells

From Owyang C, Williams JA: Pancreatic secretion. In Yamada T, editor: *Textbook of gastroenterology*, ed 3, Philadelphia, 1999, Lippincott Williams & Wilkins.

aqueous and enzyme components of pancreatic juice is separately controlled (Fig. 32-20), the protein content of the juice varies from less than 1% to as much as 10%.

Like the secretion of gastic HCl, the secretion of pancreatic juice is released during three phases: the cephalic phase, the gastric phase, and the intestinal phase.

The cephalic phase. The sight, smell, and taste of food induce the secretion of pancreatic juice with a high protein content. Vagal impulses are the major stimulus for pancreatic secretion during the cephalic phase. About 25% of the pancreatic juice secreted in response to a meal occurs in the cephalic phase.

The gastric phase. During the gastric phase of secretion, distension of the stomach elicits vagovagal reflexes and gastropancreatic reflexes that stimulate both acinar and duct cells that induce the pancreas to secrete a small volume of pancreatic juice with high enzyme concentration. Approximately 10% of the pancreatic juice is secreted during the gastric phase.

The intestinal phase. Most (about 65%) of the pancreatic juice produced in response to a meal is secreted during the intestinal phase. In the intestinal phase of secretion, certain components of the chyme in the duodenum and upper jejunum evoke pancreatic secretion. Acid in the chyme elicits the secretion of a large volume of pancreatic juice with a low enzyme concentration. *The hormone secretin is the major mediator of this response to acid.* Released by cells in the mucosa of the duodenum and upper jejunum in response to acid (pH <4.5) in the lumen, secretin directly stimulates pancreatic ductular epithelial cells to secrete the bicarbonate-rich aqueous component of the pancreatic juice.

The presence of peptides and certain amino acids (phenylalanine, valine, and methionine) in the duodenum elicits the secretion of pancreatic juice that is rich in enzyme components. Fatty acids, monoglycerides, and Ca^{2+} in the duodenum also elicit secretion of protein-rich pancreatic juice. The hormone CCK, which is released from cells in the duodenum and upper jejunum in response to these substances, is a major mediator of pancreatic secretion during the intestinal phase. Although CCK can directly stimulate acinar cells, in humans the most important effect of CCK is to stimulate the afferent arms of vagovagal reflexes that stimulate secretion by acinar cells and duct cells. Increased volume and osmolality of duodenal contents evoke pancreatic secretion

by stimulating enteropancreatic reflexes; these responses do not involve elevated levels of CCK or secretin.

Table 32-4 summarizes mechanisms of stimulation of pancreatic secretion during cephalic, gastric, and intestinal phases.

Cellular Mechanisms of Secretagogues and Inhibitors

Acinar cells. Acinar cells have receptors for several secretagogues; a simplified representation of these receptors is shown in Fig. 32-23. Occupation of receptors for acetylcholine, CCK, and bombesin stimulates the hydrolysis of inositol phospholipids and elevates the intracellular Ca^{2+} concentration. The calcium-mobilizing agonists also increase the concentration of cGMP. Although cGMP is not directly involved in enhancing secretion, it may promote growth and maintenance of acinar cells. Receptors for secretin and VIP stimulate adenylyl cyclase and increase the cellular concentrations of cAMP. Secretagogues that increase cAMP potentiate the effects of those that elevate intracellular Ca^{2+} concentrations, and vice versa. Somatostatin inhibits acinar cell secretions by inhibiting adenylyl cyclase and reducing the cAMP concentration.

Extralobular duct epithelial cells. The principal physiological agonist of pancreatic duct cell secretion, secretin, stimulates the extralobular duct cells to secrete by elevating the intracellular concentration of cAMP. VIP also has this effect on duct cells. VIP-containing neurons are present in the pancreas, but their physiological role has not been established. CCK elevates the intracellular Ca^{2+} concentration and potentiates the effects of secretion, but CCK alone is a weak secretagogue. Acetylcholine is not an effective agonist for duct epithelial cells.

Other regulatory substances. Somatostatin and glucagon, released from islet cells, inhibit secretion by both acinar and duct cells. Elevation of blood levels of glucose and amino acids inhibits pancreatic secretion; glucagon may be the mediator of these effects. Insulin significantly potentiates the effects of CCK and secretin in stimulating the enzyme and aqueous components, respectively. Pancreatic polypeptide, released from islet cells by cholinergic stimulation, inhibits pancreatic secretion; it may serve as a brake on the neuronal stimulation of pancreatic secretion.

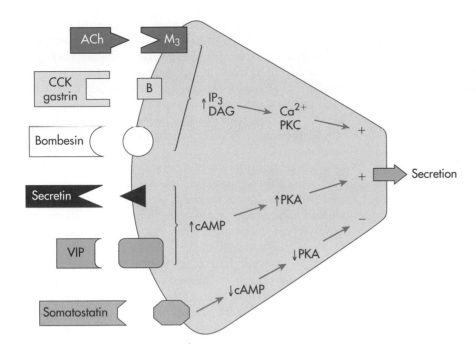

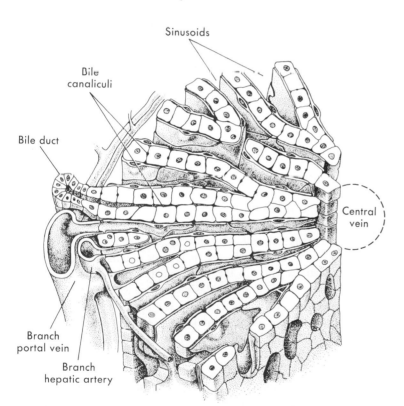

■ **Fig. 32-23** Agonists of pancreatic acinar cell secretion. Acetylcholine acting on M₃ muscarinic receptors is the major physiologic agonist in humans. CCK and gastrin act on CCK-B receptors (some other species have CCK-A receptors). Acetylcholine and CCK stimulate secretion by elevating inositol trisphosphate *(IP₃)* and diacyl glycerol *(DAG)*, which results in increased cytosolic Ca^{2+} and stimulates protein kinase C *(PKC)*. VIP and secretin stimulate secretion by elevating cytosolic cAMP, which enhances the activity of protein kinase A *(PKA)*. Somatostatin inhibits secretion by decreasing cytosolic levels of cAMP.

■ **Fig. 32-24** Diagrammatic representation of a hepatic lobule. A central vein is located in the center of the lobule, with plates of hepatocytes disposed radially. Branches of the portal vein and hepatic artery are located on the periphery of the lobule, and blood from both perfuses the sinusoids. Peripherally located bile ducts drain the bile canaliculi that run between the hepatocytes. (From Bloom W, Fawcett DW: *A textbook of histology,* ed 10, Philadelphia, 1975, WB Saunders.)

FUNCTIONS OF THE LIVER AND GALLBLADDER

Structure of the Liver

The histological appearance of the liver is shown in Fig. 32-24. Each liver **lobule** is organized around a **central vein.** At the periphery of the lobule, blood enters the **sinusoids** from branches of the **portal vein** and the **hepatic artery** (see also Chapter 23). In the sinusoids, blood flows toward the center of the lobule between plates of **hepatocytes** that are one or two cells thick. Because of the large fenestrations between the endothelial cells that line the sinusoids, each hepatocyte is in direct contact with sinusoidal blood. The intimate contact of a large portion of the hepatocyte surface with blood accounts in part for the liver's ability to clear the blood of certain classes of compounds. **Biliary canaliculi** lie between adjacent hepatocytes. These canaliculi drain into bile ducts at the periphery of the lobule.

Functions of the Liver

The liver performs many vital functions. It is essential in regulating metabolism, synthesizing proteins and other molecules, storing vitamins and iron, degrading hormones, and inactivating and excreting drugs and toxins.

The liver regulates the metabolism of carbohydrates, lipids, and proteins. Liver and skeletal muscle are the two major sites of glycogen storage in the body. When the level of glucose in the blood is high, some of this glucose is converted to glycogen, which is deposited in the liver. When the blood glucose level is low, glycogen in the liver is broken down to glucose **(glycogenolysis),** and the glucose is then released into the blood. The liver thus helps to maintain a relatively constant blood glucose level. The liver is also the major site of **gluconeogenesis,** the conversion of amino acids, lipids, or simple carbohydrates (e.g., lactate) into glucose. Carbohydrate metabolism by the liver is regulated by several hormones (see Chapters 40 and 41).

The liver is also centrally involved in lipid metabolism. As described in Chapter 33, absorbed lipids leave the intestine in **chylomicrons** in the lymph. Lipoprotein lipase on the endothelial cell surface of blood vessels hydrolyzes some of the triglycerides in the chylomicrons and releases glycerol and fatty acids. The glycerol and fatty acids are then taken up by **adipocytes.** What remains from this processing of chylomicrons are **chylomicron remnants** rich in cholesterol. These remnants are taken up by hepatocytes and degraded. Hepatocytes also synthesize and secrete **very-low-density lipoproteins (VLDLs).** VLDLs are then converted to the other types of serum lipoproteins (such as high-density lipoproteins and low-density lipoproteins). These lipoproteins are the major sources of cholesterol and triglycerides that supply most other tissues of the body. *Bile is the only route of excretion of cholesterol. Hepatocytes are thus a principal source of cholesterol in the body, and they are the major site of excretion of cholesterol. Thus, hepatocytes play a central role in the regulation of serum cholesterol levels.*

Because carbohydrate utilization is impaired in **diabetes mellitus,** β oxidation of fatty acids provides a major source of energy for the body (see Chapter 40). In the liver, the oxidation of fatty acids produces acetoacetate, β-hydroxybutyrate, and acetone. These three compounds are called **ketone bodies.** Ketone bodies are released from hepatocytes and carried in the circulation to other tissues, where they are metabolized. The levels of ketone bodies in the urine and blood can indicate the severity of diabetic acidosis.

The liver is also centrally involved in protein metabolism. When proteins are broken down (catabolized), amino acids are deaminated to form **ammonia (NH$_3$).** Ammonia cannot be further broken down by most tissues, and toxic levels of ammonia may therefore result. Ammonia is dissipated by conversion to **urea,** which takes place mainly in the liver. The liver also synthesizes all the nonessential amino acids.

In addition, *the liver synthesizes all the major plasma proteins,* including the plasma lipoproteins, albumins, globulins, fibrinogens, and other proteins involved in blood clotting.

The liver stores certain substances important in metabolism. *Next to hemoglobin in red blood cells, the liver is the most important storage site for iron. Some vitamins, most notably A, D, and B$_{12}$, are also stored in the liver.* Hepatic storage protects the body from transient deficiencies of these vitamins.

The liver transforms and excretes many hormones, drugs, and toxins. These substances are frequently converted to inactive forms by reactions that occur in hepatocytes. The smooth endoplasmic reticulum of hepatocytes contains a variety of enzymes and cofactors that are responsible for the chemical transformation of many substances. Other enzymes in the endoplasmic reticulum catalyze the conjugation of many compounds with glucuronic acid, glycine, or glutathione. The transformations that occur in the liver render many compounds more water soluble so that they are more readily excreted by the kidneys. Some liver metabolites are secreted into the bile.

Bile

The hepatic function most important to the digestive tract is the secretion of bile. Bile, produced by hepatocytes, contains **bile acids, cholesterol, phospholipids,** and **bile pigments.** All of these constituents are secreted by hepatocytes into the bile canaliculi, along with an isotonic fluid that resembles plasma in its electrolyte concentrations. The bile canaliculi merge into ever larger ducts and finally into a single large bile duct. The epithelial cells that line the bile ducts secrete a watery, bicarbonate-rich fluid that contributes to the volume of bile leaving the liver.

The secretory function of the liver resembles that of the exocrine pancreas in some ways. In both organs, the major parenchymal cell type produces a primary secretion that contains the substances that carry out the main digestive functions. In both the liver and the pancreas, the primary secretion is isotonic to plasma, and the levels of Na$^+$, K$^+$, and Cl$^-$ are close to plasma levels. The primary secretion of both pancreas and liver is stimulated by CCK. The epithelial cells that line the duct systems of these organs modify the primary secretion. When stimulated by secretin, the ductular epithelial cells in pancreas and liver contribute an aqueous secretion with a high bicarbonate concentration.

Between meals, bile is diverted into the **gallbladder.** *The gallbladder epithelium extracts salts and water from the stored bile, concentrating the bile acids 5-fold to 20-fold.* After an individual eats, the gallbladder contracts and empties its concentrated bile into the duodenum. *The most potent stimulus for emptying of the gallbladder is CCK.* From 250 to 1500 ml of bile enter the duodenum each day.

Bile acids **emulsify** lipids and thereby increase the surface area available to lipolytic enzymes. Bile acids then form **mixed micelles** (see Chapter 33) with the products of lipid digestion. Micelles increase the transport of the products of lipid digestion to the brush border plasma membrane, thereby enhancing the absorption of lipids by the epithelial cells. The epithelial cells actively absorb bile acids, mainly in the terminal ileum. Only about 10% to 20% of bile acids escapes absorption and is excreted. Bile acids that return to the liver are avidly taken up by hepatocytes, which rapidly resecrete them during the course of digestion. The entire bile acid pool is recirculated two or more times in response to a typical meal. This recirculation of the bile is known as the **enterohepatic circulation** (Fig. 32-25). Approximately 20% of the bile acid pool is excreted in the feces each day and is replenished by hepatic synthesis of new bile acids.

Bile acids lost into the feces are the only significant mechanism of cholesterol excretion. Treatment with drugs that block the reabsorption of bile acids in the ileum promotes the synthesis of new bile acids from cholesterol. These drugs can be used to lower the level of cholesterol in the blood.

Fraction of bile secreted by hepatocytes

Bile acids. Bile acids make up about 65% of the dry weight of bile. Other important compounds secreted by the hepatocytes into the bile include phospholipids (about 20%), cholesterol (about 4%), proteins (about 5%), and bilirubin and related bile pigments (about 0.3%).

Bile acids are synthesized by the hepatocytes from cholesterol (Fig. 32-26), from which they acquire their steroid nucleus. The major bile acids synthesized by the liver are called **primary bile acids.** These are **cholic acid** (3-hydroxyl groups) and **chenodeoxycholic acid** (2-hydroxyl groups). The presence of the carboxyl and hydroxyl groups makes the bile acids much more water soluble than the cholesterol from which they are synthesized.

The bacteria that normally colonize in the digestive tract dehydroxylate bile acids to form **secondary bile acids.** The major secondary bile acids are **deoxycholic acid** (from dehydroxylation of cholic acid) and **lithocholic acid** (from dehydroxylation of chenodeoxycholic acid). Bile contains both primary and secondary bile acids.

Bile acids are normally conjugated with glycine or taurine. The glycine or taurine is linked by a peptide bond between the carboxyl group of an unconjugated bile acid and the amino group of glycine or taurine (Fig. 32-26, *bottom*). At the near neutral pH of the gastrointestinal tract, conjugated bile acids are more completely ionized, and are thus more water soluble, than are unconjugated bile acids. Conjugated bile acids are present almost entirely as salts of various cations (mostly Na^+) and are often called **bile salts.**

The steroid nucleus of bile acids is almost planar. In solution, the polar (hydrophilic) groups of bile acids—the hydroxyl groups, the carboxyl moiety of glycine or taurine, and the peptide bond—are arranged on one side of the molecule (Fig. 32-27, *A*). *This arrangement makes the bile acid molecule amphipathic,* that is, having both hydrophilic and hydrophobic domains. Because they are amphipathic, bile

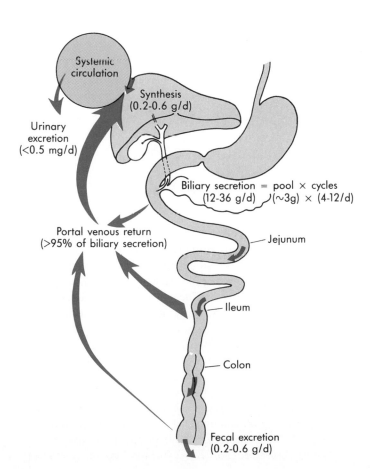

■ **Fig. 32-25**   Representation of key components of the enterohepatic circulation of bile acids in normal humans. Bile is dumped into the duodenum by contractions of the gallbladder. In the small intestine, bile acids first emulsify dietary fat and then form mixed micelles with the products of fat digestion. In the terminal ileum, bile acids are reabsorbed. Bile acids return to the liver in the portal blood, where they are avidly taken up by hepatocytes and resecreted into bile. (From Carey MC, Cahalane MJ: In Arias IM et al: *The liver: biology and pathobiology,* ed 2, New York, 1988, Raven Press.)

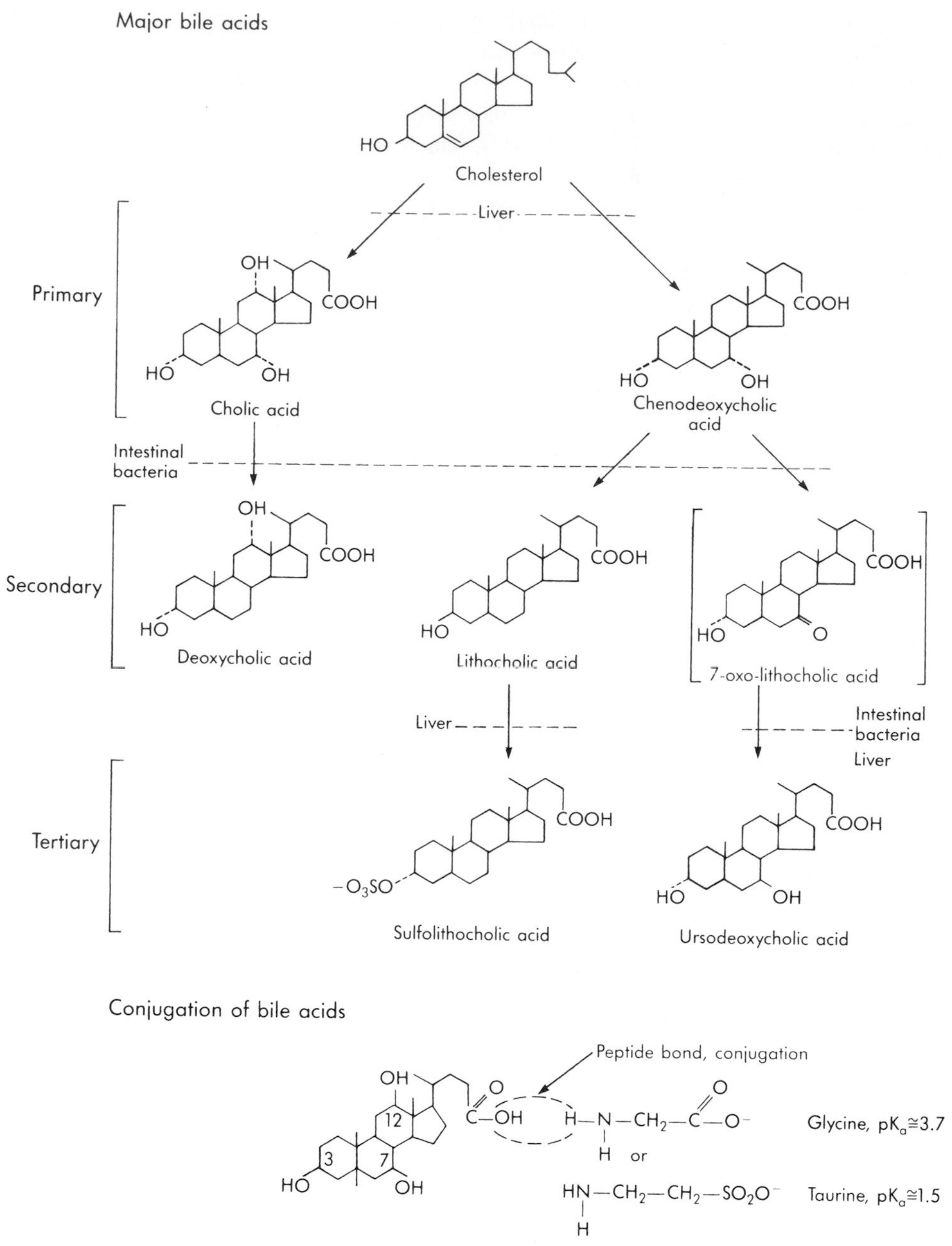

Major bile acids

■ **Fig. 32-26** Structures and sites of conversion of major primary, secondary, and tertiary bile acids in human bile. At the bottom of the figure, the conjugation of cholic acid with glycine or taurine is shown. (From Carey MC, Cahalane MJ: In Arias IM et al: *The liver: biology and pathobiology*, ed 2, New York, 1988, Raven Press.)

Conjugation of bile acids

acids tend to form molecular aggregates, called **micelles,** in a solution. In a bile acid micelle, the hydrophobic side of the bile acid faces inside and away from water, and the hydrophilic surface faces outward toward the water. Bile acid micelles form when the concentration of bile acids exceeds a certain limit, called the **critical micelle concentration.** Above this concentration, any additional bile acid will join the micelles and not form a molecular solution. Conjugated bile acids have lower critical micelle concentrations than unconjugated bile acids. Normally, the bile acid concentration in bile is much greater than the critical micelle concentration.

Phospholipids and cholesterol in bile. Hepatocytes also secrete phospholipids, especially **lecithins,** into bile. Cholesterol is also secreted into the bile, thus constituting the major route for cholesterol excretion. Hepatocytes secrete phos-

pholipids and cholesterol into the bile canaliculi as lipid bilayer vesicles. Phospholipids and cholesterol molecules partition into the bile acid micelles to form **mixed micelles** (Fig. 32-27, *B*), and the lipid vesicles gradually disappear. In the small intestine, the products of triglyceride digestion (2-monoglycerides and free fatty acids) and fat-soluble vitamins partition into these mixed micelles. The more phospholipid that is present, the greater is the amount of cholesterol that can be solubilized in the micelles.

If more cholesterol is present in the bile than can be solubilized in the micelles, bile is said to be **supersaturated** with cholesterol, and crystals of cholesterol tend to form in the bile. Cholesterol crystals in bile aid in the formation of **cholesterol gallstones** (the most common variety)

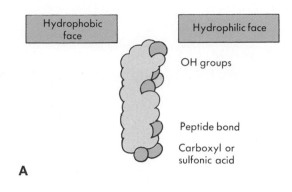

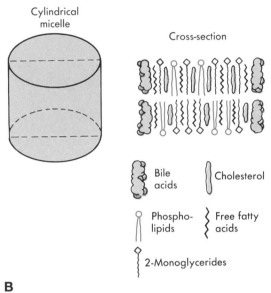

■ **Fig. 32-27** Schematic depiction of bile acids and mixed micelles. **A,** A bile acid molecule in solution. The molecule is amphipathic; it has a hydrophilic face and a hydrophobic face. The amphipathic nature of bile acids is the key to their ability to emulsify lipids and to form mixed micelles with the products of lipid digestion. **B,** A model of the structure of a bile acid lipid mixed micelle.

in the duct system of the liver or (more often) in the gallbladder. Normal individuals tend to secrete bile that is supersaturated in cholesterol only at night; the bile of individuals with cholesterol gallstones tends to be supersaturated with cholesterol throughout the entire day.

Bile pigments. When aging red blood cells are degraded in reticuloendothelial cells, the porphyrin moiety of hemoglobin is converted to **bilirubin.** Bilirubin is released into the plasma, where it is bound to albumin. Hepatocytes efficiently remove bilirubin from blood in the sinusoids and conjugate it with one or two glucuronic acid molecules. The resultant **bilirubin glucuronides** are then secreted into the bile by an adenosine triphosphate (ATP)-dependent transport protein in the canalicular membrane. Bilirubin is yellow and contributes to the color of bile.

Colonic bacteria convert bilirubin to urobilinogen, some of which is absorbed into the blood. A fraction of the urobilinogen is excreted in urine; the remainder is taken up by hepatocytes and resecreted into bile.

Secretion of the bile duct epithelium. The epithelial cells that line the bile ducts secrete an aqueous secretion that accounts for about 50% of the total volume of the bile. This aqueous secretion is isotonic and contains Na^+ and K^+ at concentrations similar to those of plasma. However, the concentration of HCO_3^- is greater and the concentration of Cl^- is less than in plasma. *The secretory activity of the bile duct epithelium is specifically stimulated by secretin.*

Cellular Mechanisms of Bile Secretion

Secretion of bile acids. As is the case for all epithelia, the apical plasma membrane of the hepatocyte (the membrane that faces the bile canaliculus) contains different transport proteins than does the basolateral plasma membrane (the membrane that faces the sinusoidal blood).

As shown in Fig. 32-28, multiple transport mechanisms are located in the hepatocyte plasma membrane for uptake of bile acids, both conjugated and unconjugated, from the sinusoidal blood. The transport proteins that take up bile acids and other organic compounds from sinusoidal blood into hepatocytes are shown in Fig. 32-28. Na^+-dependent taurocholate transporter (NTCP) is a secondary active transporter that takes up all of the conjugated bile acids, both primary and secondary. Two Na^+ ions are transported per bile acid, so that NTCP is electrogenic and thus it is powered partly by the negative membrane potential (about –45 mV) of the hepatocyte. Organic anion transport protein (OATP) transports bile acids, both conjugated and unconjugated ones, and other organic anions from sinusoidal blood into the hepatocyte. OATP is also present in renal proximal tubular epithelial cells. Organic cation transporter 1 (OCT1) takes up organic cations, such as quaternary ammonium compounds, from sinusoidal blood. OCT1 is only present in the liver.

In hepatocyte cytosol, bile acids are mostly bound to **bile acid-binding proteins.** These binding proteins prevent the concentrated bile acids from disrupting the membranes of hepatocyte organelles. Almost all deconjugated bile acids are reconjugated with glycine or taurine. Some of the secondary bile acids are rehydroxylated to primary bile acids.

Bile acids are secreted into the lumen of the secretory canaliculus, probably by facilitated transporters that are protein mediated and are located in the apical membrane. Bile acids move into bile down concentration and electrical potential gradients; the cytosol is about 35 mV negative to the lumen. The concentration gradient is maintained partly because the bile acids form micelles in the canaliculi. The formation of micelles keeps the concentration of bile acids in true solution quite low (equal to the critical micelle concentration).

In the canalicular plasma membrane there are four different proteins (Fig. 32-28) that transport organic compounds from the hepatocyte cytosol into the bile canaliculus. These

■ **Fig. 32-28** Transport proteins of hepatocytes. Bile acids are taken up by hepatocytes from sinusoidal blood by two different transporters. Na⁺-dependent taurocholate transporter *(NTCP)* is a secondary active transporter that takes up all of the conjugated bile acids, both primary and secondary. Organic anion transport protein *(OATP)* transports bile acids, both conjugated and unconjugated, and other organic anions from sinusoidal blood into the hepatocyte. Organic cation transporter 1 *(OCT1)* takes up organic cations from sinusoidal blood. There are four different transport proteins in the canalicular membrane that transport compounds from the hepatocyte cytosol into the bile canaliculus. Bile salt export protein *(BSEP)* transports bile acids into the bile canaliculus. Multidrug resistance *(MDR1)* protein transports organic cations and multidrug transporter-related protein *(MRP2)* transports organic anions. *MDR3* catalyzes the flipping of phosphatidylcholine from the inner leaflet of the plasma membrane to the outer leaflet.

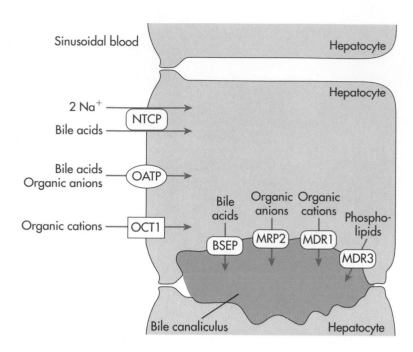

transporters are all members of the ATP-binding cassette (ABC) transport protein family that was discussed in Chapter 1 (see Fig. 1-15). Bile salt export protein (BSEP) transports monovalent anionic bile acids into the bile canaliculus. BSEP is also known as sister protein of P-glycoprotein (SPGP). Multidrug resistance (MDR1) protein transports organic cations and multidrug transporter-related protein (MRP2) transports organic anions. MDR1 is the major human protein responsible for multiple drug resistance syndrome in cancer cells. MDR1 transports cationic xenobiotics (such as drugs and drug metabolites) into bile for excretion. MRP2 is responsible for transporting anionic compounds such as sulfated bile acids and compounds that are conjugated in hepatocytes with glucuronide, sulfate, or glutathione. Bilirubin glucuronides are transported into bile by MRP2. MDR3 catalyzes the flipping of phosphatidylcholine (PC) from the inner leaflet of the canalicular plasma membrane to the outer leaflet, where domains enriched in PC and cholesterol form. Due to the high concentration of bile acids in the canaliculus the domains of PC and cholesterol vesiculate and bud off from the canalicular membrane into the lumen of the canaliculus. Bile acid micelles then take up the PC and cholesterol from the vesicles.

Secretion of water and electrolytes into bile. Water and electrolytes are present in the bile canaliculi in concentrations that equal those of plasma. The osmotic pressure of bile acids and other molecules secreted by the hepatocytes causes water to flow into the canaliculi via the leaky tight junctions that join the hepatocytes. The electrolytes are brought along by solvent drag. In addition, ionic secretory processes in the hepatocyte may contribute electrolytes to the canalicular bile.

The bile duct epithelial cells secrete a bicarbonate-rich fluid into the duct lumen. The transporters involved in secreting water and electrolytes into bile ducts are illustrated in Fig. 32-29. Cl⁻ enters the ductular epithelial cell at the basolateral membrane via the electroneutral Na/K/2Cl transporter and Cl⁻ is transported into the ductular lumen by two Cl⁻ channels: the cystic fibrosis transmembrane regulator (CFTR) and a Ca²⁺-stimulated Cl⁻ channel. Bicarbonate is actively transported from extracellular fluid into the ductular cell by a sodium-bicarbonate cotransporter. The energy of the Na⁺ gradient is used to actively take up HCO_3^-. Bicarbonate enters the ductular lumen via an anion-exchange protein (AE2) that exchanges HCO_3^- for Cl⁻. Secretin and VIP raise levels of cAMP, which increases the open time of the CFTR chloride channel, thus increasing secretion of both Cl⁻ and HCO_3^-.

Bile Concentration and Storage in the Gallbladder

Between meals, the tone of the **sphincter of Oddi,** which guards the entrance of the common bile duct into the duodenum, is high. Thus, most bile flow is diverted into the gallbladder. The gallbladder is a small organ, with a capacity of 15 to 60 ml in humans. Between meals, this volume of bile may be secreted by the liver. The gallbladder concentrates the bile by absorbing Na⁺, Cl⁻, HCO_3^-, and water from the bile, increasing the bile acid concentration 5-fold to 20-fold. The active transport of Na⁺ is the primary active process in the concentrating action of the gallbladder.

Because of its high rate of water absorption, the gallbladder serves as a model for water and electrolyte transport by epithelia connected by tight junctions. The **standing osmotic gradient mechanism** for fluid absorption was first proposed for the gallbladder (Fig. 32-30).

In the standing osmotic gradient mechanism, the active transport of Na⁺ into the lateral intercellular spaces is the primary active transport process. Na⁺,K⁺-ATPase molecules are concentrated in the basolateral membrane near the

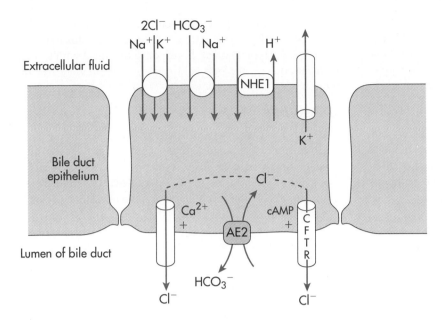

■ **Fig. 32-29** The major transport proteins of the bile duct epithelial cells (cholangiocytes). The membrane that faces the bile duct contains an anion exchanger *(AE2)* that exports HCO_3^- in exchange for Cl^- and two different chloride channels: one is the cystic fibrosis transmembrane regulator *(CFTR)* and the other is a Ca^{2+}-stimulated Cl^- channel. Cl^- is actively taken up across the basolateral membrane by the Na/K/2Cl electroneutral transporter. A basolateral Na^+, H^+ *(NHE1)* exchanger helps to maintain the alkalinity of the cytoplasm and basolateral K^+ channels help maintain the negative membrane potential that powers Cl^- secretion across the ductular membrane.

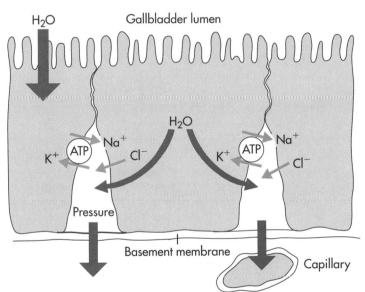

■ **Fig. 32-30** Water absorption from the gallbladder by the standing osmotic gradient mechanism. Na^+, K^+-ATPase molecules are especially concentrated in the basolateral membrane near the mucosal (apical) end of the intercellular channels. Cl^- and HCO_3^- are also transported into the intercellular space, probably because of the electrical potential created by electrogenic Na^+ transport. The high ion concentration near the apical end of the intercellular space causes the fluid there to be hypertonic. This produces an osmotic flow of water from the lumen via adjacent cells into the intercellular space. Water distends the intercellular channels because of increased hydrostatic pressure. As a result of water flow from adjacent cells, the fluid becomes less hypertonic as it flows down the intercellular channel, so that the fluid is essentially isotonic when it reaches the serosal (basal) end of the channel. Ions and water move across the basement membrane of the epithelium and are carried away by the capillaries.

mucosal (apical) end of the intercellular channels. Cl^- and HCO_3^- are also transported into the intercellular space to preserve electroneutrality. The hypertonic concentration of NaCl near the apical end of the intercellular space causes the osmotic flow of water into the intercellular space from the gallbladder lumen and from adjacent epithelial cells. Water distends the intercellular channels, and the fluid flows down the intercellular space toward the basement membrane. Ions and water then move across the basement membrane of the epithelium and are carried away in the blood.

Emptying of the Gallbladder

Emptying of the gallbladder begins several minutes after the start of a meal. Intermittent contractions of the gallbladder force bile through the partially relaxed sphincter of Oddi. During the cephalic and gastric phases of digestion, gallbladder contraction and relaxation of the sphincter are mediated by cholinergic fibers in the vagus nerves and by enteric neurons. Stimulation of sympathetic nerves to the gallbladder and duodenum inhibits emptying of the gallbladder.

The highest rate of gallbladder emptying occurs during the intestinal phase of digestion; the strongest stimulus for the emptying is CCK. CCK reaches the gallbladder via the circulation, and it causes strong contractions of the gallbladder and relaxation of the sphincter of Oddi. Substances that mimic the actions of CCK in promoting gallbladder emptying (such as gastrin) are called **cholecystagogues.**

Under normal circumstances, the rate of gallbladder emptying is sufficient to keep the concentration of bile acids in the duodenum above the critical micelle concentration.

Intestinal Absorption of Bile Acids and Their Enterohepatic Circulation

The functions of bile acids in emulsifying dietary lipid and in forming mixed micelles with the products of lipid digestion are discussed in Chapter 33. Normally, by the time chyme reaches the terminal part of the ileum, dietary fat is almost completely absorbed. Bile acids are then absorbed. *Transport mechanisms are present in the brush border of the terminal ileum for uptake of both conjugated and unconjugated bile acids.* Conjugated bile acids can be taken up against a large concentration gradient. Because bile acids are also lipid soluble, they can be taken up by simple diffusion as well. Bacteria in the terminal part of the ileum and colon deconjugate bile acids and also dehydroxylate them to produce secondary bile acids. Both deconjugation and dehydroxylation lessen the polarity of bile acids, thereby enhancing their lipid solubility and their absorption by simple diffusion.

Typically, about 0.2 to 0.6 g of bile acids escapes absorption and are excreted in the feces each day. This quantity is 15% to 35% of the total bile acid pool, which is normally replenished by synthesis of new bile acids by the liver.

Bile acids, whether absorbed by active transport or by simple diffusion, are transported away from the intestine in the portal blood, mostly bound to albumin in plasma. In the liver, hepatocytes avidly extract the bile acids from the portal blood. *In a single pass through the liver, the portal blood is cleared of the majority of bile acids.* Bile acids in all forms, primary and secondary, both conjugated and deconjugated, are taken up by the hepatocytes. The hepatocytes reconjugate almost all the deconjugated bile acids and rehydroxylate some of the secondary bile acids. These bile acids are secreted into the bile along with newly synthesized bile acids (Fig. 32-28).

Control of Bile Acid Synthesis and Secretion

The rate of return of the bile acids to the liver affects the rate of synthesis and secretion of bile acids. *Bile acids in the portal blood stimulate the uptake and resecretion of bile acids by the hepatoctyes but inhibit the synthesis of new bile acids* (Fig. 32-31). The stimulation of secretion is called the **choleretic effect** of bile acids; substances that enhance bile acid secretion are called **choleretics.** So powerful is

the stimulus to resecrete the returning bile acids that the entire pool of bile acids (1.5 to 31.5 g) recirculates twice in response to a typical meal. In response to a meal with a very high fat content, the bile acid pool may recirculate five or more times.

Gallstones

Cholesterol is essentially insoluble in water. When bile contains more cholesterol than can be solubilized in the bile acid–phospholipid micelles, crystals of cholesterol form in the bile. Such bile is said to be **supersaturated** with cholesterol. The formation of cholesterol gallstones in supersaturated bile was discussed previously.

Bile pigment gallstones are the other major class of gallstones; their main constituent is the calcium salt of unconjugated bilirubin. Conjugated bilirubin is quite soluble and does not form insoluble calcium salts in bile. In liver disease, bile may contain elevated levels of unconjugated bilirubin, because hepatocytes are deficient in forming the glucuronides of bilirubin. Individuals with liver disease have an increased likelihood of forming bile pigment stones.

INTESTINAL SECRETIONS

The mucosa of the intestine, from the duodenum through the rectum, produces secretions that contain mucus, electrolytes, and water. The total volume of intestinal secretions is about 1500 ml/day. The mucus in the secretions protects the mucosa from mechanical damage. The nature of the secretions and the mechanisms that control secretion vary in different segments of the intestine.

Duodenal Secretions

The duodenal submucosa contains branching glands that produce a secretion rich in mucus. The duodenal epithelial cells

■ **Fig. 32-31**   A reciprocal relationship exists between the rates of de novo synthesis of bile acids by hepatocytes and the rate of secretion of bile acids. When bile acids return to the liver in the portal blood, synthesis is inhibited and the energy of the hepatocyte is used to reprocess and secrete the returning bile acids. Removal of the distal ileum decreases the rate of return of bile acids in the portal blood, resulting in a much greater rate of synthesis of bile acids. Feeding bile acids results in increased levels of bile acids in portal blood and in greater inhibition of bile acid synthesis. (From Carey MC, Cahalane MJ: In Arias IM et al: *The liver: biology and pathobiology,* ed 2, New York, 1988, Raven Press.)

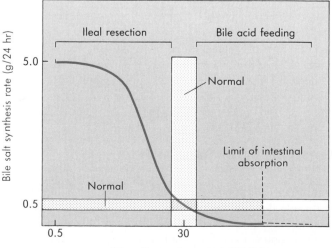

also produce a small amount of duodenal secretions. The duodenal secretion contains mucus and an aqueous component that does not differ significantly from plasma in its concentrations of the major ions.

Secretions of the Small Intestine

Goblet cells, which lie among the columnar epithelial cells of the small intestine, secrete mucus. During normal digestion, an aqueous secretion is produced by the epithelial cells at a rate only slightly less than the rate of fluid absorption by the small intestine (see Chapter 33).

Secretions of the Colon

The secretions of the colon are smaller in volume but richer in mucus than are the small intestinal secretions. The mucus is produced by numerous goblet cells in the colonic mucosa. The aqueous component of colonic secretions is rich in K^+ and HCO_3^-. Colonic secretion is stimulated by mechanical irritation of the mucosa and by activation of cholinergic pathways to the colon. Stimulation of sympathetic nerves to the colon decreases the rate of colonic secretion.

SUMMARY

1. The epithelial cells that line the gastrointestinal tract and the cells of various glands associated with the gastrointestinal tract produce secretions that contain water, electrolytes, proteins, and other substances.

2. The gastrointestinal secretions are regulated by intrinsic and extrinsic neurons, hormones, and paracrine mediators.

3. Salivary glands produce a hypotonic fluid that contains bicarbonate and potassium concentrations in excess of plasma levels. Saliva contains an α-amylase that begins the digestion of starch. Mucus in saliva lubricates food. Parasympathetic nerves are the key regulators of salivary secretion.

4. The stomach serves as a reservoir for ingested food and empties gastric contents into the duodenum at a regulated rate. Parietal cells secrete HCl and intrinsic factor into the stomach. Chief cells secrete pepsinogens.

5. The regulation of HCl secretion in the stomach involves extrinsic and intrinsic nerves, and acetylcholine is the major stimulatory neurotransmitter. Gastrin, a hormone released by G cells in the gastric antrum and in the duodenum, and histamine, a paracrine agonist released by ECL cells in the stomach, are also important physiological agonists of HCl secretion.

6. HCl catalyzes the conversion of pepsinogens to active pepsins. Pepsins convert a significant fraction of ingested protein to oligopeptides.

7. Mucus and bicarbonate secretions form the gastric mucosal barrier that protects the epithelial cells of the stomach from the effects of HCl and pepsins.

8. The pancreas produces a bicarbonate-rich fluid that contains enzymes essential for the digestion of carbohydrates, proteins, and fats. Pancreatic acinar cells produce the enzyme component of pancreatic juice; the intralobular and extralobular ducts secrete much of the aqueous component (water and electrolytes) of pancreatic juice.

9. CCK and secretin are released from the duodenal mucosa in response to digestion products of fats and proteins and pH below 4.5, respectively. CCK stimulates the afferent limbs of vagovagal reflexes that stimulate acinar cells to release enzymes. Secretin directly stimulates the duct cells to secrete bicarbonate-rich fluid.

10. The liver produces and the gallbladder concentrates a secretion called bile. Bile is a bicarbonate-rich fluid that contains bile acids, bile pigments, phospholipids, cholesterol, and numerous other components. Bile acids play a vital role in the digestion and absorption of lipids.

11. Hepatocytes are responsible for secreting the organic components of bile. The cells of the bile ducts secrete a bicarbonate-rich fluid. CCK is a secretagogue for secretion by the hepatocytes. Secretin stimulates the bile ducts to produce their bicarbonate-rich fluid.

12. Bile acids are absorbed in the terminal ileum and return to the liver in the portal vein. Hepatocytes rapidly clear the blood of bile acids and resecrete them. Bile acids in the portal blood are a powerful stimulus to the hepatocytes to resecrete bile acids. The bile acid pool may be recirculated two to five times in response to a single meal. The secretion, return, and resecretion of bile acids is known as the enterohepatic circulation of bile acids.

BIBLIOGRAPHY

Journal articles

Blaser MJ: The bacteria behind ulcers, *Sci Am* 274:104, 1996.

Chew CS: Intracellular mechanisms in control of acid secretion, *Curr Opin Gastroenterol* 7:856, 1991.

Cohen H: Peptic ulcer and *Helicobacter pylori*, *Gastrointestinal Clin North Am* 29:775, 2000.

El-Omer EM et al: *Helicobacter pylori* infection and abnormalities of gastric secretion in patients with duodenal ulcer disease, *Gastroenterology* 109:681, 1995.

Gerber JG, Payne NA: The role of gastric secretagogues in regulating gastric histamine release in vivo, *Gastroenterology* 102:403, 1992.

Hoffman AF: Bile acids: the good, the bad, and the ugly, *News Physiol Sci* 14:24, 1999.

Holzer PH: Gastroduodenal mucosal defense, *Curr Opin Gastroenterol* 16:469, 2000.

Logsdon CD: Signal transduction in pancreatic acinar cell physiology and pathophysiology, *Curr Opin Gastroenterol* 16:404, 2000.

Meier PJ, Stieger B: Molecular mechanisms in bile formation, *News Physiol Sci* 15:89, 2000.

Prall RT, LaRusso NF: Biliary tract physiology, *Curr Opin Gastroenterol* 16:432, 2000.

Putney JW Jr: Identification of cellular activation mechanisms associated with salivary secretion, *Annu Rev Physiol* 48:75, 1986.

Rabon EC, Reuben MA: The mechanism and structure of the gastric H, K-ATPase, *Annu Rev Physiol* 52:321, 1990.

Raeder M: The origin and subcellular mechanisms causing pancreatic bicarbonate secretion, *Gastroenterology* 103:1674, 1992.

Raufman J-P: Gastric chief cells: receptors and signal transduction mechanisms, *Gastroenterology* 102:699, 1992.

Schubert ML: Gastric secretion, *Curr Opin Gastroenterol* 17:481, 2001.

Zsembery A, Thalhammer T, Graf J: Bile formation: a concerted action of membrane transporters in hepatocytes and cholangiocytes, *News Physiol Sci* 15:6, 2000.

Books and monographs

Argent BE, Case RM: Pancreatic ducts: cellular mechanisms and control of bicarbonate secretion. In Johnson LR, editor: *Physiology of the gastrointestinal tract,* ed 3, New York, 1994, Raven Press.

Arias IM et al: *The liver: biology and pathobiology,* ed 4, New York, 2001, Raven Press.

Cook DI et al: Secretion by the major salivary glands. In Johnson LR, editor: *Physiology of the gastrointestinal tract,* ed 3, New York, 1994, Raven Press.

Del Valle J, Todisco A: Gastric secretion. In Yamada T, editor: *Textbook of gastroenterology,* ed 3, Philadelphia, 1999, Lippincott Williams & Wilkins.

Feldman M: Gastric secretion: normal and abnormal. In Sleisenger M, Fordtran JS, editors: *Gastrointestinal diseases,* ed 6, Philadelphia, 1998, WB Saunders.

Flemström G: Gastric and duodenal secretion of mucus and bicarbonate. In Johnson LR, editor: *Physiology of the gastrointestinal tract,* ed 3, New York, 1994, Raven Press.

Go VLW et al, editors: *The pancreas: biology, pathobiology, and disease,* ed 2, New York, 1993, Raven Press.

Gorelick FS, Jamieson JD: The pancreatic acinar cell: structure-function relationships. In Johnson LR, editor: *Physiology of the gastrointestinal tract,* ed 3, New York, 1994, Raven Press.

Hernandez DE, Glavin GB, editors: *Neurobiology of stress ulcers,* Ann NY Acad Sci, vol 299, New York, 1990, New York Academy of Sciences.

Hersey SJ: Gastric secretion of pepsins. In Johnson LR, editor: *Physiology of the gastrointestinal tract,* ed 3, New York, 1994, Raven Press.

Hoffman AF: Biliary secretion and excretion: the hepatobiliary components of the enterohepatic circulation of bile acids. In Johnson LR, editor: *Physiology of the gastrointestinal tract,* ed 3, New York, 1994, Raven Press.

Moseley RH: Bile secretion. In Yamada T, editor: *Textbook of gastroenterology,* ed 3, Philadelphia, 1999, Lippincott Williams & Wilkins.

Owyang C, Williams JA: Pancreatic secretion. In Yamada T, editor: *Textbook of gastroenterology,* ed 3, Philadelphia, 1999, Lippincott Williams & Wilkins.

Sachs G: The gastric H, K-ATPase: regulation and structure/function of the acid pump of the stomach. In Johnson LR, editor: *Physiology of the gastrointestinal tract,* ed 3, New York, 1994, Raven Press.

Scharschmidt BF: Bilirubin metabolism, bile formation, and gallbladder and bile duct function. In Sleisenger MH, Fordtran JS, editors: *gastrointestinal disease,* ed 5, Philadelphia, 1993, WB Saunders.

Siegers C-P, Watkins JB III, editors: *Biliary excretion of drugs and other chemicals,* New York, 1991, Gustav Fischer Verlag.

Soll AH, Berglindh T: Receptors that regulate gastric acid secretory function. In Johnson LR, editor: *Physiology of the gastrointestinal tract,* ed 3, New York, 1994, Raven Press.

Tavoloni N, Berk PD, editors: *Hepatic transport and bile secretion,* New York, 1993, Raven Press.

Yule DI, Williams JA: Stimulus-secretion coupling in the pancreatic acinus. In Johnson LR, editor: *Physiology of the gastrointestinal tract,* ed 3, New York, 1994, Raven Press.

chapter thirty-three

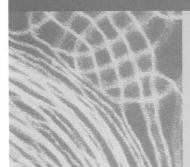

Digestion and Absorption

Most nutrients cannot be absorbed by the epithelial cells that line the gastrointestinal tract in the forms in which they are ingested. **Digestion** refers to the processes by which ingested molecules are converted to forms that can be absorbed by gastrointestinal tract epithelial cells. In digestion, ingested molecules are cleaved into smaller ones by reactions catalyzed by enzymes in the lumen or on the luminal surface of the gastrointestinal tract. **Absorption** refers to the processes by which molecules are transported through the epithelium of the gastrointestinal tract to enter the blood or lymph draining that region of the tract.

DIGESTION AND ABSORPTION OF CARBOHYDRATES

Carbohydrates in the Diet

Plant starch, **amylopectin,** is the major source of carbohydrate in most human diets. *Humans have no nutritional requirement for carbohydrate per se, but it is usually the principal source of calories.* Amylopectin is a high-molecular-weight ($>10^6$), branched molecule of glucose monomers. Another, smaller source of dietary starch is **amylose.** Amylose has a lower molecular weight ($<10^5$) than amylopectin, and it is a linear α-1,4-linked polymer of glucose. **Cellulose,** the major component of dietary fiber, is a β-1,4-linked glucose polymer. Intestinal enzymes cannot hydrolyze β-glycosidic linkages; thus, cellulose and other molecules with β-glycosidic linkages remain undigested. **Glycogen** is a branched animal starch. The amount of glycogen ingested varies widely among cultures and among individuals within a given culture. **Sucrose** and **lactose** are the principal dietary disaccharides; **glucose** and **fructose** are the major monosaccharides.

Digestion of Carbohydrates

The structure of a branched starch molecule is depicted in Fig. 33-1. Starch is a polymer of glucose, and it consists of chains of glucose units linked by α-1,4 glycosidic bonds. The α-1,4 chains have branch points formed by α-1,6 linkages, and thus the starch molecule is highly branched.

The digestion of starch begins in the mouth with the action of the α-**amylase,** formerly known as **ptyalin,** which is contained in salivary secretions. This enzyme catalyzes the hydrolysis of the internal α-1,4 links of starch, but it cannot hydrolyze the α-1,6 branching links, the terminal α-1,4 linkages, or the α-1,4 bonds that are adjacent to an α-1,6 branch point. The α-amylase secreted by the pancreas has the same specificity. The principal products of α-amylase digestion of starch are shown in Fig. 33-1. The action of the salivary α-amylase continues until the food in the stomach is mixed with gastric acid, which inactivates the enzyme. Although considerable amounts of starch may be digested by the salivary α-amylase, this enzyme is not required for complete digestion and absorption of starch. After the salivary α-amylase is inactivated by gastric acid, no further processing of carbohydrate occurs in the stomach.

The α-amylase secreted by the pancreas is highly active. Both salivary and pancreatic α-amylases produce the same products, but the total activity of the pancreatic enzyme is considerably greater than that of the salivary amylase. Pancreatic α-amylase is most concentrated in the duodenum. Within 10 minutes after entering the duodenum, starch is mostly converted to maltose, maltotriose, α-1,4 linked maltooligosaccharides (from four to nine glucose units long), and α-limit dextrins (Fig. 33-1), which contain five to nine glucose monomers.

Further digestion of these oligosaccharides is accomplished by enzymes (called **oligosaccharidases**) that reside in the brush border membrane of the epithelium of the duodenum and jejunum (Fig. 33-2). The active sites of these enzymes face the lumen; they are **ectoenzymes.** The major brush border oligosaccharidases are **lactase,** which splits lactose into glucose and galactose; **sucrase,** which splits sucrose into fructose and glucose; α-**dextrinase** (also called **isomaltase**), which "debranches" the α-limit dextrins by cleaving the α-1,6 linkages at the branch points; and **glucoamylase,** which breaks maltooligosaccharides down into single glucose units by removing one glucose at a time from the nonreducing end of the α-1, 4-linked chain.

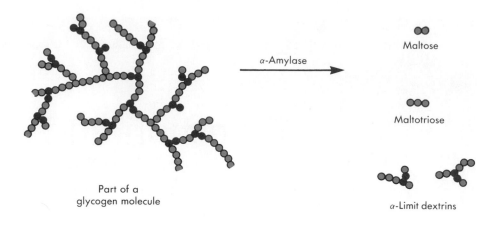

■ **Fig. 33-1** Structure of a branched starch molecule and the action of α-amylase. The colored circles represent glucose monomers linked by α-1,4 linkages. The black circles represent glucose units linked by α-1,6 linkages at the branch points. The α-1,6 linkages and terminal α-1,4 bonds cannot be cleaved by α-amylase.

Part of a glycogen molecule

Maltose

Maltotriose

α-Limit dextrins

α-Amylase

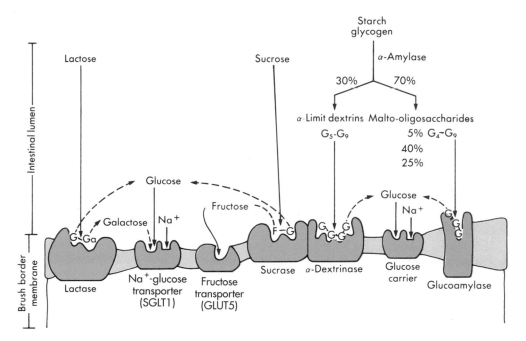

■ **Fig. 33-2** Functions of the major brush border oligosaccharidases. The glucose, galactose, and fructose molecules released by enzymatic hydrolysis are then transported into the epithelial cell by specific transport proteins. The glucose-galactose transporter is also known as SGLT1 and the fructose transporter as GLUT5. *G,* Glucose; *Ga,* galactose; *F,* fructose. (From Gray GM: *N Engl J Med* 292:1225, 1975.)

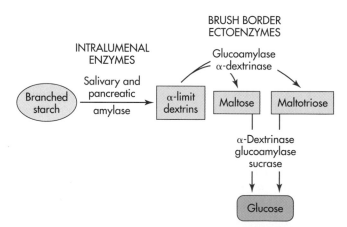

■ **Fig. 33-3** Cleavage of an α-limit dextrin by the oligosaccharidases of the brush border plasma membrane. Glucose monomers are removed in sequence, beginning at the nonreducing end of the molecule by glucoamylase. α-Dextrinase (isomaltase) is the only enzyme that cleaves the α-1,6 linkages at the branch points of the α-limit dextrins.

The activity of these four brush border oligosaccharidases is highest in the duodenum and upper jejunum. Their activity gradually declines through the rest of the small intestine. The digestion of α-limit dextrins proceeds with the sequential removal of glucose monomers from the nonreducing ends. The branch points of the oligosaccharides are then cleaved by α-dextrinase (Fig. 33-3).

Sucrase and α-dextrinase are noncovalently associated subunits of a single protein. After this protein is inserted into the brush border membrane, it is cleaved into two separate polypeptides to form the two different enzymes, which remain associated via noncovalent interactions.

Trehalase is a minor brush border disaccharidase. It cleaves trehalose, a disaccharide of glucose, into glucose units. Trehalose is present in mushrooms and yeast.

Absorption of Carbohydrates

The duodenum and upper jejunum have the highest capacity to absorb sugars. The capacities of the lower jejunum and ileum are progressively less. The only dietary monosaccharides that are well absorbed are glucose, galactose, and fructose.

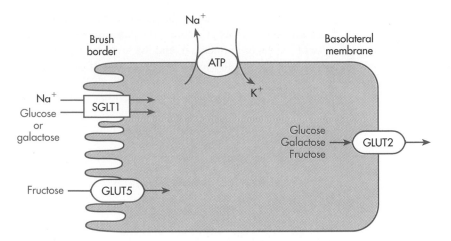

■ **Fig. 33-4** Absorption of glucose, galactose, and fructose in the upper small intestine. Glucose and galactose enter the epithelial cell at the brush border against a concentration gradient via the SGLT1 transport protein; the Na^+ gradient provides the energy for monosaccharide entry. Facilitated transport of fructose across the brush border membrane is mediated by GLUT5. Glucose, galactose, and fructose leave the cell at the basolateral membrane by facilitated transport via a common transporter, GLUT2.

Glucose and galactose are actively taken up by the brush border epithelial cells by a well-characterized transport protein (see Chapter 1) called **SGLT1** (for **sodium-glucose transport protein 1**). As its name implies, SGLT1 uses the energy of the Na^+ gradient to actively transport glucose and galactose into the intestinal epithelial cells. Glucose and galactose compete for entry; most other sugars are not effective competitors. The active entry of glucose and galactose into the intestinal epithelial cells is stimulated by the presence of Na^+ in the lumen. Similarly, the entry of Na^+ into the epithelial cell across the brush border membrane is stimulated by glucose or galactose in the lumen. SGLT1 transports two Na^+ ions and one glucose or galactose molecule across the brush border membrane. The electrochemical potential gradient for Na^+ is created by Na^+,K^+-ATPase pumps present in the basolateral plasma membranes of the intestinal epithelial cells.

Glucose and galactose leave the intestinal epithelial cell at the basal and lateral plasma membranes via facilitated transport, and they then diffuse into the mucosal capillaries. Figure 33-4 summarizes major features of glucose and galactose absorption. The transport protein responsible for efflux of glucose and galactose across the basolateral membrane is **GLUT2.** GLUT2, a member of the family of monosaccharide-facilitated transporters, is also present in liver, kidney, and pancreatic islet cells.

Fructose is not a substrate for the brush border glucose-galactose transporter. The facilitated transport of fructose across the brush border plasma membrane is mediated by a separate transport protein called **GLUT5.** GLUT5 is present only in the brush border plasma membrane of mature intestinal epithelial cells. GLUT5 is rather specific for fructose; fructose transport is not inhibited by glucose, galactose, or most other sugars. Fructose crosses the basolateral membrane of the intestinal epithelial cells via the same GLUT2 transporters used by glucose and galactose.

SGLT1, GLUT2, and GLUT5 are expressed in mature intestinal epithelial cells on the villi, but they are not present in immature intestinal epithelial cells in the crypts of Lieberkühn.

Absorption of carbohydrate from different food sources. The extent of absorption of the different forms of dietary carbohydrate—monosaccharides, disaccharides, and starch—varies in the human small intestine. Monosaccharides and disaccharides in the diet are completely absorbed in the small intestine. Dietary starch, however, is not completely absorbed. In healthy humans fed a test meal that contains 20 or 60 g of starch, about 6% to 10% escapes absorption in the small intestine. This quantity of starch is passed on to the colon, where it serves as an excellent carbon source for colonic bacteria. The failure to completely absorb carbohydrate from starch is normal and is not associated with any untoward symptoms.

The rate and extent of digestion and absorption of starch in the small intestine vary with the starch-containing foodstuff (Table 33-1). Colonic bacteria metabolize carbohydrate, producing short-chain fatty acids, such as acetate, propionate, and butyrate, which are taken up and metabolized by colonic epithelial cells. Starch-containing foods that are more rapidly absorbed result in a greater rate and quantity of insulin release from the pancreas.

Carbohydrate Malabsorption Syndromes

Malabsorption of carbohydrates is usually caused by a deficiency in one of the oligosaccharidases of the brush border.

Lactose malabsorption syndrome is a common disorder caused by a deficiency of lactase in the brush border of the duodenum and jejunum. As a result of this deficiency, undigested lactose cannot be absorbed and is instead passed on to the colonic bacteria, which avidly metabolize the lactose. The bacteria release gas and metabolic products that enhance colonic motility. Individuals with this disorder are said to be **lactose intolerant.** The symptoms of this disorder (and of the other carbohydrate malabsorption syndromes) are intestinal distension, borborygmi (gurgling noises in the intestine), flatulence, and diarrhea.

More than 50% of the adults in the world are lactose intolerant. This condition is genetically determined. In Asian societies, lactose intolerance among adults is almost universal. Most northern European adults, on the other hand, are lactose tolerant. A large proportion of African-American adults are lactose intolerant. Lactose tolerance in adults is associated with autosomal recessive mutation. Many lactose-

■ **Table 33-1**   Absorption of glucose from various carbohydrate-containing foods

Food	Glycemic index
Glucose	100
Carrots	92
Corn flakes	80
Rice, white	72
Potatoes, raw	70
Bread, white	69
Shredded wheat	67
Bananas	62
Corn	59
Pear	51
All-Bran	51
Spaghetti	50
Potatoes, sweet	48
Orange	40
Apple	39
Beans, navy	31
Beans, kidney	29
Sausages	28

Healthy adult men and women were fed amounts of the various food listed sufficient to provide 50 g of carbohydrate. Their blood glucose levels were followed for 2 hours after eating the carbohydrate. For each substance the amount of glucose that appeared in the blood over the 2 hours, expressed as a percentage of the increased amount of glucose in the blood in the 2 hours after eating 50 g of glucose, is called the glycemic index. Data are the means of 5 to 10 individuals. (Based on data from Jenkins DJA et al: *Am J Clin Nutr* 34:362, 1981.)

intolerant adults simply do not drink milk or eat certain milk products, and they therefore avoid the symptoms without being aware that they have the disorder. The presence of lactose in the diet may induce a higher level of intestinal lactase activity than would be present in the absence of dietary lactose.

Congenital lactose intolerance is rare. Infants with this disorder are deficient in jejunal lactase and have diarrhea when they are fed breast milk or formula containing lactose. The resultant dehydration and electrolyte imbalance are life threatening. Such infants must be fed a formula that contains sucrose or fructose instead of lactose.

Sucrase-isomaltase deficiency is characterized by very low levels of sucrase and isomaltase activity in the small intestinal brush border. This deficiency is an autosomal recessive, inherited disorder that results in intolerance to ingested sucrose or starch. About 10% of Greenland's Eskimos and as many as 0.2% of North Americans have sucrase-isomaltase deficiency. In this disorder, either the synthesis of the single protein that carries out both sucrase and isomaltase activities is suppressed or the protein is destroyed by antibodies. Individuals with sucrase-isomaltase deficiency do well on diets low in sucrose and starch.

Glucose-galactose malabsorption syndrome is a very rare hereditary disorder caused by a missense mutation in SGLT1, the brush border active transport protein for glucose and galactose. Ingestion of glucose, galactose, or starch leads to flatulence and severe diarrhea. Fructose is well tolerated and can be fed to infants with this disorder. The brush border oligosaccharidases are normal in this disease.

All these disorders can be diagnosed with the **oral sugar tolerance test.** In this procedure, the patient is given an oral dose of the sugar in question, and the levels of that sugar in the patient's blood and feces are monitored. If the patient is intolerant of the administered sugar, diarrhea will ensue. The sugar will fail to appear in the blood but will appear in the feces. In suspected oligosaccharidase deficiency, the definitive test involves sampling the jejunal mucosa and assaying it for the deficient enzyme.

DIGESTION AND ABSORPTION OF PROTEINS

The amount of dietary protein varies greatly among cultures and even among individuals within a culture. In poor societies, an adult may find it difficult to obtain the amount of protein (0.5 to 0.7 g/day/kg of body weight) required to balance normal catabolism of proteins. Children find it even more difficult to get the relatively greater amounts of protein they require to sustain normal growth. In wealthier societies, chiefly in industrially developed countries, a typical individual ingests protein far exceeding the nutritional requirement.

In addition to ingested protein, the gastrointestinal tract must also process the 10 to 30 g of protein per day contained in digestive secretions and a similar amount of protein in exfoliated epithelial cells. *In normal humans, essentially all ingested protein is digested and absorbed.* Most of the protein in digestive secretions and exfoliated epithelial cells is also digested and absorbed. The small amount of protein present in the feces is derived principally from colonic bacteria, exfoliated cells, and proteins in mucous secretions of the colon. In humans, ingested protein is almost completely absorbed by the time the meal has traversed the jejunum.

Digestion of Proteins

Digestion in the stomach. The chief cells of the stomach secrete inactive **pepsinogens,** proteases that are converted by hydrogen ions to active **pepsins.** There are seven different isoforms of pepsins. The extent to which pepsins hydrolyze dietary protein is significant but highly variable. The low pH in the stomach partly denatures dietary proteins, making them more susceptible to hydrolysis by pepsins. Pepsins are inactive at neutral pH, but are highly active in the acid environment of the stomach. At most, pepsins reduce about 15% of dietary protein to amino acids and small peptides. However, the duodenum and small intestine have such a high capacity to process protein that the total absence of pepsins does not impair the digestion and absorption of dietary protein.

Digestion in the lumen of the duodenum and small intestine. Proteases secreted by the pancreas play major roles in protein digestion. The most important of these proteases are **trypsin, chymotrypsin, carboxypeptidases A and B,** and **elastase.** These enzymes are present in inactive, proenzyme forms in pancreatic juice. The enzyme **enteropeptidase,** which is present on the brush border plasma

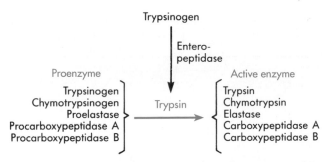

■ **Fig. 33-5** Conversion of inactive proenzymes of pancreatic juice to active enzymes by the action of trypsin. Trypsinogen of pancreatic juice is proteolytically converted to active trypsin by enteropeptidase (also known as enterokinase) secreted by the epithelial cells of the duodenum and jejunum. Trypsin then activates the other proenzymes of pancreatic juice as shown.

membrane of the duodenum and jejunum, converts trypsinogen to trypsin. Trypsin acts autocatalytically to activate trypsinogen, and it also converts the other proenzymes to active enzymes (Fig. 33-5). Within the duodenum, all the pancreatic proteases are highly active, and they rapidly convert dietary protein to small peptides. About

50% of the ingested protein is digested and absorbed in the duodenum.

Digestion on the luminal surface of the brush border. The brush border of the duodenum and the small intestine contains a number of peptidases. These peptidases are integral membrane proteins whose active sites face the intestinal lumen. The proximal jejunum contains the highest amounts of these brush border enzymes. These enzymes reduce the peptides produced by pancreatic proteases to oligopeptides and amino acids. The brush border peptidases include **aminopeptidases,** which cleave single amino acids from the N terminals of peptides; **dipeptidases,** which cleave dipeptides to amino acids; and **dipeptidyl aminopeptidases** and **dipeptidyl carboxypeptidases,** which cleave a dipeptide from the N-terminal and C-terminal end of peptides, respectively. Figure 33-6 illustrates some major proteases and peptidases present in the small intestine.

The principal products of protein digestion by pancreatic proteases and brush border peptidases are small peptides and amino acids. The small peptides (primarily dipeptides, tripeptides, and tetrapeptides) are produced in concentrations about three or four times higher than those of the single amino acids. As discussed below, small peptides and

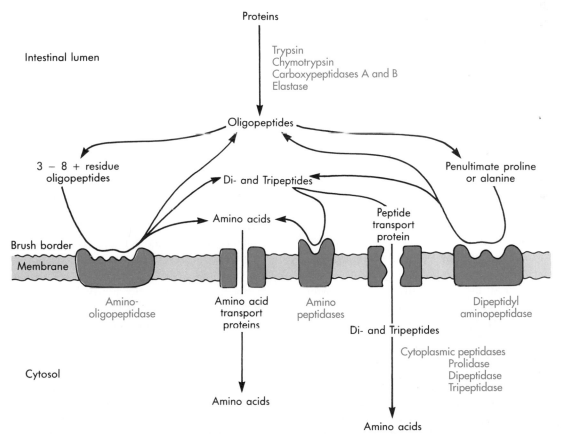

■ **Fig. 33-6** The hierarchy of proteases and peptidases that functions in the small intestine. The pancreatic proteases convert dietary proteins to oligopeptides. Brush border peptidases then convert the oligopeptides to amino acids (about 70%) and dipeptides and tripeptides (about 30%). The amino acids are taken up across the brush border membrane by amino acid transporters and the small peptides by a peptide transporter. In the cytosol of the enterocyte, dipeptides and tripeptides are cleaved to single amino acids. (From Van Dyke RW: Mechanisms of digestion and absorption of food. In Sleisenger MH, Fordtran JS, editors: *Gastrointestinal disease,* ed 4, Philadelphia, 1989, WB Saunders.)

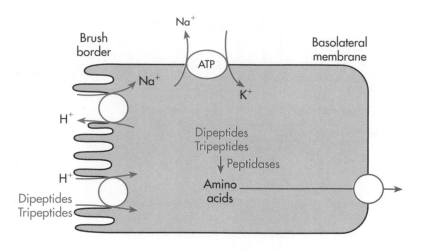

■ **Fig. 33-7**   A wide variety of dipeptides and tripeptides is taken up across the brush border plasma membrane by a single type of H⁺-powered secondary active transport protein. The H⁺ gradient is created by Na⁺-H⁺ exchangers in the brush border membrane. In the epithelial cell cytosol, peptidases cleave most of the dipeptides and tripeptides to single amino acids, which leave the cell at the basolateral membrane by facilitated transport.

amino acids are transported across the brush border plasma membrane into intestinal epithelial cells.

Digestion in the cytosol of duodenal and small intestinal epithelial cells. Small peptides are then hydrolyzed by peptidases in the cytosol of the epithelial cells to single amino acids. These cytosolic peptidases are more abundant than the brush border peptidases, and they are particularly active against dipeptides and tripeptides, which are transported with high efficiency across the brush border membrane. The brush border peptidases, on the other hand, are mainly active against peptides of four or more amino acids.

Absorption of the Products of Protein Digestion

Absorption of intact proteins and large peptides. Intact proteins and large peptides are not absorbed by humans to an extent that is nutritionally significant. Small amounts of luminal proteins are taken up by the M cells of the mucosal immune system. In ruminants and rodents, but not in humans, the neonatal intestine has a high capacity for the specific absorption by receptor-mediated endocytosis of immune proteins present in colostrum. This absorption is vital in the development of normal immune competence in ruminants and rodents.

Absorption of small peptides. After the breakdown of proteins by pancreatic proteins and brush border peptidases, the dipeptides and tripeptides produced are transported across the brush border membrane. The rate of transport of these small peptides usually exceeds the rate of transport of individual amino acids.

A single membrane transport system with broad specificity is responsible for the absorption of small peptides. This transport system apparently has a high affinity for dipeptides and tripeptides but very low affinities for peptides of four or more amino acid residues. The transport system is stereospecific, and it prefers peptides of the physiological L-amino acids. The affinity of the system is higher for peptides of amino acids with bulky side chains. The transport of dipeptides and tripeptides is powered by the electrochemical potential difference of H⁺ across the membrane (Fig. 33-7)

and is thus a secondary active process. The action of the Na⁺-H⁺ exchanger in the luminal plasma membrane creates an acidic microclimate near the surface of the brush border that facilitates the absorption of small peptides. The jejunum is more active than the ileum in uptake of dipeptides and tripeptides. The total amount of each amino acid that enters jejunal epithelial cells in the form of dipeptides or tripeptides is greater than the amount that enters as the single amino acid.

Most of the small peptides that enter the intestinal epithelial cells are cleaved to single amino acids in the cell and absorbed into the blood as single amino acids. However, recent evidence suggests that a small, but significant, amount of dipeptides and tripeptides is transported into the blood by a peptide transporter in the basolateral membrane; this transporter remains poorly characterized.

Absorption of amino acids. The ileum is more active in the uptake of single amino acids than is the jejunum; as observed in the previous section, the opposite order applies to small peptides. Amino acids are transported across the brush border plasma membrane into the epithelial cell via certain specific amino acid transport systems. Transport of amino acids out of the epithelial cell across the basolateral membrane occurs primarily by a different set of transporters. Some of the transporters in both membranes depend on the Na⁺ gradient (as previously described for glucose and galactose absorption), whereas other transport systems are independent of Na⁺. The basolateral membrane, however, is less highly differentiated than is the brush border membrane. The amino acid transporters present in the basolateral membrane occur in many nonepithelial cells, whereas the amino acid transporters in the brush border membrane are mostly unique to epithelial cells.

For some amino acids, simple diffusion may be a significant pathway across both brush border and basolateral membranes. The more hydrophobic the amino acid and the larger its concentration gradient across the membrane, the greater is the importance of diffusion.

Brush border membrane. Current knowledge of amino acid transporters present in the brush border plasma membrane is summarized in Table 33-2. Of the five transporter

■ **Table 33-2** Amino acid transporters of the brush border plasma membrane of the upper small intestine

Transporter type	Preferred substrates
Na$^+$-dependent	
B	Neutral amino acids
X$_{\overline{AG}}$	Acidic amino acids
IMINO	Imino acids (proline and hydroxyproline)
Independent of Na$^+$	
b$^{0,+}$	Neutral and basic amino acids, cystine
y$^+$	Basic amino acids

■ **Table 33-3** Amino acid transporters of the basolateral plasma membrane of the upper small intestine

Transporter type	Preferred substrates
Na$^+$-dependent	
A	Neutral amino acids, imino acids
ASC	Small neutral amino acids, especially alanine, serine, and cystine
Independent of Na$^+$	
asc	Same as for ASC
y$^+$	Basic amino acids
L	Larger and hydrophobic neutral amino acids

types present, three depend on the Na$^+$ gradient and catalyze secondary active uptake of amino acids. Two transporters are independent of Na$^+$, and their uptake of amino acids is mediated by facilitated transport.

The basolateral membrane. The five classes of amino acid transporters present in the basolateral membrane are listed in Table 33-3. The three transporters that are independent of the Na$^+$ gradient are primarily responsible for efflux of amino acids into the blood. The two Na$^+$-dependent systems mediate active uptake of amino acids across the basolateral membrane; these transporters serve to provide amino acids for protein synthesis in the epithelial cells during interdigestive periods.

There are no known basolateral transporters of acidic amino acids. Glutamine, glutamate, and aspartate are among the fuels preferred by intestinal epithelial cells. Most of the glutamine, glutamate, and aspartate that enter the cells across the brush border are probably shunted to the pathways of energy metabolism, and these amino acids are not transported across the basolateral membrane into the blood.

Defects of Amino Acid Digestion and Absorption

Trypsinogen deficiency is a rare congenital abnormality. Infants with this disease fail to thrive and have low levels of plasma protein. Feeding partially hydrolyzed protein is effective therapy.

Hartnup's disease is a rare hereditary disorder that involves defective renal and intestinal transport of neutral amino acids. Neutral amino acids are present in the urine.

Hartnup's disease is most often caused by defects in the B$^\circ$ system of the epithelial cells of the small intestine and the proximal renal tubule. Patients with Hartnup's disease are not protein deficient, but they suffer from the symptoms of niacin deficiency. Most of the needed niacin is synthesized from tryptophan, which is in inadequate supply in Hartnup's sufferers due to unusually high urinary excretion.

Cystinuria is a disorder characterized by the presence of cystine in the urine. This disease is caused by a defect in b$^{0,+}$ transporters in the brush border membrane of the epithelial cells of the small intestine and the renal proximal tubule. Individuals with cystinuria may suffer from cysteine-rich kidney stones. This is due to low rates of reabsorption of cysteine in the renal proximal tubules.

Prolinuria is a rare disorder that involves defective renal and intestinal reabsorption of proline. Proline and hydroxyproline are present in the urine. Prolinuria appears to be caused by a defect in the IMINO system in the epithelial cell brush border plasma membrane of the small intestine and the renal proximal tubule.

Because the epithelial cells are still capable of absorbing dipeptides and tripeptides, neither Hartnup's disease, cystinuria, nor prolinuria results in protein malnutrition.

INTESTINAL ABSORPTION OF SALTS AND WATER

Normally, humans absorb about 98% of the water and ions contained in ingested food and gastrointestinal secretions. The net movement of water and ions is normally from the lumen to the blood. In most cases, this net movement represents the difference between large unidirectional movements from lumen to blood and from blood to lumen.

Absorption of Water

Typically, about 2 L of water is ingested each day, and approximately 7 L/day is contained in the gastrointestinal secretions (Fig. 33-8). Only about 100 ml/day of water is lost in the feces. The gastrointestinal tract thus typically absorbs almost 9 L/day.

Very little net transport of water occurs in the duodenum. In fact, water is usually added to the chyme to bring it to isotonicity. Chyme delivered from the stomach is often hypertonic. The action of digestive enzymes creates still more osmotic activity. Usually, the net flux of water in the duodenum is from blood to lumen owing to the hypertonicity of the chyme.

Large net water absorption occurs in the small intestine; the jejunum is more active than the ileum in absorbing water. The net absorption that occurs in the colon is relatively small, about 400 ml/day. However, the colon can absorb water against a larger osmotic pressure difference than can the rest of the gastrointestinal tract. Figure 33-8 summarizes the handling of water by the gastrointestinal tract.

Absorption of Na$^+$

Na$^+$ is absorbed along the entire length of the intestine (Table 33-4).

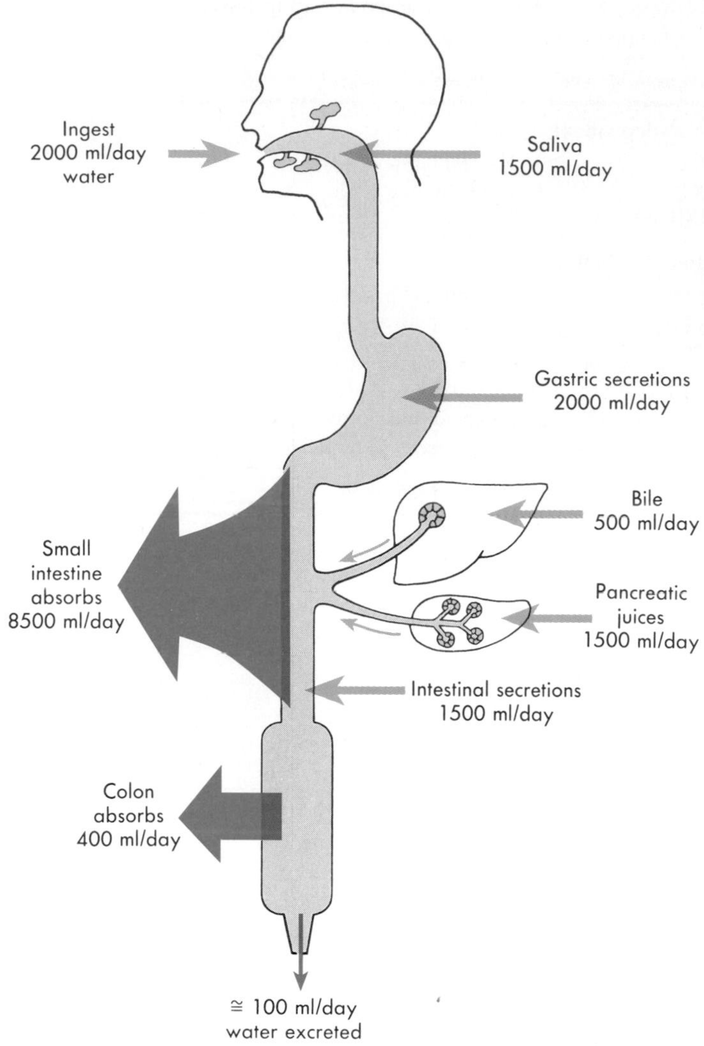

Ingest
2000 ml/day
water

Saliva
1500 ml/day

Gastric secretions
2000 ml/day

Bile
500 ml/day

Small
intestine
absorbs
8500 ml/day

Pancreatic
juices
1500 ml/day

Intestinal secretions
1500 ml/day

Colon
absorbs
400 ml/day

≅ 100 ml/day
water excreted

■ **Fig. 33-8** Overall fluid balance in the human gastrointestinal tract. About 2 L of water is ingested each day, and 7 L of various secretions enters the gastrointestinal tract. Of this total of 9 L, 8.5 L is absorbed in the small intestine. About 500 ml is passed on to the colon, which normally absorbs 80% to 90% of the water presented to it. (From Vander AJ, Sherman JII, Luciano DS: *Human physiology,* ed 6, New York, 1994, McGraw-Hill.)

■ **Table 33-4**   Transport of Na$^+$, K$^+$, Cl$^-$, and HCO$_3^-$ in the small and large intestines

Segment of intestine	Na$^+$	K$^+$	Cl$^-$	HCO$_3^-$
Jejunum	Actively absorbed; absorption enhanced by sugars, neutral amino acids	Passively absorbed when concentration rises because of absorption of water	Absorbed	Absorbed
Ileum	Actively absorbed	Passively absorbed	Absorbed, some in exchange for HCO$_3^-$	Secreted, partly in exchange for Cl$^-$
Colon	Actively absorbed	Net secretion occurs when (K$^+$) concentration in lumen <25 mM	Absorbed, some in exchange for HCO$_3^-$	Secreted, partly in exchange for Cl$^-$

Na$^+$ crosses the brush border membrane down an electrochemical gradient, and it is actively extruded from epithelial cells by the Na$^+$,K$^+$-ATPase in the basal and lateral plasma membrane. The contents of the small intestine are isotonic to plasma. Luminal contents have about the same Na$^+$ concentration as does plasma, so that Na$^+$ absorption normally takes place in the absence of a significant concentration gradient. Na$^+$ absorption is active, however, and can occur against a small electrochemical potential difference for Na$^+$.

The net rate of absorption of Na$^+$ is highest in the jejunum. Here, Na$^+$ absorption is enhanced by the presence of glucose, galactose, and neutral amino acids in the lumen. These substances and Na$^+$ cross the brush border membrane on the same transport proteins. Na$^+$ moves down its electrochemical potential gradient and provides the energy for moving the sugars (glucose and galactose) and neutral amino acids into the epithelial cells against concentration gradients. Thus, Na$^+$ enhances the absorption of sugars and amino acids, and vice versa.

The ability of glucose to enhance the absorption of Na⁺, and hence of Cl⁻ and water, is exploited in **oral rehydration therapy** for **cholera** and other secretory diarrheas. When patients with cholera drink a solution that contains glucose, NaCl, and other constituents, the absorption of glucose, salt, and water helps to counteract the secretory fluxes of salt and water that would otherwise dehydrate the patient. Despite its simplicity, oral rehydration therapy is a major advance because of its impact on world health.

The net rate of Na⁺ absorption in the ileum is smaller. Na⁺ absorption is only slightly stimulated by sugars and amino acids. The ileum can absorb Na⁺ against a larger electrochemical potential than can the jejunum.

In the colon, Na⁺ is normally absorbed against a large electrochemical potential difference. Sodium concentrations in the luminal contents can be as low as 25 mM, compared with about 120 mM in the plasma.

Absorption of Cl⁻ and HCO₃⁻

In the proximal duodenum, HCO₃⁻ is secreted into the lumen. In the jejunum, both Cl⁻ and HCO₃⁻ are absorbed in large amounts. At the end of the jejunum, most of the HCO₃⁻ in the hepatic and pancreatic secretions has been absorbed. In the ileum, Cl⁻ is absorbed, but HCO₃⁻ is normally secreted. If the HCO₃⁻ concentration in the lumen of the ileum exceeds about 45 mM, the flux from lumen to blood exceeds that from blood to lumen, and net absorption occurs. *In the colon, the transport of these ions is qualitatively similar to that in the ileum, in that Cl⁻ is absorbed and bicarbonate is usually secreted.*

Absorption and Secretion of K⁺

In the jejunum and in the ileum, the net flux of K⁺ is from lumen to blood. As the volume of intestinal contents is reduced by the absorption of water, K⁺ is concentrated. This action provides a driving force for the movement of K⁺ across the intestinal mucosa and into the blood. Evidence for active transport of K⁺ in the small intestine is lacking. *In the colon, K⁺ may be either secreted or absorbed.* Net secretion occurs when the luminal concentration is less than about 25 mM; above 25 mM, net absorption occurs. Under most circumstances, net secretion of K⁺ takes place in the colon; the secretory process is active (Table 33-4).

Most of the absorption of K⁺ in the small intestine is caused by the absorption of water, which increases the K⁺ concentration in the lumen. Hence, significant K⁺ loss may occur in diarrhea. If diarrhea is prolonged, the K⁺ level in the extracellular fluid compartment of the body falls. Because maintenance of normal extracellular levels of K⁺ is important to many body functions, especially those of the heart and other muscles, life-threatening consequences such as **cardiac arrhythmias** may ensue with a decrease in K⁺. Infants with prolonged diarrhea are particularly susceptible to **hypokalemia** (low plasma K⁺).

Mechanisms of Salt and Water Transport by the Intestine

Transcellular versus paracellular transport. Because tight junctions are leaky, some fraction of the water and ions that traverse the intestinal epithelium passes between, rather than through, the epithelial cells. Transmucosal movement achieved by passing through tight junctions and the lateral intercellular spaces of an epithelium is called **paracellular transport.** Passage through the epithelial cells is termed **transcellular transport.**

Because the tight junctions in the duodenum are very leaky, a major portion of the large unidirectional fluxes of water and ions that takes place in the duodenum occurs via the paracellular pathway. The proportions of water or a particular ion that pass through the transcellular and paracellular routes are determined by the relative permeabilities of the two pathways for a particular substance. Even in the ileum, where the junctions are much tighter than in the duodenum, significant proportions of water and electrolyte flows across the epithelium occur via the paracellular route.

Villous versus crypt cells. The highly differentiated epithelial cells near the tips of the villi are specialized for absorption of water and ions, whereas the less differentiated cells in the crypts usually produce net secretion of water and ions.

Ion Transport by Intestinal Epithelial Cells

The movement of water across the intestinal epithelium is secondary to the movement of ions and other solutes. In all regions of the intestine, the basolateral plasma membrane contains the Na⁺,K⁺-ATPase. As a result of the active extrusion of Na⁺ ions from the cytoplasm by the Na⁺,K⁺-ATPase, the electrochemical potential of Na⁺ in the cytoplasm is much less than that in the luminal fluid. Na⁺ enters the epithelial cell by moving down this large electrochemical potential gradient. Membrane transport proteins of the epithelial cells couple the influx of Na⁺ to the secondary active transport of sugars, amino acids, and other ions.

Mechanisms of Salt and Water Transport by the Intestine

NaCl absorption in the ileum and jejunum. Na⁺ and Cl⁻ are absorbed by similar mechanisms in the ileum and jejunum. Sodium is absorbed across the luminal membrane by a Na⁺-glucose cotransporter (SGLT-1) and by a Na⁺-amino acid cotransporter (Fig. 33-9). In addition, NaCl absorption across the luminal membrane occurs by the parallel operation of a Na⁺-H⁺ exchanger (NHE³) and a Cl⁻-HCO₃⁻ exchanger (downregulated in adenoma, DRA, or anion exchanger 1, AE1). The operation of these two transporters at equal rates results in the net entry of NaCl into the cell. The Na⁺ that enters the cell across the luminal membrane is pumped out of the cell into the blood via the Na⁺,K⁺-ATPase. The glucose that enters the cell is transported across the basolateral membrane into the blood via a glucose transporter, GLUT-2. The Cl⁻ that enters the cell via

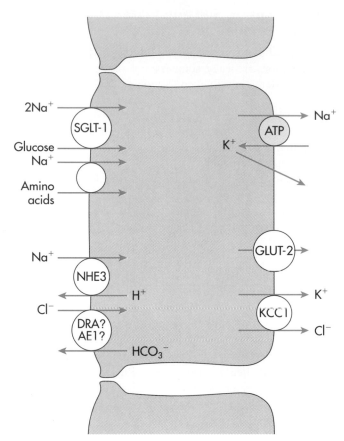

■ **Fig. 33-9**   Mechanisms of NaCl absorption in the ileum and jejunum.

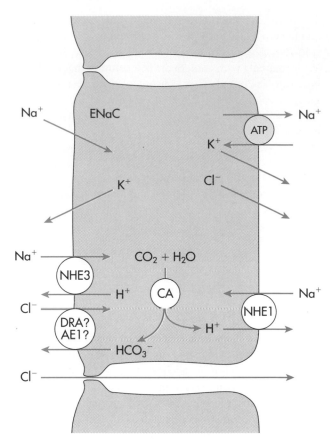

■ **Fig. 33-10**   Mechanisms of NaCl absorption and K secretion by the colon.

DRA or AE1 is transported into the blood by a K^+-Cl^- cotransporter called KCC1.

   NaCl absorption and K secretion by the colon.   In the colon, there is net absorption of NaCl and secretion of K^+ (Fig. 33-10). Na^+ is absorbed by two mechanisms. First, similar to the ileum and jejunum, it is absorbed by the parallel operation of a Na^+-H^+ exchanger (NHE_3) and a Cl^--HCO_3^- exchanger (DRA or AE1) located in the luminal membrane. Second, Na^+ enters the cell across the luminal membrane by a Na^+-selective channel called ENaC, which is the epithelial Na^+ channel. Na^+ absorption by ENaC causes the luminal fluid to be electrically negative relative to the blood and provides the electrochemical driving force for the absorption of Cl^- from the lumen to the blood between cells across the tight junctions.

   HCO_3^- secretion by the duodenum. HCO_3^- is secreted into the lumen of the duodenum by the mechanisms depicted in Fig. 33-11. First, some HCO_3^- is produced in the cell from CO_2 and H_2O. In addition, some HCO_3^- also enters the cell across the basolateral membrane by a Na^+-HCO_3^- cotransporter (Na^+-HCO_3^- transporter, NBC1). A Cl^--HCO_3^- exchanger (DRA or AE1) transports HCO_3^- from both sources from the cell into the luminal fluid. The Cl^- that enters the cell in exchange for HCO_3^- recycles back into the luminal fluid across the luminal membrane by the CFTR Cl^- channel. Thus, working together, CFTR and DRA mediate HCO_3^- secretion. The H^+ produced in the cell by the gener-

ation of HCO_3^- is transported into the blood across the basolateral membrane by a Na^+-H^+ exchanger (NHE1). The Na^+ that enters the cell in exchange for H^+ is pumped back into the blood by the Na^+,K^+-ATPase.

The Mechanism of Water Absorption

As noted, the absorption of water depends on the absorption of ions, principally Na^+ and Cl^-. Under normal circumstances, water absorption in the small intestine occurs in the absence of an osmotic pressure difference between the luminal contents and the blood in the intestinal capillaries. Water absorption by the colon typically proceeds against a transmucosal osmotic pressure gradient. Water is absorbed by a mechanism known as standing gradient osmosis (see Fig. 32-30). The major features of the standing gradient osmotic mechanism are described in Chapter 32.

   Because most water absorption takes place in the absence of a transmucosal osmotic pressure difference, the absorption of the end products of digestion, particularly sugars and amino acids, is important in water absorption. The absorption of sugars and amino acids allows more water to be absorbed. The role of aquaporins, water transport channel proteins, in intestinal water transport has not been established. It has been proposed that SGLT1, the Na-coupled glucose transporter, transports about 250 water molecules from lumen to cytosol for each glucose that passes.

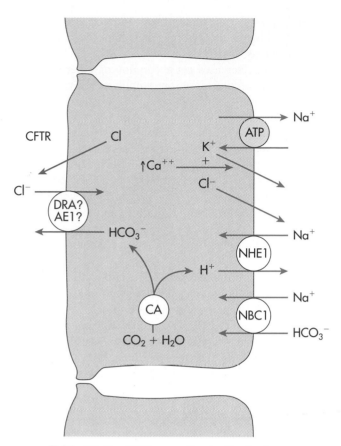

■ **Fig. 33-11** HCO_3^- secretion by the duodenum.

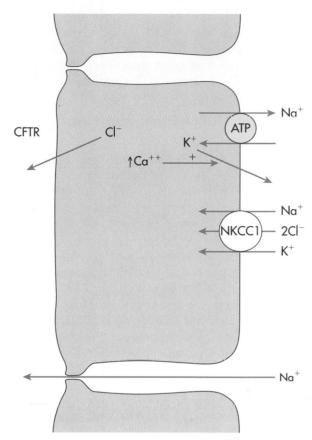

■ **Fig. 33-12** Ion transport pathways involved in secretion of NaCl. *CFTR*, Cystic fibrosis transmembrane conductance regulator.

Secretion of Electrolytes and Water by Cells in Lieberkühn's Crypts

Mature epithelial cells near the tips of the villi are usually active in net absorption, whereas more immature cells in Lieberkühn's crypts usually function as net secretors of electrolytes and water.

A current view of the ionic transport mechanisms that function in the crypt cells is shown in Fig. 33-12. In this model, Cl^- is actively taken up at the basolateral plasma membrane by the Na^+,K^+, $2Cl^-$ cotransporter (NKCC1). This transporter uses the chemical concentration gradient of Na^+ to transport Cl^- into the cell against its electrochemical gradient. Cl^- leaves the cell at the luminal membrane via the CFTR Cl^- channel. Na^+ is transported into the lumen, driven by the net luminal electronegativity produced by Cl^- secretion into the lumen. Efflux of K^+ via K^+ channels in the basolateral membrane prevents K^+ from accumulating in the cytosol of the crypt cell and maintains an electrical potential difference (cytosol negative) across the luminal and basolateral membranes. This potential difference contributes to the electrochemical driving force for efflux of Cl^-.

The amount of time that the luminal Cl^- channel remains open is enhanced by cyclic AMP (cAMP), and basolateral K^+ channels are activated by Ca^{2+} or by elevated cAMP. Thus, net secretion by the crypt cells is enhanced by agonists that elevate intracellular AMP [e.g., prostaglandins and vasoactive intestinal peptide (VIP)] and by Ca^{2+}-mobilizing

agonists (e.g., acetylcholine). The effects of agonists that elevate AMP are potentiated by agonists that increase cytosolic Ca^{2+}, and vice versa.

Agonists that elevate cAMP in the cystosol of enterocytes, in addition to the prosecretory effects just noted, also inhibit the absorption of Na^+ and Cl^- by mature enterocytes. Agonists that increase cyclic GMP (cGMP) also promote net secretion. The heat-stable toxin of *Escherichia coli* (STa) binds to a luminal receptor that is a guanylyl cyclase, thereby elevating cGMP in the enterocyte. Guanylin, a hormone produced by intestinal epithelial cells, acts on the same receptor that binds STa.

In secretory diarrheal diseases, such as **cholera,** the secretion of Cl^-, Na^+, and water into the intestinal lumen by the cells in Lieberkühn's crypts is specifically elevated. Cholera is caused by the cholera toxin that is produced by the bacterium *Vibrio cholerae*. **Cholera toxin** permanently activates adenylyl cyclase, and thereby elevates the concentration of cAMP in the crypt cells. cAMP activates the brush border Cl^- channels and thereby prolongs the secretion of Cl^- (and therefore also of Na^+ and water). Cholera patients may produce up to 20 L/day of watery stool. Such patients are likely to die unless they are promptly and adequately rehydrated.

The luminal Cl^- channel in the cells in Lieberkühn's crypts is the same protein that is defective in **cystic fibrosis (CF).** CF is by far the most common autosomal recessive disorder; about 1 in 20 American adults are CF carriers. Animal experiments show that CF carriers, who have one normal and one defective copy of the gene for the Cl⁻ channel, suffer much less severe diarrhea in response to cholera than do normal individuals. Resistance of CF carriers to secretory diarrheas may explain the unusual prevalence of this mutation.

Physiological Regulation of Salt and Water Absorption

The control of net absorption of electrolytes and water by epithelial cells near the villous tips and of net secretion of water and electrolytes by cells in the crypts of Lieberkühn is complex. Rates of absorption and secretion of electrolytes and water are influenced by hormones; sympathetic, parasympathetic, and enteric nervous systems; and cells of the gastrointestinal immune system. Moreover, interactions among these regulatory pathways are also important in the control of secretion and absorption.

Hormones, paracrine agonists, and substances released from neurons in the wall of the gastrointestinal tract regulate the absorption and secretion of water and electrolytes by intestinal epithelial cells. Some of these regulatory substances, and the cells that release them, are listed in Table 33-5.

Endocrine control of absorption and secretion. Some of the hormones that influence absorption and secretion of electrolytes and water are released by cells in the wall of the gastrointestinal tract; others come from endocrine cells located elsewhere in the body. Among the hormones that can influence intestinal absorption and secretion are mineralocorticoids, glucocorticoids, catecholamines, somatostatin, and enkephalins.

Aldosterone increases net absorption of water and electrolytes in the colon. Aldosterone stimulates the synthesis of the luminal electrogenic Na^+ channel and the basolateral Na^+,K^+-ATPase.

Glucocorticoids stimulate electrolyte and water absorption in both the small and large intestines. This stimulation is most likely the result of an increase in the number of Na^+,K^+-ATPase molecules in the basolateral membranes of enterocytes.

Epinephrine acts on α-receptors on epithelial cells to increase electroneutral NaCl absorption in the ileum and to suppress secretory fluxes. Epinephrine also acts at the level of the submucosal ganglia to inhibit secretomotor outflow to epithelial cells.

Somatostatin stimulates electrolyte and water absorption in the ileum and colon and inhibits secretion. In intestinal epithelial cells, somatostatin appears to act by decreasing cellular levels of cAMP. The ability of somatostatin to decrease secretion by crypt cells has led to the use of somatostatin analogs to treat secretory diarrheas. Somatostatin may also act on enteric neurons to suppress secretomotor outflow to enterocytes.

Opioids act on δ-receptors in the intestine to stimulate salt and water absorption. Opioids act on other receptor subtypes to inhibit intestinal motility. Both of these effects may contribute to the antidiarrheal effects of opioids.

■ **Table 33-5**   Endogenous compounds that influence intestinal absorption of electrolytes and water

Compounds	Stimulate net secretion	Promote net absorption
Released by enteric neurons	Acetylcholine Nitric oxide Serotonin VIP* Substance P	Norepinephrine Neuropeptide Y Opioids
Released by enteroendocrine cells of immunocytes in mucosa or submucosa	Histamine Calcitonin Guanylin Bradykinin Platelet-activating factor Reactive oxygen species Prostaglandins Leukotrienes Calcitonin Arachidonic acid Adenosine	Somatostatin
Hormones (reach epithelial cells via blood)	Prostaglandins Atrial natriuretic peptide Gastrin Motilin Bombesin GIP	Epinephrine Enkephalins Aldosterone Glucocorticoids Angiotensin II Peptide YY Prolactin Growth hormone
Present in the lumen	Bile salts Long-chain fatty acids	Short-chain fatty acids

VIP, Vasoactive intestinal peptide.

*Note that some compounds may be released by neurons and by enteroendocrine cells or immunocytes. For simplicity, these compounds are listed only once.

Neural regulation of absorption and secretion. Most of the direct innervation of intestinal epithelial cells comes from neurons of the enteric nervous system, especially from the submucosal ganglia. The predominant influences of parasympathetic and sympathetic neurons occur via their influences on the activities of enteric neurons. Neural reflexes, both extrinsic and intrinsic to the gastrointestinal tract, regulate the absorptive and secretory activities of intestinal epithelial cells.

Enteric nervous system. Epithelial cells are innervated by secretomotor neurons, predominantly from submucosal ganglia, but also from the myenteric ganglia. This innervation stimulates net secretion. *Submucosal secretomotor neurons release acetylcholine and/or VIP onto epithelial cells to stimulate secretion.* An array of mucosal reflexes controls and coordinates the neural outflow from the enteric nervous system to intestinal epithelial cells. Enteric neurons that inhibit secretion by intestinal epithelial cells have not been found.

In addition to those already mentioned, other neurotransmitters, putative transmitters, and neuromodulators are present in enteric neurons, and these neuroactive substances may influence absorption and secretion. They may directly act on epithelial cells, or they may exert their influences at the level of the submucosal ganglia to stimulate or inhibit outflow from secretomotor neurons.

Reflexes in the enteric nervous system modulate secretomotor outflow from submucosal ganglia to intestinal epithelial cells. Some of these reflexes are elicited by luminal stimuli, such as distension of the gut lumen; stroking the mucosal surface; or the presence in the lumen of glucose, acid pH, bile salts, ethanol, cholera toxin, or an antigen to which the gastrointestinal immune system has been previously sensitized. All of these stimuli evoke reflex stimulation of secretion. Most of these stimuli also enhance propulsive motility in the stimulated gut segment. These actions demonstrate the interplay between neural control of secretion and motility.

Parasympathetic nervous system. The enteric nervous system is heavily innervated by parasympathetic fibers, to both myenteric and submucosal ganglia. *Stimulation of the parasympathetic fibers diminishes absorptive fluxes and enhances secretion.* Parasympathetic fibers do not directly innervate epithelial cells to a significant degree. Parasympathetic tone apparently contributes to basal rates of secretion. Cholinergic input to the interneurons and secretomotor neurons, especially in the submucosal plexus, enhances secretomotor outflow to epithelial cells and perhaps to other mucosal effector cells also.

Sympathetic nervous system. Stimulation of sympathetic nerves to the gut enhances net absorption. Chemical ablation of the sympathetic nerves diminishes absorption. In diabetics, autonomic neuropathy may cause decreased sympathetic outflow to the intestine and contribute to "diabetic diarrhea."

Some adrenergic fibers directly innervate epithelial cells, where norepinephrine acts on α-receptors to enhance absorption. Sympathetic input to the enteric nervous system diminishes the secretomotor outflow by enteric neurons, especially in the submucosal ganglia, to epithelial cells. Norepinephrine, acting on α receptors, has multiple effects on neurons of submucosal ganglia. These effects decrease the secretomotor outflow to epithelial cells. Somatostatin, another transmitter known to stimulate absorption, is coreleased with norepinephrine at some nerve terminals.

Catecholamines and α-adrenergic agents can strongly inhibit intestinal secretion evoked by cholera toxin, dibutyryl cAMP, VIP, 5-hydroxytryptamine, and many other potent secretagogues.

Regulation of absorption and secretion by the gastrointestinal immune system. The cells of the gastrointestinal immune system contain numerous mediators that influence gastrointestinal salt and water transport. Most of these compounds enhance net secretion of water and electrolytes. Inflammatory mediators stimulate secretion of electrolytes and water by crypt cells, inhibit absorption by villus cells, and in some cases enhance proliferation of crypt cells. The mediators include histamine, serotonin, prostaglandins and thromboxanes, leukotrienes, platelet-activating factor, adenosine, reactive oxygen species, nitric oxide, and endothelin. The cells that contain these mediators include mast cells, phagocytes, lymphocytes, basophils, neutrophils, endothelial cells, and fibroblasts.

Primed mast cells play a central role in the gastrointestinal response to an antigen. A primed mast cell carries antibody on its surface. When the antibody recognizes its particular antigen, the mast cell degranulates and releases many different mediators. Several of these mediators induce hypersecretion of salts and water by the epithelial cells as well as hypermotility. Mast cells also release cytokines that recruit other mucosal immune cells to the response. These cells may then also release secretagogues.

Mediators released from mast cells and other gastrointestinal immunocytes evoke secretion in two ways: they (1) directly affect intestinal epithelial cells to stimulate secretion and/or inhibit absorption and (2) act on enteric neurons to increase the activity in secretomotor circuits. Histamine and prostaglandins appear to be key mediators of the effects on enteric neurons.

In addition to acting as targets of the immune mediators, enteric neurons modulate the release of these mediators from mast cells and influence the function of other gastrointestinal immunocytes. Neurons that release substance P onto mast cells stimulate degranulation of the mast cells and contribute to neurogenic inflammation and to secretion of water and electrolytes.

Inhibition of absorption and promotion of secretion of water and electrolytes by inflammatory mediators play a key role in the secretory diarrhea of **inflammatory bowel disease, Crohn's disease,** and other intestinal immune disorders. Prosecretory neural tone can enhance the responses to secretor mediators.

Pathophysiological Alterations of Salt and Water Absorption

The general causes of abnormalities in the absorption of salts and water include (1) deficiency of a normal ion transport system; (2) malabsorption of a nonelectrolyte (nutrient), which results in osmotic diarrhea; (3) hypermotility of the intestine, which leads to abnormally rapid flow of intestinal contents past the absorptive epithelium; and (4) an enhanced rate of net secretion of water and electrolytes by the intestinal mucosa. Examples of each of these classes of abnormalities follow.

Deficiency of a normal ion transport system. In **congenital chloride diarrhea,** the Cl^-, HCO_3^- exchange in the brush border plasma membrane of the ileum and colon is impaired. As a result, chloride absorption is severely impaired. Impairment of chloride absorption leads to a type of diarrhea in which the stools contain an unusually high chloride concentration; the concentration of Cl^- in the stool exceeds the sum of the concentrations of Na^+ and K^+. In addition, because the Na^+-H^+ exchanger continues to operate, H^+ is eliminated in the feces without HCO_3^- to neutralize it. The net loss of H^+, with retention of HCO_3^-, contributes to metabolic alkalosis. The protein that is mutated in this disease (DRA) has been identified, but the function of DRA is not known.

Malabsorption of a nutrient. In any of the carbohydrate malabsorption syndromes, the sugar that is retained in the lumen of the small intestine increases the osmotic pressure of the luminal contents. Water is also retained as a result, and an increased volume of chyme is passed on to the colon. The increased volume flow may overwhelm the ability of the colon to absorb electrolytes and water, and pronounced diarrhea results. In addition, the high level of carbohydrates provides a medium that supports increased growth and metabolism of colonic bacteria. The increased production of CO_2 by colonic bacteria contributes to gaseousness and borborygmi, and certain products of bacterial metabolism inhibit absorption of electrolytes by the colonic epithelium.

In some disorders the surface area of the intestinal mucosa is dramatically decreased, leading to the malabsorption of nutrients, electrolytes, and water. In these disorders, the height of small intestinal villi is markedly reduced and the number of microvilli is diminished. This occurs in celiac disease (gluten enteropathy), in response to infection by certain rotaviruses, and in a disease of uncertain etiology called **tropical sprue.** Celiac disease is also known as **celiac sprue.**

Hypermotility of the intestine. Hypermotility is common in inflammatory bowel disease. The causes of hypermotility of the intestine are not well understood. Hypermotility of the small intestine may deliver electrolytes and water to the colon at faster rates than they can be absorbed by the colonic epithelial cells. Hypermotility of the colon may result in the elimination of feces before the maximal amount of salts and water can be extracted from them. Hypermotility may add to other factors that cause diarrhea. In cases of fat malabsorption, colonic bacteria metabolize lipids and produce certain waste products, such as hydroxylated fatty acids, that enhance the motility of the colon and inhibit salt and water absorption by the colonic epithelium.

Enhanced secretion of water and electrolytes. Increased secretion of water and electrolytes is an important mechanism in serious diarrheal diseases. As mentioned previously, immature epithelial cells in Lieberkühn's crypts normally function to secrete Na^+, Cl^-, and H_2O. When the secretory activities of the crypt cells are elevated, the unidirectional secretory flux may exceed the unidirectional absorptive flux, so that net secretion prevails. Cholera, discussed previously, is the best understood type of secretory diarrhea. Other agents that elevate cAMP in intestinal epithelial cells also lead to secretion of water and electrolytes.

VIP, which is present in certain enteric neurons and also circulates as a hormone, elevates cAMP in intestinal epithelial cells. Certain individuals with islet cell tumors of the pancreas suffer from a watery diarrhea known as **pancreatic cholera.** In this disorder, elevated plasma levels of VIP cause secretory diarrhea.

The epithelial cells of the crypts of the small intestine are also stimulated to secrete electrolytes and water by elevated intracellular Ca^{2+} concentrations (Fig. 33-13). Acetylcholine, serotonin, substance P, and neurotensin elicit intestinal secretion of water and electrolytes by increasing the concentration of intracellular Ca^{2+}. All these agents are present in intrinsic neurons of the intestinal wall and thus may contribute to diarrhea in certain pathological situations.

ABSORPTION OF CALCIUM

Calcium ions are actively absorbed by all segments of the intestine. Calcium forms insoluble salts with many anions present in food such as phytate, phosphate, and oxalate. These salts are soluble at low pH, so gastric acid plays an important role in calcium absorption. Ca^{2+} ions are actively absorbed by all segments of the small intestine; the amount absorbed is greater in the proximal small intestine and less in the distal portions. The rate of absorption of Ca^{2+} is much greater than that of any other divalent ion, but still 50 times slower than Na^+ absorption.

The ability of the intestine to absorb Ca^{2+} is regulated. Animals that receive a calcium-deficient diet increase their ability to absorb Ca^{2+}. Animals that receive high-calcium diets are less able to absorb Ca^{2+}. Intestinal absorption of Ca^{2+} is markedly stimulated by vitamin D. Parathyroid hormone stimulates intestinal absorption of Ca^{2+} by promoting release of the active form of vitamin D from the kidney.

Most Ca^{2+} absorption occurs through the intestinal epithelial cells, but significant absorption also takes place across tight junctions via the paracellular pathway. This absorption is driven by the elevated concentration of Ca^{2+} in the intestinal lumen that results from the absorption of water and the transmucosal electrical potential difference, lumen negative.

Cellular Mechanism of Calcium Absorption

The brush border membrane. Cellular mechanisms of Ca^{2+} absorption by the epithelial cells of the small intestine

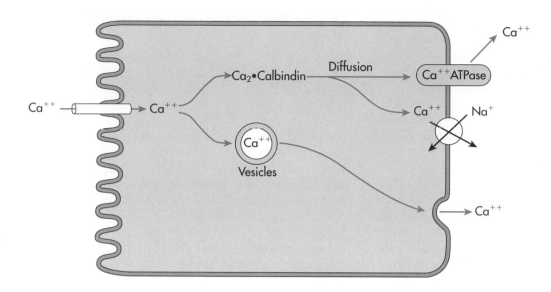

■ **Fig. 33-13** Cellular mechanisms of Ca²⁺ absorption in the small intestine. Ca²⁺ crosses the brush border plasma membrane via Ca²⁺ channels. In the cytosol of the enterocyte, Ca²⁺ is bound to calbindin. Ca²⁺ is extruded across the basolateral membrane by a Ca²⁺-ATPase and an Na⁺-Ca²⁺ exchange mechanism. Some Ca²⁺ is transported through the cytosol in membrane vesicles and released at the basolateral membrane by exocytosis.

are depicted in Fig. 33-13. Ca^{2+} moves through Ca^{2+} channels down its electrochemical potential gradient across the brush border membrane into the cytosol. A protein, called the **intestinal membrane calcium-binding protein (IMCal),** may bind Ca^{2+} at the inner face of the brush border membrane.

Epithelial cell cytosol. The cytosol of the intestinal epithelial cells contains proteins called **calbindins,** an essential component of Ca^{2+} absorption. Calbindins are also known as **intestinal calcium binding proteins (CaBP).** There are two forms of calbindin in enterocytes: calbindin-D_{9K}, which binds two Ca^{2+} ions, and calbindin-D_{28K}, which binds four Ca^{2+} ions. Calbindins allow large amounts of Ca^{2+} to traverse the cytosol, and binding of Ca^{2+} to calbindins prevents concentrations of free Ca^{2+} ions that are high enough to form insoluble salts with intracellular anions.

Ca^{2+} is also transported through the cytosol of intestinal epithelial cells in membrane vesicles. Vesicular Ca^{2+} is released across the basolateral membrane by exocytosis. Calbindins also promote Ca^{2+} transport via the vesicular pathway.

The basolateral membrane. The basolateral plasma membrane contains two transport proteins that can eject Ca^{2+} from the cell against its electrochemical potential gradient. A **Ca^{2+}-ATPase** in the basolateral membrane, a primary active transport protein, splits ATP and uses the energy to transport Ca^{2+}. The Na⁺-Ca^{2+} exchanger present in the basolateral membrane uses the energy of the Na⁺ gradient to extrude Ca^{2+} by secondary active transport. The Na⁺-Ca^{2+} exchanger is more effective when intracellular Ca^{2+} concentrations are high, whereas the Ca^{2+}-ATPase is the major mechanism for Ca^{2+} extrusion when intracellular concentrations of Ca^{2+} are low. Ca^{2+} itself, bound to calmodulin, stimulates the activity of the Ca^{2+}-ATPase, as does phosphorylation of the Ca^{2+}-ATPase by cAMP-dependent protein kinase.

Actions of Vitamin D

Vitamin D is essential for normal levels of calcium absorption by the intestine (see also Chapter 42).

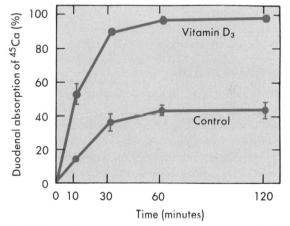

■ **Fig. 33-14** Effects of vitamin D_3 on absorption of Ca^{2+} by chick duodenum. Control animals were fed a diet deficient in vitamin D *(lower curve). Upper curve:* Ca^{2+} absorption by animals fed the same diet but administered vitamin D_3 24 hours before the experiment. (From Wasserman RH: *J Nutr* 77:69, 1962.)

In **rickets,** a disease caused by vitamin D deficiency, the rate of absorption of Ca^{2+} is very low, and thus the amount of Ca^{2+} available for bone growth is also low. In children with rickets, bone growth is abnormal. Because of the failure to deposit normal amounts of calcium salts in the bone matrix, bones are softer and more flexible than normal. These changes contribute to the characteristic "bow-legged" appearance of children with rickets.

Figure 33-14 illustrates the effects of administration of vitamin D on intestinal absorption of Ca^{2+} by chicks with rickets. Vitamin D stimulates each phase of absorption of Ca^{2+} by the epithelium of the small intestine: passage across the brush border membrane, traversal of the cytosol, and active extrusion across the basolateral membrane. Like other steroid hormones, vitamin D exerts its major effects by binding to nuclear receptors and stimulating the synthesis of messenger RNA that encodes particular proteins. Vitamin D dramatically stimulates the synthesis of both calbindin-D_{9K} and calbindin-D_{28K}. The calbindin level correlates well with the capacity of the small intestine to absorb Ca^{2+}. Vitamin D also increases the level of the brush border-associated calbindin, which may promote transport of Ca^{2+} across the brush border plasma membrane. In addition, vitamin D increases the level of the basolateral Ca^{2+}-ATPase that actively pumps calcium out of the enterocyte.

Malabsorption of Calcium

Calcium absorption decreases in elderly people. This may be due to lower levels of vitamin D or to diminished responsiveness to vitamin D in older people. The role of gastric acid in promoting Ca^{2+} absorption was mentioned previously. People, particularly elderly individuals, who chronically use drugs that suppress gastric HCl secretion are at increased risk for malabsorbing calcium. Calcium malabsorption may occur in inflammatory bowel disease and in disorders such as gluten enteropathy and tropical sprue that diminish the surface area of the brush border.

Absorption of Iron

A typical adult in Western societies ingests about 15 to 20 mg of iron daily. Only 0.5 to 1 mg of iron is absorbed by normal adult men, and 1 to 1.5 mg is absorbed by premenopausal adult women. Iron depletion, caused by hemorrhage, for example, increases iron absorption. Growing children and pregnant women also absorb increased amounts of iron. Iron deficiency is common, even in economically developed countries, and is the most prevalent nutrient deficiency in the world.

Iron absorption is limited because iron tends to form insoluble salts with anions, such as hydroxide, phosphate, and bicarbonate, that are present in intestinal secretions. Iron also tends to form insoluble complexes with other substances commonly present in food, such as phytate, tannins, and the fiber of cereal grains. These iron complexes are more soluble at low pH. Therefore, hydrochloric acid (HCl) secreted by the stomach enhances iron absorption, whereas iron absorption is commonly low in individuals deficient in acid secretion. Ascorbate effectively promotes iron absorption. Ascorbate forms a soluble complex with iron, thereby preventing iron from forming insoluble complexes. Ascorbate also reduces Fe^{3+} to Fe^{2+}. The tendency of Fe^{2+} to form insoluble complexes is much less than that of Fe^{3+}, and partly for this reason, Fe^{2+} is absorbed much better than is Fe^{3+}.

Heme iron is relatively well absorbed; about 15% of ingested heme is absorbed. Proteolytic enzymes release heme groups from proteins in the intestinal lumen. Heme is probably taken up by facilitated transport by the epithelial cells that line the upper small intestine. In the epithelial cell, iron is split from the heme by reactions that involve **heme oxygenase.** No intact heme is transported into the portal blood. The heme oxygenase reaction is the rate-limiting step in the absorption of heme iron.

Cellular Mechanism of Inorganic Iron Absorption

Our understanding of the mechanisms of absorption of inorganic or nonheme iron is incomplete; a provisional model is depicted in Fig. 33-15. Duodenal epithelial cells are principally responsible for absorption of nonheme iron. The brush border plasma membrane contains transport proteins that bind Fe^{2+} and transport it into the duodenal epithelial cells; Fe^{3+} is not transported. The brush border plasma membrane has a transport protein (**DCT1**) that cotransports H^+ and Fe^{2+} across the luminal membrane. When the pH of the lumen is more acid than that in the cytosol of the enterocyte DCT1 uses energy from the H^+ gradient to actively take up Fe^{2+} into the cells of the duodenum and upper jejunum. DCT1 cannot transport Fe^{3+}, but an **iron reductase** on the brush border surface can reduce Fe^{3+} to Fe^{2+} prior to transport. In the cytosol of the enterocytes Fe^{2+} is oxidized to Fe^{3+}. In the epithelial cell, Fe^{3+} is bound to cytosolic iron-binding proteins, which may function in a way analogous to calbindin, namely, to prevent Fe^{3+} from forming insoluble complexes with intracellular anions, and to facilitate the diffusion of Fe^{3+} through the cytosol.

Fe^{3+} is transported from the cytosol across the basolateral plasma membrane by another ion transport protein (**IREG1**). IREG1 is associated with a copper-containing oxidase (**hyphaestin**) whose activity is required for transport. In the blood, Fe^{3+} is bound to the iron carrier protein **transferrin.** Cells elsewhere that take up iron from the blood have membrane receptors for the iron-transferrin complex, which is taken up by receptor-mediated endocytosis.

Regulation of Iron Absorption

Iron absorption is regulated in accordance with the body's need for iron. In chronic iron deficiency or after hemorrhage, the duodenum and jejunum increase their capacity to absorb iron. The intestine also protects the body from the consequences of absorbing too much iron. However, the excretion of iron is limited. Thus, the absorption of more iron than is needed may lead to iron overload.

Iron overload can result from chronic ingestion of large amounts of absorbable iron. This condition is common in certain African tribes that regularly consume a home-brewed beer with a high iron content. In the genetic disorder called **idiopathic hemochromatosis,** an excessive amount of iron is absorbed from a diet that is normal in iron content. In some cases of idiopathic hemochromatosis there are increased levels of the ion transport proteins DCT1 and IREG1.

An important mechanism for preventing excess absorption of iron is the almost irreversible binding of iron to **ferritin** in the intestinal epithelial cell. *Iron bound to ferritin is not available for transport into the plasma* (Fig. 33-15) but is instead lost into the intestinal lumen and excreted in the

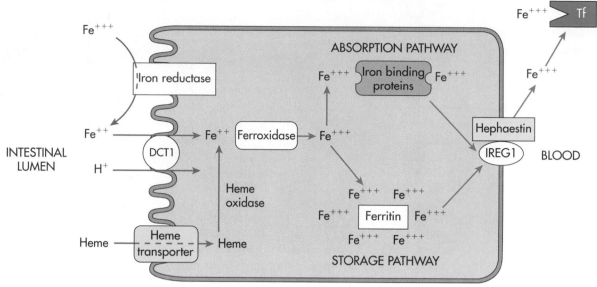

■ **Fig. 33-15** A current view of the absorption of iron by intestinal epithelial cells. See text for details.

feces when the intestinal epithelial cell exfoliates. The amount of **apoferritin** present in the intestinal epithelial cells determines how much iron can be trapped in this nonabsorbable pool. Apoferritin (MW about 19,000) is the protein part of ferritin. Ferritin is a large complex consisting of 24 apoferritins in the form of a hollow shell with up to 4000 iron atoms bound inside in the form of insoluble iron salts of hydroxide and phosphate.

After a hemorrhage, the capacity of the duodenum and jejunum to absorb iron increases, with a time lag of 3 to 4 days. During this time, the intestinal epithelial cells migrate from their sites of formation in Lieberkühn's crypts to the tips of the villi, where they are most involved in absorptive activities.

The iron absorptive capacity of enterocytes is "programmed" when the cells reside in the crypts of Lieberkühn (Fig. 33-16). The crypt cells have basolateral receptors for the transferrin-iron complex. When blood levels of transferrin-iron are high, the cytosolic level of Fe^{3+} rises and Fe^{3+} binds to an **iron regulatory protein (IRP)** in the cytosol. Bound iron prevents IRP from doing its job, which is regulating the rate of translation or the stability of particular messenger RNAs that encode proteins involved in iron transport. In an iron-depleted individual, less transferrin-iron is taken up, cytosolic levels of Fe^{3+} fall, and IRP can then bind to messenger RNAs. IRP binding to mRNAs results in increased translation of mRNAs encoding the iron transport proteins DCT1 and IREG1 and decreased translation of apoferritin mRNA, thus enhancing the ability of the enterocyte to absorb Fe^{2+}. When the level of transferrin-iron in blood is high, Fe^{3+} binds to IRG, IRG fails to have the effects just mentioned on RNA translation, and levels of DCT1 and IREG1 fall, the level of apoferritin rises, and the enterocyte has a low capacity for absorbing Fe^{2+}.

ABSORPTION OF OTHER IONS

Magnesium

Magnesium is absorbed along the entire length of the small intestine. About half of the normal dietary intake of magnesium is absorbed. The largest portion of Mg^{2+} absorption takes place in the ileum; a smaller portion is absorbed in the duodenum. The colon absorbs a still smaller, but significant, portion of Mg^{2+}. The rate of Mg^{2+} absorption is not adjusted in response to dietary loads.

The cellular mechanisms of Mg^{2+} absorption are not well understood. Much Mg^{2+} absorption may occur by the paracellular pathway, and it may be driven by the concentration of Mg^{2+} in the lumen when water is absorbed.

Phosphate

Like magnesium, phosphate is also absorbed all along the small intestine. From highest to lowest capacity for phosphate absorption per centimeter of length of the gastrointestinal tract, the order is duodenum > jejunum > ileum. Because both the length of the duodenum and its transit time are short, the jejunum is responsible for the largest portion of phosphate absorption. In response to low levels of serum phosphate, the intestinal capacity to absorb phosphate increases. This response depends on vitamin D, but the mechanisms by which vitamin D enhances phosphate absorption are not well understood. Phosphate crosses the brush border plasma membrane largely by Na^+-powered secondary active transport. Phosphate leaves the cell by moving down its electrochemical potential gradient across the basolateral membrane by means of facilitated transport.

Copper

Approximately 50% of the copper ingested in the diet is absorbed, mainly in the jejunum. When dietary copper is low,

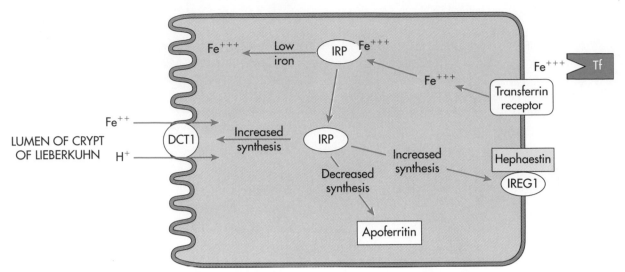

■ **Fig. 33-16**   The current view of how cells in the crypt of Lieberkuhn adjust their capacity to absorb iron in keeping with the body's iron stores. In an iron-replete individual the iron-transferrin (Tf) complex is taken up at the basolateral membrane and iron binds to a cytosolic iron regulatory protein (IRP). In iron repletion, the amount of apoferritin (the protein part of ferritin) is increased, while levels of DCT1 and IREG1 are decreased. When extracellular iron concentrations are low, less iron-transferrin is taken up, so that Fe^{+++} dissociates from IRP. IRP then causes increased synthesis of DCT1 and IREG1, but decreased synthesis of apoferritin.

the fraction of ingested copper that is absorbed increases. Copper is an essential component of certain vital enzymes, such as the superoxide dismutases. Most (70% to 95%) of the copper in plasma is bound to ceruloplasmin. Much of the remainder is bound to albumin. Many details of copper absorption in the small intestine are not known. Here we present a tentative mechanism for copper absorption that is consistent with current knowledge.

The brush border plasma membrane of the small intestine has receptors that bind ceruloplasmin; it is not known whether these receptors play a role in intestinal absorption of copper. Ceruloplasmin does not enter the epithelial cell. The luminal membrane has a transport protein that passively takes up cuprous ion, Cu^+, into the cytosol; cupric copper, Cu^{2+}, is not transported. The same Cu^+ transporter appears to take up copper from ceruloplasmin and from other sources. A brush border reductase reduces Cu^{2+} to Cu^+, permitting it to be taken up into the enterocyte. Some copper appears to be taken up by receptor-mediated endocytosis and some by transport directly into the cytosol. In the cytosol of enterocytes, Cu^+ is bound to glutathione; this copper is available for the synthetic needs of the enterocyte. Vesicles in the enterocyte have a copper-transporting ABC (ATP-binding cassette) transporter in their limiting membranes. This ABC transporter is almost certainly closely related to the ABC transport proteins that are mutated in Menkes and Wilson disease. The ABC transporter pumps copper, both Cu^+ and Cu^{2+}, into the vesicle interior. Copper is then released to the extracellular fluid from these vesicles by exocytosis at the basolateral membrane.

Copper is secreted in the bile bound to certain bile acids, and most of this copper is lost in the feces. In individuals who fail to secrete sufficient amounts of copper in the bile,

the body's copper pool grows and copper accumulates in certain tissues.

ABSORPTION OF WATER-SOLUBLE VITAMINS

Most water-soluble vitamins can be absorbed by simple diffusion if taken in sufficiently high doses. Nevertheless, specific transport mechanisms are important in the normal absorption of most water-soluble vitamins. Several water-soluble vitamins are taken up across the brush border membrane by Na^+-powered secondary active transport processes. Table 33-6 summarizes current knowledge about these transport mechanisms.

Absorption of Vitamin B$_{12}$

By vitamin B_{12} we denote cobalamin and its physiologically active derivatives, such as methylcobalamin and adenosylcobalamin. A specific transport process has also been implicated in the absorption of vitamin B_{12}. The dietary requirement for B_{12} is fairly close to the maximal absorption capacity for the vitamin. In the absence of sufficient vitamin B_{12}, the maturation of red blood cells slows and **pernicious anemia** ensues. Because of its medical importance, considerable research has focused on the absorption of vitamin B_{12}. Enteric bacteria synthesize vitamin B_{12} and other B vitamins, but the colonic epithelium lacks specific mechanisms for their absorption.

Storage in the liver. The liver contains a large store of vitamin B_{12} (2 to 5 mg). Vitamin B_{12} is normally present in the bile (0.5 to 5 µg daily), but about 70% of this vitamin B_{12} is normally reabsorbed. Because only about 0.1% of the

■ Table 33-6 Intestinal absorption of water-soluble vitamins

Vitamin	Site of absorption	Transport mechanism
Ascorbic acid (C)	Ileum	*Co-transport with Na^+
Biotin	Duodenum, jejunum	†Facilitated transport?
Choline	Small intestine	Facilitated transport
Folic acid and folate derivatives	Jejunum	Facilitated transport
Inositol	Small intestine	Co-transport with Na^+?
Nicotinic acid	Jejunum	Diffusion of acid form
Pantothenic acid	Small intestine	Co-transport with Na^+
Pyridoxine (B_6)	Duodenum, jejunum	Diffusion
Riboflavin (B_2)	Duodenum, jejunum	Facilitated transport
Thiamin (B_1)	Jejunum	Co-transport with Na^+
Vitamin B_{12}	Distal ileum	Receptor-mediated endocytosis

*Secondary active transport powered by electrochemical gradient of Na^+.
†Via a transporter not linked to energy in any way.

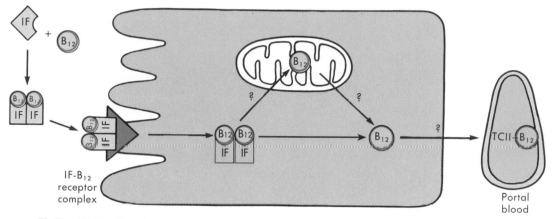

■ Fig. 33-17 Postulated mechanism of vitamin B_{12} absorption by epithelial cells of the ileum.

store is lost daily, the store will last for 3 to 6 years even if absorption totally ceases.

Gastric phase. Most of the vitamin B_{12} present in food is bound to proteins. During the gastric phase of digestion, the low pH in the stomach and the digestion of proteins by pepsin release free vitamin B_{12}. The free vitamin B_{12} is rapidly bound to a number of vitamin B_{12}-binding glycoproteins called **R proteins.** R proteins are present in saliva and in gastric juice, and bind vitamin B_{12} tightly over a wide pH range. The R proteins of saliva and gastric juice have molecular weights near 60,000 and are closely related to transcobalamins I, II, and III.

Intrinsic factor (IF) is a vitamin B_{12}-binding protein that is secreted by the gastric parietal cells. IF is a glycoprotein that contains 15% carbohydrate and has a molecular weight of about 45,000. The rate of IF secretion usually parallels the rate of HCl secretion. IF binds vitamin B_{12} with less affinity than do the R proteins. Thus, in the stomach, most of the vitamin B_{12} released from food is bound by R proteins.

Intestinal phase. During the intestinal phase of digestion, pancreatic proteases begin degradation of the complexes between R proteins and cobalamins. This degradation greatly lowers the affinities of the R proteins for cobalamins, so that cobalamins are transferred to IF. IF and IF-cobalamin complexes resist digestion by pancreatic proteases. As described

later, the normal mechanism for absorption involves brush border receptors for IF-cobalamin complexes. These receptors do not recognize the R protein-cobalamin complexes. Thus, in pancreatic insufficiency, when R proteins are not degraded, cobalamins remain bound to R proteins. These complexes are not available for absorption, and therefore vitamin B_{12} deficiency may ensue.

Absorption of vitamin B_{12}. Figure 33-17 summarizes the mechanism of vitamin B_{12} absorption. The normal absorption of cobalamins depends on the presence of IF. When IF binds vitamin B_{12}, IF undergoes a conformational change that favors the formation of dimers; each dimer binds two vitamin B_{12} molecules. The brush border plasma membranes of the epithelial cells of the ileum contain a receptor protein that recognizes and binds the IF-B_{12} dimer. Free IF does not compete for binding, and the receptor does not recognize free cobalamins. Binding to the receptor is required for uptake of vitamin B_{12} into the cell. The IF-B_{12} complex is taken up into the ileal epithelial cell across the brush border plasma membrane by receptor-mediated endocytosis.

After the uptake of the IF-B_{12} complex, vitamin B_{12} is slowly transported through the epithelial cell and into the blood. Vitamin B_{12} does not appear in the blood until 4 hours after it is ingested, and the peak B_{12} level in plasma occurs 6 to 8 hours after a meal. The reason for this delay is not well understood, but for much of the lag period B_{12} may be located predominantly in the mitochondria of the epithelial cells.

The exit of vitamin B_{12} from the cells of the ileal epithelium is poorly understood. Facilitated or active transport is presumably involved. Most of the B_{12} that is absorbed appears in the portal blood bound to **transcobalamin II,** a globulin. Transcobalamin II is synthesized in the liver, but the ileal epithelium also makes this protein. The transcobalamin II-B_{12} complex is rapidly cleared from the portal blood by the liver by means of receptor-mediated endocytosis.

Absorption in the absence of IF. In the complete absence of IF, about 1% to 2% of an ingested load of B_{12} will be absorbed. If large doses of vitamin B_{12} are taken (about 1 mg/day), enough B_{12} can be absorbed to treat pernicious anemia. The IF-independent mechanism shows no maximal absorptive capacity, does not appear to be limited to the ileum, and shows a much shorter lag time (about 1 hour) than IF-dependent absorption.

In the absence of sufficient levels of vitamin B_{12}, the maturation of red cells slows and anemia results. **Pernicious anemia,** the most common cause of malabsorption of vitamin B_{12}, usually occurs in elderly adults of European ancestry. Most individuals with pernicious anemia have circulating antibodies that prevent B_{12} from binding to IF,

antibodies that prevent the IF-B_{12} complex from binding to ileal receptors, or both of these types of antibodies. A majority of these people also have circulating antibodies against parietal cells that result in the almost complete inability to secrete HCl, pepsinogens, and IF.

Pernicious anemia in childhood is rare and has three forms: (1) an **autoimmune type of pernicious anemia** with characteristics just described; (2) **congenital IF deficiency,** in which pepsin and acid secretion are normal but IF secretion is deficient; and (3) **congenital vitamin B_{12}** malabsorption syndrome, in which gastric function and levels of IF are normal, but B_{12} absorption is deficient owing to a defect in the ileal IF-B_{12} receptors.

DIGESTION AND ABSORPTION OF LIPIDS

The primary lipids of a normal diet are triglycerides. The diet contains smaller amounts of sterols, sterol esters, and phospholipids (Fig. 33-18). Because lipids are only slightly soluble in water, each stage of their processing poses special problems to the gastrointestinal tract. In the stomach, lipids tend to separate out into an oily phase. In the duodenum and small intestine, lipids are emulsified with the aid of bile acids. The large surface area of the emulsion droplets allows

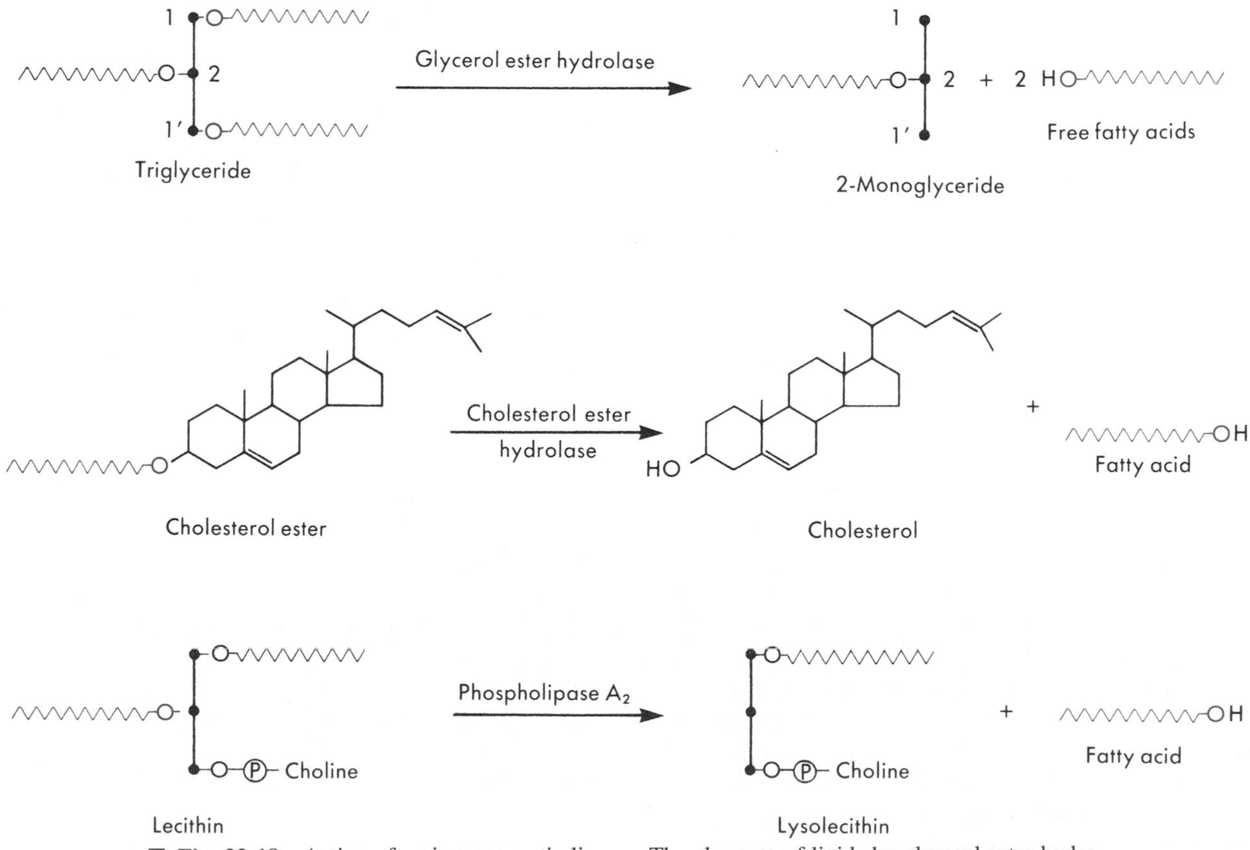

■ **Fig. 33-18**   Action of major pancreatic lipases. The cleavage of lipids by glycerol ester hydrolase (pancreatic lipase), cholesterol ester hydrolase, and phospholipase A_2 is illustrated. *P,* Phosphate.

access of the water-soluble lipolytic enzymes to their substrates. The digestion products of lipids form small molecular aggregates, known as **micelles,** with the bile acids. The micelles are small enough to diffuse among the microvilli and allow absorption of the lipids from molecular solution at the intestinal brush border. The digestion and absorption of lipids are more complex than for any other class of nutrients and are more frequently subject to malfunction.

Digestion of Lipids in the Stomach

Because fats tend to separate out into an oily phase that sits on top of the gastric contents, they are emptied from the stomach later than the other gastric contents. Formation of emulsions with phospholipids or other natural emulsifying agents is inhibited by the high acidity of the stomach. Fat in the duodenum strongly inhibits gastric emptying. This inhibition ensures that the fat is not emptied from the stomach more rapidly than it can be accommodated by the duodenal mechanisms that provide for emulsification and digestion.

Significant hydrolysis of triglycerides occurs in the stomach. The enzymes responsible for lipid hydrolysis in the stomach are known as **preduodenal lipases.** These enzymes operate most effectively at acid pHs. In rats, the principal preduodenal lipase is **lingual lipase,** which is produced by glands under the circumvallate papillae of the tongue. In humans, lingual lipase is only a minor component of preduodenal lipase; the major component is **gastric lipase** produced by gland cells in the fundus of the stomach. Normally, the amount of pancreatic lipase is so great that the absence of preduodenal lipase does not cause malabsorption of triglycerides. However, when pancreatic lipase is grossly deficient or pancreatic lipase is inactive because of high acidity in the upper small intestine (e.g., in Zollinger-Ellison syndrome), the hydrolysis of triglycerides by gastric lipase may be essential for digestion and absorption of triglycerides.

Digestion of Lipids in the Duodenum and Jejunum

The lipolytic enzymes of the pancreatic juice are water-soluble molecules and thus have access to the lipids only at the surfaces of the fat droplets. The surface area available for digestion is increased many thousand times by emulsification of the lipids. Bile acids themselves are rather poor emulsifying agents. However, with the aid of lecithin, which is present in high concentration in the bile, the bile acids emulsify dietary fats. The emulsion droplets are about 1 μm in diameter and have a large surface area on which the digestive enzymes can work.

Pancreatic lipolytic enzymes. *Pancreatic juice contains the major lipolytic enzymes responsible for digestion of lipids* (Fig. 33-18). The most important digestive enzymes are **glycerol ester hydrolase, colipase, cholesterol ester hydrolase,** and **phopholipase A.**

Glycerol ester hydrolase (also called simply **pancreatic lipase**) cleaves the 1 and 1′ fatty acids from a triglyceride to produce two free fatty acids and one 2-monoglyceride. Glycerol ester hydrolase of pancreatic juice has a molecular weight of about 50,000 and is rather specific for triglycerides. Pancreatic lipase has very low activity against triglycerides in molecular solution, but it is very active on droplets or emulsions of triglycerides. The enzyme operates at the interface between the aqueous phase and the triglyceride-containing oil phase. The activity of pancreatic lipase is proportional to the surface area of the oil phase. The amount of pancreatic lipase present in samples of duodenal contents can hydrolyze the average daily intake of triglyceride in 1 to 2 minutes.

Pancreatic lipase is essentially completely inactivated by bile salts at physiological concentrations. However, a protein of 10,000 molecular weight, known as **colipase,** present in pancreatic juice can relieve the inactivation of lipase by bile salts. Bile salts inhibit the activity of pancreatic lipase by binding to the surface of triglyceride-containing oil droplets, and thereby they prevent the pancreatic lipase from binding. Colipase displaces bile salts from the surface of oil droplets. One pancreatic lipase molecule then binds to each colipase molecule. The resultant lipase-colipase complex then cleaves the 1 and 1′ fatty acids from triglycerides at the surface of the oil droplet.

Cholesterol ester hydrolase (cholesterol esterase) cleaves the ester bond in a cholesterol ester to yield one fatty acid and free cholesterol. Cholesterol esterase is probably identical to a nonspecific enzyme, known as **nonspecific lipase** or **nonspecific esterase,** that cleaves fatty acid ester linkages in a variety of lipid substrates. In humans, nonspecific lipase has a molecular weight of about 100,000. The enzyme forms dimers in the presence of bile salts, and in this form it is protected from proteolytic digestion. The dimeric enzyme hydrolyzes fatty acids from cholesterol esters, lysophospholipids, triglycerides, 2-monoglycerides, and fatty acyl esters of vitamins A, D, and E. The total activity of nonspecific lipase in pancreatic juice is small compared with the activity of pancreatic lipase.

Phospholipase A_2 cleaves the ester bond at the 2 position of a glycerophosphatide to yield, in the case of phosphatidylcholine, one fatty acid and one lysophosphatidylcholine. Phospholipase A_2 is secreted as a proenzyme by the pancreas. Tryptic cleavage of the proenzyme activates phospholipase A_2 against phospholipids emulsified by bile salts. Phospholipase A_2 is a highly stable protein with a molecular weight of 14,000, and it requires calcium ions for activity. Neither phospholipase A_2 nor pancreatic lipase appreciably cleaves the fatty acyl ester linkage at the number 1 position of a phospholipid. Therefore, lysophosphatides are the principal form in which phospholipids are absorbed.

The formation of micelles. Bile acids form micelles with the products of fat digestion, especially 2-monoglycerides. The micelles are multimolecular aggregates, about 5 nm in diameter, and they contain about 20 to 30 lipid molecules. The hydrophobic acyl chains of 2-monoglycerides and lysophosphatides tend to be in the interior of the micelle, and the more polar portions tend to face the surrounding water (see Fig. 32-27). Bile acids are flat molecules that have a polar and a nonpolar face. Much of the surface of the micelles is covered with bile acids, with the nonpolar face of the bile acid toward the lipid interior of the micelle and the polar face toward the outside. Extremely hydrophobic molecules, such as long-chain fatty acids, cholesterol, and certain fat-soluble vitamins, tend to partition into the interior of the micelle. Micelles contain almost no intact triglyceride.

Bile acids must be present at a certain minimal concentration, called the **critical micelle concentration,** before micelles will form. Conjugated bile acids have a much lower critical micelle concentration than unconjugated forms. Normally, bile acids are present in the duodenum at concentrations greater than the critical micelle concentration.

Lipids and lipid digestion products in the micelles exchange rapidly with lipid digestion products in the aqueous solution surrounding the micelle. In this way, micelles keep the aqueous solution that surrounds them saturated with 2-monoglycerides, various fatty acids, cholesterol, and lysophosphatides. These lipids are present in the aqueous solution at low concentrations because of their limited water solubility.

Absorption of the Products of Lipid Digestion

The function of micelles in lipid absorption. Mixed micelles are important in the absorption of the products of lipid digestion and in the absorption of most other fat-soluble molecules (such as the fat-soluble vitamins). Micelles are small enough to diffuse among the microvilli that form the brush border. The presence of micelles tends to keep the aqueous solution that contacts the brush border plasma membrane saturated with fatty acids, 2-monoglycerides, cholesterol, and other micellar contents. *Thus, the*

huge surface area of the brush border is made available for the absorption of the micellar contents (Fig. 33-19).

Uptake of lipids by intestinal epithelial cells. The duodenum and jejunum are most active in fat absorption, and most ingested fat is absorbed by the midjejunum. The fat present in normal stools is not ingested fat (which is completely absorbed), but fat from colonic bacteria and exfoliated intestinal epithelial cells. Cholesterol is absorbed more slowly than most of the other constituents of the micelles. Therefore, as the micelles progress down the small intestine, they become enriched in cholesterol.

Role of the unstirred layer. Free fatty acids, 2-monoglycerides, and the other products of lipid digestion cross the brush border plasma membrane so rapidly that this step does not limit the rate of their uptake. *The main limitation to the rate of lipid uptake by the epithelial cells of the upper small intestine is the diffusion of the mixed micelles through an unstirred layer* (or diffusion boundary layer) on the luminal surface of the brush border plasma membrane (Fig. 33-19). Partly because the surface of the intestinal mucosa is convoluted, the fluid in immediate contact with the epithelial cell surface is not readily mixed with the bulk of the luminal contents. The effective thickness of this unstirred layer ranges from 200 to 500 µm. Nutrients present in the well-mixed contents of the intestinal lumen must diffuse through the unstirred layer to reach the brush border plasma membrane. A concentration gradient exists across the unstirred layer, with micelles and lipid digestion products in lower concentration at the brush border surface than in the well-mixed contents of the lumen. A pH gradient also exists across

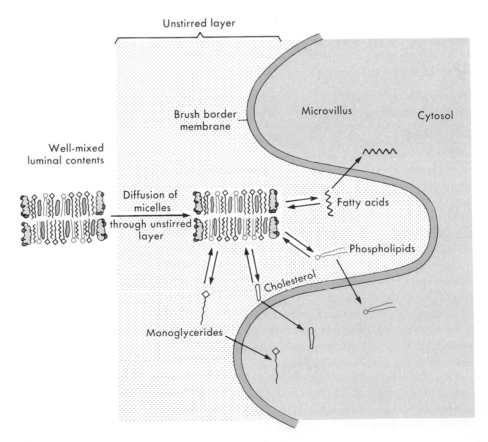

■ **Fig. 33-19**   Lipid absorption in the small intestine. Mixed micelles of bile acids and lipid digestion products diffuse through the unstirred layer and among the microvilli. As digestion products are absorbed from free solution by the enterocytes, more digestion products partition out of the micelles. The ability of micelles to diffuse among the microvilli makes the whole surface of the brush border available for lipid absorption. Transport proteins mediate the facilitated transport of fatty acids and cholesterol across the brush border plasma membrane. In the cytosol of the epithelial cell, fatty acids are bound to fatty acid-binding protein and cholesterol is bound to sterol carrier proteins.

the unstirred layer: the fluid in immediate contact with the brush border plasma membrane is about 1 pH unit more acidic than the bulk luminal contents. The lower pH at the brush border surface may enhance absorption of fatty acids, because protonated fatty acids are more lipid soluble than ionized ones.

Transport of lipids across the brush border membrane. Because of their high lipid solubility, the fatty acids, 2-monoglycerides, cholesterol, and lysolecithin can simply diffuse across the brush border membrane. Nevertheless, transport proteins in the brush border membrane have been shown to mediate the uptake of long-chain fatty acids.

Cholesterol esterase is bound to the luminal surface of the brush border plasma membrane of the upper small intestine. Hydrolysis of cholesterol esters in such close proximity to the membrane may promote cellular uptake of cholesterol.

A specific protein in the brush border plasma membrane facilitates the transport of long-chain fatty acids. This protein is called **MVM-FABP,** for **microvillous membrane fatty acid-binding protein.** MVM-FABP uses the energy of the Na^+ gradient to power the secondary active uptake of long-chain fatty acids. MVM-FABP may also mediate the uptake of lysophospholipids.

Cholesterol probably crosses the luminal plasma membrane by simple diffusion. Cholesterol present in the lumen consists of dietary cholesterol plus cholesterol ingested in food. Only about 50% of the cholesterol is absorbed. The restriction of cholesterol absorption appears to be due mainly to the function of an ABC transport protein in the brush border membrane. Functioning in a way similar to MDR, the ABC transporter responsible for multidrug resistance (Chapter 1), the cholesterol transporter uses the energy of ATP to remove cholesterol from the membrane and to pump it back into the lumen of the intestine. The cholesterol transporter limits even more strongly the absorption of plant sterols; only about 2% of plant sterols is absorbed.

Handling of Lipids Inside the Intestinal Epithelial Cell

Cytosolic lipid transport proteins. Two classes of fatty acid-binding proteins exist in the cytosol of epithelial cells of the upper small intestine. These proteins are known as **I-FABP** and **L-FABP.** I-FABP was first isolated from intestine and L-FABP was first found in liver. I-FABP binds long-chain fatty acids. L-FABP has a broader specificity and binds cholesterol, monoglycerides, and lysophosphatides as well as fatty acids.

Two isoforms of sterol carrier proteins, **SCP-1** and **SCP-2,** are also present in epithelial cell cytosol. These proteins bind cholesterol and other sterols.

Binding of lipids to intracellular binding proteins may prevent lipids from forming oil droplets in the cytosol. The binding proteins apparently function to transport lipid digestion products from the brush border plasma membrane to the smooth endoplasmic reticulum.

Resynthesis of lipids in the smooth endoplasmic reticulum. The products of lipid digestion are carried by the binding proteins to the smooth endoplasmic reticulum. In the smooth endoplasmic reticulum, which becomes engorged with lipid after a meal, considerable chemical reprocessing of lipids occurs (Fig. 33-20). The 2-monoglycerides are reesterified with fatty acids at the 1 and 1' carbons to re-form triglycerides. Lysophospholipids are reconverted to phospholipids. Cholesterol is reesterified substantially, although some free cholesterol remains. The processing of 2-monoglycerides and lysophospholipids is essentially complete. The intestinal epithelial cells are also capable of some synthesis of new lipids.

Chylomicron formation and transport. The reprocessed lipids, along with new lipids that are synthesized in the epithelial cell, accumulate in the smooth endoplasmic reticulum. Phospholipids tend to cover the external surfaces of these lipid droplets, with their hydrophobic acyl chains in the fatty interior and their polar head groups toward the aqueous exterior. These lipid droplets are known as **prechylomicrons.** About 10% of their surface is covered by apolipoproteins of the A, B, and C classes.

Prechylomicrons are transferred from the smooth endoplasmic reticulum to the Golgi apparatus of the intestinal epithelial cells. Further processing of the prechylomicrons occurs in the Golgi apparatus. The lipid droplets, now known as **chylomicrons,** are ejected from the cell by exocytosis and enter the lateral intercellular spaces (Fig. 33-20). Chylomicrons are too large to traverse the basement membrane that invests the mucosal capillaries. However, they do enter the lacteals, which have sufficiently large fenestrations for the chylomicrons to pass through. Chylomicrons leave the intestine with the lymph, primarily via the thoracic duct, and flow into the venous circulation.

In certain disorders, lipids are malabsorbed and chylomicrons do not appear in intestinal lymph. In such diseases, intestinal epithelial cells become engorged with lipid, and few chylomicrons are exported. In **abetalipoproteinemia,** apo-B is missing from serum lipoproteins. It was previously thought that a deficiency of apo-B was responsible for the lipid malabsorption, but it is now known that apo-B is present in intestinal epithelial cells in this disorder. The molecular defect responsible for the failure to produce and release chylomicrons in abetalipoproteinemia remains to be elucidated. In **chylomicron storage disease,** chylomicrons appear to mature normally in the Golgi apparatus, but the Golgi apparatus fails to release the chylomicrons by exocytosis.

Chylomicrons are approximately spherical and vary greatly in size (60 to 750 nm). When large amounts of lipid are being absorbed, large chylomicrons are formed; when little lipid is being absorbed, the chylomicrons tend to be small. Triglycerides account for about 90% of the mass of chylomicrons. Phospholipids, mainly biliary phospholipids, cover about 80% of the surface of the chylomicrons and account for about 5% of their mass. Apolipoproteins cover the remaining 20% of the chylomicron surface. Cholesterol and cholesterol esters are present in the triglyceride-rich core of the particles; each of these substances makes up about 1% of the chylomicron mass.

Many, but not all, of the apoproteins associated with chylomicrons in intestinal lymph are synthesized by intestinal

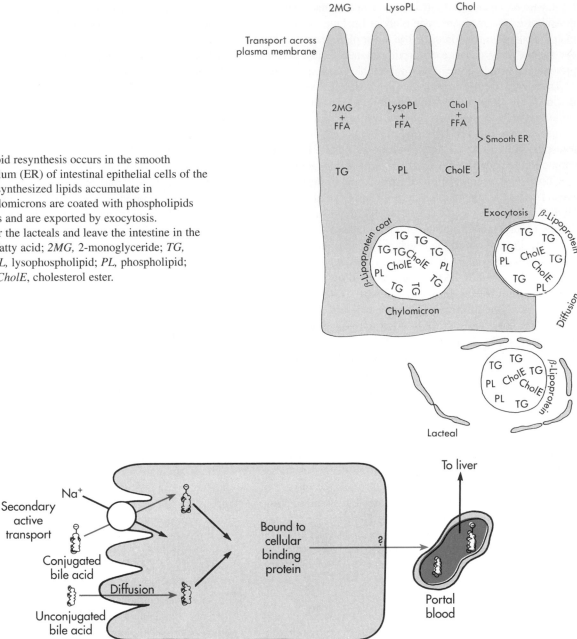

Fig. 33-20 Lipid resynthesis occurs in the smooth endoplasmic reticulum (ER) of intestinal epithelial cells of the small intestine. Resynthesized lipids accumulate in chylomicrons. Chylomicrons are coated with phospholipids and apolipoproteins and are exported by exocytosis. Chylomicrons enter the lacteals and leave the intestine in the lymph. *FFA*, Free fatty acid; *2MG*, 2-monoglyceride; *TG*, triglyceride; *LysoPL*, lysophospholipid; *PL*, phospholipid; *Chol*, cholesterol; *CholE*, cholesterol ester.

Fig. 33-21 Absorption of bile acids by epithelial cells of the terminal ileum. Bile acids are absorbed both by simple diffusion and by Na⁺-powered secondary active transport. Conjugated bile acids are absorbed avidly by active transport. Unconjugated bile acids are absorbed chiefly by simple diffusion. In the cytosol of the epithelial cells, bile acids are bound to specific binding proteins. The mechanisms of transport of bile acids across the basolateral membrane remain to be elucidated.

epithelial cells. Hepatocytes are the other major source of apolipoproteins.

When fat is absent from the intestine, the intestinal epithelial cells of the upper small intestine do not form chylomicrons, but they do synthesize **very-low-density lipoproteins (VLDLs)** and release them into intestinal lymph. VLDLs are smaller and more dense than chylomicrons. Compared with chylomicrons, VLDLs have much less triglyceride (60% of VLDL mass) and much more protein (about 10% of VLDL mass).

Absorption of Bile Acids

Absorption of dietary lipids is typically complete when these substances reach the midjejunum. Bile acids, by contrast, are absorbed largely in the terminal part of the ileum. As for other fat-soluble substances, the unstirred layer is an important barrier to bile acid absorption. Bile acids cross the brush border plasma membrane by two routes: by an active transport process and by simple diffusion (Fig. 33-21). The active process is secondary active transport, powered by the Na⁺ gradient across the brush border membrane. Conjugated bile acids are the principal substrates for active absorption; unconjugated bile acids have poor affinity for the transporter. However, because unconjugated bile acids are less polar than conjugated bile acids, they are better absorbed by simple diffusion. The fewer hydroxyl groups on a bile acid, the poorer substrate the bile acid is for active absorption and the more nonpolar is the bile acid. For these reasons, dehydroxylation of bile acids by enteric bacteria to form secondary bile acids enhances absorption of bile acids by diffusion.

Other aspects of the absorption of bile acids are less well understood. Bile acids may be bound to proteins, which remain to be identified, in intestinal epithelial cells. The process by which bile acids traverse the basolateral plasma membrane of the enterocyte has not been characterized.

Absorbed bile acids are carried away from the intestine in the portal blood, mostly bound to albumins. Hepatocytes avidly extract bile acids, essentially clearing the bile acids from the blood in a single pass through the liver. In the hepatocytes, most deconjugated bile acids are reconjugated, and some secondary bile acids are rehydroxylated. The reprocessed bile acids, together with newly synthesized bile acids, are secreted into bile.

Malabsorption of Lipids

Malabsorption of lipids occurs more frequently than malabsorption of proteins or carbohydrates. Among the general causes of lipid malabsorption are bile deficiency, pancreatic insufficiency, and the intestinal mucosal atrophy that occurs in some disease states.

In cases of **bile deficiency** and **pancreatic insufficiency,** the levels of bile acids and lipolytic enzymes, respectively, must be severely reduced before serious malabsorption occurs. In both bile deficiency and pancreatic insufficiency, the quantity of fecal fat is roughly proportional to the quantity ingested.

Even in the complete absence of bile acids, significant hydrolysis of triglyceride occurs. The rate of absorption of fatty acids from triglycerides may be 50% of normal. Cholesterol, cholesterol esters, and fat-soluble vitamins are much less water soluble than are fatty acids, and their absorption is grossly deficient in the absence of bile acids.

In the complete absence of pancreatic lipases, all lipid classes are poorly absorbed. This problem probably occurs because 2-monoglycerides and lysophosphatides (products of the action of pancreatic lipases) are required for the formation of mixed micelles with bile acids.

In **tropical sprue** and **gluten enteropathy,** the intestinal epithelium is flattened and the density of microvilli is decreased. Lipid malabsorption in these diseases is probably a consequence of the marked decrease in the surface area available for lipid absorption.

Absorption of Fat-Soluble Vitamins

Because of their solubility in nonpolar environments, the fat-soluble vitamins (A, D, E, and K) partition into the mixed micelles formed by the bile acids and lipid digestion products. Fat-soluble vitamins enter the intestinal epithelial cell by diffusing across the brush border plasma membrane. The presence of bile acids and lipid digestion products enhances the absorption of fat-soluble vitamins. In the intestinal epithelial cell, the fat-soluble vitamins enter the chylomicrons and leave the intestine in the lymph. In the absence of bile acids, a significant portion of the ingested load of a fat-soluble vitamin may be absorbed and leave the intestine in the portal blood.

SUMMARY

1. The α-amylases of saliva and pancreatic juice cleave branched starch into maltose, maltotriose, and α-limit dextrins. These digestion products are then reduced to glucose molecules by glucoamylase and isomaltase, carbohydrate-digesting enzymes on the brush border plasma membrane.

2. The brush border also contains the disaccharidases sucrase and lactase that cleave sucrose and lactose into monosaccharides. These cleavage products are transported into the epithelial cell by the monosaccharide transport proteins of the brush border membrane, the glucose-galactose transporter and the fructose transporter.

3. Protein digestion begins in the stomach with the action of pepsins. The pancreatic proteases rapidly cleave proteins in the duodenum and jejunum to oligopeptides. Peptidases on the brush border membrane reduce oligopeptides to single amino acids and to dipeptides and tripeptides.

4. Amino acids are taken into the epithelial cell by an array of amino acid-transporting proteins in the brush border membrane. Dipeptides and tripeptides are taken up by a brush border peptide transport protein with broad specificity.

5. A typical human ingests 2 L of water per day, and about 7 L enters the gastrointestinal tract in gastrointestinal secretions. About 99% of the water presented to the gastrointestinal tract is absorbed; approximately 100 ml of water escapes into feces each day. The absorption of water is powered by the absorption of ions and nutrients, predominantly in the small intestine.

6. The mature epithelial cells at the tips of small intestinal villi are active in absorption of water and electrolytes. Cells in Lieberkühn's crypts are net secretors of water and ions. The net absorption that usually occurs in the small intestine is the resultant of much larger absorptive and secretory fluxes. In secretory diarrheal diseases, such as cholera, the secretory fluxes in the crypt cells increase and the absorptive fluxes in cells at the villous tips are inhibited.

7. Calcium is actively absorbed in the small intestine. Vitamin D stimulates the absorption of Ca^{2+} by enhancing the synthesis of cytosolic calbindin, a Ca^{2+}-binding protein, and the other proteins involved in transmucosal transport of Ca^{2+}. Ca^{2+} is transported across the basolateral membrane by

the Ca^{2+}-ATPase and the Na^+-Ca^{2+} exchange protein. The capacity of the intestinal epithelial cells to absorb Ca^{2+} is regulated in accordance with the body's need for Ca^{2+}.

8. About 5% of the ingested inorganic iron is absorbed by the small intestine; approximately 15% of heme iron is absorbed. The brush border membrane of small intestinal epithelial cells has transport proteins that bind Fe^{2+} and transport it into the cytosol. Heme groups are taken up by a different transporter. In the cytosol of the intestinal epithelial cell, some of the Fe^{2+} is bound to iron-binding proteins and some is bound to ferritin.

9. Iron bound to ferritin is unavailable for absorption and is lost into the feces when the cell is exfoliated. Iron bound to cytosolic iron-binding proteins is passed on an iron-exporting protein in the basolateral membrane. Fe^{3+} is bound to transferrin in blood.

10. Most water-soluble vitamins are taken up by specific transporters in the small intestinal brush border membrane. Vitamin B_{12} is bound to R proteins in saliva and gastric juice. When R proteins are digested, vitamin B_{12} is bound by intrinsic factor (IF). Receptors on the ileal brush border membrane take up the IF-B_{12} complex into the ileal epithelial cell. Vitamin B_{12} appears in the plasma bound to transcobalamin II. Pernicious anemia is caused by a deficiency of IF.

11. Triglyceride is the principal dietary lipid. Lipids form droplets in the stomach and are emulsified in the duodenum by bile acids. Emulsification greatly increases the surface area available for the action of lipases of the pancreatic juice.

12. The products of triglyceride digestion, 2-monoglycerides and fatty acids, form mixed micelles with bile acids. Cholesterol, fat-soluble vitamins, and other lipids partition into the micelles. Mixed micelles are small enough to diffuse among the microvilli. Thus, the micelles greatly enhance the brush border surface area available for lipid absorption.

13. In the epithelial cell, triglycerides and phospholipids are resynthesized and packaged along with other lipids into chylomicrons. Chylomicrons are coated with phospholipids and apolipoproteins and released at the basolateral membrane by exocytosis. Chylomicrons leave the intestine in the lymphatic vessels and the thoracic duct.

BIBLIOGRAPHY

Journal articles

Allayee H, Lafitte BA, Lusis AJ: An absorbing study of cholesterol, *Science* 290:1709, 2000.

Cooke HJ: Neuroimmune signaling in regulation of intestinal transport, *Am J Physiol* 266:G167, 1994.

Eastwoood MA: The physiological effect of dietary fiber: an update, *Annu Rev Nutr* 12:19, 1992.

Fei Y, Ganapathy V, Liebach FH: Molecular and structural features of the proton-coupled oligopeptide transporter superfamily, *Progr Nucleic Acid Res Mol Biol* 58:239, 1998.

Gray GM: Starch digestion and absorption in nonruminants, *J Nutr* 122:172, 1992.

Jenkins DJA et al: Glycemic index of foods: a physiological basis for carbohydrate exchange, *Am J Clin Nutr* 34:362, 1981.

Mailliard ME, Stevens BR, Mann GE: Amino acid transport by small intestinal, hepatic, and pancreatic epithelia, *Gastroenterology* 108:888, 1995.

Nemere I: Vesicular calcium transport in chick intestine, *J Nutr* 122:657, 1992.

Ostlund RE Jr: Cholesterol absorption, *Curr Opin Gastroenterol* 18:254, 2002.

Rolfs A, Hediger MA: Intestinal metal ion absorption: an update, *Curr Opin Gastroenterol* 17:177, 2001.

Rose RC: Intestinal absorption of water-soluble vitamins, *Annu Rev Nutr* 212:191, 1996.

Schaefer M, Gitlin JD IV: Wilsons disease and Menkes disease, *Am J Physiol* 276:G311, 1999.

Southgate DAT: Digestion and metabolism of sugars, *Am J Clin Nutr* 62:s203, 1995.

Steel A et al: Stoichiometry and pH dependence of the rabbit proton-dependent oligopeptide transporter PEPT1, *J Physiol* 498:563, 1997.

Thompson ABR: Dietary regulation of intestinal nutrient transport in health and disease, *Dig Dis Sci* 42:453, 1997.

Ushijima K, Riber JE, Kretchmer N: Carbohydrate malabsorption, *Pedriatr Clin North Am* 42:899, 1995.

Vulpe CD, Packman S: Cellular copper transport, *Annu Rev Nutr* 15:293, 1995.

Wasserman et al: Intestinal calcium transport and calcium extrusion processes at the basolateral membrane, *J Nutr* 122:662, 1992.

Wright EM et al: Sodium cotransporters, *Curr Opin Cell Biol* 8:468, 1996.

Books and monographs

Cooke HJ, Reddix RA: Neural regulation of intestinal electrolyte transport. In Johnson LR, editor: *Physiology of the gastrointestinal tract,* ed 3, New York, 1994, Raven Press.

Davidson NO: Intestinal lipid absorption. In Yamada T, editor: *Textbook of gastroenterology,* ed 3, Philadelphia, 1999, Lippincott Williams & Wilkins.

Johnson LR, Gerwin TA, editors: *Gastrointestinal physiology,* ed 6, St. Louis, 2001, Mosby.

Lacey SW, Seidel RH Jr: Vitamin and mineral absorption. In Yamada T, editor: *Textbook of gastroenterology,* ed 3, Philadelphia, 1999, Lippincott Williams & Wilkins.

Marsh MN, Riley SA: Digestion and absorption of nutrients and vitamins. In Sleisenger MH, Fordtran JS, editors: *Gastrointestinal disease,* ed 6, Philadelphia, 1997, WB Saunders.

Montrose MH, Keely SJ, Barrett KE: Electrolyte secretion and absorption: small intestine and colon. In Yamada T, editor: *Textbook of gastroenterology,* ed 3, Philadelphia, 1999, Lippincott Williams & Wilkins.

Sellin JH: Intestinal electrolyte absorption and secretion. In Sleisenger MH, Fordtran JS, editors: *Gastrointestinal disease,* ed 6, Philadelphia, 1997, WB Saunders.

Traber PG: Carbohydrate assimilation. In Yamada T, editor: *Textbook of gastroenterology,* ed 3, Philadelphia, 1999, Lippincott Williams & Wilkins.

Wright EM et al: Intestinal sugar transport. In Johnson LR, editor: *Physiology of the gastrointestinal tract,* ed 3, New York, 1994, Raven Press.

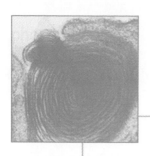

The Kidney

Bruce A. Stanton
Bruce M. Koeppen

chapter thirty-four

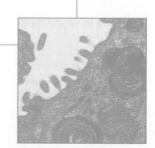

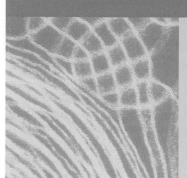

Elements of Renal Function

OVERVIEW OF RENAL FUNCTION

The kidneys are both excretory and regulatory organs. By excreting water and solutes, the kidneys rid the body of excess water and waste products. They also regulate the volume and composition of the body fluids within a very narrow range, despite wide variations in the intake of food and water. Because of the kidneys' homeostatic role, the tissues and cells of the body are able to carry out their normal functions in a relatively constant environment.

The kidneys have several major functions, including:

- Regulation of body fluid osmolality and volumes
- Regulation of electrolyte balance
- Regulation of acid-base balance
- Excretion of metabolic products and foreign substances
- Production and secretion of hormones

The control of body fluid osmolality is important for the maintenance of normal cell volume in all tissues of the body. Control of the volume of the body fluids is necessary for normal function of the cardiovascular system. The kidneys, working in concert with components of the cardiovascular, endocrine, and central nervous systems, accomplish these tasks by regulating the excretion of water and NaCl.

The kidneys play an essential role in regulating the amount of several important inorganic ions in the body, including Na^+, K^+, Cl^-, HCO_3^-, H^+, Ca^{2+}, and PO_4^{3-}. To maintain appropriate balance, the excretion of these electrolytes must be equal to their daily intake. If intake of an electrolyte exceeds its excretion, the amount of this electrolyte in the body increases and the individual is said to be in positive balance for that electrolyte. Conversely, if excretion of an electrolyte exceeds its intake, its amount in the body decreases, and the individual is in negative balance for that electrolyte. For many electrolytes the kidneys are the sole or primary route by which they are excreted.

Another important role of the kidneys is the regulation of acid-base balance. Many of the metabolic functions of the body are exquisitely sensitive to pH. Thus, the pH of the body fluids must be maintained within narrow limits. The pH is maintained by buffers within the body fluids and by the coordinated action of the lungs, liver, and kidneys.

The kidneys also excrete a number of end products of metabolism that are no longer needed by the body. These waste products include urea (from amino acids), uric acid (from nucleic acids), creatinine (from muscle creatine), end products of hemoglobin metabolism, and metabolites of hormones. The kidneys eliminate these substances from the body at a rate that matches their production. Thus, the kidneys regulate their concentrations within the body fluids. The kidneys also eliminate foreign substances from the body, such as drugs, pesticides, and other chemicals ingested in food.

Finally, the kidneys are important endocrine organs that produce and secrete renin, calcitriol, and erythropoietin. **Renin** activates the renin-angiotensin-aldosterone system, which helps regulate blood pressure and sodium and potassium balance. **Calcitriol,** a metabolite of vitamin D_3, is necessary for normal reabsorption of Ca^{2+} by the gastrointestinal tract and for its deposition in bone (see also Chapter 42). In patients with renal disease, the kidneys' ability to produce calcitriol is impaired, and levels of this hormone are reduced. As a result, Ca^{2+} reabsorption by the intestine is decreased. This reduced intestinal Ca^{2+} reabsorption contributes to the abnormalities in bone formation seen in patients with chronic renal disease. Another consequence of many kidney diseases is a reduction in erythropoietin production and secretion. **Erythropoietin** stimulates red blood cell formation by the bone marrow. Decreased erythrocyte production is a cause of the anemia seen in chronic renal failure.

In the following chapters, various aspects of these important renal functions are considered. Where information is available, these functions are considered at several levels of organization: whole kidney, single nephron, cell, membrane, and transport protein.

FUNCTIONAL ANATOMY OF THE KIDNEYS

Structure and function are closely linked in the kidneys. Consequently, an appreciation of the gross anatomical and histological features of the kidneys is necessary to understand their function.

Gross Anatomy

The kidneys are paired organs that lie on the posterior wall of the abdomen behind the peritoneum on either side of the vertebral column. In the adult human, each kidney weighs between 115 and 170 g and is approximately 11 cm in length, 6 cm in width, and 3 cm thick.

The gross anatomical features of the human kidney are illustrated in Fig. 34-1. The medial side of each kidney contains an indentation through which pass the renal artery and vein, nerves, and pelvis. If a kidney were cut in half, two regions would be evident: an outer region called the **cortex** and an inner region called the **medulla.** The cortex and medulla are composed of **nephrons** (the functional units of the kidney), blood vessels, lymphatics, and nerves. The medulla in the human kidney is divided into 8 to 18 conical masses, the **renal pyramids.** The base of each pyramid originates at the corticomedullary border and the apex terminates in a **papilla,** which lies within a **minor calyx.** Minor calyces collect the urine from each papilla. The numerous

minor calyces expand into two or three open-ended pouches, the **major calyces.** The major calyces in turn feed into the pelvis. The pelvis represents the upper expanded region of the ureter, which carries urine from the pelvis to the urinary bladder. The walls of the calyces, pelvis, and ureters contain smooth muscle that contracts to propel the urine toward the **urinary bladder.**

The blood flow to the two kidneys is equal to about 25% (1.25 L/min) of the cardiac output in resting individuals. However, the kidneys constitute less than 0.5% of the total body weight. As illustrated in Fig. 34-2 *(left panel),* the renal artery branches to form progressively the **interlobar artery,** the **arcuate artery,** the **interlobular artery** (cortical radial artery), and the **afferent arteriole,** which leads into the **glomerular capillary network** (i.e., **glomerulus**). The glomerular capillaries come together to form the **efferent arteriole,** which leads into a second capillary network, the **peritubular capillaries,** which supply blood to the nephron. The vessels of the venous system run parallel to the arterial vessels and branch progressively to form the interlobular vein (cortical radial vein), the **arcuate vein,** the **interlobar vein,** and the **renal vein,** which courses beside the ureter.

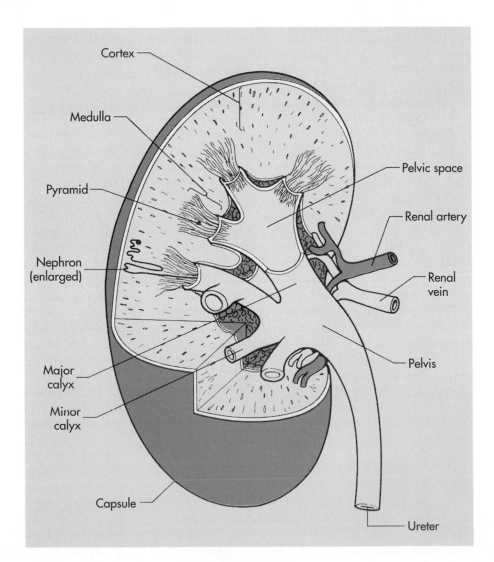

■ **Fig. 34-1**   Structure of the human kidney, cut to show internal structures. (Modified from Marsh DJ: *Renal physiology,* New York, 1983, Raven Press.)

Ultrastructure of the Nephron

The functional unit of the kidneys is the **nephron.** Each human kidney contains approximately 1.2 million nephrons, which are hollow tubes composed of a single cell layer (Fig. 34-2, *right panel*). The nephron consists of (1) a renal corpuscle, (2) a proximal tubule, (3) a loop of Henle, (4) a distal tubule, and (5) a collecting duct system.[*] The renal

---

[*]The organization of the nephron is actually more complicated than presented here. However, for simplicity and clarity of presentation in subsequent chapters, the nephron is divided into five segments. For details on the subdivisions of the five nephron segments, consult the references by Kriz and Bankir, Kriz and Kaissling, and Tisher and Madsen. The collecting duct system is not actually part of the nephron, but for simplicity we consider the collecting duct system part of the nephron.

corpuscle consists of glomerular capillaries and Bowman's capsule. The **proximal tubule** initially forms several coils followed by a straight segment that descends toward the medulla. The next segment is **Henle's loop,** which consists of the straight part of the proximal tubule, the descending thin limb (which ends in a hairpin turn), the ascending thin limb (only in nephrons with long loops of Henle), and the **thick ascending limb.** Near the end of the thick ascending limb, the nephron passes between its afferent and efferent arterioles. This short segment of the thick ascending limb is called the **macula densa.** The **distal tubule** begins a short distance beyond the macula densa and extends to the point in the cortex where two or more nephrons join to form the **cortical collecting duct.** The cortical collecting duct enters

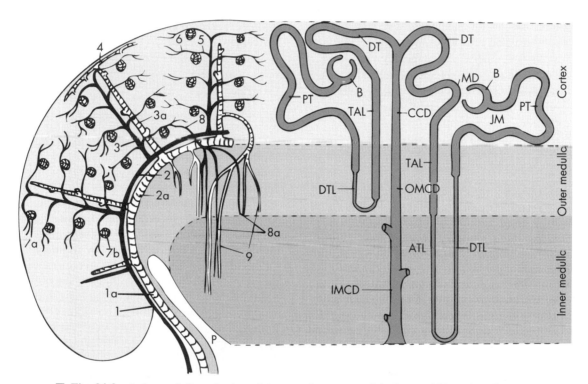

■ **Fig. 34-2** *Left panel*, Organization of the vascular system of the human kidney (not drawn to scale). The course and distribution of the intrarenal blood vessels are depicted; peritubular capillaries are not shown. The renal artery branches to form interlobar arteries *(1)*, which give rise to arcuate arteries *(2)*. Arcuate arteries lead to interlobular arteries *(3)*, which radiate toward the renal capsule and branch to form afferent arterioles *(5)*. Afferent arterioles branch to form glomerular capillary networks (i.e., glomeruli: *7a, 7b*) which then coalesce to form efferent arterioles *(6)*. The efferent arterioles of the superficial nephrons form capillary networks (not shown) that suffuse the cells in the cortex. The efferent arterioles of the juxtamedullary nephrons divide into descending vasa recta *(8)*, which form capillary networks that supply blood to the outer and inner medulla *(8a)*. Blood from the peritubular capillaries enters, consecutively, the stellate vein *(4)*, interlobular vein *(3a)*, arcuate vein *(2a)*, and interlobar vein *(1a)*. Blood from the ascending vasa recta *(9)* enters the interlobular and arcuate veins. *P*, Pelvis. (Modified from Kriz W, Bankir L: *Am J Physiol* 254:F1, 1988.) *Right panel*, Organization of the human nephron (not drawn to scale). A superficial nephron is illustrated on the left and a juxtamedullary nephron *(JM)* on the right. *B*, Bowman's capsule; *DT*, distal tubule; *PT*, proximal tubule; *CCD*, cortical collecting duct; *TAL*, thick ascending limb; *DTL*, descending thin limb; *OMCD*, outer medullary collecting duct; *ATL*, ascending thin limb; *IMCD*, inner medullary collecting duct; *MD*, macula densa. The loop of Henle includes the straight portion of the *PT*, and the *DTL*, *ATL*, and *TAL*. (Modified from Koushanpour E, Kriz W: *Renal physiology*, ed 2, Berlin, 1986, Springer-Verlag; and Kriz W, Bankir L: *Am J Physiol* 254:F1,1988.)

the medulla and becomes the **outer medullary collecting duct,** and then the **inner medullary collecting duct.**

Each nephron segment consists of cells that are uniquely suited to perform specific transport functions (Fig. 34-3). Proximal tubule cells have an extensively amplified apical membrane (the urine side of the cell) called the brush border; only cells in the proximal tubule have this **brush border.** The basolateral membrane (the blood side of the cell) of proximal tubule cells is highly invaginated. These invaginations contain many mitochondria. In contrast, cells of the descending thin limb and ascending thin limb of Henle's loop have poorly developed apical and basolateral surfaces and only a few mitochondria. The cells of the thick ascending limb and the distal tubule have abundant mitochondria and extensive infoldings of the basolateral membrane. The collecting duct is composed of two cell types: **principal cells** and **intercalated cells.** Principal cells have a moderately invaginated basolateral membrane and contain few mitochondria. Intercalated cells have a high density of mitochondria. The final segment of the nephron, the inner medullary collecting duct, is composed of inner medullary collecting duct cells. Cells of the inner medullary collecting duct have poorly developed apical and basolateral surfaces and few mitochondria.

There are two types of nephrons: **superficial** and **juxtamedullary** (Fig. 34-2, *right panel*). The renal corpuscle of each superficial nephron is located in the outer region of the cortex. Its loop of Henle is short, and its efferent arteriole branches into peritubular capillaries that surround the nephron segments of its own and adjacent nephrons. This capillary network conveys oxygen and important nutrients to the nephron segments, delivers substances to the nephron for secretion (i.e., the movement of a substance from the blood into the tubular fluid), and serves as a pathway for the return of reabsorbed water and solutes to the circulatory sys-

tem. A few species, including humans, also possess very short superficial nephrons whose loops of Henle never enter the medulla.

The renal corpuscle of each juxtamedullary nephron is located in the region of the cortex next to the medulla (Fig. 34-2, *right panel*). The juxtamedullary nephrons differ anatomically from superficial nephrons in two important ways: (1) the loop of Henle is longer and extends deeper into the medulla and (2) the efferent arteriole forms not only a network of peritubular capillaries, but also a series of vascular loops called the **vasa recta.** As illustrated in Fig. 34-2 *(left panel),* the vasa recta descend into the medulla, where they form capillary networks that surround the collecting ducts and ascending limbs of Henle's loop. The blood returns to the cortex in the ascending vasa recta. *Although less than 0.7% of the renal blood flow enters the vasa recta, these vessels perform many important functions, including conveying oxygen and important nutrients to nephron segments, delivering substances to the nephron for secretion, serving as a pathway for the return of reabsorbed water and solutes to the circulatory system, and concentrating and diluting the urine.*

Ultrastructure of the Renal Corpuscle

The first step in urine formation begins with the passive movement of a plasma ultrafiltrate, an essentially protein-free fluid, from the glomerular capillaries into Bowman's space. To appreciate the process of ultrafiltration, one must understand the anatomy of the renal corpuscle. The glomerulus consists of a network of capillaries supplied by the afferent arteriole and drained by the efferent arteriole (Figs. 34-4 to 34-7). During embryological development, the glomerular capillaries press into the closed end of the proximal tubule, forming the Bowman's capsule of a renal corpuscle. The capillaries are covered by epithelial cells, called **podocytes,**

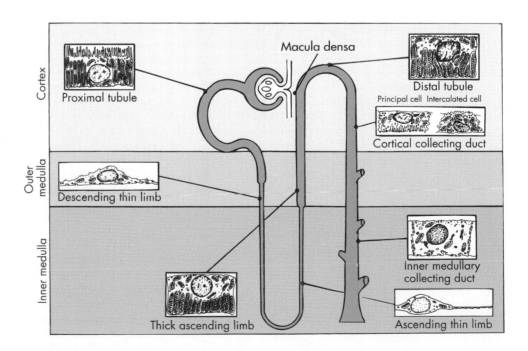

■ **Fig. 34-3** Diagram of a nephron, including the cellular ultrastructure.

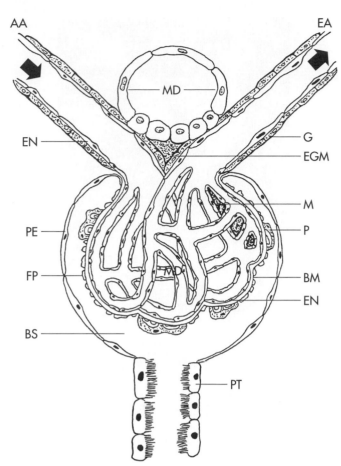

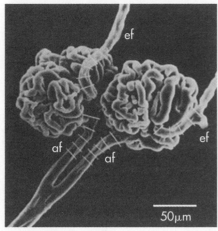

■ **Fig. 34-5** Scanning electron micrograph of interlobular artery; afferent arteriole *(af);* efferent arteriole *(ef);* and glomerulus. The white bars on the afferent and efferent arterioles indicate that they are about 15 to 20 μm in diameter. (From Kimura K et al: *Am J Physiol* 259:F936, 1990.)

■ **Fig. 34-4** Anatomy of the renal corpuscle and the juxta-glomerular apparatus. The latter is composed of the (1) macula densa of the thick ascending limb, (2) extraglomerular mesangial cells, and (3) renin-producing granular cells of the afferent arteriole. *AA,* Afferent arteriole; *EA,* efferent arteriole; *G,* granular cell of the afferent arteriole; *MD,* macula densa; *BM,* basement membrane; *FP,* foot processes of the podocyte; *P,* podocyte cell body (visceral cell layer); *M,* mesangial cells between capillaries; *EGM,* extraglomerular mesangial cells between the afferent and efferent arterioles; *EN,* endothelial cell; *PT,* proximal tubule cell; *BS,* Bowman's space; *PE,* parietal epithelium. (From Koushanpour E, Kriz W: *Renal physiology,* ed 2, Berlin, 1986, Springer-Verlag.)

which form the **visceral layer** of Bowman's capsule (Figs. 34-4 to 34-7). The visceral cells face outward at the vascular pole (i.e., where the afferent and efferent arterioles enter and exit Bowman's capsule) to form the parietal layer of Bowman's capsule. The space between the visceral layer and the parietal layer is called **Bowman's space,** which, at the urinary pole (i.e., where the proximal tubule joins Bowman's capsule) of the glomerulus, becomes the lumen of the proximal tubule.

The **endothelial cells** of glomerular capillaries are covered by a **basement membrane,** which is surrounded by podocytes (Figs. 34-6). The capillary endothelium, basement membrane, and foot processes of podocytes form the so-called filtration barrier (Figs. 34-4 to 34-7). The endothelium is fenestrated (i.e., it contains 700-Å holes where 1 Å $= 10^{-10}$ m) and is freely permeable to water; to small solutes

such as sodium, urea, and glucose; and even to small proteins, but it is not permeable to cells. Because endothelial cells express negatively charged glycoproteins on their surface, they can retard the filtration of large anionic proteins (see page 634). The basement membrane, which is a porous matrix of extracellular proteins including type IV collagen, laminin, fibronectin, and other negatively charged proteins, is an important filtration barrier to plasma proteins. The podocytes, which are **endocytic** (i.e., the process of endocytosis allows materials to enter the cell without passing through the membrane), have long, finger-like processes that completely encircle the outer surface of the capillaries (Fig. 34-7). The processes of the podocytes interdigitate to cover the basement membrane and are separated by gaps, called **filtration slits.** Each filtration slit is bridged by a thin diaphragm, which contains pores with dimensions of 40 × 140 Å. Podocalyxin is a negatively charged membrane glycoprotein in podocytes and is thought to keep the filtration slits open. Therefore, the filtration slits retard the filtration of some proteins and macromolecules that pass through the endothelium and basement membrane. *Because the endothelium, basement membrane, and filtration slits contain negatively charged glycoproteins, some molecules are held back on the basis of size and charge.* For molecules with an effective molecular radius between 20 and 42 Å, cationic molecules are filtered more readily than anionic molecules (see Fig. 34-13).

Nephrotic syndrome is produced by a variety of disorders and is characterized by an increase in the permeability of the glomerular capillaries to proteins. The augmented permeability results in an increase in urinary protein excretion **(proteinuria).** Thus the appearance of proteins in the urine can indicate kidney disease. Individuals with nephrotic syndrome may also develop edema and hypoalbuminemia as a result of proteinuria.

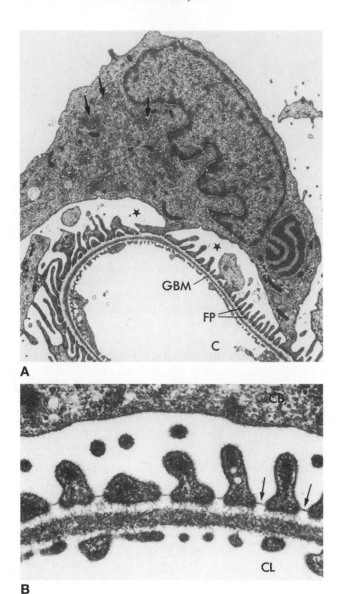

A

B

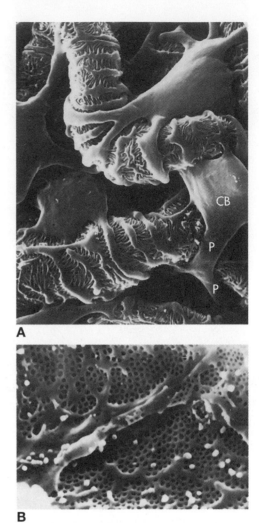

A

B

■ **Fig. 34-6   A,** Electron micrograph of a podocyte surrounding a glomerular capillary. The cell body of the podocyte contains a large nucleus with three indentations. Cell processes of the podocyte form the interdigitating foot processes *(FP).* The arrows in the cytoplasm of the podocyte indicate the well-developed Golgi apparatus. *C,* Capillary lumen; *GBM,* glomerular basement membrane. Stars indicate Bowman's space. (Magnification ~5700×.) **B,** Electron micrograph of the filtration barrier of a glomerular capillary. *CL,* Capillary lumen; *CB,* cell body of a podocyte. The filtration barrier is composed of three layers: the endothelium, the basement membrane, and the foot processes of the podocytes. Note the diaphragm bridging the floor of the filtration slits *(arrows).* (Magnification ~42,700×.) (Courtesy of Kriz W, Kaissling B: Structural organization of the mammalian kidney. In Seldin DW, Giebisch G, editors: *The kidney: physiology and pathophysiology,* ed 2, New York, 1992, Raven Press.)

■ **Fig. 34-7   A,** Scanning electron micrograph showing the outer surface of glomerular capillaries. This is the view that would be seen from Bowman's space. Processes *(P)* of podocytes run from the cell body *(CB)* toward the capillaries where they ultimately split into foot processes. Interdigitation of the foot processes creates the filtration slits. (Magnification ~2,500×.) **B,** Scanning electron micrograph of the inner surface (blood side) of a glomerular capillary. This view would be seen from the lumen of the capillary. The fenestrations of the endothelial cells are seen as small 700-Å holes. (Magnification ~12,000×.) (Courtesy of Kriz W, Kaissling B: Structural organization of the mammalian kidney. In Seldin DW, Giebisch G, editors: *The kidney: physiology and pathophysiology,* ed 2, New York, 1992, Raven Press.)

Nephrin is a transmembrane protein that is a major component of the slit diaphragm. Mutations in the nephrin gene in some individuals with congential nephrotic syndrome lead to abnormal or absent slit diaphragms, leading to massive proteinuria and renal failure. These observations suggest that nephrin plays an essential role in the formation of the normal glomerular filtration barrier.

Alport's syndrome is characterized by hematuria (i.e., blood in the urine) and progressive glomerulonephritis (i.e., inflammation of the glomerular capillaries) and accounts for 1% to 2% of cases of end-stage renal failure. Alport's syndrome is caused by defects in type IV collagen, a major component of the glomerular basement membrane. In about 85% of patients with Alport's syndrome, the disease is X-linked recessive with mutations in the COL4A5 gene. The remaining 15% of patients also have mutations in type IV collagen genes; six have been identified, but the mode of inheritance is autosomal recessive. In Alport's syndrome, the golmerular basement becomes irregular in thickness (i.e., normally 300 nm thick, the glomerular basement membrance can be as thick as 1200 nm or as thin as 100 nm) and fails to serve as an effective filtration barrier to red blood cells and protein.

Another important component of the renal corpuscle is the **mesangium,** which consists of **mesangial cells** and the **mesangial matrix** (Fig. 34-8). Mesangial cells are similar in structure to monocytes. They surround glomerular capillaries, provide structural support for the glomerular capillaries, secrete the extracellular matrix, exhibit phagocytic activity, and secrete prostaglandins and cytokines. Because they also contract and are adjacent to glomerular capillaries, mesangial cells may influence the glomerular filtration rate by regulating blood flow through glomerular capillaries or by altering the capillary surface area. Mesangial cells located outside the glomerulus (between the afferent and efferent arterioles) are called **extraglomerular mesangial cells** (or **lacis cells** or **Goormaghtigh cells**). Extraglomerular mesangial cells exhibit phagocytic activity.

Mesangial cells are involved in the development of immune complex–mediated glomerular disease. Because the glomerular basement membrane does not completely surround the glomerular capillaries (Fig. 34-8), immune complexes can enter the mesangial area without crossing the glomerular basement membrane. Accumulation of immune complexes induces the infiltration of inflammatory cells into the mesangium and prompts the production of cytokines and autocoids by cells in the mesangium. These cytokines and autocoids enhance the inflammatory response, which can lead to cell scarring and eventually obliterate the glomerulus.

Ultrastructure of the Juxtaglomerular Apparatus

The structures of the juxtaglomerular apparatus include (1) the macula densa of the thick ascending limb, (2) the extraglomerular mesangial cells, and (3) the renin-producing **granular cells** of the afferent arteriole (Fig. 34-4). The cells of the macula densa represent a morphologically distinct region of the thick ascending limb. This region passes through the angle formed by the afferent and efferent arterioles of the same nephron. The cells of the macula densa contact the extraglomerular mesangial cells and the granular cells of the afferent arteriole. Granular cells of the afferent arteriole are

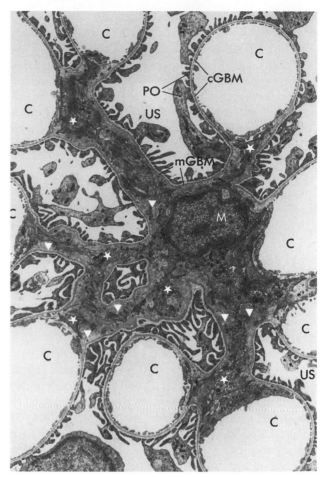

■ **Fig. 34-8** Electron micrograph of the mesangium, the area between glomerular capillaries containing mesangial cells. *C,* Glomerular capillaries; *cGBM,* capillary glomerular basement membrane surrounded by foot processes of podocytes *(PO)* and endothelial cells; *mGBM,* mesangial glomerular basement membrane surrounded by foot processes of podocytes and mesangial cells; *M,* mesangial cell that gives rise to several processes, some marked by stars; *US,* urinary space. Note the extensive extracellular matrix surrounded by mesangial cells (marked by triangles). (Magnification ~4,100×.) (From Kriz W, Kaissling B: Structural organization of the mammalian kidney. In Seldin DW, Giebisch G, editors: *The kidney: physiology and pathophysiology,* ed 2, New York, 1992, Raven Press.)

modified smooth muscle cells that manufacture, store, and release **renin.** Renin is involved in the formation of **angiotensin II** and ultimately in the secretion of **aldosterone** (see Chapters 36 and 45). The juxtaglomerular apparatus is one component of an important feedback mechanism (i.e., **tubuloglomerular feedback mechanism**) that is involved in the autoregulation of renal blood flow and of the glomerular filtration rate.

Innervation of the Kidney

Renal nerves help regulate renal blood flow, glomerular filtration rate, and salt and water reabsorption by the nephron.

The nerve supply to the kidneys consists of sympathetic nerve fibers that originate mainly in the celiac plexus. There is no parasympathetic innervation. Adrenergic fibers that innervate the kidneys release norepinephrine and dopamine. The adrenergic fibers lie adjacent to the smooth muscle cells of the major branches of the renal artery (interlobar, arcuate, and interlobular arteries) and the afferent arteriole. Moreover, the renin-producing granular cells of the afferent arteriole are innervated by sympathetic nerves. Renin secretion is stimulated by increased sympathetic activity. Nerve fibers also innervate the proximal tubule, loop of Henle, distal tubule, and collecting duct; activation of these nerves enhances sodium reabsorption by these nephron segments.

ANATOMY AND PHYSIOLOGY OF THE LOWER URINARY TRACT

Gross Anatomy and Histology

Once urine leaves the renal calyces and renal pelvis, it flows through the **ureters** and enters the **urinary bladder,** where it is stored (Fig. 34-9). The ureters are muscular tubes 30 cm long. They enter the bladder on its posterior aspect near the base, above the bladder neck. The bladder is composed of two parts: the **fundus** or body, which stores urine, and the neck, which is funnel shaped and connects with the urethra. The bladder **neck,** which is 2 to 3 cm long, is also called the posterior **urethra.** In females, the posterior urethra is the end of the urinary tract and the point where urine exits the body. In males, urine flows through the posterior urethra into the anterior urethra, which extends through the penis. Urine leaves the urethra through the external meatus.

The renal calyces, pelvis, ureter, and urinary bladder are lined with a transitional epithelium composed of several layers of cells: basal columnar cells, intermediate cuboidal cells, and superficial squamous cells. This epithelium is sur-

rounded by spiral and longitudinal smooth muscle fibers. The bladder is also lined with a transitional epithelium that is surrounded by smooth muscle fibers, called the **detrusor muscle.** Detrusor muscle fibers are arranged at random. They do not form layers except close to the bladder neck, where the fibers form three layers: inner longitudinal, middle circular, and outer longitudinal. Muscle fibers in the bladder neck form the **internal sphincter.** This is not a true sphincter but a thickening of the bladder wall formed by converging muscle fibers. *The internal sphincter is not under conscious control.* Its inherent tone prevents emptying of the bladder until appropriate stimuli trigger urination. The urethra passes through the **urogenital diaphragm,** which contains a layer of skeletal muscle called the **external sphincter.** This muscle is under voluntary control and can be used to prevent or interrupt urination, especially in males. In females, the external sphincter is poorly developed; thus, it is less important in voluntary bladder control. The smooth muscle cells in the lower urinary tract are electrically coupled, exhibit spontaneous action potentials, contract when stretched, and are under autonomic control.

The walls of the ureters, bladder, and urethra are highly folded and therefore very distensible. In the bladder and urethra, these folds are called **rugae.** As the bladder fills with urine, the rugae flatten and the volume of the bladder increases with very little change in intravesical pressure. Bladder volume can increase from a minimum of 10 ml after urination to 400 ml, yet pressure changes only 5 cm H_2O, which illustrates the highly compliant nature of the bladder.

Innervation of the Bladder

Innervation of the bladder and urethra is important in controlling urination. The smooth muscle of the bladder neck receives sympathetic innervation from the hypogastric nerves. α-Adrenergic receptors, located mainly in the bladder neck and the urethra, cause contraction. Stimulation of these

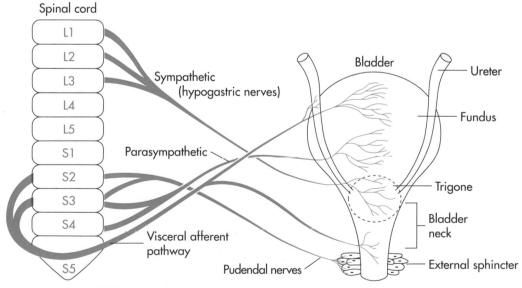

■ **Fig. 34-9** Anatomy of the lower urinary tract and its innervation.

receptors induces closure of the urethra and thus facilitates storage of urine. Sacral parasympathetic fibers (muscarinic) innervate the body of the bladder and cause a sustained bladder contraction. Sensory fibers of the pelvic nerves (visceral afferent pathway) also innervate the fundus. These sensory fibers carry input from receptors that detect bladder fullness, pain, and temperature sensation. The sacral pudendal nerves innervate the skeletal muscle fibers of the external sphincter; excitatory impulses cause the external sphincter to contract.

Passage of Urine from the Kidney to the Bladder

Renal calyces stretch as they collect urine. Stretching promotes their inherent pacemaker activity. Pacemaker activity generates action potentials, which initiate a peristaltic contraction. The peristaltic wave begins in the calyces, spreads to the pelvis and along the length of the ureter, and passes along the smooth muscle syncytium. This process thereby forces urine from the renal pelvis toward the bladder. The ureters are innervated with sensory nerve fibers (pelvic nerves).

> **Nephrolithiasis (kidney stones)** is a common medical problem: 5% to 10% of Americans develop kidney stones sometime in their life. Most stones (80% to 90%) are composed of calcium salts. The remaining stones are composed of uric acid, magnesium-ammonium acetate, or cysteine. Stones are formed by crystallization in a supersaturated urinary milieu. When the ureter is blocked with a kidney stone, reflex constriction of the ureter around the stone elicits severe flank pain.

Micturition

Micturition is the process of emptying the urinary bladder. Two processes are involved: (1) progressive filling of the bladder until the pressure rises to a critical value and (2) a neuronal reflex called the **micturition reflex,** which empties the bladder. The micturition reflex is an automatic spinal cord reflex. However, it can be inhibited or facilitated by centers in the brainstem and the cerebral cortex.

Filling of the bladder stretches the bladder wall and triggers a reflex initiated by stretch receptors, causing the bladder wall to contract. Sensory signals from the bladder fundus enter the spinal cord via pelvic nerves and return directly to the bladder through parasympathetic fibers in the same nerves. Stimulation of parasympathetic fibers causes intense stimulation of the detrusor muscle. The smooth muscle in the bladder is a syncytium; accordingly, stimulation of the detrusor also causes the muscle cells in the neck of the bladder to contract. Because the muscle fibers of the bladder outlet are oriented both longitudinally and radially, contraction opens the bladder neck and allows urine to flow through the posterior urethra. A voluntary relaxation of the external sphincter, achieved by cortical inhibition of the pudendal

nerve, permits the flow of urine through the external meatus. Voluntary relaxation of the external sphincter is required for urine to flow through it, and may be the event that initiates micturition. Interruption of the hypogastric sympathetic nerves and the pudendal nerves to the lower urinary tract does not alter the micturition reflex. In contrast, destruction of the parasympathetic nerves results in complete bladder dysfunction.

ASSESSMENT OF RENAL FUNCTION

The coordinated actions of the nephron's various segments determine the amount of a substance that appears in the urine. This represents three general processes: (1) glomerular filtration, (2) reabsorption of the substance from the tubular fluid back into the blood, and (3) (in some cases) secretion of the substance from the blood into the tubular fluid. The first step in the formation of urine by the kidneys is the production of an ultrafiltrate of plasma across the glomerulus. The process of glomerular filtration and the regulation of glomerular filtration rate and renal blood flow are discussed next. The concept of **renal clearance,** which is the theoretical basis of measurements of glomerular filtration rate and renal blood flow, is presented in the following section. Reabsorption and secretion are discussed in subsequent chapters.

> Knowledge of the **glomerular filtration rate (GFR)** is essential in evaluating the severity and course of **kidney disease.** The GFR is equal to the sum of the filtration rates of all the functioning nephrons. Thus, GFR is an index of kidney function. A fall in GFR generally means that disease is progressing, whereas an increase in GFR generally suggests recovery.

Renal Clearance

The concept of renal clearance is based on the **Fick principle** (mass balance or conservation of mass) (see also Chapter 16). Figure 34-10 illustrates the various factors required to describe the mass balance relationships of a kidney. The renal artery is the single input source to the kidney, whereas the renal vein and ureter constitute the two output routes. The following equation defines the mass balance relationship:

$$P^a_x \times RPF^a = (P^v_x \times RPF^v) + (U_x \times \dot{V}) \qquad (34\text{-}1)$$

where P^a_x and P^v_x are the concentrations of substance x in the renal artery and renal vein plasma, respectively; RPF^a and RPF^v are the renal plasma flow rates in the artery and vein, respectively; U_x is the concentration of x in the urine; and $\dot{V}$ is the urine flow rate. This relationship permits the quantification of the amount of x excreted in the urine versus the amount returned to the systemic circulation in the renal venous blood. Thus, for any substance that is neither synthesized nor metabolized, the amount that enters the kidneys is equal to the amount that leaves the kidneys in the

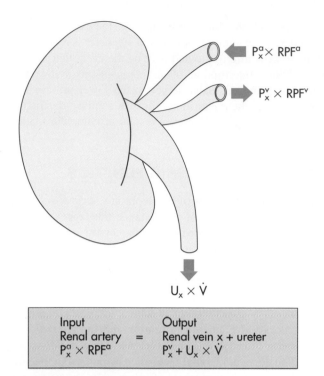

$$P_x^a \times RPF^a$$

$$P_x^v \times RPF^v$$

$$U_x \times \dot{V}$$

Input		Output
Renal artery	=	Renal vein x + ureter
$P_x^a \times RPF^a$		$P_x^v + U_x \times \dot{V}$

■ **Fig. 34-10** Mass balance relationships for the kidney. See text for definition of symbols.

urine plus the amount that leaves the kidneys in the renal venous blood.

The principle of renal clearance emphasizes the excretory function of the kidney; it considers only the rate at which a substance is excreted into the urine, and not its rate of return to the systemic circulation in the renal vein. Therefore, in terms of mass balance (equation 34-1), the urinary excretion rate of x ($U_x \times \dot{V}$) is proportional to the plasma concentration of x (P_x^a).

$$P_x^a \sim U_x \times \dot{V} \qquad (34\text{-}2)$$

To equate the urinary excretion rate of x to its renal arterial plasma concentration, one must determine the rate at which x is removed from the plasma by the kidneys. This removal rate is the clearance (C_x):

$$P_x^a \times C_x = U_x \times \dot{V} \qquad (34\text{-}3)$$

If equation 34-3 is rearranged, and if the concentration of x in the renal artery plasma (P_x) is assumed to be identical to its concentration in a plasma sample from any peripheral blood vessel, the following relationship is obtained:

$$C_x = \frac{U_x \times \dot{V}}{P_x} \qquad (34\text{-}4)$$

Clearance has the dimensions of volume/time, and it represents a volume of plasma from which all the substance has been removed and excreted into the urine per unit of time. This last point is best illustrated by considering the following example.

If a substance is present in the urine at a concentration of 100 mg/ml, and the urine flow rate is 1 ml/min, the excretion rate for this substance is calculated as

$$\begin{aligned} \text{excretion rate} &= U_x \times \dot{V} = \\ &(100 \text{ mg/ml}) \times (1 \text{ ml/min}) = 100 \text{ mg/min} \end{aligned} \qquad (34\text{-}5)$$

If this substance is present in the plasma at a concentration of 1 mg/ml, its clearance according to equation 35-4 is

$$C_x = \frac{U_x \times \dot{V}}{P_x} = (100 \text{ mg/min})/(1 \text{ mg/ml})$$

$$= 100 \text{ ml/min} \qquad (34\text{-}6)$$

That is, 100 ml of plasma will be completely cleared of substance x each minute. The definition of clearance as a volume of plasma from which all the substance has been removed and excreted into the urine per unit time is somewhat misleading. The volume of plasma in this equation is not a real volume of plasma; rather, it is an idealized volume.* Nevertheless the concept of clearance is important because it can be used to measure the GFR and renal plasma flow and to determine whether a substance is reabsorbed or secreted along the nephron.

Glomerular Filtration Rate: Clearance of Inulin

Inulin is a polymer of fructose (molecular weight about 5000) that can be used to measure the GFR. It is not produced by the body and therefore must be administered intravenously. Inulin is freely filtered across the glomerulus into Bowman's space and is neither reabsorbed, secreted, nor metabolized by the cells of the nephron. Accordingly, *the amount of inulin excreted in the urine per minute equals the amount of inulin filtered at the glomerulus each minute* (Fig. 34-11):

$$\begin{aligned} \text{amount filtered} &= \text{amount excreted} \\ \text{GFR} \times P_{in} &= U_{in} \times \dot{V} \end{aligned} \qquad (34\text{-}7)$$

where GFR is the glomerular filtration rate, P_{in} and U_{in} are the plasma and urine concentrations of inulin, and $\dot{V}$ is the rate of urine flow. If equation 34-7 is solved for the GFR:

$$GFR = \frac{U_{in} \times \dot{V}}{P_{in}} \qquad (34\text{-}8)$$

This equation is in the same form as that for clearance (see equation 34-4). Thus, determining the clearance of inulin provides a means for determining the GFR.

Inulin is not the only substance that can be used to measure GFR. Any substance that meets the following criteria will serve as an appropriate marker for the measurement of GFR. The substance must:

1. Be freely filtered across the glomerulus into Bowman's space.
2. Not be reabsorbed or secreted by the nephron.
3. Not be metabolized or produced by the kidney.
4. Not alter GFR.

*For most substances cleared from the plasma by the kidneys, only a portion is actually removed and excreted in a single pass through the kidneys.

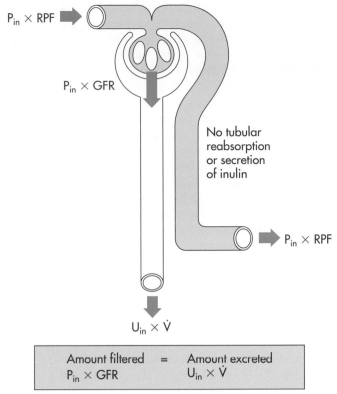

Amount filtered	=	Amount excreted
$P_{in} \times GFR$		$U_{in} \times \dot{V}$

■ **Fig. 34-11** Renal handling of inulin. Inulin is freely filtered across the glomerulus and is neither reabsorbed, secreted, nor metabolized by the nephron. P_{in}, Plasma inulin concentration; *RPF*, renal plasma flow; *GFR*, glomerular filtration rate; U_{in}, urinary concentration of inulin; $\dot{V}$, urine flow rate. Note that all inulin entering the kidney in the renal artery is not filtered at the glomerulus (normally 15% to 20% of plasma and inulin is filtered). The portion that is not filtered is returned to the systemic circulation in the renal vein.

Whereas inulin is used extensively in experimental studies, the need to administer it intravenously limits its clinical use. Consequently, **creatinine** is used to estimate GFR in clinical practice. Creatinine is a by-product of skeletal muscle creatine metabolism. It is produced at a relatively constant rate, and the amount produced is proportional to the muscle mass. Because creatinine is produced endogenously, an intravenous infusion is unnecessary. However, creatinine is not a perfect substance to use to measure GFR, because a small amount is secreted by the organic cation secretory system in the proximal tubule (see Chapter 35). The error introduced by this secretory component is approximately 10%. Thus, the amount of creatinine excreted in the urine exceeds the amount expected from filtration alone by 10%. However, the method used to quantitate the plasma creatinine concentration overestimates the true value by 10%. Consequently, the two errors cancel, and *in most clinical situations* **creatinine clearance** *provides a reasonably accurate measure of GFR.*

As illustrated in Fig. 34-11, not all the inulin (or any substance used to measure GFR) that enters the kidney in the renal arterial plasma is filtered at the glomerulus. Likewise, not all the plasma entering the kidney is filtered.* The portion of plasma that is filtered is termed the **filtration fraction** and is determined as

$$\text{filtration fraction} = GFR/RPF \qquad (34-9)$$

where, again, RPF is renal plasma flow. Under normal conditions, the filtration fraction averages 0.15 to 0.20. *This means that only 15% to 20% of the plasma that enters the glomerulus is actually filtered.* The remaining 80% to 85% continues on through the glomerulus into the efferent arterioles and peritubular capillaries, and is finally returned to the systemic circulation in the renal vein.

A fall in GFR may be the first and only clinical sign of kidney disease. Thus, measuring GFR is important when kidney disease is suspected. For example, a 50% loss of functioning nephrons will reduce the GFR only by approximately 20% to 30%. The decline in GFR is not 50% because the remaining nephrons compensate. Because measurements of GFR are cumbersome, kidney function is usually assessed in the clinical setting by measuring plasma [creatinine] (P_{cr}), which is inversely related to GFR (Fig. 34-12). However, as Fig. 34-12 shows, GFR must decline substantially before an increase in P_{cr} can be detected in a clinical setting. For example, a fall in GFR from 120 to 100 ml/min is accompanied by an increase in P_{cr} from 1.0 to 1.2 mg/dl. This does not appear to be a significant change in P_{cr}, yet GFR has actually fallen by almost 20%.

GLOMERULAR FILTRATION

In normal adults, the GFR averages 90 to 140 ml/min for males and 80 to 125 ml/min for females. Thus, in a 24-hour period, as much as 180 L/day of plasma is filtered at the glomerulus. After age 30 GFR declines with age. However, this decline in GFR usually does not adversely affect the kidneys' excretory function, nor their ability to maintain fluid, electrolyte, and acid-base balance.

The first step in the formation of urine is the production of an ultrafiltrate of the plasma at the glomerulus. The ultrafiltrate is devoid of cellular elements and is essentially protein free. The concentrations of salts and of organic molecules, such as glucose and amino acids, are similar in the plasma and ultrafiltrate. Ultrafiltration is driven by Starling forces (see Chapter 20) across the glomerular capillaries, and changes in these forces alter the GFR. GFR and RPF are normally held within narrow ranges by a phenomenon called **autoregulation** (see page 636). This section reviews the composition of the

---

*Nearly all the plasma that enters the kidney in the renal artery passes through the glomerulus. Approximately 10% does not.

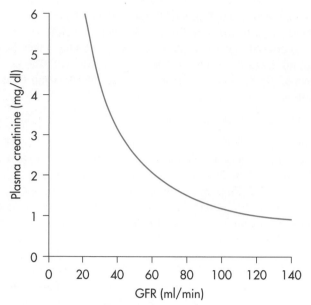

Fig. 34-12 Relationship between GFR and plasma creatinine concentration. As with inulin, the amount of creatinine filtered is essentially equal to the amount excreted (i.e., amount filtered = amount excreted, thus, GFR × P_{cr} = U_{Cr} × $\dot{V}$). Because production of creatinine is constant, excretion must be constant to maintain creatinine balance. Thus, if GFR falls from 120 to 60 ml/min, P_{cr} must increase from 1 to 2 mg/dl to keep the filtration of creatinine and thus its excretion equal to the production rate.

glomerular filtrate, the dynamics of its formation, and the relationship between RPF and GFR. In addition, the factors that contribute to the autoregulation of GFR and RBF are discussed.

Determinants of Ultrafiltrate Composition

The unique structure of the glomerular filtration barrier (capillary endothelium, basement membrane, and filtration slits

of the podocytes) determines the composition of the plasma ultrafiltrate. The glomerular filtration barrier restricts the filtration of molecules on the basis of size and electrical charge (Fig. 34-13). In general, neutral molecules with a radius less than 20 Å are filtered freely, molecules larger than 42 Å are not filtered, and molecules between 20 and 42 Å are filtered to various degrees. For example, serum albumin, an anionic protein that has an effective molecular radius of 34.5 Å, is filtered poorly: approximately 7 g of albumin is filtered each day.[*] Because albumin is reabsorbed avidly by the proximal tubule, however, almost none appears in the urine.

Figure 34-13 illustrates how electrical charge affects the filtration of macromolecules (e.g., dextrans) by the glomerulus. **Dextrans** are a family of exogenous polysaccharides that are manufactured in various molecular weights. They can be in an electrically neutral form or have negative (polyanionic) charges or positive (polycationic) charges. As the size (i.e., effective molecular radius) of a dextran increases, the rate at which it is filtered decreases. For any given molecular radius, cationic molecules are more readily filtered than are anionic molecules. The reduced filtration of anionic molecules is explained by the presence of negatively charged glycoproteins on the surface of all components of the glomerular filtration barrier. These charged glycoproteins repel similarly charged molecules. Because most plasma proteins are negatively charged, the negative charge on the filtration barrier restricts the filtration of proteins that have a molecular radius of 20 to 42 Å.

---

[*]Approximately 50,000 g/day of albumin passes through the glomeruli. Therefore, the filtration of 7 g/day represents approximately 0.01% of the albumin that passes through the glomeruli. This is well below the filtration fraction for substances that are freely filtered (15% to 20%).

Fig. 34-13 Influence of size and electrical charge of dextran on its filterability. A value of one indicates that it is filtered freely, whereas a value of zero indicates that it is not filtered. The filterability of dextrans between approximately 20 and 42 Å depends on charge. Dextrans larger than 42 Å are not filtered, regardless of charge, and polycationic dextrans and neutral dextrans smaller than 20 Å are freely filtered.

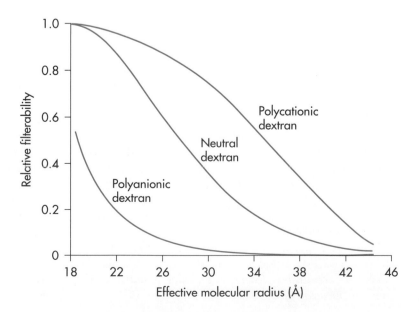

The importance of the negative charges on the filtration barrier in restricting filtration of plasma proteins is shown in Fig. 34-14. Removal of negative charges from the filtration barrier causes proteins to be filtered solely on the basis of their effective molecular radius. Hence, at any molecular radius between approximately 20 and 42 Å, the filtration of polyanionic proteins will exceed the filtration that prevails in the normal state (in which the filtration barrier has anionic charges). In a number of glomerular diseases, the negative charge on the filtration barrier is reduced because of immunological damage and inflammation. As a result, filtration of proteins is increased, and proteins appear in the urine (**proteinuria).**

Dynamics of Ultrafiltration

The forces responsible for the glomerular filtration of plasma are the same as those involved in fluid exchange across all capillary beds (see Chapter 20). Ultrafiltration occurs because Starling forces (i.e., hydrostatic and oncotic pressures) drive fluid from the lumen of glomerular capillaries, across the filtration barrier, and into Bowman's space (Fig. 34-15). The hydrostatic pressure in the glomerular capillary (P_{GC}) is oriented to promote the movement of fluid from the glomerular capillary into Bowman's space. Because the reflection coefficient (σ) for proteins across the glomerular capillary is essentially 1, the glomerular ultrafiltrate is essentially protein free and the oncotic pressure in Bowman's space (π_{BS}) is near zero. Therefore, P_{GC} is the only force that favors filtration. Filtration is opposed by the hydrostatic pressure in Bowman's space (P_{BS}) and the oncotic pressure in the glomerular capillary (π_{GC}).

The Starling forces across the glomerular capillary are difficult to measure, and only estimates have been made for humans. As shown in Fig. 34-15, a net ultrafiltration pressure (P_{UF}) of 17 mm Hg exists at the afferent end of the glomerulus, whereas at the efferent end the P_{UF} is 8 mm Hg (where $P_{UF} = P_{GC} - P_{BS} - \pi_{GC}$). Two additional points concerning Starling forces and this pressure change are important. First, P_{GC} decreases slightly along the length of the capillary because of the resistance to flow in the capillary. Second, π_{GC} increases along the length of the glomerular capillary because water is filtered and protein is retained in the glomerular capillary. As a result the protein concentration in the capillary rises and π_{GC} increases.

The GFR is proportional to the sum of the Starling forces that exist across the capillaries $[(P_{GC} - P_{BS}) - \sigma(\pi_{GC} - \pi_{BS})]$ times the ultrafiltration coefficient, K_f:

$$GFR = K_f [(P_{GC} - P_{BS}) - \sigma(\pi_{GC} - \pi_{BS})] \qquad (34\text{-}10)$$

The K_f is the product of the intrinsic permeability of the glomerular capillary and the glomerular surface area available for filtration. The rate of filtration is considerably greater in glomerular capillaries than in systemic capillaries, mainly because the K_f is approximately 100 times higher in glomerular capillaries. In addition, the hydrostatic pressure within the glomerular capillaries is approximately twice as high as that in systemic capillaries.

The GFR can be altered by changing K_f or by changing any of the Starling forces. In normal individuals GFR is regulated by alterations in P_{GC} that are mediated primarily by changes in glomerular arteriolar resistance. P_{GC} is affected in three ways.

1. Changes in afferent arteriolar resistance: A fall in resistance increases P_{GC} and GFR, whereas an increase in resistance decreases P_{GC} and GFR.
2. Changes in efferent arteriolar resistance: A fall in resistance reduces P_{GC} and GFR, whereas an increase in resistance elevates P_{GC} and GFR.
3. Changes in renal arteriolar pressure: An increase in blood pressure transiently increases P_{GC} (which enhances GFR), whereas a decrease in blood pressure transiently decreases P_{GC} (which reduces GFR).

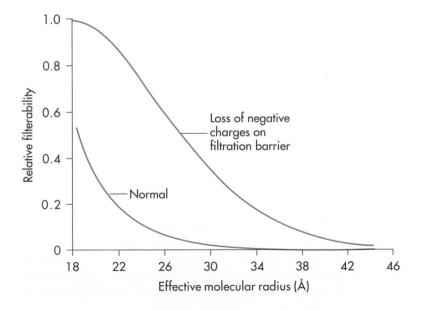

■ **Fig. 34-14** Reduction of the negative charges on the glomerular wall results in the filtration of proteins on the basis of size only. In this situation, the relative filterability of proteins is dependent only on the molecular radius. Accordingly, the excretion of polyanionic proteins (20 to 42 Å) in the urine increases because more proteins of this size are filtered.

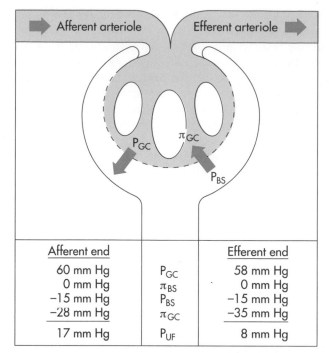

Afferent end		Efferent end
60 mm Hg	P_{GC}	58 mm Hg
0 mm Hg	π_{BS}	0 mm Hg
−15 mm Hg	P_{BS}	−15 mm Hg
−28 mm Hg	π_{GC}	−35 mm Hg
17 mm Hg	P_{UF}	8 mm Hg

■ **Fig. 34-15** Schematic representation of an idealized glomerular capillary and the Starling forces across the glomerular capillary. P_{UF}, Net ultrafiltration pressure; P_{GC}, glomerular capillary hydrostatic pressure; P_{BS}, Bowman's space hydrostatic pressure; π_{GC}, glomerular capillary oncotic pressure; π_{BS}, Bowman's space oncotic pressure. The reflection coefficient (σ) for protein across the glomerular capillary is 1.

Pathological conditions and drugs may also affect GFR. A reduction in GFR in disease states is most often due to decreases in K_f because of the loss of filtration surface area. GFR also changes in pathophysiological conditions owing to changes in P_{GC}, π_{GC}, and P_{BS}.

1. Changes in K_f: Increased K_f enhances GFR, whereas decreased K_f reduces GFR. Some kidney diseases reduce K_f by decreasing the number of filtering glomeruli (i.e., surface area). Some drugs and hormones that dilate the glomerular arterioles also increase K_f. Similarly, drugs and hormones that constrict the glomerular arterioles also decrease K_f.
2. Changes in P_{GC}: In acute renal failure, GFR declines because P_{GC} falls. As discussed above, a reduction in P_{GC} is caused by a decline in renal arterial pressure, an increase in afferent arteriolar resistance, or a decrease in efferent arteriolar resistance.
3. Changes in π_{GC}: An inverse relationship exists between π_{GC} and GFR. Alterations in π_{GC} result from changes in protein synthesis outside the kidneys. In addition, protein loss in the urine caused by some renal diseases can lead to a decrease in plasma protein concentration and thus π_{GC}.
4. Changes in P_{BS}: Increased P_{BS} reduces GFR, whereas decreased P_{BS} enhances GFR. Acute obstruction of the urinary tract (e.g., a kidney stone occluding the ureter) increases P_{BS}.

RENAL BLOOD FLOW

In resting subjects, the blood flow to the kidneys (about 1.25 L/min) is equal to about 25% of the cardiac output. However, the kidneys constitute less than 0.5% of total body weight. Blood flow through the kidneys serves several important functions:

1. Indirectly determining the GFR.
2. Modifying the rate of solute and water reabsorption by the proximal tubule.
3. Participating in the concentration and dilution of the urine.
4. Delivering oxygen, nutrients, and hormones to the cells of the nephron and returning carbon dioxide and reabsorbed fluid and solutes to the general circulation.
5. Delivering substrates for excretion in the urine.

The blood flow through any organ may be represented by the following equation:

$$Q = \Delta P/R \tag{34-11}$$

where Q equals blood flow, ΔP equals mean arterial pressure minus venous pressure for that organ, and R equals the resistance to flow through that organ (see also Chapter 18). Accordingly, RBF is equal to the pressure difference between the renal artery and the renal vein divided by the renal vascular resistance:

$$\text{RBF} = \text{aortic pressure} - \text{renal venous pressure} /$$
$$\text{renal vascular resistance} \tag{34-12}$$

Because the afferent arteriole, the efferent arteriole, and the interlobular artery are the major resistance vessels in the kidney, they determine renal vascular resistance. The kidneys, like most organs, regulate their blood flow by adjusting the vascular resistance in response to changes in arterial pressure. As shown in Fig. 34-16, these adjustments are so precise that blood flow remains relatively constant as arterial blood pressure changes between 90 and 180 mm Hg. GFR is also regulated over the same range of arterial pressures. The phenomenon that allows this relatively constant maintenance of RBF and GFR, **autoregulation** (see Chapter 21), is achieved by changes in vascular resistance, primarily within the afferent arterioles of the kidneys. Because both GFR and RBF are regulated over the same range of pressures, it is not surprising that the same mechanisms regulate both flows.

Two mechanisms are responsible for autoregulation of RBF and GFR: one mechanism that responds to changes in arterial pressure, and another that responds to changes in the NaCl concentration of tubular fluid. Both regulate the tone of the afferent arteriole. The pressure-sensitive mechanism, or **myogenic mechanism,** is related to an intrinsic property of vascular smooth muscle: the tendency to contract when it is stretched (see also Chapter 21). Accordingly, when arterial pressure rises and the renal afferent arteriole is stretched, the smooth muscle contracts. Because the increase in the resistance of the arteriole offsets the increase in

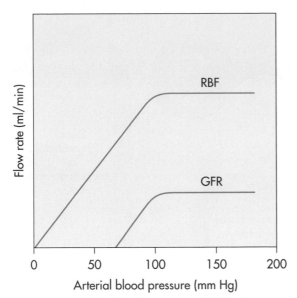

■ **Fig. 34-16**   Relationships between arterial blood pressure and renal blood flow *(RBF)* and glomerular filtration rate *(GFR)*. Autoregulation allows RBF and GFR to remain relatively constant as blood pressure changes from 90 to 180 mm Hg.

pressure, RBF, and therefore GFR, remain constant (i.e., RBF is constant if the ratio of ΔP/R is kept constant, see equation 34-11).

The second mechanism responsible for autoregulation of GFR and RBF, the NaCl concentration-dependent mechanism, is known as **tubuloglomerular feedback** (Fig. 34-17). This mechanism involves a feedback loop in which the NaCl concentration of tubular fluid (or some other factors, such as changes in the cytosolic composition of macula densa cells, changes in interstitial fluid composition surrounding macula densa cells, or changes in cellular metabolism) is sensed by the macula densa of the juxtaglomerular apparatus (JGA). The JGA sends a signal that affects afferent arteriolar resistance, and thus GFR. When GFR increases and causes the NaCl concentration of tubular fluid at the macula densa to rise, the JGA sends a signal that causes vasoconstriction to return RBF and GFR to normal levels. In contrast, when GFR and NaCl concentration at the macula densa decrease, the JGA sends a signal causing RBF and GFR to increase to normal levels. The signal affects RBF and GFR mainly by changing the resistance of the afferent arteriole, but the mediator for this effect is not entirely clear. Questions about tubuloglomerular feedback concern the variable that is sensed at the macula densa and the effector substance that alters the resistance of the afferent arteriole. It has been suggested that changes in NaCl concentration are sensed by the macula densa. The effector mechanism is most likely adenosine, which constricts the afferent arteriole (in contrast to its vasodilator effect on most other vasculature beds). Adenosine triphosphate (ATP), which selectively vasoconstricts the afferent arteriole, and metabolites of arachidonic acid may contribute to tubuloglomerular feedback (TGF).

Nitric oxide (NO), a vasodilator produced by the macula densa, endothelial cells, and angiotensin II may also play a role in TGF, but they are not essential for autoregulation. The macula densa may release both a vasoconstrictor and a vasodilator (e.g., NO), which oppose each other's action at the level of the afferent arteriole.

Because animals engage in many activities that can change arterial blood pressure, mechanisms that maintain RBF and GFR relatively constant despite changes in arterial pressure are highly desirable. Alterations in GFR influence water and solute excretion (the reason is discussed in the next chapter). If RBF and GFR were to rise or fall suddenly in proportion to changes in blood pressure, urinary excretion of fluid and solute would also change suddenly. Such changes in water and solute excretion, without comparable alterations in intake, would alter fluid and electrolyte balance. Accordingly, autoregulation of GFR and RBF is an effective means for uncoupling renal function from arterial pressure and ensures that fluid and solute excretion remain constant. Three points concerning autoregulation should be made:

1. Autoregulation is absent below arterial pressures of 90 mm Hg.
2. Autoregulation is not perfect; RBF and GFR do change slightly as arterial blood pressure varies.
3. Despite autoregulation, GFR and RBF can be changed under appropriate conditions by several hormones (Table 34-1).

Individuals with **renal artery stenosis** (a narrowing of the artery lumen), caused by atherosclerosis, for example, can have an elevated systemic blood pressure mediated by stimulation of the renin-angiotensin system (see Chapter 36 for details). The pressure in the artery proximal to the stenosis is increased, but pressure is normal or reduced distal to the stenosis. Autoregulation plays an important role in maintaining RBF, P_{GC}, and GFR in the presence of this stenosis. The administration of drugs to lower systemic blood pressure also lowers pressure distal to the stenosis; accordingly, RBF, P_{GC}, and GFR fall.

REGULATION OF RENAL BLOOD FLOW AND GLOMERULAR FILTRATION RATE

Several factors and hormones have a major effect on RBF and GFR (Table 34-1). As discussed in the previous section, the myogenic mechanism and tubuloglomerular feedback play key roles in maintaining RBF and GFR. *Sympathetic nerves, angiotensin II, prostaglandins, NO, endothelin, bradykinin, and perhaps adenosine exert the major control over RBF and GFR.* The physiological and pathophysiological roles of the other hormones discussed below are under investigation. Figure 34-18 shows how changes in afferent and efferent arteriolar resistance modulate RBF and GFR.

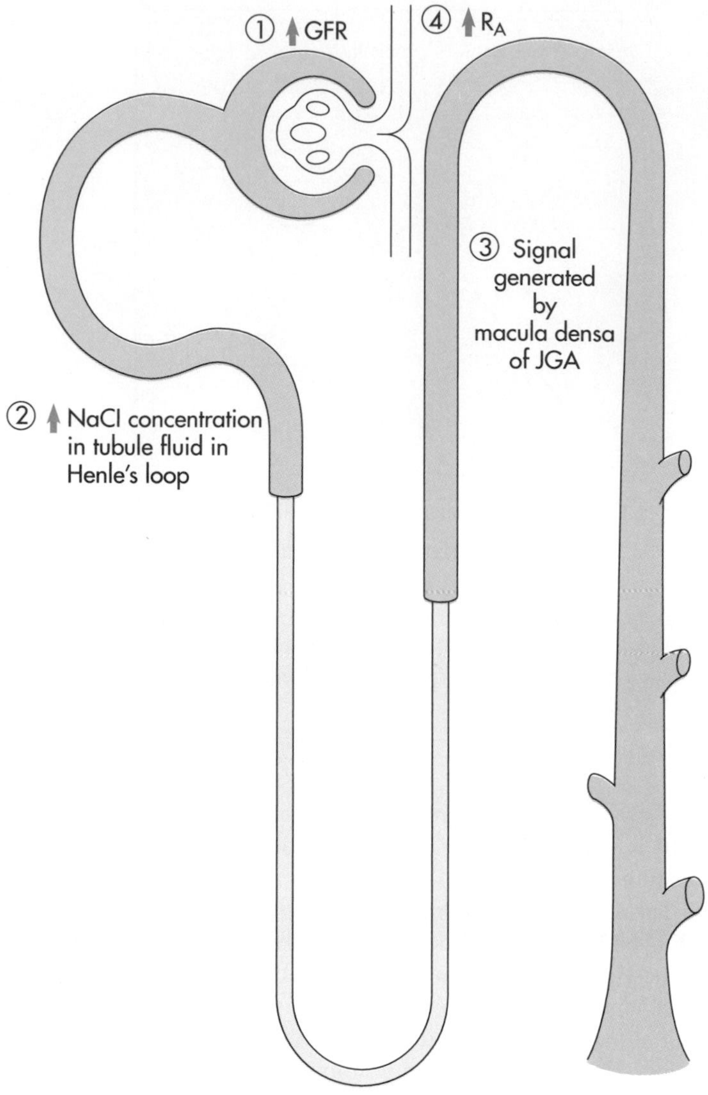

① ↑ GFR   ④ ↑ R_A

③ Signal generated by macula densa of JGA

② ↑ NaCl concentration in tubule fluid in Henle's loop

■ **Fig. 34-17** Tubuloglomerular feedback. An increase in GFR *(1)* increases NaCl concentration in tubule fluid in the loop of Henle *(2)*, which is sensed by the macula densa and converted into a signal *(3)*. This signal increases RA *(4)* the resistance of the afferent arteriole, which decreases GFR. *JGA,* Juxtaglomerular apparatus.

■ **Table 34-1** Major hormones that influence GFR and RBF

	Stimulus	*Effect on GFR*	*Effect on RBF*
Vasoconstrictors			
Sympathetic nerves	↓ ECV	↓	↓
Angiotensin II	↓ ECV	↓	↓
Endothelin	↑ Stretch, angiotensin II, bradykinin, epinephrine, ↓ ECV	↓	↓
Vasodilators			
Prostaglandins (PGI$_2$, PGE$_2$)	↓ ECV, ↑ stretch, angiotensin II	NC	↑
Nitric oxide	↑ Stretch, acetylcholine, histamine, bradykinin, adenosine triphosphate	↑	↑
Bradykinin	Prostaglandin, ↓ angiontensin converting enzyme	↑	↑
ANP	↑ ECV	↑	↑

ECV, Effective circulating volume.

Sympathetic nerves. The afferent and efferent arterioles are innervated by sympathetic neurons; however, sympathetic tone is minimal when the circulating blood volume is normal (see page 673). Norepinephrine is released by sympathetic nerves, and circulating epinephrine is secreted by the adrenal medulla. These substances cause vasoconstric-tion by binding to α_1-adrenoceptors, which are located mainly on the afferent arterioles. This binding thereby decreases RBF and GFR. A reduction in the effective circulating blood volume or strong emotional stimuli, such as fear and pain, activate sympathetic nerves and reduce RBF and GFR.

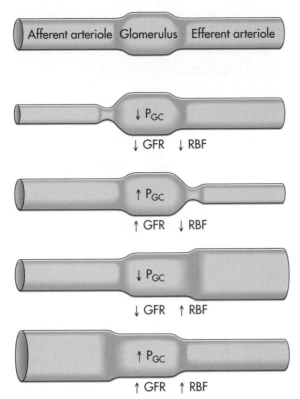

■ **Fig. 34-18** Relationship between selective changes in the resistance of either the afferent arteriole or efferent arteriole and RBF and GFR. Constriction of either the afferent or efferent arteriole increases resistance. According to equation 34-11 (Q = ΔP/R), an increase in resistance (R) will decrease flow, Q (i.e., RBF). Dilation of either the afferent or efferent arteriole will increase flow (i.e., RBF). Constriction of the afferent arteriole decreases P_{GC} (because less of the arterial pressure is transmitted to the glomerulus) and thereby reduces GFR. In contrast, constriction of the efferent arteriole elevates P_{GC} and thus increases GFR. Dilation of the afferent arteriole increases P_{GC}, because more of the arterial pressure is transmitted to the glomerulus, and thereby increases GFR. In contrast, dilation of the efferent arteriole decreases P_{GC} and thus decreases GFR. (Modified from Rose BD, Rennke HG: *Renal pathophysiology: the essentials,* Baltimore, 1994, Williams & Wilkins.)

Because **hemorrhage** decreases arterial blood pressure, it activates the sympathetic nerves to the kidneys via the baroreceptor reflex (Fig. 34-19). Norepinephrine causes intense vasoconstriction of the afferent and efferent arterioles, and thereby decreases RBF and GFR. The rise in sympathetic activity also increases the release of epinephrine and angiotensin II, which causes further vasoconstriction and a fall in RBF. The rise in the vascular resistance of the kidney and other vascular beds increases total peripheral resistance. The resultant increased blood pressure (BP = cardiac output × total peripheral resistance) offsets the fall in mean arterial blood pressure caused by hemorrhage (see also Chapter 24). Hence, this system works to preserve arterial

pressure at the expense of maintaining a normal RBF and GFR. Importantly, although autoregulatory mechanisms can prevent the effects of changes in arterial pressure on RBF and GFR, sympathetic nerves and angiotensin II have important salutary effects on RBF and GFR.

Angiotensin II. Angiotensin II is produced systemically and within the kidney. It constricts the afferent and efferent arterioles* and decreases RBF and GFR (see Chapter 36 for details on the renin-angiotensin system). Figure 34-19 shows how norepinephrine, epinephrine, and angiotensin II act together to decrease RBF and GFR, as would occur, for example, with hemorrhage.

Angiotensin-converting enzyme (ACE) degrades and thereby inactivates bradykinin and converts angiotensin I, an inactive hormone, to angiotensin II. Thus, ACE increases angiotensin II levels and decreases bradykinin levels. Drugs called **ACE inhibitors,** which reduce systemic blood pressure in patients with hypertension, reduce angiotensin II levels and elevate bradykinin levels. These effects lower systemic vascular resistance, reduce blood pressure, and decrease renal vascular resistance. ACE inhibitors therefore increase RBF and GFR (see Chapter 36).

Prostaglandins. Prostaglandins may not regulate RBF or GFR in healthy, resting people. However, during pathophysiological conditions, such as hemorrhage, prostaglandins (PGI_2, PGE_2) are produced locally within the kidneys and increase RBF without changing GFR. Prostaglandins increase RBF by dampening the vasoconstrictor effects of sympathetic nerves and angiotensin II. This effect of prostaglandins prevents severe and potentially harmful vasoconstriction and renal ischemia. Prostaglandin synthesis is stimulated by decreased effective circulating volume and stress (e.g., surgery, anesthesia), angiotensin II, and sympathetic nerves.

Nitric oxide. NO, an endothelium-derived relaxing factor, plays an important vasodilatory role in normal conditions, and counteracts vasoconstriction produced by angiotensin II and catecholamines. An increase in stretch of the endothelial cells in the arterioles, as well as a number of hormones (including acetylcholine, histamine, bradykinin, and ATP), increases the production of NO. This increased NO production causes vasodilation of the afferent and efferent arterioles in the kidneys. In addition, NO decreases total peripheral resistance, and inhibition of NO production increases blood pressure.

*The efferent arteriole is more sensitive to angiotensin II than the afferent arteriole. Therefore, with low concentrations of angiotensin II, constriction of the efferent arteriole predominates. However, with high concentrations of angiotensin II, constriction of both afferent and efferent arterioles occurs and GFR and RBF fall.

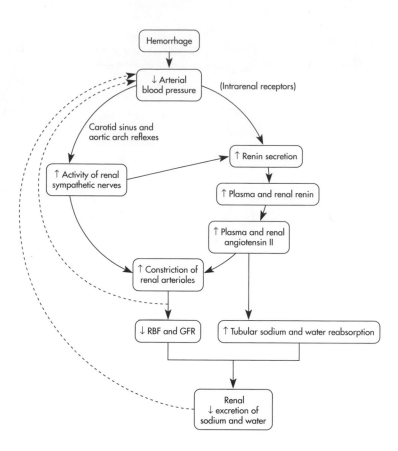

■ **Fig. 34-19**   Pathway by which hemorrhage activates renal sympathetic nerve activity and stimulates angiotensin II production. (Modified from Vander AJ: *Renal physiology,* ed 2, New York, 1980, McGraw-Hill.)

*Abnormal production of NO is observed in individuals with **diabetes mellitus** and **hypertension.*** Excess NO production in diabetes may be responsible for the glomerular hyperfiltration and damage of the glomerulus that are characteristic of this disease. Elevated NO levels increase glomerular capillary pressure secondary to a fall in afferent arteriolar resistance. The ensuing hyperfiltration is thought to cause glomerular damage. The normal response to an increase in dietary salt intake includes stimulation of NO production, which maintains blood pressure. In some individuals, NO production may not increase appropriately in response to an increase in salt intake, and therefore blood pressure rises.

Endothelin. Endothelin is a potent vasoconstrictor secreted by endothelial cells of renal vessels, mesangial cells, and distal tubular cells in response to angiotensin II, bradykinin, epinephrine, and stretch. Endothelin causes profound vasoconstriction of the afferent and efferent arterioles and decreases GFR and RBF. Although this potent vasoconstrictor may not influence GFR and RBF in normal resting subjects, endothelin production is elevated in a number of glomerular disease states (e.g., renal disease associated with diabetes mellitus).

Bradykinin. Kallikrein is a proteolytic enzyme produced in the kidneys. Kallikrein cleaves circulating kininogen to bradykinin, which is a vasodilator that acts by stimulating the release of NO and prostaglandins. Bradykinin increases GFR and RBF.

Adenosine. Adenosine is produced within the kidneys and causes vasoconstriction of the afferent arteriole, thereby reducing RBF and GFR. As previously mentioned, adenosine plays an important role in tubuloglomerular feedback.

Atrial natriuretic peptide (ANP). ANP secretion by the heart rises with hypertension and expansion of extracellular fluid volume, causing vasodilation of the afferent arteriole and vasoconstriction of the efferent arteriole. The net effect of ANP is therefore to produce a modest increase in GFR with little change in RBF.

ATP. Various cells release ATP into the renal interstitial fluid. ATP has dual effects on GFR and RBF. Under some conditions, ATP constricts the afferent arteriole, reduces RBF and GFR, and may play a role in tubuloglomerular feedback. In contrast, in other situations, ATP may stimulate NO production and increase GFR and RBF.

Glucocorticoids. Administration of therapeutic doses of glucocorticoids increases GFR and RBF.

Histamine. Local release of histamine may play a role in modulating RBF in the normal state and during inflammation and injury. Histamine increases RBF without elevating GFR by decreasing the resistance of the afferent and efferent arterioles.

Dopamine. The proximal tubule produces the vasodilator hormone dopamine. Dopamine has several actions within the kidney, such as increasing RBF and inhibiting renin secretion.

As shown in Fig. 34-20, endothelial cells are important in regulating the resistance of the afferent and efferent arterioles by producing a number of paracrine hormones, including

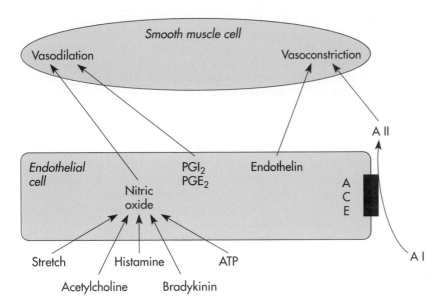

■ **Fig. 34-20** Examples of interactions of endothelial cells with smooth muscle or mesangial cells. *ACE,* Angiotensin converting enzyme; *AI,* angiotensin I; *AII,* angiotensin II; *PGI_2*, prostaglandin I_2; *PGE_2*, prostaglandin E_2. (Modified from Navar LG et al: *Physiol Rev* 76:425, 1996.)

NO, PGI_2, endothelin, and angiotensin II. These hormones regulate contraction or relaxation of smooth muscle cells in afferent and efferent arterioles or mesangial cells. Stretch, acetylcholine, histamine, bradykinin, and ATP stimulate the production of NO, which increases GFR and RBF. Angiotensin converting enzyme (primarily on the surface of endothelial cells lining the afferent arteriole and glomerular capillaries) converts angiotensin I to angiotensin II, which decreases GFR and RBF. Angiotensin II may also be produced in juxtaglomerular cells and proximal tubular cells. PGI_2 and PGE_2 secretion by endothelial cells, stimulated by sympathetic nerve activity or angiotensin II, increases GFR and RBF. Finally, endothelin release from endothelial cells decreases GFR and RBF.

SUMMARY

1. The functional unit of the kidney is the nephron. Each nephron consists of a renal corpuscle, proximal tubule, loop of Henle, distal tubule, and collecting duct.

2. The renal corpuscle is composed of glomerular capillaries and Bowman's capsule.

3. The juxtaglomerular apparatus is one component of an important feedback mechanism that regulates renal blood flow and glomerular filtration rate. The juxtaglomerular apparatus consists of the macula densa, the extraglomerular mesangial cells, and the renin-producing granular cells in the afferent arteriole.

4. The lower urinary tract consists of the ureters, bladder, and urethra. Micturition is the process of emptying the urinary bladder. The micturition reflex is an automatic spinal cord reflex. However, it can be inhibited or facilitated by centers in the brainstem and cortex.

5. The rate of glomerular filtration is calculated by measuring the clearance of inulin or creatinine. Changes in GFR can be monitored by measuring the plasma creatinine concentration.

6. Starling forces across the glomerular capillaries provide the driving force for the ultrafiltration of plasma from the glomerular capillaries into Bowman's space.

7. The glomerular ultrafiltrate is devoid of cellular elements and contains very little protein, but otherwise is identical to plasma. Proteins with a molecular radius smaller than 20 Å are readily filtered, proteins between 20 and 42 Å are filtered at rates that depend on size and charge (anionic proteins are less readily filtered), and proteins with a molecular radius greater than 42 Å are not filtered.

8. Renal blood flow (1.25 L/min) is about 25% of cardiac output, yet the kidneys constitute less than 0.5% of total body weight. RBF determines the GFR; modifies solute and water reabsorption by the proximal tubule; participates in concentration and dilution of the urine; delivers oxygen, nutrients, and hormones to the cells of the nephron; returns carbon dioxide and reabsorbed fluid and solutes to the general circulation; and delivers substrates for excretion in the urine.

9. Autoregulation allows RBF and GFR to remain constant despite changes in arterial blood pressure between 90 and 180 mm Hg. Autoregulation is achieved by changes in renal vascular resistance mediated by the myogenic reflex and tubuloglomerular feedback.

10. Sympathetic nerves, angiotensin II, prostaglandins, NO, endothelin, bradykinin, and adenosine exert the most control over RBF and GFR.

BIBLIOGRAPHY

Journal articles

Kriz W, Bankir L: A standard nomenclature for structures of the kidney, *Am J Physiol* 254:F1, 1988.
Pirson Y: Making the diagnosis in Alport's syndrome, *Kidney Int* 56:760, 1999.

Schnerman J: Juxtaglomerular cell complex in the regulation of renal salt excretion, *Am J Physiol* 274:R263, 1998.

Sun D et al: Mediation of tubuloglomerular feedback by adenosine: evidence from mice lacking adenosine A1 receptors, *Proc Natl Acad Sci USA* 98:9983, 2001.

Tryggvason K: Unraveling the mechanisms of glomerular ultrafiltration: nephrin, a key component of the slit diaphram, *J Am Soc Nephrol* 10:2440, 1999.

Books and monographs

Arendshorst WJ, Navar LG: Renal circulation and glomerular hemodynamics. In Schrier RW, Gottschalk CW, editors: *Diseases of the kidney,* ed 6, Boston, 1997, Little, Brown.

Bradley WE: Physiology of the urinary bladder. In Walsh PC et al, editors: *Campbell's urology,* ed 7, Philadelphia, 1998, WB Saunders.

Dupont MC, Steers WD: Disorder of micturition. In Schrier RW, Gottschalk CW: *Diseases of the kidney,* ed 6, Boston, 1997, Little, Brown.

Dworkin LD, Brenner BM: Biophysical basis of glomerular filtration. In Seldin DW, Giebisch G, editors: *The kidney: physiology and pathophysiology,* ed 3, Philadelphia, 2000, Lippincott, Williams & Wilkins.

Dworkin LD, Sun AM, Brenner BM: The renal circulation. In Brenner BM, editor: *The kidney,* ed 6, Philadelphia, 2000, WB Saunders.

Herbert SC, Kriz W: Structural-functional relationships in the kidney. In Schrier RW, Gottschalk WR, editors: *Diseases of the kidney,* ed 6, Boston, 1997, Little, Brown.

Koushanpour E, Kriz W: *Renal physiology,* ed 2, Berlin, 1986, Springer-Verlag. Philadelphia, 1996, WB Saunders.

Kriz W, Kaissling B: Structural organization of the mammalian kidney. In Seldin DW, Giebisch G, editors: *The kidney: physiology and pathophysiology,* ed 3, Philadelphia, 2000, Lippincott, Williams & Wilkins.

Lafayette RA, Perrone RD, Levey AS: Laboratory evaluation of renal function. In Schrier RW, Gottschalk WR, editors: *Diseases of the kidney,* ed 6, Boston, 1997, Little, Brown.

Maddox DA, Brenner BM: Glomerular ultrafiltration. In Brenner BM, editor: *Brenner and Rector's the kidney,* ed 6, Philadelphia, 2000, WB Saunders.

Tanagho EA: Anatomy of the genitourinary tract. In Tanagho EA, McAnich JW, editors: *Smith's general urology,* ed 14, Norwalk, Conn, 1995, Appleton & Lange.

Tisher CC, Madsen KM: Anatomy of the kidney. In Brenner BM, editor: *Brenner and Rector's the kidney,* ed 6, Philadelphia, 2000, WB Saunders.

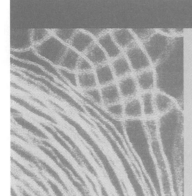

chapter thirty-five

Solute and Water Transport Along the Nephron: Tubular Function

Formation of urine involves three basic processes:

- Ultrafiltration of plasma by the glomerulus
- Reabsorption of water and solutes from the ultrafiltrate
- Secretion of selected solutes into the tubular fluid

Although 180 L of essentially protein-free fluid is filtered by the human glomeruli each day,* less than 1% of the filtered water and NaCl, and variable amounts of the other solutes, are excreted in the urine (Table 35-1). By the processes of reabsorption and secretion, the renal tubules modulate the volume and composition of the urine (Table 35-2). Consequently, the tubules precisely control the volume, osmolality, composition, and pH of the intracellular and extracellular fluid compartments.

The first part of this chapter defines basic transport mechanisms used by kidney cells to reabsorb and secrete solutes. Then, NaCl and water reabsorption and some of the factors and hormones that regulate reabsorption are discussed. Details on acid-base transport; K^+, Ca^{2+}, and P_i transport; and their regulation are provided in Chapters 37 and 38.

GENERAL PRINCIPLES OF MEMBRANE TRANSPORT

Solutes may be transported across cell membranes by passive mechanisms, by active transport mechanisms, or by endocytosis. In mammals, solute movement occurs by both passive and active mechanisms, whereas *all water movement is passive* (see Box 35-1).

Passive Mechanisms

Passive movement of a solute across a membrane develops spontaneously and does not require direct expenditure of metabolic energy. In **passive transport (diffusion),** uncharged solutes move from an area of higher concentration to an area of lower concentration (i.e., down their chemical concentration gradient). Additionally, because ions are charged, the passive diffusion of ions is affected by the electrical potential difference (i.e., electrical gradient) across cell membranes and across the renal tubules. Cations (Na^+, K^+, and so forth) move to the negative side of the membrane, whereas anions (Cl^-, HCO_3^-, and so forth) move to the positive side of the membrane. Diffusion of lipid-soluble substances, such as the gases O_2, CO_2, and NH_3, occurs across the lipid bilayer of plasma membranes. Diffusion of water (**osmosis**) occurs through channels in the cell membrane and is driven by osmotic pressure gradients. When water is reabsorbed across tubule segments, the solutes dissolved in the water are also carried along with the water. This process, called **solvent drag,** can account for a substantial amount of solute reabsorption across the proximal tubule.

In **facilitated diffusion,** transport depends on the interaction of the solute with a specific protein in the membrane that facilitates movement of the solute across the membrane. The term facilitated diffusion describes several different types of membrane transporters. For example, one form of facilitated diffusion is the diffusion of ions (such as Na^+ and K^+) across membranes. These ions move through water-filled channels created by proteins that span the plasma membrane. Another example is the movement of a single molecule across the membrane by means of a transport protein (**uniport**), as occurs with urea and glucose.*

A third form of facilitated diffusion is **coupled transport,** in which two or more solutes move across a membrane by interacting with a specific transport protein. Coupled transport of two or more solutes in the same direction is mediated by a **symport mechanism.** Examples of symport mechanisms in the kidneys include Na^+-glucose, Na^+–amino acid, and Na^+-phosphate symporters in the proximal tubule and $1Na^+$-$1K^+$-$2Cl^-$ symport in the thick ascending limb of Henle's loop. Coupled transport of two or more solutes in

---

*The normal glomerular filtration rate (GFR) averages 127-184 L/day in women and 140-197 L/day in men. Thus, the volume of the ultrafiltrate represents a volume 10 times that of the extracellular fluid volume. For simplicity, throughout the remainder of this book, we will assume that the GFR is 180 L/day.

*Some authors restrict the term facilitated diffusion to this type of transport, and use as the classic example the glucose uniporter that brings glucose into a wide variety of cells (e.g., skeletal muscle cells).

■ **Table 35-1**   Filtration, excretion, and reabsorption of water, electrolytes, and solutes

Substance	Measure	Filtered	Excreted	Reabsorbed	% Filtered load reabsorbed
Water	L/day	180	1.5	178.5	99.2
Na^+	mEq/day	25,200	150	25,050	99.4
K^+	mEq/day	720	100	620	86.1
Ca^{2+}	mEq/day	540	10	530	98.2
HCO_3^-	mEq/day	4320	2	4318	99.9
Cl^-	mEq/day	18,000	150	17,850	99.2
Glucose	mmol/day	800	0	800	100.0
Urea	g/day	56	28	28	50.0

The filtered amount of any substance is calculated by multiplying the concentration of that substance in the ultrafiltrate by the glomerular filtration rate (GFR); for example, the filtered load of Na^+ is calculated as $[Na^+]$ultrafiltrate (140 mEq/L) × GFR (180 L/day) = 25,200 mEq/day.

■ **Table 35-2**   Composition of urine

Substance	Concentration
Na^+	50-130 mEq/L
K^+	20-70 mEq/L
NH_4^+	30-50 mEq/L
Ca^{2+}	5-12 mEq/L
Mg^{2+}	2-18 mEq/L
Cl^-	50-130 mEq/L
P_i	20-40 mEq/L
Urea	200-400 mM
Creatinine	6-20 mM
pH	5.0-7.0
Osmolality	500-800 mOsm/kg H_2O
Glucose*	0
Amino acids*	0
Protein*	0
Blood*	0
Ketones*	0
Leukocytes*	0
Bilirubin*	0

Modified from Valtin HV: *Renal physiology,* ed 2, Boston, 1983, Little, Brown.

*These values represent average ranges. Asterisks indicate that the presence of these substances in freshly voided urine is measured with dipstick reagent strips. These small strips of plastic contain reagents that change color in a semiquantitative manner in the presence of specific compounds. Water excretion ranges between 0.5 and 1.5 L/day.

■ **Box 35-1**   Mechanisms of solute transport

Passive: Spontaneous, down an electrochemical gradient (no energy requirement).
  Diffusion
  Facilitated diffusion
    Channels
    Uniport
    Coupled transport: antiport or symport
  Solvent drag
Active: Against an electrochemical gradient (requires direct input of energy). Includes endocytosis.

adenosine triphosphate (ATP) (see below). Instead, the energy is derived from the gradient of the other coupled ion (in this example, Na^+).

Active Mechanisms

Transport is active if it is coupled directly to energy derived from metabolic processes (i.e., consumes ATP). In **active transport,** solutes usually move from an area of lower concentration to an area of higher concentration. In the kidney, *the most prevalent active transport mechanism is the Na^+,K^+-ATPase* (or sodium pump). Located in the basolateral membrane, the Na^+,K^+-ATPase is composed of several proteins. Together these proteins actively move Na^+ out of the cell and move K^+ into the cell. Other active transport mechanisms in the kidneys include the H^+-ATPase, H^+,K^+-ATPase, and Ca^{2+}-ATPase. H^+-ATPase and H^+,K^+-ATPase are responsible for H^+ secretion in the collecting duct system (see Chapter 38). The Ca^{2+}-ATPase is responsible for Ca^{2+} movement from the cytoplasm into the blood (see Chapter 37).

Endocytosis is another form of active transport. In endocytosis, a section of the plasma membrane invaginates. The portions around this invagination then engulf the substance being transported. Once the substance is engulfed, the membrane completely pinches off and forms a vesicle in the cytoplasm. Endocytosis is an important mechanism for reabsorbing small proteins and macromolecules by the proximal tubule and for the retrieval of water channels from the apical membrane of collecting duct cells. Because endocytosis requires ATP, it is a form of active transport.

opposite directions is mediated by an **antiport mechanism.** For example, Na^+-H^+ antiporter in the proximal tubule mediates Na^+ reabsorption and H^+ secretion. With coupled transporters, at least one of the solutes is usually transported against its chemical (and electrical) gradient. The energy for this uphill movement is derived from the passive downhill movement of at least one of the other solutes into the cell. For example, in the proximal tubule, operation of the Na^+-H^+ antiporter in the cell's apical membrane causes H^+ to move against its electrochemical gradient out of the cell into the tubular lumen. This uphill movement of H^+ is driven by the movement of Na^+ from the tubular lumen into the cell down its electrochemical gradient. The uphill movement of H^+ is termed **secondary active transport** because the movement of H^+ is not directly coupled to the hydrolysis of

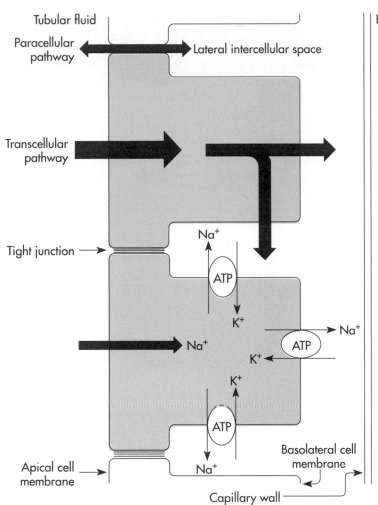

■ **Fig. 35-1**   Paracellular and transcellular transport pathways in the proximal tubule. See text for details. *ATP,* Adenosine triphosphate.

GENERAL PRINCIPLES OF TRANSEPITHELIAL SOLUTE AND WATER TRANSPORT

Renal cells are held together by **tight junctions** (Fig. 35-1). The tight junctions separate the apical membranes from the basolateral membranes. Below the tight junctions, the cells are separated by lateral intercellular spaces. A useful way to visualize the renal epithelium is to consider a six-pack of soda: the soda cans are the cells and the plastic holder represents the tight junctions.

In the nephron, a substance can be reabsorbed or secreted through cells (the transcellular pathway) or between cells (the paracellular pathway) (Fig. 35-1). Na⁺ reabsorption by the proximal tubule is a good example of transport by the **transcellular pathway.** Na⁺ reabsorption in this nephron segment depends on the operation of Na⁺,K⁺-ATPase (Fig. 35-1). Na⁺,K⁺-ATPase is located exclusively in the basolateral membrane. This pump moves Na⁺ out of the cell into the blood and moves K⁺ into the cell. Thus, Na⁺,K⁺-ATPase lowers intracellular Na⁺ concentration and increases intracellular K⁺ concentration. Because intracellular [Na⁺] is low (12 mEq/L) and the [Na⁺] in tubular fluid is high (145 mEq/L), Na⁺ moves across the apical cell membrane down a chemical concentration gradient from the tubular lumen into the cell. Na⁺,K⁺-ATPase, sensing the addition of Na⁺ to the cell, is stimulated to increase the rate of Na⁺ extrusion into the blood. This action returns intracellular Na⁺ to normal levels. Transcellular Na⁺ reabsorption by the proximal tubule is thus a two-step process:

1. Na⁺ moves across the apical membrane into the cell down an electrochemical gradient established by Na⁺,K⁺-ATPase.
2. Na⁺ moves across the basolateral membrane against an electrochemical gradient via Na⁺,K⁺-ATPasc.

The reabsorption of Ca²⁺ and K⁺ across the proximal tubule is a good example of **paracellular transport.** Some of the water reabsorbed across the proximal tubule crosses the paracellular pathway. Some solutes dissolved in this water (in particular Ca²⁺ and K⁺) are carried along with the reabsorbed fluid and are reabsorbed by the process of solvent drag.

SOLUTE AND WATER REABSORPTION ALONG THE NEPHRON

In a quantitative sense, the reabsuption of NaCl and water represents the major function of the nephrons (approximately

25,000 mEq/day of Na⁺ and 179 L/day of water are reabsorbed; Table 35-1). In addition, the transport of many other important solutes is linked either directly or indirectly to Na⁺ reabsorption. In the following sections, we discuss the NaCl and water transport properties of each nephron segment and its regulation by hormones and other factors.

Proximal Tubule

The proximal tubule reabsorbs approximately 67% of the filtered water, Na⁺, Cl⁻, K⁺, and other solutes. In addition, the proximal tubule reabsorbs virtually all the glucose and amino acids filtered by the glomerulus. *The key element in proximal tubule reabsorption is the Na⁺,K⁺-ATPase in the basolateral membrane.* The reabsorption of every substance, including water, is linked in some way to the operation of Na⁺,K⁺-ATPase.

Na⁺ reabsorption. Na⁺ is reabsorbed by different mechanisms in the early (first half) and late (second half) segments of the proximal tubule. In the early segment, Na⁺ is reabsorbed primarily with HCO_3^- and a number of organic molecules (e.g., glucose, amino acids, P_i, lactate). By contrast, in the second half of the proximal tubule, Na⁺ is reabsorbed mainly with Cl⁻. This difference exists because of differences in Na⁺ transport systems present in the early and late segments of the proximal tubule, and because of differences in the composition of tubular fluid at these sites.

As illustrated in Fig. 35-2, in the early segment of the proximal tubule, Na⁺ uptake into the cell is coupled with either H⁺ or organic solutes. Na⁺ entry into the cell across the apical membrane is mediated by specific symporter and antiporter proteins, and not by diffusion through channels. For example, Na⁺ entry is coupled with the pumping of H⁺ out of the cell by the Na⁺-H⁺ antiporter (Fig. 35-2, A). H⁺ secretion results in $NaHCO_3$ reabsorption (see also Chapter 38). Na⁺ also enters proximal cells by several symporter mechanisms, including Na⁺-glucose, Na⁺-amino acid, Na⁺-Pi, and Na⁺-lactate symporters (Fig. 35-2, B). The glucose (and other organic solutes) that enters the cell with Na⁺ leaves the

■ **Fig. 35-2** Na⁺ transport processes in the first half of the proximal tubule. The transport mechanisms depicted in **A** and **B** are present in all cells in the first half of the proximal tubule. They are separated into different cells to simplify the discussion. **A,** The operation of the Na⁺-H⁺ antiporter in the apical membrane and the Na⁺,K⁺-ATPase and the HCO_3^- transporter in the basolateral membrane mediate $NaHCO_3$ reabsorption. CO_2 and H_2O combine inside the cells to form H⁺ and HCO_3^- in a reaction facilitated by the enzyme carbonic anhydrase *(CA).* **B,** The operation of the Na⁺-glucose transporter in the apical membrane, in conjunction with the Na⁺,K⁺-ATPase and the glucose transporter in the basolateral membrane, mediate Na⁺-glucose reabsorption. Na⁺ reabsorption is also coupled with other solutes, including amino acids, P_i, and lactate. Reabsorption of these solutes is mediated by Na⁺-amino acid, Na⁺-P_i, and Na⁺-lactate symporters located in the apical membrane and the Na⁺,K⁺-ATPase and the amino acid, P_i, and lactate transporters in the basolateral membrane.

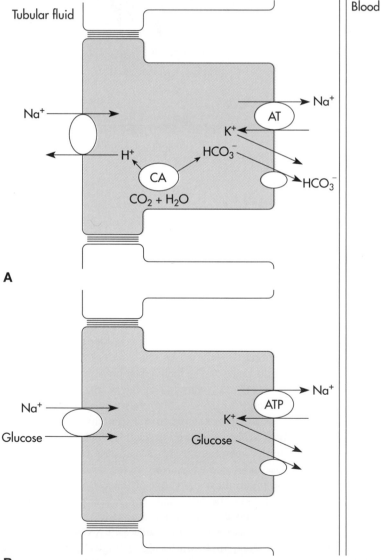

cell across the basolateral membrane by passive transporter mechanisms. Any Na^+ that enters the cell across the apical membrane leaves the cell and enters the blood via the Na^+,K^+-ATPase. *In summary, in the early segment of the proximal tubule, the reabsorption of Na^+ is coupled to that of HCO_3^- and a number of organic molecules.* Reabsorption of many organic molecules is so avid in this segment that they are almost completely removed from the tubular fluid (Fig. 35-3). The reabsorption of $NaHCO_3$ and Na^+-organic solutes across the proximal tubule establishes a transtubular osmotic gradient that provides the driving force for the passive reabsorption of water by osmosis. Because more water than Cl^- is reabsorbed in the early segment of the proximal tubule, the Cl^- concentration in tubular fluid rises along the length of the early proximal tubule (Fig. 35-3).

In the second half of the proximal tubule, Na^+ is primarily reabsorbed with Cl^- across both the transcellular and paracellular pathways (Fig. 35-4). Na^+ is reabsorbed with Cl^- rather than with organic solutes or HCO_3^- as the accompanying anion. This occurs because the cells lining the late proximal tubule have different Na^+ transport mechanisms from those in the early proximal tubule. Furthermore, the tubular fluid that enters the late proximal tubule contains very little glucose and amino acids but has a high concentration of Cl^- (140 mEq/L) compared with that in the early proximal tubule (105 mEq/L). The high Cl^- concentration is due to the preferential reabsorption of Na^+ with HCO_3^- and organic solutes in the early proximal tubule (Fig. 35-2).

The mechanism of transcellular Na^+ reabsorption in the late proximal tubule is shown in Fig. 35-4. Na^+ enters the cell across the luminal membrane by the parallel operation of Na^+-H^+ and one or more Cl^- anion antiporters. Because the secreted H^+ and anion combine in the tubular fluid and reenter the cell, the operation of the Na^+-H^+ and Cl^- anion antiporters is equivalent to NaCl uptake from tubular fluid into the cell. Na^+ leaves the cell by the action of Na^+,K^+-ATPase, and Cl^- leaves the cell by the action of a KCl symport protein in the basolateral membrane.

NaCl is also reabsorbed across the late proximal tubule by a paracellular route. *Paracellular NaCl reabsorption occurs because the rise in $[Cl^-]$ in the tubular fluid in the early proximal tubule creates a concentration gradient of Cl^- (140 mEq/L in the tubule lumen and 105 mEq/L in the interstitium). This concentration gradient favors the diffusion of Cl^- from the tubular lumen across the tight junctions into the lateral intercellular space.* Movement of the negatively charged Cl^- causes the tubular fluid to become positively charged relative to the blood. This positive transepithelial voltage causes the diffusion of positively charged Na^+ out of the tubular fluid across the tight junctions into the blood. Thus, in the late proximal tubule, some Na^+ and Cl^- is reabsorbed across the tight junctions by passive diffusion. The reabsorption of NaCl establishes a transtubular osmotic gradient that provides the driving force for the passive reabsorption of water by osmosis (as described below).

In summary, reabsorption of Na^+ and Cl^- in the proximal tubule occurs across the paracellular pathway and across the transcellular pathway. Approximately 17,000 mEq of the 25,200 mEq of NaCl filtered each day is reabsorbed in the proximal tubule (~67% of the filtered amount). Of this, two-thirds is transported across the transcellular pathway, while the remaining one-third is transported across the paracellular pathway (Tables 35-3 and 35-4).

Water reabsorption. The proximal tubule reabsorbs 67% of the filtered water (Fig. 35-5). *The driving force for water reabsorption is a transtubular osmotic gradient established by solute reabsorption (i.e., NaCl, Na^+-glucose, and so forth).* The reabsorption of Na^+ along with organic solutes HCO_3^- and Cl^- from the tubular fluid into the lateral intercellular spaces reduces the osmolality of the tubular fluid and increases the osmolality of the lateral intercellular space. Because the proximal tubule is highly permeable to water, water will flow by osmosis across both the tight junctions and the proximal tubular cells. Accumulation of fluid and solutes within the lateral intercellular space increases the hydrostatic pressure in this compartment. This increased hydrostatic pressure forces fluid and solutes to move into the capillaries. Thus, water reabsorption follows solute reabsorption in the proximal tubule. The reabsorbed fluid is slightly hyperosmotic to plasma. An important consequence of osmotic water flow across the proximal tubule is that some solutes, especially K^+ and Ca^{2+}, are carried along in the reabsorbed fluid and are thereby reabsorbed by the process

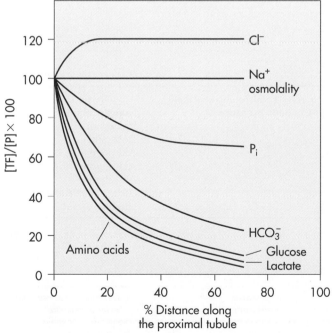

■ **Fig. 35-3** Concentration of solutes in tubular fluid as a function of length along the proximal tubule. [TF] is the concentration of the substance in tubular fluid; [P] is the concentration of the substance in plasma. Values above 100 indicate that relatively less of the solute than water was reabsorbed; values below 100 indicate that relatively more of the substance than water was reabsorbed. (Modified from Vander AJ: *Renal physiology,* ed 4, New York, 1991, McGraw-Hill.)

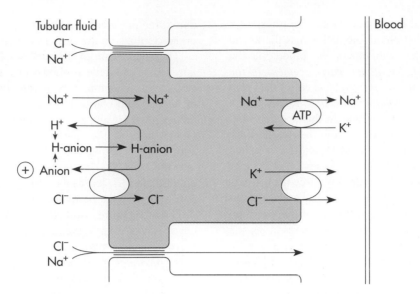

■ **Fig. 35-4** Na$^+$ transport processes in the second half of the proximal tubule. Na$^+$ and Cl$^-$ enter the cell across the apical membrane by the operation of parallel Na$^+$-H$^+$ and Cl$^-$-anion antiporters. More than one Cl$^-$ anion antiporter may be involved in this process, but only one is depicted here. The secreted H$^+$ and anion combine in the tubular fluid to form an H$^+$-anion complex that can recycle across the plasma membrane. Accumulation of H$^+$-anion in tubular fluid establishes an H$^+$-anion concentration gradient that favors H$^+$-anion recycling across the apical plasma membrane into the cell. Inside the cell H$^+$ and the anion dissociate and recycle back across the apical plasma membrane. The net result is NaCl uptake across the apical membrane. The anion may be OH$^-$, formate (HCO$_2^-$), oxalate$^-$, HCO$_3^-$, or sulfate. The lumen-positive transepithelial voltage (indicated by the plus sign inside the circle in the tubular lumen) is generated by the diffusion of Cl$^-$ (lumen-to-blood) across the tight junctions. The high [Cl$^-$] of tubular fluid provides the driving force for Cl$^-$ diffusion.

■ **Table 35-3** NaCl transport along the nephron

Segment	Percentage filtered reabsorbed	Mechanism of Na$^+$ entry across the apical membrane	Major regulatory hormones
Proximal tubule	67%	Na$^+$-H$^+$ exchange, Na$^+$-cotransport with amino acids and organic solutes, Na$^+$/H$^+$-Cl$^-$/anion exchange	Angiotensin II Norepinephrine Epinephrine Dopamine
Loop of Henle	25%	1Na$^+$-1K$^+$-2Cl$^-$ symport	Aldosterone
Distal tubule	~4%	NaCl symport	Aldosterone
Late distal tubule and collecting duct	~3%	Na$^+$ channels	Aldosterone Atrial natriuretic peptide Urodilatin

■ **Table 35-4** Water transport along the nephron

Segment	Percentage of filtered reabsorbed	Mechanism of water reabsorption	Hormones that regulate water permeability
Proximal tubule	67%	Passive	None
Loop of Henle	15%	DTL only; passive	None
Distal tubule	0%	No water reabsorption	None
Late distal tubule and collecting duct	~8%-17%	Passive	ADH, ANP*

*ANP inhibits the ADH-stimulated water permeability.

ADH, Antidiuretic hormone; *ANP*, atrial natriuretic peptide.

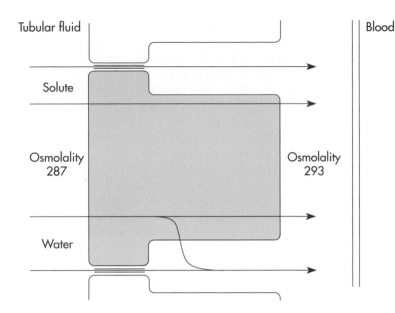

Tubular fluid

Solute

Osmolality
287

Water

Blood

Osmolality
293

■ **Fig. 35-5** Routes of water and solute reabsorption across the proximal tubule. Transport of solutes, including Na⁺, Cl⁻, and organic solutes, into the lateral intercellular space increases the osmolality of this compartment, which establishes the driving force for osmotic water reabsorption across the proximal tubule. This occurs because some Na^+,K^+-ATPase and some transporters of organic solute, HCO_3^-, and Cl⁻, are located on the lateral cell membranes and deposit these solutes between cells. Furthermore, some NaCl also enters the lateral intercellular space by diffusion across the tight junction (i.e., paracellular pathway). An important consequence of osmotic water flow across the transcellular and paracellular pathways in the proximal tubule is that some solutes, especially K⁺ and Ca^{2+}, are carried along in the reabsorbed fluid and are thereby reabsorbed by the process of solvent drag.

of solvent drag (Fig. 35-5). The reabsorption of virtually all organic solutes, Cl⁻, other ions, and water is coupled to Na⁺ reabsorption. Therefore, changes in Na⁺ reabsorption influence the reabsorption of water and other solutes by the proximal tubule.

Fanconi's syndrome is a renal disease that is either hereditary or acquired. It results from an impaired ability of the proximal tubule to reabsorb amino acids, glucose, and low-molecular-weight proteins. Because other segments of the nephron cannot reabsorb these solutes, Fanconi's syndrome causes an increase in the excretion of amino acids, glucose, P_i, and low-molecular-weight proteins in the urine.

Protein reabsorption. Proteins filtered by the glomerulus are also reabsorbed in the proximal tubule. As mentioned previously, peptide hormones, small proteins, and even small amounts of larger proteins, such as albumin, are filtered by the glomerulus. The glomerulus filters only a small amount of proteins (the concentration of proteins in the ultrafiltrate is only 40 mg/L). However, the amount of protein filtered per day is significant because the GFR is so high:

filtered protein = GFR × [protein] in the ultrafiltrate
filtered protein = 180 L/day × 40 mg/L = 7.2 g/day

Protein reabsorption in the proximal tubule begins when the proteins are partially degraded by enzymes on the surface of the proximal tubule cells. These partially degraded proteins are taken into the cell by endocytosis. Once they are inside the cell, enzymes digest the proteins and peptides into their constituent amino acids. Amino acids then exit the cell across the basolateral membrane and return to the blood. Normally, this mechanism reabsorbs virtually all of the protein filtered and hence the urine is essentially protein free.

However, because the mechanism is easily saturated, if the amount of protein filtered increases, protein will appear in the urine. Disruption of the glomerular filtration barrier to proteins will increase the filtration of proteins and result in **proteinuria** (the appearance of protein in the urine). Proteinuria is frequently seen with kidney disease.

During routine urinalysis, it is not abnormal to find traces of protein in the urine. Protein in the urine can be derived from two sources: (1) filtration and incomplete reabsorption by the proximal tubule and (2) synthesis by the thick ascending limb of Henle's loop. Cells in the thick ascending limb produce **Tamm-Horsfall glycoprotein** and secrete the protein into the tubular fluid. Because the mechanism for protein reabsorption is upstream of the thick ascending limb (i.e., proximal tubule), the secreted Tamm-Horsfall glycoprotein appears in the urine.

Organic anion and organic cation secretion. In addition to reabsorbing solutes and water, cells of the proximal tubule secrete organic cations and organic anions (Tables 35-5 and 35-6 present a partial listing). Many of these organic anions and cations are end products of metabolism that circulate in the plasma. The proximal tubule also secretes numerous exogenous organic compounds, including *p*-aminohippuric acid (PAH), drugs such as penicillin, some nonsteroidal antiinflammatory agents (e.g., ibuprofen, indomethacin, and naproxen), and the antiviral drug adefovir, which is effective in the treatment of human immunodeficiency virus (HIV)-infected patients. Many of these organic compounds can be bound to plasma proteins and are not readily filtered. Therefore, excretion by filtration alone eliminates only a small portion of these potentially toxic substances from the body. Such substances are also secreted from the peritubular capillaries into the tubular fluid. These secretory mechanisms are very powerful and

■ **Table 35-5**   Some organic anions secreted by the proximal tubule

Endogenous anions	Drugs
Cyclic adenosine monophosphate (cAMP)	Acetazolamide
Bile salts	Chlorothiazide
Hippurates	Furosemide
Oxalate	Penicillin
Prostaglandins	Probenecid
Urate	Salicylate (aspirin)
	Hydrochlorothiazide
	Bumetanide
	Adefovir
	Cidovir
	NSAID
	Enalapril

NSAID, Nonsteroidal antiinflammatory drugs.

■ **Table 35-6**   Some organic cations secreted by the proximal tubule

Endogenous cations	Drugs
Creatinine	Atropine
Dopamine	Isoproterenol
Epinephrine	Cimetidine
Norepinephrine	Morphine
	Quinine
	Amiloride
	Procainamide
	Verapamil

remove virtually all organic anions and cations from the plasma entering the kidneys. Hence, these substances are removed from the plasma by both filtration and secretion.

An example of organic anion secretion is PAH transport across the proximal tubule (Fig. 35-6). This secretory pathway has a maximal transport rate, has a low specificity (i.e., it transports a variety of organic anions), and is responsible

for the secretion of all organic anions listed in Table 35-5. PAH is taken into the cell across the basolateral membrane, against its chemical gradient, in exchange for α-ketoglutarate (αKG) via a PAH-αKG antiport mechanism. αKG accumulates inside the cells via the metabolism of glutamate and by an Na^+-αKG symporter, also present in the basolateral membrane. Thus, PAH uptake into the cell against its electrochemical gradient is coupled to the exit of αKG out of the cell down its chemical gradient; this activity is generated by the Na^+-αKG antiport mechanism and the metabolism of glutamate. The resultant high intracellular concentration of PAH provides the driving force for PAH exit across the luminal membrane into the tubular fluid via a PAH-anion antiporter and possibly a voltage-driven PAH transporter (Fig. 35-6).

Because organic anions compete for the same transporters, elevated plasma levels of one anion inhibit the secretion of the others. For example, infusing PAH can produce a reduction of penicillin secretion by the proximal tubule. Because the kidneys are responsible for eliminating penicillin, the infusion of PAH into individuals receiving penicillin reduces urinary penicillin excretion, and thereby extends the biological half-life of the drug. In World War II, when penicillin was in short supply, hippurates were given with the penicillin to extend the drug's therapeutic effect.

Figure 35-7 illustrates the mechanism of organic cation (OC^+) transport across the proximal tubule. Organic cations are taken into the cell, across the basolateral membrane, by a mechanism that involves facilitated diffusion. This uniport mechanism is driven by the magnitude of the voltage difference (negative potential) across the basolateral membrane. Organic cation transport across the luminal membrane into the tubular fluid is mediated by an OC^+-H^+ antiporter.

■ **Fig. 35-6**   Organic anion secretion [e.g., *p*-aminohippuric acid (PAH)] across the proximal tubule. PAH enters the cell across the basolateral membrane by a PAH-α-ketoglutarate *(αKG)* antiport mechanism. The uptake of αKG into the cell, against its chemical gradient, is driven by the movement of Na^+ into the cell. The αKG recycles across the basolateral membrane. PAH leaves the cell across the apical membrane down its chemical concentration gradient by a PAH-anion (A–) transporter and possibly a voltage-driven transporter.

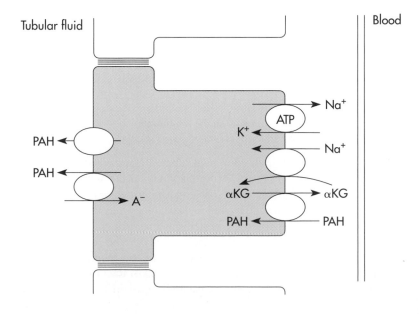

Because the transport mechanisms for organic cation secretion are nonspecific, several cations compete for the transport pathway (Table 35-6).

> The histamine H2-antagonist **cimetidine** is used to treat gastric ulcers. Cimetidine is secreted by the organic cation pathway in the proximal tubule. It reduces the urinary excretion of the antiarrhythmic drug **procainamide** (also an organic cation), by competing with procainamide for the secretory pathway. It is important to recognize that coadministration of organic cations can increase the plasma concentration of both drugs to levels much higher than those seen when the drugs are given alone. This increase can lead to drug toxicity.

P-glycoprotein and multidrug resistance (MDR)-associated protein 2 (Mrp2) may also play an important role in the renal excretion of organic compounds. P-glycoprotein and Mrp2 possess ATPase activity, are located in the apical membrane of the proximal tubule, and transfer some organic compounds from the cell interior into tubular fluid. These transporters are called MDR proteins because they facilitate the removal of cytotoxic drugs from the cell interior. Other drug-transporting ATPases, including Mrp1, are located in the basolateral membrane and move organic compounds from the blood into the cells of the proximal tubule. P-glycoprotein transports hydrophobic cationic compounds and some drugs including anticancer agents, digoxin, and immunosuppressive agents such as cyclosporin. Mrp2 transports conjugated anionic compounds such as glutathione-conjugated leukotriene C4 and the glucuronide-conjugated of bilirubin.

Henle's Loop

Henle's loop reabsorbs approximately 25% of the filtered NaCl and K+. Ca^{2+} and HCO_3^- are also reabsorbed in the loop of Henle (see Chapters 37 and 38 for more details). This reabsorption occurs almost exclusively in the thick ascending limb. By comparison, the ascending thin limb has a much lower reabsorptive capacity, and the descending thin limb does not reabsorb significant amounts of solutes. The loop of Henle reabsorbs approximately 15% of the filtered water. Water reabsorption occurs exclusively in the descending thin limb. *The ascending limb is impermeable to water.*

The key element in solute reabsorption by the thick ascending limb is the Na+,K+-ATPase in the basolateral membrane (Fig. 35-8). As with reabsorption in the proximal tubule, the reabsorption of every solute by the thick ascending limb is in some way linked to Na+,K+-ATPase. This pump maintains a low intracellular [Na+]. This low [Na+] provides a favorable chemical gradient for the movement of Na+ from the tubular fluid into the cell. The movement of Na+ across the apical membrane into the cell is mediated by the 1Na+-1K+-2Cl− symporter, which couples the movement of 1Na+ with 1K+ and 2Cl−. Using the potential energy released by the downhill movement of Na+ and Cl−, this symport drives the uphill movement of K+ into the cell. An Na+-H+ antiporter in the apical cell membrane also mediates Na+ reabsorption as well as H+ secretion (HCO_3^- reabsorption) in the thick ascending limb (Chapter 38 contains details of HCO_3^- reabsorption by the thick ascending limb). Na+ leaves the cell across the basolateral membrane via the action of Na+,K+-ATPase, and K+, Cl−, and HCO_3^- leave the cell across the basolateral membrane by separate pathways.

The voltage across the thick ascending limb is important in the reabsorption of several cations. The tubular fluid is positively charged relative to the blood because of the unique location of transport proteins in the apical and basolateral membranes. *Two points are important here: (1) increased salt transport by the thick ascending limb increases the magnitude of the positive charge in the lumen, and (2) this voltage is an important driving force for the reabsorption of several cations, including Na+, K+, and Ca^{2+} across the paracellular pathway* (Fig. 35-8). Thus, salt reabsorption across the thick

Tubular fluid

Blood

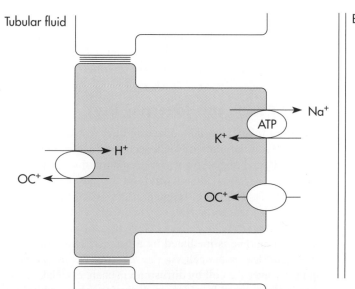

■ **Fig. 35-7** Organic cation secretion *(OC+)* across the proximal tubule. OC+ enters the cell across the basolateral membrane by facilitated diffusion. The uptake of OC+ into the cell, against its chemical gradient, is driven by the cell-negative potential difference. OC+ leaves the cell across the apical membrane in exchange with H+ by an OC+-H+ antiport mechanism.

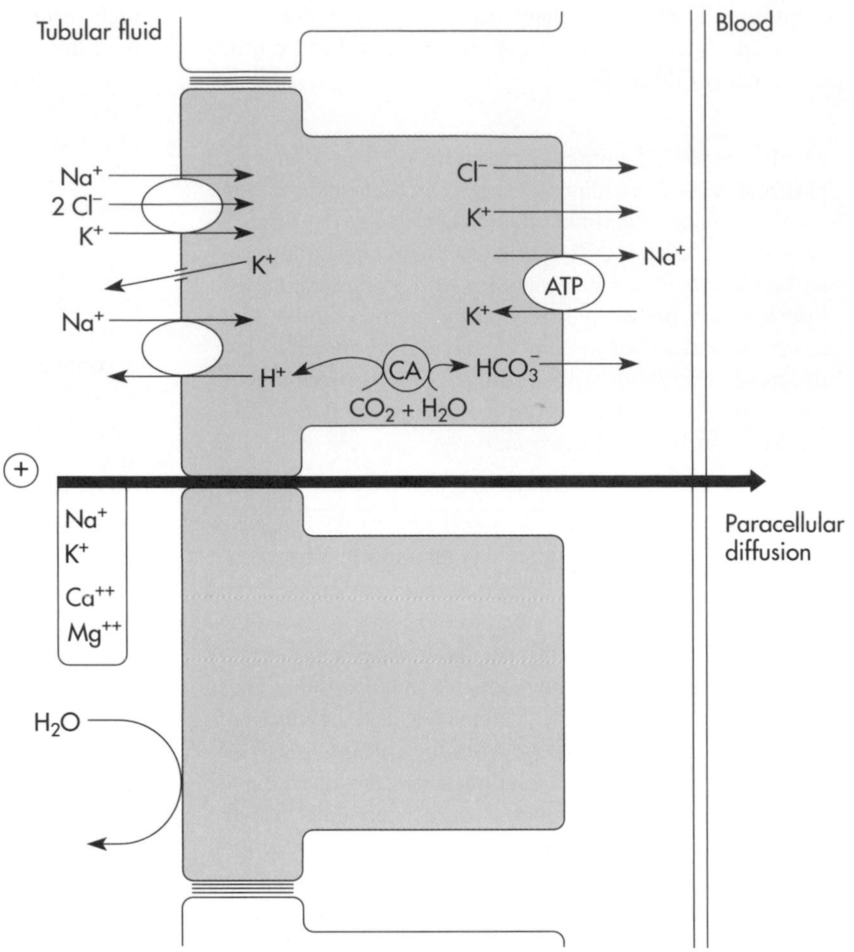

Fig. 35-8 Transport mechanisms for NaCl reabsorption in the thick ascending limb of Henle's loop. The positive charge in the lumen plays a major role in driving passive paracellular reabsorption of cations. *CA,* Carbonic anhydrase.

ascending limb occurs by transcellular and paracellular pathways. Fifty percent of solute transport is transcellular and 50% is paracellular. Because the thick ascending limb is impermeable to water, reabsorption of NaCl and other solutes reduces the osmolality of tubular fluid to less than 150 mOsm/kg H_2O.

Bartter's syndrome is a set of autosomal-recessive genetic disorders characterized by hypokalemia, metabolic alkalosis, and hyperaldosteronism (see Table 35-7). Mutations in the genes coding for the $1Na^+$-$1K^+$-$2Cl^-$ cotransporter, the apical K^+ channel, or the basolateral Cl^- channel in the thick ascending limb (Fig. 35-8) decrease NaCl and K^+ absorption by the thick ascending limb, which in turn causes hypokalemia and a decrease in the effective circulating volume (ECV), which stimulates the secretion of aldosterone.

Inhibition of the $1Na^+$-$1K^+$-$2Cl^-$ symporter in the thick ascending limb by loop diuretics, such as **furosemide,** inhibits NaCl reabsorption by the thick ascending limb and thereby increases urinary NaCl excretion. Furosemide also inhibits K^+ and Ca^{2+} reabsorption by reducing the lumen-positive voltage, which drives the paracellular reabsorption of these ions. Thus, furosemide also increases

urinary K^+ and Ca^{2+} excretion. Furosemide also increases water excretion by reducing the osmolality of the interstitial fluid in the medulla. Water reabsorption by the descending thin limb of Henle's loop is passive and driven by the osmotic gradient between the tubular fluid in the descending thin limb (which is ~290 mOsm/kg H_2O at the beginning of the limb) and the interstitial fluid (which is ~1200 mOsm/kg H_2O in the medulla). Thus, a reduction of the osmolality of the interstitial fluid will reduce water reabsorption and thereby increase excretion.

Distal Tubule and Collecting Duct

The distal tubule and the collecting duct reabsorb approximately 7% of the filtered NaCl, secrete variable amounts of K^+ and H^+, and reabsorb a variable amount of water (~8% to 17%). Water reabsorption depends on the plasma concentration of ADH. The initial segment of the distal tubule (early distal tubule) reabsorbs Na^+, Cl^-, and Ca^{2+}, and is impermeable to water (Fig. 35-9). NaCl entry into the cell across the apical membrane is mediated by a Na^+-Cl^- symporter (Fig. 35-9). Na^+ leaves the cell via the action of Na^+,K^+-ATPase, and Cl^- leaves the cell by diffusion via channels. NaCl reabsorption is reduced by **thiazide diuretics,** which inhibit the

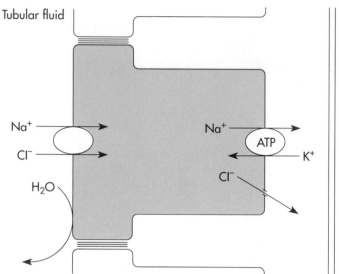

Tubular fluid

Blood

■ **Fig. 35-9** Transport mechanism for Na$^+$ and Cl$^-$ reabsorption in the early segment of the distal tubule. This segment is impermeable to water. See text for details.

Na$^+$-Cl$^-$ symporter. Thus, the dilution of the tubular fluid begins in the thick ascending limb and continues in the early distal tubule.

The last segments of the distal tubule (late distal tubule) and of the collecting duct are composed of two cell types, **principal cells** and **intercalated cells.** As shown in Fig. 35-10, *principal cells reabsorb Na$^+$ and water and secrete K$^+$. Intercalated cells either secrete H$^+$ (reabsorb HCO$_3^-$) or secrete HCO$_3$ and thus are important in regulating acid-base balance* (Chapter 38 contains details on H$^+$ and HCO$_3^-$ secretion by intercalated cells). Intercalated cells also reabsorb K$^+$. Both Na$^+$ reabsorption and K$^+$ secretion by principal cells depend on the activity of the Na$^+$,K$^+$-ATPase in the basolateral membrane (Fig. 35-10). By maintaining a low cell [Na$^+$], this pump provides a favorable chemical gradient for the movement of Na$^+$ from the tubular fluid into the cell. Because Na$^+$ enters the cell by diffusion through Na$^+$-selective channels in the apical membrane,* the negative charge inside the cell facilitates Na$^+$ entry. Na$^+$ leaves the cell across the basolateral membrane and enters the blood via the action of Na$^+$,K$^+$-ATPase. This sodium reabsorption generates a lumen-negative charge across the late distal tubule and collecting duct. Cells in the collecting duct reabsorb significant amounts of Cl$^-$, probably across the paracellular pathway. Reabsorption of Cl$^-$ is driven by the voltage differences across the late distal tubule and collecting duct.

Liddle's syndrome is a rare genetic disorder characterized by an increase in the extracellular fluid volume (ECFV), which causes an increase in blood pressure (i.e., hypertension). Liddle's syndrome is caused by mutations in the genes that encode either the β or γ subunit of ENaC.* These mutations cause Na$^+$ channels to become

overactive. Inappropriately high rates of renal Na$^+$ absorption occur, which lead to an increase in the ECFV (see Chapter 36). **Pseudohypoaldosteronism type I (PHA1)** is an uncommon and inherited disorder characterized by an increase in Na$^+$ excretion, a reduction in ECFV, and hypotension. PHA1 is due to mutations in the genes encoding the γ subunit of ENaC. These mutations inactivate the channel, resulting in inappropriately low rates of renal Na$^+$ absorption, which reduces the ECFV.

K$^+$ is secreted from the blood into the tubular fluid by principal cells in two steps (Fig. 35-10). First, K$^+$ uptake across the basolateral membrane occurs via the action of Na$^+$,K$^+$-ATPase. In the second step, K$^+$ leaves the cells by passive diffusion. Because the [K$^+$] inside the cells is high (150 mEq/L) and the [K$^+$] in tubular fluid is low (~10 mEq/L), K$^+$ diffuses down its concentration gradient across the apical cell membrane into the tubular fluid. Although the negative potential inside the cells tends to retain K$^+$ within the cell, the electrochemical gradient across the apical membrane favors K$^+$ secretion from the cell into the tubular fluid. Additional details of K$^+$ secretion and its regulation are considered in Chapter 37. The mechanism of K$^+$ reabsorption by intercalated cells is not completely understood but is thought to be mediated by an H$^+$,K$^+$-ATPase located in the apical cell membrane (see Chapters 37 and 38).

Amiloride is a diuretic that inhibits Na$^+$ reabsorption by the distal tubule and collecting duct by directly inhibiting Na$^+$ channels in the luminal cell membrane. Amiloride also inhibits Cl$^-$ reabsorption indirectly: inhibition of Na$^+$ reabsorption reduces the magnitude of the negative charge in the lumen, which is the driving force for paracellular Cl$^-$ reabsorption. Because amiloride reduces the negative charge in the lumen, it also acts to inhibit K$^+$ secretion. By inhibiting K$^+$ secretion across the distal tubule and collecting duct, amiloride reduces the amount

---

*Recently, cDNA clones for the renal Na$^+$ channel (i.e., epithelial Na$^+$ channel, or ENaC) have been isolated. ENaC is composed of three subunits, α, β, and γ, and all three subunits are required to form functional Na$^+$ channels.

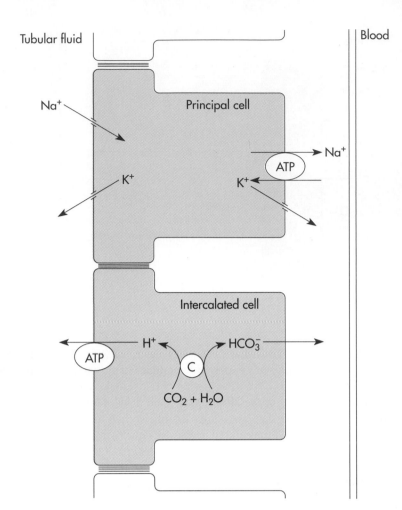

■ **Fig. 35-10**   Transport pathways in principal cells and intercalated cells of the distal tubule and collecting duct. See text for details. *CA,* Carbonic anhydrase.

of K⁺ excreted in the urine. Consequently, amiloride is frequently referred to as a **K⁺-sparing diuretic.** It is most often used in patients who excrete too much K⁺ in their urine.

Genetic Diseases and Renal Transport Proteins

Many renal diseases have a genetic component. The disease-susceptibility genes for more than 20 renal diseases have been identified, and many of these genes code for transport proteins. The disorders summarized in Table 35-7 are transmitted as single Mendelian traits and lead to clinically relevant changes in renal function and fluid and electrolyte homeostasis. The rapid development of molecular genetics and the Human Genome Project, a cooperative effort to identify the genome structure and sequence of human and animal models, will no doubt lead to the identification of additional genes responsible for renal diseases, including those that contribute to complex polygenic diseases such as nephropathies associated with hypertension, diabetes, and lupus. Moreover, it is also becoming clear that disease progression in genetic disorders is modulated by other molecular pathways such as the renin-angiotensin system and

environmental factors. Detailed information on the molecular pathogenesis of renal disease will provide new opportunities for treatment and prevention. The challenges that lie ahead include a thorough understanding of the molecular pathogenesis of renal genetic diseases and the development of novel treatments, including gene therapy and pharmacologic agents that target specific aspects of the molecular pathogenesis.

REGULATION OF NaCl AND WATER REABSORPTION

Several hormones and factors regulate NaCl reabsorption. Table 35-8 summarizes, for each hormone, the major stimulus for secretion, the nephron site of action, and the effect on transport. Angiotensin II, aldosterone, ANP, urodilatin, epinephrine, and norepinephrine released by sympathetic nerves are the most important hormones that regulate NaCl reabsorption and thereby urinary NaCl excretion. However, other hormones (including dopamine and glucocorticoids), Starling forces, and the phenomenon of glomerulotubular balance also influence NaCl reabsorption. ADH is the only major hormone that directly regulates the amount of water excreted by the kidneys.

■ Table 35-7 Monogenic renal diseases involving transport proteins

Diseases		Mode of inheritance	Gene	Transport protein	Nephron segment	Phenotype
Cystinuria	type I	AR	SLC3A1	Basic amino acid transporter (rBAT)	Proximal tubule	Increased excretion of basic amino acids, nephrolithiasis (kidney stones)
	type II and III	IAR	SLC7A9	b°, +AT	Proximal tubule	
Proximal renal tubular acidosis		AR	SLC4A4	Na+-HCO$_3^-$ cotransporter	Proximal tubule	Hyperchloremic metabolic acidosis
Bartter syndrome		AR	SLC12A1 (type I)	Na+-K+-2Cl- transporter (furosemide sensitive)	TAL	Hypokalemia, metabolic alkalosis, hyperaldosteronism
			KCNJ1 (type II) CLCNKB (type III)	Potassium channel Chloride channel		
X-linked nephrolithiasis (Dents disease)		XLR	CLC5	Chloride channel (C1C-5)	Distal tubule	Hypercalciuria, nephrolithiasis (kidney stones)
Hypomagnesemia-hypercalciuria syndrome		AR	PCCLN-1	Paracellin-1	TAL	Hypomagnesemia, hypercalciuria, nephrolithiasis
Gitelman syndrome		AR	SLC12A3	Thiazide-sensitive cotransporter	Distal tubule	Hypomagnesemia, hypokalemic metabolic alkalosis, hypocalciuria, hypotension
Pseudohypoaldosteronism, type 1a		AR	SCNN1A, SCNN1B, and SCNN1G	α, β, and γ subunit of amiloride-sensitive Na+ channel	Collecting duct	Increased excretion of Na+, hypotension
Liddle syndrome		AD	SCNN1B, SCNN1G	α, β, and γ subunit of amiloride-sensitive Na+ channel	Collecting duct	Decreased excretion of Na+, hypertension
Nephrogenic diabetes insipidus (NDI)		AR	AQP2	Aquaporin 2 water channel	Collecting duct	Polyuria, polydipsia, plasma hyperosmolality
Distal renal tubular acidosis		AD AR	SLC4A1 ATP6B1	Cl-/HCO$_3^-$ exchanger Subunit of H+-ATPase	Collecting duct	Metabolic acidosis, hypokalemia, hypercalciuria, nephrolithiasis (kidney stones)
		AR	ATP6N1A	Accessory subunit of H+-ATPase		

Modified from Guay-Woodford LM: Overview: the genetics of renal disease, *Semin Nephrol* 19(4):312, 1999 and Zelikovic I: Molecular pathophysiology of tubular transport disorders, *Pediatr Nephrol* 16:919, 2001.
AR, Autosomal recessive; *IAR*, incomplete autosomal recessive; *XLR*, X-linked recessive; *b°*, *+AT*, light subunit of rBAT; *TAL*, thick ascending limb of Henle's loop; *AD*, autosomal dominant.

■ Table 35-8 Hormones that regulate NaCl and water absorption

Hormone	Major stimulus	Nephron site of action	Effect on transport
Angiotensin II	↑ Renin	PT	↑ NaCl and H$_2$O reabsorption
Aldosterone	↑ Angiotensin II, ↑ [K+]$_p$	TAL, DT/CD	↑ NaCl and H$_2$O reabsorption*
ANP	↑ ECV	CD	↓ H$_2$O and NaCl reabsorption
Urodilatin	↑ ECV	CD	↓ H$_2$O and NaCl reabsorption
Sympathetic nerves	↓ ECV	PT, TAL, DT/CD	↑ NaCl and H$_2$O reabsorption*
Dopamine	↑ ECV	PT	↓ H$_2$O and NaCl reabsorption
ADH	↑ P$_{osm}$, ↓ ECV	DT/CD	↑ H$_2$O reabsorption*

*All the hormones listed act within minutes, except aldosterone, which exerts its action on NaCl reabsorption with a delay of 1 hour. *PT*, Proximal tubule; *TAL*, thick ascending limb; *DT/CD*, distal tubule and collecting duct; *ECV*, effective circulating volume; [K+]$_p$, plasma [K+]; *P$_{osm}$*, plasma osmolality. The asterisks indicate that the effect on H$_2$O reabsorption does not include the TAL. ↓ indicates a decrease and ↑ indicates an increase.

Angiotensin II. The hormone angiotensin II has a potent stimulating effect on NaCl and water reabsorption in the proximal tubule. A decrease in the **effective circulating volume (ECV)** activates the renin-angiotensin-aldosterone system (discussed in Chapter 36), thereby increasing plasma angiotensin II concentration.

Aldosterone. Aldosterone is synthesized by the glomerulosa cells of the adrenal cortex. It stimulates NaCl reabsorption by the thick ascending limb of Henle's loop and the distal tubule and collecting duct. Aldosterone also stimulates K+ secretion by the distal tubule and collecting duct (see Chapter 36). *The two most important stimuli for aldosterone* *secretion are an increase in angiotensin II concentration and an increase in plasma [K⁺].* By its stimulation of NaCl reabsorption in the collecting duct, aldosterone also increases water reabsorption by this nephron segment.

Some individuals with an expanded ECF volume and elevated blood pressure are treated with drugs that inhibit angiotensin converting enzyme (**ACE inhibitors,** e.g., **enalapril** and **lisinopril**). These drugs lower fluid volume and blood pressure. Inhibition of ACE blocks the degradation of angiotensin I to angiotensin II and thereby lowers plasma angiotensin II levels (see Chapter 36). The decline in plasma angiotensin II concentration has three effects: (1) NaCl and water reabsorption by the proximal tubule falls; (2) aldosterone secretion falls, which reduces NaCl reabsorption in the distal tubule and collecting duct; and (3) because angiotensin is a potent vasoconstrictor, the systemic arterioles dilate and arterial blood pressure falls. In addition, ACE degrades the vasodilating hormone bradykinin; ACE inhibitors therefore increase the concentrations of bradykinin. Thus, ACE inhibitors decrease the ECF volume and the arterial blood pressure by promoting renal NaCl and water excretion and by depressing total peripheral resistance.

Atrial natriuretic peptide and urodilatin. ANP and urodilatin are encoded by the same gene and have very similar amino acid sequences. **ANP** is a 28-amino acid hormone secreted by the cardiac atria. Its secretion is stimulated by a rise in blood pressure and an increase in the effective circulating volume. ANP reduces blood pressure by decreasing total peripheral resistance and by enhancing urinary NaCl and water excretion. The hormone also inhibits NaCl reabsorption by the medullary portion of the collecting duct, inhibits ADH-stimulated water reabsorption across the collecting duct, and reduces the secretion of ADH from the posterior pituitary.

Urodilatin is a 32-amino acid hormone that differs from ANP by the addition of four amino acids to the amino terminus. Urodilatin is secreted by the distal tubule and collecting duct and is not present in the systemic circulation; thus, urodilatin influences only the function of the kidneys. Urodilatin secretion is stimulated by a rise in blood pressure and an increase in the effective circulating volume. It inhibits NaCl and water reabsorption across the medullary portion of the collecting duct. Urodilatin is a more potent natriuretic and diuretic hormone than ANP because ANP entering the kidneys in the blood is degraded by a neutral endopeptidase that has no effect on urodilatin.

Sympathetic nerves. Catecholamines released from sympathetic nerves (norepinephrine) and the adrenal medulla (epinephrine) stimulate NaCl and water reabsorption by the proximal tubule, the thick ascending limb of Henle's loop, the distal tubule, and the collecting duct. Activation of sympathetic nerves (e.g., after hemorrhage or due to a decrease in the effective circulating volume) stimulates NaCl and water reabsorption by the proximal tubule, the thick ascending limb of Henle's loop, the distal tubule, and the collecting duct.

Dopamine. Dopamine, a catecholamine, is released from dopaminergic nerves in the kidneys and may also be synthesized by cells of the proximal tubule. The action of dopamine is opposite to that of norepinephrine and epinephrine. Dopamine secretion is stimulated by an increase in the effective circulating volume, and it directly inhibits NaCl and water reabsorption in the proximal tubule.

Antidiuretic hormone. *Antidiuretic hormone is the most important hormone that regulates water balance* (see Chapters 36 and 43). This hormone is secreted by the posterior pituitary in response to an increase in plasma osmolality or a decrease in the effective circulating volume. ADH increases the permeability of the collecting duct to water. Also, because an osmotic gradient exists across the wall of the collecting duct, ADH increases water reabsorption by the collecting duct (see Chapter 36 for details). ADH has little effect on urinary NaCl excretion.

Starling forces. Starling forces (see also Chapters 20 and 34) regulate NaCl and water reabsorption across the proximal tubule (Fig. 35-11). As described above, Na^+, Cl^-, HCO_3^-, amino acids, glucose, and water are transported into the intercellular space of the proximal tubule. Starling forces between this space and the peritubular capillaries facilitate the movement of the reabsorbed substances into the capillaries. Starling forces that favor this movement are the capillary oncotic pressure (π_c) and the hydrostatic pressure in the intercellular space (P_i). The opposing Starling forces are the interstitial oncotic pressure (π_i) and the capillary hydrostatic pressure (P_c). Normally, the sum of the Starling forces favors movement of solute and water from the intercellular space into the capillary. However, some of the solutes and fluid that enter the lateral intercellular space leak back into the proximal tubular fluid. Starling forces do not affect transport by the loop of Henle, distal tubule, and collecting duct, because these segments are less permeable to water than is the proximal tubule.

A number of forces can alter the Starling forces across the peritubular capillaries surrounding the proximal tubule. For example, dilation of the efferent arteriole increases the hydrostatic pressure in the peritubular capillaries (P_c), whereas constriction of the efferent arteriole decreases P_c. An increase in P_c inhibits solute and water reabsorption by increasing the back leak of NaCl and water across the tight junction, whereas a decrease in P_c stimulates reabsorption by decreasing back leak across the tight junction.

The oncotic pressure in the peritubular capillary is partly determined by the rate of formation of the glomerular ultrafiltrate. For example, if one assumes a constant plasma flow in the afferent arteriole, then as less ultrafiltrate is formed (i.e., as GFR decreases), the plasma proteins become less concentrated in the plasma that enters the efferent arteriole and peritubular capillary. Hence, the peritubular oncotic pressure decreases. The peritubular oncotic pressure is directly related to the filtration fraction (FF = GFR/RPF). A fall in FF, because of a decrease in GFR at constant RPF,

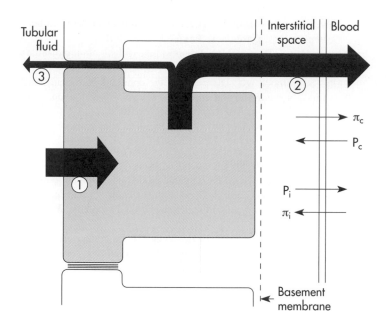

■ **Fig. 35-11**   Routes of solute and water transport across the proximal tubule and the Starling forces that modify reabsorption. *1,* Solute and water are reabsorbed across the apical membrane and then cross the lateral cell membrane. Some solute and water reenter the tubule fluid (arrow labeled *3*), and the remainder enters the interstitial space and then flows into the capillary (arrow labeled *2*). The width of the arrows is directly proportional to the amount of solute and water moving by the pathways labeled *1* to *3*. Starling forces across the capillary wall determine the amount of fluid flowing through pathways *2* versus *3*. Transport mechanisms in the apical cell membranes determine the amount of solute and water entering the cell (pathway *1*). π_c, Capillary oncotic pressure; P_c, capillary hydrostatic pressure; π_i, interstitial fluid oncotic pressure; P_i, interstitial hydrostatic pressure. Thin arrows across the capillary wall indicate the direction of water movement in response to each force.

decreases the peritubular capillary oncotic pressure. This in turn increases the back flux of NaCl and water from the lateral intercellular space into the tubular fluid, and thereby decreases net solute and water reabsorption across the proximal tubule. An increase in FF has the opposite effect.

The importance of Starling forces in regulating solute and water reabsorption by the proximal tubule is underscored by the phenomenon of **glomerulotubular (G-T) balance.** Spontaneous changes in GFR markedly alter the filtered load of sodium (filtered load = GFR × [Na⁺]). Without rapid adjustments in Na⁺ reabsorption to counter the changes, urinary Na⁺ excretion would fluctuate widely and disturb the Na⁺ balance of the whole body. However, spontaneous changes in GFR do not alter Na⁺ balance because of the phenomenon of G-T balance. *When body Na⁺ balance is normal, G-T balance refers to the simultaneous increase in Na⁺ and water reabsorption as a result of an increase in GFR and filtered load of Na⁺. Thus, a constant fraction of the filtered Na⁺ and water is reabsorbed from the proximal tubule despite variations in GFR.* The net result of G-T balance is to reduce the impact of GFR changes on the amount of Na⁺ and water excreted in the urine.

Two mechanisms are responsible for G-T balance. One is related to the oncotic and hydrostatic pressures between the peritubular capillaries and the lateral intercellular space (i.e., Starling forces). For example, an increase in GFR (at constant RPF) raises the protein concentration in the glomerular capillary plasma above normal. This protein-rich plasma leaves the glomerular capillaries, flows through the efferent arteriole, and enters the peritubular capillaries. The increased oncotic pressure in the peritubular capillaries augments the movement of solute and fluid from the lateral intercellular space into the peritubular capillaries. This action increases net solute and water reabsorption by the proximal tubule.

The second mechanism responsible for G-T balance is initiated by an increase in the filtered load of glucose and amino acids. As discussed earlier in this chapter, the reab-

sorption of Na⁺ in the early proximal tubule is coupled to that of glucose and amino acids. The rate of Na⁺ reabsorption therefore depends in part on the filtered load of glucose and amino acids. As GFR and the filtered load of glucose and amino acids increase, Na⁺ and water reabsorption also rise.

In addition to G-T balance, another mechanism minimizes changes in the filtered load of Na⁺. As discussed earlier in this chapter, an increase in GFR (and thus in the amount of Na⁺ filtered by the glomerulus) activates the tubuloglomerular feedback mechanism. This action returns GFR and the filtration of Na⁺ to normal values. Thus, spontaneous changes in GFR (e.g., those caused by changes in posture and blood pressure) increase the amount of Na⁺ filtered for only a few minutes. Until GFR returns to normal values, the mechanisms that underlie G-T balance maintain urinary Na⁺ excretion constant and thereby maintain Na⁺ homeostasis.

SUMMARY

1. The four major segments of the nephron (proximal tubule, Henle's loop, distal tubule, and collecting duct) determine the composition and volume of the urine by the processes of selective reabsorption of solutes and water and selective secretion of solutes.

2. Tubular reabsorption allows the kidneys to retain those substances that are essential and to regulate their levels in the plasma by altering the degree to which they are reabsorbed. The reabsorption of Na⁺, Cl⁻, other anions, and organic solutes together with water constitutes the major function of the nephron. Approximately 25,200 mEq of Na⁺ and 179 L of water are reabsorbed each day. The proximal tubule cells reabsorb 67% of the glomerular ultrafiltrate, and cells of the loop of Henle reabsorb about 25% of the filtered NaCl and about 15% of the filtered water. The distal segments of the nephron (distal tubule and collecting duct system) have a more limited reabsorptive capacity. However, the final

adjustments in the composition and volume of the urine, and most of the regulation by hormones and other factors, occur in distal segments.

3. Secretion of substances into tubular fluid is a means for excreting various by-products of metabolism. It also eliminates exogenous organic anions and bases (e.g., drugs) and pollutants from the body. Many organic compounds are bound to plasma proteins and are therefore unavailable for ultrafiltration. Secretion is thus their major route of excretion in the urine.

4. Various hormones (including angiotensin II, aldosterone, ADH, ANP, and urodilatin), sympathetic nerves, dopamine, and Starling forces regulate NaCl reabsorption by the kidneys. ADH is the major hormone that regulates water reabsorption.

BIBLIOGRAPHY

Journal articles

Aronson PS: Role of ion exchanges in mediating NaCl transport in the proximal tubule, *Kidney Int* 49(6):1665, 1996.

Burckhardt G, Bahn A, Wolff NA: Molcular physiology of renal p-aminohippurate secretion, *News Physiol Sci* 16:114, 2001.

De la Rosa A et al: Structure and regulation of amiloride-sensitive sodium channels, *Annu Rev Physiol* 62:573, 2000.

Guay-Woodford LM: Overview: the genetics of renal disease, *Semin Nephrol* 19:312, 1999.

Herbert SC: Molecular mechanisms, *Semin Nephrol* 19:504, 1999.

Inui KI, Masuda S, Saito H: Cellular and molecular aspects of drug transport in the kidney, *Kidney Int* 58:944, 2000.

Knepper MA, Brooks HL: Regulation of the sodium transporters NHE3, NKCC2, and NCC in the kidney, *Curr Opin Nephrol Hypertens* 10(5):655, 2001.

Meyer M, Forssmann K: The renal urodilatin system: clinical implications, *Cardiovasc Res* 51(3):450, 2001.

Murer H et al: Proximal tubular phosphate reabsorption: molecular mechanisms, *Physiol Rev* 80(4):1373, 2000.

Oh YS, Warnock DG: Disorders of the epithelial Na$^+$ channel in Liddle's syndrome and autosomal recessive pseudohypoaldosteronism type 1, *Exp Nephrol* 8(6):320, 2000.

Zelikovic I: Molecular pathophysiology of tubular transport disorders, *Pediatr Nephrol* 16:919, 2001.

Books and monographs

Burckhardt G, Pritchard JB: Organic anion and cation antiporters. In Seldin DW, Giebisch G, editors: *The kidney: physiology and pathophysiology,* ed 3, Philadelphia, 2000, Lippincott, Williams & Wilkins.

Ibrahim HN, Rosenberg ME, Hostetter TH: Proteinuria. In Seldin DW, Giebisch G, editors: *The kidney: physiology and pathophysiology,* ed 3, Philadelphia, 2000, Lippincott, Williams & Wilkins.

Lifton RP: Inherited disorders of renal salt homeostasis: insights from molecular genetic studies. In Seldin DW, Giebisch G, editors: *The kidney: physiology and pathophysiology,* ed 3, Philadelphia, 2000, Lippincott, Williams & Wilkins.

Moe OW, Berry CA, Rector RC Jr: Renal transport of glucose, amino acids, sodium, chloride, and water. In Brenner BM, editor: *Brenner and Rector's the kidney,* ed 6, Philadelphia, 2000, WB Saunders.

Reeves WB, Andreoli TE: Sodium chloride transport in the loop of Henle, distal tubule, and collecting duct. In Seldin DW, Giebisch G, editors: *The kidney: physiology and pathophysiology,* ed 3, Philadelphia, 2000, Lippincott, Williams & Wilkins.

Silbernagel S, Gekle M: Amino acids and oligopeptides, In Seldin DW, Giebisch G, editors: *The kidney: physiology and pathophysiology,* ed 3, Philadelphia, 2000, Lippincott, Williams & Wilkins.

chapter thirty-six

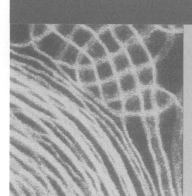

Control of Body Fluid Osmolality and Volume

The kidneys maintain the osmolality and volume of the body fluids within a narrow range by regulating the excretion of water and NaCl, respectively. This chapter discusses the regulation of renal water excretion (urine concentration and dilution) and NaCl excretion. As an introduction to this material, we will review the normal volume and composition of the various body fluid compartments.

THE BODY FLUID COMPARTMENTS

Volumes of Body Fluid Compartments

Water accounts for approximately 60% of body weight. Individual water content varies with the amount of adipose tissue; the greater the amount of adipose tissue, the smaller is the fraction of body weight attributable to water. Water content of the body also varies with age. In the newborn infant, water constitutes about 75% of body weight. This amount decreases to the adult value of 60% by the age of 1 year.

As illustrated in Fig. 36-1, **total body water** is distributed between two major compartments, which are separated by the cell membrane. The **intracellular fluid (ICF)** compartment is the larger compartment; it contains approximately two thirds of total body water. The remaining one third is contained in the **extracellular fluid (ECF)** compartment. Expressed as percentages of body weight, the volumes of total body water, ICF, and ECF can be estimated as*

$$\text{total body water} = 0.6 \times (\text{body weight})$$
$$\text{ICF} = 0.4 \times (\text{body weight}) \qquad (36\text{-}1)$$
$$\text{ECF} = 0.2 \times (\text{body weight})$$

The ECF compartment is subdivided into **interstitial fluid (ISF)** and **plasma;** these compartments are separated by the capillary wall. The interstitial fluid, which represents the

*In these and all subsequent calculations, it is assumed that 1 L of fluid (e.g., ICF and ECF) has a mass of 1 kg. This assumption allows interconversion between units of osmolality and volume.

fluid surrounding the cells in the various tissues of the body, comprises three fourths of the ECF volume. Included in this compartment is water contained within bone and dense connective tissue. The plasma volume represents the remaining one fourth of the ECF.

Composition of Body Fluid Compartments

The concentrations of the major cations and anions in the ECF and ICF are listed in Table 36-1. Na^+ is the major cation of the ECF, and Cl^- and HCO_3^- are the major anions. Because these compartments are separated only by the capillary wall, which is freely permeable to small ions, the ionic composition of the two major compartments of the ECF (interstitial fluid and plasma) is similar. *The major difference between the composition of the ISF and that of plasma is that the plasma contains significantly more protein.* Although the presence of protein in the plasma can affect the distribution of cations and anions across the capillary wall by the Gibbs-Donnan effect (see Chapter 2), this effect is normally quite small, and the ionic composition of the interstitial fluid and plasma can be considered identical.

Because of its abundance, Na^+ (and its attendant anions Cl^- and HCO_3^-) is the major determinant of the osmolality of the ECF. Accordingly, a rough estimate of the ECF osmolality can be obtained by simply doubling the sodium concentration ($[Na^+]$). For example, if the plasma $[Na^+]$ is 145 mEq/L, the osmolality of plasma and thus of the body fluids can be estimated as follows:

$$\text{plasma osmolality} = 2 \times (\text{plasma } [Na^+]) =$$
$$290 \text{ mOsm/kg } H_2O \qquad (36\text{-}2)$$

The normal plasma osmolality ranges from approximately 285 to 295 mOsm/kg H_2O. Because water is in osmotic equilibrium across the capillary wall and the plasma membrane of cells, measuring the plasma osmolality also provides a measure of the osmolality of the ECF and ICF.

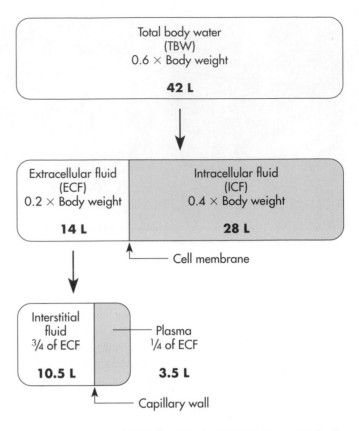

■ **Fig. 36-1** Relationship between the volumes of the major body fluid compartments. The actual values shown are calculated for a 70-kg individual.

In clinical situations, a more accurate estimate of the plasma osmolality is obtained by also considering the contribution of glucose and urea to plasma osmolality. Accordingly, plasma osmolality can be estimated as follows:

$$\text{plasma osmolality} = 2(\text{plasma}[Na^+]) + \frac{[\text{glucose}]}{18} + \frac{[\text{urea}]}{2.8} \quad (36\text{-}3)$$

The glucose and urea concentrations are expressed in units of milligrams per deciliter (if we divide glucose by 18 and urea by 2.8, we can convert from the units of mg/dl to mmol/L and thus to mOsm/kg H_2O).* This estimation of plasma osmolality is especially useful when dealing with patients who have an elevated plasma [glucose] secondary to diabetes mellitus, **and in patients with** chronic renal failure, **whose plasma [urea] is elevated. However, urea and glucose are not "effective osmoles" in the determination of the effect of changes in plasma osmolality on shifts of fluid between the ICF and ECF.† Therefore, multiplying the plasma [Na$^+$] by two provides the best estimate of the effective osmolality of the plasma. Thus effective osmolality is most important in determining the impact of changes in body fluid osmolality on ICF and ECF volumes.**

In contrast to ECF, the [Na$^+$] of ICF is low. K$^+$ is the predominant cation of this compartment. This asymmetric distribution of Na$^+$ and K$^+$ across the plasma membrane is maintained by the activity of the ubiquitous Na$^+$,K$^+$-ATPase. By its action, Na$^+$ is pumped out of the cell in exchange for K$^+$. The anion composition of ICF also differs markedly from that of ECF; [Cl$^-$] and [HCO$_3^-$] of ICF are lower than those of ECF. The major ICF anions are phosphates, organic anions, and proteins.

Fluid Exchange Between Body Fluid Compartments

Water moves freely between the various body fluid compartments. Two forces determine this movement: hydrostatic pressure and osmotic pressure. **Hydrostatic pressure** is generated by the pumping of the heart (and the effect of gravity on the column of blood in the vessels). Hydrostatic pressure together with the **osmotic pressure** of the plasma proteins (oncotic pressure) are important determinants of fluid movement across capillary walls (see Chapter 20), whereas osmotic pressure differences between the ICF and ECF are responsible for fluid movement across cell membranes. Because the plasma membranes of cells are highly permeable to water, a change in the osmolality of either the ICF or ECF results in the rapid movement of water between these compartments. Thus, except for transient changes, the ICF and ECF compartments are in osmotic equilibrium.

In contrast to the movement of water, the movement of ions across cell membranes is variable and depends on the presence of specific membrane transporters (see Chapter

---

*The [urea] in plasma is measured as the portion of nitrogen in the urea molecule, or blood urea nitrogen (BUN).

†A solute can exert an osmotic pressure only if it does not cross the cell membrane; such solutes are termed effective osmoles. Because urea and glucose freely cross many cell membranes, they are considered ineffective osmoles.

■ Table 36-1 Distribution of some cations and anions between extracellular fluid (ECF) and intracellular fluid (ICF)

		ECF	*ICF*
Na$^+$	(mEq/L)	145	12
K$^+$	(mEq/L)	4	150
Ca^{2+}	(mEq/L)	5	0.001
Cl$^-$	(mEq/L)	105	5
HCO$_3$	(mEq/L)	25	12
Pi	(mEq/L)	2	100
pH		7.4	7.1

The ICF concentrations are estimates from skeletal muscle, and include amounts bound to intracellular proteins and free within the cytosol. Intracellular phosphate (P$_i$) is primarily in the form of organic molecules [e.g., adenosine triphosphate (ATP)].

35). Consequently, a useful starting point in analyzing the fluid exchange between ICF and ECF under pathophysiological conditions is to assume that appreciable shifts of ions between the compartments do not occur. This assumption about the movement of fluids between ICF and ECF is outlined in the fluid shift analysis below. To illustrate this approach, consider what happens when solutions containing various amounts of NaCl are added to the ECF.*

Example 1: addition of isotonic NaCl to ECF. Addition of an isotonic NaCl solution (e.g., intravenous infusion of 0.9% NaCl: osmolality ≈ 290 mOsm/kg H$_2$O)† to the ECF increases the volume of this compartment by the volume of fluid administered. Because this fluid has the same osmolality as ECF, and therefore also ICF, no driving force for fluid movement exists between these compartments. Therefore there will be no movement of water, and the volume of the ICF does not change. Although Na$^+$ can cross cell membranes, it is effectively restricted to the ECF by the activity of the Na$^+$,K$^+$-ATPase, which is present in all cells. Therefore, no net movement of the infused NaCl into the cells occurs.

Principles for Analysis of Fluid Shifts between ICF and ECF

* The volumes of the various body fluid compartments can be estimated in the normal adult by the following:

(36-4)

*Fluids are usually administered intravenously. When electrolyte solutions are infused by this route, rapid (i.e., minutes) equilibration occurs between plasma and interstitial fluid, because of the high permeability of the capillary wall to water and electrolytes. Thus, these fluids are essentially added to the entire ECF.

†0.9% NaCl solution has a concentration of 154 mEq/L. Because NaCl does not dissociate completely (i.e., 1.88 osmoles/mole), the osmolality of this solution is 290 mOsm/kg H$_2$O, or essentially isoosmotic to the body fluids. Because NaCl is an effective osmole, a 0.9% solution is also isotonic.

* All exchanges of water and solutes with the external environment occur through the ECF (e.g., intravenous infusion, intake, or loss via the gastrointestinal tract). Changes in ICF are secondary to fluid shifts between ECF and ICF. Fluid shifts occur only if perturbation of the ECF alters its osmolality.
* Except for brief periods (seconds to minutes) ICF and ECF are in osmotic equilibrium. A measurement of plasma osmolality provides a measure of both ECF and ICF osmolality.
* For the sake of simplification, it can be assumed that equilibration between ICF and ECF occurs only by movement of water, and not by movement of osmotically active solutes.
* Conservation of mass must be maintained. This principle is especially important in situations in which either water and/or solutes are added to or excreted from the body.

Example 2: addition of hypotonic NaCl to ECF. Addition of a hypotonic NaCl solution to ECF (e.g., intravenous infusion of 0.45% NaCl: osmolality ≈ 145 mOsm/kg H$_2$O) decreases the osmolality of this compartment and causes water to move into the ICF. After osmotic equilibration is reached, the osmolalities of ICF and ECF are equal, but lower than before the infusion, and the volume of each compartment is increased. The increase in ECF volume is greater than the increase in ICF volume.

Example 3: addition of hypertonic NaCl to ECF. Addition of a hypertonic NaCl solution to ECF (e.g., intravenous infusion of 3% NaCl: osmolality ≈ 1000 mOsm/kg H$_2$O) increases the osmolality of this compartment and causes water to move out of cells. After osmotic equilibration is reached, the osmolalities of ECF and ICF are equal. The volume of ECF is increased, whereas that of ICF is decreased. The increase in ECF volume includes the volume of the infused solution, plus the volume of fluid that shifts out of ICF into ECF.

Intravenous solutions are available in many formulations. The type of fluid administered to a particular patient is dictated by the patient's need. For example, if the patient's vascular volume needs to be increased, a solution containing substances that have low permeability across the capillary wall is infused (e.g., 5% albumin solution). The oncotic pressure generated by the albumin molecules causes fluid to be retained in the vascular compartment, thus expanding its volume. Expansion of ECF is accomplished most often with isotonic saline solutions (e.g., 0.9% NaCl). As already noted, administration of an isotonic NaCl solution does not generate an osmotic pressure gradient across the plasma membrane of cells. Therefore, the entire volume of infused solution remains in the ECF. Patients whose body fluids are hyperosmotic may need hypotonic solutions. These solutions may be hypotonic NaCl [e.g., 0.45% NaCl or 5% dextrose in water

(D_5W)]. Administration of the D_5W solution is equivalent to infusion of distilled water, because the dextrose is ultimately metabolized to CO_2 and water. Administration of these fluids increases the volumes of both ICF and ECF. Finally, patients whose body fluids are hypotonic may need hypertonic solutions. These solutions, which are typically NaCl-containing solutions (e.g., 3% and 5% NaCl), will expand the volume of ECF but decrease the volume of ICF. Other constituents, such as electrolytes (e.g., K^+ or drugs), can be added to intravenous solutions to tailor the therapy to the patient's fluid, electrolyte, and metabolic needs.

CONTROL OF BODY FLUID OSMOLALITY: URINE CONCENTRATION AND DILUTION

The kidneys are responsible for regulating water balance, and under most conditions are the major route for elimination of water from the body (Table 36-2). Other routes of water loss from the body include evaporation from the cells of the skin and the respiratory passages. Collectively, water loss by these routes is termed **insensible water loss,** because the individual is unaware of its occurrence. Additional water can be lost by the production of sweat. Water loss by this mechanism can increase dramatically in a hot environment, with exercise, or in the presence of fever (Table 36-3). Finally, water can be lost from the gastrointestinal tract. Fecal water loss is normally small but increases with diarrhea. Gastrointestinal water losses can also occur with vomiting.

Water loss in sweat, feces, and evaporation from the lungs and skin is not regulated. In contrast, *the renal excretion of water is tightly regulated to maintain water balance.* The maintenance of water balance requires that water intake precisely match water loss from the body. If intake exceeds losses, positive water balance exists. Conversely, when intake is less than losses, negative water balance exists.

When water intake is low or water losses increase, the kidneys conserve water by producing a small volume of urine that is hyperosmotic with respect to plasma. When water intake is high, a large volume of hypoosmotic urine is produced. In a normal individual, urine osmolality can vary from approximately 50 to 1200 mOsm/kg H_2O, and the corresponding urine volume can vary from near 18 L/day to as little as 0.5 L/day.

When the maintenance of water balance is disrupted, the body fluid osmolality is altered. These alterations are usually measured by changes in plasma osmolality (P_{osm}). Because the major determinant of plasma osmolality is Na^+ (with its anions Cl^- and HCO_3^-), disorders of water balance will result in alterations in the plasma [Na^+]. When evaluating an abnormal plasma [Na^+] in an individual, it is tempting to suspect a problem in Na^+ balance. However, the problem most often relates to water balance, not Na^+ balance. Changes in Na^+ balance result in alterations in the volume of extracellular fluid, not its osmolality.

■ **Table 36-2**   Normal routes of water gain and loss in adults at room temperature (23°C)

Route	ml/day
Water intake	
Fluid*	1200
In food	1000
Metabolically produced from food	300
TOTAL	2500
Water output	
Insensible	700
Sweat	100
Feces	200
Urine	1500
TOTAL	2500

*Fluid intake varies widely for both social and cultural reasons.

■ **Table 36-3**   Effect of environmental temperature and exercise on water loss and intake in adults (in ml/day)

	Normal temperature	Hot weather	Prolonged heavy exercise
Water loss			
Insensible loss			
Skin	350	350	350
Lungs	350	250	650
Sweat	100	1400	5000
Feces	200	200	200
Urine	1500	1200	500
Total loss	2500	3400	6700
Water intake to maintain water balance	2500	3400	6700

In hot weather and during prolonged heavy exercise, water balance is maintained only if the individual increases water intake to match the increased loss of water in sweat. Decreased water excretion by the kidneys alone is insufficient to maintain water balance.

In the clinical setting, **hypoosmolality** (a reduction in plasma osmolality) shifts water into cells, and this process results in cell swelling. Symptoms associated with hypoosmolality are related primarily to swelling of brain cells. For example, a rapid fall in P_{osm} can alter neurological function and thereby cause nausea, malaise, headache, confusion, lethargy, seizures, and coma. When P_{osm} is increased (i.e., **hyperosmolality**), water is lost from cells. The symptoms of an increase in P_{osm} are also primarily neurological, and they include lethargy, weakness, seizures, coma, and even death.

The kidneys control water excretion independently of their ability to control the excretion of a number of other physiologically important substances (e.g., Na^+, K^+, H^+, urea). Indeed, this dual control is necessary for survival, because it allows the kidneys to achieve water balance without upsetting the other homeostatic functions of the kidneys.

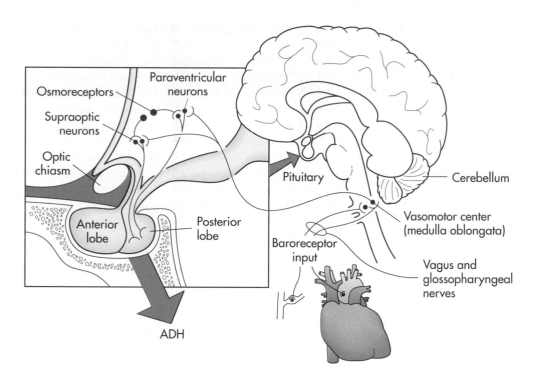

■ **Fig. 36-2** Anatomy of the hypothalamus and pituitary gland (midsagittal section) depicting the pathways for antidiuretic hormone (ADH) secretion. Also shown are pathways involved in regulating ADH secretion. Afferent fibers from the baroreceptors are carried in the vagus and glossopharyngeal nerves. The vasomotor center includes the solitary tract nucleus. The closed box gives an expanded view of the hypothalamus and pituitary gland.

The following sections discuss the mechanisms by which the kidneys excrete either hypoosmotic (dilute) or hyperosmotic (concentrated) urine. The control of antidiuretic hormone secretion and its important role in regulating the excretion of water by the kidneys are also explained (see also Chapter 43).

Antidiuretic Hormone

Antidiuretic hormone (ADH), or vasopressin, acts on the kidneys to regulate the volume and osmolality of the urine. When plasma ADH levels are low, a large volume of urine is excreted **(diuresis),** and the urine is dilute.* When plasma ADH levels are elevated, a small volume of urine is excreted **(antidiuresis),** and the urine is concentrated.

ADH is a small peptide nine amino acids in length. It is synthesized by neuroendocrine cells located within the supraoptic and paraventricular nuclei of the hypothalamus (see also Chapter 43). The synthesized hormone is packaged in granules, which are transported down the axon of the cell and then stored in the nerve terminals located in the neurohypophysis (posterior pituitary). The anatomy of the hypothalamus and pituitary gland is illustrated in Fig. 36-2.

Several factors influence the secretion of ADH by the posterior pituitary. The two physiological regulators of ADH secretion are the osmolality of the body fluids (osmotic) and the volume and pressure of the vascular system (hemodynamic). Other factors that can alter ADH secretion include nausea (stimulates), atrial natriuretic peptide (ANP) (inhibits), and angiotensin II (stimulates). A number of drugs, prescription and nonprescription, also affect ADH secretion.

For example, nicotine stimulates ADH secretion, whereas ethanol inhibits its secretion (see also Chapter 43).

Osmotic control of ADH secretion. *A change in the body fluid osmolality is the primary regulator of ADH secretion.* Changes in osmolality as small as 1% are sufficient to significantly alter ADH secretion. Cells involved in sensing changes in body fluid osmolality are located in the hypothalamus but are distinct from those that synthesize ADH.* These cells, called **osmoreceptors,** appear to behave as osmometers, and sense changes in body fluid osmolality by either shrinking or swelling. Importantly, osmoreceptors respond only to solutes that are **effective osmoles.** For example, urea does not affect the function of the osmoreceptors and is thus an **ineffective osmole.** Elevation of the plasma urea concentration alone has little effect on ADH secretion.

When the effective osmolality of the body fluids increases, osmoreceptors send signals to the ADH-synthesizing cells in the supraoptic and paraventricular nuclei of the hypothalamus, and ADH secretion is stimulated. Conversely, when the effective osmolality of the body fluid is reduced, secretion is inhibited. Because ADH is rapidly broken down in the plasma, circulating levels can be reduced to zero within minutes after secretion is inhibited. As a result, the ADH system can respond rapidly to fluctuations in body fluid osmolality.

Figure 36-3, *A* illustrates the effect of changes in body fluid osmolality (measured as plasma osmolality) on circulating ADH levels. The **set point** of the system is defined as the plasma osmolality value at which ADH secretion begins to increase. Below this set point, virtually no ADH is

---

*Diuresis is a general term for a large urinary output. Output of urine that contains primarily water is called a water diuresis.

*The osmoreceptor cells are located outside the blood-brain barrier in the anterior wall of the third ventricle (organum vasculosum of the lamina terminalis, and perhaps also the subfornical organ).

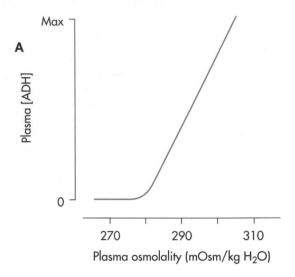

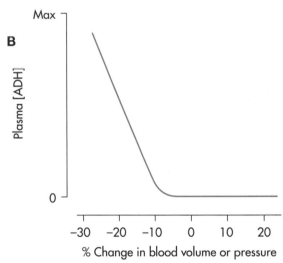

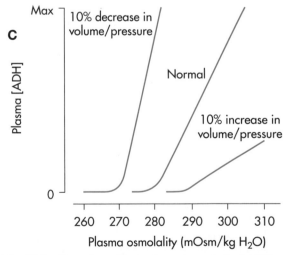

■ **Fig. 36-3** Osmotic and hemodynamic control of ADH secretion. **A,** Effect of changes in plasma osmolality (constant blood volume and pressure) on plasma ADH levels. **B,** Effect of changes in blood volume or pressure (constant plasma osmolality) on plasma ADH levels. **C,** Interactions between osmolar and blood volume and pressure stimuli on ADH secretion.

released. Above the set point, the slope of the relationship is quite steep, reflecting the sensitivity of this system. The set point varies among individuals and is genetically determined. In healthy adults, the set point varies from 280 to 295 mOsm/kg H_2O. Several physiological factors, such as alterations in blood volume and pressure, can also change the set point, as discussed below. Also, pregnancy is associated with a decrease in the set point.

Hemodynamic control of ADH secretion. A decrease in blood volume or arterial pressure also stimulates ADH secretion. The receptors activated by this response are located in both the low-pressure (left atrium and large pulmonary vessels) and the high-pressure (aortic arch and carotid sinus) sides of the circulatory system (see also Chapters 21 and 22). Because they are located in the high capacitance side of the circulatory system, low-pressure receptors respond to overall vascular volume. High-pressure receptors, on the other hand, respond to arterial pressure. Both groups of receptors are sensitive to stretch of the wall of the structure in which they are located (e.g., cardiac atrial wall, wall of aortic arch) and are thus called **baroreceptors.** Signals from these receptors are carried in afferent fibers of the vagus and glossopharyngeal nerves to the brainstem (solitary tract nucleus of the medulla oblongata), which is part of the center that regulates heart rate and blood pressure (see Chapter 22). Signals are then relayed from the brainstem to the ADH secretory cells of the supraoptic and paraventricular hypothalamic nuclei. Normally, signals from the baroreceptors tonically inhibit ADH secretion. However, when blood volume or arterial pressure decreases, this inhibitory input is overridden and ADH secretion is stimulated. The sensitivity of the baroreceptor system is less than that of the osmoreceptors; a 5% to 10% decrease in blood volume or arterial pressure is required before ADH secretion is stimulated. The response of the baroreceptor system is illustrated in Fig. 36-3, *B*.

Alterations in blood volume or arterial pressure also affect the secretion of ADH in response to changes in body fluid osmolality (Fig. 36-3, *C*). With a decrease in blood volume or arterial pressure, the set point shifts to lower osmolality values, and the slope of the relationship is steeper. In an individual with circulatory collapse, the shift in set point allows the kidney to continue to conserve water, even though the water retention will reduce the osmolality of the body fluids. With an increase in blood volume or arterial pressure, the opposite response occurs and the set point shifts to higher osmolality values and the slope of the relationship is decreased.

Inadequate release of ADH from the posterior pituitary results in excretion of large volumes of dilute urine **(polyuria).** To compensate for this loss of water, the individual must ingest large volumes of water **(polydipsia)** to maintain body fluid osmolality constant. If the individual is deprived of water, the body fluids will become hyperosmotic. This condition is called **central diabetes** insipidus, neurogenic diabetes insipidus, or **pituitary diabetes insipidus.** Rarely, central diabetes insipidus is inherited. It occurs more commonly after head trauma, with brain neoplasms, or with brain infections. Individuals with central diabetes insipidus have a urine-concentrating defect that can be corrected by administration of exogenous ADH.

The **syndrome of inappropriate ADH secretion (SIADH)** is a common clinical problem. SIADH is characterized by plasma ADH levels that are elevated above those expected on the basis of body fluid osmolality and blood volume or arterial pressure (hence the term inappropriate). Individuals with SIADH retain water (i.e., reduce renal excretion). If water intake is not reduced in parallel, their body fluids become progressively hypoosmotic. Characteristically, the urine of these individuals is more concentrated than expected on the basis of the low body fluid osmolality. SIADH can be caused by infections and neoplasms of the brain, drugs (e.g., antitumor agents), pulmonary diseases, and carcinoma of the lung.

Many different mutations in the gene encoding the ADH molecule have been shown to cause the autosomal dominant form of central diabetes insipidus. The ADH gene is located on chromosome 20, and encodes for a preprohormone, which is ultimately processed into three peptides: ADH, a glycoprotein, and neurophysin. In these patients, mutations have been found in all regions of the gene; however, the most common mutation occurs in the portion of the gene that encodes for neurophysin. With these mutations there is defective trafficking of the preprohormone, which accumulates in the rough endoplasmic reticulum. It is thought that this abnormal accumulation of the preprohormone ultimately leads to the death of the ADH secretory cells in the supraoptic and paraventricular nuclei.

ADH actions on the kidney. *The primary action of ADH on the kidneys is to increase the permeability of the collecting duct to water.* It also increases the permeability of the medullary portion of the collecting duct to urea.

The actions of ADH on the water permeability of the collecting duct have been extensively studied. ADH binds to a receptor on the basolateral membrane of the cell. This is called the V2 receptor (vasopressin 2 receptor).* Binding of ADH to this receptor, which is coupled to adenylyl cyclase via a stimulatory G protein (G_s), increases the intracellular levels of cyclic adenosine monophosphate (cAMP). The rise in intracellular cAMP activates **protein kinase A,** which prompts the insertion of intracellular vesicles containing

water channels* into the apical membrane of the cell. These water channels are preformed and reside in vesicles located beneath the cell's apical membrane. When ADH is removed, the water channels return to their original position within the cell, and the apical membrane is once again impermeable to water. The shuttling of water channels into and out of the apical membrane provides a mechanism for rapidly controlling membrane water permeability. Because the basolateral membrane is freely permeable to water, any water that enters the cell through apical membrane water channels exits across the basolateral membrane, resulting in the net absorption of water from the tubule lumen into the peritubular blood.

In addition to the action of ADH just described, it also has a long-term effect on the collecting duct by altering the expression of aquaporin 2. In states of prolonged water deprivation ADH (and perhaps other factors) increases the expression of the aquaporin 2 gene, and thereby the amount of aquaporin 2 in the collecting cell. Thus, the collecting duct has a higher water permeability, which further enhances the kidneys' ability to conserve water. Conversely, aquaporin 2 expression in the collecting duct is reduced when the kidneys must excrete water over prolonged periods of time.

The collecting ducts of some individuals do not respond normally to ADH. These individuals cannot maximally concentrate their urine. Consequently, they suffer from polyuria and polydipsia. This entity is termed **nephrogenic diabetes insipidus** to distinguish it from central diabetes insipidus (see Chapter 43). Although nephrogenic diabetes insipidus can be inherited, it is most often caused by other factors such as metabolic disorders (e.g., hypercalcemia) or certain drugs. For example, approximately 30% to 40% of individuals taking the medication lithium for bipolar disorder develop some degree of nephrogenic diabetes insipidus.

ADH also increases the permeability of the terminal portion of the inner medullary collecting duct to urea. Urea enters the collecting duct cell across the apical membrane via a specific urea transporter (UT1), and exits the cell across the basolateral membrane by a different transporter (UT4). ADH (acting through adenylyl cyclase, cAMP, and protein kinase A) phosphorylates the apical membrane transporter, and thereby increases the movement of urea into the cell and ultimately across the cell. (The urea permeability of the basolateral membrane is high, and ADH does not

---

*A different ADH receptor (V_1 receptor) is located in blood vessels. This receptor mediates the vasoconstrictor response to ADH. It is this action of ADH that accounts for its alternative name of vasopressin.

*The water channels involved in the collecting duct response to ADH are part of a family of integral membrane proteins called **aquaporins.** The aquaporin-2 channel is inserted into the apical membrane of collecting duct principal cells in response to ADH. Different channels (aquaporin-3 and aquaporin-4) mediate the movement of water across the basolateral membrane of the principal cell. Water movement across the proximal tubule and descending thin limb of Henle's loop is mediated by yet another water channel (aquaporin-1).

appear to alter the activity of the urea transporter in this membrane.) Increased osmolality of the renal medulla also increases the urea permeability of the collecting duct. This effect is separate and additive to that of ADH.

The inherited forms of nephrogenic diabetes insipidus result from mutations in either the ADH receptor (V_2) or aquaporin 2. The gene for the V_2 receptor is located on the X chromosome. Thus this inherited form is X-linked. Most of the mutations in the V_2 receptor result in defective trafficking and trapping of the receptor in the rough endoplasmic reticulum; only a few mutations result in the expression of a receptor on the membrane of the cell that will not bind ADH. The gene encoding for aquaporin 2 is located on chromosome 12, and is inherited as an autosomal recessive defect. This is a much less common form of nephrogenic diabetes insipidus (<10% of all inherited forms of the disease), and the mutations usually result in a protein that is trapped in the rough endoplasmic reticulum.

Many of the aquired forms of nephrogenic diabetes insipidus are the result of decreased expression of aquaporin 2 in the collecting duct. Decreased expression of aquaporin 2 has been documented in the urine concentration defects associated with hypokalemia, lithium ingestion, ureteral obstruction, and hypercalcemia. Conversely, increased expression of aquaporin 2 is seen in states of renal water retention (e.g., congestive heart failure and pregnancy).

Thirst

In addition to affecting the secretion of ADH, *changes in plasma osmolality, blood volume, or arterial pressure alter the perception of thirst.* When body fluid osmolality is increased or the blood volume and pressure are reduced, the individual perceives thirst. Of these stimuli, hyperosmolality is the most potent. An increase of only 2% to 3% in plasma osmolality will produce a strong desire to drink, whereas decreases of 10% to 15% in blood volume and arterial pressure are required to produce the same response.

The neural centers involved in regulating water intake (the thirst center) are located in the anterolateral region of the hypothalamus (subfornical organ and organum vasculosum of the lamina terminalis). Even though they are located in the same region of the hypothalamus, the cells of the thirst center appear to be distinct from the osmoreceptors involved in ADH secretion. However, like the osmoreceptors involved in ADH secretion, thirst center cells respond only to effective osmoles (e.g., NaCl). Even less is known about the pathways involved in the thirst response to decreased blood volume or arterial pressure, but it is believed that the pathways are the same as those involved in regulation of ADH secretion. Angiotensin II, acting on cells of the thirst center (subfornical organ), also evokes the sensation of thirst. Because angiotensin II levels are increased when blood volume and pressure are reduced (see page 675), this effect of angiotensin II contributes to the homeostatic response that restores and maintains the body fluids at their normal volume.

The sensation of thirst is satisfied by the act of drinking even before sufficient water is absorbed from the gastrointestinal tract to correct the plasma osmolality. Oropharyngeal and upper gastrointestinal receptors appear to be involved in this response. However, relief of the thirst sensation via these receptors is short-lived. Thirst is completely satisfied only when the plasma osmolality, blood volume, and arterial pressure are corrected.

The ADH and thirst systems work in concert to maintain water balance. An increase in plasma osmolality invokes drinking and, via ADH action on the kidneys, conservation of water. Conversely, when plasma osmolality is decreased, thirst is suppressed and, in the absence of ADH, renal water excretion is enhanced.

With adequate access to water, the thirst mechanism can prevent the development of hyperosmolality. Indeed, this mechanism is responsible for the polydipsia that occurs in response to the polyuria of both **central and nephrogenic diabetes insipidus.**

Water intake is also influenced by social and cultural factors. Thus, individuals ingest water even in the absence of the thirst sensation. Normally, the kidneys are able to excrete this excess water, since they can excrete up to 18 L/day of urine. However, in some instances the volume of water ingested exceeds the capacity of the kidneys to excrete water. Body fluids then become hypoosmotic.

The maximum amount of water that can be excreted by the kidneys depends on the amount of solute excreted, which in turn depends on food intake. For example, with maximally dilute urine (U_{osm} = 50 mOsm/kg H_2O), the maximum urine output of 18 L/day will be achieved only if the solute excretion rate is 900 mmol/day.

$$U_{osm} = \text{Solute excretion/volume excretion} = $$
$$50 \text{ mOsm/kg } H_2O = 900 \text{ mmol/18 L} \qquad (36\text{-}5)$$

If solute excretion is reduced, as commonly occurs in the elderly with reduced food intake, the maximum urine output will decrease. For example, if solute excretion is only 400 mmol, then a maximum urine output (at U_{osm} = 50 mOsm/kg H_2O) of only 8 L/day can be achieved. Thus, individuals with reduced food intake have a reduced capacity to excrete water.

Renal Mechanisms for Dilution and Concentration of Urine

Under normal circumstances, the excretion of water is regulated separately from the excretion of solutes (e.g., NaCl). For this separate regulation to occur, the kidneys must excrete urine that is either hypoosmotic or hyperosmotic with respect to the body fluids. This ability to excrete urine of varying osmolality in turn requires that solute be separated from water at some point along the nephron. As discussed in Chapter 35, reabsorption of solute in the proximal tubule results in the reabsorption of a proportional amount of water. Hence, solute and water are not separated in this portion of the nephron. Moreover, separation does not occur regardless of whether the kidneys excrete dilute or concentrated urine. *Henle's loop, in particular the thick ascending limb, is the major nephron site where the separation of solute and water occurs.* Thus, the excretion of both dilute and concentrated urine requires normal function of Henle's loop.

The production of hypoosmotic urine is conceptually easy to understand. The nephron must simply reabsorb solute from the tubular fluid and not allow water to follow. As just noted, and as described in greater detail below, reabsorption of solute occurs primarily in the thick ascending limb of Henle's loop. Under appropriate conditions (i.e., in the absence of ADH), the distal tubule and the collecting duct also participate in this process.

The excretion of a hyperosmotic urine is conceptually more difficult to understand. This process requires the removal of water from the tubular fluid, leaving solute behind. Because water can only move passively (driven by an osmotic gradient), the kidneys must generate a hyperosmotic environment that drives water removal from the tubular fluid. Such an environment is generated in the interstitial fluid of the renal medulla. Henle's loop, and especially the thick ascending limb, is critical for generating this hyperosmotic medullary environment. Once this hyperosmotic environment is established in the medullary interstitium, it drives water reabsorption from the collecting duct, and thereby concentrates the urine.

Figure 36-4 summarizes the essential features of the mechanisms whereby the kidneys excrete either a dilute *(A)* or a concentrated *(B)* urine. First, we consider how the kidneys excrete a dilute urine **(water diuresis),** when ADH levels are low or absent. The following numbers refer to those encircled in Fig. 36-4, *A*.

1. Fluid entering the descending thin limb of Henle's loop from the proximal tubule is isoosmotic with respect to plasma. This isoosmotic fluid reflects the essentially isoosmotic nature of solute and water reabsorption in the proximal tubule (see Chapter 35).
2. The descending thin limb is highly permeable to water but much less so to solutes such as NaCl and urea.* Consequently, as the fluid descends deeper into the hyperosmotic medulla, water is reabsorbed owing to the osmotic gradient that is set up across the descending thin limb. By this process, fluid at the bend of the loop has an osmolality equal to that of the surrounding interstitial fluid. However, although the osmolality of the tubular and interstitial fluids are similar at the bend of the loop, their compositions differ. The tubular fluid [NaCl] is greater than that of the surrounding interstitial fluid, but the [urea] of the tubular fluid is less than that of the interstitial fluid (see page 669).

---

*Urea is an ineffective osmole for many cells within the body, because it freely crosses the plasma membrane of these cells. However, in many portions of the nephron, urea permeability is quite low (Table 36-4). In these regions of the nephron, urea serves as an effective osmole and causes osmotic water movement.

3. The ascending thin limb is impermeable to water but permeable to NaCl and urea. Consequently, as tubular fluid moves up the ascending limb, NaCl is passively reabsorbed (because tubular fluid [NaCl] > interstitial fluid [NaCl]), while urea passively diffuses into the tubular fluid (because tubular fluid [urea] < interstitial fluid [urea]). The net effect is that the volume of the tubular fluid remains unchanged along the length of the thin ascending limb, but the [NaCl] decreases and the [urea] increases. Overall, the movement of NaCl out of the lumen of the thin ascending limb is greater than the movement of urea into the lumen, and the tubular fluid becomes diluted.
4. The thick ascending limb of Henle's loop is impermeable to water and urea. This portion of the nephron actively reabsorbs NaCl, thereby diluting the tubular fluid. Dilution occurs to such a degree that this segment is often referred to as the diluting segment of the kidney. Fluid leaving the thick ascending limb is hypoosmotic with respect to plasma (approximately 150 mOsm/kg H_2O).
5. The distal tubule and cortical portion of the collecting duct actively reabsorb NaCl but are impermeable to urea. In the absence of ADH, these segments are not permeable to water. Thus, when ADH is absent or present at low levels (i.e., decreased P_{osm}), the distal tubule and the cortical collecting duct are impermeable to water. Accordingly, the osmolality of tubule fluid in these segments is reduced further because NaCl is reabsorbed without water. Fluid entering the cortical portion of the collecting duct is hypoosmotic with respect to plasma (approximately 100 mOsm/kg H_2O).
6. The medullary collecting duct actively reabsorbs NaCl. Even in the absence of ADH, this segment is slightly permeable to water and urea. Consequently, some urea enters the collecting duct from the medullary interstitium, and a small volume of water is reabsorbed.
7. The urine will have an osmolality of $\approx$ 50 mOsm/kg H_2O and will contain low concentrations of NaCl and urea. The volume of urine excreted can be as much as 18 L/day, or approximately 10% of the glomerular filtration rate (GFR).

Next, we consider how the kidneys excrete a concentrated urine **(antidiuresis),** when P_{osm} and plasma ADH levels are high. The following numbers refer to those encircled in Fig. 36-4, *B*.

1–4. Steps 1 to 4 are similar when either a dilute or a concentrated urine is produced. An important point in understanding how a concentrated urine is produced is that while reabsorption of NaCl by the ascending thin and thick limbs of Henle's loop dilutes the tubular fluid, the reabsorbed NaCl accumulates in the medullary interstitium and raises its osmolality. The accumulation of NaCl in the medullary interstitium is critically important for the production of urine hyperosmotic to plasma, because it provides the osmotic driving force for water reabsorption by the collecting duct. The overall process by which Henle's

■ Fig. 36-4 A, Mechanism for the excretion of dilute urine (water diuresis). ADH is absent, and the collecting duct is essentially impermeable to water. Note that the osmolality of the medullary interstitium is reduced during water diuresis. **B,** Mechanism for the excretion of a concentrated urine (antidiuresis). Plasma ADH levels are maximal, and the collecting duct is highly permeable to water. Under this condition, the medullary interstitial gradient is maximal. The circled numbers correlate with the description in the text.

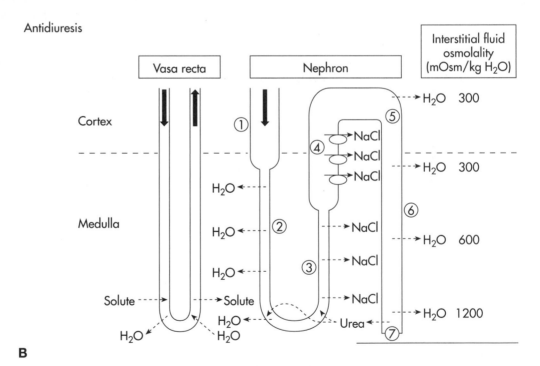

loop, and in particular the thick ascending limb, generates the hyperosmotic medullary interstitial gradient is termed **countercurrent multiplication.**[*]

5. Owing to NaCl reabsorption by the thick ascending limb of Henle's loop, fluid reaching the collecting duct is hypoosmotic with respect to the surrounding interstitial fluid. Thus, an osmotic gradient is established across the collecting duct. In the presence of ADH, which increases the water permeability of the collecting duct, water diffuses out of the tubule lumen, and the tubule fluid osmolality increases. This diffusion of water begins the process of urine concentration. The maximal osmolality that the fluid in the cortical collecting duct can attain is approximately 300 mOsm/kg H_2O, which is the osmolality of the surrounding interstitial fluid and plasma. Although the fluid at this point has the same osmolality as the fluid that entered the descending thin limb, its composition has been altered dramatically. Because of NaCl reabsorption by the preceding nephron segments, NaCl accounts for a much smaller portion of the total tubular fluid osmolality. Instead, the tubule fluid osmolality is accounted for by urea (filtered urea, plus urea added in the descending thin and ascending thin limbs of Henle's loop) and other nonreabsorbed solutes (e.g., K^+, creatinine).

6. The osmolality of the interstitial fluid in the medulla progressively increases from the corticomedullary junction, where it is approximately 300 mOsm/kg H_2O, to the papilla, where it is approximately 1200 mOsm/kg H_2O. Thus, an osmotic gradient exists between tubular fluid and the interstitial fluid along the entire medullary collecting duct. In the presence of ADH, which renders the medullary collecting duct permeable to water, the osmolality of tubular fluid increases as water is reabsorbed. Because the initial portion of the collecting duct is impermeable to urea, it remains in the tubular fluid, and its concentration in the tubular fluid increases. In the presence of ADH, the urea permeability of the last portion of the medullary collecting duct is increased. Because the urea concentration of the tubular fluid has been increased by

water reabsorption in the cortex and outer medulla, its concentration in the tubular fluid is greater than its concentration in the interstitial fluid, and some urea diffuses out of the tubule lumen into the medullary interstitium. The maximal osmolality that the fluid in the medullary collecting duct can attain is equal to that of the surrounding interstitial fluid. The major components of the tubular fluid within the medullary collecting ducts are substances that have either escaped reabsorption or have been secreted into the tubular fluid. Of these, urea is the most abundant.

7. The urine has an osmolality of 1200 mOsm/kg H_2O and contains high concentrations of urea and other nonreabsorbed solutes. Because urea in the tubular fluid equilibrates with urea in the medullary interstitial fluid, its concentration in the urine will be similar to that of the interstitium. Urine volume under this condition can be as low as 0.5 L/day.

Table 36-4 summarizes the transport and passive permeability properties of the nephron segments involved in the process of concentrating and diluting the urine. Water reabsorption by the proximal tubule (67% of filtered load) and the descending limb of Henle's loop (15% of filtered load) is relatively constant. Depending on the plasma ADH concentration, a variable amount of water is reabsorbed by the late distal tubule and collecting duct, such that water excretion ranges from 0.3% to 10% of the filtered load. During antidiuresis the largest volume of water is reabsorbed in the cortex (late distal tubule and cortical collecting duct). Much less is reabsorbed by the medullary collecting duct. This distribution of water reabsorption between cortical and medullary nephron segments helps maintain the hyperosmotic interstitial environment in the inner medulla, which in turn allows maximal urinary concentration.

Medullary interstitium. The interstitial fluid of the medulla is critically important in concentrating the urine, because the osmotic pressure of this fluid provides the driving force for reabsorbing water from both the descending thin limb of Henle's loop and the collecting duct. The principal components of the medullary interstitial fluid are NaCl and urea, but the concentration of these solutes is not uniform throughout the medulla (i.e., a gradient exists from cortex to papilla). Other solutes also accumulate in the medullary interstitium (e.g., NH_4^+ and K^+), but the most abundant solutes are NaCl and urea. For simplicity, we can assume that NaCl and urea are the only solutes. At the junction of the medulla with the cortex, the interstitial fluid has an osmolality of approximately 300 mOsm/kg H_2O, with virtually all osmoles attributable to NaCl. The concentrations of both NaCl and urea increase progressively as the tubular fluid moves deeper into the medulla. When a maximally concentrated urine is excreted, the medullary interstitial fluid osmolality is approximately 1200 mOsm/kg H_2O at the papilla (Fig. 36-4, *B*). Of this value, approximately 600 mOsm/kg H_2O is attributed to NaCl and 600 mOsm/kg H_2O to urea.

The medullary gradient for NaCl is created when NaCl reabsorbed by the nephron segments accumulates in the

---

[*]The term countercurrent multiplication derives from both the form and function of Henle's loop. Henle's loop consists of two parallel limbs with tubular fluid flowing in opposite directions (countercurrent flow). Fluid flows into the medulla in the descending limb, and out of the medulla in the ascending limb. The ascending limb is impermeable to water and reabsorbs solute from the tubular fluid. Thus, fluid within the ascending limb becomes diluted. This separation of solute and water by the ascending limb is termed the **single effect** of the countercurrent multiplication process. The solute removed from the ascending limb tubular fluid accumulates in the surrounding interstitial fluid and raises its osmolality. Because the descending limb is highly permeable to water, the increased osmolality of the medullary interstitium causes water to be absorbed and thereby concentrates the tubular fluid. The countercurrent flow within the descending and ascending limbs of Henle's loop magnifies, or "multiplies," the osmotic gradient between the tubular fluid in the descending and ascending limbs of Henle's loop.

■ Table 36-4   Transport and permeability properties of nephron segments involved in urine concentration and dilution

Tubule segment	Active transport	Passive permeability*			Effect of ADH
		NaCl	Urea	H₂O	
Henle's loop					
Descending thin limb	0	+	+	+++	
Ascending thin limb	0	+++	+	0	
Thick ascending limb	+++	+	0	0	
Distal tubule	+	+	0	0	
Collecting duct					
Cortex	+	+	0	0	↑ H₂O permeability
Medulla	+	+	++	+	↑ H₂O and urea permeability

*Permeability is proportional to the number of plus signs indicated: +, low permeability; +++, high permeability; 0, impermeable.

medulla during the process of countercurrent multiplication. The most important segment in this regard is the ascending limb (thick limb > thin limb) of Henle's loop. Urea accumulation within the medullary interstitium is more complex and occurs most effectively when a hyperosmotic urine is excreted (i.e., antidiuresis). When a dilute urine is produced, especially over extended periods of time, the osmolality of the medullary interstitium declines (compare panels *A* and *B* of Fig. 36-4). This reduced osmolality is almost entirely due to a decrease in the concentration of urea. This decrease in urea concentration reflects washout by the vasa recta and diffusion of urea from the interstitium into the tubular fluid within the medullary portion of the collecting duct (recall that the medullary collecting duct has a significant permeability to urea even in the absence of ADH; see Table 36-4).

Urea is generated by the liver as a result of protein metabolism, and enters the tubular fluid by glomerular filtration. As indicated in Table 36-4, the permeability to urea of most nephron segments involved in urinary concentration and dilution is relatively low, with the exception of the medullary collecting duct (especially in the presence of ADH). As fluid moves along the nephron, and as water is reabsorbed in the collecting duct (i.e., antidiuresis), the urea concentration in the tubular fluid increases. When this urea-rich tubular fluid reaches the medullary collecting duct, where the permeability to urea not only is high but is increased by ADH, urea diffuses down its concentration gradient into the medullary interstitial fluid, where it accumulates. When ADH levels are elevated, the urea within the collecting duct and the interstitium equilibrate. The resultant urea concentration of the urine will be equal to that of the medullary interstitium at the papilla, or approximately 600 mOsm/kg H₂O.

Some of the urea within the interstitium enters the descending thin and ascending thin limbs of Henle's loop. This urea is then trapped in the nephron until it again reaches the medullary collecting duct, where it can reenter the medullary interstitium. Thus, *urea recycles from the interstitium to the nephron, and back into the interstitium. This process of recycling serves to facilitate the accumulation of urea in the medullary interstitium.*

To summarize, the hyperosmotic medullary interstitium is essential for concentrating the tubular fluid within the collecting duct. Because water reabsorption is a passive process

driven by an osmotic gradient, the maximal concentration that the urine can attain is equal to that of the medullary interstitium at the papilla (approximately 1200 mOsm/kg H₂O). Because a hyperosmotic medullary interstitium is essential for urine concentration, any condition that reduces this gradient impairs the ability of the kidneys to maximally concentrate the urine.

It is apparent that the concentration of urea in the medullary interstitial fluid plays an important role in determining the osmolality of the urine. However, urea is not an effective osmole across the medullary collecting duct, because this part of the nephron has a high permeability to urea, especially in the presence of ADH. The role of effective and ineffective osmoles (e.g., urea) in the maintenance of whole body water balance is considered in more detail on page 659. The main point to remember about the role of urea within the medullary interstitium is that urea does not drive water reabsorption from the lumen of the collecting duct into the medullary interstitium. Instead, the urea in the tubular fluid and medullary interstitium equilibrates, especially at the slow tubular flow rates associated with the excretion of a concentrated urine. Thus, urine with a high urea concentration is excreted. It is the medullary interstitial NaCl concentration that is responsible for the reabsorption of water from the medullary collecting duct and thus for the concentration of nonurea solutes (e.g., NH₄⁺-salts, K⁺-salts, creatinine) in the urine.

Vasa recta function: countercurrent exchange. *The vasa recta, the capillary networks that supply blood to the medulla, are highly permeable to solute and water.* As with Henle's loop, the vasa recta form a parallel set of hairpin loops within the medulla (see Chapter 34). The vasa recta not only bring nutrients and oxygen to the tubules within the medulla, but more importantly remove excess water and solute, which are continuously added to the medullary interstitium by the nephron segments in this region. The ability of the vasa recta to maintain the medullary interstitial gradient is flow dependent. A substantial increase in blood flow through the vasa recta will ultimately dissipate the medullary gradient (i.e., "wash out" the medullary interstitial gradient). Alternatively, if blood flow is reduced, the nephron segments within the medulla will receive inadequate oxygen. Under conditions of reduced blood flow, tubular transport, especially by the thick ascending limb of Henle's loop, is impaired. As a result, the medullary interstitial osmotic gradient cannot be maintained.

Assessment of Renal Diluting and Concentrating Ability

Assessment of the dilution and concentration processes involves measurements of urine osmolality and the volume of urine excreted. Urine osmolality ranges from 50 mOsm/kg H_2O to 1200 mOsm/kg H_2O. The corresponding urine volume ranges from 18 L to as little as 0.5 L per day. These ranges are not fixed; rather, they vary from individual to individual, and as noted previously, depend on the amount of the solute excreted.

Traditionally, the handling of water by the kidneys has been quantitated by measuring what has been termed the **free-water clearance.** As noted previously, the central process in the dilution or concentration of urine is the single effect of separating solute from water. Through this separation, the kidneys in a sense generate a volume of water that is "free of all solute." When the urine is dilute, this **solute-free water** is excreted from the body. When the urine is concentrated, the solute-free water is returned to the systemic circulation. The concept of free-water clearance is merely a means for quantitating the ability of the kidneys to generate solute-free water. The free-water concept follows directly from renal clearance, as described in Chapter 34.

The clearance of total solute (i.e., all osmoles, whether effective or ineffective) from plasma by the kidneys can be calculated as

$$C_{osm} = \frac{U_{osm} \times \dot{V}}{P_{osm}} \qquad (36\text{-}6)$$

where C_{osm} is the **osmolar clearance,** U_{osm} is the urine osmolality, $\dot{V}$ is the urine flow rate, and P_{osm} is the plasma osmolality. C_{osm} is expressed in units of volume/unit time. Free-water clearance (C_{H_2O}) is then calculated as

$$C_{H_2O} = \dot{V} - C_{osm} \qquad (36\text{-}7)$$

By rearranging equation 36-3, it should be apparent that

$$\dot{V} = C_{H_2O} + C_{osm} \qquad (36\text{-}8)$$

In other words, we can divide total urine output ($\dot{V}$) into two hypothetical components. One component contains all the urine solutes and has an osmolality equal to that of plasma (i.e., $U_{osm} = P_{osm}$). This component is defined by C_{osm}, and represents a volume from which there has been no net separation of solute and water. The second component (C_{H_2O}) is a volume of solute-free water.

When dilute urine is produced, the value of C_{H_2O} is positive, indicating that solute-free water is excreted from the body. When concentrated urine is produced, the value of C_{H_2O} is negative, indicating that solute-free water is retained in the body. By convention, negative C_{H_2O} values are expressed as $T^c_{H_2O}$ **(tubular conservation of water).**

Calculating C_{H_2O} and $T^c_{H_2O}$ can provide important information about the function of those portions of the nephron involved in producing dilute and concentrated urine. *Whether the kidneys excrete or reabsorb free water depends on the presence of ADH.* When ADH is absent or ADH levels are low, solute-free water is excreted. When ADH levels are high, solute-free water is reabsorbed.

The following factors are necessary for the kidneys to excrete a maximal amount of solute-free water (C_{H_2O}):

1. ADH must be absent. Without ADH, the collecting duct does not reabsorb water.
2. The tubular structures, which separate solute from water (i.e., dilute the luminal fluid), must function normally. In the absence of ADH, the following nephron segments can dilute the luminal fluid:
   - Ascending thin limb of Henle's loop
   - Thick ascending limb of Henle's loop
   - Distal tubule
   - Collecting duct

   Because of its high transport rate, the thick ascending limb is quantitatively the most important of these segments involved in the separation of solute and water.
3. An adequate amount of tubular fluid must be delivered to the above nephron sites for maximal separation of solute and water. Factors that reduce delivery (e.g., decreased GFR or enhanced proximal tubule reabsorption) impair the ability of the kidneys to maximally excrete C_{H_2O}.

Similar requirements also apply to the conservation of water by the kidneys ($T^c_{H_2O}$). For the kidneys to conserve water maximally, the following conditions must exist:

1. Maximal levels of ADH must be present and the collecting duct must respond normally to ADH.
2. Reabsorption of NaCl by the nephron segments must be normal; again, the most important segment is the thick ascending limb of Henle's loop.
3. An adequate amount of tubular fluid must be delivered to those nephron segments in which separation of solute and water occurs. The important segment in the separation of solute and water is the thick ascending limb of Henle's loop. Delivery of tubular fluid to Henle's loop depends in turn on GFR and proximal tubule reabsorption.
4. A hyperosmotic medullary interstitium must be present. The interstitial osmolality is maintained by NaCl reabsorption by Henle's loop.

The concept of free-water clearance as just described does not distinguish between effective and ineffective osmoles, either in the plasma or in the urine. However, urea, which can account for half of total urine osmoles, is not an effective osmole when the movement of water between the ICF and ECF is considered. Accordingly, to understand how the handling of water by the kidneys contributes to the maintenance of whole body water balance, it is more appropriate to consider only those solutes that are effective osmoles. For plasma (i.e., ECF), the effective osmoles are Na^+ and its attendant anions. For urine, they are the nonurea solutes.

The importance of using effective osmoles in determining the impact of renal water handling on whole body water balance (i.e., body fluid osmolality) is illustrated by the following example. A patient has an elevated plasma [urea], and his plasma $[Na^+]$ is also increased. His total plasma osmolality (including urea) is 320 mOsm/kg H_2O, but his effective plasma osmolality (calculated as $2 \times [Na^+]$) is only 300 mOsm/kg H_2O. His urine osmolality is 600 mOsm/kg H_2O: 300 mOsm/kg H_2O due to urea and 300 mOsm/kg H_2O due to nonurea solutes. His urinary flow rate is 3 L/day.

According to equations 36-4 and 36-5, his total osmolar clearance (C_{osm}) and free-water clearance (C_{H_2O}) are

$$C_{osm} = \frac{600 \text{ mOsm/kg } H_2O \times 3 \text{ L/day}}{320 \text{ mOsm/kg } H_2O} = 5.6 \text{ L/day} \quad (36\text{-}9)$$

$$C_{H_2O} = 3 \text{ L/day} - 5.6 \text{ L/day} = -2.6 \text{ L/day } (T^c_{H_2O}) \quad (36\text{-}10)$$

Thus, it would appear that the kidneys are conserving 2.6 L/day of solute-free water, which would be an appropriate response to correct the elevated plasma osmolality and hypernatremia. However, when C_{osm} and C_{H_2O} are analyzed from the perspective of effective osmoles, the following results are obtained:

$$C_{osm} = \frac{300 \text{ mOsm/kg } H_2O \times 3 \text{ L/day}}{300 \text{ mOsm/kg } H_2O} = 3 \text{ L/day} \quad (36\text{-}11)$$

$$C_{H_2O} = 3 \text{ L/day} - 3 \text{ L/day} = 0 \text{ L/day} \quad (36\text{-}12)$$

Thus, when viewed from the more appropriate perspective of effective osmoles, it is apparent that the kidneys are not reabsorbing solute-free water, and the patient's kidneys will not correct the hyperosmolality and hypernatremia.

CONTROL OF EXTRACELLULAR FLUID VOLUME AND REGULATION OF RENAL NaCl EXCRETION

The major solutes of the ECF are the salts of Na^+. Of these, NaCl is the most abundant. Because NaCl is also the major determinant of the osmolality of ECF, it is commonly assumed that alterations in Na^+ balance disturb ECF osmolality. However, under normal conditions, this is not the case. Changes in Na^+ balance do not normally alter ECF osmolality, because the ADH and thirst systems maintain body fluid osmolality within a narrow range. For example, addition of NaCl to ECF (without water) increases the $[Na^+]$ and osmolality of this compartment (ICF osmolality also increases because of osmotic equilibration with ECF). This increase in osmolality in turn stimulates thirst and the release of ADH from the posterior pituitary. The increased ingestion of water in response to thirst, together with the ADH-induced decrease in water excretion by the kidneys, quickly restores ECF osmolality to normal. However, the volume of ECF increases in proportion to the amount of water ingested, which in turn depends on

the amount of NaCl added to ECF. Thus, in the new steady state, addition of NaCl to ECF is equivalent to adding an isoosmotic solution. Conversely, a decrease in the NaCl content of ECF results in a decrease in the volume of this compartment.

The kidneys are the major route of NaCl excretion from the body. As such, they play an important role in regulating the volume of ECF. *Under normal conditions, the kidneys keep the volume of ECF constant by adjusting the excretion of NaCl to match the amount ingested in the diet.* If ingestion exceeds excretion, ECF volume increases above normal; the opposite occurs if excretion exceeds ingestion. To defend itself against changes in ECF volume, the body relies on a system that monitors the volume of this compartment (actually the pressure in the vascular system, which changes as a function of volume) and sends signals to the kidneys to make appropriate adjustments in NaCl excretion.

> The typical diet contains approximately 140 mEq/day of Na^+ (≈ 8 g of NaCl), and thus daily Na^+ excretion is also about 140 mEq/day. However, the kidneys can vary the excretion of Na^+ over a wide range. Excretion rates as low as 10 mEq/day can be attained when individuals are placed on a low-salt diet. Conversely, the kidneys can increase their excretion rate to more than 1000 mEq/day when challenged by the ingestion of a high-salt diet. These changes in Na^+ excretion occur with only modest changes in the steady-state Na^+ content of the body.
>
> The response of the kidneys to abrupt changes in NaCl intake typically takes several hours to several days, depending on the magnitude of the change. During this transition period, intake and excretion of Na^+ are not matched as they are in the steady state. Thus, the individual experiences either **positive Na^+ balance** (intake > excretion) or **negative Na^+ balance** (intake < excretion). By the end of the transition period, a new steady state is established and intake once again equals excretion. Provided that the ADH and thirst systems are normal, alterations in Na^+ balance result in changes in the volume of ECF but not the serum $[Na^+]$ or plasma osmolality. Changes in ECF volume can be monitored by measuring body weight, since 1 L of ECF equals 1 kg of body weight.

This section reviews the physiology of the volume receptors and explains the various signals that act on the kidneys to regulate NaCl excretion, and thereby ECF volume, along with the responses of the various portions of the nephron to these signals.

Concept of Effective Circulating Volume

As noted, Na^+ and its salts are the major constituents of the ECF, and changes in Na^+ balance lead to alterations in ECF volume. Changes in ECF volume can also influence Na^+ balance by altering the amount of NaCl excreted by the kidneys. However, the relationship between ECF volume, renal

NaCl excretion, and whole body Na⁺ balance is complex, especially in certain pathological conditions. Therefore, to understand the relationship among these factors, one must consider the concept of **effective circulating volume.**

The effective circulating volume is not a measurable and distinct body fluid compartment, and it is defined physiologically not anatomically. *The effective circulating volume refers to the portion of ECF volume that is contained within the vascular system and is "effectively" perfusing the tissues.* In this regard, it reflects, and is dependent on, the volume of and "pressure" within the vascular system. In addition, it is related to cardiac output. However, as illustrated below, the effective circulating volume cannot simply be equated with the volume of fluid within the vascular tree.

In a normal individual, the effective circulating volume varies directly with the volume of ECF and in particular the vascular system (arterial and venous), the arterial blood pressure, and the cardiac output. Thus, a decrease in ECF and vascular volume, arterial pressure, or cardiac output will be sensed by the body as a decrease in effective circulating volume. Conversely, an increase in ECF and vascular volume, arterial pressure, or cardiac output will be sensed as an increase in effective circulating volume.

ECF volume, vascular volume, arterial blood pressure, and cardiac output all depend on the effective circulating volume, which in turn is related to Na⁺ balance. Consequently, the kidneys alter NaCl excretion in response to changes in the effective circulating volume. When the effective circulating volume is decreased, renal NaCl excretion is reduced. This adaptive response restores the effective circulating volume to normal and thereby maintains adequate tissue perfusion. Conversely, an increase in the effective circulating volume results in enhanced renal NaCl excretion, termed **natriuresis.** Again, this is an adaptive response to restore the effective circulating volume to its normal set point.

In a normal individual, Na⁺ balance determines the effective circulating volume, the ECF volume, and the vascular volume, which in turn influence arterial blood pressure and cardiac output. However, under some important pathological conditions, the effective circulating volume can vary independently from the ECF and vascular volumes, arterial blood pressure, or even cardiac output. Regardless of the condition, the kidneys adjust their excretion of NaCl in response to perceived changes in the effective circulating volume, and thus how effectively the tissues of the body are perfused.

Patients with **congestive heart failure** frequently have an increase in ECF and vascular volumes, which is manifested as accumulation of fluid in the lungs **(pulmonary edema)** and peripheral tissues **(generalized edema).** This excess fluid is the result of NaCl and water retention by the kidneys. The kidneys' response (i.e., retention of NaCl and water) seems paradoxical, because both the ECF and vascular volumes in such patients are increased. However, the effective circulating volume is decreased in congestive heart failure because of poor cardiac performance, and thus decreased cardiac output. As a result of this decreased effective circulating volume, and by mechanisms described below, the kidneys retain NaCl and water. Hence, the kidneys' response is directed at increasing the effective circulating volume and thereby tissue perfusion. Unfortunately, in the setting of poor cardiac performance, this adaptive response increases ECF volume above its normal set point, and results in the development of pulmonary and generalized edema.

Advanced **hepatic cirrhosis** further illustrates how the effective circulating volume can vary independently of ECF volume, vascular volume, and cardiac output. Patients with advanced hepatic cirrhosis accumulate large volumes of fluid in the peritoneal cavity **(ascites).** This fluid is a component of ECF. These patients' vascular volume is also increased because of pooling of blood in the venous side of the splanchnic circulation (the damaged liver impedes drainage of blood from the splanchnic circulation via the portal vein). Finally, these patients develop multiple **arteriovenous fistulas** throughout the body. These fistulas shunt blood from the arterial to the venous side of the circulation (i.e., bypass the capillary beds) and have the effects of increasing cardiac output but impairing tissue perfusion. Thus, these patients have an increase in ECF volume, vascular volume, and cardiac output. However, their tissues are not effectively perfused. Consequently, the body senses a decreased effective circulating volume, and the kidneys respond by retaining NaCl and water. It is the retention of NaCl and water by the kidneys that results in the increase in ECF volume (i.e., ascites) and vascular volume.

The remaining portions of this section will examine the relationship between the effective circulating volume and renal NaCl excretion in normal adults (i.e., those free of disease). In this setting, changes in the effective circulating volume parallel those of ECF volume, vascular volume, arterial blood pressure, and cardiac output. First, the maintenance of a normal effective circulating volume **(euvolemia)** is reviewed. This is followed by consideration of the renal response to an increase in the effective circulating volume **(volume expansion or hypervolemia),** and the renal response to a decrease in the effective circulating volume **(volume contraction or hypovolemia).**

Volume-Sensing System

The various sensors involved in monitoring the effective circulating volume are listed in Table 36-5. A number of the sensors are located in the vascular system and monitor its fullness by responding to changes in pressure. Although we refer to these as volume receptors, they are also called baroreceptors because they respond to pressure-induced stretch of the vessel walls in which they are located. The sensors within the liver and central nervous system (CNS) are less well understood and do not seem to be as important as the vascular sensors in monitoring the effective circulating volume.

■ **Table 36-5**　Volume sensors

I. Vascular
   A. Low pressure
     1. Cardiac atria
     2. Pulmonary vasculature
   B. High pressure
     1. Carotid sinus
     2. Aortic arch
     3. Juxtaglomerular apparatus of kidneys
II. Hepatic
III. Central nervous system

Vascular low-pressure volume sensors. Baroreceptors are located within the walls of the cardiac atria and large pulmonary vessels, and respond to distension of these structures (see also Chapters 21 and 22). Because the low-pressure side of the circulatory system has a high capacitance, the atrial and pulmonary vascular sensors respond prmarily to the "fullness" of the vascular system, and these baroreceptors send signals to the brainstem (solitary tract nucleus of the medulla oblongata) via afferent fibers in the vagus nerve. The activity of these sensors modulates both sympathetic nerve outflow and ADH secretion. For example, a decrease in filling of the pulmonary vessels and cardiac atria increases sympathetic nerve activity and stimulates ADH secretion. Conversely, distension of these structures decreases sympathetic nerve activity. In general, 5% to 10% changes in blood volume and pressure are necessary to evoke a response.

The cardiac atria possess an additional mechanism related to control of renal NaCl excretion. The myocytes of the atria synthesize and store a peptide hormone, termed **atrial natriuretic peptide (ANP),** that is released when the atria are distended. By mechanisms outlined in subsequent sections, ANP reduces blood pressure and increases the excretion of NaCl and water by the kidneys (see page 675).

Vascular high-pressure volume sensors. Baroreceptors are also present in the arterial side of the circulatory system, located in the wall of the aortic arch, the carotid sinus (see also Chapter 21), and the afferent arterioles of the kidneys. These baroreceptors respond primarily to blood pressure. The aortic arch and carotid baroreceptors also send input to the brainstem (solitary tract nucleus of the medulla oblongata) via afferent fibers in the vagus and glossopharyngeal nerves. The response to this input also involves alterations in sympathetic outflow and ADH secretion. Thus, a decrease in blood pressure will increase sympathetic nerve activity and ADH secretion. An increase in pressure tends to reduce sympathetic nerve activity. The sensitivity of the high-pressure baroreceptors is similar to that of those in the low-pressure side of the vascular system, with 5% to 10% changes in pressure needed to evoke a response.

The **juxtaglomerular apparatus** of the kidneys (see Chapter 34), particularly the afferent arterioles, responds directly to changes in pressure. If perfusion pressure of the afferent arterioles is reduced, renin is released from the myocytes. Renin secretion is suppressed when perfusion pressure is increased. As described in subsequent sections, renin determines blood levels of angiotensin II and aldosterone, both of which play an important role in regulating renal Na$^+$ excretion.

> Constriction of a renal artery (**renal artery stenosis**) by an atherosclerotic plaque, for example, reduces perfusion pressure to that kidney. This reduced perfusion pressure is sensed by the afferent arterioles and results in the secretion of renin. The elevated renin levels increase production of angiotensin II, which in turn increases systemic blood pressure by its constrictor effect on arterioles throughout the vascular system. The increased systemic blood pressure is sensed by the afferent arterioles of the contralateral kidney (i.e., the kidney without stenosis of its renal artery), and renin secretion from that kidney is suppressed.

Hepatic sensors. The liver also contains volume sensors that although not as important as the vascular sensors in monitoring the effective circulating volume, can modulate renal NaCl excretion. One type of hepatic sensor responds to pressure within the hepatic vasculature and therefore functions in a manner similar to the low- and high-pressure baroreceptors just described. A different type of sensor also appears to exist in the liver; it responds to the concentration of Na$^+$ in the portal vein blood. Afferent signals from both types of sensors are carried to the CNS in the hepatic nerves. These afferent signals are sent to the same region of the brainstem (solitary tract nucleus of the medulla oblongata), where afferent fibers from the low- and high-pressure baroreceptors also converge. Increased pressure within the hepatic vasculature, or an increase in portal vein [Na$^+$], results in a decrease in renal sympathetic nerve activity.[*] As described subsequently, this decrease in renal sympathetic tone leads to an increase in renal NaCl excretion.

Central nervous system Na$^+$ sensors. Like the hepatic sensors, the CNS sensors are not as important as the vascular sensors in monitoring the effective circulating volume. Nevertheless, alterations in the [Na$^+$] of blood carried to the brain by the carotid arteries, or the [Na$^+$] of the cerebrospinal fluid (CSF), modulate renal NaCl excretion. For example, if the [Na$^+$] in either the carotid artery blood or the CSF is increased, there is a decrease in renal sympathetic nerve activity, which in turn leads to an increase in renal NaCl excretion. The precise location of the Na$^+$ receptors involved in this response is not known, although they are thought to be in the hypothalamus.

Volume Sensor Signals

The kidneys play an important role in Na$^+$ homeostasis. Both neural and hormonal signals have been identified.

---

[*]The hepatic sensors also appear to be involved in the regulation of gastrointestinal NaCl absorption. For example, when the [Na$^+$] of the portal vein blood is increased, there is a reflex reduction in jejunal NaCl absorption.

■ **Table 36-6** Signals involved in the control of renal NaCl and water excretion

Renal sympathetic nerves (↑ activity: ↓ NaCl excretion)

↓ Glomerular filtration rate
↑ Renin secretion
↑ Proximal tubule, thick ascending limb of Henle's loop, distal tubule, and collecting duct NaCl reabsorption

Renin-angiotensin-aldosterone (↑ secretion: ↓ NaCl excretion)

↑ Angiotensin II levels stimulate proximal tubule NaCl reabsorption
↑ Aldosterone levels stimulate thick ascending limb of Henle's loop, distal tubule, and collecting duct NaCl reabsorption
↑ Angiotensin II levels stimulate ADH secretion

Atrial natriuretic peptide (↑ secretion: ↑ NaCl excretion)

↑ Glomerular filtration rate
↓ Renin secretion
↓ Aldosterone secretion
↓ NaCl and water reabsorption by the collecting duct*
↓ ADH secretion and action of ADH on the collecting duct

ADH (↑ secretion: ↓ H₂O excretion)

↑ H₂O absorption by the collecting duct

*Urodilatin contributes to this effect.

These signals are summarized in Table 36-6, as are their effects on renal NaCl and water excretion.

Renal sympathetic nerves. As described in Chapter 34, sympathetic nerve fibers innervate the afferent and efferent arterioles of the glomerulus, as well as nephron cells. With negative Na^+ balance (i.e., volume depletion), the volume sensors (especially the low- and high-pressure vascular baroreceptors) stimulate renal sympathetic nerve activity. This stimulation has the following effects:

1. The afferent and efferent arterioles are constricted by activation of α-adrenergic receptors. This vasoconstriction (the effect appears to be greater on the afferent arteriole) decreases the hydrostatic pressure within the glomerular capillary lumen, and thereby reduces the GFR. With this decrease in GFR, the filtered load of Na^+ to the nephrons is reduced (filtered load = GFR × plasma $[Na^+]$).
2. Renin secretion by the cells of the afferent arteriole is stimulated via activation of β-adrenergic receptors. As described below, renin ultimately increases circulating levels of angiotensin II and aldosterone.
3. NaCl reabsorption along the nephron is directly stimulated via activation of α-adrenergic receptors (in some species β-adrenergic receptors mediate this response). Quantitatively, the most important segment influenced by sympathetic nerve activity is the proximal tubule.

The combined effect of these actions contributes to an overall decrease in NaCl excretion, an adaptive response that works to restore euvolemia. Conversely, with positive Na^+ balance (i.e., volume expansion), renal sympathetic nerve activity is reduced. This response generally reverses the effects just described.

Renin-angiotensin-aldosterone system. Smooth muscle cells in the afferent arteriole are the site of synthesis, storage, and release of **renin.** Three factors play an important role in stimulating renin secretion:

1. *Perfusion pressure.* The afferent arteriole is a high-pressure baroreceptor. When perfusion pressure to the kidneys is reduced, renin secretion is stimulated. Conversely, an increase in perfusion pressure inhibits renin release.
2. *Sympathetic nerve activity.* Activation of the sympathetic nerve fibers innervating the afferent arteriole results in an increase in renin secretion. Renin secretion is decreased as renal sympathetic nerve activity is decreased.
3. *Delivery of NaCl to the macula densa.* This regulates the GFR by a process called *tubuloglomerular feedback* (see Chapter 34). By this feedback mechanism, increased NaCl delivery to the macula densa results in a decrease in GFR. Conversely, decreased NaCl delivery increases GFR. In addition to its role in regulating GFR, the macula densa plays a role in renin secretion. When NaCl delivery to the macula densa is decreased, renin secretion is enhanced. Conversely, an increase in NaCl delivery inhibits renin secretion. This macula densa-mediated secretion of renin does not appear to be involved in the alterations in glomerular hemodynamics that underlie the phenomenon of tubuloglomerular feedback.*

Figure 36-5 summarizes the essential components of the renin-angiotensin-aldosterone system. Renin alone does not have a physiological function; it functions solely as a proteolytic enzyme. Its substrate is a circulating protein, **angiotensinogen,** which is produced by the liver. Angiotensinogen is cleaved by renin to yield a 10-amino acid peptide, **angiotensin I.** Angiotensin I also has no known physiological function, and is further cleaved to an 8-amino acid peptide, **angiotensin II,** by a converting enzyme [**angiotensin-converting enzyme (ACE)**] found on the surface of vascular endothelial cells (pulmonary and renal endothelial cells are important sites for the conversion of angiotensin I to angiotensin II). Angiotensin II has several important physiological functions, including

1. Stimulation of aldosterone secretion by the adrenal cortex.
2. Arteriolar vasoconstriction, which increases blood pressure.
3. Stimulation of ADH secretion and thirst.
4. Enhancement of NaCl reabsorption by the proximal tubule.

*It is thought that macula densa–mediated renin secretion may play a role in maintaining systemic arterial pressure under conditions of a reduced vascular volume. For example, when vascular volume is reduced, perfusion of the body tissues (including the kidneys) will decrease. This in turn will result in a decrease in GFR and the filtered load of NaCl. The reduced delivery of NaCl to the macula densa will then stimulate renin secretion, which through angiotensin II (a potent vasoconstrictor) will act to increase blood pressure and thereby maintain tissue perfusion.

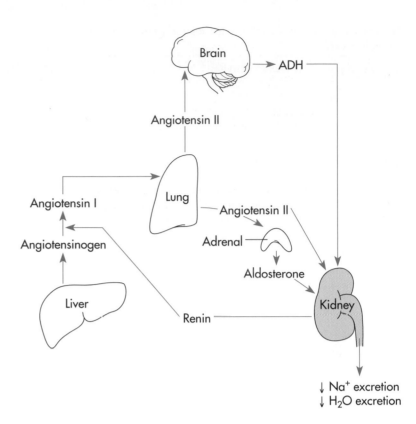

■ **Fig. 36-5** Schematic representation of the essential components of the renin-angiotensin-aldosterone system. Activation of this system results in a decrease in the excretion of Na$^+$ and water by the kidneys. *Note:* Angiotensin I is converted to angiotensin II by angiotensin-converting enzyme (ACE), which is present on all vascular endothelial cells. The endothelial cells within the lungs play a significant role in this conversion process. See text for details.

Angiotensin II is an important secretagogue for **aldosterone** (an increase in plasma [K$^+$] is the other important stimulus for aldosterone secretion; see Chapter 37). Aldosterone is a steroid hormone produced by the glomerulosa cells of the adrenal cortex (see also Chapter 45). It acts in a number of ways on the kidneys (see also Chapters 37 and 38). With regard to regulation of the effective circulating volume, aldosterone reduces NaCl excretion by stimulating its reabsorption by the thick ascending limb of Henle's loop, the distal tubule, and the collecting duct. The effect of aldosterone on renal NaCl excretion depends primarily on its ability to stimulate Na$^+$ reabsorption in the distal tubule and collecting duct. Because the transcellular reabsorption of Na$^+$ by the principal cell generates a lumen-negative transepithelial voltage (see Chapter 35), the enhanced Na$^+$ reabsorption from the luminal fluid increases the magnitude of this voltage. As a result of the increased magnitude of the transepithelial voltage, the passive movement of Cl$^-$ from the lumen to blood via the paracellular pathway is enhanced. Thus, aldosterone increases the reabsorption of NaCl from the tubular fluid. Reduced levels of aldosterone result in a decrease in the amount of NaCl reabsorbed by the principal cell.

The effects of aldosterone on Na$^+$ reabsorption by the late portion of the distal tubule and the collecting duct can be separated into an early phase (minutes to hours) and a late phase (hours to days). The most important early phase effect is an activation (i.e., increased opening) of the amiloride-sensitive Na$^+$ channel (ENaC) present in the apical membrane of the principal cells. This allows increased entry of Na$^+$ into the cell, which together with aldosterone, results in the late phase effects. The specific late phase effects of aldosterone are a result of alteration in DNA transcription. Aldosterone enters the cell and binds to an intracellular receptor, and the hormone-receptor complex regulates DNA transcription. A number of aldosterone-induced proteins are synthesized. With regard to Na$^+$ reabsorption, there is increased synthesis of ENaC, as well as the basolateral membrane Na$^+$,K$^+$-ATPase. The net effect of all these changes is increased entry of Na$^+$ into the cell across the apical membrane, and increased extrusion from the cell across the basolateral membrane.

Aldosterone also enhances NaCl reabsorption by cells of the thick ascending limb of Henle's loop. The precise cellular mechanisms involved in aldosterone's action on the thick ascending limb cells have not yet been elucidated. However, it is likely that both Na$^+$ entry into the cell (perhaps via the apical membrane 1Na$^+$-1K$^+$-2Cl$^-$ symporter) and its extrusion from the cell (via the basolateral membrane Na$^+$,K$^+$-ATPase) are stimulated.

Diseases of the adrenal cortex can alter aldosterone levels and thereby impair the ability of the kidneys to maintain Na$^+$ balance and euvolemia. With decreased secretion of aldosterone **(hypoaldosteronism),** Na$^+$ reabsorption, primarily by the collecting duct, is reduced. The result is a loss of Na$^+$ in the urine. Because urinary Na$^+$ loss can exceed the amount ingested in the diet, negative Na$^+$ balance will ensue, and volume contraction occurs. In response, sympathetic tone is increased, leading to elevated levels of renin, angiotensin II, and ADH. With increased aldosterone secretion **(hyperaldosteronism),** the opposite effects occur. Na⁺ reabsorption, especially by the collecting duct, is enhanced, resulting in reduced excretion of Na⁺. Consequently, volume expansion results; sympathetic tone is decreased; and levels of renin, angiotensin II, and ADH are decreased. As described below, ANP levels are also elevated in this setting.

As summarized in Table 36-6, *activation of the renin-angiotensin-aldosterone system, as occurs with volume depletion, results in decreased excretion of NaCl by the kidneys.* This system is suppressed with volume expansion, and renal NaCl excretion is therefore enhanced.

Atrial natriuretic peptide. Atrial myocytes produce and store a peptide hormone, atrial natriuretic peptide (ANP), that relaxes vascular smooth muscle and promotes NaCl and water excretion by the kidney. ANP is released with atrial stretch, as would occur with volume expansion. The circulating form of ANP is 28 amino acids in length. In general, ANP actions, as they relate to renal NaCl and water excretion, antagonize those of the renin-angiotensin-aldosterone system. They include the following:

1. Vasodilation of the afferent and vasoconstriction of the efferent arterioles of the glomerulus, increasing GFR and the filtered load of Na⁺.
2. Inhibition of renin secretion by the afferent arteriole.
3. Inhibition of aldosterone secretion by the glomerulosa cells of the adrenal cortex. ANP reduces aldosterone secretion by two mechanisms: it inhibits renin secretion, thereby reducing angiotensin II–induced aldosterone secretion, and it acts directly on the glomerulosa cells of the adrenal cortex to inhibit aldosterone secretion.
4. Inhibition of NaCl reabsorption by the collecting duct. This effect is due in part to reduced levels of aldosterone; however, ANP also acts directly on the collecting duct cells. Through its second messenger, cyclic guanine monophosphate (cGMP), ANP inhibits Na⁺ channels in the apical membrane of the cell, and thereby NaCl reabsorption. This effect is predominantly in the medullary portion of the collecting duct.
5. Inhibition of ADH secretion by the posterior pituitary and ADH action on the collecting duct. This results in a reduction in water reabsorption by the collecting duct and thus increased excretion of water in the urine.

Taken together, these effects of ANP increase the excretion of NaCl and water by the kidneys. Hypothetically, a reduction in circulating levels of ANP would be expected to decrease NaCl and water excretion. However, no convincing evidence for this effect has been found.

Atrial natriuretic peptide (ANP) is one member of a family of peptides that plays a role in the regulation of the cardiovascular and renal systems, and especially the effective circulating volume. All of these peptides are thought to be involved to varying degrees in the body's response to an increased effective circulating volume. Urodilation, also called renal natriuretic peptide (RNP), is produced by, and has effects within, the kidney. Like ANP it increases GFR and reduces collecting duct Na⁺ reabsorption, and thereby contributes to the ANP-induced natriuresis and diuresis. However, it does not appear to affect ADH action on the collecting duct as ANP does. The cardiac myocytes also secrete brain natriuretic peptide (BNP), so named because it is also found in the CNS. The actions of BNP are not well dilineated, but are likely similar to those of ANP. Yet another peptide is found in the brain (CNP), however, its physiological role in regulating the effective circulating volume remains to be defined.

Antidiuretic hormone. As already discussed, with volume depletion, ADH secretion by the posterior pituitary is stimulated. The elevated levels of ADH cause decreased water excretion by the kidneys, which serves to reestablish euvolemia.

Control of Na⁺ Excretion During Euvolemia

The maintenance of Na⁺ balance and therefore euvolemia requires a precise balance between the amount of NaCl ingested and that excreted from the body. In a euvolemic individual, daily urine NaCl excretion equals daily NaCl intake.

The kidneys can vary the amount of NaCl they excrete over a wide range. Under conditions of salt restriction (e.g., low-NaCl diet), virtually no NaCl appears in the urine. Conversely, in individuals who ingest large quantities of salt, renal Na⁺ excretion can exceed 1000 mEq/day. The kidneys' response to variations in dietary salt intake may take several days. During the transition period, excretion does not match intake, and the individual will be in either positive (intake > excretion) or negative (intake < excretion) Na⁺ balance. When Na⁺ balance is altered during these transition periods, the ECF volume changes in parallel (water excretion, regulated via the ADH system, is also adjusted to keep plasma osmolality constant, resulting in an isoosmotic change in ECF volume). Thus, with positive balance, volume expansion occurs (detected as an increase in body weight), whereas with negative balance, volume contraction occurs (detected as a decrease in body weight). Ultimately, renal excretion will reach a new steady state, and euvolemia will be reestablished as NaCl excretion is once again matched to intake. The time course for adjustment of renal NaCl excretion to intake is variable and depends on the magnitude of the change in NaCl intake. Adaptation to large changes in NaCl intake requires a longer time than does the adaptation to small changes in intake.

To comprehend how renal Na⁺ excretion is regulated, the general features of Na⁺ handling along the nephron must be understood. Figure 36-6 summarizes the contribution of each nephron segment to the reabsorption of the filtered load of Na⁺ under euvolemic conditions (the specific cellular

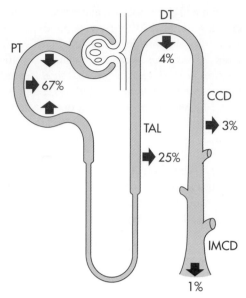

Fig. 36-6 Segmental Na⁺ reabsorption. The percentage of the filtered load of Na⁺ reabsorbed by each nephron segment is indicated. *PT,* Proximal tubule; *TAL,* thick ascending limb; *DT,* distal tubule; *CCD,* cortical collecting duct; *IMCD,* inner medullary collecting duct.

mechanisms of Na⁺ transport are explained in Chapter 35). Most of the filtered load of Na⁺ (67%) is reabsorbed by the proximal tubule. An additional 25% is reabsorbed by the thick ascending limb of Henle's loop, and the remainder by the distal tubule and collecting duct.

The following discussion considers only the renal handling of Na⁺. Although not specifically addressed, Cl⁻ reabsorption is regulated in parallel.

In a normal adult, the filtered load of Na⁺ can be calculated as

$$
\begin{aligned}
\text{filtered load of Na}^+ &= \text{(GFR)(plasma [Na}^+\text{])} \\
&= (180 \text{ L/day})(140 \text{ mEq/L}) \quad (36\text{-}13) \\
&= 25,200 \text{ mEq/day}
\end{aligned}
$$

With a typical diet, less than 1% of this filtered load is excreted in the urine (approximately 140 mEq/day). Because of the large filtered load of Na⁺, it is important to recognize that small changes in Na⁺ reabsorption by the nephron can profoundly affect Na⁺ balance and thus the volume of ECF. For example, an increase in Na⁺ excretion from 1% to 3% of the filtered load represents an additional loss of approximately 500 mEq/day. Because ECF [Na⁺] is 140 mEq/L, Na⁺ loss of this magnitude would decrease ECF volume by more than 3 L (water excretion would parallel the loss of Na⁺ to maintain body fluid osmolality constant; 500 mEq/day ÷ 140 mEq/L = 3.6 L/day of fluid loss).

In euvolemic subjects the collecting duct is the main nephron segment where Na⁺ reabsorption is adjusted to maintain excretion at a level appropriate for dietary intake. However, other portions of the nephron also play a role in this process. Because the reabsorptive capacity of the collecting duct is limited, these other portions of the nephron must reabsorb the bulk of the filtered load of Na⁺. Thus, during euvolemia, Na⁺ handling by the nephron can be explained by two general processes:

1. Na⁺ reabsorption by the proximal tubule, Henle's loop, and the distal tubule is regulated so that a relatively constant portion of the filtered load of Na⁺ is delivered to the collecting duct. As indicated in Fig. 36-6, the combined action of these nephron segments reabsorbs 96% of the filtered load of Na⁺. The remaining 4% of the filtered load is delivered to the beginning of the collecting duct.

2. Reabsorption of this remaining portion of the filtered load of Na⁺ by the collecting duct is regulated so that the amount of Na⁺ excreted in the urine matches the amount ingested in the diet. Thus, the collecting duct makes final adjustments in Na⁺ excretion to maintain the euvolemic state.

Mechanisms for maintaining constant Na⁺ delivery to the collecting duct. A number of mechanisms maintain delivery of a constant fraction of the filtered load of Na⁺ to the beginning of the collecting duct. These mechanisms are autoregulation of GFR, and thus the filtered load of Na⁺; glomerulotubular balance; and load dependency of Na⁺ reabsorption by Henle's loop and the distal tubule.

Autoregulation of GFR (see Chapter 34) allows for the maintenance of a relatively constant filtration rate over a wide range of mean arterial pressures. Because the filtration rate is constant, the amount of the filtered load of Na⁺ delivered to the nephrons is also constant.

Despite the autoregulatory control of GFR, small variations do occur. If these changes were not compensated for by an appropriate adjustment in Na⁺ reabsorption by the nephron, marked changes in Na⁺ excretion would result. However, Na⁺ reabsorption in the euvolemic state, especially by the proximal tubule, does change parallel to changes in GFR. This phenomenon is called **glomerulotubular (G-T) balance.** By this process, reabsorption of Na⁺, primarily by the proximal tubule, is adjusted to match the GFR. Thus, if GFR increases, the amount of Na⁺ reabsorbed by the proximal tubule also increases. The opposite occurs if GFR decreases. (G-T balance is further described in Chapter 35).

The final mechanism that helps maintain the constant delivery of Na⁺ to the beginning of the collecting duct involves the ability of Henle's loop and the distal tubule to increase their Na⁺ reabsorptive rates in response to increased delivery. Of these two segments, Henle's loop, particularly the thick ascending limb, has the greater capacity to increase Na⁺ reabsorption in response to increased delivery. The mechanism by which the thick ascending limb increases its Na⁺ reabsorptive rate in response to an increased delivered load is not completely understood, although there is increased abundance of the apical membrane NaCl symporter.

Regulation of collecting duct Na⁺ reabsorption. When the delivery rate of Na⁺ is constant, small adjustments in collecting duct reabsorption are sufficient to balance excretion with intake. (Recall that a 2% change in the fractional excretion of Na⁺ would produce more than a 3 L change in the volume of ECF.) Aldosterone is the primary regulator of col-

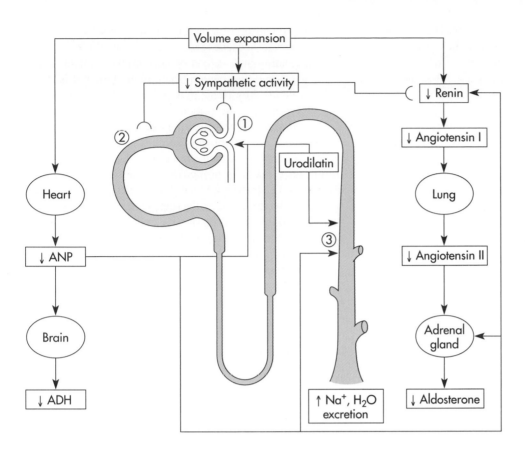

■ **Fig. 36-7** Integrated response to volume expansion. Numbers refer to the description of the response in the text. *ANP,* Atrial natriuretic peptide. $U_{Na^+}\dot{V}$, Na^+ excretion rate; *GFR,* glomerular filtration rate; P_{Na^+}, plasma $[Na^+]$; R, tubular reabsorption of Na^+.

$$\uparrow U_{Na^+}\dot{V} = \uparrow GFR \times P_{Na^+} - \downarrow R$$

lecting duct Na^+ reabsorption, and thus of Na^+ excretion, under this condition. When aldosterone levels are elevated, Na^+ reabsorption by the principal cells of the collecting duct is increased (excretion decreased). When aldosterone levels are suppressed, Na^+ reabsorption is decreased (excretion increased).

In addition to aldosterone, a number of other factors alter collecting duct Na^+ reabsorption, including ANP, prostaglandin, urodilatin, and sympathetic nerves. However, at present, the relative roles of these other factors in the regulation of collecting duct Na^+ reabsorption during euvolemia are not clear.

As long as variations in the dietary intake of NaCl are minor, the mechanisms described above can regulate renal Na^+ excretion appropriately, thereby maintaining euvolemia. However, these mechanisms cannot effectively handle significant changes in NaCl intake. When NaCl intake significantly increases, volume expansion or contraction occurs. In such cases, additional factors are called into play that act on the kidneys to adjust Na^+ reabsorption to reestablish the euvolemic state.

Control of Na^+ Excretion with Volume Expansion

During volume expansion, the volume sensors send signals to the kidneys, resulting in an increase in the excre-

tion of NaCl and water. The signals acting on the kidneys include

1. Decreased activity of the renal sympathetic nerves.
2. Release of ANP from atrial myocytes as well as other natriuretic peptides (e.g., urodilatin in the kidney).
3. Inhibition of ADH secretion from the posterior pituitary.
4. Decreased renin secretion, and thus decreased production of angiotensin II.
5. Decreased secretion of aldosterone, due to reduced angiotensin II levels, and elevated ANP levels.

The integrated response of the nephron to these signals is illustrated in Fig. 36-7. The important difference between a situation during volume expansion and that during the euvolemic state is that the renal response is not limited to the collecting duct; rather, it involves the entire nephron.

Three general responses to volume expansion occur (Fig. 36-7). The numbers correlate to those encircled in the figure.

1. *GFR increases.* GFR increases primarily as a result of the decrease in sympathetic nerve activity. Sympathetic fibers innervate the afferent and efferent arterioles of the glomerulus and control their diameter. Decreased sympathetic nerve activity leads to their dilation. Because this effect appears to be greater on the afferent arteriole, the hydrostatic

pressure within the glomerular capillary is increased, and GFR increases. ANP and urodilatin also increase GFR by dilating the afferent and constricting the efferent arterioles. With the increase in GFR, the filtered load of Na⁺ increases.

2. *Reabsorption of Na⁺ decreases in the proximal tubule.* Several mechanisms appear to be involved in reducing Na⁺ reabsorption by the proximal tubule, but the precise role of each of these mechanisms remains controversial. Because activation of the sympathetic nerve fibers innervating this nephron segment stimulates Na⁺ reabsorption, the decreased sympathetic nerve activity resulting from volume expansion may contribute to the decreased Na⁺ reabsorption that occurs. In addition, angiotensin II directly stimulates Na⁺ reabsorption by the proximal tubule. Because angiotensin II levels are also reduced under this condition, it is possible that proximal tubule Na⁺ reabsorption is decreased as a result. The increased hydrostatic pressure within the glomerular capillaries also leads to an increase in the hydrostatic pressure within the peritubular capillaries. This alteration in the capillary Starling forces reduces the absorption of solute (e.g., NaCl) and water from the lateral intercellular space, thus reducing tubular reabsorption (see Chapter 35 for the mechanism).

3. *Na⁺ reabsorption decreases in the collecting duct.* Both the increase in the filtered load and the decrease in proximal tubule NaCl reabsorption result in the delivery of large amounts of NaCl to Henle's loop and the distal tubule. Because increased activity of both sympathetic nerves and aldosterone stimulates NaCl reabsorption by Henle's loop, the reduced nerve activity and low aldosterone levels seen with volume expansion could in theory reduce

NaCl reabsorption by this nephron segment. However, because reabsorption by the thick ascending limb is load dependent, these effects are offset, and the fraction of the filtered load of Na⁺ reabsorbed by Henle's loop is actually increased. Nevertheless, the amount of Na⁺ delivered to the beginning of the collecting duct is increased compared with the euvolemic state (Fig. 36-8).

The amount of Na⁺ delivered to the beginning of the collecting duct varies in proportion to the degree of volume expansion. This increased load of Na⁺ overwhelms the reabsorptive capacity of the collecting duct, which is even further reduced by the actions of ANP and urodilatin and by the decrease in the circulating levels of aldosterone.

The final component in the response to volume expansion is the excretion of water. As Na⁺ excretion increases, plasma osmolality begins to fall. This results in decreased secretion of ADH. ADH secretion is also decreased in response to the elevated levels of ANP. In addition, ANP inhibits the action of ADH on the collecting duct. Together, these effects decrease water reabsorption by the collecting duct, thereby increasing water excretion by the kidneys. Thus, the excretion of Na⁺ and water occurs in concert; euvolemia is restored, and body fluid osmolality remains constant. As already noted, the time course of this response (hours to days) depends on the magnitude of the volume expansion. Thus, if the degree of volume expansion is small, the mechanisms just described will restore euvolemia within 24 hours. However, with large degrees of volume expansion, the response can take several days.

In summary, the nephron's response to volume expansion involves the integrated action of all its parts. The filtered load is increased, proximal tubule reabsorption is reduced (GFR is increased, whereas proximal reabsorption is decreased; thus, G-T balance does not occur under this con-

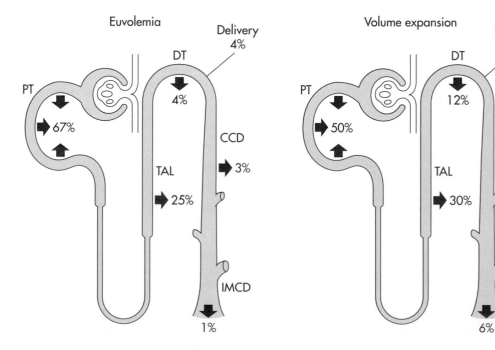

■ **Fig. 36-8** Segmental Na⁺ reabsorption during euvolemia and during volume expansion. Note that with volume expansion, delivery of Na⁺ to the collecting duct is increased from 4% to 8%. With inhibition of Na⁺ reabsorption by the collecting duct, Na⁺ excretion is increased from 1% to 6%. *PT,* Proximal tubule; *TAL,* thick ascending limb; *DT,* distal tubule; *CCD,* cortical collecting duct; *IMCD,* inner medullary collecting duct.

dition), and the delivery of NaCl to the beginning of the collecting duct is increased. This increased delivery, along with inhibition of collecting duct reabsorption, results in the excretion of a larger fraction of the filtered load of Na⁺, thus restoring euvolemia.

Control of Na⁺ Excretion with Volume Contraction

During volume contraction, the sensors send signals to the kidneys, which reduce Na⁺ and water excretion. The signals acting on the kidneys include

1. Increased renal sympathetic nerve activity.
2. Increased secretion of renin, which results in elevated angiotensin II levels and thus increased secretion of aldosterone by the adrenal cortex.
3. Inhibition of ANP secretion by the atrial myocytes and urodilatin production by the kidneys.
4. Stimulation of ADH secretion by the posterior pituitary.

The integrated response of the nephron to these signals is illustrated in Fig. 36-9.

The nephron's response to ECV contraction involves all nephron segments. The general response is as follows. The numbers correlate to those encircled in Fig. 36-9.

1. *GFR decreases.* Afferent and efferent arteriolar constriction occurs as a result of increased renal

sympathetic nerve activity. The effect appears to be greater on the afferent arteriole, causing the hydrostatic pressure in the glomerular capillary to fall, and thereby decreasing the GFR. This decrease in GFR in turn reduces the filtered load of Na⁺.

2. *Na⁺ reabsorption by the proximal tubule is increased.* Several mechanisms appear to be involved in augmenting Na⁺ reabsorption in this segment. For example, increased sympathetic nerve activity and angiotensin II directly stimulate proximal tubule Na⁺ reabsorption. The decreased hydrostatic pressure within the glomerular capillaries also leads to a decrease in the hydrostatic pressure within the peritubular capillaries. This alteration in the capillary Starling forces facilitates the movement of fluid from the lateral intercellular space into the capillary, thereby stimulating proximal tubule reabsorption of solute and water (see Chapter 35 for a complete description of this mechanism).

3. *Na⁺ reabsorption by the collecting duct is enhanced.* The reduction in filtered load and enhanced proximal tubule reabsorption result in decreased delivery of Na⁺ to Henle's loop and the distal tubule. Increased sympathetic nerve activity and aldosterone stimulate Na⁺ reabsorption by the thick ascending limb and distal tubule. Because sympathetic nerve activity is increased and aldosterone levels are elevated during volume

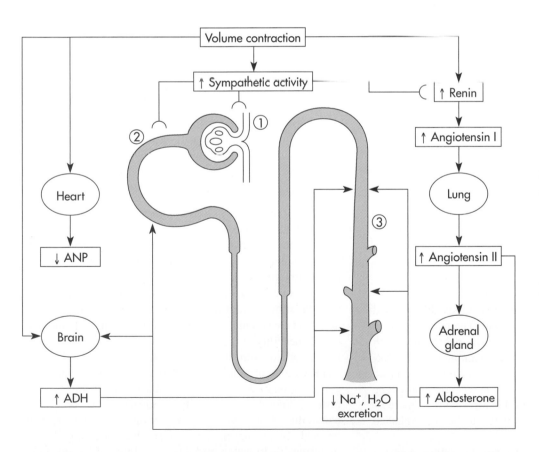

■ **Fig. 36-9** Integrated response to volume contraction. The circled numbers correlate with the description in the text. Urodilatin levels are also decreased but are not depicted. *ANP,* Atrial natriuretic peptide, $U_{Na^+}\dot{V}$, Na⁺ excretion rate; *GFR,* glomerular filtration rate; P_{Na^+}, plasma [Na⁺]; *R,* tubular reabsorption of Na⁺.

$$\downarrow U_{Na^+}\dot{V} = \downarrow GFR \times P_{Na^+} - \uparrow R$$

■ **Fig. 36-10** Segmental Na⁺ reabsorption during euvolemia and during volume contraction. Note that with volume contraction, delivery of Na⁺ to the collecting duct is reduced from 4% to 2%. The collecting duct reabsorbs virtually all the Na⁺ it receives, and Na⁺ excretion is reduced to near zero. *PT,* Proximal tubule; *TAL,* thick ascending limb; *DT,* distal tubule; *CCD,* collecting duct; *IMCD,* inner medullary collecting duct.

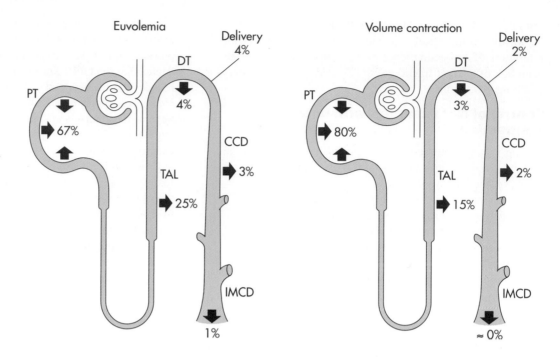

contraction, the potential for increased Na⁺ reabsorption by these segments exists. However, because Na⁺ transport by the thick ascending limb and distal tubule is load dependent, the stimulatory effects of increased sympathetic nerve activity and aldosterone are offset. Therefore, the fraction of the filtered load of Na⁺ reabsorbed by these segments is actually less than that seen in the euvolemic state. Nevertheless, the net result is that less Na⁺ is delivered to the beginning of the collecting duct. This process is illustrated in Fig. 36-10.

The small amount of Na⁺ delivered to the collecting duct is almost completely reabsorbed, because transport in this segment is enhanced. This stimulation of collecting duct Na⁺ reabsorption is primarily due to increased aldosterone levels. Additionally, ANP and urodilatin, which inhibit collecting duct reabsorption, are not present.

Finally, water reabsorption by the collecting duct is enhanced by ADH, the levels of which are elevated owing to activation of the low- and high-pressure vascular baroreceptors, as well as by the elevated levels of angiotensin II. As a result, water excretion is reduced and, together with the Na⁺ retained by the kidneys, euvolemia is reestablished and body fluid osmolality remains constant. The time course of this reexpansion (hours to days) and the degree to which euvolemia is attained depend on the magnitude of the volume contraction as well as the dietary intake of Na⁺. Thus, the kidneys can reduce Na⁺ excretion, and euvolemia will be restored to its normal level as NaCl is ingested (i.e., increasing NaCl intake will allow euvolemia to be reestablished more quickly).

In summary, the nephron's response to volume contraction involves the integrated action of all its segments. The filtered load of Na⁺ is decreased, proximal tubule reab

sorption is enhanced (GFR is decreased, whereas proximal reabsorption is increased; thus, G-T balance does not occur under this condition), and the delivery of Na⁺ to the beginning of the collecting duct is reduced. This decreased delivery, together with enhanced Na⁺ reabsorption by the collecting duct, virtually eliminates Na⁺ from the urine.

SUMMARY

1. The osmolality and volume of the body fluids are maintained within a narrow range, despite wide variation in water and solute intake. The kidneys play the central role in this regulatory process by virtue of their ability to vary the excretion of water and solutes.

2. Regulation of body fluid osmolality requires that water intake matches water loss from the body. Regulation of body fluid osmolality involves the integrated interaction of the ADH secretory and thirst centers of the hypothalamus, and the ability of the kidneys to excrete urine that is either hypoosmotic or hyperosmotic with respect to the body fluids. When body fluid osmolality increases, ADH secretion and thirst are stimulated. ADH acts on the kidneys to increase the permeability of the collecting duct to water. Hence, water is reabsorbed from the lumen of the collecting duct, and a small volume of hyperosmotic urine is excreted. This renal conservation of water, together with increased water intake, restores body fluid osmolality to normal. When body fluid osmolality decreases, ADH secretion and thirst are suppressed. In the absence of ADH, the collecting duct is impermeable to water, and a large volume of hypoosmotic urine is excreted. With this increased excretion of water, and with a decreased intake of water caused by suppres

sion of thirst, the osmolality of the body fluids is restored to normal.

3. Central to the process of concentrating and diluting the urine is Henle's loop. The reabsorption of NaCl by Henle's loop allows the separation of solute and water, which is essential for the formation of hypoosmotic urine. By this same mechanism, the interstitial fluid in the medullary portion of the kidney is rendered hyperosmotic. This hyperosmotic medullary interstitial fluid in turn provides the osmotic driving force for the reabsorption of water from the lumen of the collecting duct when ADH is present.

4. Disorders of water balance alter body fluid osmolality. Changes in body fluid osmolality are manifest by a change in plasma [Na^+]. Positive water balance (intake > excretion) results in a decrease in body fluid osmolality and hyponatremia. Negative water balance (intake < excretion) results in an increase in body fluid osmolality and hypernatremia.

5. Maximal excretion of solute-free water by the kidneys requires normal nephron function (especially the thick ascending limb of Henle's loop), adequate delivery of tubular fluid to the nephrons, and the absence of ADH. Maximal reabsorption of solute-free water by the kidneys requires normal nephron function (especially the thick ascending limb of Henle's loop), adequate delivery of tubular fluid to the nephrons, a hyperosmotic medullary interstitium, the presence of ADH, and responsiveness of the collecting duct to ADH.

6. The volume of ECF is determined by Na^+ balance. When intake of Na^+ exceeds excretion, positive Na^+ balance exists and volume expansion occurs. Conversely, when excretion of Na^+ exceeds intake, negative Na^+ balance exists and volume depletion occurs. The kidneys are the primary route for Na^+ excretion from the body.

7. The coordination of Na^+ intake and excretion, and thus the maintenance of euvolemia, requires the integrated action of the kidneys, the cardiovascular system, and the sympathetic nervous systems. Sensors throughout the body (most importantly the low- and high-pressure vascular volume sensors) monitor the effective circulating volume. Neural and hormonal signals then modulate renal NaCl excretion to match it to intake.

8. During euvolemia, Na^+ excretion by the kidneys is matched to the amount of Na^+ ingested in the diet. The kidneys accomplish this matching by reabsorbing virtually all the filtered load of Na^+ (typically less than 1% of the filtered load is excreted). During euvolemia, the collecting duct adjusts urinary NaCl excretion to effect Na^+ balance. The major factor that regulates collecting duct Na^+ reabsorption is aldosterone, which acts to stimulate Na^+ reabsorption.

9. With volume expansion, low- and high-pressure volume sensors initiate a response that ultimately leads to increased excretion of Na^+ by the kidneys and the reestablishment of euvolemia. The components of this response include a decrease in sympathetic neural outflow to the kidney, a sup-

pression of the renin-angiotensin-aldosterone system, and release of atrial natriuretic peptide from the cardiac atria. At the level of the kidneys, the GFR is enhanced, thereby increasing the filtered load of Na^+. Na^+ reabsorption by the proximal tubule and collecting duct is reduced. Together, these changes in renal Na^+ handling enhance Na^+ excretion. With volume contraction, the above sequence of events is reversed.

BIBLIOGRAPHY

Journal articles

Agree P: Aquaporin channels in kidney, *J Am Soc Nephrol* 11:764, 2000.

Bankir LT, Trinh-Trang-Tan MM: Renal urea transporters: direct and indirect regulation by vasopressin, *Exp Physiol* 85:243s, 2000.

Birnbaumer M: Vasopressin receptors, *Trends Endocrinol Metab* 11:406, 2000.

Deen PM et al: Nephrogenic diabetes insipidus, *Curr Opin Nephrol Hypertens* 9:591, 2000.

Farman N, Rafestin-Oblin ME: Multiple aspects of mineralocorticoid selectivity, *Am J Physiol* 280:F181, 2001.

Forssmann W et al: The renal urodilatin system: clinical implications, *Cardiovasc Res* 51:450, 2001.

Greger R: Physiology of renal sodium transport, *Am J Med Sci* 319:51, 2000.

Inoue T et al: Physiological effects of vasopressin and atrial natriuretic peptide in the collecting duct, *Cardiovasc Res* 51:470, 2001.

Lumbers ER: Angiotensin and aldosterone, *Regul Pept* 80:91, 1999.

Morello JP, Bichet DR: Nephrogenic diabetes insipidus, *Annu Rev Physiol* 63:607, 2001.

Oh MS, Halperin ML: The mechanism of urine concentration in the inner medulla, *Nephron* 75:384, 1997.

Sands JM: Regulation of urea transporters, *J Am Soc Nephrol* 10:635, 1999.

Suzuki T et al: The role of natriuretic peptides in the cardiovascular system, *Cardiovasc Res* 51:489, 2001.

Verkman AS, Mitra AK: Structure and function of aquaporin water channels, *Am J Physiol* 278:F13, 2000.

Vesley DL: Atrial natriuretic peptides in pathophysiological diseases, *Cardiovasc Res* 51:647, 2001.

Books and monographs

Agree P et al: Aquaporin water channels in mammalian kidney. In Seldin DW, Giebisch G, editors: *The kidney: physiology and pathophysiology*, ed 3, Philadelphia, 2000, Lippincott, Williams & Wilkins.

Bankir L, Trinh-Trangi-Tan MM: Urea and the kidney. In Brenner BM, editor: *The kidney*, ed 6, Philadelphia, 2000, WB Saunders.

Berl T, Robertson GL: Pathophysiology of water metabolism. In Brenner BM, editor: *The kidney*, ed 6, Philadelphia, 2000, WB Saunders.

Bichet DG: Polyuria and diabetes insipidus. In Seldin DW, Giebisch G, editors: *The kidney: physiology and pathophysiology*, ed 3, Philadelphia, 2000, Lippincott, Williams & Wilkins.

Brown D, Neilsen E: Cell biology of vasopressin action. In Brenner BM, editor: *The kidney*, ed 6, Philadelphia, 2000, WB Saunders.

Chan L, Wang W: Hypernatremic states. In Seldin DW, Giebisch G, editors: *The kidney: physiology and pathophysiology,* ed 3, Philadelphia, 2000, Lippincott, Williams & Wilkins.

DiBona GF, Kopp UC: Neural control of renal function. In Seldin DW, Giebisch G, editors: *The kidney: physiology and pathophysiology,* ed 3, Philadelphia, 2000, Lippincott, Williams & Wilkins.

Fitzsimmons JT: Physiology and pathophysiology of thirst and sodium appetite. In Seldin DW, Giebisch G, editors: *The kidney: physiology and pathophysiology,* ed 3, Philadelphia, 2000, Lippincott, Williams & Wilkins.

Hall JE, Brands MW: The renin-angiotensin-aldosterone systems: renal mechanisms and circulatory homeostasis. In Seldin DW, Giebisch G, editors: *The kidney: physiology and pathophysiology,* ed 3, Philadelphia, 2000, Lippincott, Williams & Wilkins.

Humphreys MH, Valentin JP: Natriuretic humoral agents. In Seldin DW, Giebisch G, editors: *The kidney: physiology and pathophysiology,* ed 3, Philadelphia, 2000, Lippincott, Williams & Wilkins.

Masilamani S et al: Urine concentration and dilution. In Brenner BM, editor: *The kidney,* ed 6, Philadelphia, 2000, WB Saunders.

Palmer BF et al: Physiology and pathophysiology of sodium retention. In Seldin DW, Giebisch G, editors: *The kidney: physiology and pathophysiology,* ed 3, Philadelphia, 2000, Lippincott, Williams & Wilkins.

Robertson GL: Vasopressin. In Seldin DW, Giebisch G, editors: *The kidney: physiology and pathophysiology,* ed 3, Philadelphia, 2000, Lippincott, Williams & Wilkins.

Sands JM, Layton HE: Urine concentrating mechanism and its regulation. In Seldin DW, Giebisch G, editors: *The kidney: physiology and pathophysiology,* ed 3, Philadelphia, 2000, Lippincott, Williams & Wilkins.

Schnermann J, Briggs JP: Function of the juxtaglomerular apparatus: control of glomerular hemodynamics and renin secretion. In Seldin DW, Giebisch G, editors: *The kidney: physiology and pathophysiology,* ed 3, Philadelphia, 2000, Lippincott, Williams & Wilkins.

Sterns RH et al: Hyponatremia. In Seldin DW, Giebisch G, editors: *The kidney: physiology and pathophysiology,* ed 3, Philadelphia, 2000, Lippincott, Williams & Wilkins.

Verrey F et al: Control of Na^+ transport by aldosterone. In Seldin DW, Giebisch G, editors: *The kidney: physiology and pathophysiology,* ed 3, Philadelphia, 2000, Lippincott, Williams & Wilkins.

Winaver J et al: Control of extracellular fluid volume and the pathophysiology of edema formation. In Brenner BM, editor: *The kidney,* ed 6, Philadelphia, 2000, WB Saunders.

chapter thirty-seven

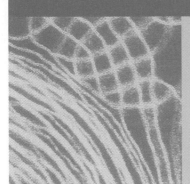
Potassium, Calcium, and Phosphate Homeostasis

K⁺ HOMEOSTASIS

Potassium (K⁺) is one of the most abundant cations in the body and is critical for many cell functions. Despite wide fluctuations in dietary K⁺ intake, its concentration in cells and extracellular fluid (ECF) remains constant. Two sets of regulatory mechanisms safeguard K⁺ homeostasis. First, certain mechanisms regulate the potassium [K⁺] in the ECF.* Second, other mechanisms keep the amount of K⁺ in the body constant by adjusting renal K⁺ excretion to match dietary K⁺ intake. It is the kidneys that regulate K⁺ excretion. In this chapter we focus on the hormones and the factors that influence the [K⁺] in the ECF compartment and those that regulate the amount of K⁺ excreted in the urine.

Total body K⁺ constitutes 50 mEq/kg of body weight, or 3500 mEq for a 70-kg individual. Ninety-eight percent of the K⁺ in the body is located within cells, where its average concentration is 150 mEq/L. A high intracellular concentration of K⁺ is required for many cell functions, including cell growth and division and volume regulation. Only 2% of total body K⁺ is located in the ECF, where its normal concentration is approximately 4 mEq/L. When the [K⁺] of the ECF exceeds 5.0 mEq/L, **hyperkalemia** exists. Conversely, **hypokalemia** exists when the [K⁺] of the ECF is less than 3.5 mEq/L.

The large concentration difference of K⁺ across cell membranes (≈ 146 mEq/L) is maintained by the operation of Na⁺,K⁺-ATPase. This K⁺ gradient is important in maintaining the potential difference across cell membranes (see also Chapters 2 and 15). Thus, K⁺ is critical for the excitability of nerve and muscle cells, as well as for the contractility of cardiac, skeletal, and smooth muscle cells (Fig. 37-1).

Cardiac arrhythmias are produced by both hypokalemia and hyperkalemia. Figure 37-2 illustrates several electro-cardiograms (ECGs) from patients with various levels of plasma [K⁺]. The first sign of hyperkalemia is the appearance of tall, thin T waves. Further increases in plasma [K⁺] prolong the PR interval, depress the ST segment, and lengthen the QRS interval. Finally, as plasma [K⁺] approaches 10 mEq/L, the P wave disappears, the QRS interval broadens, the ECG appears as a sine wave, and the ventricles fibrillate (i.e., manifest rapid, unco-ordinated contractions of muscle fibers). Hypokalemia prolongs the QT interval, inverts the T wave, and lowers the ST segment. The ECG is a fast and easy way to determine whether changes in plasma [K⁺] are influencing the heart and other excitable cells. In contrast, measurements of plasma [K⁺] by the clinical laboratory require a blood sample, and values are often not immediately available.

Internal K⁺ Distribution

After a meal, the K⁺ absorbed by the gastrointestinal tract enters the ECF within minutes (Fig. 37-3). If the K⁺ ingested during a normal meal (≈ 33 mEq) were to remain in the ECF compartment, plasma [K⁺] would increase by a potentially lethal 2.4 mEq/L (33 mEq added to 14 L of ECF = ~2.4 mEq/L). This rise in plasma [K⁺] is prevented by the rapid uptake of K⁺ into cells. *Because the excretion of K⁺ by the kidneys after a meal is relatively slow (hours), the buffering of K⁺ by cells is essential to prevent life-threatening hyperkalemia.* To maintain total body K⁺ constant, all the K⁺ absorbed by the gastrointestinal tract must eventually be excreted by the kidneys. K⁺ excretion is slow; after 6 hours it is completely eliminated from the body.

Several hormones promote the uptake of K⁺ into cells after a rise in plasma [K⁺], and this increased uptake prevents dangerous hyperkalemia. As illustrated in Fig. 37-3 and summarized in Table 37-1, these hormones include epinephrine, insulin, and aldosterone. All these hormones increase K⁺ uptake into skeletal muscle, liver, bone, and red blood cells by stimulating the Na⁺,K⁺-ATPase pump. Acute stimulation of K⁺ uptake (i.e., within minutes) is mediated by increased

---

*The [K⁺] in the ECF is monitored in the clinical setting by measuring the plasma [K⁺]. For simplicity, in this book we use plasma [K⁺] interchangeable with ECF [K⁺].

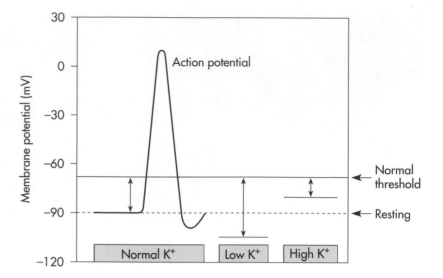

■ **Fig. 37-1** Effects of variations in plasma [K⁺] on the resting membrane potential of skeletal muscle. Hyperkalemia causes the membrane potential to become less negative, which decreases the excitability by inactivating fast Na⁺ channels. Hypokalemia hyperpolarizes the membrane potential, thereby reducing excitability.

turnover rate of existing Na⁺,K⁺-ATPase, whereas the chronic increase in K⁺ uptake (i.e., within hours to days) is mediated by an increase in Na⁺,K⁺-ATPase. A rise in plasma [K⁺] that follows K⁺ absorption by the gastrointestinal tract stimulates insulin secretion from the pancreas, aldosterone release from the adrenal cortex, and epinephrine secretion from the adrenal medulla. In contrast, a decrease in plasma [K⁺] inhibits release of these hormones. Whereas insulin and epinephrine act within a few minutes, aldosterone requires about 1 hour to stimulate K⁺ uptake into cells.

Epinephrine. Catecholamines affect the distribution of K⁺ across cell membranes by activating α- and β₂-adrenergic receptors. Stimulation of α receptors releases K⁺ from cells, especially in the liver, whereas stimulation of β₂ receptors causes K⁺ uptake by cells.

> α-Adrenoceptor activation is important in preventing hypokalemia after exercise. The importance of β₂ receptors is illustrated by two observations. First, the rise in plasma [K⁺] after a K⁺-rich meal is greater if the subject has been treated with **propranolol,** a β-adrenergic blocker. Second, the release of epinephrine during stress (e.g., myocardial ischemia) can rapidly lower plasma [K⁺].

Insulin. Insulin also stimulates K⁺ uptake into cells. The importance of insulin in stimulating K⁺ uptake is illustrated by two observations. First, the rise in plasma [K⁺] after a K⁺-rich meal is greater in individuals with diabetes mellitus (i.e., insulin deficiency) than in normal people. Second, infusion of insulin (and glucose to prevent insulin-induced hypoglycemia) can be used to correct hyperkalemia. *Insulin is the most important hormone that shifts K⁺ into cells after ingestion of K⁺ in a meal.*

Aldosterone. Aldosterone, like catecholamines and insulin, also promotes K⁺ uptake into cells. A rise in aldosterone levels (e.g., **primary aldosteronism**) causes hypokalemia, while a fall in aldosterone levels (e.g., **Addison's disease**) causes hyperkalemia. As discussed below, aldosterone also

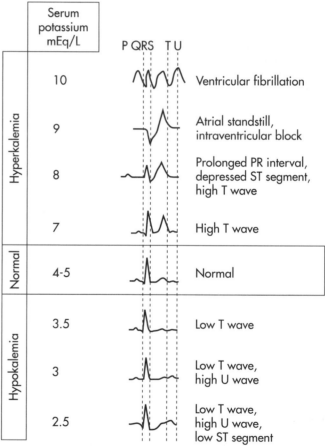

■ **Fig. 37-2** Electrocardiograms from individuals with varying plasma [K⁺]. Hyperkalemia increases the height of the T wave; hypokalemia inverts the T wave. See text for details. (Modified from Barker L, Burton J, Zieve P: *Principles of ambulatory medicine,* Baltimore, 1999, Williams & Wilkins.)

stimulates urinary K⁺ excretion. Thus, aldosterone alters plasma [K⁺] by acting on K⁺ uptake into cells and by altering urinary K⁺ excretion.

Thus far, our discussion has focused on hormones that keep the distribution of K⁺ across cell membranes constant.

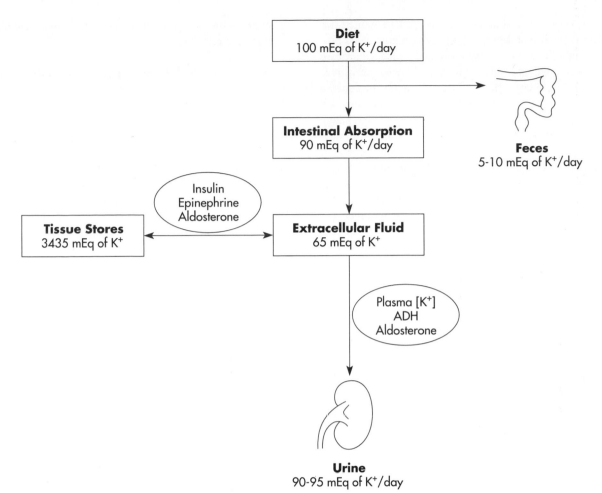

■ **Fig. 37-3** Overview of potassium (K⁺) homeostasis. An increase in plasma insulin, epinephrine, and aldosterone stimulates the movement of K⁺ into cells and decreases plasma [K⁺], whereas a fall in the plasma concentration of these hormones increases plasma [K⁺]. The amount of K⁺ in the body is determined by the kidneys. An individual is in K⁺ balance when dietary intake and urinary output (plus output by the gastrointestinal tract) are equal. The excretion of K⁺ by the kidneys is regulated by plasma [K⁺], aldosterone, and antidiuretic hormone (ADH).

Other factors and some drugs are not homeostatic mechanisms, because they displace normal plasma [K⁺] levels. Table 37-1 summarizes these factors and drugs.

Acid-base balance. In general, metabolic acidosis increases plasma [K⁺], whereas metabolic alkalosis decreases plasma [K⁺]. In contrast, respiratory acid-base disorders have little or no effect on plasma [K⁺]. A metabolic acidosis produced by the addition of inorganic acids (e.g., HCl, H_2SO_4) increases plasma [K⁺] to a much greater extent than does a similar acidosis produced by the accumulation of organic acids (e.g., lactic acid, acetic acid, keto acids). The reduced pH promotes movement of H⁺ into cells and the reciprocal movement of K⁺ out of cells. Metabolic alkalosis has the opposite effect; plasma [K⁺] decreases as K⁺ moves into cells and H⁺ exits cells. The mechanism responsible for this shift is not fully understood. It has been proposed that the movement of H⁺ occurs as the cells buffer changes in the [H⁺] of the ECF. As H⁺ moves across the cell membranes, K⁺ moves in the

■ **Table 37-1** Major factors, hormones, and drugs influencing the distribution of K⁺ between the intracellular and extracellular fluid compartments

Physiological: keep plasma [K⁺] constant

Epinephrine
Insulin
Aldosterone

Pathophysiological: displace plasma [K⁺] from normal

Acid-base balance
Plasma osmolality
Cell lysis
Exercise

Drugs that induce hyperkalemia

Potassium supplements
ACE inhibitors
K-sparing diuretics
Heparin

opposite direction, and thus cations are neither gained nor lost across the cell membranes. Although organic acids produce a metabolic acidosis, they do not cause significant hyperkalemia. Two possible explanations have been suggested for the reduced effect of organic acids in causing hyperkalemia. First, the organic anion may enter the cell with H^+, thereby eliminating the need for K^+/H^+ exchange across the membrane. Second, organic anions may stimulate insulin secretion, which moves K^+ into cells. This movement may counteract the direct effect of the acidosis, which moves K^+ out of cells.

Plasma osmolality. The osmolality of the plasma also influences the distribution of K^+ across cell membranes. An increase in the osmolality of the ECF enhances K^+ release by cells and thus increases extracellular $[K^+]$. The plasma K^+ level may increase by 0.4 to 0.8 mEq/L for a 10 mOsm/kg H_2O elevation in plasma osmolality. Hypoosmolality has the opposite action. The alterations in plasma $[K^+]$ associated with changes in osmolality are related to changes in cell volume. For example, as plasma osmolality increases, water will leave cells because of the osmotic gradient across the plasma membrane. Water leaves cells until the intracellular osmolality equals that of the ECF. This loss of water shrinks cells and causes the $[K^+]$ to rise. The rise in intracellular $[K^+]$ provides a driving force for the exit of K^+ from the cells. This sequence increases plasma $[K^+]$. A fall in plasma osmolality has the opposite effect.

Cell lysis. Cell lysis causes hyperkalemia. The hyperkalemia results from the addition of intracellular K^+ to the ECF.

Severe trauma (e.g., burns) and some diseases such as **tumor lysis syndrome** and **rhabdomyolysis** (i.e., destruction of skeletal muscle) cause cell destruction and release of K^+ (and other cell solutes) into the ECF. In addition, **gastric ulcers** may cause seepage of red blood cells into the gastrointestinal tract. The blood cells are digested, and the K^+ released from the cells is absorbed and can cause hyperkalemia.

Exercise. During exercise, more K^+ is released from skeletal muscle cells than during rest. Release of K^+ during the recovery phase of the action potential and the ensuing hyperkalemia depends on the degree of exercise. In subjects walking slowly the plasma $[K^+]$ increases by 0.3 mEq/L, and levels may increase by up to 2.0 mEq/L or more above normal with more vigorous exercise.

Exercise-induced changes in plasma $[K^+]$ usually do not produce symptoms and are reversed after several minutes of rest. However, in individuals (1) with certain endocrine disorders that affect the release of insulin, epinephrine, or aldosterone; (2) whose ability to excrete K^+ is impaired (e.g., in renal failure); or (3) who take certain medications, such as β-adrenergic blockers, exercise can lead to potentially life-threatening hyperkalemia. For example, during exercise, plasma $[K^+]$ may increase by 2 to 4 mEq/L or more in individuals taking β-adrenergic blockers for hypertension.

Because acid-base balance, plasma osmolality, cell lysis, and exercise do not maintain plasma $[K^+]$ at a normal value, they therefore do not contribute to K^+ homeostasis. The extent to which these pathophysiological states alter plasma $[K^+]$ depends on the integrity of the homeostatic mechanisms that regulate plasma $[K^+]$ (e.g., secretion of epinephrine, insulin, and aldosterone).

Drug-induced hyperkalemia. Drugs are responsible for one third of the cases of clinically significant hyperkalemia and are contributory factors in more than 60% of hyperkalemia in hospitalized patients. Potassium supplements, angiotensin-converting enzyme (ACE) inhibitors, K^+ sparing diuretics, heparin, and prostaglandin-suppressing drugs that cause hyporeninemic hypoaldosteronism account for the majority of these cases. The risk for drug-induced hyperkalemia is increased in patients with diabetes mellitus and renal insufficiency, and in the elderly.

K^+ Excretion by the Kidneys

The kidneys play the major role in maintaining K^+ balance. As illustrated in Fig. 37-3, the kidneys excrete 90% to 95% of the K^+ ingested in the diet. Excretion equals intake even when intake increases by as much as 10-fold. This balance of urinary excretion and dietary intake underscores the importance of the kidneys in maintaining K^+ homeostasis. Although small amounts of K^+ are lost each day in the stool and sweat ($\approx$ 5% to 10% of the K^+ ingested in the diet), this amount is essentially constant, is not regulated, and therefore is relatively much less important than is the K^+ excreted by the kidneys.[*] *The main event in determining urinary K^+ excretion is K^+ secretion from the blood into the tubular fluid by the cells of the distal tubule and collecting duct system.* The transport pattern of K^+ by the major nephron segments is illustrated in Fig. 37-4.

Because K^+ is not bound to plasma proteins, it is freely filtered by the glomerulus. When normal individuals ingest an average diet, urinary K^+ excretion is 15% of the amount filtered. Accordingly, K^+ must be reabsorbed along the nephron. When dietary K^+ intake increases, however, K^+ excretion can exceed the amount filtered. Thus, K^+ can also be secreted.

The proximal tubule reabsorbs 67% of the filtered K^+ under most conditions. Approximately 20% of the filtered K^+ is reabsorbed by Henle's loop and, as with the proximal tubule, the amount reabsorbed is a constant fraction of the amount filtered. In contrast to these segments, which are capable of only reabsorbing K^+, the distal tubule and the collecting duct are able to either reabsorb or secrete K^+. The rate of K^+ reabsorption or secretion by the distal tubule and the collecting duct depends on a variety of hormones and

---

[*]Loss of K^+ in the feces can become significant during periods of diarrhea.

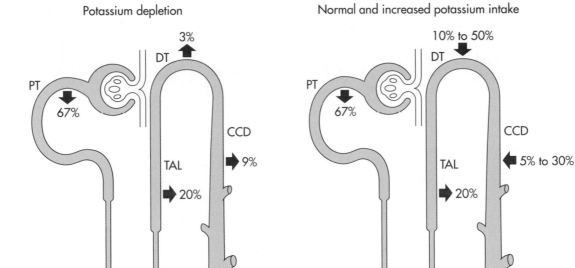

Potassium depletion

Normal and increased potassium intake

■ **Fig. 37-4** K⁺ transport along the nephron. K⁺ excretion depends on the rate and direction of K⁺ transport by the distal tubule and the collecting duct. Percentages refer to the amount of filtered K⁺ reabsorbed or secreted by each nephron segment. *Left panel,* Dietary K⁺ depletion. An amount of K⁺ equal to 1% of the filtered load of K⁺ is excreted. *Right panel,* Normal and increased dietary K⁺ intake. An amount of K⁺ equal to 15% to 80% of the filtered load is excreted. *PT,* Proximal tubule; *TAL,* thick ascending limb; *DT,* distal tubule; *CCD,* collecting duct; *IMCD,* inner medullary collecting duct.

factors. When K⁺ intake is normal (100 mEq/day), K⁺ is secreted. A rise in dietary K⁺ intake increases K⁺ secretion. K⁺ secretion can increase the amount of K⁺ appearing in the urine so that it approaches 80% of the amount filtered (Fig. 37-4). In contrast, a low K⁺ diet activates K⁺ reabsorption along the distal tubule and collecting duct, so that urinary excretion falls to 1% of the K⁺ filtered by the glomerulus (Fig. 37-4). The kidneys are not able to reduce K⁺ excretion to the same low levels as they can for Na⁺ (0.2%). Therefore, hypokalemia can develop in individuals placed on a K⁺-deficient diet.

Because the magnitude and direction of K⁺ transport by the distal tubule and collecting duct are variable, the overall rate of urinary K⁺ excretion is determined by these tubular segments.

In individuals with **advanced renal disease,** the kidneys are unable to eliminate K⁺ from the body. Plasma [K⁺] therefore rises. The resultant hyperkalemia reduces the resting membrane potential (i.e., the voltage becomes less negative), which decreases the excitability of neurons, cardiac cells, and muscle cells by inactivating fast Na⁺ channels in the membrane. Severe, rapid increases in plasma [K⁺] can lead to cardiac arrest and death. In contrast, in patients taking diuretic drugs for hypertension, urinary K⁺ excretion often exceeds dietary K⁺ intake. Accordingly, negative K⁺ balance exists and hypokalemia develops. This decline in extracellular [K⁺] hyperpolarizes the resting cell membrane potential (i.e., the voltage

becomes more negative), which reduces the excitability of neurons, cardiac cells, and muscle cells. Severe hypokalemia can lead to paralysis, cardiac arrhythmia, and death. Hypokalemia can also impair the ability of the kidneys to concentrate the urine and stimulate renal production of NH₄⁺. Therefore, maintenance of a high intracellular [K⁺], a low extracellular [K⁺], and a high K⁺ concentration gradient across cell membranes is essential for a number of cellular functions.

Cellular Mechanisms of K⁺ Transport by the Distal Tubule and Collecting Duct

Figure 37-5 illustrates the cellular mechanism of K⁺ secretion by principal cells in the distal tubule and collecting duct. Secretion from blood into tubular fluid is a two-step process involving (1) K⁺ uptake across the basolateral membrane by Na⁺,K⁺-ATPase and (2) diffusion of K⁺ from the cell into the tubular fluid. The operation of the Na⁺,K⁺-ATPase creates a high intracellular [K⁺], which provides the driving force for K⁺ exit across the apical membrane through K⁺ channels. Although K⁺ channels are also present in the basolateral membrane, K⁺ preferentially leaves the cell across the apical membrane and enters the tubular fluid. K⁺ transport follows this route for two reasons. First, the electrochemical gradient of K⁺ across the apical membrane favors its downhill movement into the tubular fluid. Second,

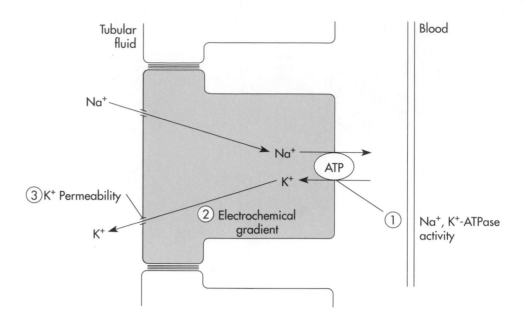

■ **Fig. 37-5** Cellular mechanism of K⁺ secretion by a principal cell in the distal tubule and collecting duct. The numbers indicate the sites where K⁺ secretion is regulated: *1,* Na⁺,K⁺-ATPase; *2,* electrochemical gradient of K⁺ across the apical membrane; *3,* K⁺ permeability of the apical membrane.

the permeability of the apical membrane to K⁺ is greater than that of the basolateral membrane. Therefore, K⁺ preferentially diffuses across the apical membrane into the tubular fluid. The three major factors that control the rate of K⁺ secretion by the distal tubule and the collecting duct (Fig. 37-5) are as follows:

1. The activity of the Na⁺,K⁺-ATPase
2. The driving force (electrochemical gradient) for K⁺ movement across the apical membrane
3. The permeability of the apical membrane to K⁺

Any change in K⁺ secretion results from an alteration in one or more of these factors.

In contrast, the cellular pathways and mechanisms of K⁺ reabsorption in the distal tubule and collecting duct are not completely understood. Intercalated cells may reabsorb K⁺ by a H⁺,K⁺-ATPase transport mechanism located in the apical membrane. This transporter mediates K⁺ uptake in exchange for H⁺. However, the pathway of K⁺ exit from intercalated cells into the blood is unknown. As we have seen, reabsorption of K⁺ is activated by a low-K⁺ diet.

Bartter's syndrome is a set of autosomal-recessive genetic disorders characterized by hypokalemia, metabolic alkalosis, and hyperaldosteronism. Mutations in the genes coding for the 1Na⁺-1K⁺-2Cl⁻ cotransporter, the apical K⁺ channel, or the basolateral Cl⁻ channel in the thick ascending limb (see Fig. 35-8) decrease NaCl and K⁺ absorption by the thick ascending limb, which in turn causes hypokalemia and a decrease in the effective circulating volume (ECV), which stimulates the secretion of aldosterone.

Regulation of K⁺ Secretion by the Distal Tubule and Collecting Duct

Regulation of K⁺ excretion is achieved mainly by alterations in K⁺ secretion by principal cells of the distal tubule and collecting duct. *Plasma [K⁺] and aldosterone are the major physiological regulators of K⁺ secretion. Antidiuretic hormone (ADH) also stimulates K⁺ secretion; however, it is less*

■ **Table 37-2**   Major factors and hormones influencing K⁺ excretion

Physiological: keep K⁺ balance constant
Plasma [K⁺]
Aldosterone
Antidiuretic hormone
Pathophysiological: displace K⁺ balance
Flow rate of tubular fluid
Acid-base balance

important than plasma [K⁺] and aldosterone. Other factors, including the flow rate of tubular fluid and acid-base balance, influence K⁺ secretion by the distal tubule and collecting duct. However, they are not homeostatic mechanisms because they disturb K⁺ balance (Table 37-2).

Hormones and Factors That Regulate Urinary K⁺ Excretion

Plasma [K⁺]. Plasma [K⁺] is an important determinant of K⁺ secretion by the distal tubule and collecting duct (Fig. 37-6). Hyperkalemia (e.g., resulting from a high K⁺ diet or rhabdomyolysis) stimulates secretion within minutes. Several mechanisms are involved. First, hyperkalemia stimulates the Na⁺,K⁺-ATPase and thereby increases K⁺ uptake across the basolateral membrane. This uptake raises intracellular [K⁺] and increases the electrochemical driving force for K⁺ exit across the apical membrane. Second, hyperkalemia also increases the permeability of the apical membrane to K⁺. Third, hyperkalemia stimulates aldosterone secretion by the adrenal cortex, which, as discussed below, acts synergistically with plasma [K⁺] to stimulate K⁺ secretion. Fourth, hyperkalemia also increases the flow rate of tubular fluid, which, as discussed below, stimulates K⁺ secretion by the distal tubule and collecting duct.

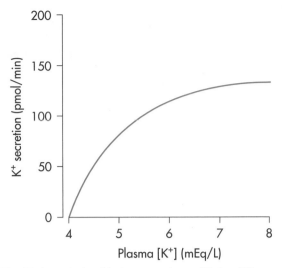

■ **Fig. 37-6** Relationship between plasma [K⁺] and K⁺ secretion by the distal tubule and cortical collecting duct.

Hypokalemia (e.g., caused by a low-K⁺ diet or diarrhea) decreases K⁺ secretion by mechanisms opposite to those described for hyperkalemia. Hence, hypokalemia inhibits Na⁺,K⁺-ATPase, decreases the electrochemical driving force for K⁺ efflux across the apical membrane, reduces the permeability of the apical membrane to K⁺, and causes a reduction in plasma aldosterone levels.

Chronic hypokalemia (plasma [K⁺] <3.5 mEq/L) occurs most often in patients receiving diuretic therapy for hypertension. Hypokalemia also occurs in individuals who vomit, have nasogastric suction, have diarrhea, abuse laxatives, or have **hyperaldosteronism.** Hypokalemia occurs because the excretion of K⁺ by the kidneys exceeds dietary intake of K⁺. Vomiting, nasogastric suction, diuretics, and diarrhea can all cause volume contraction, which in turn stimulates aldosterone secretion (see Chapters 36 and 45). Because aldosterone stimulates K⁺ excretion by the kidneys, its action contributes to the development of hypokalemia.

Chronic hyperkalemia (plasma [K⁺] >5.0 mEq/L) occurs most frequently in individuals with a reduced urinary flow or a low plasma aldosterone level, or in individuals with renal disease whose glomerular filtration rate (GFR) falls to less than 20% of normal. In these individuals, hyperkalemia occurs because the excretion of K⁺ by the kidneys is less than dietary intake of K⁺. Less common causes for hyperkalemia include deficiencies of insulin, epinephrine, or aldosterone secretion, or metabolic acidosis caused by inorganic acids.

Aldosterone. A chronic (i.e., ≥24-hour) elevation in plasma aldosterone concentration enhances K⁺ secretion across the distal tubule and collecting duct by increasing the amount of Na⁺,K⁺-ATPase in principal cells (Fig. 37-7). This uptake elevates cell [K⁺]. Aldosterone also increases the driving force for K⁺ exit across the apical membrane and increases the permeability of the apical membrane to K⁺. Aldosterone secretion is increased by hyperkalemia and by angiotensin II (after activation of the renin-angiotensin system); aldosterone secretion is decreased by hypokalemia and atrial natriuretic peptide (ANP).

Although an acute increase in aldosterone (i.e., within hours) enhances the activity of the Na⁺,K⁺-ATPase, K⁺ excretion does not increase. The reason for this lack of increase relates to the effect of aldosterone on Na⁺ reabsorption and tubular flow. Aldosterone stimulates Na⁺ and thereby water reabsorption and thus decreases tubular flow. The decrease in flow in turn decreases K⁺ secretion (this process is discussed in more detail later). However, chronic stimulation of Na⁺ reabsorption results in volume expansion, and thereby returns tubular flow to normal. These actions allow the direct stimulatory effect of aldosterone on the distal tubule and collecting duct to increase K⁺ excretion.

Glucocorticoids. Glucocorticoids also stimulate K⁺ excretion. However, this effect is indirect and mediated by an increase in GFR, which increases tubular flow.

Antidiuretic hormone. ADH increases the electrochemical driving force for K⁺ exit across the apical membrane of principal cells by stimulating Na⁺ uptake across the apical membrane. The increased Na⁺ uptake reduces the electrical potential difference across the apical membrane (i.e., the interior of the cell becomes less negatively charged). Despite this effect, ADH does not change K⁺ secretion by these nephron segments. The reason for this relates to the effect of ADH on tubular fluid flow. ADH decreases tubular fluid flow by stimulating water reabsorption. The decrease in tubular flow in turn decreases K⁺ secretion (see below for a discussion). The inhibitory effect of decreased tubular flow offsets the stimulatory effect of ADH on the electrochemical driving force for K⁺ exit across the apical membrane (Fig. 37-8). If ADH did not increase the electrochemical gradient favoring K⁺ secretion, urinary K⁺ excretion would fall as ADH levels increase and urinary flow rates decrease. Hence, K⁺ balance would change in response to alterations in water balance. Thus, these effects of ADH on the electrochemical driving force for K⁺ exit across the apical membrane and tubule flow enable urinary K⁺ excretion to be maintained constant despite wide fluctuations in water excretion.

Factors That Perturb K⁺ Excretion

Flow of tubular fluid. A rise in the flow of tubular fluid (e.g., with diuretic therapy, ECF volume expansion) rapidly (within minutes) stimulates K⁺ secretion, whereas a fall in flow (e.g., ECF volume contraction caused by hemorrhage or severe vomiting or diarrhea) reduces K⁺ secretion by the distal tubule and collecting duct (Fig. 37-9). Increments in tubular fluid flow are more effective in stimulating K⁺ secretion as dietary K⁺ intake is increased. Alterations in tubular fluid flow influence K⁺ secretion by changing the driving force for K⁺ exit across the apical membrane. As K⁺ is secreted into the tubular fluid, the [K⁺] of the fluid increases. The

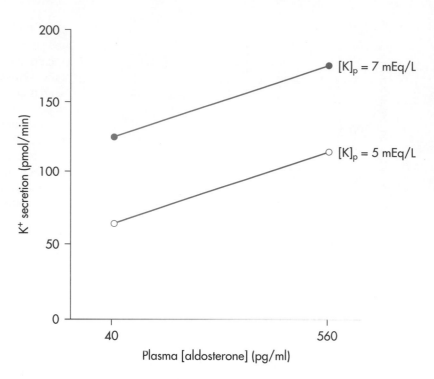

Fig. 37-7   Relationship between plasma aldosterone and K⁺ secretion by the distal tubule and cortical collecting duct. Note that K⁺ secretion is further increased when plasma [K⁺] ($[K]_p$) is increased.

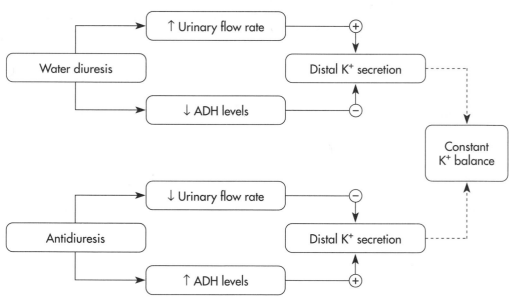

■ **Fig. 37-8**   Opposing effects of ADH on K⁺ secretion by the distal tubule and cortical collecting duct. Secretion is stimulated by an increase in the magnitude of the electrochemical gradient for K⁺ across the apical membrane and perhaps by an increase in the K⁺ permeability of the apical membrane. In contrast, secretion is reduced by a fall in the flow rate of tubular fluid. Because these effects oppose each other, ADH has no net effect on net K⁺ secretion.

increase in [K⁺] of the tubular fluid reduces the electrochemical driving force for K⁺ exit across the apical membrane, thereby reducing the rate of secretion. An increase in tubular fluid flow minimizes the rise in tubular fluid [K⁺] as the secreted K⁺ is washed downstream. A second mechanism responsible for flow-dependent stimulation of K⁺ secretion is related to Na⁺ reabsorption. A rise in tubular flow increases the amount of Na⁺ entering the distal tubule and collecting duct, which in turn enhances Na⁺ reabsorption. The increase in Na⁺ reabsorption stimulates K⁺ uptake across the basolateral membrane by increasing the activity of the Na⁺,K⁺-ATPase, which promotes K⁺ secretion. *Because diuretic drugs increase the flow of tubular fluid through the distal tubule and collecting duct, they also enhance urinary*

K⁺ excretion. In contrast, a decline in tubular fluid flow inhibits K⁺ secretion. This occurs because a decline in tubular fluid flow facilitates the rise in tubular fluid [K⁺], thereby reducing secretion.

Acid-base balance. Another factor that modulates K⁺ secretion is the [H⁺] of the ECF (Fig. 37-10). Acute alterations (over a period of minutes to hours) in the pH of the plasma affect K⁺ secretion by the distal tubule and collecting duct. **Alkalosis** (a plasma pH above normal) increases H⁺ secretion, whereas **acidosis** (a plasma pH below normal) decreases K⁺ secretion. Acute acidosis reduces K⁺ secretion by two mechanisms: (1) it inhibits Na⁺,K⁺-ATPase, thereby reducing cell [K⁺] and the electrochemical driving force for K⁺ exit across the apical membrane; and (2) it reduces the

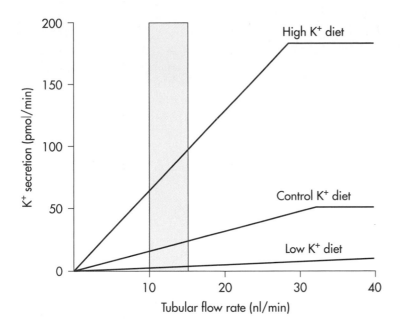

■ **Fig. 37-9** Relationship between tubular flow rate and K+ secretion by the distal tubule and cortical collecting duct. A diet high in K+ increases the slope of the relationship between flow rate and secretion and increases the maximal rate of secretion. A diet low in K+ has the opposite effects. The shaded bar indicates the flow rate under most physiological conditions.

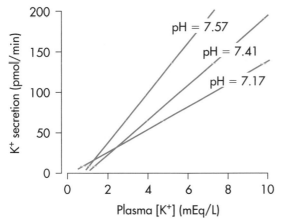

■ **Fig. 37-10** Effect of plasma pH on the relationship between plasma [K+] and K+ secretion by the distal tubule and collecting duct.

permeability of the apical membrane to K+. Alkalosis has the opposite effects.

The effect of metabolic acidosis on K+ excretion is time dependent. When a metabolic acidosis lasts for several days, urinary K+ excretion is stimulated (Fig. 37-11). This occurs because chronic metabolic acidosis decreases water and NaCl reabsorption by the proximal tubule by inhibiting Na+,K+-ATPase in the proximal tubular cells. Hence, the flow of tubular fluid is augmented through the distal tubule and collecting duct. The inhibition of proximal tubular water and NaCl reabsorption also causes a decrease in ECF, thereby stimulating aldosterone secretion. In addition, chronic acidosis caused by inorganic acids increases plasma [K+], which stimulates aldosterone secretion. The rise in tubular fluid flow, plasma [K+], and aldosterone offsets the effects of acidosis on cell [K+] and apical membrane permeability, and K+ secretion rises. Thus, metabolic acidosis may either inhibit or stimulate K+ excretion, depending on the duration of the disturbance.

The flow of tubular fluid and acid-base balance do not maintain K+ balance at a normal value and therefore do not contribute to K+ homeostasis. The extent to which changes in flow and acid-base balance alter K+ balance and plasma [K+] depends on the integrity of the homeostatic mechanisms that regulate K+ balance and plasma [K+].

Frequently, as discussed above, the rate of urinary K+ excretion is determined by simultaneous changes in hormone levels, acid-base balance, or tubular flow (Table 37-3). The powerful effect of tubular flow often enhances or opposes the response of the distal tubule and collecting duct to hormones and changes in acid-base balance. This interaction can be beneficial, as in the case of hyperkalemia, in which the change in flow enhances K+ excretion and thereby restores K+ homeostasis. However, this interaction can also be detrimental, as in the case of alkalosis, in which changes in flow and acid-base status perturb K+ homeostasis.

OVERVIEW OF Ca²⁺ AND Pᵢ HOMEOSTASIS

Ca²⁺ and inorganic phosphate (Pᵢ)* are multivalent ions that subserve many complex and vital functions. In a normal adult, the renal excretion of these ions is balanced by gastrointestinal absorption. If the plasma concentrations decline substantially, gastrointestinal absorption, bone resorption, and renal tubular reabsorption increase and return plasma concentrations of Ca²⁺ and Pᵢ to normal levels. During growth and pregnancy, intestinal absorption exceeds urinary excretion, and these ions accumulate in newly formed fetal tissue and bone. In contrast, bone disease (e.g., **osteoporosis**) or a decline in lean body mass increases urinary multivalent ion loss without a change in intestinal absorption. In these conditions, there is net loss of Ca²⁺ and Pᵢ from the body. *The*

---

*At physiological pH, inorganic phosphate exists as HPO_4^{2-} and $H_2PO_4^-$ (pK = 6.8). For simplicity, we collectively refer to these ion species as P_i.

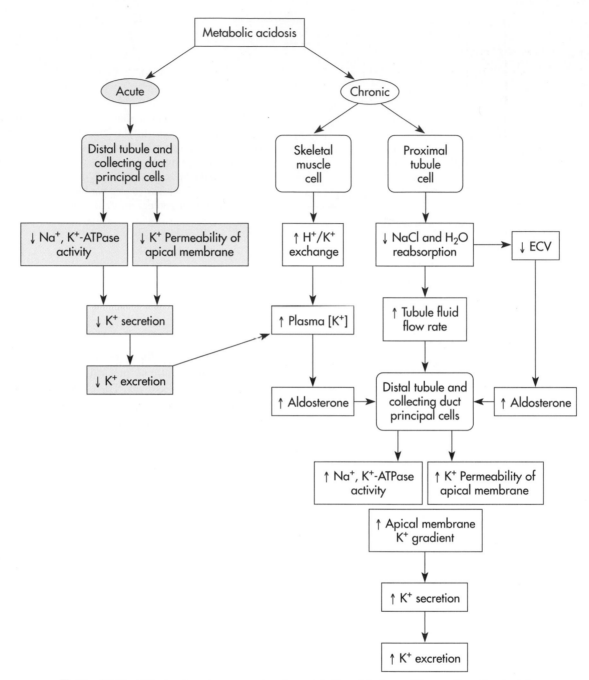

■ **Fig. 37-11** Effects of acute versus chronic metabolic acidosis on K⁺ excretion. See text for details. *ECV,* Effective circulating volume.

kidneys, in conjunction with the gastrointestinal tract and bone, play a major role in maintaining plasma Ca²⁺ and P_i levels.

Calcium

Calcium ions play a major role in many processes, including bone formation, cell division and growth, blood coagulation, hormone-response coupling, and electrical stimulus-response coupling (e.g., muscle contraction and neurotransmitter release). Ninety-nine percent of Ca²⁺ is stored in bone, 1% is found in the intracellular fluid (ICF), and 0.1% is in the ECF (Table 37-4). The total [Ca²⁺] in plasma is 10 mg/dl

(2.5 mM or 5 mEq/L), and its concentration is normally maintained within narrow limits. A low ionized plasma [Ca²⁺], called **hypocalcemia,** increases the excitability of nerve and muscle cells and can lead to **hypocalcemic tetany,** which is characterized by skeletal muscle spasms. An elevated ionized plasma [Ca²⁺], called **hypercalcemia,** may produce decreased neuromuscular excitability, cardiac arrhythmias, lethargy, disorientation, and even death (see Chapter 42).

Overview of Ca²⁺ homeostasis. Ca²⁺ homeostasis depends on two factors: (1) the total amount of Ca²⁺ in the body and (2) the distribution of Ca²⁺ between bone and the ECF compartment. Total body Ca²⁺ is determined by the relative

■ **Table 37-3** Interaction between the direct/indirect effects of hormones and factors on K⁺ secretion by the distal tubule and collecting duct and flow of tubular fluid

	Direct or indirect	Flow	Urinary excretion
Hyperkalemia	↑	↑	↑↑
Aldosterone			
Acute (<1 hr)	↑	↓	NC
Chonic (>1 hr)	↑	NC	↑
Glucocorticoids	NC	↑	↓
ADH	↑	↓	NC
Acidosis			
Acute	↓	NC	↓
Chronic	↓	↑↑	↑
Alkalosis	↑	↑	↑↑

Modified from Field MJ et al: Regulation of renal potassium metabolism. In Narins R, editor: *Textbook of nephrology: clinical disorders of fluid and electrolyte metabolism,* ed 5, New York, 1994, McGraw-Hill. *NC,* No change; *ADH,* antidiuretic hormone.

■ **Table 37-4** Body content and distribution of Ca^{2+} and P_i

| | | | Compartment | |
Ion	*Body content*	*Bone*	*Intracellular*	*Extracellular*
Ca^{2+}	1300 g	99%	1%	0.10%
P_i	700 g	86%	14%	0.03%

amounts of Ca^{2+} absorbed by the gastrointestinal tract and excreted by the kidneys (Fig. 37-12). Ca^{2+} is absorbed by the gastrointestinal tract through an active, carrier-mediated transport mechanism that is stimulated by **calcitriol,** a metabolite of vitamin D_3 (see also Chapter 42).* Net Ca^{2+} absorption is normally 200 mg/day, but it can increase to 600 mg/day when calcitriol levels rise. In adults, Ca^{2+} excretion by the

*Vitamin D_3 is ingested in the diet and can be synthesized in the skin in the presence of ultraviolet light. Vitamin D_3 is converted in the liver to calcifediol and then in the kidney, primarily in the proximal tubule, to the active metabolite calcitriol [1,25-(OH)₂-D_3].

kidneys is equal to the amount absorbed by the gastrointestinal tract (200 mg/day), and it changes in parallel with the reabsorption of Ca^{2+} by the gastrointestinal tract. Thus, in adults, Ca^{2+} balance is maintained because the amount of Ca^{2+} ingested in an average diet (1500 mg/day) is equal to the amount lost in the feces (1300 mg/day: the amount that escapes absorption by the gastrointestinal tract) plus the amount excreted in the urine (200 mg/day).

The second factor that controls Ca^{2+} homeostasis is the distribution of Ca^{2+} between bone and the ECF. Three hormones—**parathyroid hormone (PTH),** calcitriol, and **calcitonin**—are the most important hormones that regulate the distribution of Ca^{2+} between bone and the ECF and thereby regulate plasma $[Ca^{2+}]$. PTH is secreted by the parathyroid glands. Secretion of PTH is stimulated by a decline in plasma $[Ca^{2+}]$ (i.e., in hypocalcemia). PTH increases plasma $[Ca^{2+}]$ by the following:

1. Stimulating bone resorption
2. Increasing Ca^{2+} reabsorption by the kidneys
3. Stimulating the production of calcitriol, which in turn increases Ca^{2+} absorption by the gastrointestinal tract and stimulates bone resorption

Hypercalcemia reduces PTH secretion, which leads to actions opposite to those described above. The production of calcitriol by the proximal tubule cells of the kidneys is stimulated by hypocalcemia and hypophosphatemia. The effect of hypocalcemia is secondary to increased levels of PTH, which are elevated as a result of the decrease in plasma $[Ca^{2+}]$. The effect of hypophosphatemia is direct, because the decrease in plasma $[P_i]$ stimulates the production of calcitriol by the proximal tubule cells. Calcitriol increases plasma $[Ca^{2+}]$ by actions similar to those of PTH (see above).

Calcitonin is secreted by the parafollicular cells of the thyroid gland, and its secretion is stimulated by hypercalcemia. Calcitonin decreases plasma $[Ca^{2+}]$ mainly by stimulating bone formation (i.e., the deposition of Ca^{2+} in bone). Figure 37-13 illustrates the relationship between plasma $[Ca^{2+}]$ and plasma levels of PTH and calcitonin.

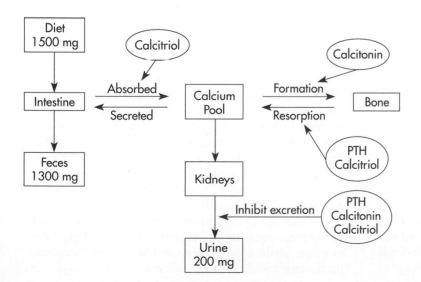

■ **Fig. 37-12** Overview of Ca^{2+} homeostasis. See text for details. *PTH,* Parathyroid hormone.

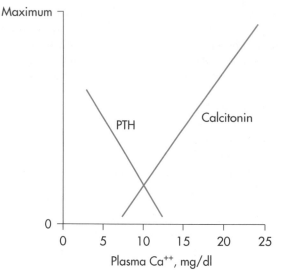

■ **Fig. 37-13**   Effect of plasma [Ca²⁺] on plasma levels of PTH and calcitonin. (Modified from Azria M: *The calcitonins: physiology and pharmacology,* Basel, Switzerland, 1989, Karger.)

■ **Table 37-5**   Forms of Ca²⁺ and Pᵢ in plasma

Ion	mg/dl	Ionized	Percentage of total Protein-bound	Complexed
Ca²⁺	10	50%	45%	5%
Pᵢ	4	84%	10%	6%

Ca²⁺ is bound (i.e., complexed) to various anions in the plasma, including HCO_3^-, citrate, P_i, and SO_4^{2-}. P_i is complexed to various cations, including Na^+ and K^+.

In patients with **acidosis,** the [H⁺] of plasma is increased. This increase in [H⁺] causes more H⁺ to bind to plasma proteins, HCO_3^-, citrate, P_i, and SO_4^{2-}, thereby displacing Ca²⁺. This displacement of Ca²⁺ in turn increases the plasma concentration of ionized Ca²⁺. In contrast, in patients with **alkalosis,** the [H⁺] of plasma decreases. Some H⁺ ions dissociate from plasma proteins, HCO_3^-, citrate, P_i, and SO_4^{2-}, in exchange for Ca²⁺, thereby decreasing the plasma concentration of ionized Ca²⁺.

Conditions that lower PTH levels (e.g., postsurgical hypoparathyroidism following parathyroidectomy caused by adenoma) reduce plasma [Ca²⁺] and can cause **hypocalcemic tetany** (intermittent muscular contraction), which is characterized by skeletal muscle spasms. In severe cases, hypocalcemic tetany can cause death by asphyxiation. Hypercalcemia can also cause cardiac arrhythmia and decreased neuromuscular excitability, both of which can be lethal. Clinically, the most common causes of hypercalcemia are **primary hyperparathyroidism and malignancy-associated hypercalcemia.** Primary hyperparathyroidism results from the overproduction of PTH caused by a tumor of the parathyroid glands. In contrast, malignancy-associated hypercalcemia occurs in 10% to 20% of all patients with cancer and is caused by secretion of PTH-related peptide (PTHRP), a PTH-like hormone secreted by carcinomas in a variety of organs. Increased levels of PTH and PTHRP cause hypercalcemia and hypercalciuria.

Approximately 50% of the Ca²⁺ in plasma is ionized, 45% is bound to plasma proteins (mainly albumin), and 5% is complexed to several anions, including HCO_3^-, citrate, P_i, and SO_4^{2-} (Table 37-5). The pH of the plasma influences this distribution. Acidosis increases the percentage of ionized calcium at the expense of Ca²⁺ bound to proteins, whereas alkalosis decreases the percentage of ionized calcium, again by altering Ca²⁺ bound to proteins. Thus, individuals with alkalosis are susceptible to tetany, whereas individuals with acidosis are less susceptible to tetany, even when total plasma Ca²⁺ levels are reduced. The Ca²⁺ available for filtration consists of the ionized fraction and that complexed with anions. Thus, about 55% of the Ca²⁺ in the plasma is available for glomerular filtration.

Ca²⁺ transport along the nephron. Normally, 99% of filtered Ca²⁺ (i.e., ionized and complexed) is reabsorbed by the nephron. The proximal tubule reabsorbs 70% of filtered Ca²⁺. Another 20% is reabsorbed in Henle's loop (mainly the thick ascending limb), another 9% is reabsorbed in the distal tubule, and <1% is reabsorbed by the collecting duct. About 1% (200 mg/day) is excreted in the urine. This fraction is equal to the net amount absorbed daily by the gastrointestinal tract. Figure 37-14 summarizes the handling of Ca²⁺ by the different portions of the nephron.

Cellular mechanisms of Ca²⁺ reabsorption. Ca²⁺ reabsorption by the proximal tubule occurs via two pathways: transcellular and paracellular (Fig. 37-15). Ca²⁺ reabsorption across the cellular pathway (i.e., transcellular) accounts for 20% of proximal reabsorption. Ca²⁺ reabsorption through the cell is an active process that occurs in two steps. First, Ca²⁺ diffuses across the apical membrane into the cell down its electrochemical gradient. This gradient is exceptionally steep because the Ca²⁺ concentration in the cell is only 0.4 μM, about 10,000-fold less than that in the tubular fluid (~1.5 mM). The cell interior is electrically negative with respect to the luminal side of the apical membrane; this electrical gradient also favors Ca²⁺ entry into the cell, via Ca²⁺ channels. Ca²⁺ leaves the cell across the basolateral membrane against its electrochemical gradient. The mechanism for the exit of Ca²⁺ occurs by Ca²⁺-ATPase and a 3Na⁺-Ca²⁺ antiporter. Eighty percent of Ca²⁺ is reabsorbed between cells across the tight junctions (i.e., paracellular pathway). This passive, paracellular reabsorption of Ca²⁺ occurs by solvent drag along the entire length of the proximal tubule, and is also driven by the positive luminal voltage in the second half of the proximal tubule. Thus, in the proximal tubule, approximately 80% of Ca²⁺ reabsorption is paracellular and 20% is transcellular.

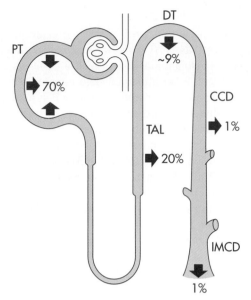

■ **Fig. 37-14** Transport pattern of Ca^{2+} along the nephron. Percentages refer to the amount of filtered Ca^{2+} reabsorbed by each nephron segment. Approximately 1% of filtered Ca^{2+} is excreted. *PT,* Proximal tubule; *TAL,* thick ascending limb; *DT,* distal tubule; *CCD,* cortical collecting duct; *IMCD,* inner medullary collecting duct.

Ca^{2+} reabsorption by Henle's loop is restricted to the thick ascending limb. Ca^{2+} is reabsorbed via a cellular and a paracellular route by mechanisms similar to those described for the proximal tubule, with one difference. Ca^{2+} is not reabsorbed by solvent drag in this segment (recall that the thick ascending limb is impermeable to water). In the thick ascending limb, Ca^{2+} and Na^+ reabsorption parallel each other because of the significant amount of Ca^{2+} reabsorption that occurs by passive, paracellular mechanisms secondary to Na^+ reabsorption and by the generation of the lumen-positive transepithelial voltage. Therefore, *changes in Na^+*

reabsorption will also cause parallel changes in Ca^{2+} reabsorption by the proximal tubule and the thick ascending limb of Henle's loop.

In the distal tubule, where the voltage in the tubule lumen is electrically negative with respect to the blood, Ca^{2+} reabsorption is entirely active because Ca^{2+} is reabsorbed against its electrochemical gradient. Ca^{2+} reabsorption by the distal tubule is exclusively transcellular, and the mechanism is similar to that in the proximal tubule and thick ascending limb: uptake across the apical membrane by a Ca^{2+}-permeable ion channel and exit across the basolateral membrane by a Ca^{2+}-ATPase and a $3Na^+$-Ca^{2+} antiporter. *Na^+ and Ca^{2+} excretion in the urine usually change in parallel. However, this is not always the case because reabsorption of Ca^{2+} and Na^+ by the distal tubule are independent and are differentially regulated. For example, thiazide diuretics inhibit Na^+ reabsorption by the distal tubule and stimulate Ca^{2+} reabsorption by this segment. Accordingly, the net effect of thiazide diuretics is to increase urinary Na^+ excretion and reduce urinary Ca^{2+} excretion.*

As noted in Chapter 35, Gitelman's syndrome is caused by an inactivating mutation in the gene that codes for the NaCl cotransporter, which is expressed in the apical membrane of the distal tubule. Gitelman's syndrome is characterized by an increase in urinary NaCl excretion, hypotension, hypokalemic metabolic alkalosis, and hypocalciuria (i.e., a reduction in urinary calcium excretion). Because the direction and magnitude of sodium and calcium transport are inversely related in the distal tubule, a reduction in NaCl reabsorption increases calcium reabsorption, thereby reducing urinary calcium excretion.

Regulation of urinary Ca^{2+} excretion. Urinary Ca^{2+} excretion is regulated by PTH, calcitonin, and calcitriol. *PTH exerts the most powerful effect on renal Ca^{2+} excretion and is responsible for maintaining Ca^{2+} homeostasis.* Overall,

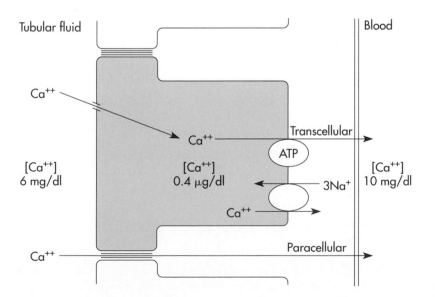

■ **Fig. 37-15** Cellular mechanisms of Ca^{2+} reabsorption by the proximal tubule. Ca^{2+} is reabsorbed by both transcellular and paracellular routes.

this hormone stimulates Ca^{2+} reabsorption by the kidneys (i.e., reduces Ca^{2+} excretion). Although PTH inhibits the reabsorption of NaCl and fluid, and therefore of Ca^{2+}, by the proximal tubule, PTH dramatically stimulates Ca^{2+} reabsorption by the thick ascending limb of Henle's loop and the distal tubule. As a result, urinary Ca^{2+} excretion declines. Calcitonin and calcitriol also stimulate Ca^{2+} reabsorption by the kidneys. Calcitonin stimulates Ca^{2+} reabsorption by the thick ascending limb of Henle's loop and the distal tubule, but it is quantitatively less important than PTH. Calcitriol, either directly or indirectly, enhances Ca^{2+} reabsorption by the distal tubule. It is also quantitatively less important than PTH.

Several factors disturb Ca^{2+} excretion. An increase in plasma $[P_i]$ (e.g., increased dietary intake of P_i) elevates PTH levels, thereby decreasing Ca^{2+} excretion. A decline in the plasma $[P_i]$ (e.g., dietary P_i depletion) has the opposite effect. Changes in ECF volume alter Ca^{2+} excretion mainly by affecting NaCl and fluid reabsorption in the proximal tubule. Volume contraction increases NaCl and water reabsorption by the proximal tubule, thereby enhancing Ca^{2+} reabsorption (Table 37-6). Accordingly, urinary Ca^{2+} excretion declines. Volume expansion has the opposite effect. Acidosis increases Ca^{2+} excretion, whereas alkalosis decreases excretion. The regulation of Ca^{2+} reabsorption by pH occurs in the distal tubule by an unknown mechanism.

■ **Table 37-6**   Hormones and factors that influence renal calcium transport

Tubule segment	↑ Calcium reabsorption	↓ Calcium reabsorption
Proximal tubule	↓ECV, P_i loading	↑ ECV, P_i depletion
Loop of Henle	PTH, calcitonin	↑ $[Ca^{2+}]_p$, PTH
Distal tubule	PTH, calcitonin, thiazides, P_i loading, alkalosis	Furosemide, bumetanide, acidosis

ECV, Effective circulating volume.

Phosphate

P_i is an important component of many organic molecules, including DNA, RNA, ATP, and intermediates of metabolic pathways. It is also a major constituent of bone. Its concentration in plasma is an important determinant in bone formation and resorption. In addition, urinary P_i is an important buffer (titratable acid) in the maintenance of acid-base balance (see Chapter 38). Eighty-six percent of P_i is located in bone, 14% is in the ICF, and 0.03% is in the ECF (Table 37-4). Normal plasma $[P_i]$ is 4 mg/dl (Table 37-5). Approximately 10% of the P_i in plasma is protein bound and therefore unavailable for ultrafiltration by the glomerulus. According, the $[P_i]$ in the ultrafiltrate is 10% less than in plasma.

Overview of P_i homeostasis. A general scheme of P_i homeostasis is shown in Fig. 37-16. P_i homeostasis depends on two factors: (1) the amount of P_i in the body and (2) the distribution of P_i between the ICF and ECF compartments. Total body P_i is determined by the relative amount of P_i absorbed by the gastrointestinal tract minus the amount excreted by the kidneys. P_i absorption by the gastrointestinal tract occurs by both active and passive mechanisms; P_i absorption increases as dietary P_i rises and it is stimulated by calcitriol. Despite variations in P_i intake of between 800 and 1500 mg/day, the kidneys keep total body P_i constant by excreting an amount of P_i in the urine equal to the amount absorbed by the gastrointestinal tract. Thus, *the kidneys play a vital role in P_i homeostasis.*

The second factor in P_i homeostasis is the distribution of P_i among bone and the ICF and ECF compartments. PTH, calcitriol, and calcitonin regulate the distribution of P_i between bone and ECF. The release of P_i from intracellular stores is stimulated by the same hormones (PTH and calcitriol) that release Ca^{2+} from this pool. Thus, the release of P_i is always accompanied by a release of Ca^{2+}. In contrast, calcitonin increases bone formation, thereby decreasing plasma $[P_i]$.

The kidneys also play an important role in the regulation of plasma $[P_i]$. A small increase in plasma $[P_i]$ increases the

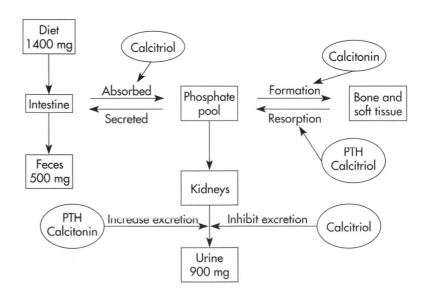

■ **Fig. 37-16**   Overview of P_i homeostasis. See text for details.

amount of P_i filtered by the glomerulus. Because the kidneys normally reabsorb P_i at a maximal rate, any increase in the amount filtered leads to a rise in urinary P_i excretion. In fact, urinary P_i excretion increases to a value above P_i absorption by the gastrointestinal tract, resulting in a net loss of P_i from the body. This loss of P_i causes plasma $[P_i]$ to fall. In this way, *the kidneys regulate plasma $[P_i]$.* The maximal reabsorptive rate for P_i is variable and is regulated by dietary P_i intake. A high P_i diet decreases the maximal reabsorptive rate of P_i by the kidneys, and a low P_i diet increases the maximal reabsorptive rate. This effect of dietary P_i intake on the maximal P_i transport rate of the kidneys is *independent* of changes in PTH levels.

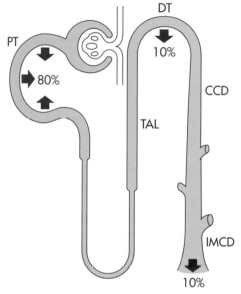

Fig. 37-17 Transport pattern of P_i along the nephron. P_i is reabsorbed primarily by the proximal tubule. Percentages refer to the amount of filtered P_i reabsorbed by each nephron segment. Approximately 10% of filtered P_i is excreted. *PT,* Proximal tubule; *TAL,* thick ascending limb; *DT,* distal tubule; *CCD,* collecting duct; *IMCD,* inner medullary collecting duct.

In patients with **chronic renal failure,** the kidneys cannot excrete P_i and, because of continued P_i absorption by the gastrointestinal tract, P_i accumulates in the body, thereby elevating plasma $[P_i]$. The increased P_i complexes with Ca^{2+}, thereby reducing plasma $[Ca^{2+}]$. P_i accumulation also decreases the production of calcitriol, which reduces Ca^{2+} absorption by the intestine, an effect that further decreases plasma $[Ca^{2+}]$. The fall in plasma $[Ca^{2+}]$ increases PTH secretion and Ca^{2+} release from bone, resulting in **osteitis fibrosa cystica** (i.e., increased bone resorption with replacement by fibrous tissue, which makes bone more susceptible to fracture). Chronic **hyperparathyroidism** (i.e., elevated PTH levels) during chronic renal failure can lead to metastatic calcifications in which Ca^{2+} and P_i precipitate in arteries, soft tissues, and viscera. Deposition of Ca^{2+} and P_i in heart and lung tissue may cause myocardial failure and pulmonary insufficiency, respectively. Prevention and treatment of hyperparathyroidism and P_i retention include a low-P_i diet or the administration of a "phosphate binder" (an agent that renders the P_i unavailable for reabsorption by the gastrointestinal tract by forming insoluble P_i salts). Supplemental Ca^{2+} and calcitriol are also used.

P_i **transport along the nephron.** Figure 37-17 summarizes P_i transport by the various portions of the nephron. The proximal tubule reabsorbs 80% of the P_i filtered by the glomerulus, and the distal tubule reabsorbs 10%. In contrast, Henle's loop and the collecting duct reabsorb only small amounts of P_i. Therefore, 10% of the filtered load of P_i is excreted.

P_i reabsorption by the proximal tubule occurs mainly, if not exclusively, by a transcellular route. As shown in Fig. 37-18, P_i uptake across the apical membrane occurs by a $2Na^+$-P_i symport mechanism. P_i exits across the basolateral membrane, most likely by a P_i-anion antiporter. The cellular mechanism of P_i reabsorption by the distal tubule has not been characterized.

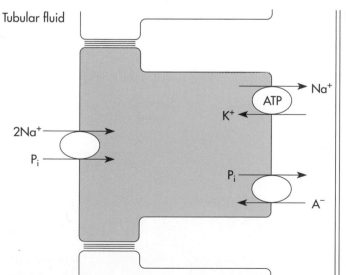

Fig. 37-18 Cellular mechanism of P_i reabsorption by the proximal tubule. The apical transport pathway is a $2Na^+/P_i$ symporter. P_i leaves the cell across the basolateral membrane via a P_i-anion antiporter and possibly via a Na^+/P_i symporter (not shown). A^- indicates an anion.

Regulation of urinary P_i excretion. Table 37-7 summarizes the major hormones and factors that regulate urinary P_i excretion. All act on the proximal tubule and either stimulate or inhibit P_i reabsorption. *PTH is the most important hormone that controls P_i excretion.* PTH stimulates cyclic adenosine monophosphate (cAMP) production and inhibits P_i reabsorption by the proximal tubule, thereby increasing P_i excretion. Dietary P_i intake also regulates P_i excretion by mechanisms independent of changes in PTH levels. P_i loading increases excretion, whereas P_i depletion decreases excretion. These changes in dietary P_i intake modulate P_i transport by altering the transport rate of each $2Na^+$-P_i symporter and by increasing the number of transporters.

ECF volume also affects P_i excretion. Volume expansion increases excretion and volume contraction decreases excretion. The effect of the ECF volume of P_i excretion is indirect and may involve changes in hormone levels other than PTH. Acid-base balance also influences P_i excretion: acidosis increases and alkalosis decreases P_i excretion. Glucocorticoids increase the excretion of P_i. Glucocorticoids increase the delivery of P_i to the distal tubule and collecting ducts by inhibiting proximal tubular P_i reabsorption. This inhibition enables the distal tubule and collecting duct to secrete more H^+ and generate more HCO_3^- because P_i is an important urinary buffer (see Chapter 38 for an explanation). Finally, growth hormone decreases P_i excretion.

■ **Table 37-7**   Hormones and factors that influence urinary P_i excretion

Increased excretion	*Decreased excretion*
Increase of PTH	Decrease of PTH
P_i loading	P_i depletion
↑ECV	↓ECV
Acidosis	Alkalosis
Glucocorticoids	Growth hormone

In the absence of glucocorticoids (e.g., in **Addison's disease**), P_i excretion is depressed, as is the ability of the kidneys to excrete titratable acid and to generate new HCO_3^-. Growth hormone increases the reabsorption of P_i by the proximal tubule. As a result, growing children have a plasma $[P_i]$ that is elevated above that found in adults. This higher level of P_i is important for the formation of bone.

INTEGRATED REVIEW OF PTH, CALCITRIOL, AND CALCITONIN ON Ca^{2+} AND P_i HOMEOSTASIS

Hypocalcemia is the major stimulus of PTH secretion. As summarized in Fig. 37-19, PTH has numerous effects on Ca^{2+} and P_i homeostasis. PTH stimulates bone resorption (i.e., release of Ca^{2+} and P_i from bone), increases urinary P_i excretion, decreases urinary Ca^{2+} excretion, and stimulates the production of calcitriol, which stimulates Ca^{2+} and P_i absorption by the intestine. *Because changes in P_i handling in bone, intestine, and the kidneys tend to cancel each other out, PTH increases plasma $[Ca^{2+}]$ but has little effect on plasma $[P_i]$. Overall, a rise in plasma PTH levels increases plasma $[Ca^{2+}]$ and decreases plasma $[P_i]$. A decline in plasma PTH levels has the opposite effect.*

Calcitriol also plays an important role in Ca^{2+} and P_i homeostasis (Fig. 37-20). Calcitriol stimulates Ca^{2+} and P_i absorption by the intestine and Ca^{2+} and P_i release from bone, but decreases Ca^{2+} and P_i excretion by the kidneys. The net effect of calcitriol is to increase plasma $[Ca^{2+}]$ and $[P_i]$. *Thus, the major stimuli of calcitriol production are hypocalcemia via PTH and hypophosphatemia (i.e., a low plasma $[P_i]$).*

Calcitonin is also an important hormone in Ca^{2+} homeostasis because it blocks bone resorption and stimulates

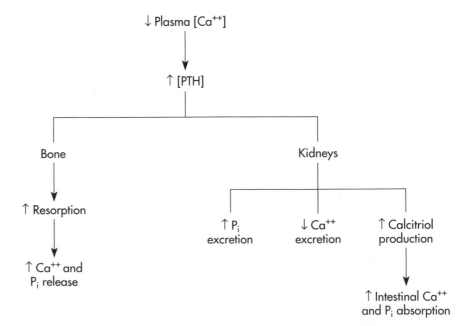

■ **Fig. 37-19**   Effect of PTH on Ca^{2+} and P_i homeostasis. The major stimulus of PTH secretion is hypocalcemia.

Ca^{2+} deposition in bone (Fig. 37-21). Calcitonin's modest direct effect on decreasing urinary Ca^{2+} excretion is a relatively minor action of the hormone. The major stimulus of calcitonin secretion is increase in plasma $[Ca^{2+}]$. *Because changes in P_i handling in bone, intestine, and the kidneys tend to cancel each other out, calcitonin decreases plasma $[Ca^{2+}]$ but has little effect on plasma $[P_i]$.*

Estrogens defend against PTH-mediated resorption of bone. In estrogen-deficient conditions, such as that after menopause, the unabated effect of PTH on bone contributes to the development of osteoporosis.

Calcium-Sensing Receptor

The **calcium-sensing receptor (CaSR)** is a receptor expressed in the plasma membrane of cells involved in regulating Ca^{2+} homeostasis. The CaSR senses small changes in extracellular $[Ca^{2+}]$. Ca^{2+} binds to CaSRs in PTH-secreting cells of the parathyroid gland, calcitonin-secreting parafollicular cells in the thyroid gland, and calcitriol-producing cells in the proximal tubule. An increase in plasma $[Ca^{2+}]$ is converted to intracellular signals that inhibit the secretion of PTH and the production of calcitriol and stimulates the secretion of calcitonin. Moreover, the reduction in PTH also contributes to decreased production of calcitriol because PTH is a potent stimulus of calcitriol synthesis. By contrast, a fall in plasma $[Ca^{2+}]$ has the opposite effect on PTH, calcitriol, and calcitonin secretion. These three hormones act on the kidneys, intestine, and bone to regulate plasma $[Ca^{2+}]$ by mechanisms described elsewhere in this chapter.

The CaSR also maintains Ca^{2+} homeostasis by directly regulating Ca^{2+} excretion by the kidneys. CaSRs in the thick ascending limb and distal tubule respond directly to changes in plasma $[Ca^{2+}]$ and regulate Ca^{2+} absorption by these nephron segments. An increase in plasma $[Ca^{2+}]$ activates CaSR in the thick ascending limb and distal tubule and inhibits Ca^{2+} absorption in these nephron segments, thereby stimulating urinary Ca^{2+} excretion. By contrast, a fall in plasma $[Ca^{2+}]$ leads to an increase in Ca^{2+} absorption by the thick ascending limb and distal tubule and a corresponding decrease in urinary Ca^{2+} excretion. Thus the direct effect of plasma $[Ca^{2+}]$ on CaSRs in the thick ascending limb and distal tubule acts in concert with changes in PTH to regulate urinary Ca^{2+} excretion and thereby maintain Ca^{2+} homeostasis.

Mutations of the gene coding for the CaSR cause disorders in calcium homeostasis. Familial hypocalciuric hypercalcemia (FHH) is an autosomal-dominant disease caused by an inactivating mutation of CaSR. The hypercalcemia is caused by deranged Ca^{2+}-regulated PTH

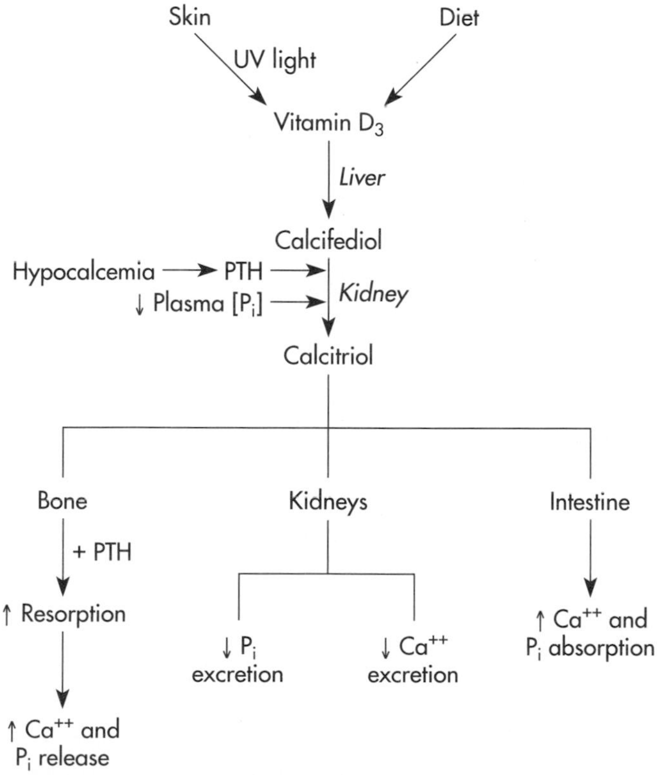

Fig. 37-20 Activation of vitamin D_3 and its effect on Ca^{2+} and P_i metabolism. Hypocalcemia, via PTH, and hypophosphatemia are the major stimuli of the metabolism of calcifediol to calcitriol in the kidneys. The net effect of calcitriol is an increase in plasma $[Ca^{2+}]$ and $[P_i]$.

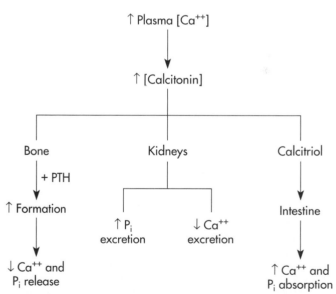

■ **Fig. 37-21** Effect of calcitonin on Ca^{2+} and P_i homeostasis. The major stimulus of calcitonin secretion is hypercalcemia. The net effect of calcitonin is a reduction in plasma $[Ca^{2+}]$. Quantitatively, therefore, the most important effects of calcitonin are to stimulate bone formation and decrease bone resorption. Although calcitonin reduces urinary Ca^{2+} excretion and intestinal Ca^{2+} absorption, these effects are relatively minor and have little effect on plasma $[Ca^{2+}]$. The effects of calcitonin on the kidneys and calcitriol production are relatively minor versus its effect on bone.

secretion (i.e., PTH levels are elevated at any level of plasma [Ca^{2+}]) and the hypocalciuria is caused by enhanced Ca^{2+} absorption by the thick ascending limb and distal tubule owing to elevated PTH levels and defective CaSR regulation of Ca^{2+} transport in these nephron segments. Autosomal-dominant hypocalcemia is caused by an activating mutation in CaSR. Activation of CaSRs causes deranged Ca^{2+}-regulated PTH secretion (i.e., PTH levels are decreased at any level of plasma [Ca^{2+}], thereby decreasing plasma [Ca^{2+}]) and the hypercalciuria is caused by decreased PTH levels and defective CaSR-regulated Ca^{2+} absorption by the thick ascending limb and distal tubule.

SUMMARY

1. K$^+$ is one of the most abundant cations in the body. It is crucial for many cellular functions, including cell growth and division and the excitability of nerve and muscle.

2. K$^+$ homeostasis is maintained by hormones that regulate plasma [K$^+$] and by the kidneys, which adjust K$^+$ excretion to match dietary K$^+$ intake. Plasma [K$^+$] is maintained by insulin, epinephrine, and aldosterone. In contrast, cell lysis, exercise, and changes in acid-base balance and plasma osmolality disturb plasma [K$^+$].

3. K$^+$ excretion by the kidneys is determined by the rate of K$^+$ secretion by the distal tubule and collecting duct. K$^+$ secretion by these tubular segments is regulated by plasma [K$^+$], aldosterone, and ADH. In contrast, changes in tubular fluid flow and acid-base disturbance disturb K$^+$ excretion by the kidneys.

4. Ca^{2+} and inorganic phosphate (P$_i$) are multivalent ions that perform many important functions. The kidneys, in conjunction with the gastrointestinal tract and bone, play a vital role in regulating plasma Ca^{2+} and P$_i$ levels.

5. Plasma [Ca^{2+}] is regulated by PTH, calcitriol, and calcitonin. Ca^{2+} excretion by the kidneys is determined by the net amount of intestinal Ca^{2+} absorption, the balance between bone formation and resorption, and the net amount of Ca^{2+} reabsorption by the distal tubule and thick ascending limb of Henle's loop. Ca^{2+} reabsorption by the thick ascending limb is regulated by PTH, calcitriol, and calcitonin, which stimulate Ca^{2+} reabsorption.

6. Plasma [P$_i$] is regulated by the kidney's maximal reabsorptive capacity of P$_i$. A fall in plasma [P$_i$] stimulates production of calcitriol, which causes the release of P$_i$ from bone into the ECF. Calcitriol also increases P$_i$ absorption by the intestine and decreases urinary P$_i$ excretion.

BIBLIOGRAPHY

Journal articles

Brown EM, MacLeod RJ: Extracellular calcium sensing and extracellular calcium signaling, *Physiol Rev* 81(1):239, 2001.

Friedman PA: Mechanisms of renal calcium transport, *Exp Nephrol* 8(6):343, 2000.

Giebisch G: Renal potassium channels: function, regulation, and structure, *Kidney Int* 60(2):436, 2001.

Murer H et al: Proximal tubular phosphate reabsorption: molecular mechanisms, *Physiol Rev* 80(4):1373, 2000.

Books and monographs

Agarwal R, Knochel JP: Hypophosphatemia and hyperphosphatemia. In Brenner BM, editor: *The kidney,* ed 6, Philadelphia, 2000, WB Saunders.

Friedman PA: Renal calcium metabolism. In Seldin DW, Giebisch G, editors: *The kidney: physiology and pathophysiology,* ed 3, Philadelphia, 2000, Lippincott, Williams & Wilkins.

Malnic G, Muto S, Giebisch G: Regulation of potassium excretion. In Seldin DW, Giebisch G, editors: *The kidney: physiology and pathophysiology,* ed 3, Philadelphia, 2000, Lippincott, Williams & Wilkins.

Mujais SK, Katz AI: Extrarenal potassium metabolism. In Seldin DW, Giebisch G, editors: *The kidney: physiology and pathophysiology,* ed 3, Philadelphia, 2000, Lippincott, Williams & Wilkins.

Murer H et al: Cellular mechanisms in proximal tubular handling of phosphate. In Seldin DW, Giebisch G, editors: *The kidney: physiology and pathophysiology,* ed 3, Philadelphia, 2000, Lippincott, Williams & Wilkins.

Silve C, Friedlander G: Renal regulation of phosphate excretion. In Seldin DW, Giebisch G, editors: *The kidney: physiology and pathophysiology,* ed 3, Philadelphia, 2000, Lippincott, Williams & Wilkins.

Suki WN, Lederer ED, Rouse D: Renal transport of calcium, magnesium and phosphate. In Brenner BM, editor: *The kidney,* ed 6, Philadelphia, 2000, WB Saunders.

Veestra TD, Kumar R: The hormonal regulation of calcium metabolism. In Seldin DW, Giebisch G, editors: *The kidney: physiology and pathophysiology,* ed 3, Philadelphia, 2000, Lippincott, Williams & Wilkins.

chapter thirty-eight

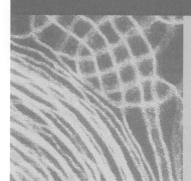

Role of the Kidneys in the Regulation of Acid-Base Balance

The concentration of H⁺ in the body fluids is low compared with that of many other ions. For example, Na^+ is present at a concentration some 3 million times greater than that of H⁺ ($[Na^+]$ = 140 mEq/L; $[H^+]$ = 40 nEq/L). Because of the low $[H^+]$ of the body fluids, $[H^+]$ is commonly expressed as the negative logarithm, or pH.

Many of the body's metabolic functions are exquisitely sensitive to pH, and normal function can occur only within a very narrow pH range. The pH range of 6.8 to 7.8 (160 to 16 nEq/L of H⁺) in the extracellular fluid (ECF) is generally compatible with life. Normally, the pH of the ECF is maintained between 7.35 and 7.45.

Each day, acid and alkali are ingested in the diet. Also, cellular metabolism produces a number of substances that have an impact on the pH of body fluids. Without appropriate mechanisms to deal with this daily acid and alkali load and thereby maintain acid-base balance, many processes necessary for life could not occur. This chapter reviews the maintenance of whole-body acid-base balance. Although the emphasis is on the role of the kidneys in this process, the role of lungs and liver are also considered. In addition, the impact of diet and cellular metabolism on acid-base balance is presented. Finally, disorders of acid-base balance are considered, primarily to illustrate the physiological processes involved. Throughout this chapter, **acid** is defined as any substance that adds H⁺ to the body fluids, whereas **alkali** is defined as a substance that removes H⁺ from the body fluids.

THE HCO₃⁻ BUFFER SYSTEM

Bicarbonate (HCO_3^-) is an important buffer of the ECF. Given a plasma $[HCO_3^-]$ of 23 to 25 mEq/L and a plasma volume of 14 L, the bicarbonate within the ECF can potentially buffer 350 mEq of H⁺. The HCO_3^- buffer system differs from the other buffer systems of the body (e.g., phosphate) because it is regulated by both the lungs and the kidneys. This difference is best appreciated by considering the following reaction:

$$CO_2 + H_2O \xrightarrow{\text{CA}} H_2CO_3 \longleftrightarrow H^+ + HCO_3^- \qquad (38\text{-}1)$$

The first reaction (hydration/dehydration of CO_2) is the rate-limiting step. This reaction would proceed at a very slow rate without the presence of the enzyme **carbonic anhydrase (CA),** which greatly accelerates the reaction. The second reaction, the ionization of H_2CO_3 to H⁺ and HCO_3^-, is virtually instantaneous.

The **Henderson-Hasselbalch equation** (equation 38-2) is used to quantitate the impact of changes in CO_2 and HCO_3^- on pH.

$$pH = pK' + \log \frac{[HCO_3^-]}{\alpha P_{CO_2}} \qquad (38\text{-}2)$$

or

$$pH = 6.1 + \log \frac{[HCO_3^-]}{0.03 P_{CO_2}} \qquad (38\text{-}3)$$

The amount of CO_2 in plasma depends on the partial pressure of CO_2 (P_{CO_2}) and its solubility (α). For plasma at 37° C, α = 0.03 and the pK = 6.1. The partial pressure of CO_2 is expressed in mm Hg.

Inspection of equation 38-3 shows that the pH of the plasma varies when either $[HCO_3^-]$ or P_{CO_2} is altered. Disturbances of acid-base balance that result from a change in the plasma $[HCO_3^-]$ are termed *metabolic acid-base disorders,* whereas those resulting from a change in P_{CO_2} are termed *respiratory acid-base disorders.* These disorders are considered in more detail in a subsequent section. The kidneys are primarily responsible for regulating the $[HCO_3^-]$ of the plasma and ECF, whereas the lungs control the P_{CO_2}.

DIETARY AND METABOLIC PRODUCTION OF ACID AND ALKALI

The diet of humans contains many constituents that are either acid or alkali. In addition, cellular metabolism produces acid and alkali. Finally, alkali is normally lost in the feces. As described later, the net effect of these processes is the addition of acid to the body fluids. So that acid-base balance can be maintained, acid must be excreted from the body at a rate equivalent to its addition. If acid addition exceeds excretion,

acidosis results. Conversely, if acid excretion exceeds addition, **alkalosis** results.

In the normal individual, the metabolism of dietary foodstuffs produces a number of substances that can have an impact on acid-base status. The major constituents of the diet are carbohydrates and fats. When tissue perfusion is adequate, O_2 is available to tissues, and insulin is present at normal levels, carbohydrates and fats are metabolized to CO_2 and H_2O. Daily, 15 to 20 moles of CO_2 are generated through this process. Normally, this large quantity of CO_2 is effectively eliminated from the body by the lungs, so this metabolically derived CO_2 has no impact on acid-base balance. CO_2 is usually termed **volatile acid,** reflecting the fact that it has the potential to generate H^+ after hydration with H_2O. Acid not derived from the hydration of CO_2 is termed **nonvolatile acid** (e.g., lactic acid).

The cellular metabolism of other dietary constituents also has an impact on acid-base balance. For example, cysteine and methionine, sulfur-containing amino acids, yield sulfuric acid when metabolized, whereas hydrochloric acid results from the metabolism of lysine, arginine, and histidine. A portion of this nonvolatile acid load is offset by the production of bicarbonate (HCO_3^-) through the metabolism of the amino acids aspartate and glutamate. On average, the metabolism of dietary amino acids yields net nonvolatile acid production. Finally, the metabolism of certain organic anions (e.g., citrate) results in the production of HCO_3^-, which offsets nonvolatile acid production to some degree. On balance, in individuals ingesting a meat-containing diet, acid production exceeds HCO_3^- production. In addition to the metabolically derived acids and alkalis, the foods ingested contain acid and alkali. For example, the presence of phosphate ($H_2PO_4^-$) in ingested food increases the dietary acid load. Finally, during digestion, some HCO_3^- is normally lost in the feces. This loss is equivalent to the addition of nonvolatile acid to the body. Together, dietary intake, cellular metabolism, and fecal HCO_3^- loss result in the addition of approximately 1 mEq/kg body weight of nonvolatile acid to the body each day (50 to 100 mEq/day for most adults). It should be emphasized that the production of nonvolatile acids is highly dependent on the diet. For example, a vegetarian diet can result in lessened acid production. In the remainder of this chapter, it is assumed that there is net production of nonvolatile acid. The term used for this acid is "net acid load," and it has a value of 50 to 100 mEq/day.

When insulin levels are normal, carbohydrates and fats are completely metabolized to $CO_2 + H_2O$. However, if insulin levels are abnormally low (e.g., **diabetes mellitus**), the metabolism of carbohydrates leads to the production of several organic ketoacids (e.g., β-hydroxybutyric acid).

In the absence of adequate levels of O_2 (**hypoxia**), anaerobic metabolism by cells can also lead to the production of organic acids (e.g., lactic acid) rather than $CO_2 + H_2O$. This often occurs in normal individuals during vigorous exercise. Poor tissue perfusion, such as occurs with reduced cardiac output, can also lead to anaerobic metabolism by cells and thus to acidosis.

In these conditions, the organic acids accumulate and the pH of the body fluids decreases (acidosis). Treatment (e.g., administration of insulin in the case of diabetes) or improved delivery of adequate levels of O_2 to the tissues (e.g., in the case of poor tissue perfusion) results in the metabolism of these organic acids to $CO_2 + H_2O$ and thereby helps correct the acid-base disorder.

The nonvolatile acids produced during metabolism do not circulate as free acids, but are immediately buffered:

$$H_2SO_4 + 2NaHCO_3 \longleftrightarrow Na_2SO_4 + 2CO_2 + 2H_2O \quad (38\text{-}4)$$
$$HCl + NaHCO_3 \longleftrightarrow NaCl + CO_2 + H_2O \quad (38\text{-}5)$$

This buffering process yields Na^+ salts and removes HCO_3^- from the ECF. Buffering of strong acids by HCO_3^- minimizes the tendency for strong acids to lower the pH of the ECF. To maintain acid-base balance, the kidneys must excrete these acid salts and replenish the HCO_3^- lost by neutralization of the H^+.

OVERVIEW OF RENAL ACID EXCRETION

To maintain acid-base balance, the kidneys must excrete an amount of acid equal to the net acid load. In addition, the kidneys must prevent the loss of HCO_3^- in the urine. This latter task is quantitatively more important, because the filtered load of HCO_3^- is approximately 4320 mEq/day (24 mEq/L × 180 L/day = 4320 mEq/day) compared with only 50 to 100 mEq/day needed to excrete the net acid load.

Both the reabsorption of filtered HCO_3^- and the excretion of acid are accomplished through the process of H^+ secretion by the nephrons. Thus, in a single day the nephrons secrete approximately 4380 mEq of H^+ into the tubular fluid. Most of this H^+ does not leave the body in the urine, but serves to reabsorb the filtered HCO_3^-, and only 50 to 100 mEq is excreted. As a result of this acid excretion, the urine is normally acidic.

Theoretically, the kidneys could excrete the nonvolatile acids and replenish the HCO_3^- lost during titration by reversing the reactions shown in equations 38-4 and 38-5. However, because the pKs of these acids are low, this process would require a urine pH of 1.0, and the minimal urine pH attainable by the kidneys is only 4.0 to 4.5. Consequently, the kidneys cannot excrete the free acids. Instead, they excrete the acid anion (A^-) with various cations (Na^+, K^+, NH_4^+, etc.). At a urine pH of 4.0 only 0.1 mEq/L of H^+ can be excreted. Additional H^+ is excreted with urinary buffers. The primary urinary buffer is phosphate ($HPO_4^{2-}/H_2PO_4^-$). Other constituents of the urine can also serve as buffers (e.g., creatinine), although their roles are less important than that of phosphate. Collectively, the various urinary buffers are called **titratable acid.**[*]

---

[*]The term titratable acid is derived from the method by which these buffers are quantitated in the laboratory. Typically, alkali (OH^-) is added to a urine sample to titrate its pH to that of plasma (i.e., 7.4). The amount of alkali added is equal to the H^+ titrated by these urine buffers, and is thus called titratable acid.

Titratable acid excretion is approximately 30 mEq/day, which is insufficient to balance the daily net acid load (50 to 100 mEq/day). An additional and important mechanism by which the kidneys contribute to the maintenance of acid-base balance is through the synthesis and excretion of **ammonium (NH$_4^+$).**[*] The mechanisms involved in this process are discussed in more detail later in this chapter. With regard to the renal regulation of acid-base balance, each NH$_4^+$ excreted in the urine results in the return of an HCO$_3^-$ to the systemic circulation, which replenishes the HCO$_3^-$ lost during neutralization of the nonvolatile acid. Thus, the production and excretion of NH$_4^+$ are equivalent to the excretion of acid by the kidneys.

In brief, *the kidneys contribute to acid-base homeostasis by reabsorbing the filtered load of HCO$_3^-$ and excreting an amount of acid equivalent to the daily net acid load.* This overall process is termed **net acid excretion (NAE)** and can be quantitated as follows:

$$NAE = [(U_{NH_4^+} \times \dot{V}) + (U_{TA} \times \dot{V})] - (U_{HCO_3^-} \times \dot{V}) \quad (38\text{-}6)$$

where $U_{NH_4^+} \times \dot{V}$ and $U_{TA} \times \dot{V}$ are the rates of excretion (mEq/day) of NH$_4^+$ and titratable acid (TA); and $U_{HCO_3^-} \times \dot{V}$ is the amount of HCO$_3^-$ lost in the urine (equivalent to adding H$^+$ to the body). Again, to maintain acid-base balance, the amount of net acid excretion must equal the daily net acid load. Under most conditions very little HCO$_3^-$ is excreted in the urine. Thus NAE essentially reflects titratable acid and NH$_4^+$ excretion. Quantitatively, titratable acid accounts for approximately two-thirds of NAE.

HCO$_3^-$ Reabsorption along the Nephron

Glomerular filtration delivers 4320 mEq/day of HCO$_3^-$ to the nephrons. Figure 38-1 illustrates the contribution of the various nephron segments to the reabsorption of this HCO$_3^-$. The reabsorption of HCO$_3^-$ is critically important for the prevention of its loss in the urine. Under normal conditions, virtually all the filtered HCO$_3^-$ is reabsorbed, and none appears in the urine.

Approximately 80% of the filtered load of HCO$_3^-$ is reabsorbed in the proximal tubule. The cellular mechanisms involved in this reabsorption are illustrated in Fig. 38-2. The apical membrane of the proximal tubule cell contains an Na$^+$-H$^+$ antiporter that uses the energy in the lumen-to-cell Na$^+$ gradient to secrete H$^+$ into the tubular fluid. In addition, some H$^+$ is secreted via an H$^+$-ATPase. Within the cell, H$^+$ and HCO$_3^-$ are produced in a reaction catalyzed by carbonic anhydrase (see equation 38-1). H$^+$ is secreted into the tubular fluid, whereas HCO$_3^-$ exits the cell across the basolateral membrane and returns to the peritubular blood.

Although the electrochemical gradient for HCO$_3^-$ favors its passive movement out of the cell across the basolateral membrane, simple diffusion does not appear to occur to a

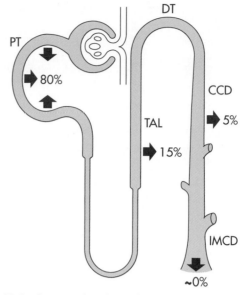

■ **Fig. 38-1** Segmental reabsorption of HCO$_3^-$. The fraction of the filtered load of HCO$_3^-$ reabsorbed by the various segments of the nephron is shown. Normally, the entire filtered load of HCO$_3^-$ is reabsorbed. *PT,* Proximal tubule; *TAL,* thick ascending limb; *DT,* distal tubule; *CCD,* collecting duct; *IMCD,* inner medullary collecting duct.

significant degree. Instead, HCO$_3^-$ movement out of the cell across the basolateral membrane is coupled to that of other ions. Most of the HCO$_3^-$ exits via a symporter that couples the exit of one Na$^+$ to three HCO$_3^-$. Additionally, some of the HCO$_3^-$ exits in exchange for Cl$^-$ (via a Cl$^-$-HCO$_3^-$ antiporter).

Within the tubular fluid, the secreted H$^+$ combines with the filtered HCO$_3^-$ to form H$_2$CO$_3$. This H$_2$CO$_3$ is rapidly converted to CO$_2$ and H$_2$O. Carbonic anhydrase present in the apical membrane and exposed to the tubular fluid contents facilitates the conversion of H$_2$CO$_3$ to H$_2$O and CO$_2$. Because the tubule is highly permeable to both CO$_2$ and H$_2$O, these are rapidly reabsorbed. The net effect of this process is that for each HCO$_3^-$ removed from the tubular fluid, one HCO$_3^-$ appears in the peritubular blood.

An additional 15% of the filtered load of HCO$_3^-$ is reabsorbed by Henle's loop. Most of this HCO$_3^-$ is reabsorbed by the cells of the thick ascending limb. The cellular mechanism for HCO$_3^-$ reabsorption by the ascending limb of Henle's loop is virtually identical to that described for the proximal tubule. The only difference is that carbonic anhydrase is not present in the apical membrane of thick ascending limb cells.

The distal tubule and collecting duct reabsorb the small amount of HCO$_3^-$ that escapes reabsorption by the proximal tubule and Henle's loop (5% off the filtered load). This reabsorption does not depend on Na$^+$ (i.e., apical membrane Na$^+$-H$^+$ antiporter), as is the case in the earlier nephron segments. Figure 38-3 shows the mechanism of HCO$_3^-$ reabsorption by the collecting duct. Here, H$^+$ secretion occurs via the intercalated cell (see Chapter 34). Within the cell, H$^+$ and HCO$_3^-$ are produced by the hydration of CO$_2$; this reaction is

---

[*]Traditionally, ammonia (NH$_3$) was considered a urinary buffer. However, as described later in this chapter, this designation is not consistent with what is currently known about ammonium production and excretion. Consequently, we do not refer to ammonia/ammonium as a urinary buffer.

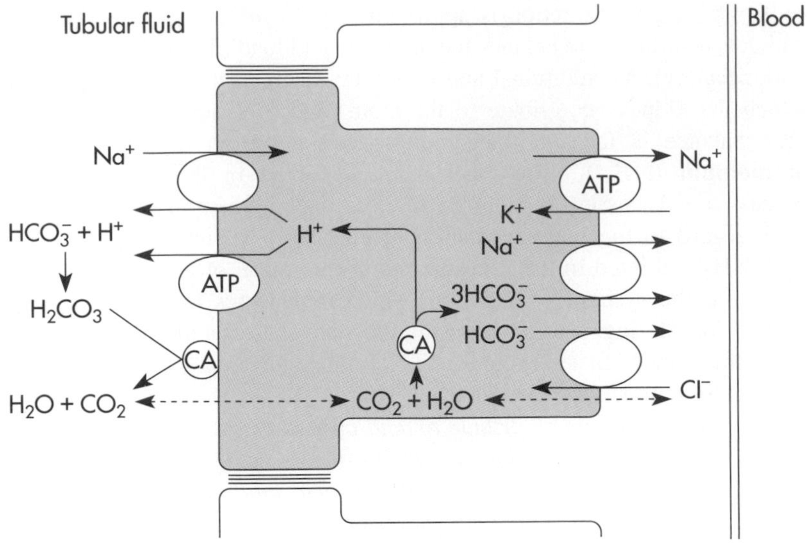

■ **Fig. 38-2**   Cellular mechanism for reabsorption of filtered HCO_3^- by cells of the proximal tubule. *CA,* Carbonic anhydrase; *ATP,* adenosine triphosphate. See text for details.

catalyzed by carbonic anhydrase. The H^+ is secreted into the tubular fluid by two mechanisms. The first mechanism involves an apical membrane H^+-ATPase. The second mechanism couples the secretion of H^+ to the reabsorption of K^+ via an H^+,K^+-ATPase. The HCO_3^- exits the cell across the basolateral membrane in exchange for Cl^- (via a Cl^--HCO_3^- antiporter) and enters the peritubular capillary blood.

A second population of intercalated cells within the collecting duct secrete HCO_3^- rather than H^+ into the tubular fluid. These cells appear to have the H^+-ATPase located in the basolateral membrane and a Cl^--HCO_3^- antiporter in the apical membrane (Fig. 38-3). Their activity can be increased during metabolic alkalosis when the kidneys must excrete excess HCO_3^-. However, under normal conditions, H^+ secretion predominates in the collecting duct.

The apical membrane of the cells of the collecting duct has a low permeability to H^+, and the pH of the tubular fluid can become quite acidic. Indeed, the most acidic tubular fluid along the nephron (pH = 4.0 to 4.5) is produced here. By comparison, the permeability of the proximal tubule to H^+ and HCO_3^- is much higher, and the tubular fluid pH falls to only 6.5 in this segment. As explained below, the ability of the collecting duct to lower the pH of the tubular fluid is critically important for the excretion of urinary buffers and ammonium.

The Na^+-H^+ antiporter present in the apical membrane of both the proximal tubule and thick ascending limb cells is the NHE-3 isoform of this membrane transporter. The H^+-ATPase provides a parallel pathway for H^+ secretion across the apical membrane of these nephron segments and is a major mechanism for H^+ secretion by the intercalated cells of the collecting duct. The isoform of this transporter in the proximal tubule and thick ascending limb is different from the isoform found in the intercalated cells of the collecting duct. The H^+,K^+-ATPase found in the apical membrane of the intercalated cells is similar to, but distinct from, the isoform found in gastric parietal cells.

Regulation of HCO_3^- Reabsorption

A number of factors regulate the secretion of H^+ by the cells of the nephron (Table 38-1). From a physiological perspective, the primary factor that regulates H^+ secretion by the nephron is changes in systemic acid-base balance. At the cellular level, this reflects changes in the cell-to-tubular fluid gradient for H^+. Whether produced by a decrease in the HCO_3^- in plasma or by an increase in P_{CO_2}, acidosis decreases the pH of the cells of the nephron, creating a move favorable cell-to-tubular fluid H^+ gradient and thereby stimulating H^+ secretion along the entire nephron. Conversely, alkalosis secondary to an increase in the $[HCO_3^-]$ or a decrease in the P_{CO_2}, inhibits H^+ secretion secondary to an increase in the intracellular pH of the nephron cells. Although alterations in the intracellular pH of nephron cells directly influence H^+ secretion across the apical membrane, there is evidence that these changes in pH, perhaps mediated by other intracellular messengers, also alter the activity and expression of key H^+ and HCO_3^- transporters. For example, the intercalated cells of the collecting duct insert more H^+-ATPase into their apical membranes in response to acidosis. In the proximal tubule, acidosis also increases the abundance and activity of the apical membrane Na^+-H^+ antiporter as well as the Na^+-$3HCO_3^-$ symporter in the basolateral membrane. It is likely that the effects of inhibited H^+ secretion caused by systemic alkalosis are also mediated in part by the reduced activity and expression of these H^+ and HCO_3^- transporters.

Table 38-1 also lists other factors that influence the secretion of H^+ by the cells of the nephron. However, these factors are not directly related to the maintenance of acid-base balance. Because H^+ secretion in the proximal tubule and thick ascending limb of Henle's loop is linked to the reabsorption of Na^+ (via the Na^+-H^+ antiporter), factors that alter Na^+ reabsorption secondarily effect H^+ secretion. For example, the process of glomerulotubular balance ensures that the reabsorption rate of the proximal tubule is matched to the glomerular filtration rate (see Chapter 35). Thus, when the glomerular fil-

H$^+$-secreting cell

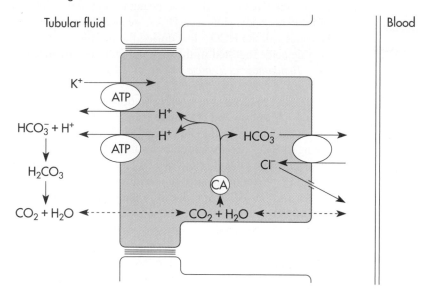

HCO$_3^-$-secreting cell

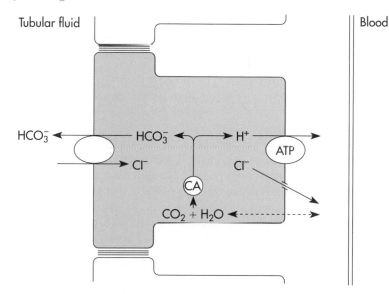

■ **Fig. 38-3** Cellular mechanisms for reabsorption and secretion of HCO$_3^-$ by intercalated cells of the collecting duct. *CA,* Carbonic anhydrase; *ATP,* adenosine triphosphate. See text for details.

tration rate is increased, the filtered load to the proximal tubule is increased, and more fluid (including HCO$_3^-$) is reabsorbed. Conversely, a decrease in the filtered load results in the decreased reabsorption of fluid and thus HCO$_3^-$.

Alterations in Na$^+$ balance, through changes in the ECF volume, also have an impact on H$^+$ secretion. With volume depletion (negative Na$^+$ balance), H$^+$ secretion is enhanced. This occurs via several mechanisms. First, the renin-angiotensin-aldosterone system is activated by volume depletion, and Na$^+$ reabsorption by the nephron is enhanced (see Chapter 36). Angiotensin II acts on the proximal tubule and thick ascending limb of Henle's loop to stimulate the apical membrane Na$^+$-H$^+$ antiporter and thereby stimulate H$^+$ secretion. Aldosterone's primary action on the collecting duct is to stimulate Na$^+$ reabsorption. However, it also stim-

ulates the intercalated cells to secrete H$^+$. Second, the peritubular Starling forces across the proximal tubule are altered during volume depletion to enhance overall proximal tubule reabsorption (see Chapter 36). With volume expansion (positive Na$^+$ balance), H$^+$ secretion is reduced because of low levels of angiotensin II and aldosterone, as well as because of alterations in the peritubular Starling forces (reduced reabsorption by the proximal tubule).

Parathyroid hormone (PTH) also inhibits HCO$_3^-$ reabsorption by the proximal tubule. PTH is mainly involved in the maintenance of Ca^{2+} and phosphate balance (see Chapter 37). However, PTH inhibits the Na$^+$-H$^+$ antiporter in the apical membrane of proximal tubule cells. Finally, K$^+$ balance influences the secretion of H$^+$ by the proximal tubule, with hypokalemia stimulating and hyperkalemia inhibiting

■ Table 38-1 Factors that regulate H⁺ secretion (HCO₃⁻ reabsorption) by the nephron

Factor	Principal site of action
Increased H⁺ secretion	
Primary	
Decrease in plasma HCO₃⁻ concentration (↓ pH)	Entire nephron
Increase in partial pressure of arterial carbon dioxide	Entire nephron
Secondary (not directed at maintaining acid-base balance)	
Increase in filtered load of HCO₃⁻	Proximal tubule
Decrease in ECF volume	Proximal tubule
Increase in angiotensin II	Proximal tubule
Increase in aldosterone	Collecting duct
Hypokalemia	Proximal tubule
Decreased H⁺ secretion	
Primary	
Increase in plasma HCO₃⁻ concentration (↑ pH)	Entire nephron
Decrease in partial pressure of arterial carbon dioxide	Entire nephron
Secondary (not directed at maintaining acid-base balance)	
Decrease in filtered load of HCO₃⁻	Proximal tubule
Increase in ECF volume	Proximal tubule
Decrease in aldosterone	Collecting duct
Hyperkalemia	Proximal tubule

ECF, Extracellular fluid.

secretion. It is thought that K⁺-induced changes in intracellular pH are responsible for this effect, with hypokalemia acidifying and hyperkalemia alkalinizing the cells.

Formation of New HCO₃⁻: The Role of Ammonium

As discussed previously, reabsorption of the filtered load of HCO₃⁻ by the kidneys is important for the maintenance of acid-base balance. HCO₃⁻ loss in the urine would decrease the plasma [HCO₃⁻] and would be equivalent to the addition of H⁺ to the body. However, HCO₃⁻ reabsorption alone does not replenish the HCO₃⁻ lost during the titration of the nonvolatile acids ingested in the diet and produced by metabolism. *To maintain acid-base balance, the kidneys must replace this lost HCO₃⁻ with new HCO₃⁻.* A portion of the new HCO₃⁻ is produced during the titration of urinary buffers such as phosphate and creatinine (Fig. 38-4). In the collecting duct, where tubular fluid contains little or no HCO₃⁻ owing to HCO₃⁻ reabsorption in upstream tubular segments, H⁺ secreted into tubular fluid combines with a urinary buffer. Thus, H⁺ secretion results in excretion of the H⁺ with a buffer, and the HCO₃⁻ produced in the cell from the hydration of CO₂ is added back to the blood.

As noted previously, the primary urinary buffer is phosphate (HPO₄²⁻/H₂PO₄⁻). The amount of phosphate excreted each day, and therefore available to serve as a urinary buffer, is derived solely from the diet. Moreover, the amount of P$_i$ excreted is regulated in response to the need to maintain Ca²⁺ and P$_i$ balance (see Chapters 37 and 42), and not in response to the need to maintain acid-base balance. However, NH₄⁺ is produced by the kidneys, and its synthesis and subsequent excretion are regulated in response to the body's acid-base requirements. Because NH₄⁺ excretion is tied to acid-base requirements, it is critically involved in new HCO₃⁻ formation.

Ammonium is produced in the kidneys by the metabolism of the amino acid glutamine. Glutamine (primarily from the liver) and the Na⁺ salts of the nonvolatile acids (e.g., Na₂SO₄) are delivered to the kidneys in the renal arterial plasma. The kidneys metabolize the glutamine, excrete NH₄⁺ with the acid anion (e.g., SO₄²⁻), and return NaHCO₃ to the body in the renal vein plasma. An important point to recognize is that the formation of new HCO₃⁻ by this process depends on the kidney's ability to excrete the NH₄⁺ in the urine. If NH₄⁺ is not excreted in the urine, but instead enters the systemic circulation, it will titrate plasma HCO₃⁻, thus negating the

■ Fig. 38-4 General scheme for the excretion of H⁺ with non-HCO₃⁻ urinary buffers. The primary urinary buffer is HPO₄²⁻. Other buffers include creatinine. Collectively, the urinary buffers are called titratable acid. For simplicity, only the H⁺-ATPase is shown. H⁺ secretion by the H⁺,K⁺-ATPase also titrates luminal buffers. *CA,* Carbonic anhydrase; *ATP,* adenosine triphosphate.

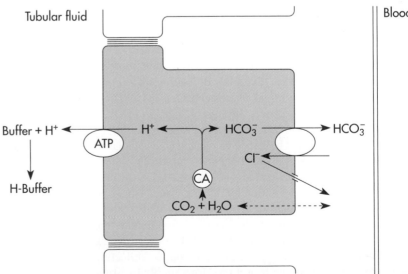

process of generating new HCO_3^-.* The process by which the kidneys excrete NH_4^+ is complex (Fig. 38-5).

Ammonium is produced in proximal tubule cells from glutamine. Each glutamine molecule produces two molecules of NH_4^+ and a divalent anion. Metabolism of this anion ultimately provides two molecules of HCO_3^-:

$$\text{Glutamine} \longleftrightarrow 2NH_4^+ + \text{anion}^{2-} \longleftrightarrow 2HCO_3^- + 2NH_4^+ \quad (38\text{-}7)$$

The HCO_3^- exits the proximal tubule cell across the basolateral membrane and enters the peritubular blood as new HCO_3^-. NH_4^+ exits the cell across the apical membrane and enters the tubular fluid. A major mechanism for the secretion of NH_4^+ into the tubular fluid involves the Na^+-H^+ antiporter, with NH_4^+ substituting for H^+. In addition, ammonia (NH_3) can diffuse out of the cell into the tubular lumen, where it is protonated to NH_4^+. A significant portion of the NH_4^+ secreted by the proximal tubule is reabsorbed by Henle's loop. The thick ascending limb is the primary site of this NH_4^+ reabsorption. NH_4^+ substitutes for K^+ on the $1Na^+$-$1K^+$-$2Cl^-$ symporter. In addition, the lumen-positive transepithelial

---

*The mechanism by which NH_4^+ titrates HCO_3^- is indirect and occurs as a result of the synthesis of urea from NH_4^+ by the liver (i.e., the urea cycle). When urea is synthesized from NH_4^+, H^+ is generated. This H^+ is rapidly buffered by HCO_3^-.

voltage in this segment drives paracellular reabsorption of NH_4^+.

The reabsorbed NH_4^+ accumulates in the medullary interstitium, where it exists in chemical equilibrium with NH_3.* NH_4^+ then reenters the tubular fluid of the collecting duct. The mechanism by which NH_4^+ reappears in the collecting duct involves the processes of nonionic diffusion and diffusion trapping. The collecting duct does not have a specific transport mechanism for the secretion of NH_4^+, nor do the cells have a significant passive permeability to NH_4^+. However, the cells of the collecting duct are permeable to NH_3, which can diffuse from the medullary interstitium into the lumen of the collecting duct. As described previously, H^+ secretion by the collecting duct intercalated cells results in acidification of the luminal fluid (luminal fluid pH as low as 4.0 to 4.5 can be achieved). Consequently, NH_3 diffusing from the medullary interstitium into the collecting duct lumen (nonionic diffusion) is protonated to NH_4^+ by the acidic tubular fluid. Because the collecting duct is less permeable to NH_4^+ than to NH_3, NH_4^+ is trapped in the tubule lumen (diffusion trapping) and eliminated from the body in the urine.

---

*Ammonia is a weak base that is present as both NH_4^+ and NH_3, with the relative amounts of each species determined by the pK_a ($pK_a = 9.0$).

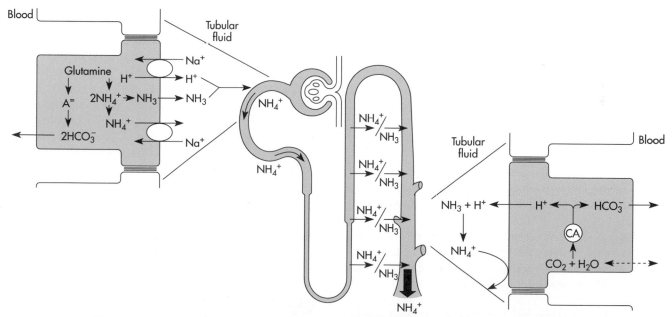

■ **Fig. 38-5** Production, transport, and excretion of NH_4^+ by the nephron. Glutamine is metabolized in the proximal tubule to NH_4^+ and HCO_3^-. The NH_4^+ is secreted into the lumen, and the HCO_3^- enters the blood. The secreted NH_4^+ is reabsorbed in Henle's loop primarily by the thick ascending limb, and accumulates in the medullary interstitium, where it exists as both NH_4^+ and NH_3. NH_3 diffuses into the tubular fluid of the collecting duct, and H^+ secretion by the collecting duct leads to accumulation of NH_4^+ in the lumen by the processes of nonionic diffusion and diffusion trapping. For every NH_4^+ excreted in the urine, a "new HCO_3^-" is returned to the systemic circulation. Therefore, the excretion of NH_4^+ can be used as a marker of proximal tubule glutamine metabolism, which in turn determines new HCO_3^- formation.

H⁺ secretion by the collecting duct is critical for the excretion of NH₄⁺. If collecting duct H⁺ secretion is inhibited, the NH₄⁺ reabsorbed by the thick ascending limb will not be excreted in the urine. Instead, it will be returned to the systemic circulation, where as described previously, it will be converted to urea by the liver and consume HCO_3^- in the process. Thus, new HCO_3^- is produced during the metabolism of glutamine by cells of the proximal tubule. However, the overall process is not complete until the NH₄⁺ is excreted (i.e., the production of urea from NH₄⁺ by the liver is prevented). Thus, NH₄⁺ excretion can be used as a marker of proximal tubule glutamine metabolism. Because of the stoichiometry of this reaction, one new HCO_3^- is returned to the systemic circulation for each NH₄⁺ excreted in the urine.

An important feature of the NH₄⁺ system is that it can be regulated. Alterations in ECF pH, presumably by affecting intracellular pH, cause changes in glutamine metabolism (NH₄⁺ production) in the proximal tubule cells. During systemic acidosis, the enzymes in the proximal tubule cell, which are responsible for the metabolism of glutamine, are stimulated. This stimulation involves the synthesis of new enzyme and requires several days for complete adaptation. With increased levels of this enzyme, NH₄⁺ production is increased, thus allowing enhanced production of new HCO_3^-. Conversely, glutamine metabolism is reduced with alkalosis.

Assessing NH₄⁺ excretion by the kidneys is done indirectly because assays of urine NH₄⁺ are not routinely available. Consider, for example, the situation of metabolic acidosis. In the setting of metabolic acidosis, the appropriate renal response is to increase net acid excretion. Accodingly, little or no HCO_3^- will appear in the urine, the urine will be acidic, and NH₄⁺ excretion will be increased. To assess this, and especially the amount of NH₄⁺ excreted, the "urinary net charge" or "urine anion gap" can be calculated by measuring the urinary concentration of Na⁺, K⁺, and Cl⁻.

$$\text{Urine anion gap} = [Na^+] + [K^+] - [Cl^-] \qquad (38\text{-}8)$$

The concept of urine anion gap assumes that the major cations in the urine are Na⁺, K⁺, and NH₄⁺ and that the major anion is Cl⁻ (with urine pH <6.5, virtually no HCO_3^- is present). As a result, the urine anion gap will yield a negative value when adequate amounts of NH₄⁺ are being excreted. Indeed, the absence of a urine anion gap or the existence of a positive value indicates a renal defect in NH₄⁺ production and excretion.

Plasma [K⁺] also alters NH₄⁺ production. In hyperkalemia, NH₄⁺ production is inhibited, whereas hypokalemia stimulates its production. The mechanism by which plasma K⁺ alters NH₄⁺ production is not fully understood. Alterations in plasma [K⁺] may change intracellular [H⁺] by exchanging H⁺ for K⁺ (see Chapter 37), and the change in intracellular pH may then control glutamine metabolism. By this mechanism, exchange of extracellular K⁺ for intracellular H⁺ during hyperkalemia would raise intracellular pH, thereby inhibiting glutamine metabolism. The opposite would occur during hypokalemia.

Renal tubule acidosis (RTA) refers to conditions in which urine acidification is impaired. Under these conditions, the kidneys are unable to excrete a sufficient amount of net acid to balance the daily net acid load, and metabolic acidosis results. RTA can occur either by a defect in proximal tubule H⁺ secretion (proximal RTA), by a defect in distal tubule H⁺ secretion (distal RTA), or by inadequate production of NH₄⁺.

Proximal RTA can be caused by many hereditary and acquired conditions (e.g., cystinosis, Fanconi's syndrome, administration of carbonic anhydrase inhibitors). H⁺ secretion by proximal tubule cells is impaired and results in a decrease in the reabsorption of the filtered load of HCO_3^-. Consequently, HCO_3^- is lost in the urine, plasma $[HCO_3^-]$ decreases, and metabolic acidosis ensues.

Distal RTA also occurs in a number of hereditary and acquired conditions (e.g., with medullary sponge kidney, with the use of certain drugs such as amphotericin B, and secondary to urinary tract obstruction). Depending on the cause, secretion of H⁺ by intercalated cells of the collecting duct is impaired or the permeability of the collecting duct to H⁺ may be increased. In either case, the ability to acidify the tubular fluid is impaired. Consequently, titratable acid excretion is reduced and nonionic diffusion and diffusion trapping of NH₄⁺ is reduced. This in turn decreases NAE, with the subsequent development of metabolic acidosis.

Failure to produce sufficient quantities of urinary NH₄⁺ can also reduce the amount of net acid excreted by the kidneys. In this situation, proximal tubule H⁺ secretion is normal, as is H⁺secretion by the distal tubule and collecting duct, and the urine pH is maximally acidic. However, because of the lack of sufficient quantities of NH₄⁺, net acid excretion is less than net acid production, and metabolic acidosis develops. This form of RTA is usually seen in individuals who have a reduced number of nephrons (i.e., mild to moderate renal failure). If the acidosis that results from any of these forms of RTA is severe, individuals must ingest alkali (e.g., $NaHCO_3$) to maintain acid-base balance. In this way, the HCO_3^- lost each day in the buffering of nonvolatile acid is replenished by new HCO_3^- ingested in the diet.

RESPONSE TO ACID-BASE DISORDERS

The pH of the ECF is maintained within a very narrow range (7.35 to 7.45).* Acidosis exists when the blood pH falls

---

*For simplicity, the value of 7.40 will be used as normal, and deviations from this single value are deemed abnormal. Similarly, the normal range for P_{CO_2} is 33 to 44 mm Hg. However, a P_{CO_2} of 40 mm Hg is used as the normal reference value. Finally, a value of 24 mEq/L is considered a normal ECF $[HCO_3^-]$, even though the normal range is 22 to 28 mEq/L.

below this range, whereas alkalosis exists when the blood pH exceeds this range. When the acid-base disorder results from a primary change in [HCO_3^-], it is called a *metabolic disorder.* When the primary disturbance is an alteration in blood P_{CO_2}, it is called a *respiratory disorder.*

When an acid-base disturbance develops, the body employs a series of mechanisms to defend against the change in the pH of the ECF. *These defense mechanisms do not correct the acid-base disturbance but merely minimize the change in pH imposed by the disturbance.* Restoration of the blood pH to its normal value requires correction of the underlying process or processes that produced the acid-base disorder. For example, metabolism of carbohydrates and fats in the absence of insulin leads to the accumulation of ketoacids (a nonvolatile acid) in the blood. As a result of this accumulation, metabolic acidosis develops. The acid-base defense mechanisms minimize the fall in pH that occurs in this condition, but normal acid-base balance is not restored until insulin is administered and ketoacid production ceases.

The body has three general mechanisms to defend against changes in body fluid pH produced by acid-base disturbances: (1) extracellular and intracellular buffering, (2) adjustments in blood P_{CO_2} by alterations in the ventilatory rate of the lungs, and (3) adjustments in renal acid excretion.

Extracellular and Intracellular Buffering

The first line of defense against acid-base disorders is extracellular and intracellular buffering. The response of the extracellular buffers is virtually instantaneous, whereas intracellular buffering is somewhat slower and can take several minutes to complete.

Metabolic disorders that result from the addition of nonvolatile acid or alkali to the body fluids are buffered in both the ECF and intracellular fluid (ICF). The HCO_3^- buffer system is the principal ECF buffer (see equation 38-1). When nonvolatile acid is added to the body fluids or alkali is lost from the body, HCO_3^- is consumed during the process of neutralizing the acid load, and the plasma [HCO_3^-] is reduced. Conversely, when nonvolatile alkali is added to the body fluids or acid is lost from the body, H^+ is consumed. This causes more HCO_3^- to be produced from the dissociation of H_2CO_3, and consequently [HCO_3^-] increases.

Although the HCO_3^- buffer system is the principal ECF buffer, phosphate and plasma protein provide additional extracellular buffering:

$$H^+ + HPO_4^{2-} \longleftrightarrow H_2PO_4^- \qquad (38\text{-}9)$$
$$H^+ + protein \longleftrightarrow H\text{-}Protein$$

The combined action of the HCO_3^-, phosphate, and plasma protein buffering processes accounts for approximately 50% of the buffering of a nonvolatile acid load and 70% of a nonvolatile alkali load. The remainder of the buffering under these two conditions occurs intracellularly. Intracellular buffering involves the movement of H^+ into cells (during buffering of nonvolatile acid) or the movement of H^+ out of cells (during buffering of nonvolatile

alkali). H^+ is titrated inside the cell by HCO_3^-, phosphate, and the histidine groups on protein.

Bone represents an additional source of extracellular buffer (e.g., $NaHCO_3$, $KHCO_3$, $CaCO_3$, $CaHPO_4$). In chronic acidosis, buffering by bone results in demineralization; in other words Ca^{2+} is released from bone as Ca^{2+}-containing buffers bind H^+ in exchange for Ca^{2+}.

In respiratory acid-base disorders, body fluid pH changes as a result of alterations in [H_2CO_3], which is determined directly by the P_{CO_2} (see equation 38-1). Virtually all buffering in respiratory acid-base disorders occurs intracellularly. When P_{CO_2} rises (respiratory acidosis), CO_2 moves into cells, where it combines with H_2O to form H_2CO_3. H_2CO_3 dissociates to H^+ and HCO_3^-. Some of the H^+ is buffered by cellular proteins, and HCO_3^- exits the cell and raises the plasma [HCO_3^-].

This process is reversed when P_{CO_2} is reduced (respiratory alkalosis). Under this condition, the hydration reaction ($H_2O + CO_2 \longleftrightarrow H_2CO_3$) is shifted to the left by the decrease in P_{CO_2}. As a result, the dissociation reaction ($H_2CO_3 \longleftrightarrow H^+ + HCO_3^-$) also shifts to the left, thereby reducing the plasma [HCO_3^-].

Respiratory Defense

The lungs are the second line of defense against acid-base disorders. As indicated by the Henderson-Hasselbalch equation (see equation 38-3), changes in P_{CO_2} alter blood pH. An increase in P_{CO_2} decreases pH; a decrease in P_{CO_2} increases pH.

The ventilatory rate determines the P_{CO_2}. Increased ventilation decreases P_{CO_2}, whereas decreased ventilation increases P_{CO_2}. The blood P_{CO_2} and pH are important regulators of the ventilatory rate. Chemoreceptors located in the brain (ventral surface of the medulla) and in the periphery (carotid and aortic bodies) sense changes in P_{CO_2} and [H^+] and alter the ventilatory rate (see Chapter 29). In metabolic acidosis, an increase in [H^+] (decrease in pH) increases the ventilatory rate. Conversely, during metabolic alkalosis, a decrease in [H^+] (increase in pH) leads to a decrease in the ventilatory rate.* The respiratory response to metabolic acid-base disturbances may take effect within several minutes but may require several hours to complete.

> Individuals with insulin-dependent diabetes can develop a metabolic acidosis (secondary to the production of keto-acids) if insulin dosages are not adequate. As a compensatory response to this acidosis, the individual develops deep and rapid breathing. This breathing pattern is termed **Kussmaul respiration.** With prolonged Kussmaul respiration, the respiratory muscles can become fatigued. Respiratory compensation can then be impaired and the acidosis can become severe.

---

*With maximal hyperventilation, P_{CO_2} can be reduced to approximately 10 mm Hg. Because hypoxia, which is a potent stimulator of ventilation, also develops with hypoventilation, the degree to which P_{CO_2} can be increased by hypoventilation is limited. In an otherwise normal individual, hypoventilation cannot raise P_{CO_2} above 60 mm Hg.

Renal Defense

The third and final line of defense against acid-base disorders is the kidneys. In response to a change in the plasma pH and P_{CO_2}, the kidneys make appropriate adjustments in the excretion of HCO_3^- and net acid. The increase in net acid excretion is primarily the result of increased synthesis and excretion of NH_4^+. The renal response requires several days to complete because it takes hours to days to increase the synthesis and activity of the enzymes involved in NH_4^+ production.

In acidosis (increase in $[H^+]$ or P_{CO_2}), secretion of H^+ by the nephron is stimulated, and the entire filtered load of HCO_3^- is reabsorbed. The production and excretion of NH_4^+ are also stimulated, thus increasing net acid excretion by the kidneys (see equation 38-6). The new HCO_3^- generated during the process of net acid excretion is returned to the body, and plasma $[HCO_3^-]$ increases.

In alkalosis (decrease in $[H^+]$ or P_{CO_2}), secretion of H^+ by the nephron is inhibited. As a result, net acid excretion and HCO_3^- reabsorption are reduced. HCO_3^- will appear in the urine, thereby reducing the plasma $[HCO_3^-]$.

Loss of gastric contents from the body (e.g., during vomiting or nasogastric suction) produces a metabolic alkalosis secondary to the loss of HCl. If the volume of gastric fluid loss is significant, volume contraction will occur. Under this condition, the kidneys cannot excrete sufficient quantities of HCO_3^- to compensate for the metabolic alkalosis. HCO_3^- excretion does not occur, because volume contraction results in enhanced proximal tubule Na^+ reabsorption and increased levels of aldosterone (see Chapter 36). These responses in turn limit HCO_3^- excretion, because Na^+ reabsorption in the proximal tubule is coupled to H^+ secretion via the Na^+-H^+ antiporter (i.e., HCO_3^- is reabsorbed because of the need to reduce Na^+ excretion). In addition, the elevated aldosterone levels stimulate H^+ secretion by the collecting duct. Thus, individuals who experience significant gastric fluid loss typically have a metabolic alkalosis and a paradoxically acidic urine. Correction of the alkalosis occurs only when euvolemia is restored. With restoration of euvolemia, HCO_3^- reabsorption by the proximal tubule will decrease, as will H^+ secretion by the collecting duct. As a result, HCO_3^- excretion will increase and the plasma $[HCO_3^-]$ will return to normal.

SIMPLE ACID-BASE DISORDERS

Table 38-2 summarizes the primary alterations and the subsequent defense mechanisms for the various simple acid-base disorders. These respiratory and renal defense mechanisms are commonly referred to as **compensatory responses.** Note again that these compensatory mechanisms do not correct the underlying disorder but simply reduce the magnitude of the change in blood pH. Complete recovery from the acid-base disorder requires correction of the underlying cause of the disturbance.

Types of Acid-Base Disorders

Metabolic acidosis. Metabolic acidosis is characterized by a low plasma $[HCO_3^-]$ and a low plasma pH. This condition can develop through the addition of nonvolatile acid to the body (e.g., in diabetic ketoacidosis), the loss of nonvolatile alkali (e.g., with diarrhea), or the failure of the kidneys to excrete sufficient net acid to replenish the HCO_3^- used to titrate the net daily acid load (e.g., in renal tubular acidosis or renal failure). As described above, buffering of H^+ occurs in both the ECF and ICF. When pH falls, the respiratory centers are stimulated and the ventilatory rate is increased (respiratory compensation). This increase in respiratory rate reduces P_{CO_2}, which further minimizes the fall in plasma pH. In general, there is a 1.2 mm Hg decrease in P_{CO_2} for every 1 mEq/L fall in plasma $[HCO_3^-]$. Thus, if plasma $[HCO_3^-]$ were reduced to 14 mEq/L from a normal value of 24 mEq/L, the expected decrease in P_{CO_2} would be 12 mm Hg, and the measured P_{CO_2} would be 28 mm Hg (normal P_{CO_2} = 40 mm Hg).

Finally, renal excretion of net acid is increased. This increased excretion occurs through eliminating all HCO_3^- from the urine (enhanced reabsorption of filtered HCO_3^-) and increasing NH_4^+ excretion (enhanced production of new HCO_3^-). If the process that initiated the acid-base disturbance is corrected, the kidneys' enhanced excretion of acid will ultimately return the pH and $[HCO_3^-]$ to normal. With correction of the pH, the ventilatory rate will also return to normal.

When nonvolatile acid is added to the body fluids, the $[H^+]$ increases (pH decreases) and the $[HCO_3^-]$ decreases. In addition, the concentration of the anion, which is associated with the nonvolatile acid, will increase. This change in the [anion] provides a convenient way to analyze and help determine the cause of a metabolic acidosis, and is known as calculating the anion gap. The anion rep-

■ Table 38-2   Characteristics of simple acid-base disorders

Disorder	Plasma pH	Primary alteration	Defense mechanisms
Metabolic acidosis	↓	↓ plasma $[HCO_3^-]$	ICF and ECF buffers, hyperventilation (↓ P_{CO_2}), ↑ renal NAE excretion
Metabolic alkalosis	↑	↑ plasma $[HCO_3^-]$	ICF and ECF buffers, hypoventilation (↑ P_{CO_2}), ↓ renal NAE excretion
Respiratory acidosis	↓	↑ P_{CO_2}	ICF buffers, ↑ renal NAE excretion
Respiratory alkalosis	↑	↓ P_{CO_2}	ICF buffers, ↓ renal NAE excretion

NAE, Net acid excretion; *ICF,* intracellular fluid; *ECF,* extracellular fluid.

resents the difference between the concentration of the major plasma cation (Na^+) and the major plasma anions (Cl^- and HCO_3^-).

$$\text{Anion gap} = [Na^+] - ([Cl^-] + [HCO_3^-]) \qquad (38\text{-}10)$$

Under normal conditions, the anion gap is in the range of 8 to 16 mEq/L.* If the anion of the nonvolatile acid is Cl^-, the anion gap will be normal (i.e., the decrease in $[HCO_3^-]$ is matched by an increase in $[Cl^-]$). The metabolic acidosis associated with diarrhea or renal tubular acidosis has a normal anion gap. In contrast, if the anion of the nonvolatile acid is not Cl^- (e.g., lactate, β-hydroxybutyrate), the anion gap will increase (i.e., the decrease in $[HCO_3^-]$ is not matched by an increase in the $[Cl^-]$, but rather by an increase in the concentration of the unmeasured anion). The anion gap is increased in the metabolic acidosis associated with renal failure, diabetes (ketoacidosis), lactic acidosis, or the ingestion of large quantities of aspirin. Thus, *calculation of the anion gap is a useful way to identify the cause of a metabolic acidosis.*

Metabolic alkalosis. Metabolic alkalosis is characterized by an elevated plasma $[HCO_3^-]$ and an elevated plasma pH. This condition can be caused by the addition of nonvolatile alkali to the body (e.g., ingestion of antacids), as a result of volume contraction (e.g., hemorrhage), or more commonly from loss of nonvolatile acid (e.g., loss of gastric HCl with vomiting). Buffering occurs in the ECF and ICF compartments. The increase in pH inhibits the respiratory centers and the ventilatory rate is reduced, thus elevating P_{CO_2} (respiratory compensation). With appropriate respiratory compensation, P_{CO_2} increases 0.7 mm Hg for every 1 mEq/L rise in plasma $[HCO_3^-]$.

The renal compensatory response to metabolic alkalosis is to increase the excretion of HCO_3^- by reducing its reabsorption along the nephron. Normally, this response occurs quite rapidly and effectively. However, as already noted, when the alkalosis occurs in the setting of decreased volume contraction (e.g., vomiting where fluid loss occurs with the H^+ loss), HCO_3^- excretion does not occur. Renal excretion of HCO_3^- will increase, and the alkalosis will be corrected only if euvolemia is reestablished. Enhanced renal excretion of HCO_3^- will eventually return the pH and $[HCO_3^-]$ to normal, provided that the underlying cause of the initial acid-base disturbance is corrected. With correction of the pH, the ventilatory rate also returns to normal.

Respiratory acidosis. Respiratory acidosis is characterized by elevated P_{CO_2} and reduced plasma pH. It results from decreased gas exchange across the alveoli, as a result of either inadequate ventilation (e.g., drug-induced depression of the respiratory centers) or impaired gas diffusion (e.g., pulmonary edema, as may occur in cardiovascular dis-

ease or lung disease). In contrast to the metabolic disorders, buffering during respiratory acidosis occurs almost entirely in the intracellular compartment. The increase in P_{CO_2} and decrease in pH stimulate both HCO_3^- reabsorption by the nephron and NH_4^+ excretion (renal compensation). Together, these responses increase net acid excretion and generate new HCO_3^-.

The renal compensatory response takes several days to occur. Consequently, respiratory acid-base disorders are commonly divided into acute and chronic phases. In the acute phase, not enough time has elapsed for the renal compensatory response to occur, and the body relies on intracellular buffering to minimize the change in pH. During this phase, and because of the intracellular buffering, plasma $[HCO_3^-]$ increases 1 mEq/L for every 10 mm Hg rise in P_{CO_2}. In the chronic phase, renal compensation occurs, and plasma $[HCO_3^-]$ increases 3.5 mEq/L for each 10 mm Hg rise in P_{CO_2}. Correction of the underlying disorder returns P_{CO_2} to normal, and the renal excretion of acid will decrease to its initial level.

Respiratory alkalosis. Respiratory alkalosis is characterized by reduced P_{CO_2} and elevated plasma pH. It results from increased gas exchange in the lungs, usually due to increased ventilation from stimulation of the respiratory centers (e.g., by drugs or disorders of the central nervous system). Hyperventilation can also occur as a response to anxiety or fear or at high elevation. As noted, buffering is primarily intracellular. In the acute phase of respiratory alkalosis, plasma $[HCO_3^-]$ decreases 2 mEq/L for every 10 mm Hg fall in P_{CO_2}. The elevated pH and reduced P_{CO_2} inhibit HCO_3^- reabsorption by the nephron and reduce NH_4^+ excretion (renal compensation). As a result of these two effects, net acid excretion is reduced. This response takes several days to complete and results in a 5 mEq/L decrease in plasma $[HCO_3^-]$ for every 10 mm Hg reduction in P_{CO_2}. Correction of the underlying disorder will return P_{CO_2} to normal, and renal excretion of acid will increase to its initial level.

Analysis of Acid-Base Disorders

Analysis of an acid-base disorder is directed at identifying the underlying cause so that appropriate therapy can be initiated. The patient's medical history and associated physical findings often provide valuable clues about the nature and origin of an acid-base disorder. Additionally, analysis of an arterial blood sample is frequently required. Such an analysis is straightforward if approached in a systematic fashion. For example, consider the following data:

$$\text{pH} = 7.35$$
$$[HCO_3^-] = 16 \text{ mEq/L}$$
$$P_{CO_2} = 30 \text{ mm Hg}$$

The acid-base disorder represented by these values, or any other set of values, can be determined by the following three-step approach (Fig. 38-6).

1. *Examination of the pH.* By first considering the plasma pH, one can classify the underlying disorder as either an acidosis or an alkalosis. Note that the body's defense mechanisms, by themselves, cannot correct an acid-base

---

*An anion gap (i.e., a difference between the concentration of cations and anions) does not actually exist. All cations are balanced by anions. The gap simply reflects the parameters that are measured. In reality:

$$[Na^+] + [\text{unmeasured cations}] = [Cl^-] + [HCO_3^-] + [\text{unmeasured anions}]$$

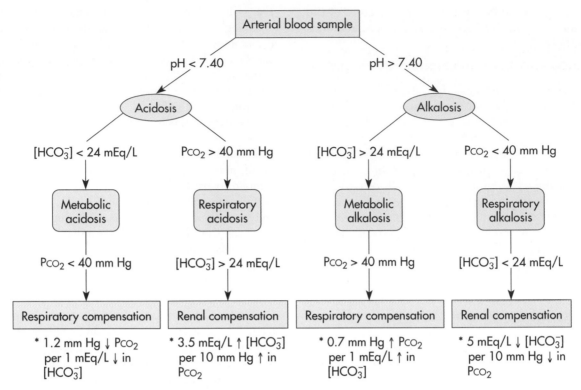

■ **Fig. 38-6** An approach to the analysis of simple acid-base disorders.

disorder. Thus, even if the defense mechanisms are completely operative, the pH still indicates the origin of the initial disorder. In the example shown above, the pH of 7.35 indicates acidosis.

2. *Determination of metabolic vs. respiratory disorder.* Simple acid-base disorders are either metabolic or respiratory. To determine which disorder is present, the $[HCO_3^-]$ and PCO_2 must next be examined. As indicated by the Henderson-Hasselbalch equation (see equation 38-3), acidosis could be the result of a decrease in the $[HCO_3^-]$ (metabolic) or an increase in the PCO_2 (respiratory). Alternatively, alkalosis could be the result of an increase in the $[HCO_3^-]$ (metabolic) or a decrease in the PCO_2 (respiratory). For the above example, the $[HCO_3^-]$ is reduced from normal (normal = 24 mEq/L), as is the PCO_2 (normal = 40 mm Hg). The disorder must therefore be a metabolic acidosis; it cannot be a respiratory acidosis, because the PCO_2 is reduced.

3. *Analysis of compensatory response.* Metabolic disorders result in compensatory changes in ventilation and thus in PCO_2, whereas respiratory disorders result in compensatory changes in renal acid excretion and thus in plasma $[HCO_3^-]$. In an appropriately compensated metabolic acidosis, PCO_2 will be decreased, whereas it is elevated in a compensated metabolic alkalosis. In respiratory acidosis, complete renal compensation results in an elevation of $[HCO_3^-]$. Conversely, $[HCO_3^-]$ is reduced in response to respiratory alkalosis. In the

above example, PCO_2 is reduced from normal, and the magnitude of this reduction (10 mm Hg decrease in PCO_2 for an 8 mEq/L increase in $[HCO_3^-]$) is as expected. Therefore, the acid-base disorder is a simple metabolic acidosis with appropriate respiratory compensation.

If the appropriate compensatory response is not present, a mixed disorder should be suspected. A **mixed acid-base disorder** reflects the presence of two or more underlying causes of the acid-base disturbance. A mixed disorder should be suspected when analysis of the arterial blood gas indicates that appropriate compensation has not occurred. For example, consider the following data:

$$pH = 6.96$$
$$[HCO_3^-] = 12 \text{ mEq/L}$$
$$PCO_2 = 55 \text{ mm Hg}$$

Following the three-step approach outlined above, it is evident that the disturbance is an acidosis that has both a metabolic component ($[HCO_3^-] < 24$ mEq/L) and a respiratory component ($PCO_2 > 40$ mm Hg). Thus, this disorder is mixed. An example of such a disorder is seen in an individual with a history of chronic pulmonary disease (e.g., emphysema with respiratory acidosis), who develops an acute gastrointestinal illness with diarrhea. Because diarrhea fluid contains HCO_3^-, its loss from the body results in the development of a metabolic acidosis.

A mixed acid-base disorder is also indicated in a patient who has abnormal PCO_2 and plasma $[HCO_3^-]$ but in whom the plasma pH is normal. Such a situation can be seen in a patient who has ingested a large quantity of aspirin. The salicylic acid (the active ingredient in aspirin) produces a metabolic acidosis, and at the same time stimulates the respiratory centers, causing hyperventilation and a respiratory alkalosis. Thus, the patient has a reduced plasma $[HCO_3^-]$ and a reduced P_{CO_2}.

SUMMARY

1. The pH of the body fluid is maintained within a narrow range by the coordinated function of the lungs and kidneys. The amount of volatile (CO_2-derived) and nonvolatile acids produced by metabolism, together with any acid or alkali ingested in the diet, must be excreted for acid-base balance to be maintained.

2. The lungs are the excretory route for CO_2, whereas the kidneys are the route for excretion of nonvolatile acids.

3. The body uses buffer systems to minimize changes in body fluid pH. The HCO_3^- buffer system of the ECF is the most important because it is regulated by both the lungs and the kidneys.

4. The kidneys maintain acid-base balance by excreting an amount of acid equal to the daily net acid load. The kidneys also prevent the loss of HCO_3^- in the urine by reabsorbing virtually all the HCO_3^- that is filtered at the glomerulus. Both the reabsorption of filtered HCO_3^- and the excretion of acid are accomplished by secretion of H^+ by the nephrons.

5. Urinary buffers are necessary for effective excretion of acid, because the minimum pH of the urine is only 4.0 to 4.5. Phosphate is the primary urinary buffer.

6. Ammonium excretion results in new HCO_3^- formation. Renal NH_4^+ production and excretion are regulated in response to acid-base disturbances.

7. Respiratory acid-base disorders result from primary alterations in the blood P_{CO_2}. Elevation of P_{CO_2} produces acidosis, and the kidneys respond by increasing excretion of acid. Conversely, reduction of P_{CO_2} produces alkalosis, and renal acid excretion is reduced. The kidneys respond to respiratory acid-base disorders over several hours to days.

8. Metabolic acid-base disorders result from primary alterations in the plasma $[HCO_3^-]$, which in turn result from addition of acid to, or loss of alkali from, the body. In response to metabolic acidosis, pulmonary ventilation is increased, which decreases the P_{CO_2}. An increase in the $[HCO_3^-]$ causes alkalosis. Alkalosis decreases pulmonary ventilation, which elevates the P_{CO_2}. The pulmonary response to metabolic acid-base disorders occurs in a matter of minutes.

BIBLIOGRAPHY

Journal articles

Battle D et al: Hereditary distal renal tubular acidosis: new understandings, *Annu Rev Med* 52:471, 2001.

DuBose TD Jr: H$^+$-K$^+$-ATPase, *Curr Opin Nephrol Hyperten* 8:597, 1999.

Nelson N, Harvey WR: Vacuolar and plasma membrane proton-adenosinetriphosphatase, *Physiol Rev* 79:361, 1999.

Shayakul C, Alper SL: Inherited renal tubular acidosis, *Curr Opin Nephrol Hyperten* 9:541, 2000.

Silver RB, Soleimani M: H$^+$-K$^+$-ATPases: regulation and role in pathophysiological states, *Am J Physiol* 276:F799, 1999.

Soleimani M, Burnham CE: Physiologic and molecular aspects of the Na$^+$:HCO$_3^-$ cotransporter in health and disease, *Kidney Int* 57:371, 2000.

Books and monographs

Alpern RJ: Renal acidification mechanisms. In Brenner BM, editor: *The kidney,* ed 6, Philadelphia, 2000, WB Saunders.

Brown D, Breton S: Structure, function and cellular distribution of the vacuolar H$^+$ATPase (H$^+$V-ATPase/proton pump). In Seldin DW, Giebisch G, editors: *The kidney: physiology and pathophysiology,* ed 3, Philadelphia, 2000, Lippincott, Williams & Wilkins.

Counillon L, Pouyssegur J: The members of the Na$^+$/H$^+$ exchanger gene family: their structure, function, expression, and regulation. In Seldin DW, Giebisch G, editors: *The kidney: physiology and pathophysiology,* ed 3, Philadelphia, 2000, Lippincott, Williams & Wilkins.

DuBose TD Jr: Acid-base disorders. In Brenner BM, editor: *The kidney,* ed 6, Philadelphia, 2000, WB Saunders.

Gennari RJ, Maddox DA: Renal regulation of acid-base homeostasis integrated response. In Seldin DW, Giebisch G, editors: *The kidney: physiology and pathophysiology,* ed 3, Philadelphia, 2000, Lippincott, Williams & Wilkins.

Hamm LL, Alpern RJ: Cellular mechanisms of renal tubular acidification. In Seldin DW, Giebisch G, editors: *The kidney: physiology and pathophysiology,* ed 3, Philadelphia, 2000, Lippincott, Williams & Wilkins.

Krapf R et al: Clinical syndromes of metabolic acidosis. In Seldin DW, Giebisch G, editors: *The kidney: physiology and pathophysiology,* ed 3, Philadelphia, 2000, Lippincott, Williams & Wilkins.

Madias NE, Androgue HJ: Respiratory alkalosis and acidosis. In Seldin DW, Giebisch G, editors: *The kidney: physiology and pathophysiology,* ed 3, Philadelphia, 2000, Lippincott, Williams & Wilkins.

Nagami GT: Renal ammonia production and excretion. In Brenner BM, editor: *The kidney,* ed 6, Philadelphia, 2000, WB Saunders.

Wesson DE et al: Clinical syndromes of metabolic alkalosis. In Brenner BM, editor: *The kidney,* ed 6, Philadelphia, 2000, WB Saunders.

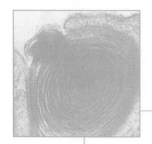

The Endocrine System

Saul M. Genuth

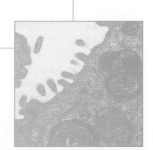

chapter thirty-nine

General Principles of Endocrine Physiology

Endocrinology has classically been defined as a discipline concerned with the "internal secretions of the body." The original concept—that a chemical substance called a hormone, liberated by a specialized type of cell, is carried by the bloodstream to act on distant target cells—represented a major advance in physiological understanding. The concept suggested a basic mechanism for maintaining the stability of the internal milieu in the face of irregular nutrient, mineral, and water fluxes, as well as physical alterations in the environment. Secretion of the hormone was evoked by a specific change in that milieu; as a result of the hormone's subsequent action on its target cells, the change was counteracted, and chemical or physical **homeostasis** (the desired status quo) was restored. However, from this basic homeostatic notion has grown an increasingly complex picture of the mission and very concept of the endocrine system. The mission includes regulation of cellular proliferation and differentiation, growth and total body maturation, body mass and its components, reproduction, senescence, and behavior.

A diversity of classic endocrine cell types (pituitary, thyroid, adrenal, gonadal, parathyroid, pancreatic islet), locations, glandular organization, and molecular species of hormones has been found. These cells and glands have evolved specifically to perform their endocrine functions. However, it has also been discovered that a number of tissues and organs, whose primary function appears to be nonendocrine, produce and secrete substances that act upon other cells that are nearby or at a distance (via the bloodstream). These cells and their hormones include renal cells (erythropoietin), cardiac atrial and ventricular cells (natriuretic hormones), gastrointestinal cells (secretin, glucagon-like peptides, cholecystokinin), endothelial cells (endothelin, nitric oxide), various lymphocytes, monocytes, and macrophages (interleukins, interferons, tumor necrosis factors), platelets and mesenchymal cells (growth factors, annexins, integrins), and adipose cells (leptin, resistin). Thus, the number and molecular variety of hormones have multiplied, and the basic premise of endocrinology has been adapted to other disciplines.

Target cells of hormone action are also diverse and include

other hormone-producing cells. Some hormones require chemical modification at intermediate sites between the gland or cell of origin and the target cells before their mission can be accomplished. A complementary group of target cell substances—hormone receptors—is also essential in mediating hormone action, which in addition involves multiple intracellular second messengers and mechanisms. Much of the control of hormone secretion depends on the feedback principle described below. Finally, important functional interrelationships between the endocrine, the neural, and the immune systems have been found. Because of this complexity and diversity, students may be overwhelmed unless they can relate the functional characteristics of each component of the endocrine system to a set of unifying principles. The major purpose of this chapter is to provide such a framework for the subsequent chapters.

RELATIONSHIP BETWEEN ENDOCRINE AND NEURAL PHYSIOLOGY

In a conceptual sense, the nervous system and the endocrine system have important functional similarities. Each is basically a system for signaling. Each operates in a stimulus-response manner. Each transmits signals that in some cases are highly localized, narrow, and unitary in purpose, and in other cases are widespread, broad, and diverse in purpose. Each system is crucial to the cooperative physiological functioning of the highly differentiated cells, tissues, and organs that make up the human organism. Therefore, *the nervous system and the endocrine system often respond together to incoming stimuli so as to integrate the organism's response to changes in its external and internal environment.* Recent advances in immunohistochemistry, cellular physiology, and molecular biology reveal increasingly intimate relationships between neural function and hormone secretion. The very distinction between a hormone and a neurotransmitter has become blurred. It may not be fanciful either to think of a circulating hormone as a signal molecule freed from the confines of a single axon to reach all responsive cells, or to think of a neurotransmitter as a signal molecule captured from the circulation to provide a restricted chemical connection between two specific cells separated in space.

This close relationship between the nervous and endocrine systems is illustrated by several common characteristics:

1. Neurons and endocrine cells can both secrete substances into the bloodstream.
2. Some endocrine cells and neurons generate electrical potentials and can be depolarized.
3. Peptides originally discovered as products of endocrine cells have neurotransmitter functions as well. Likewise, molecules nominally considered to be neurotransmitters can act as hormones.
4. A single cell can produce both biogenic amine neurotransmitters and peptide hormone molecules.
5. A single gene can be transcribed and translated to yield either a peptide neurotransmitter, a peptide hormone, or both.
6. Molecules, such as nerve growth factor and neurogenin, play roles in the development of certain endocrine cells, as well as in the development of the nervous system.
7. Receptors for hormones and neurotransmitters have structural similarities.

Two examples illustrate the coordinated function of the endocrine and nervous systems. (1) A fall in the plasma glucose to a dangerously low level is sensed in the brain and liver. The sympathetic nervous system, neurohormones from the hypothalamus, and hormones from the anterior pituitary gland, the adrenal cortex, the adrenal medulla, and the pancreatic islets all act on target cells in liver, muscle, and adipose tissue to restore plasma glucose to normal. (2) A significant decrease in the circulating blood volume is sensed by baroreceptors, the cardiac atria, the kidney, and the brain. The sympathetic nervous system, a neurohormone from the posterior pituitary gland, and hormones from the cardiac atria and ventricles, the adrenal medulla, the adrenal cortex, and the kidney act on target cells in blood vessels and kidneys to restore blood volume.

A close relationship between the endocrine and immune systems has also emerged. Immune cells secrete **cytokines,** and these molecules act on target cells through mechanisms analogous to those of hormones. Endocrine cells may themselves be targets of these cytokines in such a way that immune responses and endocrine responses to a stress are coordinated, or hormonal actions are reinforced. A number of classic hormones have been found, and are likely synthesized in immune cells, where they may act locally, even on their cells of origin.

The spectrum of hormonal signaling encompasses endocrine, neurocrine, paracrine, and autocrine effects (Fig. 39-1). **Endocrine** function is the transmission of a molecular signal from a classic endocrine cell through the bloodstream to a distant target cell. **Neurocrine** function is the transmission of a molecular signal from a neuron down its axon and then into the bloodstream to a distant target cell. **Paracrine** function is the transmission of a molecular signal from one cell type to a neighboring different cell type by diffusion through intercellular fluid channels or gap junctions.

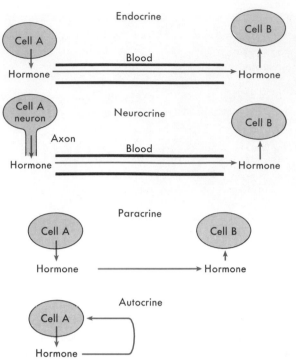

■ **Fig. 39-1** Schematic representation of mechanisms for cell-to-cell signaling via hormone molecules. In *endocrine* function the signal is carried to a distant target via the bloodstream. In *neurocrine* function the hormone signal originates in a neuron, and after axonal transport to the bloodstream it is carried to a distant target cell. In *paracrine* function the hormone signal is carried to an adjacent target cell over short distances via the interstitial fluid. In *autocrine* function the hormone signal acts back on the cell of origin or adjacent identical cells.

Autocrine function is the transmission of a molecular signal through the intercellular fluid or gap junctions to neighboring identical cells or even back to the cell of origin.

According to the route by which it is transmitted, the same messenger molecule may function as an endocrine hormone (bloodstream conveyance), as a neurotransmitter (axonal conveyance), as a neurohormone (combined axonal and bloodstream conveyance), or as a paracrine or autocrine hormone (local conveyance). The effect produced by the signaling molecule then depends on the target cell and the intracellular mechanisms that are activated. For example, a hypothalamic cell (see Chapter 43) may secrete the neurohormone **somatostatin** into blood, by which it reaches the pituitary gland and inhibits the release of growth hormone from that gland; a brain cell may transmit somatostatin to a second brain cell so as to alter behavior; and a delta cell in the pancreatic islets may release somatostatin into the fluid bathing adjacent cells and inhibit their release of insulin (see Chapter 41). The hormone insulin is secreted by beta cells in the pancreatic islets. Released into the bloodstream, insulin acts on adipose tissue, muscle, liver, and brain to regulate energy stores, carbohydrate, fat, and protein metabolism (endocrine function); released into the islet interstitial fluid, insulin inhibits the secretion of glucagon by neighboring alpha cells of the islets (paracrine function); and because beta cells possess insulin receptors, islet interstitial fluid insulin can regulate growth and function of beta cells themselves (autocrine function).

The close relationship between the neural and endocrine systems is well illustrated by some endocrine diseases. For example, in families with the **multiple endocrine adenoma syndrome–type 2,** neoplasms of the parathyroid glands that secrete parathyroid hormone and cause hypocalcemia and neoplasms of the adrenal medulla (a sympathetic nervous system component) that secrete norepinephrine and cause hypertension coexist in the same individual. In other instances, a single bronchial neoplasm may secrete the neurotransmitter serotonin and the pituitary hormone adrenocorticotropin, and these substances cause vascular flushes and a syndrome of cortisol excess, respectively, in the affected individual.

TYPES OF HORMONES

Hormone molecules fall into several chemical classes. The amines—thyroid hormones and catecholamines—both originate from the amino acid tyrosine and retain the aliphatic α-amino group. Introduction of a second hydroxyl group in the benzene ring is characteristic of the catecholamines, whereas iodination of the benzene ring distinguishes thyroid hormone. Melatonin arises from the amino acid tryptophane, and the aliphatic amino group is acetylated and the indole ringe is hydroxylated. Another chemical group is formed by the steroids, which include adrenal cortical and reproductive gland hormones and the active metabolites of vitamin D. Cholesterol is the common precursor in this class. Modification of side chains, hydroxylation at various sites, and ring aromatization confer individual biological activities on various members of this group. A third group, prostanoids, arises from the unsaturated fatty acid, arachidonic acid, and undergoes addition of oxygen atoms and cyclization to create rings. A fourth group is composed of proteins and peptides. In some instances, protein hormones with similar basic structures, but with different missions, have evolved from a common ancestral gene. In other instances a single progenitor protein gives rise to several different-sized hormone offspring, some with differing and some with overlapping actions.

HORMONE SYNTHESIS

A protein or peptide hormone is synthesized on the rough endoplasmic reticulum in the same biochemical manner as other proteins. The appropriate amino acid sequence is dictated by a specific messenger RNA that results from transcription of the hormone gene. In the simplest case, a single gene determines the structure and synthesis of a single protein or peptide hormone. However, multiple genes containing the same exon nucleotide sequence or only slightly

■ **Table 39-1**   Protein/peptide gene superfamilies

Gene	Peptide hormone products	Amino acids
A	Secretin	27
B	Pituitary adenylyl cyclase–activating polypeptide (PACAP)	27
		38
C	Peptide histidine methionine (PMH)	27
	Vasoactive intestinal polypeptide (VIP)	28
D	Glucagon	29
	Glucagon-like peptide-1	30
	Glucagon-like peptide-2	35
E	Glucose-dependent insulinotropic polypeptide (GIP)	42
F	Growth hormone-releasing hormone (GHRH)	44

varied sequences may direct the synthesis of a single peptide hormone in different cells. Alternatively, a unique gene may give rise to more than one primary RNA message by inclusion or exclusion of particular exons in the processes of excision and splicing. Thus one gene may direct the synthesis of different peptides in various cells.

Based on structural homologies, and descent from a probable common ancestor gene, many protein/peptide genes can be grouped into superfamilies. An example is shown in Table 39-1. The six genes in this superfamily give rise to nine human peptide hormones containing 27 to 44 amino acids, with as much as 70% homology between pairs of peptides. These molecules function as neurohormones in the brain, gastrointestinal tract regulators of pancreatic exocrine and endocrine function, and they have diverse paracrine roles in gonadal and placental tissue. The receptor molecules for eight of these nine hormones are also members of a single plasma membrane receptor class.

The DNA molecules for protein hormones are now readily cloned and structured. Such techniques allow the structure of the primary gene product to be deduced. This sometimes leads to the discovery of previously unknown peptide products whose function remains to be ascertained. Recombinant DNA technology is used to synthesize authentic human protein hormones, such as insulin and growth hormone, or therapeutically useful analogues with desired pharmacological properties.

The process of peptide hormone synthesis is illustrated in Fig. 39-2. A single premessenger RNA molecule is the initial unique gene product. Alternative splicing, which occurs with a frequency of 30% in humans, can give rise to multiple messenger RNAs (mRNAs) that include or exclude exons in various combinations. The varied protein products can have opposite functions, for example, they can be transcription factors that suppress or induce expression of other target genes. A striking example occurs in *Drosophila,* where alternative splicing of the *double sex gene* can yield either male- or female-specific proteins and characteristics. Splicing is itself a process that is subject to regulation by hormones, cytokines, and the ionic environment.

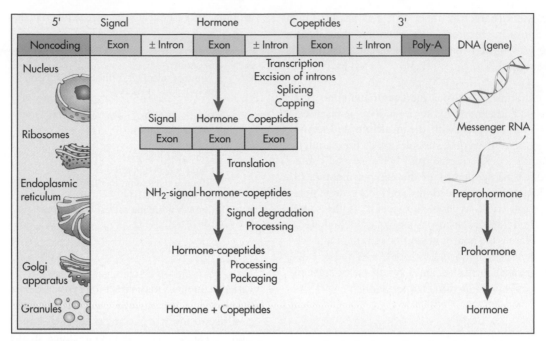

■ **Fig. 39-2** Schematic representation of peptide hormone synthesis. In the nucleus the primary gene transcript, a premessenger RNA molecule, undergoes excision of introns, splicing of the exons, capping of the 5′ end, and addition of poly(A) at the 3′ end. The resultant mature messenger RNA enters the cytoplasm, where it directs the synthesis of a preprohormone peptide sequence on ribosomes. In this process the N-terminal signal is removed, and the resultant prohormone is transferred vectorially into the endoplasmic reticulum. The prohormone undergoes further processing and packaging in the Golgi apparatus. After final cleavage of the prohormone within the granules, they contain the hormone and copeptides ready for secretion by exocytosis.

Translation of the mature RNA message begins with an N-terminal signal peptide sequence. When this is complete, translation temporarily ceases, while the signal peptide attaches the message to the endoplasmic reticulum receptors via "docking proteins." Translation then resumes until the entire encoded peptide sequence, known at this stage as a **preprohormone,** is formed. The signal peptide is then cleaved, resulting in a **prohormone,** which is simultaneously directed into the cisternal space for transport to the Golgi apparatus. Along with the hormone, the prohormone contains other peptide sequences, some of which may function to ensure proper folding of the hormone peptide chain, so as to permit formation of intramolecular linkages. Other peptide sequences within the prohormone may have related or independent functions and are cosecreted with the hormone. During transport to and within the Golgi apparatus, prohormone and hormone molecules are sorted into those that will be constitutively secreted at a basal rate and those that will be acutely secreted by exocytosis in response to stimuli. Such sorting may involve "chaperone" protein molecules and receptive sites within the endoplasmic reticulum and early Golgi. Most of the prohormone and hormone molecules accumulate in vesicles, where they are packaged for storage in **secretory granules.** The latter may also contain proteolytic enzymes, such as carboxypeptidases, that are necessary for subsequent conversion of the prohormone to the hormone or for elimination of copeptide products of translation. Golgi processing of prohormones to hormones may also

involve glycosylation, phosphorylation, palmitoylation, and isoprenylation of accessible amino groups (e.g., on lysine) or hydroxyl groups (e.g., on serine). In addition, many secretory granules of peptide hormones contain a soluble acidic protein of still unknown function—**chromogranin.**

The synthesis of amine and steroid hormones requires a sequential series of discrete enzymatic reactions. Further alterations that increase or modify the biological activity of these hormones may occur outside of the gland of origin. This multiplicity of distinctive steps means that various defects in hormone generation can and do arise from single gene–single enzyme mutations or from selective drug-induced enzyme inhibition.

Genetic diseases involving deficient or abnormal synthesis of peptide or protein hormones (e.g., insulin) usually involve the hormone gene itself. Single base substitutions or deletions can cause the mutant gene to express a product that cannot be processed or secreted normally or that has reduced biological activity. Mutant genes for proteins involved in processing or sorting hormones also exist. In the case of thyroid or steroid hormones or vitamin D, the product of the mutant gene is usually an enzyme that catalyzes one of the reactions in the biosynthetic sequence for the affected hormone. The resultant clinical state may reflect both the deficiency of the hormone product (e.g., cortisol) and the excess accumulation of a precursor that leads to overproduction of another product (e.g., an androgen).

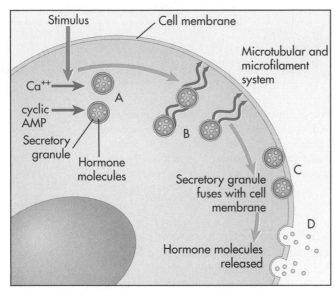

■ **Fig. 39-3** **A,** Secretion of peptide hormones via exocytosis is initiated *(A)* by application of a stimulus that raises intracellular Ca²⁺ levels and also usually raises cytosolic cAMP. The secretory granules are lined up and translocated to the plasma membrane *(B)* via activation of a microtubular and microfilament system. The membrane of the secretory granule fuses with that of the cell *(C).* The common membrane is lysed *(D),* releasing the hormone into the interstitial space. **B,** Insulin secretory granules in a β cell being stimulated by glucose. The *arrow* indicates a granule undergoing exocytosis. (From Lacy PE: *Diabetes* 19:895, 1970.)

HORMONE RELEASE

Both protein and catecholamine hormones are stored in secretory granules. Hormone release is then accomplished by the process of **exocytosis** (Fig. 39-3). The extracellular stimulus to secretion is usually followed by an immediate rise in cytosolic calcium first mobilized from intracellular bound stores and then taken up from extracellular fluid through plasma membrane channels. This initiates movement of secretory vesicle organelles (granules) to appropriate sites in the plasma membrane. This process is facilitated by specific vesicle-associated proteins, a **guanosine triphosphate (GTP)**-binding protein, and microtubule and microfilament elements. A secondary rise in **cyclic adenosine monophosphate (cAMP)** often follows. After fusion of the granule and plasma membranes, gap junctions and small pores form and the hormone is released into the extracellular fluid along with any stored copeptides, cleavage enzymes, chromogranin, and other granule contents. The membrane material from the empty core may then be reprocessed. In addition to this stimulated release of protein hormones from storage granules by exocytosis, there is a low basal rate of constitutive secretion of newly synthesized prohormones, of partially processed prohormones, or of the hormones themselves.

In the case of thyroid and steroid hormones, storage does not take place in discrete granules, although the hormones may be compartmentalized in the cell. Once the hormones have appeared in free form within the cytoplasm, they apparently leave the cell by simple transfer through the plasma membrane.

These modes of hormone synthesis and release are essentially unicellular. However, more complicated patterns of hormone production are also encountered. Two adjacent cell types in a single gland may interact so that hormone A from cell A is modified in cell B to produce hormone B, with an entirely different spectrum of biological effects. In this manner, for example, estrogens are produced from androgens in the ovaries. Furthermore, peripheral tissues, such as adipose tissue, may carry out similar conversions. A second mode of hormone production involves modification of a low activity precursor to a hormone of higher activity. For example, a sterol synthesized in the skin requires actions by the liver and kidney to produce the most potent vitamin D hormone. Lastly, peptide hormones can even be produced in the circulation itself from a protein precursor. A prototype for this pattern is the synthesis of angiotensin—a peptide hormone—from a protein secreted by the liver and acted on sequentially by enzymes released from the kidney and the lung.

REGULATION OF HORMONE SECRETION

General mechanisms that govern the secretion of hormones include the following:

Feedback control
Hormone-hormone
Substrate-hormone
Mineral-hormone

Neural control	Chronotropic control
Adrenergic	Oscillating
Cholinergic	Pulsatile
Dopaminergic	Diurnal rhythm
Serotoninergic	Sleep-wake cycle
Endorphinergic	Menstrual rhythm
enkephalinergic	Seasonal rhythm
Gabaergic	Developmental rhythm

The feedback principle is universally operative. **Negative feedback** *is most common and acts to limit the excursions in output of each partner in the pair* (Fig. 39-4). In the simplest instance, hormone A, which stimulates secretion of hormone B, in turn will be inhibited by an excess of hormone B. This straightforward mechanism characterizes the usual relationship between hormones of the pituitary gland and its target glands. Secretion of a hormone that either accelerates the production of or retards the utilization of a particular substrate will increase the concentration of that substrate in plasma; the resultant circulating excess of that substrate will then inhibit further secretion of the hormone. Conversely, a circulating deficit of that substrate from any cause will stimulate secretion of the hormone. On the other hand, a hormone that impedes the production or accelerates the utilization of a particular substrate will decrease the plasma concentration of that substrate. Secretion of such a hormone

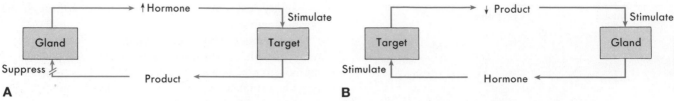

■ Fig. 39-4   Negative feedback principle. **A,** A primary increase in hormone secretion stimulates a greater output of product from the target cell. The product then feeds back on the gland to suppress further hormone secretion. In this fashion hormone excess is limited or prevented. **B,** A primary decrease in output of product from the target cell stimulates the gland to secrete hormone. The hormone then stimulates a greater output of product from the target cell. In this fashion the product deficiency is limited or corrected.

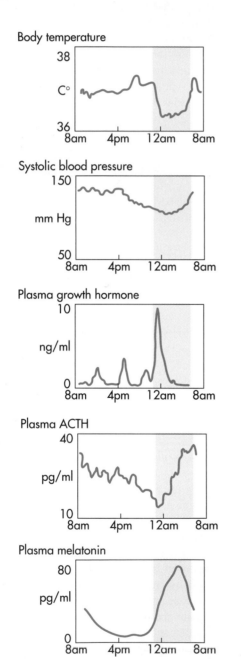

■ Fig. 39-5   A circadian pacemaker directs numerous endocrine and body functions, each with its own daily profile. The nighttime rise in plasma melatonin may mediate certain other circadian patterns. (Data from Schwartz WJ: *Adv Intern Med* 38:81, 1994.)

will be stimulated by a circulating excess, but inhibited by a circulating deficit of that substrate. The net result of negative feedback is to restore homeostasis.

Positive feedback, which is less common, *acts to amplify* the initial biological effect of the hormone. Thus hormone A, which stimulates secretion of hormone B, in turn may be initially stimulated to greater secretion rates by hormone B, but only through a limited dose-response range. Once the biological momentum for secretion of hormone B is sufficient, other influences, including negative feedback, will reduce the response of hormone A to fit the final biological purpose.

Neural control acts to evoke or suppress hormone secretion in response to both external and internal stimuli. Hormone secretion may arise from visual, auditory, olfactory, gustatory, tactile, or pressure stimuli and may be perceived consciously or unconsciously. Pain, emotion, sexual excitement, fright, injury, stress, and changes in blood volume all can modulate hormone secretion through neural mechanisms. Examples include (1) the release of **oxytocin,** which fills the milk ducts in response to the stimulus of suckling, (2) the release of **aldosterone,** which augments the circulatory volume in response to upright posture, and (3) the release of melatonin in response to darkness.

Many hormones are secreted in distinct pulses. Furthermore, certain secretory patterns are dictated by circadian (24-25 hour) rhythms, diurnal (day-night) rhythms, or ultradian (multiple within a day) rhythms. These rhythms may be genetically encoded or acquired. Circadian or daily rhythms can be demonstrated even within certain individual cells in culture. For example, pineal gland cells show regular and coordinated 24-hour variation in synthesis of the hormone **melatonin.** A coordinated intrinsic 24-hour cycle can be demonstrated for several endocrine, metabolic, and behavioral rhythms (Fig. 39-5), even in a timeless environment lacking day or night. Modifications of the intrinsic cycle occur via light signals from the retina and signals from the thalamus, midbrain, hippocampus, and pineal gland (Fig. 39-6).

The source of regular oscillatory cycles is a pulse generator(s) in the suprachiasmatic nucleus (SCN) of the hypothalamus (Fig. 39-6). The intrinsic circadian clock is also located in the SCN, which in vitro demonstrates a spontaneous peak of electrical activity at the same time every 24 to

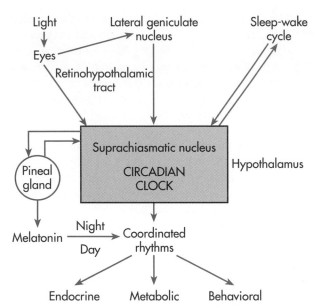

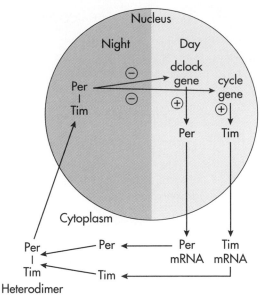

■ **Fig. 39-6** The origin of circadian rhythms in endocrine gland secretion, metabolic processes, and behavioral activity. A clock with an intrinsic 24-25–hour cycle is located in the suprachiasmatic nucleus (SCN) of the hypothalamus. This free running clock is entrained by environmental light signals to the external 24-hour day. It is also influenced by and, in turn, can influence the sleep-wake cycle, which also has independent effects on hormone secretion. The pineal gland with its hormone, melatonin, is both an agent and regulator of the SCN. (Modified from Turek FW: *Rec Prog Horm Res* 49:43, 1994.)

■ **Fig. 39-7** A cyclic pattern of functioning is created in the suprachiasmatic nucleus of the hypothalamus by an intracellular negative feedback system involving four genes. The Per-Tim heterodimeric protein represses expression of the Per and Tim genes by repressing expression of the D clock and cycle genes whose products are transactivators of the Per and Tim genes. (From Seghal A et al: *Rec Prog Horm Res* 54:61, 1999.)

25 hours. All SCN neurons synthesize the neurotransmitter γ-aminobutyric acid; some also express neurohormones, such as vasopressin, vasoactive intestinal peptide (Table 39-1), and somatostatin.

The 24- to 25-hour cycle can be "entrained" by the normal environmental light-dark cycle created by the earth's rotation, so that the periodicity of the clock appears to be environmentally controlled. Neural input is generated from specialized light-sensitive retinal cells that are distinct from rods and cones. These signals, via the retinohypothalamic tract (Fig. 39-6), with norepinephrine as the neurotransmitter, create the entrainment. Under constant conditions of light or dark, however, the SCN clock becomes "free running." Entrainment, that is shifting the phase of SCN activity so that it correlates with a regular external cycle of similar frequency, is mediated by cAMP and pituitary adenylyl cyclase-activating peptide (PACAP) (Table 39-1) during subjective daytime and by acetylcholine and cyclic guanosine monophosphate (cGMP) during subjective nighttime.

Genes that "keep time" intrinsically in the SCN were first discovered in *Drosophila* to account for circadian variation in their locomotor activity. However, these genes, *timeless* (Tim) and *period* (Per), are present in mammals along with the genes *dclock* and *cycle* (Fig. 39-7). In the daytime, Per and Tim genes are expressed in the nucleus, and the protein products of Per and Tim form a heterodimer in the cytoplasm. In the nighttime, the Per-Tim heterodimer is translocated to the nucleus where it suppresses expression of the genes

dclock and *cycle*. The products of these latter two genes are, respectively, transcriptional activators of Tim and Per. Thus, the periodicity of the SCN results from a complex intracellular negative feedback system, by which Per and Tim proteins control expression of their own genes. Light causes rapid degradation of the Per-Tim heterodimer; this is probably also a component in the day-night entrainment process.

The pineal gland forms an endocrine link between the SCN and various physiological processes that require circadian control. This tiny gland, close to the hypothalamus, synthesizes the hormone *melatonin* from the neurotransmitter *serotonin*, of which tryptophane is the precursor (Fig. 39-8). Melatonin synthesis is circadian, and the rate-limiting enzyme is *N*-acetyltransferase. The content and activity of this enzyme in the pineal gland vary markedly in cyclic fashion, which accounts for the cycling of melatonin secretion and its plasma levels (Fig. 39-5). Melatonin synthesis is also inhibited by light and markedly stimulated by darkness; the stimulating messenger is cAMP. Thus melatonin may transmit the information that nighttime has arrived, and body functions are entrained accordingly. Melatonin feedback to the SCN at dawn or dusk may also help evoke day-night entrainment of the SCN 24 to 25 hour clock. Melatonin has numerous other actions, including induction of sleep and inhibition of puberty. Its mechanism of action is initiated by binding to a plasma membrane receptor linked to G-proteins that inhibit the formation of cAMP, but that stimulate the formation of phosphoinositides as second messengers (see below).

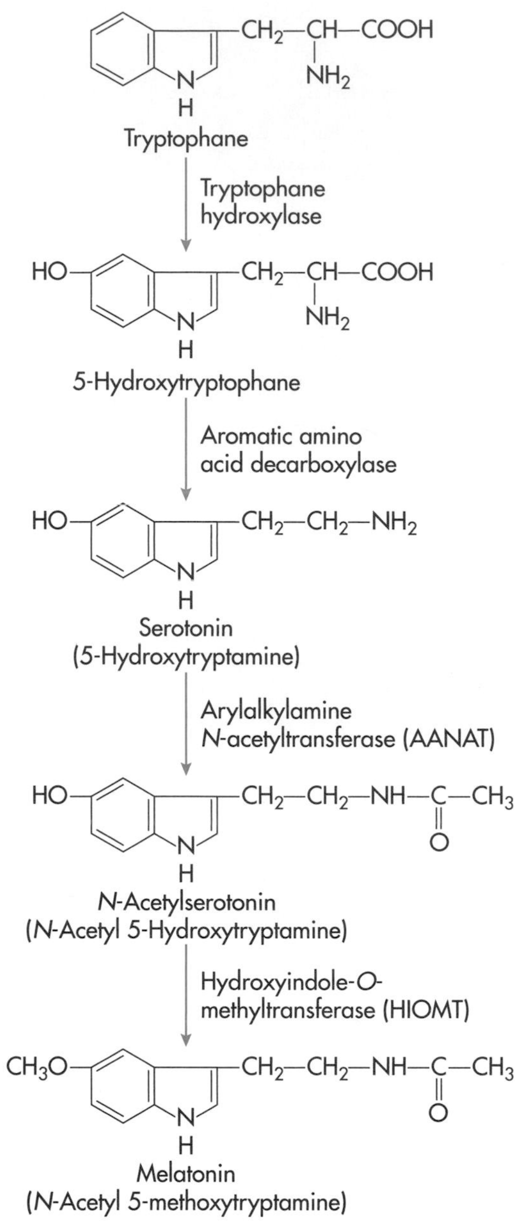

■ **Fig. 39-8** The synthesis of melatonin by the pineal gland. The acetyltransferase reaction is rate limiting.

Endocrine and related rhythms are also affected by the sleep-wake cycle via the circadian clock. In addition, input from the reticular activating substance and sleep centers to hypothalamic neurons that govern specific pituitary hormones (Chapter 43) mediate sleep-wake effects independently from the circadian clock.

Jet lag is a state in which a sudden artificial change in clock time abruptly shifts the phase of day-night and sleep-wake cycles of secretion of various hormones, including melatonin and cortisol. Reestablishment of normal cycles that are cued by the new clock time and that reflect entrainment of the intrinsic circadian clock to the altered environment often requires several days. Administration of melatonin at the proper time can facilitate the process of adaptation.

Major medical or surgical stress overrides the circadian clock and causes a pattern of persistent and exaggerated hormone release and metabolism that mobilizes endogenous fuels, for example, glucose and free fatty acids, and augments their delivery to critical organs. By contrast, growth and reproductive processes are suppressed (see Chapter 45).

Seasonal variation in the rhythm of hormone secretion also occurs. Such behavior may reflect the influence of temperature, tides, sunshine, and variation in the length of daylight on the circadian clock. Some of these secretory rhythms appear atavistic in humans, and they have probably served to fulfill the biological needs of evolutionary ancestors. Most intriguing are those patterns of hormone secretion that coincide with and are unique to a certain developmental stage, such as the onset of puberty. A diverse and still growing number of neurotransmitter molecules carries these signals to the endocrine cells.

HORMONE ACTION

Three major sequential steps are involved in eliciting the response of a target cell to a hormonal stimulus (Fig. 39-9):
1. The hormone must be recognized and bound by a specific cell receptor.
2. The hormone receptor complex must then be coupled to a signal-generating mechanism or it must act as one itself.
3. The generated signal (second messenger) then changes intracellular processes quantitatively by altering the activity or concentration of enzymes, of other functional proteins, and of structural proteins.

Two basic schemes accomplish these steps. In the first scheme, the receptor for the hormone and the signal-generating system are located within or immediately adjacent to the plasma membrane of the cell. This first scheme is classically employed by peptide/protein and catecholamine hormones, but it now extends to other signaling molecules. In this case, the essential information for triggering the response actually lies in the receptor molecule. By its occupancy, the hormone changes the receptor's conformation and allows transmission of the information contained in the receptor. The hormone is primarily only an extracellular signal. This type of hormone response is elicited within seconds to minutes.

In the second case, largely employed by steroid and thyroid hormones, the hormone must enter the cell, occupy the receptor, and in combination with the receptor, interact with DNA molecules in the nucleus to alter expression of genes. In this situation, the DNA molecules act as second messengers, and the essential information for triggering a response lies in the hormone and the receptor, coupled together. The hormone acts as a true intracellular signal. This type of hormonal action requires minutes to hours or even days for its full expression.

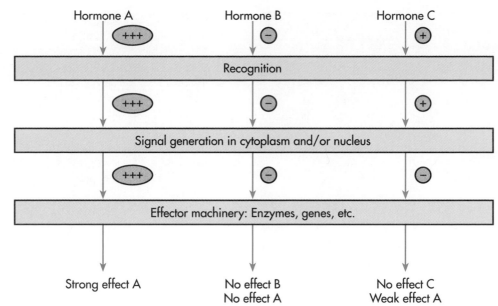

■ **Fig. 39-9** Hormone-cell interaction. Hormone A is recognized by this cell through binding with its specific receptor. An intracellular signal is generated that stimulates the appropriate enzymatic machinery, and effect A is produced. Hormone B is not recognized because the cell lacks a receptor for it. Thus hormone B cannot produce effect A in this cell even though it might operate through an identical enzymatic machinery in its own target cell. Hormone C may be slightly recognized by this cell through individual overlap with the receptor to hormone A. Although a weak intracellular signal may be generated, no effect of C results because the cell lacks the appropriate enzymatic machinery. To a minor extent, however, hormone C may produce effect A.

Receptor Kinetics

A given hormone may act through different receptor molecules in different target cells. However, multiple actions of a given hormone in the same target cell are usually initiated by binding to a sole receptor molecule. The large number of receptor molecules per cell often guarantees that receptor availability will not be rate limiting for hormone action.

Receptors are protein molecules that associate with their cognate hormones or other ligands in reversible reactions that appear to obey the following molecular chemical kinetics:

$$H + R = HR \tag{39-1}$$

$$K_{assoc} = \frac{HR}{[H][R]} \tag{39-2}$$

$$\frac{[HR]}{[H]} = K_{assoc} \times [R] \tag{39-3}$$

where

H = free hormone in solution
R = unoccupied receptor
HR = bound hormone = occupied receptor
R_0 = initial receptor capacity = [R] + [HR]
K_{assoc} = affinity constant

If a constant amount of receptor is incubated in vitro with increasing concentrations of hormone, the amount of bound hormone increases until receptor occupancy reaches 100%. At this point the number of bound hormone molecules

equals the total number of originally available receptor molecules, that is, the initial receptor capacity (R_0). At the same time, as the free hormone concentration approaches infinity and the receptor occupancy approaches 100%, the ratio of bound hormone to free hormone progressively decreases and approaches zero. That is, as

$$[H] \rightarrow Infinity$$
$$[HR] \rightarrow R_0 \tag{39-4}$$
$$\frac{[HR]}{[H]} \rightarrow 0$$

The data obtained by incubating receptors with increasing amounts of hormone can be plotted in a meaningful way by simple substitution in equation 39-3. Since

$$[R] = R_0 - [HR]$$
$$\frac{[HR]}{[H]} = K_{assoc} \times (R_0 - [HR]) \tag{39-5}$$

$$\frac{[HR]}{[H]} = K_{assoc} [HR] + K_{assoc} R_0 \tag{39-6}$$

$$\frac{Bound\ hormone}{Free\ hormone} = K_{assoc} \times Bound\ hormone + K_{assoc} \times Receptor\ capacity$$

A graph of the ratio of bound hormone to free hormone, plotted as a function of bound hormone, is called a **Scatchard plot.** This graph theoretically yields a straight line (Fig. 39-10, *A*). The slope of the line equals the negative of the association constant (K_{assoc}), and the × intercept equals R_0 (the receptor capacity).

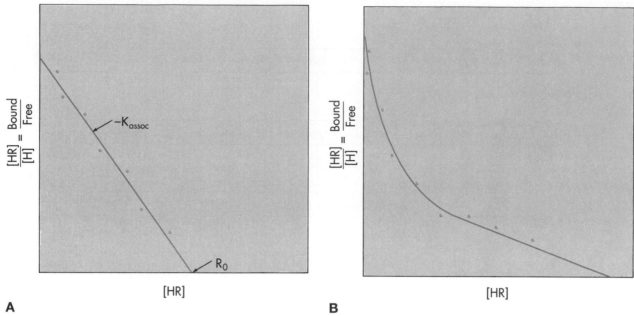

■ Fig. 39-10   Scatchard plot. **A,** A linear plot results when the hormone reacts with a single receptor class and no cooperativity is present. The negative of the association constant, K_{assoc}, equals the slope of the line. The receptor number, R_0, equals the intercept with the x axis. **B,** An exponential plot results when hormone occupancy of one receptor molecule alters the local affinity of a second nearby molecule for the hormone. This phenomenon is called negative cooperativity.

In practice many Scatchard plots of hormone binding to receptor yield exponential curves (Fig. 39-10, *B*). This suggests that hormone occupancy of a relatively small number of receptors decreases the affinity of nearby unoccupied receptor molecules for the hormone. However, in many instances, occupancy of only 5% to 10% of the total available receptor molecules is enough to yield full (i.e., maximum) biological action of the hormone. Therefore, the declining affinity of receptor for hormone does not impede hormone action quantitatively, but it may reduce the duration of hormone effect or protect the cell from a sudden massive excess of hormone.

Regulation of its hormone receptor provides another mechanism for regulating hormone action. Rearrangement of equation 39-5 to provide an expression for HR yields

$$[HR] = R_0 \times \frac{K_{assoc}\,[H]}{K_{assoc}\,[H] + I} \qquad (39\text{-}7)$$

It is evident, therefore, that HR is directly proportional to R_0, the initial receptor number. An increase in receptor number (R_0) raises the maximal [HR] level obtainable at saturating concentrations of hormone. This would raise the maximal responsiveness of the cell for those hormone effects in which receptor binding is rate limiting, rather than a later step in hormone action. This is generally the case for steroid and thyroid hormones. At submaximal hormone concentrations the increase in [HR] produced by an increase in R_0 would enhance the sensitivity of the cell. This is commonly seen with peptide hormones.

Receptor capacity often is regulated by its own hormone. In many instances the regulation is inverse, that is, a sustained excess of hormone decreases the number of its receptors per cell; this process, called **downregulation,** acts to lessen the effect of chronic exposure to excess hormone. However, in some instances, intermittent exposure of the target cells to low concentrations of the hormone creates a direct relationship, that is, the hormone appears to recruit its own receptors. This amplifies the cell's response to the hormone.

An increase in receptor affinity (K_{assoc}) will also increase [HR] and the sensitivity of the cell to hormone stimulation. Affinity can be altered by phosphorylation of the receptor, and by factors such as ambient pH, osmolality, ion concentrations, and substrate levels.

Plasma Membrane Receptor Systems

Plasma membrane receptors are large glycoproteins of molecular weight 50,000 to 200,000. They are often composed of subunits. Each molecule extends completely through the plasma membrane. A specific extracellular site(s) in the N-terminus portion of the receptor binds the hormone. The intramembranous portion may simply span the plasma membrane once or wind in and out of it a number of times. The latter configuration anchors the receptor and/or allows an interaction with more than one signal-generating mechanism within the plasma membrane. The intracellular C-terminus tail of the receptor may contain a separate signal-generating mechanism.

The receptors tend to be concentrated in cellular microvilli. Hormone binding to these receptors may change their conformation and their distribution within the plasma membrane. These changes lead to clustering of the hormone-receptor complexes. After receptor activation is completed, internalization of the complexes occurs at these sites by **endocytosis.** Within the cell, lysosomal degradation of the complex occurs. Consequently either the individual hormone and receptor molecules are destroyed or the receptor molecules are recycled back into the plasma membrane. It is possible that some internalized hormone-receptor complexes can also mediate intracellular actions of the hormone before they are disrupted.

Some plasma membrane receptors resemble immunoglobulins in structure. Certain individuals susceptible to **autoimmune diseases** develop antibodies to their own hormone receptors. When such antibodies react with the receptor molecules, they may simply block access of the hormone to the receptor and diminish the function of the target cells (e.g., the **"resistant ovary" syndrome**). Alternatively, the antibody receptor combination mimics the hormone-receptor interaction and enhances the function of the target cells (e.g., hyperthyroidism caused by **Graves' disease;** see Chapter 44).

Coupling by G-Proteins

For many hormones, occupancy of the plasma membrane receptor initiates a sequence of reactions within the membrane bilayer. *Nearly 20 families of coupling molecules, known as G-proteins* (see Chapter 5), *functionally link various receptors to nearby effector molecules. The latter, in turn, generate second messengers that mediate the hormones' intracellular actions* (Fig. 39-9).

There are three classes of plasma membrane receptors that exert their hormonal actions via G-proteins (Fig. 39-11). These receptors vary in the length and complexity of the N-terminal extracellular hormone-binding portion and in the length of the intracellular C-terminal portion. All receptors wind in and out of the plasma membrane by means of seven transmembrane segments and all have disulfide bridges (between cysteines) that connect extracellular loops 2 and 3 (Fig. 39-11). Class 2 receptors also have several disulfide bridges in the N-terminal extracellular segment. These various intramolecular features prevent the receptors from linking with G-proteins in the absence of hormone or ligand. Phosphorylation of G-protein–coupled receptors by kinase enzymes may switch them from G-protein signaling to signaling cascades that are normally initiated by growth factor receptors.

G-proteins are trimers; each has a unique α-subunit but a β-γ-dimer subunit that is similar among family members. The α-subunits bind to receptors, to effector molecules, and to guanosine diphosphate (GDP) and guanosine triphosphate (GTP). The β-γ-dimeric subunit may serve to attach the G-protein to the plasma membrane.

In its inactive state the G-protein is bound to GDP (Fig. 39-12). Creation of a hormone-receptor complex causes the appropriate adjacent G-protein α-subunit to bind to the occupied receptor. The G-protein then releases its bound GDP and binds instead to GTP. The displacement of GDP

by GTP activates the G-protein by causing the α-subunit to dissociate from both the hormone receptor and from its own β-γ-subunit. The α-subunit-GTP complex then moves to and binds to a nearby membrane effector molecule, such as the enzymes **adenylyl cyclase** and **phospholipase C** or to an ion channel carrier protein. The activity of the effector molecule is either stimulated or inhibited by the specific α-subunit–GTP complex. In this process, the α-subunit then catalyzes the hydrolysis of its bound GTP to GDP and inorganic phosphate. The α-subunit-GDP complex then reassociates with its β-γ-dimer, and thereby reconstitutes the original inactive G-protein. The latter is again free to interact with another hormone-occupied receptor molecule and start another cycle.

This coupling cycle is repeated with the G-protein α-subunit shuttling between receptor and effector molecules until the hormone dissociates from its receptor or is internalized and degraded. Mg^{2+} is required for the G-protein cycle, which is driven by the energy derived from the hydrolysis of the high-energy terminal P-O-P bond of GTP to yield GDP. Because the effector generates many intracellular second messenger molecules, the G-protein mechanism of signal transduction amplifies greatly the original extracellular hormone signal.

The plasma membrane receptor/G-protein signaling systems are regulated by other hormones that act via nuclear receptors. Expression of genes for plasma membrane receptors and G-proteins can be increased or decreased, and their mRNA molecules can be stabilized or more rapidly degraded. And they can be posttranslationally modified by phosphorylation, ADP-ribosylation, lipid or carbohydrate molecule additions, and/or proteolysis.

Second Messengers

G-proteins couple hormone-receptor complexes to at least three main effector systems: the adenylyl cyclase–cAMP system, the calcium-calmodulin system, and the membrane phospholipase-phospholipid system.

The **adenylyl cyclase–cAMP** system was the first to be described and initiated the concept of a second messenger (Fig. 39-13). The plasma membrane enzyme adenylyl cyclase catalyzes formation of cAMP from adenosine triphosphate (ATP) with Mg^{2+} as cofactor. A stimulatory G-protein (G_s) therefore increases intracellular cAMP levels, whereas an inhibitory G-protein (G_i) decreases cAMP levels.

An increase in cAMP stimulates the activation of **protein kinase A** (Fig. 39-13). This, in turn, activates a number of enzymes in numerous metabolic pathways by phosphorylating their individual enzyme kinases. Alternatively, cAMP-stimulated phosphorylation may deactivate other enzymes. Thus, after hormone binding to receptor, this system generates a cascade of effects that ultimately changes the flux of metabolites in the cell. In the end, either the storage or the release of an important metabolite may be facilitated. Activation and deactivation of reciprocal pathways by the same hormone can augment the result, for example, by simultaneously inhibiting the release pathway while stimulating

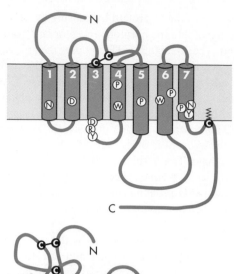

Family A. Rhodopsin/β2 adrenergic receptor-like

Biogenic amine receptors (adrenergic, serotonin, dopamine, muscarinic, histamine)

CCK, endothelin, tachykinin, neuropeptide Y, TRH, neurotensin, bombesin, and growth hormone secretagogues receptors plus opsins

Bradykinin receptors

Adenosine, melanocortin, olfactory, cannabinoid receptors.

Chemokine, GnRH, eicosanoid, leukotriene, FSH, LH, TSH, fMLP, galanin, nucleotide, opioid, oxytocin, vasopressin, somatostatin receptors plus others.

Melatonin receptors

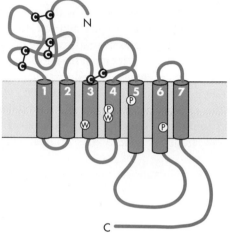

Family B. Glucagon/VIP/Calcitonin receptor-like

Calcitonin, CGRP and CRH receptors

PTH and PTHrP receptors

Glucagon, glucagon-like peptide, GIP, GHRH, PACAP, VIP, and secretin receptors

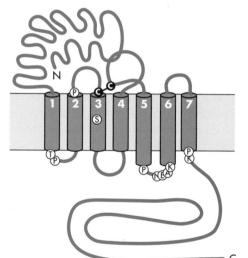

Family C. metabotropic neurotransmitter/Calcium receptors

Metabotropic glutamate receptors

Metabotropic GABA receptors

Calcium receptors

Vomeronasal pheromone receptors

■ **Fig. 39-11** Snake diagrams for the three families of plasma membrane G-protein–linked receptors. Not all members of each family are listed. (From Gether U: *Endocr Rev* 21:90, 2000.)

the storage pathway. Adenylyl cyclase and cAMP are ubiquitously distributed. Therefore, the specificity of enzyme responses to a particular hormone also may depend on the compartmentalization of increase in cAMP within the cell or on the proximity of the activated adenylyl cyclase to target enzyme(s).

cAMP may also act as a hormone second messenger by altering gene expression. Target DNA molecules have a **cAMP regulatory element (CRE)** that binds a protein transcription factor known as **cAMP response element binding protein (CREB)** (Fig. 39-13). cAMP activates protein kinase A; the catalytic subunit of the enzyme is then free to be translocated into the nucleus, where it phosphorylates CREB. The phosphorylated CREB can then bind to CRE in a complex with another transcription protein, such as activated transcription factor-1. The result is to stimulate or inhibit RNA

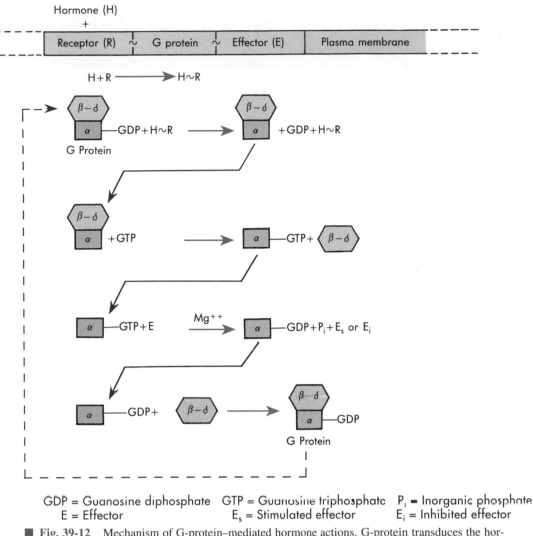

GDP = Guanosine diphosphate   GTP = Guanosine triphosphate   P$_i$ = Inorganic phosphate
E = Effector   E$_s$ = Stimulated effector   E$_i$ = Inhibited effector

■ **Fig. 39-12**   Mechanism of G-protein–mediated hormone actions. G-protein transduces the hormone-receptor complex message to either stimulate or inhibit the effector in the plasma membrane. A GDP-GTP cycle fuels the sequence. See text for detailed description.

polymerase and transcription of the target gene, and thereby to stimulate or inhibit synthesis of a specific protein.

Another molecule, **cAMP response element modulator (CREM),** also mediates cAMP effects in the nucleus. Prior to puberty, CREM is present in low levels and acts as a gene *repressor.* At puberty, CREM concentration increases markedly in the testis and by alternate splicing of the transcribed CREM gene, the CREM molecule now *activates* CREs on genes essential for producing mature sperm.

The actions of cAMP are terminated by its hydrolysis; this reaction is catalyzed by the enzyme **phosphodiesterase.** Because the activity of phosphodiesterase is also modulated by hormones via a G-protein, the level of cAMP is under dual regulation. Two hormones can function antagonistically if one stimulates adenylyl cyclase and the other stimulates phosphodiesterase.

A second system for transduction of the hormone signal is the **calcium-calmodulin system** (Fig. 39-14). As a result of hormone occupancy of its receptor, a specific G-protein activates channels in the plasma membrane through which extra-

cellular calcium can enter the cytoplasm. Calcium may also be mobilized from intracellular reservoirs in the endoplasmic reticulum and possibly the mitochondria. As a second messenger, Ca^{2+} may then transiently interact with hundreds of binding proteins and target effector molecules. The overall results are influenced by (1) restriction of calcium diffusion in the cytosol, (2) the spatial localization of target molecules, (3) a broad spectrum of protein affinities for Ca^{2+} ranging from 10 to 1000 nM, and (4) the duration of hormone-receptor interaction. Increased cytosolic calcium particularly combines with a ubiquitous and specific binding protein, **calmodulin,** in various proportions. The different calcium-calmodulin complexes activate or deactivate various calcium-dependent enzymes. In this fashion, metabolite levels within the cell are ultimately altered.

A third system for transduction of the initial hormone receptor signal is through intermediates generated from specific **plasma membrane phospholipids** (Fig. 39-15). The key phospholipid is **phosphatidylinositol,** which undergoes further phosphorylation to phosphatidylinositol-4,5-bisphosphate. Hormone occupancy of its receptor initiates

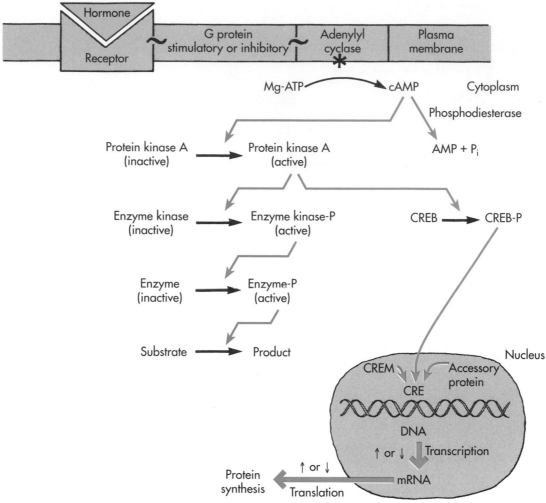

■ **Fig. 39-13** Mechanism of hormone action via cAMP as second messenger. The hormone-receptor complex, via a G-protein, either stimulates or inhibits adenylyl cyclase. If stimulated, cAMP is synthesized from ATP. cAMP activates protein kinase A, leading to a cascade of phosphorylations that ultimately activates or inactivates target enzymes. The latter regulate metabolic pathways. In addition, activated protein kinase A phosphorylates a cAMP-binding protein *(CREB),* which acts as a transcription factor by interacting with a cAMP regulatory element *(CRE)* on target DNA molecules.

a G-protein activation of the membrane-bound enzyme **phospholipase C,** which splits phosphatidyl-4,5-bisphosphate to a **diacylglycerol** and **inositol-1,4,5-trisphosphate.** The diacylglycerols are potent activators of the enzyme, **protein kinase C.** The latter is calcium dependent, and the diacylglycerol markedly increases the enzyme's affinity for calcium. Inositol trisphosphate (IP$_3$), released simultaneously with the diacylglycerol, binds to a specific IP$_3$ receptor on the endoplasmic reticulum. This leads to formation of a channel through which sequestered calcium flows into the cytosol. Therefore, the combined products of the action of phospholipase C on phosphatidylinositol bisphosphate greatly amplify protein kinase C activity. In turn, the latter phosphorylates and thereby activates or deactivates numerous enzymes involved in hormone actions. Finally, arachidonic acid, which is derived from subsequent hydrolysis of the diacylglycerol, serves as a substrate for the rapid synthesis of **prostaglandins** (see below).

Although rare, diseases caused by mutant genes for receptors or for G-proteins have provided much insight into mechanisms of hormone action. For example, the reduced activity of a mutant α-subunit of a stimulatory G-protein leads to diminished cAMP levels and results in deficient action of parathyroid hormone and **hypocalcemia** (see chapter 42). Another mutant G-protein, which is constitutively overactive, is associated with continuous hypersecretion of growth hormone causing the disease **acromegaly** (see Chapter 43). Activating mutants of G-protein–linked receptors have involved protonation of aspartic and glutamic acid residues or movements of the third and sixth transmembrane segments. Although these observations may seem esoteric, they lead to detailed understanding of structure/function relationships that permit designing of receptor agonists and antagonists for therapeutic use in much more common diseases.

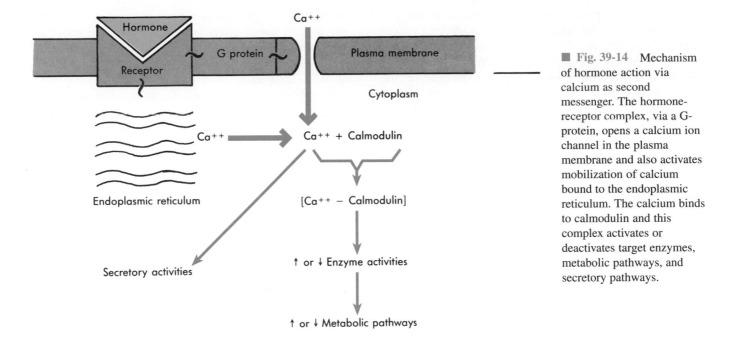

■ **Fig. 39-14** Mechanism of hormone action via calcium as second messenger. The hormone-receptor complex, via a G-protein, opens a calcium ion channel in the plasma membrane and also activates mobilization of calcium bound to the endoplasmic reticulum. The calcium binds to calmodulin and this complex activates or deactivates target enzymes, metabolic pathways, and secretory pathways.

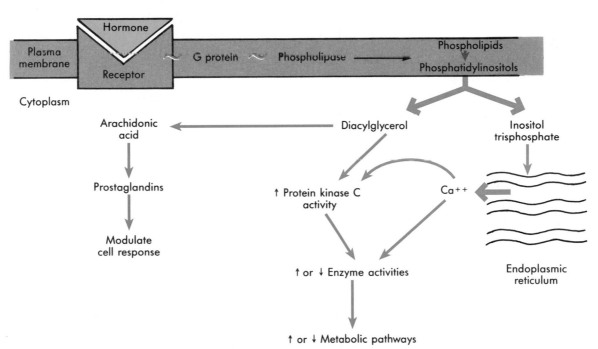

■ **Fig. 39-15** Mechanism of hormone action via membrane phospholipids. The hormone-receptor complex, via a G-protein, activates phospholipase C, which then releases diacylglycerol and inositol trisphosphate from membrane-bound phosphoinositides. Inositol trisphosphate mobilizes calcium from the endoplasmic reticulum. Calcium with diacylglycerol activates protein kinase C, which phosphorylates target enzymes, increasing or decreasing metabolic pathways. Diacylglycerol also yields arachidonic acid for synthesis of modulating prostaglandins.

Two other mechanisms of signal generation from plasma membrane receptors do not require G-protein intermediaries. These receptors have an extracellular hormone-binding portion, a single transmembrance portion, and an intracytoplasmic C-terminal portion. These components may be composed of S–S-bonded subunits. In each, the transducer(s) lie in the intracytoplasmic tail of the receptor (Fig. 39-11). In one type, exemplified by the insulin receptor, binding of the protein hormone changes the conformation of the receptor and exposes sites on its intracellular portion that are capable of receptor autophosphorylation at specific tyrosine sites. As a result, the receptor itself becomes a **tyrosine kinase** that phosphorylates tyrosine residues on intracellular protein substrates (Fig. 39-16). The latter initiate a cascade of serine and threonine phosphorylations of enzyme kinases and protein phosphatases that leads to multiple other intracellular events. These include alterations in cellular metabolism as well as in cellular proliferation and differentiation. In the second analogous mechanism, hormone binding of the extracellular portion changes the intracytoplasmic tail of the receptor. Such changes expose sites to which cytoplasmic tyrosine kinases (JAK kinases and STAT kinases) are docked and are then activated. The sequence that follows is similar to that in the example just described, in which the receptor itself becomes a tyrosine kinase. Growth hormone is an example of this type of hormone action.

Another second messenger that results from hormone interaction with the plasma membrane and with soluble forms of the enzyme *guanylyl cyclase* is **cyclic guanosine monophosphate (cGMP),** which arises from the action of guanylyl cyclase on GTP. The soluble form of guanylyl cyclase binds **nitric oxide (NO),** and cyclic GMP mediates the actions of this ubiquitous signaling molecule with potent vasodilator effects. A plasma membrane-bound form of guanylyl cyclase binds cardiac and brain natriuretic hormones, and cGMP mediates their actions as well. A G-protein that modulates cGMP phosphodiesterase activity also regulates cGMP levels. cGMP activates **protein kinase G** and thereby initiates a cascade of subsequent enzyme activations that is characteristic of this signaling system.

Hormones and other ligands that react with G-protein–linked receptors can activate still other kinases that promote growth. Mitogen-activated protein kinase (MAPK) and its precursor kinases (MAPKK and MAPKKK), when activated, begin a cascade of phosphorylations of plasma membrane and cytoplasmic proteins, as well as of cytoskeletal proteins and nuclear transcription factors. MAPKs are important mediators that are involved in embryogenesis, cell proliferation (hyperplasia), cell differentiation, and even regulated cell death (apoptosis).

Peptide and protein hormones also increase or decrease the cellular content (mass) concentration of enzymes and their mRNAs. This involves modification of gene expression and/or stabilization of mRNA levels. Because the cAMP mechanism described earlier cannot explain all these effects, other mechanisms must exist for transmitting signals from the hormone-occupied plasma membrane receptor to specific target DNA molecules.

As complex as each of these plasma membrane receptor initiated systems seem individually, it is necessary to appreciate that a single hormone may operate through one or more of the systems simultaneously or in sequence. Each messenger may subserve a different function of the hormone. Moreover, the systems can interact with each other in important ways. For example, calcium-calmodulin can stimulate not only adenylyl cyclase activity itself, but also the activity of phosphodiesterase, the enzyme that hydrolyzes cAMP. Thus, cAMP levels, initially increased by a rapid hormone activation of adenylyl cyclase, may be subsequently dampened by a later response to the same hormone that activates phosphodiesterase. Likewise, in some situations, cAMP and protein kinase A products can inhibit the activity of the phospholipid messenger system by decreasing the generation of diacylglycerols. Thus, an early stimulation of cell processes by hormone action through protein kinase C may later be dampened by hormone action through protein

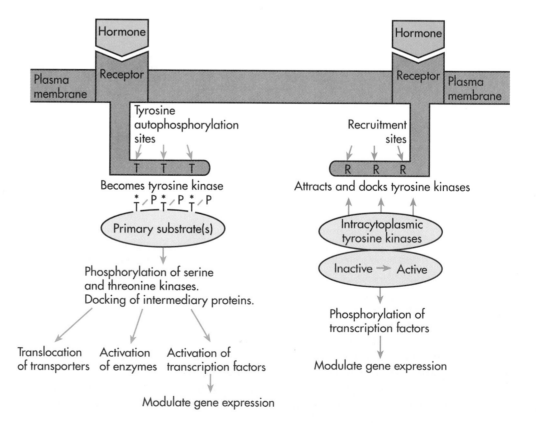

■ **Fig. 39-16** Mechanism of hormone action via tyrosine kinase activation. In one case, shown on the left, occupancy of a site on the extracellular portion of the receptor activates autophosphorylation of tyrosine residues in the intracellular tail of the receptor. This creates tyrosine kinase activity of the receptor itself. The receptor then phosphorylates multiple sites in an intracellular protein substrate, setting into motion a cascade of events leading to enzyme activations and gene transcriptions. In the case shown on the right, the intracellular tail of the receptor attracts and docks other nearby tyrosine kinases, which then phosphorylate cytoplasmic substrates such as transcription factor proteins, ultimately modulating gene expression.

kinase A. Finally, cAMP-activated phosphorylation of plasma membrane receptors themselves may decrease their affinity for hormones. This constitutes still another negative feedback mechanism for limiting the magnitude or duration of hormone action.

Intracellular Receptor Systems

An entirely different mechanism of signal transduction is characteristic of thyroid hormones, adrenal and gonadal steroid hormones, and vitamin D. In contrast to peptide and catecholamine hormones, these other hormones enter the cell and bind within minutes to receptors that usually are located in the nucleus. In some instances, receptors in the cytoplasm first bind to these hormones, and the complexes are transferred to the nucleus (Fig. 39-17). These receptors are large oligomeric proteins that are often phosphorylated. They are all coded for by an ancient superfamily of genes related to the *cis* oncogenes

Six subfamilies are currently recognized on the basis of structural similarities. One subfamily consists of receptors for thyroid hormone, retinoic acid, vitamin D, pregnane, and peroxisome proliferator activator receptors (PPAR). A second subfamily consists of glucocorticoid, progesterone, androgen, and estrogen receptors. A third subfamily contains receptors for retinoid X and hepatic nuclear factor-4. The other three subfamilies contain "orphan receptors," for which natural ligands have not yet been identified.

Figure 39-18 represents the typical structure of a nuclear receptor. The N-terminal A/B region has constitutive *ligand-independent* transactivating functions and is highly variable from receptor to receptor. The C region is the DNA-binding domain and it is quite conserved, with up to 50% homology among the receptors. The D region is a variable hinge region, which links the C and E/F regions in a manner that permits axial rotation of the DNA-binding domain around the ligand-binding domain. The C-terminal E/F region is the ligand-binding domain. The E region contains *ligand-dependent* transactivating functional sequences, and the F

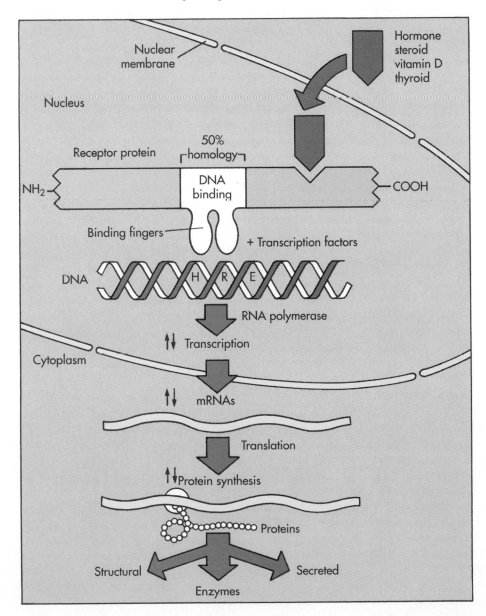

■ **Fig. 39-17**   Mechanism of action of vitamin D, steroid, and thyroid hormones. The hormone combines with the C-terminus of a specific intracellular receptor protein. The DNA-binding midportion of the receptor protein changes conformation permitting it to interact with a hormone regulatory element in target DNA molecules. Gene transcription and synthesis of protein products are thereby stimulated or repressed.

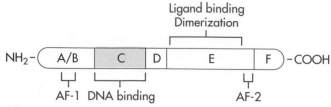

■ **Fig. 39-18** Schematic structure of a nuclear receptor that regulates gene expression. *N,* Amino terminus; *C,* carboxy terminus; *AF-1,* ligand-independent transactivating functional segment; *AF-2,* ligand-dependent transactivating functional segment. (From Aranda A, Pascual A: *Physiol Rev* 81:1269, 2001.)

region facilitates dimerization of the receptor. Either two identical receptor molecules form homodimers or two different receptor molecules form heterodimers. Retinoid X receptors are frequent and important partners in heterodimer formation. Serine, threonine, and tyrosine sites on nuclear receptors may be phosphorylated by MAP kinase. Such phosphorylations in the N-terminal region can modify function in the C-terminal region.

The hormone-binding domain of the receptor contains a specific pocket of variable size, into which the appropriate hormone or ligand fits. The DNA-binding domain consists of two zinc fingers or boxes, each containing one zinc atom bound by four cysteine residues. One box recognizes correct DNA targets and the other box forms a receptor dimerization surface. Hormone regulatory elements (HREs) of DNA molecules consist of 6 base pairs, usually in the 5′ flanking region of the gene, and relatively close to the TATA box core promoter. AGAACA and AGGTCA are consensus sequences for many receptors but there is also some variability. There can also be enhancer regions located several kilobases upstream from the transcription start site. Typically there are two HRE half sites, configured as either palindromes, inverted palindromes, or direct repeats, which bind a receptor homodimer or heterodimer. The spacing between the two zinc fingers may vary from 0 to 5 base pairs, and the spacing can confer selectivity. An unoccupied receptor bound to a target DNA molecule may repress gene transcription constitutively. Hormone binding may relieve this repression, and thus activate the gene.

In addition to transactivation of gene expression, transrepression can also occur by several mechanisms. An unoccupied receptor may constitutively transactivate a gene and hormone binding to the receptor may inhibit the transactivation. A hormone-bound receptor may compete with a transactivator and passively inhibit the transactivation, or it may form a heterodimer with a transactivating receptor resulting in loss of transactivating function. Coactivator and corepressor proteins also exist. A corepressor may interact with an unoccupied receptor at the HRE site and thereby silence that gene's expression. Occupation of the receptor by its hormone or by another ligand may disrupt the interaction with the corepressor and thus permit DNA replication to begin.

Within nuclei, *nucleosomes* that contain *histones* interact with chromatin and prevent its DNA from being transcribed.

Acetylation of lysine residues in the histones releases transcriptional activity in the impeded genes, whereas deacetylation or hypoacetylation increases the impedance to gene transcription. Some coactivators are histone-acetylating enzymes, whereas some corepressors are histone-deacetylating enzymes or cofactors, respectively, for these opposing enzyme activities. Hormones and other ligands can activate gene transcription by augmenting histone acetylation or by decreasing histone deacetylation, and thereby loosen target DNA bonds to nucleosome histones.

> The rapidly expanding knowledge of the regulation of gene expression by hormones and other ligands has widened our vistas for understanding the pathogenesis and treatment of many disorders. Mutant genes for nuclear receptors, coactivators, corepressors, and histone acetylators may explain certain classic genetic diseases, the susceptibility to or protection from cancers (e.g., breast cancer), the liability to atherosclerosis, the responsiveness or resistance to hormone or drug actions, and even the familial proclivity to longer or shorter life spans.

In addition to these direct effects of hormone receptors of the steroid, thyroid, and vitamin D classes on specific target genes, another important mechanism of hormone action involves the protooncogenes, *c-Jun* and *c-Fos.* These two peptides form a heterodimer known as AP-1 (activating protein-1), which has its own cognate regulatory site on numerous DNA molecules. Nuclear hormone-receptor complexes can interact with AP-1 bound to genes, and thereby stimulate or repress their transcription. The unoccupied or hormone-complexed receptor may also interact with c-Jun or c-Fos molecules individually. In this manner, the proliferation of target cells can be turned on or off by this class of hormones. Finally, steroid and similar hormones can also produce cascade effects within the cell. The gene that expresses a regulatory protein or a transcription factor, such as c-Jun or c-Fos, can itself be activated rapidly by the hormone-receptor complex. This early product of hormone action can then facilitate subsequent activation of more specific target genes, as described above.

Once transactivated by hormone receptors, promoter nucleotide sequences in the DNA molecule initiate transcription at the start site of the specific gene message by RNA polymerase II. The resultant "immature" RNA or pre-mRNA then undergoes maturation to messenger RNA by capping, by excision of untranslated nucleotide sequences, or by splicing. Translation of the RNA message in the cytoplasm results in synthesis of specific target proteins of the hormone.

The magnitude of gene transcriptional effects of these hormones depends on several factors: (1) the intracellular concentration of active hormone molecules, which may require conversion of a hormone precursor to the active molecule in situ; (2) the concentration and affinity of hormone receptor molecules and transcription factors; (3) the concentrations of other necessary factors, such as RNA polymerase, the enzymes of protein synthesis or processing, of transfer RNA, and of amino acid substrates; and (4) the stage of the cell cycle.

The specificity of these hormone effects on target cells depends on (1) the presence of target genes that have not been "closed" during differentiation of the cell; (2) the presence of hormone receptors, some of which exist as isoforms specific to certain cells; and (3) the presence of cell-specific transcription factors, coactivators, or corepressors in the nucleus. Although each hormone has its own subset of target genes, the nuclear actions of two different hormones can overlap.

The importance of the nuclear effects of steroid and thyroid hormone is illustrated by the fact that each regulates about 1% of all the genes expressed by some cells. Proteins whose synthesis is regulated up or down by these hormones may be enzymes, structural proteins, receptor proteins, transcriptional proteins that will regulate the expression of other genes, or proteins that are exported by the cell. By this hormone mechanism, enzymes are either induced or repressed rather than rapidly activated or inactivated. Response of metabolic pathways can either be accelerated or retarded. Other consequences of hormone action include alterations in excision and splicing of the primary RNA product, in the turnover of messenger RNA molecules, or in posttranslational modification of proteins. The transcription mechanism of steroid and thyroid hormones explains why hours are usually required for many of their biological effects to become evident or to disappear.

NONGENOMIC STEROID ACTIONS

Evidence exists and is growing for actions of steroid and thyroid hormones and vitamin D that are nongenomic and do not require protein synthesis. These actions are not blocked by inhibitors of gene expression or protein synthesis, and they can be demonstrated within 1 to 2 minutes of exposure to the hormone. Although binding sites on plasma membranes have been detected, no plasma membrane receptors have been cloned as yet. Involvement of G-proteins in these rapid actions is suspected. Examples of probable nongenomic actions by estrodiol, progesterone, aldosterone, cortisol, and vitamin D will be detailed in later sections.

Prostanoids

Prostanoids, also known as prostaglandins (PGs), are physiologically important hormone-like signaling molecules. They are produced in a variety of cells and tissues throughout the body, rather than in an exclusive endocrine organ. Although prostanoids are released from their cells of origin immediately after synthesis, and they can gain access to the bloodstream, their chemical instability and rapid metabolism limit prostanoids' actions to neighboring cells at the sites of release. Thus, the prostanoids function almost exclusively as paracrine hormones. Actions of special importance are to increase contraction or relaxation of specific smooth muscles (e.g., in the uterus during labor or in blood vessels), to

modulate neurotransmitter release, to sensitize sensory nerve fibers to pain stimuli, to generate fever, to facilitate immune responses, and to induce sleep. They also help regulate gastrointestinal motility and the transport of ions by renal tubules. They are involved in cell differentiation, apoptosis (programmed cell death), oncogenesis, and platelet activity.

PGs are synthesized from unsaturated fatty acids, predominantly from arachidonic acid in humans. PGs form a series labeled "2," because the fatty acids have two double bonds in their side chains (Fig. 39-19). PGs A, B, and C probably do not occur naturally; hence, only subtypes of D through I are represented above. Phospholipase A_2 is the enzyme that releases arachidonic acid from membrane phospholipids, and cyclooxygenase converts the arachidonic acid to the precursor prostaglandin, PGG_2. Both of these enzymes are targets for inhibitory drugs that are used to reduce fever, pain, and other aspects of inflammation in numerous diseases. Such pharmacological agents include glucocorticoids, such as prednisone (Chapter 45), aspirin, and many so called nonsteroidal antiinflammatory drugs, such as ibuprophen and "cox 2 inhibitors," such as rofecoxib or celecoxib.

PGs act through plasma membrane rhodopsin-type receptors that have seven transmembrane segments (Fig. 39-11) and that are coupled to G-proteins. PGE_2 and PGI_2 are the most important prostaglandins involved in the inflammatory reaction and in sensitization to pain. PGI_2 is an abundant product of endothelial cells that causes vasodilation, whereas thromboxane A_2 causes vasoconstriction. Likewise, PGI_2 inhibits, whereas thromboxane A_2 stimulates, platelet activity and aggregation. The balance between these two prostanoids facilitates vascular stability and maintains blood flow by preventing undue vasospasm and thrombosis. The balance is flexible enough to allow essential hemostatic functions to be carried out when bleeding seriously threatens the individual's life or well-being.

Vasodilator PGs such as PGE_1 are responsible for keeping the ductus arteriosus (Chapter 23) open in fetal life, thereby shunting venous blood to the heart without passing through the nonoxygenating lungs. Withdrawal of vasodilating PG effects causes closure of the ductus arteriosus right after birth, permitting respiration to deliver oxygen by passage of blood through the now functional lungs. The critical role of PGs in female reproduction is detailed in Chapter 46.

Endocrine Cell and Target Cell Turnover

Hormone actions often include alterations in target cell size and number. Moreover, endocrine diseases associated with excess or deficiency of a particular hormone usually involve accompanying gain or loss in mass of that hormone's cell of origin. Thus endocrine interest in the regulation of cell turnover has increased sharply, justifying a brief review of the most important aspects of that process. Cells in a static phase enter into and proceed through mitosis and the subsequent growth of daughter cells in a regular fashion, but at variable rates. Endocrine cells can respond to various growth factors that arrive from the circulation or are generated in situ, often under the influence of pituitary *trophic*

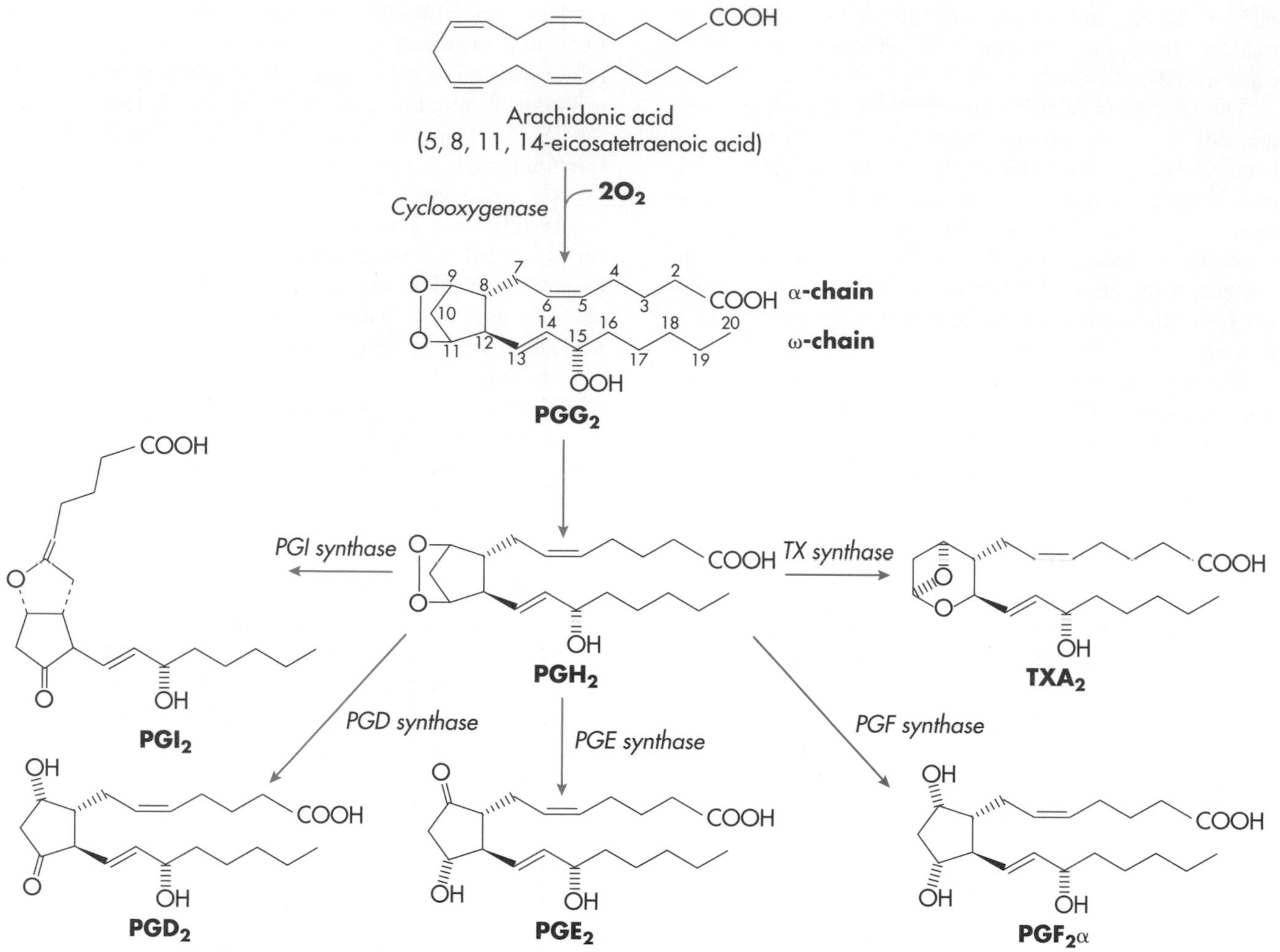

■ **Fig. 39-19**   The structures and synthesis of prostanoids (prostaglandins), which are paracrine acting hormone-like molecules (From Narumiya S et al: *Physiol Rev* 79:1193, 1999.)

hormone action on their respective target thyroid, adrenal, and gonadal glands.

A series of *cyclins* is specifically induced when a cell is stimulated by external factors to leave the quiescent G_0 phase, enter the G_1 phase, and subsequently pass through the S, M, and G_2 phases. At key points, various cyclins activate cyclin-dependent protein kinases, which phosphorylate key proteins required for DNA synthesis and mitosis. Various steps in this sequence are subject to hormonal regulation by induction of the expression of cyclin genes. In addition, protooncogenes such as *c-Fos* and *c-Jun,* as well as the growth suppressor gene *p53,* are present in endocrine cells.

At the other end of a cell's life cycle, programmed cell death (apoptosis) occurs, initiated by binding of the *fas ligand* to the *fas receptor* on a target cell's plasma membrane. As a consequence, a series of actions is stimulated that involves *capsaces,* which are cysteine proteases that cleave cytoskeletal proteins. Capsaces also activate endonucleases, which fragment DNA molecules into segments that are 185 base pairs long. The enzymes of DNA repair are simultaneously inhibited. Shrinkage and condensation of the cytoplasm, the appearance of dense pyknotic chromatin, and "budding" of plasma cell membranes resembling pseudopods

are easily visible signs of apoptosis. Each of these many steps in apoptosis is also a target for action of various hormones.

Thus the number of target cells (including other endocrine cells) can be increased by a hormone that stimulates movement through key points of the mitotic cycle, or by a hormone that inhibits apoptosis. Target cell number can be decreased by the opposite actions.

RESPONSIVITY TO HORMONES

The final outcome of the interaction of any hormone with its target cells depends on a number of factors. These include hormone concentration, receptor number, duration of exposure, intervals between consecutive exposures, intracellular conditions such as concentrations of rate-limiting enzymes, cofactors or substrates, and the concurrent effects of antagonistic or synergistic hormones. Hormonal effects are not "all or none" phenomena. The dose-response curve for the action of a hormone is generally complex and often exhibits a sigmoidal shape (Fig. 39-20, *A*). An intrinsic basal level of activity may be observed independent of added hormone and long after any previous exposure. A certain minimal threshold concentration of hormone is required to elicit a measurable response. *The effect that is obtained at saturating doses of hormone defines the maximal responsiveness of the target cell. The concentration of hormone required to elicit a half-maximal response is an index of the sensitivity of the target cell.*

Alterations in the dose-response curve in vivo can take two general forms (Fig. 39-20, *B*). (1) A decrease in maximal responsiveness could be caused by a decrease in the number of functional target cells, in the total number of receptors per cell, in the concentration of an enzyme being activated by the hormone, or in the concentration of a precursor essential to the final product of hormone action. The diminished responsiveness could also be caused by an increase in the concentration of a *noncompetitive* inhibitor. (2) A decrease in hormone sensitivity could be caused by a decrease in the number or affinity of hormone receptors, alterations in the concentration of modulating cofactors, an increase in the rate of hormone degradation, or increases in antagonistic hormones. The diminished sensitivity can also be caused by an increase in the concentration of a *competitive* inhibitor.

The normal human population range of responsiveness to a hormone is usually broad, and it is partly a result of the physiological variability created by the aforementioned factors within and among normal individuals. However, the exquisiteness with which hormonal effects can be modulated in an individual is an important component in achieving one major objective of hormonal regulation: metabolic stability.

Obesity is a good example of a condition in which sensitivity to a hormone, insulin, is considerably diminished. Moreover, in **type 2 diabetes** (non–insulin-dependent diabetes), both sensitivity and maximal responsiveness to insulin are reduced, and this plays a major role in causing high plasma glucose levels.

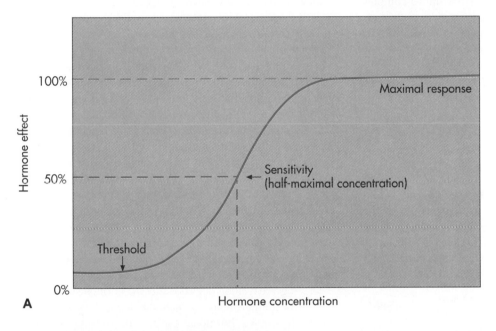

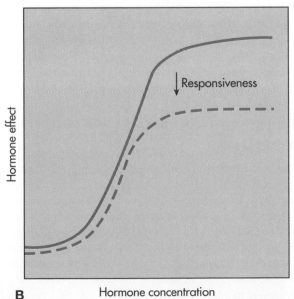

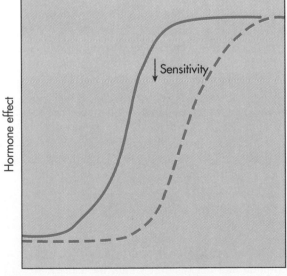

■ **Fig. 39-20** **A,** The general shape of a hormone dose-response curve. Sensitivity is most often expressed as the concentration of the hormone that produces a half-maximal response. **B,** Alterations in the dose-response curve can take the form of a change in maximal responsiveness *(left panel),* a change in sensitivity *(right panel),* or both.

HORMONE TRANSPORT

After secretion, hormones enter pools characterized by widely varying size, volume of distribution, degree of compartmentalization, and fractional turnover rates. Hormones that enter the plasma pool may circulate either as free molecules or bound to specific carrier proteins. Catecholamines and most peptide and protein hormones circulate unbound. In contrast, steroid and thyroid hormones and vitamin D circulate bound to specific globulins that are synthesized in the liver. The extent of protein binding markedly influences the exit rates of hormones from plasma into interstitial fluid, and hence to target cells. As noted in Table 39-1, the plasma half-life of a hormone is directly correlated with the percentage of protein binding. For example, thyroxine is 99.95% protein bound, and it has a plasma half-life of 6 days, whereas aldosterone is only 15% bound and has a plasma half-life of 25 minutes. Larger and more complex protein hormones tend to have longer half-lives than do smaller proteins and peptides. Hormone exit from plasma need not be entirely irreversible. In some instances hormone molecules may return to plasma from other compartments, possibly after dissociation from cell membrane receptors. The return to plasma can occur by way of the lymphatic channels.

HORMONE DISPOSAL

Irreversible removal of hormone is a result of target cell uptake, metabolic degradation, and urinary or biliary excretion. The sum of all removal processes is expressed by the term **metabolic clearance rate (MCR).** In a steady state, this is defined as the volume of plasma cleared/unit time, which equals mass removed/unit time divided by circulating mass/unit volume, that is,

$$MCR = \frac{mg/minute \ removed}{mg/ml \ of \ plasma} = \frac{ml \ cleared}{minute} \qquad (39\text{-}8)$$

MCR is one expression of the efficiency with which a hormone is removed from plasma. The ratio of MCR to the volume of distribution of a hormone is a measure of its fractional turnover rate (K). The plasma half-life, which is inversely related to K, is a cruder but more conveniently determined index of hormone disappearance. As shown in Table 39-1, MCR is inversely correlated with plasma half-life.

The kidney and liver are the major sites of hormone extraction and degradation. Renal clearance of hormone is reduced greatly by protein binding in the plasma, for example, less than 1% of secreted cortisol appears unchanged in the urine, because only the small, free fraction of plasma cortisol is filtered by the glomerulus. On the other hand, about 30% of cortisol metabolites are excreted in the urine, because they are generally unbound or only loosely bound to protein. Peptide and smaller protein hormones are filtered to some degree by the glomerulus. However, they may subsequently undergo tubular reabsorption and degradation within the kidney, so that only a small fraction appears in the final urine.

Metabolic degradation occurs by enzymatic processes that include proteolysis, oxidation, reduction, hydroxylation, decarboxylation, and methylation. Virtually all hormones are extracted from the plasma and are degraded to some extent by the liver. In addition, glucuronidation and sulfation of hormones or their metabolites may be carried out, and the conjugates are subsequently excreted in the bile or the urine. Some hormonal degradation appears to take place during interaction with target tissues. As noted previously, a portion of the hormone–plasma membrane receptor complex does internalize, and hormone may be degraded within the target cell. Hormone action and hormone degradation may be quantitatively linked in these situations.

HORMONE MEASUREMENT

The most common and useful method for measuring hormones is by immunoassay. Monoclonal antibodies can be raised that react with protein and peptide hormones, as well as with steroid, thyroid, and vitamin D molecules, after they are chemically conjugated to a protein such as albumin. These antibodies react with the respective hormones at concentrations in the picomolar range, and various techniques, including radioactive labeling, enzyme reactions and chemiluminescence, are used to quantitate the results. Immunoassays can usually be made sensitive enough to detect low plasma hormone levels, and specific enough to distinguish plasma hormones from circulating precursor molecules and products of hormone metabolism. However, very sensitive biological assays may also be required to obtain correct physiological or diagnostic information. The bioactivity of protein hormones may vary with the degree of their glycosylation and at different physiological times. For example, an immunoassay of a particular pituitary hormone may show little change in molecular concentration at some point during the menstrual cycle because glycosylation does not alter the hormone epitope with which the immunoassay antibody is reacting. Nevertheless, the concentration of hormone capable of exerting biological effects is, in fact, different. Another example is seen in diseases in which a mutant hormone is secreted, one that has low biological activity, but that retains the critical antigenic sequence. An immunoassay would show normal or even high plasma levels (from negative feedback) of the hormone, when there is actually a deficiency of hormone actions on target tissues.

ESTIMATES OF HORMONE SECRETION
Secretion Rate

Absolute quantitation of the output of a single hormone by an individual gland can be accomplished in vivo only by catheterization of the blood supply to the gland. The arterial (A) and venous (V) concentrations of hormone, in mass per unit volume, and the blood flow (BF) across the gland, in volume per unit time, must be measured. The rate of secretion in mass per unit time is then $(V - A) \times BF$. This method for assessing secretion rate is suitable for animal studies, but is not applicable to clinical circumstances.

Sampling of veins that drain glands can be used diagnostically to localize the source of excess hormone production. This is true for multiple glands, such as the parathyroid glands, or for hormones, such as steroids, that may be secreted from either the adrenal glands or the gonads. A microtumor that secretes excess amounts of a hormone may exist within the already small pituitary gland. Its presence can be identified, and it can be localized to the correct side of the gland by sampling blood from veins draining the right and left sides, respectively. This procedure is helpful in cases in which radiological methods cannot detect such a small tumor.

Production Rate

A less direct, but frequently satisfactory, method to estimate hormone secretion in physiological investigations is the measurement of the production rate (PR), in mass per unit time. This is the total amount of the hormone entering the peripheral circulation per unit time; in a steady state it will equal the total amount of hormone leaving the circulation. Therefore, production rate is determined by measuring plasma concentration (P) and the MCR:

$$PR = P \times MCR \qquad (39\text{-}9)$$

Plasma Levels

A simple plasma concentration provides a valid index of hormone production rate when the metabolic clearance of the hormone is within normal limits and it can be taken as a constant; since $PR = P \times MCR$, PR is proportional to P if MCR is taken to be a constant. This is the theoretical basis for employing plasma hormone measurements alone as an index of activity of the gland of origin. However, the release of many hormones is characterized by episodic spurts and diurnal variation. In such cases it may be hazardous to conclude too much from a single plasma value, and multiple measurements, taken at different times of the day, may be needed.

Urinary Excretion

Measurement of urinary hormone excretion is cumbersome, because it requires accurately timed collections. However, it offers the advantage of, in effect, averaging plasma fluctuations over the collection period. Furthermore, the quantity of a hormone metabolite in the urine may exceed substantially the plasma or urinary level of the hormone itself, and it is therefore more easily measurable.

Urinary excretion of a hormone or a metabolite is a valid index of production rate (and hence secretion rate) when the following two conditions are fulfilled: (1) the kidney must contribute its usual fraction of the total metabolic clearance; and (2) within the kidney itself, the usual proportioning of hormone between intrarenal degradation and urinary excretion must be maintained. The chief sources of error in employing urinary excretion as a reflection of hormone secretion are general impairment in renal function, a change in the pattern of degradation to a metabolic product excreted differently by the kidney, and incomplete collections of urine. When hormone secretion or metabolism does not vary diurnally, incomplete or untimed collections can be compensated for by indexing the urinary hormone concentration to the urinary creatinine concentration in the sample.

SUMMARY

1. The function of the endocrine system is to regulate metabolism, fluid volume and content, growth, maturation, sexual development, senescence, and behavior. The endocrine and nervous systems work conjointly to maintain homeostasis.

2. Hormones are signaling molecules that are conveyed by the bloodstream (endocrine), by neural axons and the bloodstream (neurocrine), or by local diffusion (paracrine, autocrine).

3. Hormone molecules may be proteins, peptides, catecholamines, steroids, amino acid derivatives, or prostanoids.

4. Protein and peptide hormone synthesis involves gene transcription, primary mRNA splicing and excision, translation, and further processing of a primary gene product, called a prohormone. Such further processing includes proteolytic cleavage, glycosylation, and phosphorylation. Thyroid and steroid hormones, catecholamines, and prostanoids are synthesized from precursors by multiple enzyme reactions.

5. Peptide and protein hormones and catecholamines are stored in granules and secreted by exocytosis. Thyroid hormone is stored within protein molecules in large quantities; steroid hormones are not stored at all. Both are released by diffusion.

6. Proteins and peptides, catecholamines, and prostanoids act on target cells via specific protein receptors located in the plasma membranes. The hormone-receptor complexes transduce signals through second messengers. Stimulatory or inhibitory G-proteins often link the receptor to membrane mechanisms that generate cAMP, Ca^{2+}, diacylglycerols, and inositol trisphosphate. These molecules act intracellularly to increase or decrease enzyme activities. Other receptors activate tyrosine kinase sites that subsequently phosphorylate enzymes and other key molecules. All of these effects are rapid.

7. Thyroid and steroid hormones and vitamin D act by means of specific protein receptors located in the cell nucleus. The hormone-receptor complex interacts with promoter/ elements or inhibitory elements in DNA molecules, and with transcription factors to induce or repress expression of target genes. This leads to increases or decreases in the concentration of enzymes and other cell proteins. These effects are slower than those of hormones interacting with plasma membrane receptors.

8. The sensitivity of an organism to hormone action is expressed as the hormone concentration that produces half-maximum activity. The sensitivity can be influenced by changes in receptor number, affinity, hormone degradation rate, or competitive antagonists. The maximum effect produced

by saturating concentrations of hormone can be influenced by the number of target cells, receptor number, concentration of target enzymes, or noncompetitive antagonists.

9. Hormone secretion is measured directly by arterial-venous concentration gradients and flow rates across the gland. Clinically, plasma levels and urinary excretion rates are used as indirect indices of hormonal secretion rates. These indices are valid as long as metabolic or renal clearance of the hormone is normal.

BIBLIOGRAPHY

Journal articles

Alford FP et al: Temporal patterns of circulating hormones as assessed by continuous blood sampling, *J Clin Endocrinol Metab* 36:108, 1973.

Aranda A, Pascual A: Nuclear hormone receptors and gene expression, *Physiol Rev* 81:1269, 2001.

Birnbaumer L et al: Molecular basis of regulation of ionic channels by G proteins, *Rec Prog Horm Res* 45:121, 1989.

Carson-Jurica MA et al: Steroid receptor family: structure and function, *Endocr Rev* 11:201, 1990.

Chen JD: Steroid/nuclear receptor coactivators, *Vit Horm* 58:391, 2000.

Christ M et al: Nongenomic steroid actions: fact or fantasy? *Vit Horm* 57:325, 1999.

Combarnous Y: Molecular basis of the specificity of binding of glycoprotein hormones to their receptors, *Endocr Rev,* 13:670, 1992.

Czeisler CA, Klerman EB: Circadian and sleep-dependent regulation of hormone release in humans, *Rec Prog Horm Res* 54:97, 1999.

Freedman LP: Anatomy of the steroid receptor zinc finger region, *Endocr Rev,* 13:129, 1992.

Gether U: Uncovering molecular mechanisms involved in activation of G protein-coupled receptors, *Endocr Rev,* 21:90, 2000.

Gillette MU, Tischkau SA: Suprachiasmatic nucleus: the brain's circadian clock, *Rec Prog Horm Res,* 54:33, 1999.

Glass CK: Differential recognition of target genes by nuclear receptor monomers, dimers, and heterodimers, *Endocr Rev,* 15:391, 1994.

Gordon P et al: Internalization of polypeptide hormones: mechanism, intracellular localization and significance, *Diabetologia* 18:263, 1980.

Inagami T, Naruse M, Hoover R: Endothelium as an endocrine organ, *Annu Rev Physiol,* 57:171, 1995.

Klein DC et al: The melatonin rhythm-generating enzyme: molecular regulation of serotonin *N*-acetyltransferase in the pineal gland, *Rec Prog Horm Res,* 52:307, 1997.

Lacy PE: Beta cell secretion—from the standpoint of a pathobiologist, *Diabetes* 19:895, 1970.

Lefkowitz R et al: Mechanisms of membrane-receptor regulation: biochemical, physiological, and clinical insights derived from studies of the adrenergic receptors, *N Engl J Med* 310:1570, 1984.

Lou H, Gagel RF: Alternative ribonucleic acid processing in endocrine systems, *Endocr Rev* 22:205, 2001.

Morris AJ, Malbon CC: Physiological regulation of G protein-linked signaling, *Physiol Rev* 79:1373, 1999.

Mountz JD et al: Apoptosis and cell death in the endocrine system, *Rec Prog Horm Res,* 54:235, 1999.

Nagata S: Apoptosis by death factor, *Cell,* 88:355, 1997.

Narumiya S, Sugimoto Y, Ushikubi F: Prostanoid receptors: structures, properties, and functions, *Physiol Rev,* 79:1193, 1999.

Nurse P: Ordering S phase and M phase in the cell cycle, *Cell* 79:547, 1994.

Pearson G et al: Mitogen-activated protein (MAP) kinase pathways: regulation and physiological functions, *Endoc Rev* 22:153, 2001.

Ralff CJ, Kushner PJ, Baxter JD: The nuclear hormone receptor gene superfamily, *Annu Rev Med* 46:443, 1995.

Sehgal A et al: What makes the circadian clock tick: genes that keep time? *Rec Prog Horm Res* 54:61, 1999.

Sherr CJ: Mammalian G_1 cyclins, *Cell* 73:1059, 1993.

Sherwin RS et al: A model of the kinetics of insulin in man, *J Clin Invest* 53:1481, 1974.

Spiegel AM: Guanine nucleotide binding protein and signal transduction, *Vit Horm* 44:47, 1988.

Spiegel AM, Shenker A, Weinstein LS: Receptor-effector coupling by G proteins: implications for normal and abnormal signal transduction, *Endocr Rev* 13:536, 1992.

Tait JF: The use of isotopic steroids for the measurement of production rates in vivo, *J Clin Endocrinol* 23:1285, 1963.

Thompson CB: Apoptosis in the pathogenesis and treatment of disease, *Science* 267:1456, 1995.

Wedel BJ, Garbers DL: The guanylyl cyclase family at Y2K, *Annu Rev Physiol* 63:215, 2001.

Wittenderby PA, Li PK: Melatonin receptors and ligands, *Vit Horm* 58:321, 2000.

Young MW: Molecular control of circadian behavioral rhythms, *Rec Prog Horm Res* 54:87, 1999.

Zor U: Role of Cytoskeletal organization in the regulation of adenylate cyclase-cyclic adenosine monophosphate by hormones, *Endocr Rev* 4:1, 1984.

Books and monographs

Arendt J: The pineal gland: basic physiology and clinical implications. In LJ, editor: *Endocrinology 1,* ed 4, Philadelphia, 2001, WB Saunders.

Baulieu EE, Mester J, Redeuilh G: Nuclear receptor superfamily. In DeGroot LJ, Jameson LJ, editors: *Endocrinology,* ed 4, Philadelphia, 2001, WB Saunders.

Gershengorn MC, Hinkle PM: Second messenger signaling pathways: phospholipids and calcium. In DeGroot LJ, Jameson JL, editors: *Endocrinology,* ed 4, Philadelphia, 2001 WB Saunders.

Habener JF: Genetic control of hormone formation. In Wilson JD et al, editors: *Williams textbook of endocrinology,* ed 9, Philadelphia, 1998, WB Saunders.

Habener JF: The cyclic AMP second messenger signaling pathway. In DeGroot LJ, and Jameson JL, editors: *Endocrinology,* ed 4, Philadelphia, 2001, WB Saunders.

Jameson JL: Applications of molecular biology and genetics in endocrinology. In DeGroot LJ, Jameson JL, editors: *Endocrinology,* ed 4, Philadelphia, 2001, WB Saunders.

Kahn CR, Smith RJ, Chin WW: Mechanism of action of hormones that act at the cell surface. In Wilson JD et al, editors: *Williams textbook of endocrinology,* ed 9, Philadelphia, 1998, WB Saunders.

Quirk CC, Nilson JH: Hormones and gene expression basic principals. In DeGroot LJ, Jameson JL, editors: *Endocrinology,* ed 4, Philadelphia, 2001, WB Saunders.

Shenker A: Hormone signaling via G protein-coupled receptors. In DeGroot LJ, Jameson JL, editors: *Endocrinology,* cd 4, Philadelphia, 2001, WB Saunders.

Tsai MJ et al: Mechanisms of action of hormones that act as transcription-regulatory factors. In Wilson JD et al, editors: *Williams textbook of endocrinology,* ed 9, Philadelphia, 1998, WB Saunders.

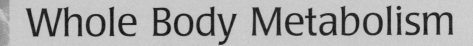

chapter forty

Whole Body Metabolism

Metabolism may be broadly defined as the sum of all the chemical processes involved in (1) producing energy from exogenous and endogenous sources, (2) synthesizing and degrading structural and functional tissue components, and (3) disposing of resultant waste products. Regulating the rate and direction of many basic aspects of metabolism is one of the major functions of the endocrine system. Therefore, a firm grasp of the fundamentals of metabolism is essential to understand the important influence of hormones on body functions.

ENERGY METABOLISM

Balance

The laws of thermodynamics require that overall energy balance be constantly maintained in living organisms when they are at a stable weight. However, energy may be obtained in various forms, may be stored in other forms, and may be expended in many different ways. Therefore, numerous interconversions of chemical, mechanical, and thermal energy are possible within the basic rule that *in the steady state, energy input must always equal energy output.* Figure 40-1 illustrates this overall flow of energy through the human organism.

Energy Input

Energy input consists of food. Of ingested calories 90% to 95% are available for oxidation or storage; the small remainder is lost in the stool or in urinary excretion of metabolic products. Foodstuffs are classified into three major chemical categories: carbohydrate, fat, and protein. The complete combustion of each chemical type yields characteristic amounts of energy, expressed as joules or kilocalories per gram (1 kcal = 4184 joules). Combustion requires characteristic amounts of oxygen, depending on the proportions of carbon, hydrogen, and oxygen in the substance. However, for each class of foodstuff, the energy yield per liter of oxygen used is quite similar, because the ratio of carbon to hydrogen atoms is also similar in each class (Table 40-1). Within the body the carbon skeletons of carbohydrate and protein can be converted to fat, and their potential energy can be stored

more efficiently in that manner. The carbon skeletons of protein can be converted to carbohydrate when that energy source is specifically needed. However, there is no significant conversion of carbon skeletons from fat to carbohydrate.

Energy Output

Energy output can be divided into several distinct and measurable components.

1. At rest, energy is expended (a) in a myriad of synthetic and degradative chemical reactions; (b) in generating and maintaining gradients of ions and other molecules across cell and organelle membranes; (c) in the creation and conduction of signals, particularly in the nervous system; (d) in the mechanical work of respiration and circulation of the blood; and (e) in obligate heat loss to the environment. This absolute minimal energy expenditure is called the **basal** or **resting metabolic rate** (**BMR** or **RMR**). In the adult human, BMR amounts to an average daily expenditure of 20 to 25 kcal (84 to 105 kjoules)/kg body weight (or 1.0 to 1.2 kcal/min), and it requires the use of approximately 200 to 250 ml oxygen/min. About 40% of the BMR is accounted for by the central nervous system and 20% to 30% by the skeletal muscle mass. Of the interindividual variance in BMR 80% is accounted for by fat-free mass, fat mass, age, and gender. The BMR is linearly related to lean body mass and to body surface area. It declines in the elderly, partly because lean body mass declines with age. Women have slightly lower BMRs than do men. Studies in identical twins and families suggest that some of the remaining variation in BMR is genetically determined. During sleep, BMR falls 10% to 15%. BMR is increased by raising environmental temperature.

During a febrile illness, BMR also increases because a high body temperature accelerates enzyme-catalyzed reactions. The increase in BMR entails an increase in respiratory rate to supply the needed oxygen and to dispose of extra carbon dioxide. An increase in caloric intake is also required to prevent weight loss if the illness is prolonged.

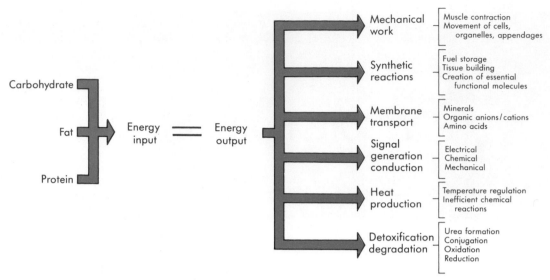

■ **Fig. 40-1**   Overview of energy balance. In a steady state, input as caloric equivalents of food equals output as caloric equivalents of various forms of mechanical and chemical work and heat.

■ **Table 40-1**   Energy equivalents of foodstuffs

	Kilocalories produced per gram	*O_2 used (L/g)*	*Kilocalories produced per liter of O_2*	*Respiratory quotient*
Carbohydrate	4.2	0.84	5.0	1.00
Fat	9.4	2.00	4.7	0.70
Protein	4.3*	0.96*	4.5	0.80
Typical fuel mix	—	—	4.8	0.85

* Each gram of protein oxidized yields 0.16 g of urinary nitrogen. Thus, these values should be multiplied by 6.25 to express them per gram of urinary nitrogen.

2. Ingestion of food causes a small obligate increase in energy expenditure, referred to as **diet-induced thermogenesis.** This is partly explained by the cost of digestion and the increased rate of reactions involved in the disposition of the ingested calories, such as storage of glucose in the large molecule, glycogen, or as degradation of amino acids to urea.

3. **Nonshivering thermogenesis** refers to energy expended for the purpose of producing heat: in an *obligatory* manner to maintain a constant thermoneutral state, or in a *facultative* manner when an individual is acutely exposed to cold. All tissues contribute to the obligatory thermogenic process. Such energy expenditure may also be evoked and may increase to compensate for prolonged exposure to caloric excess, as a means of limiting weight gain.

4. Energy is also expended by sedentary individuals in spontaneous physical activity, such as "fidgeting," at least some of which is unconscious and seemingly purposeless.

5. The additional energy expended in occupational labor and purposeful exercise (Table 40-2) varies greatly among individuals, as well as from day to day and from season to season. This component generates the greatest need for variation in daily caloric intake and underscores

the importance of energy stores to buffer temporary discrepancies between energy output and intake.

Of a total average daily expenditure of 2300 kcal (9700 kjoules) in a sedentary adult, basal metabolism accounts for 60% to 70%, dietary and obligatory thermogenesis for 5% to 15%, and spontaneous physical activity for 20% to 30%. As much as an additional 4000 kcal may be used in daily physical work. During short periods of occupational or recreational exercise, energy expenditure can increase more than tenfold over basal levels.

ENERGY GENERATION

The basic chemical currency of energy in all living cells consists of the two high-energy phosphate bonds contained in **adenosine triphosphate (ATP).** To a much lesser extent, other purine and pyrimidine nucleotides (guanosine triphosphate, cytosine triphosphate, uridine triphosphate, and inosine triphosphate) also serve as energy sources after the energy from ATP is transferred to them. In muscle, creatine phosphate is a high-energy-containing molecule of particular importance.

The two terminal P–O bonds of ATP each contains about 12 kcal of potential energy per mole under physiological conditions. These P–O bonds are in constant flux. They are

■ **Table 40-2** Estimates of energy expenditure in adults

Activity	Calorie expenditure (kcal/min)
Basal	1.1
Sitting	1.8
Walking, 2.5 miles/hr	4.3
Walking, 4.0 miles/hr	8.2
Climbing stairs	9.0
Swimming	10.9
Bicycling, 13 miles/hr	11.1
Household domestic work	2–4.5
Factory work	2–6
Farming	4–6
Building trades	4–9

Data from Kottke FJ: Animal energy exchange. In Altman PL, editor: *Metabolism,* Bethesda, Md, 1968, Federation of American Society for Experimental Biology.

generated by oxidative reactions and are consumed as the energy is either (1) transferred into other high-energy bonds involved in synthetic reactions (e.g., amino acid + ATP → amino acyl AMP), (2) expended in creating lower-energy phosphorylated metabolic intermediates (e.g., glucose + ATP → glucose-6-phosphate), or (3) converted to mechanical work (e.g., propulsion of spermatozoa). Because the production and transfer of energy are only 65% efficient, about 18 kcal of oxidative substrate is required to generate each terminal P–O bond of ATP. At any moment, the total body content of ATP would suffice for a little more than 1 minute of energy use. In a normal day when 2300 kcal is turned over, about 128 mol, or 63 kg, of ATP (a mass approximating body weight) is generated and expended. An overview of energy production with the generation of ATP from the major substrates is shown in Fig. 40-2.

The combustion of carbohydrates (chiefly glucose, with lesser amounts of fructose and galactose) includes two major phases:

1. During the cytoplasmic anaerobic phase, known as **glycolysis** (Embden-Meyerhof pathway), each partially oxidized glucose molecule has yielded two molecules of pyruvate, but only 8% of its energy content. Glycolysis can serve as a sole source of energy only briefly, because (a) the body supply of glucose is limited, and (b) the accumulated pyruvate must be syphoned off by reduction to lactate, a metabolite that in excess is noxious.

2. During the mitochondrial aerobic phase, the two pyruvate molecules are oxidized to CO_2 by the **citric acid cycle (Krebs cycle),** and the remaining energy is liberated. In this pathway, acetyl-coenzyme A (acetyl-CoA), initially formed by oxidative decarboxylation of pyruvate, is condensed with oxaloacetate to form citrate. Through a cyclic series of reactions, the acetyl carbons of acetyl-CoA appear as CO_2, and oxaloacetate is regenerated.

The combustion of fatty acids, the major energy component of fats, begins with their activation in the cytoplasm to CoA derivatives, e.g., palmitoyl-CoA. To enter the mitochondria, palmitoyl-CoA must first be converted to palmitoyl-carnitine by the outer mitochondrial membrane enzyme,

carnitine palmitoyltransferase (CPT-1). After traversing the membrane, the palmitoyl-carnitine is reconverted to palmitoyl-CoA in the inner mitochondrial membrane by CPT-2. The palmitoyl-CoA is then oxidized within the mitochondria by a repetitive biochemical sequence known as β-oxidation. This process releases two carbons at a time as acetyl-CoA until the entire fatty acid molecule is broken down. The acetyl-CoA is disposed of by way of the citric acid cycle, as already described. A variable portion of fatty acid oxidation in the liver stops at the last four carbons and yields acetoacetic and β-hydroxybutyric acids. The production of these ketoacids results from an imbalance between the flow of fatty acids into the liver mitochondria and the capacity of the Krebs cycle to dispose of acetyl-CoA. The water-soluble ketoacids are normally released by the liver in small amounts, to be oxidized in other tissues as additional energy substrates.

> Accelerated production of ketoacids occurs when carbohydrate intake is low or when fasting is prolonged beyond the usual overnight period. **Ketosis** can produce severe metabolic acidosis in humans deprived of the key hormone, *insulin,* as in insulin-dependent or type 1 diabetes mellitus.

The combustion of protein first requires hydrolysis to its component amino acids. Each of these undergoes degradation by individual pathways, which ultimately leads to intermediate compounds of the citric acid cycle and then to acetyl-CoA and CO_2.

The combustion of all foodstuffs yields large numbers of hydrogen atoms. These hydrogens are oxidized to H_2O in the mitochondrion in linkage with the phosphorylation of adenosine diphosphate (ADP) to ATP (Fig. 40-2). In this process, three high-energy P–O bonds are formed for each atom of oxygen used. This yields an overall efficiency of 60% to 65% for the recovery of usable chemical energy.

Respiratory Quotient

In the process of oxidizing substrates to meet basal energy needs, the proportion of carbon dioxide produced (Vco_2) to oxygen used (Vo_2) varies according to the fuel mix. The ratio of Vco_2 to Vo_2 is known as the **respiratory quotient (RQ).** As indicated by the following equations, RQ equals 1.0 for oxidation of carbohydrate (e.g., glucose), whereas RQ equals 0.70 for oxidation of fat (e.g., palmitic acid). For carbohydrates:

$$C_6H_{12}O_6 + 6\ O_2 \rightarrow 6\ CO_2 + 6\ H_2O$$
Glucose

$$RQ = \frac{6\ CO_2}{6\ O_2} = 1.0 \qquad (40\text{-}1)$$

For fats:

$$C_{15}H_{31}COOH + 23\ O_2 \rightarrow 16\ CO_2 + 16\ H_2O$$
Palmitic acid

$$RQ = \frac{16\ CO_2}{23\ O_2} = 0.70 \qquad (40\text{-}2)$$

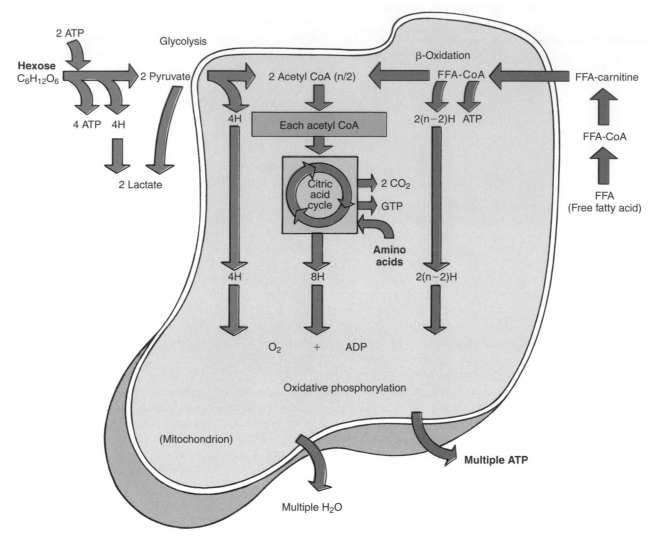

Fig. 40-2   An overview of energy production. Glycolysis and each turn of the citric acid cycle supply only two net ATP equivalents apiece. ATP is generated mainly when hydrogens removed from carbohydrate, fat, or protein substrates are oxidized in the mitochondria. *ATP,* Adenosine triphosphate; *ADP,* adenosine diphosphate; *GTP,* guanosine triphosphate.

The RQ for protein reflects that of the individual RQs of the amino acids, and it averages 0.80. Ordinarily, protein is a minor energy source. The small contribution of protein oxidation to the overall RQ can be corrected for by measuring the urinary excretion of the nitrogen that results from the metabolism of amino acids.

Determining the RQ corrected for protein allows the proportion of carbohydrate and fat in the fuel mix being oxidized to be calculated.

For example, when the O_2 consumed = 210 ml/min and the CO_2 produced = 174 ml/min:

$$RQ = \frac{174}{210} = 0.83$$

If C is the proportion of energy produced by carbohydrate oxidation and F is the remaining proportion of energy produced by fat oxidation, then

$$1 \times C + 0.7 \times F = 0.83$$

Since C + F = 1:

$$1 \times C + 0.7 \times (1 - C) = 0.83$$
$$C = 0.43$$
$$F = 0.57$$

That is, 43% of the calories are being provided by carbohydrate oxidation, and 57% of the calories are being provided by fat oxidation.

With a knowledge of the actual rate of energy expenditure in kilocalories per minute and the standard values of 4 kcal/g of carbohydrate and 9 kcal/g of fat, the actual rates of oxidation of carbohydrate and fat, respectively, in grams per minute can be calculated:

210 ml of O_2 consumed per minute = 1.05 kcal/min
4 × a gram of carbohydrate = 0.43 × 1.05

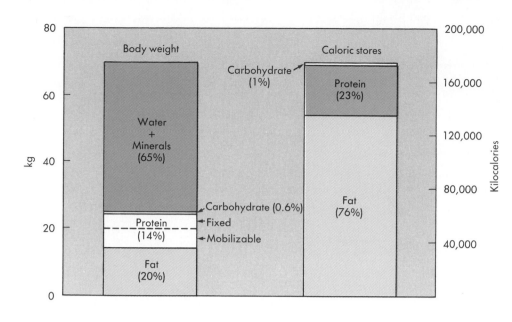

■ **Fig. 40-3**   The composition of an average 70-kg human shown in terms of weight *(left)* and caloric stores *(right)*. Note the trivial proportion of carbohydrate stores relative to fat stores.

Therefore, a gram of carbohydrate = 0.113/min

$$9 \times \text{a gram of fat} = 0.57 \times 1.05$$

Therefore, a gram of fat = 0.067/min

From the above considerations, the fuel mix can be altered advantageously to compensate for clinically impaired respiratory function. By increasing the proportion of fat, a lesser amount of CO_2 is produced for the same quantity of O_2 expended; that is, the demand on the individual's ventilation is reduced (see Chapter 29).

In the resting adult the rate of glucose oxidation is approximately 120 mg/min (170 g/day), whereas the rate of fat oxidation is approximately 60 mg/min (90 g/day). Thus in caloric equivalents glucose supplies about 45% of the energy required for basal metabolism. The central nervous system is an obligate glucose consumer, and it uses the major portion of this fuel. Estimates of cerebral glucose use are 125 to 150 g/day. In contrast, the large muscle mass oxidizes primarily fatty acids in resting individuals. However, like all tissues, the muscle mass uses at least some glucose, and thereby maintains sufficient concentrations of Krebs cycle intermediates for efficient disposal of acetyl-CoA and completion of fatty acid oxidation.

ENERGY STORAGE AND TRANSFERS

In humans, the intake of energy in the form of food is periodic. Neither the amount of calories per meal nor meal frequency exactly matches either the constant rate of energy expenditure in the basal state or that expended during intermittent muscle work. Therefore, the organism must have efficient mechanisms for storing ingested energy for future use, when the food supply may be scant or absent. The greatest part of these energy reserves (75%) is in the form of fat as triglycerides, stored in adipose tissue (Fig. 40-3). In normal-weight humans, fat constitutes 10% to 30% of body weight, but it can reach 80% in very obese individuals. Fat is a particularly efficient storage fuel because of its high caloric density (i.e., 9 kcal/g) and because it engenders little additional weight as intracellular water. Less than 10% of adipose cell weight is metabolically active cytoplasm, whereas more than 90% is inert triglyceride. Fat stores can supply energy needs for up to 2 months in totally fasted individuals of normal weight. Triglycerides are formed by esterification of free fatty acids (largely derived from the diet) with α-glycerol phosphate derived from glucose. However, free fatty acids can also be synthesized from acetyl-CoA derived from oxidation of glucose. Thus, carbohydrate can be converted to fat in liver and adipose tissue, and its energy can be stored in that more efficient form (Fig. 40-4). In humans, however, this process accounts for very little glucose use and no more than 10 to 12 g of fat is synthesized from glucose in 24 hours.

Protein (4 kcal/g) constitutes almost 25% of the potential energy reserves (see Fig. 40-3), and the component amino acids can contribute to the supply of essential glucose. However, virtually all proteins serve some vital structural or functional role. Therefore, protein use as a major source of energy is deleterious, and occurs only as a last resort before death from fasting.

Carbohydrate (4 kcal/g) in the form of a glucose polymer, **glycogen,** forms less than 1% of total energy reserves (see Fig. 40-3). However, this portion is critical for support of central nervous system metabolism and for short bursts of intense muscle work. Approximately one fourth of the glycogen stores (75-100 g) is in the liver, and about three fourths (300-400 g) is in the muscle mass. Liver glycogen can be made available to other tissues by the process of **glycogenolysis** and glucose release. Muscle glycogen can be used only by muscle, because this tissue lacks the enzyme

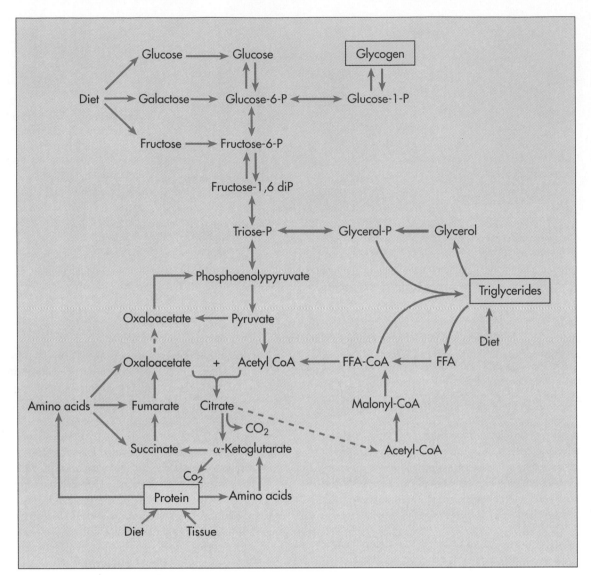

■ **Fig. 40-4**   Chemical pathways of energy transfer and storage. Carbohydrates funnel through glucose-6-phosphate to be stored as glycogen, oxidized in the Krebs cycle, or undergo glycolysis to pyruvate and be used for synthesis of fatty acids. The latter are esterified with glycerol-phosphate and stored as triglycerides. Amino acids arising from protein are converted to glucose via Krebs cycle intermediates and pyruvate, in a process known as gluconeogenesis.

glucose-6-phosphatase, which is required for release of glucose into the bloodstream.

Glycogen can be formed from all three major dietary sugars. In addition, in the liver (and to a much lesser extent in the kidney) glucose itself can also be synthesized de novo from the three carbon precursors pyruvate, lactate, and glycerol, and from parts of the carbon skeleton of all 20 amino acids in protein, except leucine and lysine. This process, known as **gluconeogenesis,** converts two pyruvate molecules to glucose, but it is not a simple reversal of all the reactions of glycolysis (see Fig. 40-4). The chemical free energy change is too large to permit efficient backward flow of the glycolytic reactions at three steps: (1) pyruvate to phosphoenolpyruvate, (2) fructose-1,6-biphosphate to fructose-6-phosphate, and (3) glucose-6-phosphate to glucose.

Substitution of simple phosphatase reactions reverses the last two steps. However, the first step requires energy input in the form of ATP and of guanosine triphosphate. It is also important to realize that *net glucose synthesis cannot occur from acetyl-CoA,* even though carbon atoms from acetyl-CoA can become part of oxaloacetate and then part of glucose molecules, by means of the citric acid cycle. Thus fat can contribute to carbohydrate stores only by way of the 3-carbon glycerol moiety of triglycerides.

The processes of energy storage and transfer themselves expend energy. This partly accounts for the stimulation of oxygen use after a meal (i.e., diet-induced thermogenesis). The cost of storing dietary fatty acids as triglycerides in adipose tissue is only 1% to 2% of the original calories, and the cost of storing glucose as glycogen is only 7% of the original calories. In contrast, conversion of carbohydrate to fat uses up 23% of the original calories, and a similar amount is expended in storing dietary amino acids as protein or in converting them to glycogen.

Because glucose and fatty acids are alternative and in effect competing energy substrates, some relationship between their use and their synthesis and storage within cells could be expected. Under circumstances in which fatty acid supply and plasma free fatty acid levels are increased, glucose transport into cells and subsequent metabolism is decreased by enhanced oxidation of fatty acids and ketoacids (Randle fatty acid–glucose cycle). Fatty acid oxidation increases the ratio of acetyl-CoA/CoA and the level of citrate. These in turn inhibit three key enzymes in glucose metabolism by glycolysis and entry into the Krebs cycle, that is, hexokinase, phosphofructokinase, and pyruvate dehydrogenase. Glucose transport into cells is thereby decreased. Furthermore, intermediates of fatty acid oxidation retard glycolysis and promote gluconeogenesis. Thus, increased use of fatty acids as fuel shifts glucose metabolism away from oxidation in liver and muscle. Also, in liver the increased use of fatty acids shifts glucose metabolism from storage as glycogen to release into the bloodstream.

Conversely, when dietary glucose is plentiful, glycolysis is augmented, more acetyl-CoA is generated from pyruvate, and more citrate is formed in the mitochondria (see Fig. 40-3). The citrate diffuses back into the cytoplasm, where it is a potent activator of the first step in the synthesis of fatty acids (acetyl-CoA → malonyl-CoA), catalyzed by the enzyme acetyl-CoA carboxylase. The product, malonyl-CoA, inhibits carnitine palmitoyl transferase and thus the entry into mitochondria and the oxidation of fatty acids. Citrate is also split back into oxaloacetate and acetyl-CoA; the latter provides the substrate for fatty acid synthesis. Furthermore, other glucose molecules are oxidized via the pentose shunt pathway, which generates NADPH, also needed for fatty acid synthesis. Thus, when the supply of glucose is plentiful, some glucose carbon is converted to fatty acid carbon, with the following stoichiometry:

$$4^1/_2 \text{ glucose} + 4 \text{ O}_2 \rightarrow \text{Palmitic acid} + 11 \text{ CO}_2$$

The resultant RQ is $11 \div 4 = 2.75$. Therefore, whenever the RQ in a human is greater than 1.0, **lipogenesis** from glucose is likely occurring. In addition, glycolysis will produce more glycerol phosphate from triose phosphates. The combination of increased fatty acid synthesis and glycerol phosphate availability increases the synthesis of triglycerides and reduces the oxidation of fat. Thus, increased carbohydrate utilization shifts fat metabolism from oxidation to storage. *Many of these intrinsic chemical checks and balances are also reinforced by hormonal effects, particularly those of insulin and glucagon.*

In addition to these intracellular relationships, transfer of energy between organs is another important aspect of metabolism. The stored energy contained within adipose tissue triglycerides is transported as free fatty acids to the liver. There, part of their energy (not their carbon atoms) is effectively transferred to glucose molecules, because as fatty acids are oxidized, gluconeogenesis is stimulated concurrently, as previously described. The newly synthesized glucose molecules in turn can then be transported to muscle tissue, where their energy is released during glycolysis and is then applied to muscle contraction. Furthermore, if the lactate produced exceeds the ability of the muscle to oxidize it rapidly enough in the citric acid cycle, the lactate can be returned to the liver, where it may again be built back up into glucose molecules. *From this viewpoint, the liver is a flexible and versatile organ that can transmute and transfer energy from fuel depots to working tissues.*

Within the larger context of equalizing total energy input and output, the above processes contribute to another objective of metabolism. The intake and expenditure of each energy source, that is, carbohydrate, fat, and protein, are individually kept in balance.

CARBOHYDRATE METABOLISM

Dietary carbohydrates give rise to various sugars (hexoses), the most important of which are glucose, fructose, and galactose. In addition to serving as energy sources, sugars are also components of glycoproteins, glycopeptides, and glycolipids. These have structural and functional roles in basement membrane collagen, mucopolysaccharides, nerve cell myelin, hormones, and hormone receptors.

Glucose is the central molecule in carbohydrate metabolism. Other sugars are metabolized through the glucose pathways. The initial step in glucose metabolism is transport of the hexose across the cell membrane down a normally large concentration gradient from extracellular fluid to cytoplasm. This process is called **facilitated diffusion,** as opposed to active transport against a concentration gradient (see Chapter 1). Facilitated diffusion is carried out by a family of glucose transport proteins that is encoded by closely related genes. Each transport protein spans the plasma membrane 12 times and both its amino and carboxy termini are located within the cytoplasm. The Glut-1 transporter is expressed constitutively and is responsible for the low level of basal glucose uptake required to sustain the energy generation process by all cells. This transporter is increased by fasting and decreased by an excess of glucose. The Glut-4 transporter is expressed exclusively in cardiac and skeletal muscle and adipose tissue, and it is specifically responsible for the glucose utilization that is stimulated by the hormone insulin (see later discussion). Glut-2 is expressed by hepatic and renal tubular cells that transfer glucose out of the cell and into the extracellular fluid and plasma and by small intestinal epithelial cells that transport glucose from the gut lumen into the plasma. Glut-2 is also present in insulin-secreting cells of the pancreatic islets, where it maintains a virtual equilibrium between the glucose concentrations in the extracellular fluid and cytoplasm. Glut-3 is a high-affinity glucose transporter expressed in neurons and the placenta.

Basal plasma glucose levels are tightly regulated around an average concentration of 80 mg/dl (4.5 μmol/L), with a range of 60 to 110 mg/dl.

When the plasma glucose level falls progressively below 60 mg/dl, the uptake of glucose and the utilization of oxygen decrease in parallel in the brain. If the homeostatic mechanisms described in Chapter 39 fail, central nervous system function becomes progressively impaired. Convulsions, coma, and death may ensue.

The major products of glycolysis, lactate and pyruvate, circulate at average concentrations of 0.7 and 0.07 mM, respectively. This 10:1 ratio of lactate to pyruvate ordinarily prevails, even when the glycolytic rate changes, as long as oxygen is plentiful.

When tissues are deprived of oxygen because of impaired circulation or respiration, the equilibrium between lactate and pyruvate shifts greatly toward the reduced molecule lactate. Plasma concentrations of lactate may rise as high as 30 mM and produce severe metabolic acidosis (blood pH may fall to as low as 6.8). Gastrointestinal symptoms may be followed by progressive loss of consciousness and total systems failure, and may often eventuate in death.

In a subject in the basal state, glucose turnover is about 2 mg/kg/min (11 μmol/kg/min), which is equivalent to about 9 g/hr or 216 g/day in adults. Approximately 55% of glucose use results from terminal oxidation, of which the brain accounts for the greatest part (Fig. 40-5). Another 20% results from glycolysis; the resulting lactate then returns to the liver for resynthesis into glucose (Cori cycle). Reuptake by the liver and other splanchnic tissues accounts for the remaining 25% of glucose use. Most of glucose use (about 70%) in the basal state is independent of insulin, a hormone with otherwise important regulatory effects on glucose metabolism.

The circulating pool of glucose is only slightly larger than the liver output in 1 hour of fasting. This pool is only sufficient to maintain brain oxidation for several hours, even if all other glucose use has ceased. This emphasizes the crucial importance of continuous hepatic production of glucose in fasting subjects. About 75% of this production results from glycogenolysis and 25% from gluconeogenesis. Hepatic uptake and use of circulating lactate account for more than half the glucose supplied by gluconeogenesis. The remainder is largely accounted for by amino acids, especially alanine. The supply of lactate comes from glycolysis in muscle, red blood cells, white blood cells, and a few other tissues. The amino acid precursors come from proteolysis of muscle. Despite the importance of the precursors, however, simply increasing their supply does not increase the rate of gluconeogenesis. The necessary enzymes (Fig. 40-4) must be upregulated by hormonal modulation or by hepatic autoregulatory responses to the falling glucose concentrations.

When an individual ingests glucose after overnight fasting, a significant proportion of the load is assimilated by peripheral tissues, mainly muscle, and the rest by splanchnic tissues, mainly liver. Only 20% to 30% of a glucose load is oxidized during the 3 to 5 hours required for its absorption

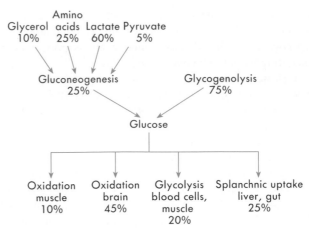

■ **Fig. 40-5** Quantitative overview of glucose turnover in overnight fasted humans. The disposal of circulating glucose *(lower portion)* is largely by oxidation and glycolysis, with the brain acting as the single largest consumer. The production of glucose in the circulation *(upper portion)* is largely from glycogenolysis. The proportionate contribution of glucose precursors to gluconeogenesis, with lactate predominating, is also shown. The average overall rate of glucose turnover is 2.0 mg/kg/min or 11 μmol/kg/min.

from the gastrointestinal tract. The remaining glucose is stored as glycogen, partly in muscle and partly in liver. Glucose initially stored as muscle glycogen can later be transferred to the liver by undergoing glycolysis to lactate, which is released into the circulation. The lactate is then taken up by the liver, rebuilt into glucose, and stored as glycogen in that organ. During the period of peak absorption of exogenous glucose, hepatic output of the sugar is largely unnecessary and is greatly reduced from basal levels. These metabolic adaptations are facilitated by coordinated secretion of the pancreatic islet hormones, insulin and glucagon.

Although glycolysis, oxidation, and storage as glycogen are the main routes of glucose metabolism, other pathways exist. The pentose phosphate pathway or hexose monophosphate shunt is active in tissues in which generation of reduced nicotine adenine nucleotide–phosphate (NADPH) is required for reductive synthesis, for example, in adipose tissue where free fatty acid (FFA) is synthesized from acetyl-CoA. When glucose concentrations are high, the enzyme *aldose reductase* reduces glucose to sorbitol, which can subsequently be oxidized to fructose by the enzyme *sorbitol dehydrogenase* (polyol pathway). Also in the presence of hyperglycemia, glucosamine-6-phosphate can be formed by the enzyme *glutamine–fructose-6-phosphate amidotransferase* (hexosamine pathway).

Diabetes is characterized by long-term complications involving the retina of the eyes, the kidneys, the nerves, and early development of atherosclerosis. The excessive operation of the polyol pathway may be involved in hyperglycemic tissue damage. Hyperglycemia also leads to functional resistance to the action of insulin in muscle and reduced glucose uptake by that tissue.

PROTEIN METABOLISM

The average adult body contains about 10 kg of protein, of which about 6 kg is metabolically active. This pool turns over continuously at a rate of 3 to 5 g/kg body weight/day; the degradative and synthetic reactions involved account for about 20% of the BMR. Of the amino acids released daily by proteolysis from muscle, the main endogenous repository, a large part cycles back into protein synthesis. However, as much as 50 g is irreversibly degraded. Therefore, the daily dietary intake of 50 g of protein (or 0.8 g/kg) is ordinarily sufficient to replace what is lost. When accretion of lean body mass is taking place (e.g., in growing children, pregnant women, persons recovering from prior weight loss), daily protein requirements increase to 1.5 to 2.0 g/kg.

All proteins are composed of the same 20 amino acids. Half of these are called **essential amino acids** because their carbon skeletons, the corresponding α-ketoacids, cannot be synthesized by humans. (The essential amino acids are threonine, methionine, valine, leucine, isoleucine, phenylalanine, tyrosine, tryptophane, lysine, and, in infants, histidine.) However, once the carbon skeletons are present they can be converted to the essential amino acids by transamination. The other half, the **nonessential amino acids,** can be synthesized endogenously, because the appropriate carbon skeletons can be built from glucose metabolites in the citric acid cycle. The essential amino acids must be supplied in the diet; the minimal requirements range from 0.5 to 1.5 g/day. All 20 amino acids are required for normal protein synthesis; therefore a deficiency of even one essential amino acid disrupts this process.

Protein sources vary greatly in their biological effectiveness, depending in part on the ratio of essential to nonessential amino acids. Milk and egg proteins are of the highest quality in this regard. During infancy and childhood, about 40% of the protein intake should consist of essential amino acids in order to support growth. In adults, this requirement falls to 20%. In addition to their incorporation into proteins, many of the amino acids, including some essential ones, are precursors for important molecules, such as purines, pyrimidines, polyamines, phospholipids, creatine, carnitine, methyl donors, certain hormones (Chapter 39), and neurotransmitters.

The plasma concentrations of the individual amino acids range widely from 20 μmol/L to 500 μmol/L. All 20 amino acids are completely oxidizable to CO_2 and H_2O after the amino group has been removed. Each amino acid traverses a specific degradative pathway. (Refer to standard biochemistry textbooks for details.) However, all these pathways converge into three general metabolic processes: **gluconeogenesis, ketogenesis,** and **ureagenesis.** Except for leucine and lysine, all the amino acids can contribute carbon atoms for the synthesis of glucose. Five ketogenic amino acids give rise either to acetoacetate or to its CoA precursors. In the degradation of all amino acids, ammonia is released. Ammonia, incorporated mainly into glutamine and alanine molecules, is then transported to the liver. In the liver

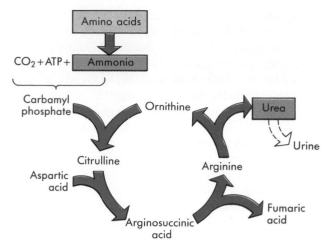

■ **Fig. 40-6** The Krebs-Henseleit urea cycle for disposal of ammonia generated by the metabolism of amino acids.

ammonia is "detoxified" by incorporation into urea, a metabolically inert molecule. The synthesis of urea by the Krebs-Henseleit cycle is depicted in Fig. 40-6. The urea resulting from protein degradation is excreted by the kidney (see Chapter 36).

In the healthy adult under steady-state conditions, the total daily nitrogen excreted in the urine as urea plus ammonia, along with minor losses of nitrogen in the feces (0.4 g/day) and skin (0.3 g/day), is equal to the nitrogen released during metabolism of exogenous and endogenous protein. Such an individual is said to be in **nitrogen balance.** When protein is not ingested, the sum of urea plus ammonia nitrogen in the urine reflects almost quantitatively the rate of endogenous protein degradation. *When protein breakdown is greatly accelerated by tissue trauma or by disease, urinary urea plus ammonia nitrogen may exceed protein nitrogen intake.* In these two cases, the individual is said to be in **negative nitrogen balance.** In a growing child or in a previously malnourished individual undergoing protein repletion with a gain in body mass, urinary urea plus ammonia nitrogen excretion is less than the intake of protein nitrogen. Such an individual is said to be in **positive nitrogen balance.**

Protein deficiency can occur in varied settings, ranging from poor "third world" countries to hospitals and nursing homes in the United States. In the former case, the available protein supply is either too low or too expensive. In the latter case, insufficient attention has been paid to nutritional considerations during a period of assisted or artificial feeding. Selective protein deficiency, but with sufficient caloric intake, leads to **kwashiorkor.** This condition is manifest by low plasma albumin levels, edema (fluid retention), fragile hair and skin, reduced healing of wounds, and depressed cellular immune function leading to increased infections.

Measurements of external nitrogen balance do not themselves quantitate the dynamic internal equilibrium between protein synthesis and protein degradation. The latter must be estimated by labeling body protein with an isotopic amino acid tracer, such as ^{15}N-glycine, and determining the flux of protein from measurements of ^{15}N-specific activity (Fig. 40-7). Such studies show that healthy adults, receiving isocaloric diets containing adequate protein, degrade and synthesize protein at a rate of 3 to 4 g/kg/day. Individual synthesis rates for most proteins are not known, but the hepatic synthesis of albumin accounts for about 5% of the above total. The rate of total body protein synthesis is diminished when the diet is severely deficient in energy, in total protein, or in one of the essential amino acids. In such situations, the rate of protein degradation usually also diminishes, but not to the same extent as the rate of synthesis, so that net loss of body protein results.

In addition to the flux of total body protein, each individual amino acid undergoes its own unique turnover. It is

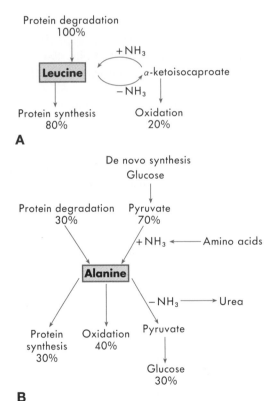

A

B

■ **Fig. 40-7 A,** Quantitative turnover of leucine, *an essential amino acid,* in overnight fasted humans. Protein degradation is the only source for this amino acid, whose carbon skeleton (α-ketoisocaproate) cannot be synthesized. The majority of leucine disposal is via reincorporation into protein synthesis. The leucine that is lost daily by oxidation must be replaced by dietary intake. **B,** Quantitative turnover of alanine, *a nonessential amino acid,* in overnight fasted humans. Alanine production is mostly by de novo synthesis from pyruvate, with a lesser contribution from protein degradation. Alanine disposal takes place via reincorporation into protein, oxidation, and gluconeogenesis. Alanine molecules, which arise from pyruvate and are reconverted to pyruvate, act as carriers for ammonia transferred from other amino acids. (Data in **A** from Matthews D et al: *Am J Physiol* 238:473, 1980; data in **B** from Chochinov R et al: *Diabetes* 27:287, 1978.)

instructive to contrast two: leucine, an essential amino acid, and alanine, a nonessential amino acid. The only source of leucine in subjects in the postabsorptive state is endogenous protein degradation (Fig. 40-7, *A*). Oxidation accounts for 20% of leucine disappearance from plasma, whereas 80% is reincorporated into new protein molecules. From a knowledge of the rate of leucine production (0.2 mg/kg/min) and the average leucine content of protein (8%), the rate of proteolysis can be estimated to be 2.5 mg/kg/min. Hormonal effects on protein breakdown can then be assessed in this way. After a subject ingests food, leucine oxidation diminishes and more leucine is used for protein synthesis. *However, because leucine oxidation is continuous and irreversible, a daily dietary intake of approximately 1 g of leucine must be provided.* During prolonged fasting, oxidation of leucine contributes slightly to energy needs. More important, leucine produced by proteolysis of dispensable proteins helps maintain the synthesis of other more critical proteins.

The turnover of alanine in the postabsorptive state is more complex (Fig. 40-7, *B*). About 30% of alanine is produced from protein degradation. The other 70% of alanine arises from de novo synthesis: the carbon skeleton from glucose by way of pyruvate and the nitrogen by transamination from other amino acids. The disposal of plasma alanine reflects three major routes and processes; about 40% is oxidized via the citric acid cycle after reconversion to pyruvate, about 30% reappears as glucose via gluconeogenesis from pyruvate, and the remaining 30% is reused for protein synthesis. Figure 40-7, *B* shows that a glucose-alanine cycle, analogous to the glucose-lactate (Cori) cycle, can be envisioned. In this cycle, alanine functions as a carrier of amino groups from muscle to liver. Except for glutamine, alanine is the predominant amino acid released by muscle. It is formed there from pyruvate by transamination from other amino acids released during muscle proteolysis. Alanine is then extracted by the liver, where the amino group is removed for urea synthesis and thereby regenerates pyruvate for gluconeogenesis. Figure 40-7, *B,* also shows that although alanine is a gluconeogenic amino acid, no *net* synthesis of glucose from protein results from this particular pathway. Carbon atoms are merely shuttling from one glucose molecule to another via pyruvate and alanine.

FAT METABOLISM

Fat usually represents almost half of the total daily substrate for oxidation (about 100 g, or 900 kcal). The usual daily intake in the United States is also approximately 100 g, or 40% of total calories. The major component of both dietary and storage fat is triglycerides. Exogenous triglycerides from the diet are absorbed as chylomicrons, whereas endogenous triglycerides are synthesized largely in the liver. Both types of triglycerides consist of long-chain, saturated, largely palmitic C-16 and stearic C-18, and monounsaturated oleic C-18:1 fatty acids esterified to glycerol. Because these fatty acids can also be synthesized in the liver and adipose tissue, in an overall sense, no strict dietary requirement exists for fat. (De novo synthesis of free fatty acids from carbohydrate ordinarily occurs only to a small degree, however.) About 3% to 5% of fatty acids are polyunsaturated and cannot be synthesized in the body. These are termed **essential dietary fatty acids** (linoleic, linolenic, and arachidonic), because they are required as precursors for certain membrane phospholipid and glycolipid substances, as well as for prostaglandins (Chapter 39). Another component of fat is the steroid molecule, cholesterol, which serves various specific functions in membranes and is the precursor for bile acids and steroid hormones. Cholesterol is both ingested and synthesized by most cells.

Table 40-3 presents the average basal concentrations of the most important plasma lipids. Although free (nonesterified) fatty acids circulate bound to albumin and at the lowest concentration, their plasma half-life is by far the shortest (2 minutes), and their rate of turnover is the greatest (up to 200 g/day). Thirty percent to 40% of plasma FFA molecules are oxidized, largely by muscle, where they are the major fuel; 50% to 70% are reesterified, cycling back to triglycerides. The rate of oxidation is largely proportional to the plasma FFA concentration. Plasma FFA derived from dietary fat or adipose tissue stores is the direct source of 50% of total lipid oxidation; the remainder represents mainly oxidation of intracellular lipids prestored in heart, muscle, and liver. A series of fatty acid-binding proteins facilitate the entry of FFA into cells and intracellular organelles. Plasma ketoacids, derived from β-oxidation, can also be oxidized by muscle, but during prolonged fasting they become an important fuel only in muscle and in the central nervous system.

Fat metabolism is greatly influenced by a family of nuclear receptors known as peroxisome proliferator acti-

vated receptors (PPARs). PPARα is found in brown adipose tissue (see below) and to lesser extent in skeletal and cardiac muscle, whereas PPARγ is found in adipose tissue generally. The gene targets of PPARα are involved in the uptake, binding, and oxidation of fatty acids and PPARα expression is increased by fasting. The gene targets of PPARγ stimulate differentiation of adipose cells from mesenchymal precursors as well as synthesis, binding, transport, and storage of FFAs. Natural ligands for PPARs include polyunsaturated fatty acids, prostanoids, and at least one leukotriene.

Pharmacological ligands for PPARα are fibric acid derivatives that are used to lower serum triglycerides in patients with dyslipidemias. Glucose metabolism is enhanced and responsiveness to the hormone insulin is increased by thiazolidine drugs, which activate PPARα. These drugs are used to lower plasma glucose in patients with type 2 diabetes.

The production, transport, and fate of plasma lipoproteins are very complex. Triglycerides and cholesterol, which form the major components of plasma lipids (see Table 40-3), circulate as complex lipoprotein particles ranging in size from 75 to 1500 μm. The nonpolar, hydrophobic core of these particles contains triglyceride and cholesterol esters, whereas their polar, hydrophilic surfaces consist of phospholipid, cholesterol, and apoproteins. The plasma lipoproteins are classified according to their physical densities (Table 40-4). As would be expected, the lowest density particles contain primarily triglycerides. As the particles increase in density, the triglyceride proportion decreases, whereas that of phospholipid and protein increases. Numerous apoproteins, varying in size and charge, are found among the lipoprotein classes. *The varied functions of apoproteins include facilitation of triglyceride transport out of the intestine and liver, activation of the enzymes of lipoprotein metabolism, and attachment of the lipoprotein particles to specific cell surface receptors.* Apoproteins also can be exchanged by lipoprotein particles, a process that facilitates the normal traffic of lipids through the blood.

Chylomicrons circulate after a meal. They are formed from dietary fat and transported across the intestinal wall into the blood, as detailed in Chapter 33. The chylomicrons are rapidly cleared from plasma, with a half-life of 5 minutes. On the capillary endothelial surfaces of adipose tissue,

■ **Table 40-3**   Average lipid concentrations in postabsorptive plasma

	mg/dl	*μmol/L*
Ketoacids	10	0.1
Free fatty acids	10	0.4
Triglycerides	100	1.2
Cholesterol (total)	185	4.8
Low density	120	
High density	50	
Very low density	15	

■ **Table 40-4**   Major lipoprotein classes

			Cholesterol			
	Density	*Triglyceride (%)*	*Free (%)*	*Esters (%)*	*Phospholipid (%)*	*Protein (%)*
Chylomicrons	<0.94	85	2	4	8	2
VLDL	0.94–1.006	60	6	16	18	10
IDL	1.006–1.019	30	8	22	22	18
LDL	1.019–1.063	7	10	40	20	25
HDL	1.063–1.21	5	4	15	30	50

muscle, and heart, chylomicron triglyceride is partly hydrolyzed by the enzyme **lipoprotein lipase** (Fig. 40-8). The latter is activated by apoprotein CII. The liberated free fatty acids are transported across the endothelial cells and taken up for resynthesis and storage as intracellular triglycerides. The remaining particles, known as **chylomicron remnants,** now contain less triglyceride and are subsequently enriched with cholesterol esters by interaction with **high-density lipoprotein (HDL) particles.** These remnants have also acquired apoprotein E, which, with apoprotein

B48, directs their uptake by the liver via specific hepatic receptors. There the remnants are degraded to free fatty acids, glycerol, and free cholesterol, and the protein portion is degraded to amino acids. Thus, the net result of chylomicron metabolism is to transfer most of the dietary triglycerides to adipose tissue and the dietary cholesterol to the liver.

Very-low-density lipoprotein (VLDL) particles are the major source of plasma triglycerides in subjects in the postabsorptive state. VLDL particles are synthesized and secreted largely by the liver, with a smaller contribution from the

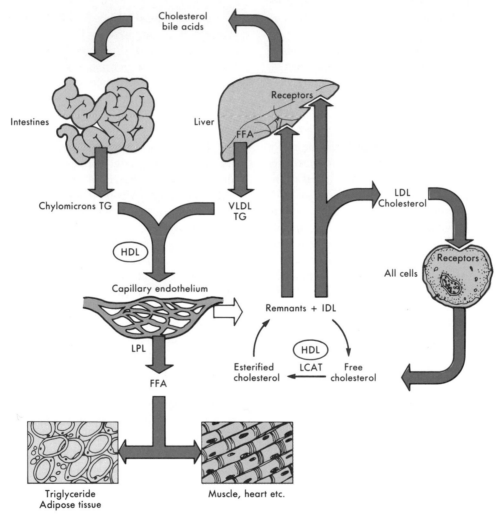

■ **Fig. 40-8** A schematic overview of lipoprotein metabolism and major aspects of lipid turnover in humans. Exogenous triglycerides (*TG,* chylomicrons absorbed from the intestine) and endogenous triglycerides (very-low-density lipoproteins, *VLDL,* produced in the liver) both give rise to free fatty acids *(FFA)* for storage in adipose tissue, oxidation in muscle, and oxidation or reconversion to TG in the liver. High-density lipoprotein particles *(HDL)* facilitate, and the enzyme lipoprotein lipase *(LPL)* directly catalyzes liberation of the free fatty acids from triglycerides. The resultant particles, called remnants from chylomicrons and intermediate-density lipoproteins *(IDL)* from VLDL, undergo further change in the circulation, which is also facilitated by HDL. The ratio of esterified cholesterol to free cholesterol is increased in the remnant and IDL particles by the enzyme lecithin-cholesterol acyltransferase *(LCAT).* The remnant particles are then taken up by the liver for further metabolism. The IDL particles are partly taken up by the liver and partly converted to cholesterol-rich low-density lipoprotein *(LDL)* particles in a process known as reverse cholesterol transport. The latter are then taken up by virtually all cells after interaction with specific LDL receptors. Cholesterol, either synthesized in the liver or extracted from remnant and IDL particles, is also excreted into the intestine, partly as bile acids.

intestine. Under normal dietary circumstances about 15 g of VLDL is produced per day. However, this can increase 3-fold to 6-fold to accommodate high-calorie or high-carbohydrate diets. VLDL particles have a plasma half-life of about 2 hours. The initial phase of VLDL metabolism follows the same route as chylomicrons (see Fig. 40-8). After lipolysis by lipoprotein lipase and interaction with HDL particles, the partially triglyceride-depleted and cholesterol-enriched particle is called **intermediate-density lipoprotein (IDL)** (Table 40-4). About half of the IDL particles are taken up by the liver; the process is directed by apoprotein E and apoprotein B100. However, the other 50% is converted to **low-density lipoprotein (LDL)** particles in the blood and liver. These latter particles transfer exogenous and endogenous cholesterol to other tissues.

LDL is the major cholesterol-containing fraction in plasma (Table 40-3), and it turns over with a half-life of 2.5 days. The average daily amount of cholesterol absorbed from the diet (300 mg), plus the average amount synthesized (600 mg), is balanced by the daily cholesterol excretion in the form of bile salts and neutral steroids. Absorption of cholesterol from the gut and excretion of cholesterol into the bile are controlled by transporters that are composed of ATP binding cassettes. Hepatic synthesis of cholesterol varies inversely with the dietary intake, and therefore a relatively constant input of cholesterol into the plasma is maintained. The cholesterol esters in the LDL particles, generated as described earlier, are taken up by numerous tissues after interaction with specific LDL receptors that recognize their apoprotein E and apoprotein B100 (see Fig. 40-8). The internalized cholesterol esters are hydrolyzed in lysosomes to free cholesterol, which is then used by different cells for various purposes. The cholesterol also may be reesterified (a reaction catalyzed by acyl-CoA-cholesterol acyltransferase) and then stored. The free cholesterol level within the cell regulates itself. Cholesterol diminishes its own further uptake into the cell by downregulating the LDL receptor, and it reduces its own intracellular de novo synthesis by suppressing the rate-limiting enzyme, hydroxymethylglutaryl-CoA (HMG-CoA) reductase.

HDL particles (Table 40-4) perform crucial functions in transferring lipid components between other lipoprotein particles and ultimately between organs. They also facilitate enzyme activities in the metabolism of lipoproteins. HDL particles synthesized in the liver contain primarily apoprotein C and apoprotein E; those that are synthesized in the intestine contain primarily apoprotein A. Nascent HDL is released as small, dense spherical particles. Shortly afterward, they acquire phospholipids and a bilayer discoid shape and equilibrate their apoprotein contents. The plasma half-life of HDL is 5 to 6 days.

HDL assists in the previously described hydrolysis of chylomicron and VLDL triglycerides to FFA (see Fig. 40-8) by providing apoprotein C for the activation of lipoprotein lipase. HDL also facilitates the flow of excess plasma triglycerides back to the liver, the flow of cholesterol to peripheral cells, and reverse transport of cholesterol back to the liver (see Figs. 40-8 and 40-9). Thus, the smaller and denser subfraction HDL$_3$ accepts free cholesterol from peripheral cells,

and from remnant and IDL particles. Esterification of this cholesterol by the plasma enzyme **lecithin-cholesterol acyltransferase (LCAT)** is activated by HDL apoprotein A$_1$. The cholesterol ester is then exchanged for triglycerides in other particles by the cholesterol-ester transfer protein; in the process, the HDL changes to the larger, less dense, more bouyant HDL$_2$ subfraction. The exchanged cholesterol esters then can either be delivered to the peripheral cells as LDL particles or taken up by the liver as part of remnant, IDL, and LDL particles, that is, reverse cholesterol transport. The HDL$_2$ can itself cycle back to HDL$_3$, as the triglycerides acquired in these exchanges are hydrolyzed by hepatic lipase (see Fig. 40-9). The process of reverse cholesterol transport contributes significantly to the maintenance of physiologically appropriate and "healthy" lipoprotein levels.

Each of the major lipoprotein fractions described above can now be further subdivided into smaller classes by new analytical techniques, for example, using nuclear magnetic resonance. The relationship between these individual subclasses and human diseases is an active area of investigation.

The factors that influence the relative proportions of LDL and HDL particles are of great public health importance, because cholesterol taken up from plasma as LDL particles by macrophages is an essential component of atherosclerotic plaques in major blood vessels. HDL particles help prevent this first pathogenic step by facilitating LDL uptake by other cells. LDL levels are higher in males than in females, and the levels are increased by androgens, smoking, obesity, a sedentary life style, a high saturated fat intake, and certain drugs. HDL levels are lower in males than in females, and they are decreased by androgens, smoking, obesity, a high polyunsaturated fat diet, and type 2 (non-insulin-dependent) diabetes. HDL levels are increased by estrogens, exercise conditioning, and moderate alcohol intake. *These effects partly explain the fact that male gender, a lack of physical fitness, obesity, and smoking are strong risk factors for premature atherosclerotic cardiovascular disease and death.* After the menopause, the relative protection enjoyed by females disappears. Strenuous public health efforts are underway (1) to screen for individuals with a high LDL/HDL ratio (> 4.0) and (2) to lower the ratio by decreased intake of saturated fat to less than 30% of total calories, weight reduction, cessation of smoking, and increased exercise.

Major abnormalities in lipoprotein levels are also caused by genetic defects in the pathways of lipid metabolism. A deficiency in lipoprotein lipase activity leads to excessive and prolonged chylomicron and triglyceride levels after fat-containing meals; this can cause severe inflammation of the pancreas. Mutations that cause deficient or low affinity cell-surface LDL receptors lead to extremely high plasma LDL cholesterol levels, visible deposits of cholesterol in skin and tendons, and premature coronary artery disease (**familial hypercholesterolemia).** Synthesis of an abnormal apoprotein E, which cannot efficiently direct lipoprotein particles to interact with cell

Reverse Cholesterol Transport

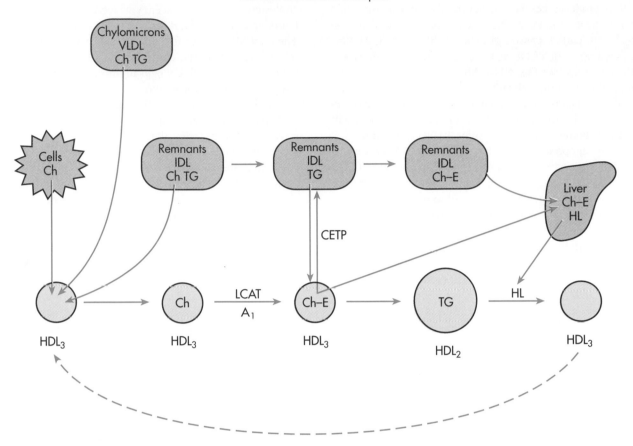

Ch = Cholesterol
A₁ = Apoprotein A₁
CETP = Cholesterol ester transfer protein
TG = Triglycerides
VLDL = Very–low–density lipoproteins

Ch–E = Cholesterol esters
LCAT = Lecithin–cholesterol acyltransferase
HL = Hepatic lipase
IDL = Intermediate–density lipoproteins

■ **Fig. 40-9** Functioning of high-density lipoprotein *(HDL)*. HDL₃ particles accept and esterify cholesterol from cells and from other lipoprotein particles. Apoprotein A₁ activates the key enzyme LCAT. The resultant particles exchange cholesterol esters for triglycerides with chylomicrons and VLDL, becoming more buoyant HDL₂ particles. These in turn are relieved of the triglycerides by the action of hepatic lipase and cycle back to HDL₃ particles.

receptors, leads to accumulation of chylomicron remnants and IDL in plasma. In this situation, both triglyceride and cholesterol levels are elevated, and they increase the risk of coronary artery disease. Another cause of this dual abnormality is excessive production of apoprotein B100 **(familial-combined hyperlipidemia).** Conversely, a deficiency of apoprotein B leads to very low levels of chylomicrons, VLDL, and LDL in plasma, but to pathological accumulation of triglycerides in the intestines and the liver.

An important class of drugs (statins) has emerged for treatment of individuals with elevated LDL cholesterol levels. These drugs inhibit the rate-limiting step in cholesterol synthesis, an action that upregulates plasma membrane LDL receptors. Serum cholesterol and triglyceride levels fall and atherosclerotic events decline in frequency.

METABOLIC ADAPTATIONS

Fasting

An individual in the fasting state totally depends on endogenous substrates for energy (Fig. 40-10). Mobilization of glucose provides essential fuel for the central nervous system; release of free fatty acids provides for the oxidative needs of the other tissues. An increase in protein degradation to amino acids is also a fundamental feature of this response. The fasting individual is said to be in a state of **catabolism,** because carbohydrate, fat, and protein stores are all decreasing.

The liver is the key organ in the metabolic response to fasting. Glucose is supplied to the circulation initially by augmenting glycogenolysis. After 12 to 15 hours of fasting, however, hepatic glycogen stores are greatly depleted, and

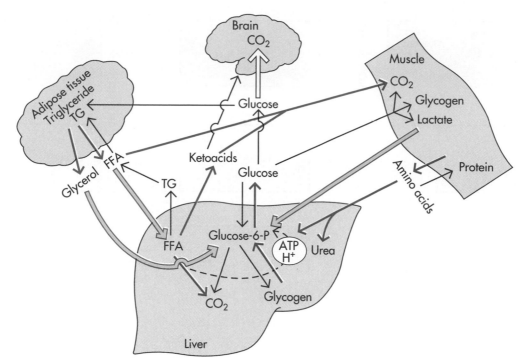

■ **Fig. 40-10**   Pattern of substrate flow in the fasting state. Adipose tissue increases free fatty acid supply to the liver, where free fatty acid is used for energy, ketogenesis, and to generate ATP and reducing equivalents for gluconeogenesis. In muscle free fatty acid oxidation spares glucose use. Muscle increases amino acid flow to the liver for use in gluconeogenesis. The ammonia released from the amino acids is detoxified by incorporation into urea. Glycerol released by adipose tissue and lactate by muscle are used for glucose production. Hepatic glucose production from glycogenolysis and gluconeogenesis is augmented. Glucose uptake by the liver, adipose tissue, and muscle is diminished, but uptake by the brain is sustained. Keotacid production by the liver and eventually ketoacid use by peripheral tissues is increased. *TG,* Triglycerides, *FFA,* free fatty acids; *colored arrows,* increased flow of fuel; *black arrows,* decreased flow of fuel.

continuing enhancement of gluconeogenesis fills the void. The kidney is also a gluconeogenetic organ that may contribute 5% to 15% of glucose production after an overnight fast. To supply glucose precursors, 75 to 100 g of muscle protein is broken down daily during the first few days. This is reflected in a rising excretion of urea in the urine. Gluconeogenesis is also supported by the provision of 15 to 20 g of glycerol daily, which is released during the accelerated lipolysis of triglycerides in adipose tissue. Glucose oxidation in muscle and liver is spared as increasing quantities of free fatty acids become available. Muscle lipoprotein lipase activity increases to facilitate the uptake of triglycerides for oxidation; adipose lipoprotein lipase activity decreases to dampen the uptake of triglyceride for storage.

A portion of fatty acid oxidation in liver yields the ketoacids β-hydroxybutyrate and acetoacetate, which spare the use of glucose by muscle cells. The shift away from glucose and toward fatty acid oxidation lowers the respiratory quotient. These adaptations are reflected in changing plasma concentrations of substrates (Fig. 40-11). Glucose and the major gluconeogenic amino acid, alanine, decrease, whereas free fatty acids, glycerol, and branch-chain amino acids, such as leucine, increase. High levels of the strong ketoacids produce a tendency to metabolic acidosis with a slight reduction in blood pH. Much of this pattern of adaptation is mediated by hormonal modification, particularly by decreasing insulin production and by increasing glucagon production (Fig. 40-11).

After a few days, other important adaptations occur. Total energy expenditure, reflected in the BMR, decreases 10% to 20% and limits the drain on energy stores. The central nervous system no longer depends entirely on glucose as an energy source, and two-thirds of its needs are eventually met by the ketoacids. As less glucose is needed for oxidation, gluconeogenesis diminishes, protein breakdown declines to 25 to 30 g/day, and the contribution of the kidney to glucose production may increase to 25%. Protein synthesis also decreases. In long-term fasting, body weight diminishes by an average of 300 g/day, two-thirds of which is accounted for by fat and one-third by lean tissue. As long as sufficient fluid is ingested, an individual of normal weight can survive up to 60 days. About that time fat stores are almost exhausted, protein degradation rapidly accelerates, and death follows. This flow of substrates, shown in Fig. 40-10, is reversed after feeding. Glucose enters the plasma from dietary carbohydrate, free fatty acids enter from dietary triglycerides, and amino acids enter from protein. Each substrate is stored as described, and the individual is said to be in a state of **anabolism.**

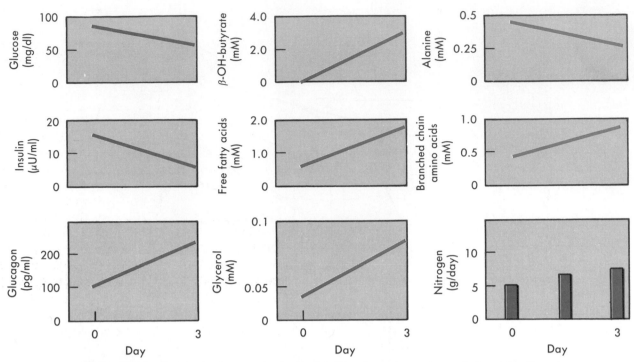

■ **Fig. 40-11** Changes in plasma substrate levels, urine nitrogen excretion, and plasma insulin and glucagon during 3 days of fasting in humans. Note the rise in lipid-derived fuels and products of proteolysis. These changes are mediated in part by a fall in insulin and a rise in glucagon (hormones from the pancreatic islets). (From Felig P et al: *J Clin Invest* 48:584, 1969.)

Exercise

The metabolic response to exercise resembles the response to fasting, in that the mobilization and generation of fuels for oxidation are dominant factors. The type and amounts of expended substrate vary with the intensity and duration of the exercise (Fig. 40-12). For very intense, short-term exercise (e.g., a 10- to 15-second sprint), stored creatine phosphate and ATP provide the energy at a rate of approximately 50 kcal/min. When these stores are depleted, additional intensive exercise for up to 2 minutes can be sustained by breakdown of muscle glycogen to glucose-6-phosphate, with glycolysis yielding the necessary energy (at a rate of 30 kcal/min). This **anaerobic** phase is not limited then by depletion of muscle glycogen, but rather by the rapid accumulation of lactic acid in the exercising muscles and the circulation.

After several minutes of exhaustive anaerobic exercise, an oxygen debt of 10 to 12 L can be built up. This must be repaid before the exercise can be repeated. From 6 to 8 L of oxygen is required either to rebuild the accumulated lactic acid back into glucose in the liver or to oxidize it to CO_2. About 2 L of oxygen is required to replenish normal muscle ATP and creatine phosphate content. An additional 2 L of oxygen will replenish the oxygen normally present in the lungs and body fluids and the oxygen bound to myoglobin and hemoglobin.

For less intense but longer periods of exercise, **aerobic** oxidation of substrates is required to produce the necessary energy (at a maximum of about 12 kcal/min). Substrates from the circulation are added to muscle glycogen (Fig. 40-12). After a few minutes, glucose uptake from the plasma increases dramatically, up to 30-fold in some muscle groups. Although resting glucose uptake by muscle is regulated by insulin, and this effect increases somewhat with exercise, the major increase in glucose transport into muscle comes about by an entirely separate insulin-independent factor. During exercise, intracellular glucose and ATP levels initially fall and AMP (adenosine monophosphate) levels rise. AMP then markedly stimulates glucose transport, probably by activating an AMP-stimulated protein kinase (AMPK). To offset this drain on extracellular glucose and to maintain a normal plasma glucose level, hepatic glucose production must increase up to 5-fold. Initially, this occurs largely from glycogenolysis. Indeed, endurance can be improved by high-carbohydrate feedings for several days before prolonged exercise (e.g., a marathon run), because this increases both liver and muscle glycogen stores. With exercise of longer duration, however, gluconeogenesis becomes increasingly important as liver glycogen stores become depleted. To support gluconeogenesis, amino acids are increasingly released by muscle proteolysis, and their fractional uptake by the liver is enhanced. The activities of key gluconeogenic enzymes, such as **phosphoenolpyruvate carboxykinase (PEPCK),** are increased, and transcription of their genes is induced. These events are coordinated by increased sympathetic neural activity and by the relative effects of the hormones glucagon and insulin (see Chapter 41).

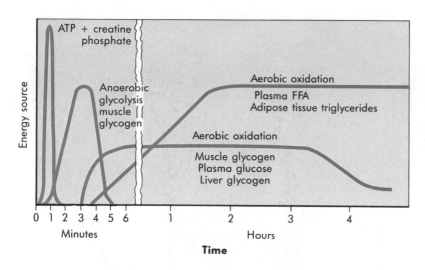

■ **Fig. 40-12** Energy sources during exercise. Note the sequential use of stored high-energy phosphate bonds, glycogen, circulating glucose, and circulating free fatty acids *(FFA)*. The latter dominate in sustained exercise.

REGULATION OF ENERGY STORES

Eventually, fatty acids liberated from adipose tissue triglycerides form the predominant energy substrate and they supply two-thirds of the needs during sustained exercise. Increased AMP levels noted above activate AMPK, which phosphorylates and thereby greatly reduces the activity of the enzyme acetyl-CoA carboxylase. Thus, levels of malonyl-CoA, the product of acetyl-CoA carboxylation, fall. This releases inhibition of carnitine palmitoyl transferase by malonyl-CoA and thereby promotes the entry of fatty acids into the mitochondria, where their oxidation provides energy for sustained muscle work. Except for increases in the circulating levels of pyruvate and lactate, which result from greatly enhanced glycolysis, the pattern of change in the other plasma substrates is similar to that induced by fasting (Fig. 40-11), but it occurs over a much shorter time frame. During recovery from exercise, muscle and liver glycogen stores must be rebuilt; this requires energy input. Some energy is also needed during this period to recycle the unexpended FFA back into triglycerides.

Several diseases that affect muscle function and exercise capacity result from genetic defects in energy-generating steps. (1) In **McArdle's disease** or **muscle phosphorylase deficiency,** glycogen cannot be rapidly broken down to glucose-6-phosphate (Fig. 40-4), and hence pain and weakness occur even during brief exercise. The impairment in glycolysis from lack of substrate is demonstrated by a failure of lactate levels to rise in a draining vein after anaerobic forearm muscle exercise with arterial inflow occluded. (2) In **Von Gierke's disease** or **glucose-6-phophatase deficiency,** hepatic glucose release is impaired, and this limits the supply of glucose during the early phase of exercise. (3) Deficiencies of β-oxidation enzymes (Fig. 40-2) or of **carnitine** or **carnitine palmitoyl transferase** (required to transfer FFA into the mitochondria) prevent efficient use of FFA. This restricts exercise capacity and produces muscle weakness and pain. Conditions (2) and (3) also lead to hypoglycemia during fasting, because hepatic glucose production is decreased.

The preponderance of stored energy consists of fat, and individuals vary greatly in the amounts and percentages of body weight that are accounted for by adipose tissue. Obesity per se is a risk factor for type 2 diabetes and cardiovascular disease, but abdominal visceral (omental) fat poses a particularly high risk. It is important to note that adipose tissue is not an inert repository of triglycerides. Adipose cells are metabolically active, and their number is not fixed. Preadipocytes in the stromal tissue can be induced to differentiate into mature adipocytes, even in adult life, and this process itself is under hormonal regulation. Moreover, adipocytes synthesize and secrete numerous peptide-signaling molecules that affect metabolism or that function in distant tissues. Among these molecules are (1) *tumor necrosis factor α* and *resistin,* both of which reduce the responsiveness of target tissues to insulin, a key hormonal regulator of glucose and fat metabolism; (2) *adiponectin,* which decreases hepatic glucose production by repressing transcription of the genes for PEPCK and glucose-6-phosphatase; and (3) *plasminogen activator inhibitor-1,* which impedes lysis of freshly formed thrombi in blood vessels and thereby increases the hypoxic tissue damage that such clots can cause. PPARγ (see above) is also expressed in adipose tissue, where this protein regulates the number of adipocytes, their metabolism of fat, and their ability to respond to insulin.

What determines the physiologically proper quantity of the adipose tissue energy reserve, and what regulates it? Does an ideal relationship exist between total fat mass and either total body weight or total lean body mass? Do all adipose tissue sites function similarly as storage depots? About 25% of the variance in total body fat and about 30% to 35% of the variance in subcutaneous truncal and abdominal fat appear to be accounted for by genetic factors. A genetic influence on fat mass is supported by (1) the tendency for body mass of adopted children to correlate better with that of their biological parents than with that of their adoptive parents; (2) the much greater similarity of adipose stores in identical (monozygotic) twins, whether reared together or apart, than in fraternal (dizygotic) twins; (3) the greater correlation between the gains in body weight and in abdominal fat in identical twins than in fraternal twins when they are fed a caloric excess; and (4) the discovery in mice and rats of several genes that cause obesity; such genes are present in analogous forms on human chromosomes, and in rare families, mutations of these genes cause inexorable obesity.

Environmental and cultural influences on energy stores, specifically the quality and quantity of the food available, are suggested by the excessive weight gain of certain laboratory animals in response to presentation of high-fat or "junk food" diets. Furthermore, obesity is much more prevalent in affluent (and relatively sedentary) westernized societies than in other populations. Also, the human species has more energy-storage adipose cells per unit body mass than do most other species, and this high adipose cell content may contribute to the propensity for larger fat masses. In addition, human fat cell number is not fixed for life; preadipocytes in mesenchymal connective tissue can be induced by hormonal influences to differentiate into mature adipocytes with a full complement of triglyceride.

Some data suggest the existence of a particular set point for energy stores in each individual. Once adult weight is reached, it tends to be relatively constant, at least until middle age, at which point most humans incur at least a modest weight gain that leads to a higher proportion of body fat. Abdominal fat particularly increases with age, especially in men. Normal and genetically obese laboratory rodents, subjected to forced overfeeding or underfeeding experiments, will return to their previous weight and degree of fatness when they are again allowed free access to food. In rodents, this compensatory control of appetite (caloric and nutrient intake) appears to reside in clusters of neurons in the lateral hypothalamus (a hunger "center") and in the ventromedial hypothalamus (a satiety "center"). Comparable clusters of neurons likely exist in humans.

Food intake is obviously influenced by a number of "nonbiological" factors that include social circumstances, cultural customs, cost, convenience, time of day, and emotions. However, physical and biological factors, such as the sight, smell, taste, sweetness, and palatability of food, and perhaps most importantly, the metabolic state and the size of energy stores of the organism, basically regulate appetite. Thus, a modest reduction in systemic plasma glucose levels, a decrease in fat oxidation in the liver, and shrinkage of adipose tissue mass stimulate hunger. Conversely, a raised level of plasma glucose in the portal vein (signaling glucose-sensitive cells that carbohydrate is entering from the diet) and overexpansion of the adipose tissue mass inhibit food-seeking behavior. The absence of a feeling of hunger, that is, satiety—a feeling of sufficiency or fullness—is an important mechanism for limiting food intake to what is needed for energy expenditures and for maintenance of proper energy stores. Satiety arises from glucose-sensing cells in the hypothalamus.

A large and steadily increasing number of neuropeptides located in the gastrointestinal tract and in the brain, and a

■ **Table 40-5**   Modulators of feeding behavior

Stimulate orexigenic	*Inhibit anorexigenic*
Neuropeptide Y (NPY)	Leptin
Agouti-related peptide (AGRP)	Insulin
Melanin concentrating hormone (MCH)	α-Melanocyte-stimulating hormone (α-MSH)
Orexin A and B (hypocretin 1 and 2)	Corticotropin-releasing hormone (CRH)
Galanin	Urocortin
Norepinephrine	Cocaine-amphetamine-regulated transcript (CART)
Ghrelin	Glucagon-like peptide-1 (GLP-1)
Cortisol	Cholecystokinin (CCK)
	Interleukin-1β
	Serotonin
	Enterostatin
	Calcitonin
	Bombesin

variety of neural pathways and neurotransmitters appear to regulate appetite and energy expenditure (Table 40-5). This bewildering array of molecules and putative pathways have been difficult to integrate into a cohesive regulatory framework until recently. The breakthrough discovery of the obese gene and its product, named *leptin*, in the hereditary obese mouse, combined with detailed immunohistochemical analysis of neuroanatomical areas and powerful molecular biological techniques, have begun to provide a firmer understanding of energy homeostasis.

Figure 40-13 presents an overall view in which leptin, a secretory peptide product of adipose cells, "reports" by its plasma level, the size of the adipose mass to leptin receptors in the hypothalamus. Leptin also signals the recent (over several days) states of fasting or feeding. However, a single meal has little effect on plasma leptin. Leptin is synthesized in adipose tissue and the plasma leptin level and messenger RNA content of leptin in fat cells correlate well with the BMI and estimated fat mass of humans. Leptin reacts with a plasma membrane receptor in hypothalamic (and other brain) cells, and it releases a jak-STAT-3 tyrosine kinase intracellular second messenger (Fig. 40-13). However, before it reaches its target cells, leptin must first cross the blood-brain barrier. This step is facilitated by a transporter that is an alternatively spliced, shortened product of the leptin receptor gene present in brain endothelial cells. Leptin actions are clearly demonstrated in the leptin-deficient obese mouse strain and in rare humans that possess this condition. Without leptin, the organism is extremely obese, overeats, has a low BMR and body temperature, and is physically very inactive. Replacement therapy with leptin causes weight loss, decreases food consumption, and increases energy expenditure and body temperature. In another congenital mouse model, the leptin receptor is mutant and functionally inactive; this results in obesity and a similar abnormal metabolism, but the plasma leptin

Feedback Regulation of Energy Stores

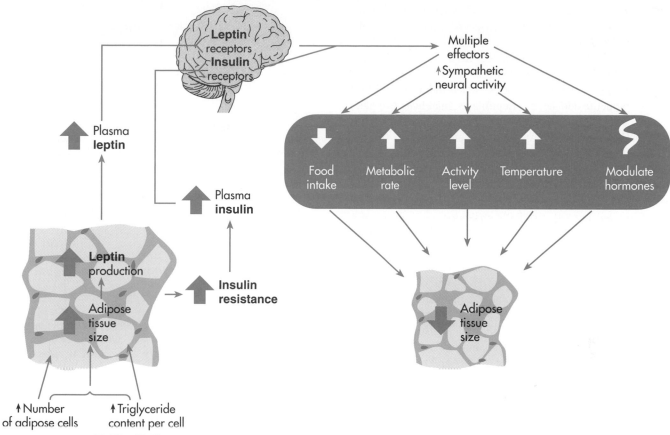

■ **Fig. 40-13**   An overview of a current concept of regulation of energy stores. Leptin production, release, and plasma levels are proportional to adipose mass and "report" the size of the latter to the hypothalamus and other brain areas. The occupied leptin receptor initiates a series of effector mechanisms that adjust the adipose mass downward when it increases beyond a set point that is physiologically optimal. Effector mechanisms decrease food intake, increase energy expenditure, and modulate secretion of hormones so as to decrease lipogenic and increase lipolytic activity of adipose tissue.

levels are high. In this mouse, treatment with leptin is ineffective.

Note that insulin, a pancreatic islet hormone (see Chapter 41), in some respects acts like leptin and reinforces leptin action. Thus, plasma insulin levels rise when adipose tissue mass increases. Insulin also enters the CNS via a transport system by which it acts to induce satiety and to increase energy expenditure by increasing sympathetic nervous system activity.

Thus, adipose tissue cells and hypothalamic cells form a negative feedback loop, with leptin acting as the primary signal molecule. The overall result is to stabilize energy stores in adipose tissue by coordinating the hypothalamic cell regulation of caloric intake and of energy expenditure. Leptin action in rodents increases the catecholaminergic outflow from the hypothalamus; the neurotransmitter norepinephrine stimulates the β_3-adrenergic receptor in the brown adipose tissue (BAT) of rodents. The liganded receptor, via cAMP as second messenger, increases expression of an uncoupling protein (UCP-1) that inserts as a channel in the mitochondrial membrane. This channel permits protons, which were pumped out of the mitochondria in the process of electron transport down the electron receptor chain, to "leak" back in, rather than to be used actively in the mitochondrial synthesis of ATP. The net result is an uncoupling of ATP synthesis from oxygen utilization and a wastage *as heat* of the energy generated by aerobic oxidation. Thus BAT, with its very large mitochondria, facilitates facultative thermogenesis and the disposal of excess calories. Although BAT is present in human newborns, and it functions to adapt them to the sudden lowering of environmental temperature at birth, BAT is difficult to detect in adult humans and exists, if at all, in quantities likely too small to contribute significantly to energy homeostasis. However, a set of homologous uncoupling proteins (UCP-2 and UCP-3) has been found in white adipose tissue and muscle of adult humans. The role of UCPs in adaptive energy expenditure and in regulation of body energy stores is still under investigation. Overexpression of UCP-3 in muscle of mice leads to increased energy expenditure and weight loss, and to a compensatory increase in food intake, as predicted by the model in Fig. 40-13. On the other hand, fasting, which brings about a compensatory *reduction* in energy expenditure, is associated with an *increase,* rather than the expected decrease, in UCP-2 and UCP-3 mRNA in tissues.

How is leptin action mediated in the hypothalamus? Figure 40-14 diagrams one current view, which encompasses several of the neuropeptides listed in Table 40-5 that regulate appetite and satiety. Leptin acts on at least two neuron types in the *arcuate nucleus* of the hypothalamus. In the first, leptin represses the production of neuropeptide Y (NPY), a very potent stimulator of food seeking (energy intake) and an inhibitor of energy expenditure. Norepinephrine, another appetite stimulator, colocalizes with NPY in some of these neurons. At the same time, leptin represses the production of agouti-related peptide (AGRP), an endogenous antagonist that acts on MC4R, a hypothalamic receptor for the anorexigenic peptide α-MSH, which inhibits food intake. In another type of arcuate neuron, leptin stimulates the production of proopiomelanocortin (POMC) products, one of which is α-MSH, and the production of cocaine amphetamine-regulated transcript (CART) (Table 40-5), both of which inhibit food intake. Thus leptin decreases food consumption and increases energy expenditure by simultaneously inhibiting NPY and the α-MSH antagonist AGRP, and by stimulating α-MSH and CART (Fig. 40-14). These second-order neuropeptides are transmitted to and interact with receptors in neurons of the *paraventricular* hypothalamic nucleus ("satiety" neurons) and lateral hypothalamic nucleus ("hunger" neurons). In turn, these hypothalamic neurons generate outputs that coordinate feeding behavior and autonomic nervous system activity (especially sympathetic outflow), with diverse endocrine actions on thyroid gland function, reproduction, and growth.

Another regulator of food intake and body energy stores is melanin-concentrating hormone (MCH). This neuropeptide increases food seeking and adipose tissue by antagonizing the satiety effect of α-MSH, downstream from the interaction of α-MSH with its MC4R receptor. The likely importance of this molecule is demonstrated by the fact that it is the only regulator whose ablation by gene knockout actually results in leanness.

In addition to maintaining overall energy homeostasis, the system must also balance specific nutrient intake and expenditure, for example, CHO intake with CHO oxidation. This may account for some specificity in neuropeptide and neurotransmitter responses to meals. Serotonin produces satiety after glucose ingestion, whereas enterostatin selectively decreases fat intake. Gastrointestinal hormones, such as CCK and GLP-1 (Table 40-5), produce satiety by humoral effects, but their local production in the brain may participate in nutrient and caloric regulation. The recently discovered hormone ghrelin is an acylated peptide with potent orexigenic activity that arises in cells of the oxyntic glands in the stomach. Plasma levels of ghrelin rise in humans in the 1 to 2 hours that precede their normal meals. The plasma levels of ghrelin fall drastically to minimum

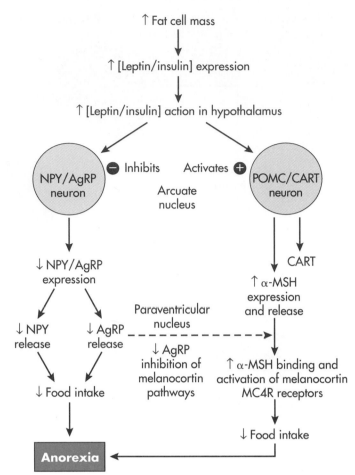

■ **Fig. 40-14** A current concept of leptin effects in the brain. One target neuron transmits the preexigenic peptide NPY and the peptide AGRP, which antagonizes the anorexigenic peptide α-MSH. The neuronal expression of these two genes is inhibited by leptin. Another target neuron transmits α-MSH, synthesized by expression of the POMC gene, and CART. This neuron's activity is stimulated by leptin. The cumulative effect of all four actions is to decrease food intake. (From Schwartz MW et al: *Nature* 404:661, 2000.)

values about 1 hour after eating. Ghrelin appears to stimulate food intake by reacting with its receptor in hypothalamic neurons that express NPY.

Humans who suffer damage to the hypothalamus from neoplasms or infiltrative disorders, such as **sarcoidosis,** sometimes gain large amounts of weight. Conversely, in the hypothalamic dysfunction of **anorexia nervosa,** weight is maintained at very low, life-threatening levels.

Pathological accumulation of fat (i.e., obesity) is a major health problem in many countries. In the United States, one third of the population now meets the definition of overweight or obesity. A body weight 20% above ideal increases the risk of disorders such as diabetes, hypertension, and cardiovascular disease; a body weight 40% to 50% above ideal greatly increases the risk of death. An excess of body weight is better expressed by the body mass index (BMI), defined as body weight in kg ÷ (height in meters)^2. A BMI > 25 is defined as overweight and a BMI > 27 as obesity. Morbidity and mortality increase steeply at BMI > 30. Accumulation of fat in abdominal and particularly in visceral depots confers an especially high risk. The prevalence of diabetes is increasing in an epidemic fashion in the United States and in other countries as the prevalence of obesity goes up.

The exact causes of human obesity are not known. Some obese individuals overeat and they are aware of binges of caloric excess, often in a diurnal pattern. However, most obese individuals report lower caloric intakes than they actually ingest. Because of the tight physiological control on how many calories can be stored as carbohydrate or as protein, an excessive intake of fat is easier to envision as the source of calories, if obesity results from an abnormality on the input side of the energy equation. Fatty acid oxidation is independent of fat intake, whereas carbohydrate and protein oxidation are stimulated by their respective intakes.

Many obese individuals behave as if they have an elevated set point for energy stores; they defend this set point tenaciously by disproportionately decreasing energy expenditure when caloric intake is reduced by dieting and weight is lost. In some studies, nonobese infants or adults with low BMRs are at greater risk for future weight gain. However, once obesity is present and static, BMR, which remains proportional to lean body mass, is generally equal to or greater than the BMR of normal-weight individuals, as are diet-induced thermogenesis, and the energy cost of exercise. Furthermore, the thermogenic response to an excess of calories is limited to 25% of the caloric intake in massive overfeeding experiments. Thus, a continuous deficit in energy expenditure is an unlikely single explanation for obesity.

In obese humans, the profile of certain hormones (increased insulin and decreased growth hormone) generally favors fat deposition rather than its mobilization. Endorphin levels are elevated, and this finding may indicate the involvement of that neuropeptide in central appetite stimulation. Furthermore, adipose tissue of obese humans contains elevated levels of lipoprotein lipase, the key enzyme that transfers circulating triglycerides via FFA into cells. However, none of these abnormalities has been proved to be the primary cause of common human obesity.

The initial studies of leptin in obese humans have suggested that absolute leptin deficiency is an extremely rare cause of their obesity. Their plasma leptin levels are elevated and correlate with their increased fat mass, as do messenger RNA levels for leptin in their adipose cells. Hence, it appears that a peripheral signal indicating that energy stores are too large is being generated, but that is is not being received or acted upon normally in the hypothalamus. Thus, resistance to leptin action appears to be a more likely cause of human obesity. Defective leptin transport into the brain, the initial step in CNS leptin action, has not yet been explored adequately as a cause of obesity. A functionally inactive leptin receptor has been reported to be a rare cause of human obesity. Resistance in one leptin target cell (Fig. 40-14) accounted for either by a defective POMC gene or by a defective prohormone convertase-1 gene, either one leading to loss of α-MSH and its anorexic effect, has been identified. Resistance at a secondary hypothalamic cell, namely a mutant defective MC$_4$R α-MSH receptor gene, has also been reported. All these rare examples are very important because they confirm the importance of leptin and the leptin-POMC-MSH-MC$_4$R pathway in normally restraining caloric intake. However, a trial of leptin therapy in common obesity, hoping to overcome resistance to leptin even if it originates in a downstream pathway, has not yielded satisfactory results in the doses tried.

Treatment of obesity by dieting, by disciplined exercise, by behavior modification, and by drugs (e.g., serotonin reuptake inhibitors, amphetamine analogs), which may act favorably at some point in the complex system that sets energy stores, is, essentially, palliation but not a cure. Gastric volume reduction or bypass surgery is effective in reducing body weight by one-third over a 1- to 2-year period. With this weight loss, the frequently accompanying diabetes, hypertension, and atherogenic serum lipid patterns usually improve greatly. Surgical complications and a low but definite mortality rate have limited the popularity of this therapeutic approach. Its use is currently indicated only in very obese individuals with BMI > 35–40 and with concomitant medical complications of obesity.

SUMMARY

1. Energy input as carbohydrate, fat, and protein calories must equal energy expenditure if body weight is to remain constant. Energy expenditure is composed of basal, diet-induced thermogenesis and of sedentary activity components, plus voluntary exercise and heavy labor needs. Basal metabolic rate (60%-70% of total) is proportional to body mass, is in part genetically determined, and declines with aging.

2. Fatty acids are the major fuel in most tissues, except for the central nervous system and red blood cells, where glucose is ordinarily the obligatory oxidative substrate. Depending on availability, fatty acids and glucose are competitive substrates in muscle and liver. Use of one substrate spares use of and may increase production of the other substrate.

3. β-Oxidation of fatty acids and disposal of acetyl-CoA by the Krebs cycle are the main biochemical mechanisms that generate ATP by oxidative phosphorylation. The overall efficiency of energy yield is 65%. Anaerobic glycolysis can support energy expenditure by exercising muscle for only minutes.

4. Energy is primarily stored as adipose tissue triglycerides. Less readily mobilizable amounts of energy are stored as

protein. Carbohydrate stores are trivial, and hence efficient glucose production by the liver (gluconeogenesis) is needed to maintain a supply for the brain.

5. During long-term fasting, gluconeogenesis from amino acids, glycerol, and lactate is required to sustain central nervous system metabolism and other critical functions that are dependent on glucose. The pathway of gluconeogenesis is partly a reversal of glycolysis, but it requires special steps from pyruvate. Increased use of fatty acids during fasting greatly increases the production of the ketoacids β-hydroxybutyrate and acetoacetate.

6. Endogenous protein turnover obligates a daily ingestion of protein, in particular, essential amino acids, such as leucine. Essential amino acids are irreversibly degraded, and their carbon skeletons cannot be synthesized. The carbon skeletons of nonessential amino acids, such as alanine, are degraded and resynthesized daily. Protein synthesis requires the availability of all 20 amino acids.

7. Fat metabolism involves various circulating lipoprotein particles that transfer triglycerides and cholesterol, originating either in the diet or from hepatic synthesis, to and from peripheral tissues and the liver. Low-density lipoprotein particles, rich in cholesterol, play a role in the development of atherosclerosis, whereas high-density lipoprotein particles have a protective effect.

8. Energy needs during exercise are met in sequence by stored muscle creatine phosphate plus ATP, stored muscle glycogen, anaerobic glycolysis, and, finally, aerobic oxidation of glucose and then fatty acids, which are taken up from the plasma. These substrates are supplied by hepatic glycogenolysis and gluconeogenesis and by adipose tissue lipolysis, respectively.

9. Correlation of energy intake and expenditure with energy stores is a complex process, controlled in the hypothalamus. This process involves numerous amine and peptide neurotransmitters and neuromodulators. The hypothalamus senses adipose tissue mass (energy stores), primarily by reception of leptin, a circulating signal generated in adipose cells. Obesity can result from an altered set point of energy stores, from unregulated caloric intake, or from decreased energy use. Resistance to the action of leptin could be one cause of obesity.

BIBLIOGRAPHY

Journal articles

Barsh GS, Farooqi IS, O'Rahilly S: Genetics of body-weight regulation, *Nature* 404:644, 2000.

Bogardus C et al: Familial dependence of the resting metabolic rate, *N Engl J Med* 315:96, 1986.

Bouchard C, Després J-P, Mauriège P: Genetic and nongenetic determinants of regional fat distribution, *Endocr Rev* 14:72, 1993.

Cahill GF: Starvation in man, *N Engl J Med* 282:668, 1970.

Caro JF et al: Leptin: the tale of an obesity gene, *Diabetes* 45:1455, 1996.

Challis BG et al: The CART gene and human obesity: mutational analysis and population genetics, *Diabetes* 49:872, 2000.

Combs TP et al: Endogenous glucose production is inhibited by the adipose-derived protein Acrp30, *J Clin Invest* 108:1875, 2001.

Cummings DE et al: A preprandial rise in plasma Ghrelin levels suggests a role in meal initiation in humans, *Diabetes* 50:1714, 2001.

Exton JH: Gluconeogenesis, *Metabolism* 21:945, 1972.

Felig P et al: Amino acid metabolism during prolonged starvation, *J Clin Invest* 48:584, 1969.

Ferrannini E et al: The disposal of an oral glucose load in healthy subjects: a quantitative study, *Diabetes* 34:580, 1985.

Foster D: From glycogen to ketones—and back (Banting Lecture 1984), *Diabetes* 33:1188, 1984.

Giesecke K et al: Protein and amino acid metabolism during early starvation as reflected by excretion of urea and methylhistidines, *Metabolism* 38:1196, 1989.

Groop LC et al: Role of free fatty acids and insulin in determining free fatty acid and lipid oxidation in man, *J Clin Invest* 87:83, 1991.

Hardie DG, Carling D, Carlson M: the AMP-activated/SNF1 protein kinase subfamily: metabolic sensors of the eukaryotic cell? *Annu Rev Biochem* 67:821, 1998.

Harris RBS: Role of set-point theory in regulation of body weight, *FASEB J* 4:3310, 1990.

Jansky L: Humoral thermogenesis and its role in maintaining energy balance, *Phys Rev* 75:237, 1995.

Jequier E, Tappy L: Regulation of body weight in humans, *Am Physiol Soc* 79:451, 1999.

Katz L et al: Splanchnic and peripheral disposal of oral glucose in man, *Diabetes* 32:675, 1983.

Kristensen P et al: Hypothalamic CART is a new anorectic peptide regulated by leptin, *Nature* 393:72, 1998.

Lowell BB, Spiegelman BM: Towards a molecular understanding of adaptive thermogenesis, *Nature* 404:652, 2000.

Ludwig DS et al: Melanin-concentrating hormone: a functional melanocortin antagonist in the hypothalamus. *Am J Physiol* 274:E627, 1998.

Maeda N et al: PPAR γ ligands increase expression and plasma concentrations of adiponectin, an adipose-derived protein, *Diabetes* 50:2094, 2001.

Matsuda M et al: Altered hypothalamic function in response to glucose ingestion in obese humans, *Diabetes* 48:1801, 1999.

Randle PJ: Regulatory interactions between lipids and carbohydrates: the glucose fatty acid cycle after 35 years, *Diabetes Metab Rev* 14:263, 1998.

Ravussin E, Swinburn BA: Energy expenditure and obesity, *Diabetes Rev.* 4:403, 1996.

Ravussin E et al: Determinants of 24-hour energy expenditure in man: methods and results using a respiratory chamber, *J Clin Invest* 78:1568, 1986.

Roberts SB et al: Dietary energy requirements of young adult men, determined by using the doubly labeled water method, *Am J Clin Nutr* 54:499, 1991.

Roden M et al: Effects of free fatty acid elevation on postabsorptive endogenous glucose production and gluconeogenesis in humans, *Diabetes* 49:701, 2000.

Rolfe DFS, Brown GC: Cellular energy utilization and molecular origin of standard metabolic rate in mammals, *Am Physiol Soc* 77:731, 1997.

Ruderman NB et al: Malonyl-CoA, fuel sensing, and insulin resistance, *Am J Physiol* 273:E1, 1999.

Schwartz MW et al: Central nervous system control of food intake, *Nature* 404:661, 2000.

Segal KR, Landt M, Klein S: Relationship between insulin sensitivity and plasma leptin concentration in lean and obese men, *Diabetes* 45:988, 1996.

Sims EAH: Energy balance in human beings: the problems of plentitude, *Vit Horm* 43:1, 1986.

Small CJ et al: Effects of chronic central nervous system administration of agouti-related protein in pair-fed animals, *Diabetes* 50:248, 2001.

Spiegelman BM, Flier JS: Obesity and the regulation of energy balance, *Cell* 104:531, 2001.

Steppan CM et al: The hormone resistin links obesity to diabetes, *Nature* 409:307, 2001.

Wasserman DH: Regulation of glucose fluxes during exercise in the postabsorptive state, *Annu Rev Physiol* 57:191, 1995.

Wasserman DH, Cherrington AD: Hepatic fuel metabolism during muscular work: role and regulation, *Am J Physiol* 260:E811, 1991.

Wolfe BM et al: Effect of elevated free fatty acids on glucose oxidation in normal humans, *Metabolism* 37:323, 1988.

Monograph and books

Cryer PE, Polonsky KS: Glucose homeostasis and hypoglycemia. In Wilson JD et al, editors: *Williams textbook of endocrinology,* ed 9, Philadelphia, 1998, WB Saunders.

DeFronzo RA, Ferrannini E: Regulation of intermediary metabolism during fasting and feeding. In DeGroot LJ, Jameson JL, editors: *Endocrinology,* ed 4, Philadelphia, 2001, WB Saunders.

Flatt JP: The biochemistry of energy expenditure. In Bray G, editor: *Recent advances in obesity research, II.* Proceedings of the Second International Congress on Obesity, Los Angeles, 1978, Newman Publishing.

Kimball SR et al: Protein metabolism. In Rifkin H, Porte D, editors: *Diabetes mellitus,* ed 4, New York, 1990, Elsevier Science.

Mahley RW, Weisgraber KH, Farese RV: Disorders of lipid metabolism. In Wilson JD et al, editors: *Williams textbook of endocrinology,* ed 9, Philadelphia, 1998, WB Saunders.

McGarry JD, Foster DW: Ketogenesis. In Porte D Jr, Sherwin RS, editors: *Ellenberg & Rifkin's diabetes mellitus,* ed 5, Stamford CT, 1996, Appleton & Lange.

Seifter S, Englard S: Carbohydrate metabolism. In Rifkin H, Porte D Jr, editors: *Diabetes mellitus,* ed 4, New York, 1990, Elsevier Science.

Shulman GI, Barrett EJ, Sherwin RS: Integrated fuel metabolism. In Porte D Jr, Sherwin RS, editors: *Ellenberg & Rifkin's diabetes mellitus,* ed 5, Stamford CT, 1996, Appleton & Lange.

Woods SC et al: Food intake and energy balance. In Porte D Jr, Sherwin RS, editors: *Ellenberg & Rifkin's diabetes mellitus,* ed 5, Stamford CT, 1996, Appleton & Lange.

chapter forty-one

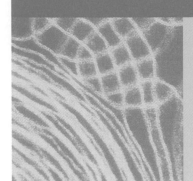

Hormones of the Pancreatic Islets

ANATOMY OF THE PANCREATIC ISLETS

The islets of the pancreas secrete two major hormones, insulin and glucagon. These hormones are rapid and powerful regulators of metabolism. *Together they coordinate the flow and metabolic fate of endogenous glucose, free fatty acids (FFAs), amino acids, and other substrates to ensure that energy needs are met in the basal state and during exercise. In addition, they coordinate the efficient disposition of the nutrient input from meals.* They accomplish these functions primarily by actions on the liver, muscle mass, and adipose tissue. Other secretory peptide products of islet cells (including amylin, pancreastatin, somatostatin, and pancreatic polypeptide) play subsidiary, if any, roles in the regulation of metabolism outside the gastrointestinal tract.

The strategic location of the pancreatic islets reflects these functions. Insulin and glucagon are released in response to nutrient inflow from the gut and to gastrointestinal secretagogues. The products of the exocrine pancreas required for digestion of the incoming nutrients are also released in response to such stimuli. The proximity of the islets to the pancreatic acini may also permit them to have local effects on exocrine pancreatic function. Islet hormones are secreted into the pancreatic vein and then into the portal vein, where they join the nutrient stream after meals. This arrangement preferentially exposes the liver, which is the central organ in substrate traffic, to islet hormone concentrations higher than those the peripheral tissues receive. In addition, the liver can extract variable amounts of insulin and glucagon on their first pass through this organ. In this manner, the liver can modulate the hormones' availability to other tissues. *Insulin and glucagon are often secreted and act in reciprocal fashion; when one is needed, the other usually is not. Therefore, the ratio of their concentrations may be more critical than their actual concentrations.*

There are approximately 1 million islets in the pancreas, and they constitute 1% to 1.5% of the human pancreatic mass. Each islet contains, on average, 2500 cells composed of four types: (1) the β cells, the unique source of insulin, make up 60% to 70%; (2) the α cells, the source of glucagon, 20% to 25%; (3) the δ cells, the source of somatostatin, 10%; and (4) mostly PP cells, the source of pancreatic polypeptide; the microscopic structure, vascular supply, and distribution of the islets are important to islet function. Each islet consists of a core of β cells (Fig. 41-1, *A*) with either a mantle of α and/or δ cells or a mantle of δ and PP cells. If islets are disaggregated experimentally and the individual cells dispersed, these cells spontaneously reaggregate into islets if the cells are brought back together again in culture. Gap junctions exist between neighboring islet cells (Fig. 41-1, *B*) and permit the flow of molecules (that exert possible paracrine effects) and electrical currents between them.

The endocrine cells of the islets arise from common endodermal ancestors, originally in the duodenal portion of the foregut and later localized in the pancreatic ducts. A transcription factor called insulin promoter factor-1 (IPF-1) is required for the specific differentiation of β cells and for the induction of insulin synthesis. Other transcription factors vital to pancreatic endocrine cell development also play roles in neuronal development. In addition, islet cells display other features characteristic of neuroectodermal cells, such as membrane polarization/depolarization and synthesis of certain neurotransmitter amines [e.g., γ-aminobutyric acid (GABA)]. Developmental factors lead to the selective expression of different hormone genes in these cells. The islets are identifiable by the fourth week of human gestation and are able to secrete insulin by the tenth week.

Renewal of adult β cells is ordinarily a slow process, with only 1% of the cells undergoing cell division by entering the sequential mitotic phases of G_1, S, G_2, and M from the quiescent G_0 phase at any one time. New β cells arise from precursors in the pancreatic ducts that transiently express IPF-1. Renewal and growth of β cells are stimulated by various growth factors, including epidermal growth factor, transforming growth factor α, growth hormone, and insulin growth factor-1. Glucose itself can stimulate β cell mitogenesis, as can glucagon-like peptide-1; both of these are also stimulators of insulin secretion. β cells express Fas-ligand, an initiator of apoptosis, but only express the Fas receptor in the presence of

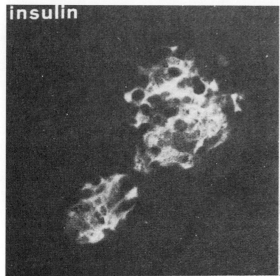

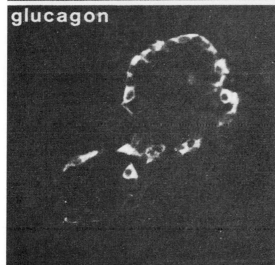

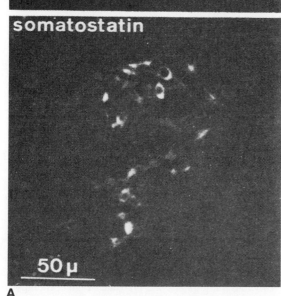

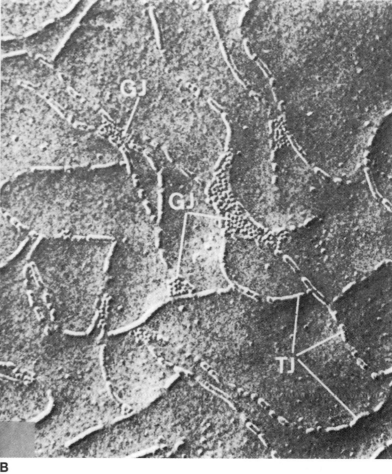

B

■ **Fig. 41-1** **A,** Human islet stained by immunohistochemical methods shows the predominance and central core location of β cells and the peripheral distribution of α cells and β cells. (From Unger RH et al: *Annu Rev Physiol* 40:307, 1978.) **B,** Electron micrograph of adjacent β and α cells in an islet showing the presence of gap junctions *(GJ)* and tight junctions *(TJ)* between them. (From Orci L et al: *J Clin Endocrinol Metab* 41:841, 1975.)

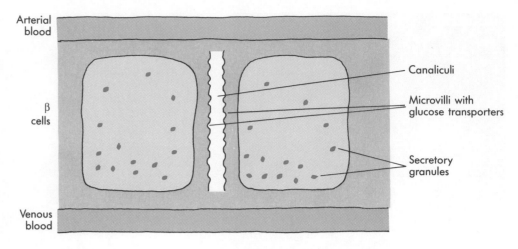

■ **Fig. 41-2**   Orientation of islet β cells to their circulatory supply. Secretory granules are concentrated on the venous face of the cell. Glucose transporters are concentrated in microvilli on the lateral surfaces in contact with channels (canaliculi) that contain intercellular fluid and connect arterial and venous vessels.

high glucose levels. Thus, glucose stimulates both proliferation and death of β cells, and likely maintains a proper level of β cell mass for normal insulin regulation of metabolism.

> Both type 1 and ultimately type 2 diabetes are marked by a deficiency of β cells. Therefore, there is great interest in understanding the processes that regulate β cell turnover, in hopes of developing therapy that would replenish and maintain a normal complement of these vital cells.

The islets are exceedingly well vascularized; they receive a pancreatic blood supply that is disproportional to their mass. Small arterioles enter the core of the islet and break up into a network of capillaries with fenestrated endothelium. These capillaries then converge into venules, which carry the blood to the mantle of the islet. This portal arrangement allows high concentrations of insulin from the β cell core to bathe the α, δ, and PP cells of the respective mantles. This type of vascular pattern also suggests the possible paracrine effects of insulin on the outer islet cell types. Each β and α cell has a basal (arterial) and an apical (venous) face. Between the lateral surfaces of neighboring β cells run canaliculi that span the distance between the arteriolar and venous ends of the cell. These canaliculi carry interstitial fluid in a venous direction and they permit selective exposure of the lateral cell surfaces to regulatory molecules, such as glucose (Fig. 41-2).

The islets are innervated by parasympathetic, sympathetic, and peptidergic nerves. The δ cells in the mantle are dendritic in shape, and they send granule-containing processes into the β cell core; these features suggest an additional neurocrine pathway of intraislet regulation by somatostatin.

Within the islet cells, hormones are stored in secretory granules with smooth membranes. These secretory granules are more heavily distributed in the apical venous (secretory) side of the cell (Fig. 41-2). Islet cells also contain a system of microtubules that are often arranged in parallel bundles that separate linear rows of secretory granules. In addition, microfilaments containing myosin and actin form a web adjacent to the plasma membrane and in association with the microtubules. These structures probably facilitate active movement of the secretory granules to the plasma membrane.

INSULIN

Structure and Synthesis

The structure of insulin and the process by which insulin is synthesized are presented in some detail as an example of how a complex protein or peptide hormone is made.

Structure.   Insulin consists of two straight peptide chains (called the A and B chains) that are linked together (Fig. 41-3). The molecular weight of insulin is 6000. The A chain, containing 21 amino acids, and the B chain, containing 30 amino acids, are connected by two disulfide bridges. In addition, the A chain contains an intrachain disulfide ring (Fig. 41-3). The tertiary structure of insulin is determined by the N-terminal and C-terminal amino acids of the A chain and the hydrophobic character of the amino acids at the C terminal of the B chain. This tertiary structure is critical to the biological activity of insulin, which resides within the B chain. Insulin monomers readily form a crystalline hexameric unit with two zinc atoms.

> Crystalline zinc insulin (CZI) was, until recently, the most important pharmaceutical preparation used in the management of **diabetes mellitus.** It is a relatively "fast-acting" insulin that is injected subcutaneously to obtain the prompt effect needed in diabetic emergencies or to prevent excessive hyperglycemia after meals. Slower acting insulins were made by altering buffers, pH, and/or zinc concentrations or by adding other substances, like protamine, to CZI. These pharmaceutical insulin preparations are absorbed more slowly from the skin and provide a longer-acting supply of insulin that partially mimics basal insulin delivery. Knowledge of the amino acid sequences and three-dimensional structure of insulin (and related insulin growth factors) has now permitted the design of insulin analogs that are made by substituting, deleting, or changing the sequence of amino acids at strategic sites in the molecule. Such new insulin analogs provide pharmacological therapy that more closely mimics normal insulin secretion patterns (see below). They act by very rapid absorption as insulin monomers before meals, or by exceedingly slow absorption, to provide the necessary continuous exposure of target tissues to the hormone.

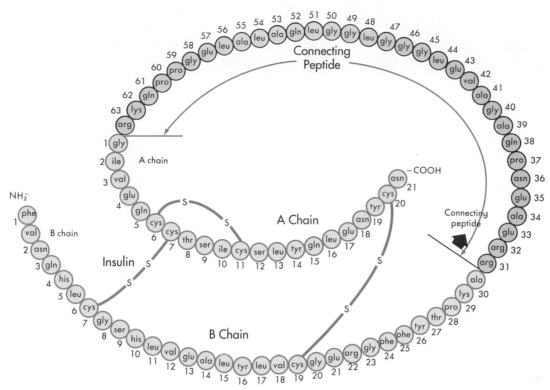

■ Fig. 41-3 The structure of human proinsulin. The solid area is the insulin molecule released by cleavage of the connecting peptide. (From Shaw WN, Chance RE: *Diabetes* 17:737, 1968.)

Synthesis. The process of insulin synthesis is diagrammed in Fig. 41-4. The insulin gene is the ancestral member of a superfamily of genes that encodes a variety of insulin-like growth factor molecules. The gene is composed of four exons and two introns. The gene directs the synthesis of preproinsulin, an insulin precursor with a molecular weight of 11,500. Preproinsulin contains four sequential peptides: an N-terminal signal peptide, the B chain of insulin, a connecting peptide (C peptide), and the A chain of insulin (Fig. 41-3). The N-terminal signal peptide is rapidly cleaved from the molecule at the site of synthesis while the proinsulin chain is being completed. As the proinsulin molecule, containing the A and B chains of insulin and C peptide, is guided to the Golgi apparatus, disulfide linkages are established that yield the "folded" proinsulin molecule, which has a molecular weight of 9000. The disulfide bonded A and B chains of insulin are linked by C peptide through two basic residues, each of which is located at the C-terminal of the B chain and the N-terminal of the A chain (Fig. 41-3). During its packaging into granules by the Golgi apparatus, proinsulin is slowly cleaved by proconvertase-1 and carboxypeptidase-H enzymes that split off the Arg-Arg and Lys-Arg residues, respectively. The resultant insulin molecule, along with the C peptide molecule, is retained in the granules and released by exocytosis in equimolar amounts. Insulin becomes associated with zinc as the secretory granules mature. The zinc insulin crystals form the dense central core of the granule, whereas C peptide is present in the clear space between the granule membrane and the core.

In the trans-Golgi region, 99% of proinsulin is processed in a manner that results in storage granules for regulated insulin release. The remaining 1% of proinsulin escapes storage in granules; this "free" proinsulin maintains a low rate of constitutive insulin secretion. *Insulin synthesis is stimulated by glucose or feeding and is decreased by fasting.* Glucose increases the expression of many β cell genes necessary for protein synthesis, for example, the signal recognition particle receptor that docks preproinsulin to the endoplasmic reticulum. Glucose also upregulates enzyme genes that promote glycolysis and downregulates those that promote gluconeogenesis in β cells. Glucose rapidly increases translation of the insulin mRNA and more slowly increases transcription of the insulin gene. A cyclic AMP (cAMP) regulatory element and a separate glucose regulatory element have been identified in the insulin gene. *In general, synthesis and secretion of insulin are closely linked.*

Insulin Secretion

A large number of factors stimulate or inhibit insulin release (Table 41-1). Because of the preeminent importance of glucose in metabolism, the mechanism whereby this substrate acutely stimulates insulin secretion has been intensively investigated. The following sequence occurs during this stimulation (Fig. 41-5):

1. A specific transporter **(Glut-2),** concentrated in the microvilli of the canaliculi between β cells (Fig. 41-2), facilitates diffusion of glucose into the β cell. This helps maintain the glucose concentration in the β cell at a

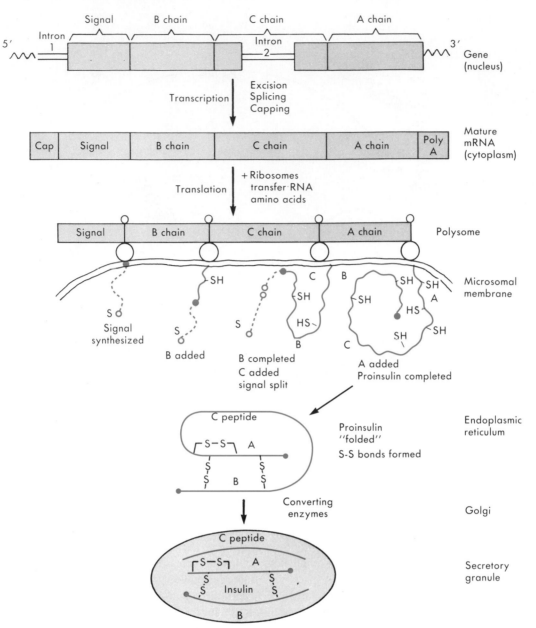

■ **Fig. 41-4**   Insulin synthesis; the insulin gene codes for preproinsulin. The mature messenger RNA initiates synthesis of the N-terminal signal peptide *(S)* in the ribosomes, followed by the B, C, and A chains. The signal is degraded during the course of completion of the proinsulin molecule. The latter is folded into a conformation that permits the disulfide linkages between the A and B chains to form. Within the Golgi and secretory granule, converting enzymes cleave off the C chain, known as the C peptide, completing the synthesis of insulin. The insulin molecules are concentrated in the electron-dense core of the granule, whereas the C peptide molecules are in the peripheral halo areas of the granule. (From Permutt M et al: *Diabetes Care* 7:386, 1984; and from Steiner DF et al: In Degroot LJ et al, editors: *Endocrinology,* vol 2, New York, 1979, Grune & Stratton.)

level that is essentially equal to that of the interstitial fluid.

2. The enzyme glucokinase appears to function as the fundamental glucose sensor that controls the subsequent β cell response. The enzyme has a K_m for glucose of 5 mM, which is in the physiological range. Phosphorylation of glucose by glucokinase is the first and rate-limiting step in islet glucose use. Subsequent glycolysis yields pyruvate. An insulin-releasing signal is then generated downstream from pyruvate, and the subsequent rate of insulin secretion parallels that of glucose oxidation. Although pyruvate and lactate, formed intracellularly from glucose, are stimulators of insulin secretion, pyruvate and lactate provided exogenously from the plasma are not. This is because β cells have very low levels of the plasma membrane

■ **Table 41-1**   Insulin secretion

Increased by	Decreased by
d-Glucose	Fasting
Galactose	Exercise
Mannose	Endurance training
Glyceraldehyde	Somatostatin
Protein	Galanin
Arginine	Pancreastatin
Lysine	Leptin
Leucine	Interleukin-1
Alanine	α-Adrenergic activity
Ketoacids	Prostaglandin E_2
Free fatty acids	Diazoxide
Potassium	
Calcium	
Glucagon	
Glucagon-like peptide 1	
Gastric inhibitory polypeptide	
Secretin	
Cholecystokinin	
Vagal activity	
Acetylcholine	
β-Adrenergic activity	
Sulfonylurea drugs	
Meglitinides	

carriers necessary for the efficient intracellular transport of these organic acids.

3. The oxidation of glucose leads to rapid increases in the intracellular ATP concentration; the ATP/ADP ratio; and concentrations of NADH, NADPH, and H^+. The critical importance of ATP generation is illustrated by the recent discovery that uncoupling protein-2 (UCP-2), which dissociates ATP generation from glucose oxidation, is present in β cells. When UCP-2 is upregulated and less ATP is produced from glucose oxidation, insulin secretion is decreased.

4. An ATP-sensitive K^+ channel closes, K^+ efflux from the β cell is suppressed, and the cell depolarizes. Depolarization opens a voltage-regulated Ca^{2+} channel, and the concentration of intracellular Ca^{2+} rapidly increases. The elevated Ca^{2+} concentration activates the mechanism for secretory granule movement along the microtubules (see Fig. 41-3), perhaps via a myosin light chain kinase. A monomeric G protein (GTPase), attached to the secretory vesicle, interacts with special plasma membrane proteins (fusins). This interaction leads to the fusion of the granule with the membrane. Exocytosis of insulin as hexamers follows. In the portal vein, the hexamers rapidly dissociate to insulin dimers and then more slowly to the biologically active monomers.

All the above processes occur within 1 minute of exposure to glucose. A similar sequence with specific transporters and enzymatic steps probably underlies the less prominent stimulatory action of other fuels, such as amino acids and ketoacids (Fig. 41-5). In addition, a secondary rise in cAMP levels in β cells also follows exposure to glucose; this stimulates insulin release via a cAMP-dependent protein kinase, possibly by phosphorylating proteins involved in exocytosis and also by

facilitating GTP-GDP exchange. Stimulatory G proteins mediate the insulin-releasing effects of such peptides as glucagon, whereas inhibitory G proteins mediate the insulin-suppressive effects of such peptides as somatostatin (Fig. 41-5). A stimulatory G protein linked to phospholipase C mediates the ability of acetylcholine to stimulate insulin release via generation of phosphatidylinositol second messengers and increased protein kinase C activity.

The mechanism for glucose sensing by glucokinase and for generation of a signal by glucose oxidation described above is present in other endocrine cells in the gut and islets, and in various hypothalamic nuclei. These cells are also important in maintaining glucose homeostasis as well as in regulating feeding behavior and energy reserves (see Chapter 40).

A class of **sulfonylurea drugs** stimulates insulin release by binding to a receptor (SUR) that forms one component of the K^+ channel and directly closes it. Two other drug classes bind to different sites on SUR and close the K^+ channel. All these drugs are used in the treatment of **type 2 non–insulin-dependent diabetes** by increasing insulin secretion. In contrast, the drug **diazoxide** opens the K^+ channel and thereby inhibits insulin release. Diazoxide is useful in the treatment of hyperinsulinism.

Many nuances exist in glucose-stimulated insulin release. For example, newly synthesized insulin molecules are preferentially secreted. In addition, individual β cells differ in their sensitivity to glucose, and only some of them respond at any one time. Those at the center of the islet show greater and faster responsiveness. If β cells are dispersed or their gap junctions are functionally blocked, insulin secretion is markedly reduced; these observations demonstrate the importance of cell-to-cell signaling in insulin secretion. Finally, an intrinsic, nonneural oscillation of β cell membrane potential, cytoplasmic Ca^{2+} concentration, ATP/ADP ratio, and insulin release exists, with a cycle of 13 to 15 minutes. Because plasma insulin levels follow a similar cycle, an unidentified pacemaker must coordinate islet function throughout the pancreas. The amplitude of insulin pulses is increased by electrical stimulation of intrapancreatic ganglia.

In rare instances, mild diabetes mellitus is caused by genetic abnormalities in the structure of proinsulin, insulin, proinsulin processing enzymes, or other molecules involved in insulin release. Some mutant genes express insulin molecules with reduced biological activity or proinsulin molecules that cannot be processed correctly. Other mutant genes express Glut-2 transporters or glucokinases with reduced affinity for glucose, and thus impair glucose uptake or sensing by β cells.

Regulation of Insulin Secretion

In the broadest sense, insulin secretion is governed by a feedback relationship with exogenous nutrient supply

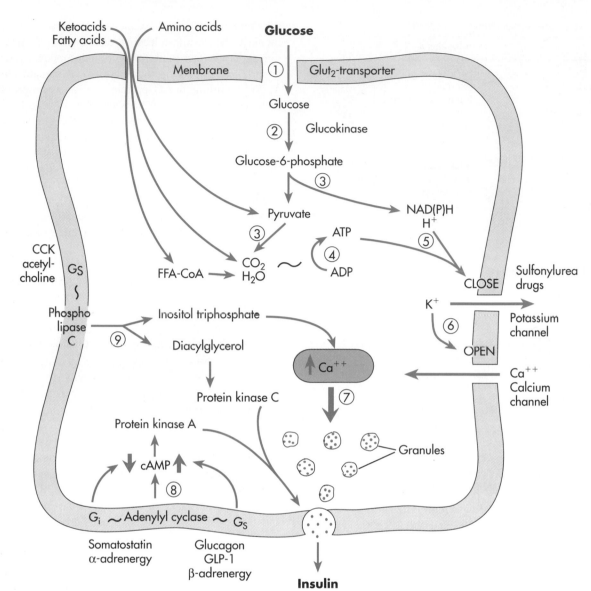

■ **Fig. 41-5**   Current concepts of regulation of insulin secretion by the β cell. Glucose transport *(1)* and glucokinase-catalyzed phosphorylation *(2)* raise glucose-6-phosphate levels. Metabolism *(3)* subsequently leads to increased adenosine triphosphate (ATP) levels *(4)* and NAD(P)H levels *(5)* that inhibit or close a potassium channel *(6)* and open a calcium channel *(6)*. Increased calcium levels then trigger exocytosis of insulin granules *(7)*. Other modulators of secretion act via the adenylyl cyclase–cAMP–protein kinase pathway *(8)* and the phospholipase-phosphoinositide pathway *(9)*. *GLP-1*, Glucagon-like peptide-1; *CCK*, cholecystokinin; *NAD(P)H*, reduced nicotine adenine dinucleotide phosphate; *ADP*, adenosine diphosphate.

(Fig. 41-6). *When substrate supply is abundant, insulin is secreted in response. Insulin then stimulates the use of these incoming nutrients and simultaneously inhibits the mobilization of analogous endogenous substrates. When nutrient supply is low or absent, insulin secretion is dampened and mobilization of endogenous fuels is enhanced.*

Glucose is the insulin stimulant of greatest importance in humans. Because insulin in turn stimulates the use of glucose, this substrate-hormone pair forms a feedback system for close regulation of plasma glucose levels. The relationship between plasma insulin and plasma glucose is sigmoidal (Fig. 41-7). Virtually no insulin is secreted below a plasma

glucose threshold of about 50 mg/dl. A half-maximal insulin secretory response occurs at a plasma glucose level of about 150 mg/dl; a maximal insulin response occurs at a level of about 300 mg/dl.

Both in vitro and in vivo, insulin secretion exhibits a biphasic response to a continuous glucose stimulus (Fig. 41-8). Within seconds of exposure to glucose, an immediate pulse of insulin is released that peaks at 1 minute and then returns toward baseline. After 10 minutes of continuous stimulation, a second phase of secretion begins. During this phase, plasma levels of insulin rise more slowly and reach a second plateau, which can be maintained for many hours in normal

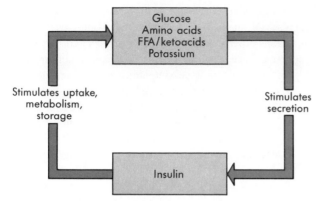

■ **Fig. 41-6** Feedback relationship between insulin and nutrients. Those nutrients that stimulate insulin secretion are the same nutrients whose disposal is facilitated by insulin, demonstrating a hormonally regulated metabolic feedback loop. *FFA,* Free fatty acids.

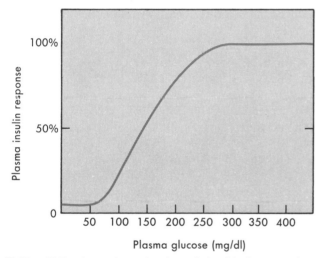

■ **Fig. 41-7** Approximate in vivo relationship between plasma glucose and insulin secretion, the latter being assessed by the plasma insulin response to stepwise infusion of glucose in humans. No insulin is secreted below a plasma glucose level of 50 mg/dl. Half-maximal secretion occurs at 125 to 150 mg/dl. (Redrawn from Karam JH et al: *Diabetes* 23:763, 1974.)

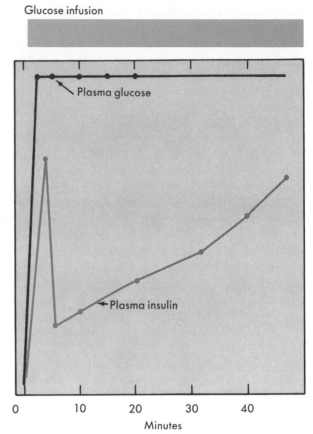

■ **Fig. 41-8** Insulin response to glucose infusion shows a rapid first phase of insulin release followed by a fall and a later, slower second phase.

individuals. This biphasic response may result from (1) rapid insulin generation, followed by the slow removal of a substance that is formed after glucose stimulation and acts as a feedback inhibitor of insulin release, (2) granules with different sensitivities to glucose, and (3) glucose stimulation of insulin synthesis that sustains the later secretory phase.

When glucose is given orally, a greater insulin response is elicited than when plasma glucose is elevated comparably by intravenous administration. This augmented insulin response to oral glucose is accounted for by one or more gastrointestinal hormones that are released in response to meals and that are capable of potentiating glucose-stimulated insulin secretion (Table 41-1). Glucagon-like peptide 1 (GLP-1) and gastric inhibitory polypeptide (GIP) are the most important of these insulinogogues. The prompt gastroin-testinal mechanism of insulinogenesis moderates the early rise in plasma glucose that follows the ingestion and absorption of a carbohydrate meal. In contrast, somatostatin released within pancreatic islets (**paracrine** or **neurocrine**) and from intestinal cells (**endocrine**) may dampen insulin responses to meals.

Insulin secretion is also stimulated by amino acids that result from digestion of protein in a meal. The basic amino acids, arginine and lysine, are the most potent stimulants; leucine, alanine, and other amino acids contribute modestly to this effect. Glucose and amino acids are synergistic stimulators of insulin release, so that the plasma insulin rise that follows a meal represents more than the additive effects of its carbohydrate and protein content. Triglycerides exert only a small stimulatory effect on insulin release in humans. In fact, this small effect may be mostly indirect and exerted by means of GIP. Ketoacids at concentrations that prevail during prolonged fasting (see Fig. 40-11) modestly stimulate insulin secretion; this effect may help sustain a critical low level of insulin when β cell stimulation by ingested nutrients is absent.

The role of free fatty acids (FFA) in insulin secretion has been recently reexamined. FFA, especially the longer chain and more saturated molecules such as stearate, enhance insulin response to glucose during total fasting when plasma

FFA rises and the β cell content of FFA-CoA increases. Even in nonfasting states, the operation of the Randle glucose-FFA cycle (see Chapter 40) within β cells raises intracellular FFA-CoA derivatives, as a result of glucose oxidation and formation of acetyl-CoA and malonyl-CoA. FFA-CoA increase can lead to increased plasma membrane phospholipids, which in turn give rise to increased diacylglycerol and more activation of protein kinase C (Fig. 41-5).

However, long-term exposure of β cells to elevated FFA can have deleterious effects on insulin secretion. This occurs because FFA also stimulates apoptosis of β cells.

Both potassium and calcium are essential for normal insulin responses to glucose. Thus, relative insulin deficiency occurs in subjects depleted of potassium, calcium, or the calcitropic hormone, vitamin D. Magnesium exerts at least a modulatory effect. Sympathetic nerves and epinephrine stimulate insulin secretion via β-adrenergic receptors, but they inhibit insulin secretion via α-adrenergic receptors. Parasympathetic activity via the vagus nerve increases insulin release. In addition, a cephalic phase of insulin secretion precedes the entrance of food into the gastrointestinal tract.

An increase in the number of β cells (hyperplasia) can also lead to an increase in insulin secretion. A variety of other hormones, directly or indirectly, cause hyperplasia of the β cells and a subsequent increase in insulin secretion, largely by antagonizing insulin action and increasing insulin need by peripheral tissues. These hormones include cortisol, growth hormone, human placental lactogen, and thyroid hormones. The β cell has insulin receptors, and insulin has a negative feedback effect on its own secretion; this effect is independent of any effect on plasma glucose concentration. The binding of insulin to its own receptors in β cells can also initiate mitogenic actions of insulin on its own cell of origin; this constitutes a form of positive feedback. Leptin also inhibits insulin synthesis and insulin release, the latter by opening the ATP-dependent K+ channel. This action closes a negative feedback loop between the two hormones (see Chapter 40), because insulin stimulates leptin secretion, independent of insulin's ability to increase adipose mass.

The net result of these many influences on insulin secretion is to maintain an average basal peripheral plasma insulin level of 10 μU/ml (7×10^{-11} M) in humans. After several days of fasting, this value declines over 50%. A similar decrease occurs during prolonged exercise. Plasma insulin levels increase 3-fold to 10-fold after a typical meal, and they usually peak 30 to 60 minutes after eating is initiated (Fig. 41-9). Plasma C peptide, coreleased with insulin, fluctuates similarly (Fig. 41-9). In addition to the intrinsic, low-level, 15-minute cycles and the bursts of insulin secretion stimulated by meals, a higher amplitude insulin cycle exists. This cycle has pulses lasting 2 hours that are entrained by glucose and that represent feedback regulation. The liver is regularly exposed to insulin concentrations two or three times higher than those of other organs in the basal state, and that are transiently 5 to 10 times higher after β cell stimulation.

Obesity markedly increases insulin secretion (Fig. 41-9), whereas sustained physical conditioning decreases it. These alterations at least partly reflect decreases and increases, respectively, in responsiveness to insulin action. The hyperinsulinemia that accompanies excess weight gain and a sedentary life style is a risk factor (though not necessarily a causative agent) for the later development of **type 2 non–insulin-dependent diabetes mellitus,** as well as for cardiovascular disease and mortality. During exercise, insulin levels decline, a response that facilitates mobilization of fuels.

In addition to resistance to insulin action and compensatory hyperinsulinemia (and accompanying hyperproinsulinemia), more subtle abnormalities in insulin secretion occur in the early phase of type 2 diabetes. These abnormalities, which include altered cyclicity, diminished pulse frequency, and a delayed response to rising glucose levels, evolve later into a complete loss of recognition of glucose as a stimulus for insulin secretion. Finally, other nutrient and pharmacological stimuli also become ineffective, and therapy with insulin is required.

Because aging is associated with a decreased ability to metabolize glucose, any effect of age on insulin availability would be important. In a large population cross-sectional study, increasing age (range 18–85) was associated with a 25% decline in posthepatic insulin delivery to the systemic circulation. A similar decline was found in the metabolic clearance rate of the hormone. Therefore, the net effect of age on systemic basal plasma insulin levels (and likely on glucose-stimulated levels) was neutral. Overall, the insulin delivery rate was directly correlated with body mass index, visceral adiposity, and fasting plasma glucose.

Insulin circulates unbound to any carrier protein. Its half-life in plasma is 5 to 8 minutes and its metabolic clearance rate is about 1000 ml/min. Basal insulin delivery rates to the peripheral circulation in humans are about 0.5 to 1 unit/hr (20 to 40 μg/hr). During meals, the delivery rate increases up to 10-fold, and the total daily peripheral delivery of insulin is about 30 units. If the amount of insulin removed during its first pass through the liver is accounted for (approximately 50% of portal vein insulin), the actual β cell secretory rate becomes approximately 60 units/day. The liver decreases its extraction of insulin in response to glucose and meals. As a result, a greater amount of insulin escapes to the periphery for stimulation of nutrient uptake.

Insulin is metabolized largely in the kidneys and liver by specific enzymes that split the disulfide bonds and separate the A and B chains. Very little insulin is excreted unchanged in the urine. Degradation of insulin also occurs in association with its plasma membrane receptor after it is internalized by target cells.

Although C peptide is secreted in amounts that are equimolar to insulin, its basal peripheral plasma levels are approximately 5-fold higher, averaging 1 ng/ml (3×10^{-10} M). This difference is caused by a lower rate of metabolic clearance

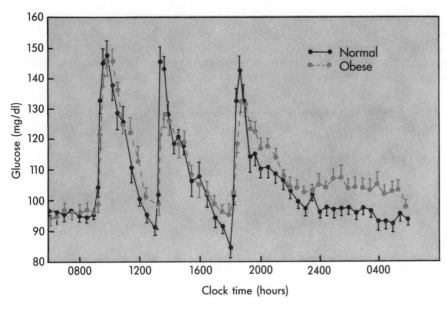

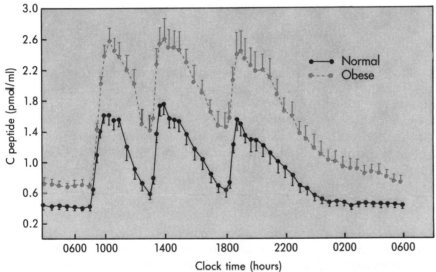

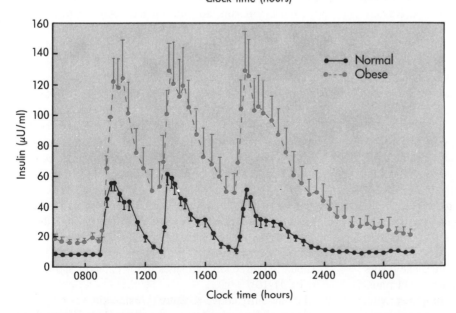

■ **Fig. 41-9** Twenty-four-hour profiles of plasma glucose, C peptide, and insulin in normal weight *(solid lines)* and obese *(dotted lines)* humans. Note the parallel increases with each meal, the rapid return toward baseline, and the exaggerated β cell responses in obesity. (Redrawn from Polonsky K et al: *J Clin Invest* 81:442, 1988.)

for C peptide. In contrast to insulin, C peptide is not extracted appreciably by the liver. Therefore, plasma (and even urine) C peptide measurements can actually provide more accurate information about β cell function than do insulin measurements in some circumstances. Proinsulin is also constitutively released by the β cell in the basal state. During glucose stimulation, proinsulin levels increase more slowly and to a lesser degree than insulin. Although proinsulin exhibits some biological insulin activity (about 5%-10% that of insulin), no physiological function can presently be ascribed to it or to C peptide.

Hypersecretion of insulin is usually caused by a tumor of the β cells. The cardinal manifestation is a low plasma glucose level (<50 mg/dl) in the fasting state. Because the sympathetic nervous system is quickly activated by abrupt hypoglycemia, bursts of insulin hypersecretion produce episodes of rapid heart rate, nervousness, sweating, and hunger. With sustained insulin excess and persistent hypoglycemia, disturbed central nervous system function is manifested by bizarre behavior, defects in cerebration, loss of consciousness, or convulsions. The need to ingest large amounts of carbohydrate, combined with the stimulating effect of insulin on fat storage, produces weight gain. The diagnosis of a β cell tumor is established by demonstrating fasting plasma insulin and C peptide levels that are inappropriately high for the prevailing glucose levels. Removal of the tumor cures the condition. Failing that, drugs that inhibit insulin secretion palliate the hypoglycemia.

Insulin Actions

The effects of insulin are broad in scope, involve many organs and intracellular pathways, and are metabolically critical. In the following discussion, the cellular mechanisms of insulin action are presented first. Tissue and interorgan effects are then discussed. Finally, the total body effects of insulin are correlated with its secretion.

Insulin action on cells. Many steps are involved in the series of events that culminate in insulin actions. The proximal steps are well defined. The distal steps are less well defined, and they grow in complexity as their interactive and web-like characteristics are revealed. The first and overall rate-limiting step in insulin action is the transport of insulin through the capillary wall. Once it arrives at the target cell, insulin combines with a plasma membrane glycoprotein receptor of the type shown in Fig. 39-12. This tetramer contains an extracellular α subunit with 731 amino acids. This α subunit is disulfide-bonded to a larger β subunit, which traverses the plasma membrane and resides largely within the cytoplasm. Two such identical α-β dimers are joined extracellularly by another disulfide (Fig. 41-10). The β subunit has 194 extracellular residues, a 23-amino acid transmembrane anchor, and an intracytoplasmic component with 403 residues. There are 200,000 to 300,000 insulin receptor molecules per target cell.

The insulin receptor gene is a member of a superfamily that codes for other growth factor receptors. Its structure is shown in Fig. 41-11. The insulin receptor gene illustrates how the many functions of a receptor can be packaged in a DNA molecule. The gene, which contains 22 exons (Fig. 41-11), codes for a proreceptor molecule. This proreceptor contains, in sequence, a signal peptide, the α subunit, a proreceptor processing site, and the β subunit. After translation and removal of the signal peptide, two proreceptor molecules associate into a disulfide dimer. After this disulfide dimer is formed, a basic amino acid site on each dimer is cleaved. This cleavage yields the discrete α and β subunits of the insulin receptor, linked by the preformed disulfide bonds. Of great importance to receptor function are exons 17 to 21, which code for its tyrosine kinase activity.

Alternate splicing yields insulin receptor A, which lacks exon 11 and is preferentially expressed initially in fetal cells and later in all cells. Insulin receptor A is expressed uniquely in brain, lymphocytes, and spleen. Insulin receptor B contains exon 11 (coding for 12 amino acids in the α-subunit) and is predominantly expressed in muscle, adipose tissue, liver, and kidney. The location of key sites of function and of key tyrosines is shown in Fig. 41-12.

After insulin binds to the insulin receptor on a target cell, a conformational change occurs that leads to aggregation of receptors. The hormone-receptor complex is subsequently internalized by endocytosis; the hormone is degraded; and the receptor is either degraded, stored, or recycled back to the plasma membrane. Insulin downregulates the insulin receptor by increasing its rate of degradation and by suppressing its synthesis. This phenomenon is one reason why obese subjects have a decreased sensitivity to insulin (Fig. 41-9). For some actions, full biological activity of insulin is expressed when only 5% of its receptor sites are occupied.

Insulin binding to its receptor causes multiple events to occur at several locations, including the plasma membrane itself, the cytoplasm, and the nucleus. All the intervening molecules and mechanisms that lead from the insulin-receptor complex to the full panoply of insulin's final biological actions have yet to be fully elucidated. The following steps are well documented. The reader is referred to recent reviews for more details (see references by Kido and by White).

1. Initial signal transduction occurs via the receptor tyrosine kinase activity that resides in the intracytoplasmic portion of the β subunit. This kinase is kept inactive when the extracellular α subunit of the receptor is unoccupied by insulin. When a single molecule of insulin binds to its α-subunit site, this kinase is activated. The process of activation possibly takes place via a conformational change transmitted through the receptor molecule. Once the receptor kinase activity is stimulated by binding ATP, it autophosphorylates its β subunit at three key tyrosines in the catalytic domain (Fig. 41-10).

2. The now fully active receptor tyrosine kinase phosphorylates tyrosines on four homologous specific insulin receptor substrates (IRS). IRS-1 and IRS-2 are

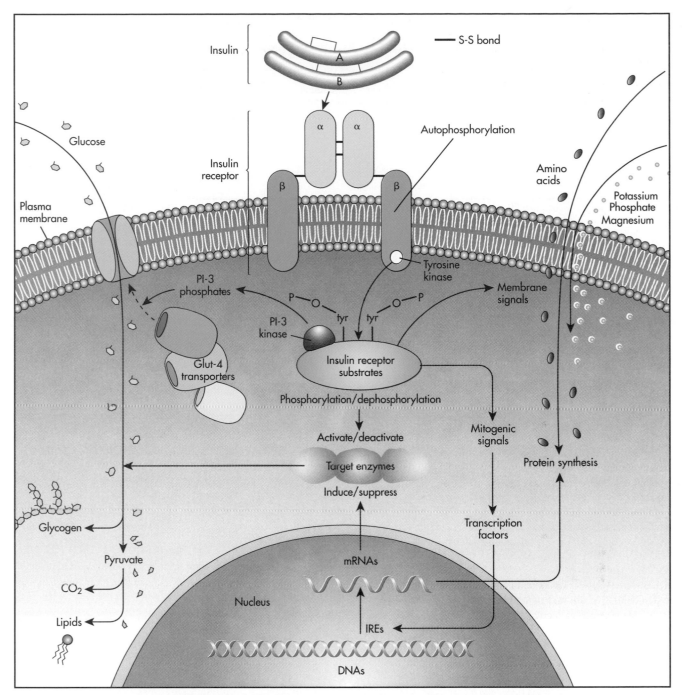

■ **Fig. 41-10** Mechanisms of insulin action on cells. Binding of insulin to the α subunit of its receptor causes autophosphorylation by ATP of intracellular β-subunit receptor tyrosine sites. This generates tyrosine kinase activity. The receptor tyrosine kinase then phosphorylates insulin receptor substrates. The latter begin a cascade of serine and threonine phosphorylations, which activate or deactivate target enzymes of glucose metabolism. Activation of phosphoinositide phosphate-3 kinase (PIP-3K) generates inositol 3,4,5-trisphosphate (PI-3 phosphates), which causes translocation of glucose transporters to the plasma membrane, where they facilitate glucose entry. Also independently, amino acid, potassium, magnesium, and phosphate entries into the cell are facilitated. Docking of other regulatory proteins to the insulin receptor substrates initiates other cascades that stimulate or repress gene transcription via insulin response elements (IREs) in DNA molecules. Mitogenic proteins are also activated that increase transcription factors required to stimulate gene expression concerned with cell growth. (From Scientific American Medicine, WebMD Corp. 9 Metab, August 2001.)

Insulin receptor gene

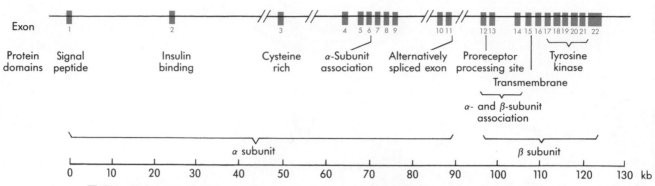

■ **Fig. 41-11** The anatomy of the insulin receptor gene. The final gene product contains two sulfhydryl-bonded subunits. Two of these monomers associate to form the receptor molecule (see Fig. 41-10). (Modified from Seino S, Seino M, Bell GI: *Diabetes* 39:129, 1990.)

■ **Fig. 41-12** The structure and functional domains of the insulin receptor. The location of key functional sites and the particular tyrosines that undergo phosphorylation on the insulin receptor are shown. The extracellular α subunit binds the insulin molecule causing conformational changes in the intracellular tail of the β subunit. ATP is bound by a specific site in the β subunit catalytic domain causing autophosphorylation of tyrosine molecules 965 and 972 in the juxtamembrane domain, 1158, 1162, and 1163 in the catalytic domain, and 1328 and 1334 in the C-terminus. The alternative form of the receptor has undergone removal of exon 11 in the α subunit. The left and right hand sides of the receptor molecule are identical. (Modified from Kido Y, Makae J, Accili D: *J Clin Endocrinol Metab* 86:972, 2001.)

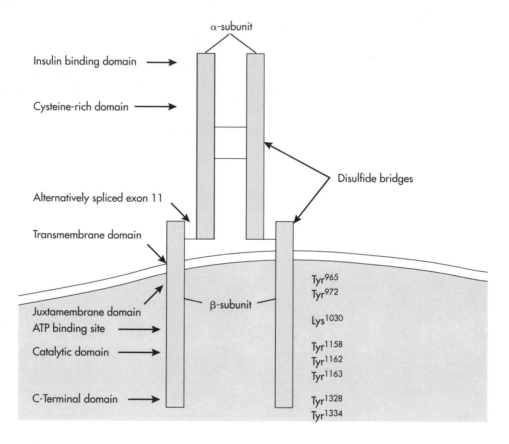

expressed in muscle, adipose, and β cells, and IRS-3 is expressed in the brain. Each of these IRS phosphotyrosines serves as a docking site and possibly an activating site for numerous other protein kinases, protein phosphatases, and facilitatory proteins that link to membrane G proteins, phospholipases, and ion channels. Many of these subsidiary steps involve serine and threonine phosphorylation.

3. IRS tyrosine phosphorylations are followed by various cascades of events that (a) ultimately translocate glucose transport proteins to the plasma membrane, (b) activate or deactivate numerous enzymes in glucose and fatty acid metabolism, and (c) repress or transcribe genes in the nucleus of the target cell. One cascade begins with activation of **phosphatidylinositol-3-kinase** (PI-3-kinase), an enzyme that generates phosphatidylinositol-3,4 and -3,4,5-phosphates. (The resulting inositol-3,4,5-trisphosphate is distinct from the second messenger, inositol-1,4,5-trisphosphate.) The PI-3 phosphates stimulate synthesis and translocation of glucose transporters to the plasma membrane, possibly through activation of protein kinase B (also called Akt) and of protein kinase C isoforms. Other downstream products of PI-3 kinase are S6 kinases that

phosphorylate nuclear accessory proteins involved in gene transcription and that also regulate translation of mRNA.

4. Another IRS-1-initiated **step involves growth receptor binding protein-2 (GRB-2).** This intermediary facilitates the binding of GTP to *ras,* a protooncogene product that resides in the plasma membrane. When thus activated, *ras* starts another series of reactions that stimulate cell growth and differentiation via mitogen-activated protein kinase (MAP kinase). The proto-oncogene c-*Jun* is a factor in this pathway. Other *ras* products participate in insulin activation of the enzyme glycogen synthase. In this context, an additional action of insulin is to inhibit apoptosis of target cells.

5. Serine/threonine phosphorylation of either the insulin receptor or of IRS-1 hastens their degradation and thereby decreases insulin action. Phosphotyrosine protein phosphatases inhibit insulin action by dephosphorylating tyrosines on IRSs. By contrast, vanadium (in the form of vanadyl ions) inhibits phosphotyrosine protein phosphatases; thus vanadyl ions mimic insulin actions.

6. For certain insulin actions, phospholipase C–generated second messengers (i.e., inositol-1,4,5-trisphosphate and diacylglycerol) are needed to produce the full hormone effect.

7. In some target cells, insulin action lowers cAMP levels by activating phosphodiesterase (see Chapter 39) and it reduces cAMP effectiveness by inhibiting its binding to protein kinase A.

8. Insulin also ultimately stimulates phosphorylation of serine-307 in IRS-1. This inhibits further tyrosine phosphorylation of IRS-1. This action of insulin is mediated by PI-3 kinase, and it constitutes still another form of negative feedback, which prevents excessive intracellular effects of the hormone.

The physiological result of many of the above effects is a rapid shift of metabolic directions in the cytoplasm and mitochondria. This shift is brought about by activating or deactivating critical enzymes through either their phosphorylation or their dephosphorylation. Such shifts are reinforced and prolonged, however, by the nuclear effects that emanate from the initial receptor and plasma membrane steps. Although no single consensus DNA sequence acts as an insulin regulatory element (IRE) that accounts for all insulin effects on gene transcription, numerous target DNA molecules exist. Both induction (e.g., glucokinase) and repression (e.g., phosphoenolpyruvate carboxykinase) of gene expression occur. These effects are likely mediated by various insulin-activated transcriptional proteins that bind to one or more DNA molecules.

The insulin signal rapidly stimulates many processes (Fig. 41-10). Within 1 minute, glucose transport into muscle and adipose cells is increased up to 20-fold by activation of a glucose carrier system in the plasma membrane. Insulin rapidly recruits the glucose transporter **Glut-4,** which is specifically expressed in muscle and adipose tissue, from a cytoplasmic pool of vesicles to the plasma membrane. This effect probably comes about by insulin-stimulated remodeling of actin filaments below the plasma membrane and by the consequent ruffling of that membrane. These actions are a necessary step in translocation of the vesicles. The snare proteins (syntax-4 in the plasma membrane and VAMP-2 in the vescicles) are essential intermediates in effectuating translocation. Insulin also increases the activity of the glucose transporter. Transcription of the Glut-4 gene is stimulated more slowly.

Glut-4 facilitates diffusion of glucose down its concentration gradient by increasing the maximum velocity of that movement. This process does not require energy. The importance of this insulin action is underscored by the fact that at low physiological insulin concentrations, glucose transport is the rate-limiting step in glucose use. At high physiological insulin concentrations, such as after a meal, the rate-limiting step may shift to an unknown downstream point in intracellular glucose metabolism. Insulin also facilitates independently the cellular uptake of the amino acids that utilize transporter system A (see Chapter 1), as well as the uptake of potassium, magnesium, and phosphate (Fig. 41-10).

After glucose and amino acids are transported into the cytoplasm, insulin also directs the disposition of these substances. Conversion of glucose to glycogen, to pyruvate, to lactate, and to fatty acids is all stimulated to varying degrees. Glycogen synthesis is increased by dephosphorylation of glycogen synthase, through insulin inhibition of glycogen synthase kinase and stimulation of a protein phosphatase. Synthesis of specific proteins, such as albumin, casein, and various enzymes from amino acids, is selectively enhanced. Inhibition of proteolytic and lipolytic enzymes protects protein and triglyceride stores. Another insulin-stimulated action of metabolic importance is the translocation of Na^+,K^+-ATPase to the plasma membrane, which thus increases energy expenditure. Finally, insulin inhibits the translocation of its own receptor to the plasma membrane, and thereby limits the extent of the hormone's actions.

An estimated 15 million people in the United States have **type 2 non–insulin-dependent diabetes mellitus,** and the incidence is increasing worldwide. In the United States, the prevalence of type 2 diabetes is expected to double by the year 2025. Because a major cause of this form of diabetes is resistance to insulin, much research into mechanisms of insulin action is motivated by the need to pinpoint the defects and to find specific remedies. With uncommon individual or family exceptions, mutations in the insulin receptor, its kinase activity, IRS-1, PI-3 kinase, Glut-4, glycogen synthase, and several other enzymes and receptors involved in glucose metabolism have thus far been eliminated as the primary cause of hyperglycemia in the usual patient. In patients with various mutant insulin receptors, diabetes ranges from mild (in which the defect merely decreases the receptor affinity for insulin) to lethal in infancy (in which the defect completely prevents the receptor from being properly processed or translocated to the plasma membrane).

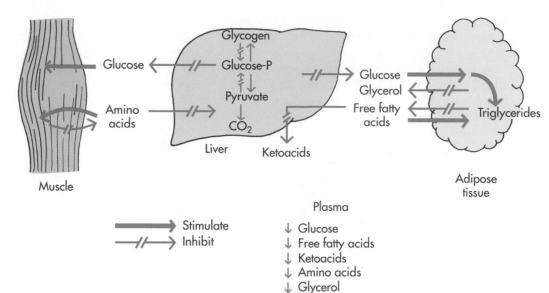

■ **Fig. 41-13** The effect of insulin on the overall flow of fuels results in tissue uptake and sequestration of glucose, free fatty acids, and amino acids, with a resultant decrease in their plasma levels. Glucose, free fatty acid, glycerol, and amino acids release is inhibited. There is a resultant decrease in the plasma levels of these substrates.

Actions on flow of fuels. *Insulin is the hormone of abundance. When the influx of nutrients exceeds concurrent energy needs and rates of anabolism, insulin induces efficient storage of the excess nutrients while suppressing mobilization of endogenous substrates.* The stored nutrients can then be made available during subsequent fasting periods to maintain glucose delivery to the central nervous system and free fatty acid delivery to the muscle mass and viscera. *The major targets for insulin action are the muscle mass, the liver, and adipose tissue.* Figure 41-13 displays the general flow of substrates produced by insulin; Fig. 41-14 shows the important metabolic control points at which insulin acts directly or indirectly in the liver.

Carbohydrates. Insulin stimulates glucose oxidation and storage while simultaneously inhibiting glucose production. Therefore, insulin either lowers the basal circulating glucose concentration or limits the rise in plasma glucose that results from a dietary carbohydrate load. These actions are accomplished by a number of insulin effects.

Liver. In the liver, extracellular glucose levels equilibrate rapidly with intracellular levels by means of the Glut-2 transporter. Insulin enhances inward movement of glucose by inducing hepatic glucokinase, which catalyzes phosphorylation of the incoming glucose to glucose-6-phosphate. Insulin then promotes storage of glucose as glycogen, by activating the glycogen synthase enzyme complex. At the same time, insulin stimulates glycolysis, which converts glucose to pyruvate and lactate, by increasing the activities of the committed enzymes, phosphofructokinase and pyruvate kinase. Oxidation of the pyruvate and lactate is stimulated by increased pyruvate dehydrogenase activity. Insulin also rapidly inhibits hepatic glycogenolysis, and therefore hepatic glucose output, by decreasing glycogen phosphorylase activity and also by decreasing glucose-6-phosphatase levels (Fig. 41-14). The suppression of hepatic glucose output by insulin during assimilation of ingested carbohydrates is an important factor in preventing undue hyperglycemia.

In addition, insulin inhibits gluconeogenesis. This inhibition is accomplished by decreasing the hepatic uptake of precursor amino acids and their availability from muscle (Fig. 41-13). Insulin also decreases the levels or activities of the committed gluconeogenic enzymes, namely pyruvate carboxylase, phosphoenolpyruvate carboxykinase, and fructose-1,6-bisphosphatase. Thus, pyruvate is shunted toward acetyl-CoA in the mitochondria; the acetyl-CoA can be returned to the cytoplasm via citrate, regenerated as acetyl-CoA, and directed into fatty acid synthesis.

Many hepatic effects of insulin require concurrent administration of glucose, and they represent amplification of biochemical events that are induced by glucose itself. Some of these effects are also augmented, because insulin inhibits the secretion of glucagon, a hormone with effects that are antagonistic to those of insulin.

If plasma insulin is raised by continuously infusing insulin into subjects in the basal state, the plasma glucose level declines as hepatic glucose output falls. However, hepatic glucose production quickly recovers from its low point. This recovery reflects three counterregulatory processes: (1) an autoregulatory response of the liver to a lowered plasma glucose concentration, probably mediated by the direct effects of glucose on phosphorylase and other enzymes; (2) a sensing of hypoglycemia by glucose sensors in the portal vein and in the hypothalamus, which stimulates glucose output via activation of the sympathetic nervous system; and (3) a sensing of hypoglycemia by the cells of the pancreatic islets, which then secrete the insulin antagonist, glucagon. These mechanisms protect the central nervous system from glucose deprivation caused by the unchecked action of insulin.

Muscle. Insulin stimulates the transport of glucose into muscle cells. Depending on the insulin concentration, 20% to 50% of the glucose that enters undergoes oxidation, mainly caused by the activation of pyruvate dehydrogenase. The remainder is specifically directed into storage as glycogen

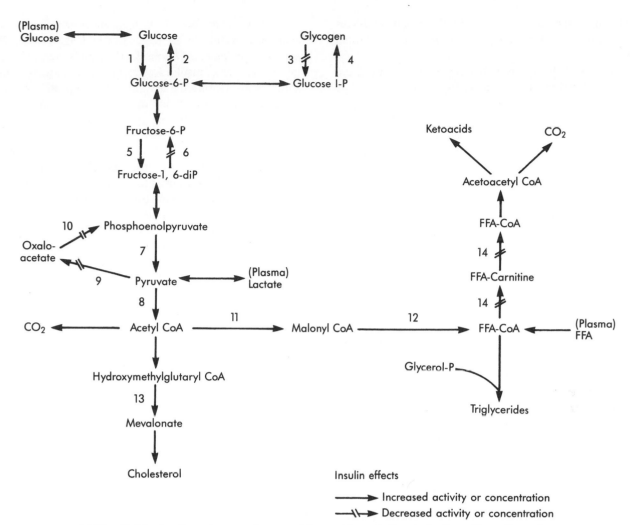

Fig. 41-14 Insulin actions on glucose and fatty acid metabolism in the liver. The pathway from pyruvate to glucose via oxaloacetate constitutes gluconeogenesis. Acetyl-CoA generated from pyruvate can be converted to fatty acids via malonyl-CoA. The key enzymes involved that are influenced by insulin are as follows: *1,* glucokinase; *2,* glucose-6-phosphatase; *3,* phosphorylase; *4,* glycogen synthase; *5,* phosphofructokinase; *6,* fructose-1,6-bisphosphatase; *7,* pyruvate kinase; *8,* pyruvate dehydrogenase; *9,* pyruvate carboxylase; *10,* phosphoenolpyruvate carboxykinase; *11,* acetyl-CoA carboxylase; *12,* fatty acid synthase; *13,* hydroxy-methylglutaryl-CoA reductase; and *14,* carnitine acyltransferase.

by insulin activation of glycogen synthase. Muscle blood flow also increases as a consequence of insulin action. Slow twitch "high oxidative" type I fibers, which depend more on fatty acid fuel, are actually more sensitive to insulin action on glucose uptake than are the fast twitch "glycolytic" and more glucose-dependent type II muscle fibers.

Adipose tissues. In adipose tissue also, insulin stimulates the transport of glucose into the cells. Much of this glucose is then converted to α-glycerophosphate, which is used in the esterification of fatty acids and permits their storage as triglycerides. To a minor extent, glucose can also be converted to fatty acids (Fig. 41-14).

Fat metabolism. The metabolism of both endogenous and exogenous fat is profoundly influenced by insulin. *The net overall effect of insulin is to enhance storage and to block mobilization and oxidation of fatty acids* (Fig. 41-13). Insulin

rapidly lowers the circulating levels of FFAs and ketoacids and may eventually reduce the level of triglycerides.

In adipose tissue, the storage of fat is stimulated by insulin in several ways. Most important, insulin profoundly inhibits **hormone-sensitive lipase activity in adipose tissue.** It accomplishes this inhibition by decreasing the levels of cAMP and by inhibiting protein kinase A. By suppressing lipolysis and the release of stored fatty acids and glycerol, insulin diminishes their delivery to the liver and peripheral tissues. It is noteworthy that abdominal visceral fat is less sensitive to insulin than is subcutaneous fat. This promotes a greater flow of FFA and glycerol from the visceral fat depots that drain into the portal vein, and thereby supports hepatic gluconeogenesis, as previously described.

A major consequence of decreased FFA flow to the liver is a marked reduction in the generation of ketoacids. Insulin also stimulates the use of ketoacids by the peripheral tissues. *Thus, insulin is the major and perhaps the sole antiketogenic hormone.*

Insulin also actively promotes deposition of circulating fat into adipose tissue by activating the key enzymes necessary for this process. The enzyme, adipose tissue lipoprotein lipase, which catalyzes hydrolysis of very-low-density lipoprotein (VLDL) and chylomicron triglycerides to FFA (see Chapter 40), is induced by insulin. The action of this enzyme makes FFAs available for transfer into adipose cells (Fig. 41-13). α-Glycerophosphate, needed for esterification of the FFAs, is generated from glyceraldehyde phosphate; the necessary enzyme, glyceraldehyde phosphate dehydrogenase, is also induced by insulin.

Muscle. Within muscle, insulin suppresses the enzyme lipoprotein lipase in inverse proportion to its stimulation of glucose uptake. Insulin also inhibits lipolysis of triglyceride stores contained within muscle. The sensitivity equals that which inhibits this process in adipose tissue. Thus in muscle, FFA uptake, release from triglycerides, and oxidation are inhibited by insulin. This occurs especially in the type I oxidative fibers that depend most on FFAs. These overall actions of insulin on fat metabolism within muscle reinforce the principle that glucose and FFAs are competitive energy substrates.

Liver. *Within the liver, insulin is also antiketogenic and lipogenic.* Under the influence of insulin, FFAs that enter from the circulation are shunted away from β oxidation and ketogenesis (Figs. 41-13 and 41-14). They are instead reesterified with D-glycerophosphate, derived either from glucose via insulin-stimulated glycolysis or from glycerol via the enzyme glycerophosphate kinase, to form triglycerides. Fatty acids are also synthesized from glucose under the influence of insulin. Mitochondrial acetyl-CoA generated from pyruvate by the action of pyruvate dehydrogenase is transferred to the cytoplasm, where it is converted to malonyl-CoA by the action of acetyl-CoA carboxylase. This rate-limiting step in fatty acid synthesis is activated by insulin, which also induces the final enzyme involved, namely fatty acid synthase. Moreover, insulin increases the activity of the hexose monophosphate shunt by inducing the enzyme, glucose-6-phosphate dehydrogenase. This shunt generates the supply of reduced NADP, which is also needed for fatty acid synthesis.

The antiketogenic action of insulin in the liver may also be mediated by stimulation of malonyl-CoA formation, because malonyl-CoA inhibits the enzyme, carnitine acyltransferase (Fig. 41-14). The latter enzyme is responsible for transferring FFAs from the cytoplasm into the mitochondria for oxidation and conversion to ketoacids (Chapter 40).

Insulin also favors hepatic synthesis of cholesterol from acetyl-CoA by activating the rate-limiting enzyme, hydroxymethylglutaryl-CoA reductase. In parallel with increasing hepatic triglyceride storage, insulin decreases apolipoprotein B synthesis; the net result is an acute suppression of VLDL release. However, under conditions of continuous, long-term hyperinsulinemia, the high rate of triglyceride synthesis ultimately elevates circulating VLDL levels.

Protein metabolism. Insulin enhances protein and amino acid sequestration in all target tissues (Fig. 41-13). *Thus, insulin is an anabolic hormone.* If administered to subjects in the basal state, insulin lowers the plasma levels of many amino acids. During the assimilation of a protein meal, the increase in insulin secretion limits the rise of plasma amino acid levels, especially of the essential branched-chain amino acids, leucine, valine, and isoleucine. In muscle, insulin stimulates the sodium-dependent transport of neutral amino acids across the muscle cell membrane. Although insulin stimulates the general rate of protein synthesis in vitro, this stimulation is evident in vivo mostly when amino acids are in abundance after a meal. (In the basal state, insulin limits the availability of endogenous amino acids for new protein synthesis.) The mechanisms include increases in gene transcription for numerous proteins (e.g., albumin and the growth hormone receptor), in rates of mRNA translation, in general RNA synthesis, and in ribosome synthesis. RNA degradation is decreased by insulin.

Even more dramatically, *insulin inhibits proteolysis.* This action is manifested by suppression of the release of branched-chain and aromatic amino acids from muscle and inhibition of their oxidation. In contrast, insulin has little effect on the flux of alanine.

As already noted, the genes for insulin and its receptor are related to genes that encode a variety of tissue growth factors. These growth factors include somatomedins [insulin-like growth factors 1 and 2 (IGF-1 and IGF-2)], epidermal growth factor, nerve growth factor, and relaxin. Insulin is not only a general anabolic hormone, but it also stimulates the synthesis of macromolecules in tissues such as cartilage and bone and thereby directly contributes to body growth. It also indirectly contributes to growth by stimulating the transcription of other related gene growth factors, such as IGF-1, and by suppressing the gene for one of the IGF-1-binding proteins. The insulin-deprived young animal or human has a reduced lean body and bone mass, and it may be profoundly retarded in height and maturation.

Other actions. Both protein anabolism and the storage of glucose as glycogen require the concurrent cellular uptake of potassium, phosphate, and magnesium. Insulin stimulates translocation of all three minerals into muscle cells and of potassium and phosphate into the liver. Therefore, insulin, secreted in response to a carbohydrate load, lowers serum potassium, phosphate, and magnesium levels, and this hormone is considered to be one of the normal regulators of potassium balance. Another effect of insulin on electrolyte balance is to increase reabsorption of potassium, phosphate, and sodium by the tubules of the kidney. These renal effects contribute to anabolism by conserving these vital electrolytes. Sodium is necessary for formation of the additional extracellular fluid required when lean body mass is expanding. Insulin likely regulates the extent to which the kidney may contribute to endogenous glucose production during fasting (Chapter 40), because insulin decreases renal gluconeogenesis.

The overall consumption of glucose by the central nervous system is independent of insulin. However, selected areas of the brain, particularly the hypothalamus and its adjacent capillary endothelium, contain insulin receptors and are insulin responsive. Insulin also reaches the cerebrospinal fluid from plasma, and when it is injected into the cerebral ventricles of primates, it decreases food intake. This action is partly mediated by a direct suppressive effect on neuropeptide Y release (see Chapter 40). In addition, continuous insulin excess increases body weight and adipose mass, and with the latter, leptin levels increase to induce satiety. If endogenous or exogenous insulin causes hypoglycemia, food intake will be stimulated by other pathways and will contribute to weight gain.

Insulin also affects blood flow in skeletal muscle and adipose tissue. An overall vasodilator effect is mediated by an increase in nitric oxide synthesis. However, this is partially counterbalanced by insulin augmentation of the action of the vasoconstrictor, endothelin-1.

Note that the β cells, which secrete insulin, also possess insulin receptors and IRS molecules. Thus insulin can have autocrine effects. Gene knockout studies have demonstrated that the insulin responsiveness pathway in β cells is essential for development of normal-size islets (which are predominately β cells) and for glucose-stimulated insulin release. This pathway may also be responsible for the ability of insulin to suppress its own release when glucose levels are kept constant.

Correlation of insulin secretion and action. The insulin sensitivity of tissues relates well to prevailing plasma insulin levels in subjects in various physiological states (Fig. 41-15). Suppression of lipolysis and FFA mobilization and consequent ketogenesis are the most sensitive insulin actions. Slightly less sensitive insulin actions are inhibition of hepatic glucose production and of muscle proteolysis, as exemplified by the release of branched-chain amino acids (Fig. 41-15). Stimulation of glucose uptake by muscle requires considerably higher insulin concentrations.

The normal postabsorptive plasma insulin concentration of about 10 µU/ml permits a finely regulated flow of FFA substrates for energy, with minimal ketogenesis during the daily nocturnal fasting period. In addition, sufficient glycogenolysis is permitted to sustain the plasma glucose level. Shortly after a person eats, insulin concentrations rise to 30 µU/ml and hepatic glucose output is greatly suppressed. When postprandial levels rise to 50 to 100 µU/ml, muscle proteolysis is completely inhibited, and glucose and amino acid uptake by peripheral tissues are strongly stimulated. These processes facilitate the use of substrates when they are abundant. Under maximal insulin stimulation at concentrations of approximately 200 µU/ml, peripheral glucose use increases from 2 to 12 mg/kg/min. Of this total increase, two-thirds is accounted for by storage as glycogen. *Thus, the β cell responds to the physiological need of the moment by delivering insulin at rates that provide appropriate hormone concentrations for regulating substrate fluxes.*

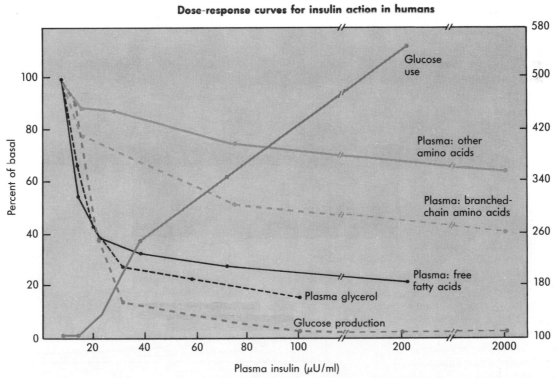

Dose-response curves for insulin action in humans

■ **Fig. 41-15**   Dose-response curves for insulin actions in humans. Note the marked sensitivity of inhibition of lipolysis and glucose production by insulin, with lesser sensitivity for insulin stimulation of glucose uptake by muscle. The effects on amino acid metabolism are intermediate.

Note that when the response of each individual's β cells to glucose is compared with that person's peripheral glucose uptake in response to insulin (Fig. 41-16), the least insulin-sensitive individuals secrete the greatest amount of insulin, and vice versa. The hyperbolic relationship dictates an exponential increase in insulin secretion as insulin sensitivity moves to its lowest point, that is, when insulin resistance is greatest (left side of Fig. 41-16). The coordination between insulin sensitivity and insulin secretion is also modulated in the CNS. Insulin sensitivity is increased by the α-MSH/MC4R pathway (Chapter 40), which decreases food intake and thereby decreases insulin secretion. This fine coordination between insulin availability (β cell function) and insulin need (tissue responsiveness) maintains the plasma glucose concentration in a narrow range.

The feedback between insulin responsiveness and insulin availability operates in obese individuals, in whom insulin secretion rates rise to accommodate decreased tissue sensitivity. Such feedback also occurs in physically trained individuals, in whom insulin secretion falls as tissue sensitivity to the hormone increases. During puberty, a *selective resistance* to insulin action on glucose metabolism leads to an increase in insulin secretion. This response facilitates insulin-sensitive cellular amino acid uptake for tissue growth. Individuals with type 2 diabetes are also insulin resistant, but they become hyperglycemic when the feedback control of insulin secretion fails to compensate sufficiently.

The complete lack of insulin action causes a major, life-threatening metabolic disturbance. Primary deficiency of insulin as a consequence of selective β cell destruction is known as **type 1 diabetes mellitus.** The disease usually results from a genetically conferred vulnerability to a probable environmental insult that triggers a destructive autoimmune process. As a consequence of the lack of insulin, hepatic glucose production is uninhibited, and the efficiency of peripheral glucose use is reduced. A new equilibrium between these processes is reached at a very high plasma glucose level of 300 to 1000 mg/dl. An increased rate of gluconeogenesis is supported by uninhibited proteolysis. Uninhibited lipolysis and ketogenesis elevate the plasma levels of FFAs and of the strong ketoacids, acetoacetic and β-OH-butyric acids. As they are neutralized by sodium bicarbonate, carbonic acid is formed, which dissociates to carbon dioxide and water. Compensatory pulmonary hyperventilation lowers P_{CO_2}, but despite this compensation, the blood pH may finally fall to less than 6.8, and death from diabetic ketoacidosis ensues.

Before this terminal point is reached in type 1 diabetes mellitus, a classic constellation of symptoms is observed. Because of the high plasma glucose levels, the filtered load of glucose exceeds the renal tubular capacity for glucose reabsorption. Glucose is therefore excreted in the urine in large quantities, and its osmotic effect causes increased excretion of water and salts and frequent urination. Thirst is stimulated by the hyperosmolality of the plasma and by the hypovolemia. The loss of glucose is also a caloric drain, which the patient attempts to recoup by eating more. This response adds to hyperglycemia, as the insulin-deficient individual is unable to store carbohydrate efficiently. Exercise capacity may be impaired because of the reduction in muscle and liver glycogen stores. The end result is a catabolic state manifested by loss of lean body mass, adipose tissue, and body fluids. Negative balances of nitrogen, potassium, phosphate, magnesium, and other intracellular components develop as these substances are excreted in the urine.

Osmotic fluid shifts secondary to the high plasma glucose level, and its conversion to other sugars, such as sorbitol, may cause swelling of the lens of the eye, blurred vision, and even formation of cataracts. Numerous proteins, including hemoglobin, albumin, and collagen, are nonenzymatically glucosylated by formation of an adduct between the aldehyde group of glucose and the N-terminus or other free amino groups in these proteins. End products

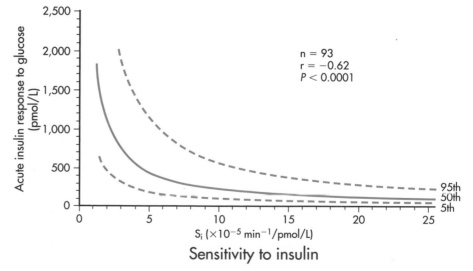

■ **Fig. 41-16** Relationship between responsiveness of peripheral tissue glucose uptake to insulin (i.e., insulin sensitivity) and responsiveness of β cells, measured by acute glucose stimulated insulin secretion. The median and 95th and 5th percentiles are shown. Note that the less sensitive tissues are to insulin, the greater is the amount of insulin secreted when glucose is administered to humans. This feedback system helps to maintain plasma glucose in the physiological range. (From Kahn SE et al: *Diabetes* 42:1663, 1993.)

n = 93
r = −0.62
P < 0.0001

Acute insulin response to glucose (pmol/L)

S_i (×10⁻⁵ min⁻¹/pmol/L)

Sensitivity to insulin

of protein glycosylation contribute to long-term tissue damage in the retina, kidneys, nerves, and cardiovascular system.

Insulin therapy systematically lowers plasma levels of glucose, FFAs, and ketoacids to normal and reduces urine nitrogen losses (Fig. 41-17). This result is achieved by the direct actions of insulin, as well as by normalizing the unrestrained secretion of glucagon that results from insulin deficiency and contributes to the hyperglycemia and ketoacidemia (Fig. 41-17). In diabetic ketoacidosis, fluid volume replacement along with potassium (to prevent hypokalemia from insulin action) is also essential to recovery.

Other β cell products. In addition to insulin, the β cell granule also contains peptides that are structurally unrelated to insulin. Although these peptides are synthesized by expression of other genes, they are packaged with insulin and coreleased during exocytosis. **Amylin** is a 37–amino acid peptide synthesized from a precursor that is expressed

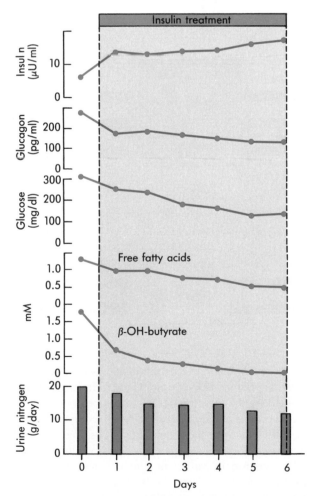

■ **Fig. 41-17** The effects of insulin replacement on plasma hormone and substrate levels and on urine losses of nitrogen in insulin-deficient diabetic humans. Note that this is a mirror image of the changes in substrates that characterize the adaptation to fasting shown in Fig. 40-11.

by a calcitonin-related gene (see Chapter 42). The granule content and the plasma levels of amylin, both in the basal state and after stimulation, are approximately 1% to 2% of those of insulin. Amylin is a noncompetitive antagonist to insulin, especially by decreasing glucose uptake and metabolism in muscle. Amylin also tends to polymerize, and fibrils containing this peptide accumulate extracellularly within the islets of individuals with type 2-dependent diabetes mellitus. The physiological and pathophysiological roles of amylin remain to be better elucidated.

Pancreastatin is a 49-amino acid peptide that is structurally related to, and may be a product of, the processing of chromogranin A (see Chapter 39). This peptide inhibits insulin secretion. Because it is coreleased with insulin from the β cell granule, pancreastatin may participate in an autofeedback regulation of insulin secretion.

GLUCAGON

Structure and Synthesis

Glucagon is a single, straight-chain peptide hormone of 29 amino acids, and its molecular weight is 3500. The N-terminal residues 1 to 6 are essential for receptor binding and for biological activity.

Glucagon is synthesized from a preproglucagon precursor by islet α cells (Fig. 41-18). The gene that encodes glucagon is a member of a superfamily that is described in Chapter 39 (Table 1). The functions of the copeptides produced by the α cells (Fig. 41-18) are unknown. In specific intestinal cells, processing of preproglucagon yields glucagon-like peptides of several types (see below), instead of glucagon (Fig. 41-18). Both glucose and insulin decrease α cell glucagon synthesis by repressing transcription of the glucagon gene. Both a cAMP-responsive element and an insulin-responsive element are present in the gene. The directional blood flow in the islets promotes the bathing of mantle α cells with high concentrations of inhibitory insulin from the core β cells. Glucagon is stored in dense granules and is released by exocytosis. This process is inhibited if α cell Ca^{2+} levels are decreased.

Regulation of Secretion

The most important principle governing glucagon secretion is the maintenance of normoglycemia in the face of increased tissue glucose demand. Exactly opposite to insulin secretion, glucagon is secreted in response to glucose deficiency and it acts to increase circulating glucose levels (Fig. 41-19). Hypoglycemia causes a 2-fold to 4-fold increase in plasma glucagon levels, whereas hyperglycemia lowers them by approximately 50%. Although glucose directly regulates glucagon secretion in vitro, its effect is strongly modulated by insulin. Glucagon secretion is stimulated much more by low glucose levels if insulin is absent. Conversely, the presence of insulin greatly potentiates the suppressive effect of high glucose levels on the α cell.

Glucagon secretion is also stimulated by a protein meal and, most effectively, by amino acids such as arginine and

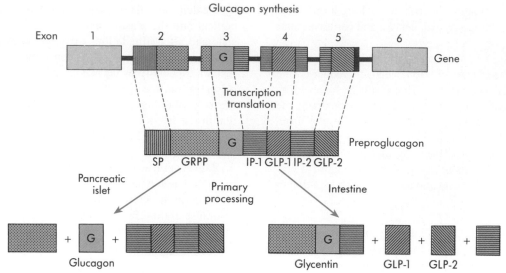

■ **Fig. 41-18** Glucagon synthesis. The gene is composed of six exons that yield preproglucagon. After elimination of the signal peptide *(SP)*, the α cells of the pancreas process proglucagon to glucagon, a glucagon-related polypeptide *(GRPP),* and a C-terminal peptide. In the intestinal L cells, glucagon itself is not produced, but glucagon-like peptides 1 and 2 *(GLP-1* and *GLP-2)* are secreted along with a larger glucagon-containing peptide called glycentin. *IP-1,* Intervening peptide-1; *IP-2,* intervening peptide-2. (Modified from Phillipe J: *Endocr Rev* 12:252, 1991.)

■ **Fig. 41-19** Feedback relationship between glucagon and nutrients. Glucagon stimulates production and release of glucose, free fatty acids *(FFA),* and ketoacids, which in turn suppress glucagon secretion. Amino acids stimulate glucagon secretion, and glucagon in turn stimulates the conversion of amino acids to glucose.

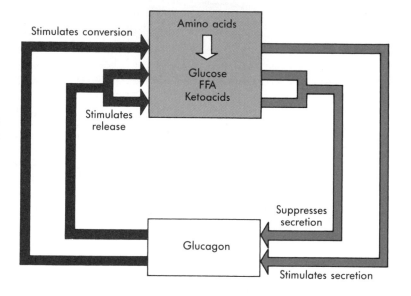

alanine. However, this α cell response to protein is greatly dampened if glucose is administered concurrently. This interaction partly occurs via insulin; positive glucagon responses to amino acids are restrained by insulin excess and are augmented by insulin deficiency. FFAs and glucose exert a suppressive effect on the glucagon response. Glucagon responses to orally ingested nutrients (as opposed to the responses to intravenous delivery) may also be reinforced by the release of gastrointestinal secretagogues that augment insulin secretion. Important exceptions are GLP-1 (a proglucagon product of the intestine) (Fig. 41-18) and secretin, both of which inhibit α cell glucagon release. The sum of all these individual influences is that the ingestion of ordinary

meals produces much less variation in plasma glucagon levels than in plasma insulin levels. These differences are partly explained by the offsetting effects of the carbohydrate and protein portions of the meal on the α cell, compared with the synergistic effects of these nutrients on the β cell.

Fasting for several days increases plasma glucagon levels 2-fold. Exercise of sufficient intensity and duration also increases plasma glucagon levels. Neural mechanisms may mediate some of these responses. In particular, vagal stimulation and acetylcholine release acutely increase glucagon secretion. The neurohormone, somatostatin, inhibits the secretion of glucagon, probably by paracrine or neurocrine effects made possible by the islet microarchitecture (Fig. 41-1).

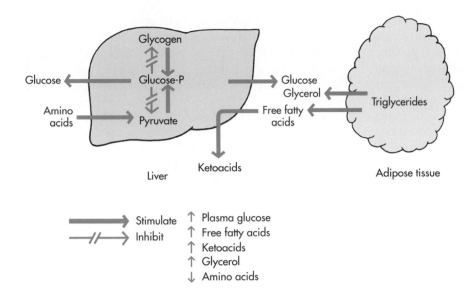

■ **Fig. 41-20** The effect of glucagon on the overall flow of fuels results in tissue release of glucose, fatty acids, and ketoacids into the circulation and hepatic uptake of amino acids for gluconeogenesis. Plasma levels of the energy fuels increase and levels of amino acids decrease.

■ **Table 41-2** Contrasting effects of insulin and glucagon on key enzymes in hepatic glucose metabolism

		Activity		Gene Expression	
	Enzyme	*Insulin*	*Glucagon*	*Insulin*	*Glucagon*
Gluconeogenesis and glucose export ↑	Glucose-6-phosphatase Fructose 1,6 bisphosphatase Phosphoenolpyruvate carboxykinase	↓	↑	↓	↑
Pyruvate ↓	Glucokinase 6-Phosphofructo-1-kinase Pyruvate kinase	↑	↓	↑	↓
Glycolysis and glucose oxidation					

A variety of stresses, including infection, burns, tissue infarction, and major surgery, rapidly increase glucagon secretion. This increased secretion is probably mediated by the sympathetic nervous system via outflow from the ventromedial hypothalamus to α-adrenergic receptors in the α cells. The excess glucagon often leads to clinically significant hyperglycemia, particularly in individuals who have diabetes mellitus.

Monomeric α cell glucagon circulates unbound in plasma at a basal concentration of 50 to 100 pg/ml (2×10^{-11} M). It has a half-life of 6 minutes. The daily secretion rate of glucagon is estimated to be 100 to 150 μg. The ratio of portal vein to peripheral vein glucagon concentrations is about 1.5 in the basal state, and about 50% of glucagon is extracted by the liver during a single passage. The kidney is the other major site of glucagon degradation. Less than 1% of the glucagon filtered by the glomerulus is excreted in the urine.

Hormone Actions

In almost all respects, the actions of glucagon are exactly opposite to those of insulin. Glucagon promotes mobilization rather than storage of fuels, especially glucose (Fig. 41-20). Both hormones act at similar control points in the liver (Table 41-2, Fig. 41-14). Glucagon may even be viewed as the primary hormone that regulates hepatic glucose production and ketogenesis, and insulin's role may be that of a glucagon antagonist.

Glucagon binds to a hepatic plasma membrane glycoprotein receptor; the resultant signal is transduced via a stimulatory G protein, adenylyl cyclase, and cAMP as second messenger (see Figs. 39-8 and 39-9). cAMP-activated protein kinase A initiates a cascade of phosphorylations that activate or deactivate a number of enzyme kinases or phosphatases by covalent modification of the enzyme structures. The first and best-studied example is phosphorylase, the enzyme that degrades glycogen. Activated protein kinase A converts inactive phosphorylase kinase to active phosphorylase kinase. The latter then converts inactive phosphorylase to active phosphorylase, and the rate of glycogenolysis increases. In contrast, phosphorylation of the enzymes phosphofructokinase and pyruvate kinase decreases their activity, and hence the rate of glycolysis is decreased.

The dominant effect of glucagon is on the liver. (Its actions on adipose tissue and muscle are minor, unless insulin is virtually absent.) In the liver, glucagon exerts an immediate and profound glycogenolytic effect through activation of glycogen phosphorylase. The glucose-1-phosphate released as a result of glycogen phosphorylase activation is prevented from undergoing resynthesis to glycogen by the simultaneous inhibition of glycogen synthase. Glucagon also stimulates gluconeogenesis by several mechanisms. The hepatic extraction of amino acids, especially alanine, is increased. The activities and concentrations of gluconeogenic enzymes are increased, whereas those of glycolysis are decreased.

The enzyme pair, phosphofructokinase and fructose-1,6-bisphosphatase, determine the direction and magnitude of the flow between fructose-6-phosphate and fructose-1,6-bisphosphate, and therefore the relative rates of glycolysis and gluconeogenesis (Fig. 41-14). The activities of these two enzymes in turn are reciprocally related to the level of fructose-2,6-bisphosphate. The concentration of this important metabolite is regulated by the unique bidirectional enzyme, 6-phosphofructo-2-kinase/fructose-2,6-bisphosphatase, which is very sensitive to the islet hormones (Fig. 41-21). This enzyme either catalyzes synthesis of fructose-2,6-bisphosphate from fructose-6-phosphate, or catalyzes hydrolysis of fructose-2,6-bisphosphate to fructose-6-phosphate.

When phosphorylated, this bidirectional enzyme is a phosphatase that decreases fructose-2,6-bisphosphate levels; when dephosphorylated, the enzyme is a kinase that increases fructose-2,6-bisphosphate levels. Glucagon action phosphorylates the enzyme and lowers fructose-2,6-bisphosphate levels; this in turn decreases phosphofructokinase and increases fructose-1,6-bisphosphatase activities (Fig. 41-21). The result is an increase in gluconeogenesis and a decrease in glycolysis. Insulin action dephosphorylates the bidirectional enzyme and has exactly the opposite effect, namely increasing fructose-2,6-bisphosphate levels (Fig. 41-21). The result is a decrease in gluconeogenesis and an increase in glycolysis.

The crucial importance of glucagon to the maintenance of basal hepatic glucose output is shown by the marked decline that follows the selective inhibition of glucagon secretion. The powerful glycogenolytic and hyperglycemic action of glucagon is exhibited at plasma hormone concentrations of 150 to 500 pg/ml, and it occurs even in the presence of insulin somewhat above basal levels (20 to 30 µU/ml). However, this action is transient; the acute stimulation of hepatic glucose output, which occurs during continuous glucagon administration, wanes after about 30 minutes because of hepatic autoregulation by hyperglycemia and stimulation of insulin release. However, if glucagon is given in a more physiological, fluctuating pattern, each increase in the hormone causes a pulse of glucose output.

Glucagon has little or no influence on glucose use by peripheral tissues. Thus, hyperglucagonemia has no effect on the plasma glucose levels that are generated by an exogenous glucose load, as long as the insulin response to the glucose stimulus is normal. The gluconeogenic action of glucagon is also reflected in the ability of the hormone to increase the rate of disposal of amino acids and of their degradation to urea. However, glucagon has no particular influence on branched-chain amino acid levels, which suggests that it has little or no effect on muscle proteolysis.

Another important intrahepatic action of glucagon is to direct incoming FFAs away from triglyceride synthesis and toward β-oxidation. Thus, glucagon is a ketogenic as well as a hyperglycemic hormone. Glucagon inactivates acetyl-CoA carboxylase, which catalyzes the rate-limiting step in FFA synthesis from cytoplasmic acetyl-CoA (Fig. 41-14). This inactivation results in lower levels of malonyl-CoA, an allosteric inhibitor of carnitine acyltransferase. In turn, lower levels of malonyl-CoA allow a faster rate of influx of fatty acyl-CoA into the mitochondrion for conversion to ketoacids.

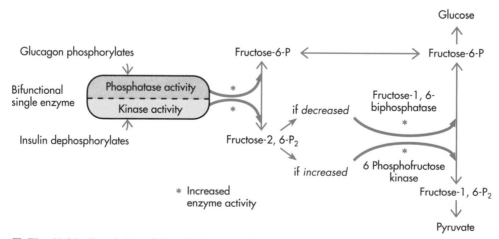

■ **Fig. 41-21** Regulation of the relative rates of gluconeogenesis and glycolysis by the actions of islet hormones on a single bifunctional enzyme. Insulin causes dephosphorylation of the enzyme, making it a kinase, which raises the level of fructose-2,6-bisphosphate. This intermediate stimulates the activity of 6-phosphofructose kinase and shifts metabolism toward pyruvate (glycolysis). Glucagon phosphorylates the bifunctional enzyme, making it a phosphatase, which lowers the level of fructose-2,6-bisphosphate, thereby increasing the activity of fructose-1,6-bisphosphatase and shifting metabolism toward glucose (gluconeogenesis).

Glucagon also activates adipose tissue lipase, and thereby increases lipolysis and the delivery of FFAs to the liver. Although the ketogenic actions of glucagon are physiologically very relevant, they are easily nullified by rather small amounts of insulin, particularly at the adipose tissue locus. Finally, hepatic hydroxy-methylglutaryl-CoA reductase activity is inhibited by glucagon, thereby decreasing hepatic cholesterol synthesis.

Other actions of glucagon include inhibition of renal tubular sodium resorption; thus, glucagon causes natriuresis. Activation of myocardial adenylyl cyclase causes a modest increase in cardiac output. Glucagon may also be synthesized in the central nervous system, and it may act locally in the regulation of appetite.

INSULIN:GLUCAGON RATIO

It should now be apparent that the direction of substrate fluxes is very sensitive to the relative availability of insulin and glucagon (compare Figs. 41-13 and 41-20). The usual molar ratio of insulin to glucagon in plasma is about 2.0. Under circumstances that require mobilization and increased use of endogenous substrates, the insulin:glucagon ratio drops to 0.5 or less. This decreased ratio is seen in fasting and in prolonged exercise, and is caused by both decreased insulin secretion and increased glucagon secretion. A low insulin:glucagon ratio facilitates increased glycogenolysis, amino acid mobilization, and gluconeogenesis, and thereby maintains glucose supply to the central nervous system. Lipolysis is also enhanced, which increases FFA flow to muscle and liver for oxidation. During exercise, the low insulin:glucagon ratio still permits muscle glucose uptake, which is stimulated by an exercise-specific mechanism that is independent of insulin.

Maintenance of a low insulin:glucagon ratio is critical in the neonatal period, when the infant is abruptly cut off from maternal fuel supplies but is not yet able to assimilate efficiently exogenous fuel from its gastrointestinal tract. When this ratio is excessive—as may occur in infants born of diabetic mothers—hypoglycemia may result.

Conversely, under circumstances in which substrate storage is advantageous, such as after a pure carbohydrate load or a mixed meal, the insulin:glucagon ratio rises to 10 or more, mainly because of increased insulin secretion. The high ratio enhances glucose uptake, oxidation, and conversion to liver and muscle glycogen, while it suppresses unneeded proteolysis and lipolysis. An interesting example of only a small change in the insulin:glucagon ratio occurs after a subject ingests a pure protein meal. In this situation, insulin secretion increases, preventing unneeded proteolysis and facilitating muscle uptake of some amino acids and their incorporation into proteins. At the same time, glucagon secretion also increases. This increase in glucagon prevents the decrease in hepatic glucose output and hypoglycemia that would ensue if the extra insulin action were completely unopposed.

Ingestion of pure fat has little influence on the insulin: glucagon ratio. After a mixed meal, however, the increase in the ratio facilitates clearance of chylomicrons by activation of adipose tissue lipoprotein lipase.

Primary glucagon excess is produced by α cell tumors. Plasma levels of glucose and of ketoacids are only modestly elevated. The marked increase in gluconeogenesis causes a generalized reduction of plasma amino acids and an increase in urinary nitrogen. The catabolic action of the hormone is exhibited by loss of weight and by a peculiar, destructive skin lesion. Severe diabetes mellitus is uncommon because of the compensatory increase in insulin secretion.

The predictable consequence of glucagon deficiency would be fasting hypoglycemia. In fact, cases of fasting hypoglycemia caused by glucagon deficiency have rarely been documented. Other hormonal adjustments likely sustain plasma glucose when glucagon is deficient. However, glucagon secretion in response to insulin-induced hypoglycemia can become greatly impaired in type 1 diabetes. The lack of glucagon increases the risk of severe "insulin reactions" if such a patient injects too much insulin, misses a meal, or exercises heavily.

GLUCAGON-LIKE PEPTIDE-1 (GLP-1)

GLP-1 is a 37-amino acid peptide product of the preproglucagon gene that is expressed predominantly in intestinal L cells (Fig. 41-18), particularly in the ileum and colon, and is secreted by those cells into the bloodstream. GLP-1 is freed from preproglucagon by the action of the enzyme proconvertase-1. Further posttranslation processing leads to the major circulating forms, which are the N-terminal peptides 7-37 and 7-36 amide. GLP-1 is secreted in response to intake of nutrients, oral but not intravenous glucose and galactose, amino acids, and cholinergic and β-adrenergic stimuli. Fasting plasma values are 7×10^{-12} M and they rise 100% with meals. GLP-1 is cleaved very quickly by the plasma enzyme, dipeptidyl peptidase, and thus the plasma half-life is less then 2 minutes.

GLP-1 acts on its plasma membrane receptor, which is linked to adenylyl cyclase by a G protein; cAMP levels then increase. Important actions of GLP-1 include stimulation of insulin release by augmenting the amplitude of β cell responses to glucose, stimulation of insulin synthesis, and stimulation of β cell neogenesis by increasing expression of IPF-1 (see above). Other actions of GLP-1 are to decrease glucagon secretion and gastric emptying. Together, all these actions tend to lower the plasma glucose concentration and to limit plasma glucose rises with meals.

GLP-1 is another gastrointestinal hormone that is also expressed in the hypothalamus and brainstem. Its CNS actions are to decrease food intake, decrease water intake, and increase diuresis.

Because of the array of its actions, GLP-1 has evoked interest as a therapeutic agent for treatment of diabetes, especially type 2. It does indeed lower plasma glucose in diabetic patients, but its very short half-life limits its usefulness. Synthesizing GLP-1 analogues resistant to dipeptidyl peptidase action or simultaneously administering inhibitors of the peptidase with GLP-1 is currently being explored to enhance the therapeutic effectiveness of GLP-1.

SOMATOSTATIN SECRETION AND ACTION

Somatostatin was discovered as a hypothalamic neuropeptide that inhibits growth hormone secretion (see Chapter 42), but it is also synthesized by the δ cells of the pancreatic islets and by intestinal cells. In the δ cells, the processing of the primary somatostatin gene product, prosomatostatin, yields mostly a 14-amino acid peptide (SS-14). In intestinal cells, a 28-amino acid peptide with an N-terminal extension is probably the major product (SS-28). Many of the biological actions of these products are similar. Somatostatin secretion is stimulated by glucose, amino acids, FFAs, various gastrointestinal hormones, glucagon, and β-adrenergic and cholinergic neurotransmitters. Somatostatin secretion is inhibited by insulin and α-adrenergic neurotransmitters. Exocytosis of somatostatin granules is stimulated by cAMP. Plasma levels of SS-28, but not of SS-14, increase with mixed meals.

Somatostatin is a profound inhibitor of both insulin and glucagon secretion. The administration of somatostatin also decreases the assimilation rate of all nutrients from the gastrointestinal tract. This effect is accomplished by inhibitory actions on gastric, duodenal, and gallbladder motility; on the secretion of hydrochloric acid, pepsin, gastrin, secretin, and intestinal juices; and on pancreatic exocrine function. Somatostatin also inhibits the absorption of glucose, xylose, and triglycerides across the mucosal membrane. SS-14 and SS-28 may participate in a feedback arrangement, whereby entrance of food into the gut stimulates their release in order to prevent rapid nutrient overload. SS-14 may be released locally and may act in neurocrine and paracrine fashion to limit insulin and glucagon responses to meals. SS-28, which is released particularly after ingestion of fat, may function as a true hormone: that is, it may reach the pancreatic islets via the bloodstream. The interaction among the α cells, β cells, δ cells, and intestinal cell products may coordinate the rates of bulk movement, digestion, and absorption of nutrients with the rates of nutrient uptake by the liver and peripheral tissues (Fig. 41-22).

Somatostatin analogs are now used therapeutically to alleviate diarrhea caused by unregulated gastrointestinal hormone secretion. They are also employed to inhibit unregulated release of various peptide and protein hormones by neoplasms. Tumors of the δ cells produce somatostatin excess. Signs and symptoms of somatostatin excess include inhibition of nutrient absorption, excess stool fat, and weight loss. Plasma insulin and glucagon levels are low, and the low insulin level may lead to modest hyperglycemia.

PANCREATIC POLYPEPTIDE

Pancreatic polypeptide is a specific product of the PP cells. It has 36 amino acids and a distinctive C-terminal tyrosineamide residue. It belongs to a family of similar molecules, including neuropeptide Y in the hypothalamus. PP is secreted in response to food ingestion via gastrointestinal secretagogues and cholinergic stimulation. PP is also stimulated by hypoglycemia and inhibited by glucose administration. Its best defined action is to inhibit exocrine pancreatic secretion, partly by inhibiting the uptake of precursor amino acids by the acinar cells. Its true physiological importance is unclear, but elevated plasma levels of PP serve as markers for the presence of islet cell tumors and their response to

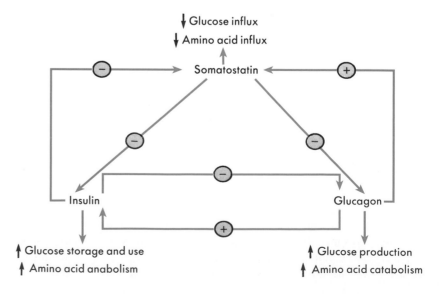

■ **Fig. 41-22** Schema interrelating the effects of somatostatin, insulin, and glucagon on each other's secretion with their effects on glucose and amino acid metabolism. (From Unger RH et al: *Annu Rev Physiol* 40: 307, 1978.)

treatment. A failure of plasma PP to increase when plasma glucose is sharply reduced suggests loss of cholinergic pancreatic islet innervation.

SUMMARY

1. The pancreatic islets are composed of insulin-secreting β cells (the majority), glucagon-secreting α cells, somatostatin-secreting δ cells, and pancreatic polypeptide (PP)-secreting cells. The microarchitecture and blood flow arrangements permit paracrine and neurocrine functioning, as well as direct cell-to-cell communication through gap junctions.

2. Insulin is a major glucoregulatory, antilipolytic, antiketogenic, and anabolic hormone. It consists of two straight-chain peptides held together by disulfide bonds, and it is synthesized from a single-chain precursor (proinsulin).

3. Insulin secretion is stimulated primarily by glucose and food intake, but also by other fuels, gastrointestinal peptides, and cholinergic and β-adrenergic stimuli. Release is decreased during fasting and by exercise, both circumstances that require fuel mobilization.

4. Insulin promotes fuel storage. Its effects in the order of increasing insulin doses required are inhibition of adipose tissue lipolysis and of ketogenesis; inhibition of hepatic glycogenolysis, gluconeogenesis, and glucose release; inhibition of muscle proteolysis; and stimulation of muscle glucose uptake and storage as glycogen.

5. Insulin also stimulates cellular uptake of amino acids, potassium, phosphate, and magnesium, as well as synthesis of numerous proteins.

6. Insulin acts through a plasma membrane receptor that binds insulin, and then phosphorylates itself at specific tyrosine residues, and thereby acquires external tyrosine kinase activity. The activated receptor phosphorylates four insulin receptor substrates. From this phosphorylation flows a cascade of modulation of the activities of numerous enzymes involved in glucose and fatty acid metabolism. In addition, gene transcription of numerous enzymes and proteins essential to cell growth is induced or repressed.

7. Insulin decreases plasma levels of glucose, free fatty acids (FFAs), ketoacids, glycerol, and branched-chain and other amino acids. Insulin deficiency leads to hyperglycemia, loss of lean body and adipose tissue mass, growth retardation, and ultimately metabolic ketoacidosis.

8. Glucagon is a straight-chain peptide released in response to hypoglycemia and to amino acids. Its secretion is suppressed by glucose, FFAs, and insulin. Glucagon secretion increases during prolonged fasting and exercise.

9. Glucagon is an insulin antagonist that promotes mobilization of glucose. It acts primarily on the liver to stimulate glycogenolysis and gluconeogenesis, as well as fatty acid oxidation and ketogenesis. cAMP is its second messenger,

and covalent modification of enzyme activities by phosphorylation is the main mechanism of action. Glucagon increases the plasma levels of glucose, FFAs, and ketoacids, but it decreases amino acid levels.

10. The insulin:glucagon ratio controls the relative rates of glycolysis and gluconeogenesis by altering hepatic fructose-2,6-bisphosphate levels. This metabolite in turn regulates the rate and direction of flow between fructose-1-phosphate and fructose-1,6-bisphosphate. The two hormones have antagonistic effects at numerous other liver enzyme steps in glucose and fatty acid metabolism.

11. Somatostatin is a neuropeptide of islet and intestinal cell origin. It decreases the motility of the gastrointestinal tract, gastrointestinal secretions, digestion and absorption of nutrients, and secretion of both insulin and glucagon. Somatostatin is secreted in response to meals; its actions, along with those of insulin and glucagon, probably coordinate nutrient input with substrate disposal.

BIBLIOGRAPHY

Journal articles

Amiel SA et al: Insulin resistance of puberty: a defect restricted to peripheral glucose metabolism, *J Clin Endocrinol Metab* 72:277, 1991.

Bavenholm PN et al: Insulin sensitivity of suppression of endogenous glucose production is the single most important determinant of glucose tolerance, *Diabetes* 50:1449, 2001.

Boden G et al: Role of glucagon in disposal of an amino acid load, *Am J Physiol* 259:E225, 1990.

Bonadonna RC et al: Dose-dependent effect of insulin on plasma free fatty acid turnover and oxidation in humans, *Am J Physiol* 259:E726, 1990.

Bonadonna RC et al: Effect of insulin on system amino acid transport in human skeletal muscle, *J Clin Invest* 91:514, 1993.

Bonner-Weir S: Islet growth and development in the adult, *J Mol Endocrinol* 24:297, 2000.

Burcelin R et al: Glucose competence of the hepatoportal vein sensor requires the presence of an activated glucagon-like peptide-1 receptor, *Diabetes* 50:1720, 2001.

Cahill GF: Starvation in man, *N Engl J Med* 282:668, 1970.

Cardillo C et al: Insulin stimulates both endothelin and nitric oxide activity in the human forearm, *Circulation* 100:820, 1999.

Cersosimo E et al: Insulin regulation of renal glucose metabolism in humans, *Am Physiol Soc* 276:E78, 1999.

Cline GW et al: Impaired glucose transport as a cause of decresed insulin-stimulated muscle glycogen synthesis in type 2 diabetes, *N Engl J Med* 341:240, 1999.

Dobbins RL et al: Circulating fatty acids are essential for efficient glucose-stimulated insulin secretion after prolonged fasting in humans, *Diabetes* 47:1613, 1998.

Drucker DJ: Glucagon-like peptides, *Diabetes* 47:159, 1998.

Edlund H: Developmental biology of the pancreas, *Diabetes* 50:S5, 2001.

Fehmann H-C, Gôke R, Gôke B: Cell and molecular biology of the incretin hormones glucagon-like peptide-I and glucose-dependent insulin releasing polypeptide, *Endocr Rev* 16:390, 1995.

Fukagawa NK et al: Insulin dose-dependent reductions in plasma amino acids in man, *Am J Physiol* 250:E13, 1986.

Inoue H et al: Isolation, characterization, and chromosomal mapping of the human insulin promoter factor 1 (IPF-1) gene, *Diabetes* 45:789, 1996.

Iozzo P et al: Independent influence of age on basal insulin secretion in nondiabetic humans, *J Clin Endocrinol Metab* 84:863, 1999.

Kahn CR: Insulin action, diabetogenes, and the cause of type II diabetes, *Diabetes* 43:1066, 1994.

Kahn SE: Regulation of β-cell function in vivo, *Diabetes Metab Rev* 4:372, 1996.

Kahn SE et al: Quantification of the relationship between insulin sensitivity and β-cell function in human subjects: evidence for a hyperbolic function, *Diabetes* 42:1663, 1993.

Katz L et al: Splanchnic and peripheral disposal of oral glucose in man, *Diabetes* 32:675, 1983.

Kido Y et al: Clinical review 125: The insulin receptor and its cellular targets, *J Clin Endocrinol Metab* 86:972, 2001.

Kimball SR, Vary TC, Jefferson LS: Regulation of protein synthesis by insulin, *Annu Rev Physiol* 56:321, 1994.

King DS et al: Insulin secretory capacity in endurance-trained and untrained young men, *Am J Physiol* 259:E155, 1990.

Krasinski SD et al: Pancreatic polypeptide and peptide YY gene expression, *Ann NY Acad Sci* 611:73, 1990.

Kulkarni RN et al: Tissue-specific knockout of the insulin receptor in pancreatic β cells creates an insulin secretory defect similar to that in type 2 diabetes, *Cell* 96:329, 1999.

Langin D: Diabetes, insulin secretion, and the pancreatic beta-cell mitochondrion, *N Engl J Med* 345:1772, 2001.

Maedler K et al: Glucose induces β-cell apoptosis via upregulation of the fas receptor in human islets, *Diabetes* 50:1683, 2001.

Marchetti P et al: Pulsatile insulin secretion from isolated human pancreatic islets, *Diabetes* 43:827, 1994.

Matschinsky FM: Glucokinase as glucose sensor and metabolic signal generator in pancreatic beta cells and hepatocytes, *Diabetes* 39:647, 1990.

Matschinsky FM, Sweet IR: Annotated questions and answers about glucose metabolism and insulin secretion of β-cells, *Diabetes Metab Rev* 4:130, 1996.

McGarry JD, Dobbins RL: Fatty acids, lipotoxicity and insulin secretion, *Diabetologia* 42:128, 1999.

Mueckler M: Family of glucose-transporter genes: implications for glucose homeostasis and diabetes, *Diabetes* 39:6, 1990.

Nair S et al: Effect of intravenous insulin treatment on in vivo whole body leucine kinetics and oxygen consumption in insulin deprived type I diabetic patients, *Metabolism* 36:491, 1987.

Nielsen JH et al: Regulation of β-cell mass by hormones and growth factors, *Diabetes* 50:S25, 2001.

Nurjhan N et al: Insulin dose-response characteristics for suppression of glycerol release and conversion to glucose in humans, *Diabetes* 35:1326, 1986.

Olefsky JM, Treatment of insulin resistance with peroxisome proliferators-activated receptor γ agonists, *J Clin Invest* 106:467, 2000.

Orskov C et al: Proglucagon products in plasma of noninsulin-dependent diabetics and nondiabetic controls in the fasting state and after oral glucose and intravenous arginine, *J Clin Invest* 87:415, 1991.

Pederson TM et al: Serine/threonine phosphorylation of IRS-1 triggers its degradation: possible regulation by tyrosine phosphorylation, *Diabetes* 50:24, 2001.

Philippe J: Structure and pancreatic expression of the insulin and glucagon genes, *Endocr Rev* 12:252, 1991.

Polonsky KS, Given BD, Van Cauter E: Twenty-four-hour profiles and pulsatile patterns of insulin secretion in normal and obese subjects, *J Clin Invest* 81:442, 1988.

Rhodes CJ: IGF-I and GH post-receptor signaling mechanisms for pancreatic β-cell replication, *J Mol Endocrinol* 24:303, 2000.

Ritzel R et al: Glucagon-like peptide 1 increases secretory burst mass of pulsatile insulin secretion in patients with type 2 diabetes and impaired glucose tolerance, *Diabetes* 50:776, 2001.

Saltiel AR, Kahn CR: Insulin signaling and the regulation of glucose and lipid metabolism, *Nature* 414:799, 2001.

Schuit FC et al: Glucose sensing in pancreatic β-cells: a model for the study of other glucose-regulated cells in gut, pancreas, and hypothalamus, *Diabetes* 50:1, 2001.

Schwartz MW et al: Insulin in the brain: a hormonal regulator of energy balance, *Endocr Rev* 13:387, 1992.

Seino S, Seino M, Bell GI: Human insulin receptor gene, *Diabetes* 39:129, 1990.

Seufert J et al: Leptin suppression of insulin secretion and gene expression in human pancreatic islets: implications for the development of adipogenic diabetes mellitus, *J Clin Endocrinol Metab* 84:670, 1999.

Sha L et al: Amplitude modulation of pulsatile insulin secretion by intrapancreatic ganglion neurons, *Diabetes* 50:51, 2001.

Shepherd PR: Glucose transporters and insulin action, *N Engl J Med* 249:248, 1999.

Stein DT et al: The insulinotropic potency of fatty acids is influenced profoundly by their chain length and degree of saturation, *J Clin Invest* 100:398, 1997.

Steiner DF, Rubenstein AH: Proinsulin C peptide-biological activity? *Science* 277:531, 1997.

Stephens JM, Pilch PF: The metabolic regulation and vesicular transport of GLUT4, the major insulin-responsive glucose transporter, *Endocr Rev* 4:529, 1995.

Stoffers DA et al: Insulinotropic glucagon-like peptide 1 agonists stimulate expression of homeodomain protein IDX-1 and increase islet size in mouse pancreas, *Diabetes* 49:741, 2000.

Sturis J et al: Entrainment of pulsatile insulin secretion by oscillatory glucose infusion, *J Clin Invest* 87:439, 1991.

Thiebaud D et al: The effect of graded doses of insulin on total glucose uptake, glucose oxidation, and glucose storage in man, *Diabetes* 31:957, 1982.

Unger RH et al: Insulin, glucagon, and somatostatin secretion in the regulation of metabolism, *Annu Rev Physiol* 40:307, 1978.

Vilsboll T et al: Reduced postprandial concentrations of intact biologically active glucagon-like peptide 1 in type 2 diabetic patients, *Diabetes* 50:609, 2001.

Webb GC et al: Expression profiling of pancreatic β cells: glucose regulation of secretory and metabolic pathway genes, *Diabetes* 50:S135, 2001.

Weir GC, Bonner-Weir S: Islets of Langerhans: the puzzle of intraislet interactions and their relevance to diabetes, *J Clin Invest* 85:983, 1990.

White MF: The IRS-signaling system: a network of docking proteins that mediate insulin and cytokine action, *Recent Progr Hormone Res* 53:119, 1998.

Wollheim CB, Lang J, Regazzi R: The exocytotic process of insulin secretion and its regulation by Ca++ and G-proteins, *Diabetes Metab Rev* 4:276, 1996.

Books and monographs

Cook DL, Taborsky GJ: β-cell function and insulin secretion. In Porte D, Sherwin RS, editors: *Diabetes mellitus*, Stamford, 1997, Appleton & Lange.

Czech MP, Erwin JL, Sleeman MW: Insulin action on glucose transport. In LeRoith D, Taylor SI, Olefsky JM, editors: *Diabetes mellitus*, Philadelphia, 2000, Lippincott Williams & Wilkins.

Drucker DJ: Glucagon secretion, α cell metabolism, and glucagon action. In DeGroot LJ, Jameson JL, editors: *Endocrinology*, ed 4, Philadelphia, 2001, WB Saunders.

Flakoll PJ, Carlson MG, Cherrington AD: Physiologic action of insulin. In LeRoith D, Taylor SI, Olefsky, JM editors: *Diabetes mellitus*, Philadelphia, 2000, Lippincott Williams & Wilkins.

O'Brien RM, Granner DK: Gene regulation. In LeRoith D, Taylor SI, Olefsky JM, editors: *Diabetes mellitus*, Philadelphia, 2000, Lippincott Williams & Wilkins.

Polonsky KS, O'Meara NM: Secretion and metabolism of insulin, proinsulin, and C peptide. In DeGroot LJ, Jameson JL, editors: *Endocrinology*, ed 4, Philadelphia, 2001, WB Saunders.

Steiner DF et al: Chemistry and biosynthesis of the islet hormones: insulin, islet amyloid polypeptide (amylin), glucagon, somatostatin, and pancreatic polypeptide. In DeGroot LJ, Jameson JL, editors: *Endocrinology*, ed 4, Philadelphia, 2001, WB Saunders.

Ueki K, Kahn CR: The biochemistry of insulin action. In LeRoith D, Taylor SI, Olefsky JM, editors: *Diabetes mellitus*, Philadelphia, 2000, Lippincott Williams & Wilkins.

chapter forty-two

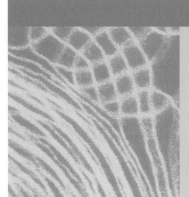

Endocrine Regulation of Calcium and Phosphate Metabolism

A complex regulatory system maintains the normal amounts of calcium, phosphate, and the related mineral, magnesium, in the body. The key hormones that regulate the amounts of calcium and phosphate are **parathyroid hormone (PTH),** a peptide, and **vitamin D,** a sterol. *These hormones act on three organ systems—the intestinal tract, the bone, and the kidneys—to maintain calcium and phosphate levels in the face of environmental changes (e.g., diet) and of internal demands (e.g., pregnancy).* Before detailing these hormonal mechanisms of regulation, an overview is presented of calcium and phosphate metabolism, as well as of the related structural and functional aspects of bone mass. This introduction attempts to explain how the individual endocrine components of the system work together.

OVERVIEW OF CALCIUM AND PHOSPHATE METABOLISM

Calcium

The calcium ion is fundamentally important to all biological systems. Therefore, the concentration of calcium must be maintained within specific limits of physiological tolerance in several compartments. The resting intracellular cytosolic concentration of free calcium is only 10^{-7} M. This value can transiently increase 10- to 100-fold when the calcium ions are involved in the creation or maintenance of action potentials, contraction, motility, cytoskeletal rearrangements, cell division, secretion, and modulation of enzyme activities. In absolute terms, however, this transient increase represents the movement of exquisitely small amounts of calcium into the cell cytoplasm from either extracellular fluid or intracellular reservoirs. Both the initial entry and subsequent extrusion of calcium into and out of these reservoirs take place very rapidly, and the amounts exchanged are balanced. Despite the small amount of calcium involved in these processes, calcium ions constitute a cellular ionic signal of unusual speed and of a large dynamic range of amplitude and sensitivity.

The total pool of intracellular free calcium is estimated to be only 0.2 mg. An additional 9 g of intracellular calcium is present in a bound form in the endoplasmic reticulum, the mitochondria, and the plasma membrane. This intracellular calcium constitutes an immediately accessible storage pool, and it also contributes to the structural integrity of the cell.

The extracellular concentration of free calcium is approximately 10^{-3} M, or four orders of magnitude higher than the intracellular concentration. This large gradient is maintained by specialized membranes and calcium pumps (see Chapter 1). Maintenance of the proper extracellular concentration is essential for generation of normal membrane potentials and neurotransmission, for calcium uptake into the cells in the course of contraction and exocytosis, for normal blood clotting, and for modulation of plasma enzyme activities. The total extracellular pool of calcium amounts to about 1 g. The skeleton and teeth contain 1 to 2 kg of calcium, depending on body size. This constitutes 99% of the total amount. This pool of bound calcium functions in skeletal structure, protection of internal organs, and locomotion.

The level of total calcium (free and bound) in the plasma ranges from 8.6 to 10.6 mg/dl (2.15-2.65 mmol/L = 4.3 to 5.3 mEq/L).* For any individual, however, the variation in the plasma calcium level from day to day is generally less than 10%. Approximately 50% of plasma calcium is in the ionized, biologically active form. Normal variation in the plasma ionized calcium level is only 1% to 2%. Ten percent of the plasma calcium is complexed in nonionic but ultrafilterable forms, such as calcium bicarbonate: much of the plasma calcium (40%) is bound to proteins, mainly albumin. Because of this binding, total plasma calcium rises and falls with the albumin concentration, even into abnormal ranges. These fluctuations have no adverse biological consequences, as long as the ionized calcium concentration remains normal. As the pH of the blood increases, however, the equilibrium between ionized and protein-bound calcium shifts toward the latter state. *Thus, alkalosis decreases and acidosis increases the plasma ionized calcium concentration.*

---

*The normal limits vary by as much as 0.5 mg/dl from laboratory to laboratory, depending on the method employed.

The plasma ionized calcium concentration can drop below normal when (1) there is a total body calcium deficit, (2) a sudden shift in internal balance causes calcium to be taken up into bone faster than the extracellular calcium pool can be replenished, or (3) plasma protein binding to calcium increases, for example, in response to respiratory alkalosis secondary to hyperventilation. A decreased concentration of ionized calcium in the plasma causes neuromuscular irritability, manifested by numbness and tingling sensations, tetanic muscle contractions in the hands and feet, and, most dangerously, spasm of muscles in the larynx and consequent airway obstruction. Central nervous system irritability can cause seizures. When plasma ionized calcium is high, reduced neurotransmission causes muscle weakness, decreased intestinal motility, impaired mentation, and even coma.

Figure 42-1 details the normal turnover of calcium in the body. Although daily dietary calcium intake can range from 200 to 2000 mg, the calcium intake of many adults is below the recommended minimum of 800 mg. The percentage of dietary calcium absorbed from the intestine is inversely related to intake, but the relationship is curvilinear. An adaptive increase in fractional absorption is one important mechanism for maintaining normal body calcium stores when the diet does not contain adequate calcium. Conversely, an adaptive decrease in absorption prevents overload when the diet supplies too much calcium. At a daily intake of 1000 mg of calcium, about 35% is absorbed, approximately half passively and half stimulated by vitamin D. The same amount of calcium, 350 mg, must ultimately be excreted to maintain balance. About 150 mg is secreted back into the intestine and excreted in the stools, along with the unabsorbed fraction from the diet. The remaining 200 mg is excreted in the urine. The kidneys filter about 10,000 mg of calcium per day (non–protein-bound calcium concentration × glomerular filtration rate = 60 mg/L × 170 L/day). However, approximately 98% is reabsorbed in the tubules. Adjustment of the small fraction of filtered calcium that is finally excreted provides a sensitive means of maintaining calcium balance. *Both the dietary calcium intake and the absorption of calcium from the intestine are diminished in elderly individuals. This decreased calcium input contributes to a declining bone mass and the increased risk of fracture in the aged (osteoporosis).*

Calcium enters and exits from an extracellular pool of 1000 mg, which is in equilibrium with a rapidly exchanging pool of several times that size. The latter pool is probably located in the surface of recently or partially mineralized bone. Approximately 500 mg of calcium is "irreversibly" removed from the extracellular space by bone formation, and the same amount is returned to it by bone resorption in the steady-state process that constitutes normal **bone remodeling.**

Calcium Sensing

The homeostatic regulation of calcium levels in extracellular fluids and in various local cellular environments is under both indirect endocrine control and direct feedback control by the calcium level itself. Both forms of control are mediated by a calcium sensing plasma membrane receptor of the G-protein–linked type (see Fig. 39-11C). The calcium receptor is located in endocrine and other cells that have principal roles in calcium homeostasis including cells secreting parathyroid hormone and calcitonin, and vitamin D-producing cells, bone-forming and bone-resorbing cells, renal tubular calcium-reabsorbing cells, and intestinal calcium-absorbing cells. The extracellular N-terminus portion of the receptor contains

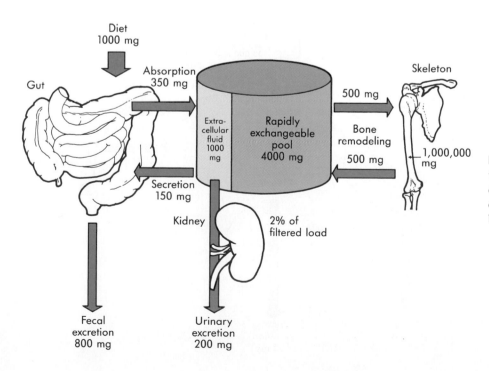

■ **Fig. 42-1** Average daily calcium turnover in humans. Note both the external balance between intake and excretion and the internal balance between entry into and exit from bone.

600 amino acids, the 7 transmembrane loops contain 250 amino acids, and the C-terminus intracellular tail contains 200 amino acids. Ca^{2+} binds to the extracellular domain at two serine residues. The intracellular portion contains sites that can be phosphorylated by protein kinase A and protein kinase C; in the latter case, the function of the calcium receptor is reduced by such phosphorylation.

The calcium receptor is coupled via G-proteins to adenylyl cyclase, phospholipases A_2, C, and D, and to MAP kinase and tyrosine kinases. The overall effect of all these actions mediated by the calcium receptor is to alter the rates of entry into or the rates of exit from the extracellular fluid, in order to protect against hypercalcemia or hypocalcemia.

Three rare clinical syndromes of genetic origin have helped to establish the essential nature of the calcium receptor to calcium metabolism in humans. Familial hypocalciuric hypercalcemia is a heterozygous state and severe neonatal hyperparathyroidism is a homozygous state of inactivating mutations in the extracellular portion of the calcium receptor. These mutations reduce the affinity of the receptor for calcium. They reset the system so that mild or severe degrees of hypercalcemia, respectively, are maintained with inappropriately low urine excretion. By contrast, mutations in the transmembrane domain of the receptor are hyperactivating, and they enhance the signal generated by calcium. This results in maintenance of hypocalcemia by inappropriately high urinary calcium excretion caused by impaired tubular resorption of calcium.

Phosphate

The phosphate ion is also critically important to all biological systems. Phosphate is an integral component of numerous intermediates in the metabolism of carbohydrates, lipids, and proteins. It forms part of the structure (1) of high-energy transfer and storage compounds, such as adenosine triphosphate (ATP) and creatine phosphate; (2) of cofactors, such as NAD, NADP, and thiamine pyrophosphate; (3) of second messengers, such as cAMP and inositol trisphosphate; and (4) of DNA and RNA. Phosphate functions as a covalent modifier of many enzymes. Inside cells, phosphate is an important anion that balances the cations K^+ and Mg^{2+}, and it is a major constituent of the crystalline structure of bone and teeth. Of the total body phosphate content, 85% is contained in the skeleton, and 6% in muscle.

The normal concentration of phosphate in the plasma is 2.5 to 4.5 mg/dl (0.81 to 1.45 mmol/L). Because the valence of phosphate changes with pH, it is less convenient to express phosphate concentration in milliequivalents per liter, as was done for calcium. The turnover of phosphate is shown in Fig. 42-2. About 70% of the phosphate ingested is absorbed by the intestine. In contrast to calcium, this absorbed amount remains relatively constant. Thus, the relationship between the intake and absorption of phosphate from the intestine is more linear than that for calcium. Also, although adaptive regulation of phosphate absorption exists, it is less important than the regulation of calcium absorption. Therefore, urinary excretion provides the major mechanism for preserving phosphate balance. Of the daily filtered load of approximately 6000 mg (plasma concentration × glomerular filtration rate = 35 mg/L × 170 L/day), the renal tubules can reabsorb from 70% to 100%, with an average of 90%. Regulation of phosphate absorption by the renal tubules provides the flexibility necessary to compensate for large swings in dietary intake.

Soft tissue stores of phosphate, such as those in the muscle mass, undergo rapid transfer with the extracellular fluid

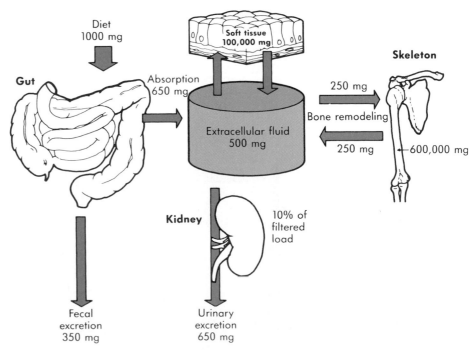

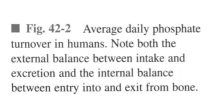

■ **Fig. 42-2** Average daily phosphate turnover in humans. Note both the external balance between intake and excretion and the internal balance between entry into and exit from bone.

pool of phosphate. This transfer process is an important factor in the minute-to-minute regulation of plasma phosphate concentration. About 250 mg, or half the total extracellular fluid pool of 500 mg, enters and leaves the bone mass daily in the process of bone remodeling. Growing evidence supports the existence of a specific phosphate receptor, "phosphatonin," but its structure and second messengers remain to be established conclusively.

Severe phosphate depletion can lead to skeletal muscle weakness, cardiac and respiratory muscle dysfunction, loss of red blood cell membrane integrity, and abnormal formation of bone.

The divalent cation, magnesium (Mg^{2+}), is related in some metabolic respects to calcium and phosphate. Magnesium is essential in neuromuscular transmission, and it serves as a cofactor in numerous enzyme reactions, most notably those involving energy transfers via ATP and those involved in protein synthesis. The normal range of magnesium in plasma is 1.8 to 2.4 mg/dl (1.5-2.0 mEq/L). One third of plasma magnesium is bound to protein. The body contains a total of about 25 g of magnesium, of which 50% is present in the skeleton, and almost all the rest is present in the intracellular fluid. The usual daily intake of magnesium ranges from 300 to 500 mg. On average, 40% of this ingested magnesium is absorbed. In a steady state, the same amount, 120 to 200 mg, is excreted in the urine. Mg^{2+} can regulate its own concentration, probably at least in part by interacting with the calcium receptor. However, the sensitivity of Mg^{2+} binding to this receptor is 2- to 3-fold lower than that of calcium.

Serious magnesium depletion results from intestinal malabsorption, alcoholism, or diuretic overuse. Neuromuscular irritability, as described for calcium depletion, may result. In rare cases, dangerous ventricular arrhythmias may occur.

BONE DYNAMICS

A detailed account of the development of the skeleton, its structural properties, and its mechanical function is beyond the scope of endocrine physiology. However, a brief review of the organization and turnover of bone in relation to its function as a mineral reservoir is essential to an understanding of the regulation of calcium and phosphate metabolism.

About 75% to 80% of the bone mass consists of **cortical bone.** The dense, concentric outer layers of the appendicular skeleton (long bones) and the thinner outer layer of the flat bones are the major components of cortical bone. About 20% to 25% of the bone mass consists of **trabecular bone,** which are bridges of bone spicules that make up the larger inner parts of the axial skeleton (skull, ribs, vertebrae, and pelvis) and the smaller interior of the shafts of long bones (Fig. 42-3). *Although of lesser mass, trabecular bone has five times as much total surface area as does cortical bone. Because of its greater accessibility, trabecular bone is more important than cortical bone in calcium turnover.*

Throughout life, the bone mass is continuously being renewed by the well-regulated coupling of the processes of bone formation and resorption. This coupling occurs within individual microscopic units, called **osteons** or **bone modeling**

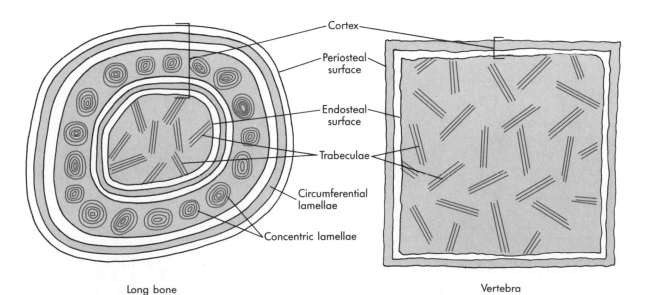

Long bone   Vertebra

■ **Fig. 42-3** Schematic cross-sectional representations of a long bone, primarily cortical, and a vertebra, primarily trabecular. The long bone is distinguished by a thick outer cortex containing circumferential rings (lamellae) within which concentric lamellae known as haversian canals are present. These contain nutrient vessels. The inner portions of long bones and vertebrae consist of bridging spicules of bone or trabeculae in organized lamellar arrays. Between the trabeculae are bone marrow elements and connective tissue cells.

units, that are present in all types of bone. During embryogenesis and the growth years, formation exceeds resorption, and skeletal mass increases. Linear growth occurs at the ends of long bones by replacement of cartilage (endochondral bone formation) in specialized areas, known as **epiphyseal plates.** Initial recruitment of chondrocytes is stimulated by hormones, as is their progression through cartilage formation and their ultimate disappearance. The growth plates are closed off by endocrine mechanisms at the end of puberty when adult height is reached. Increase in bone width occurs by addition to the periosteum, which is the outer surface of the cortical bone located under the connective tissue covering. Once adult bone mass is achieved, equal rates of formation and resorption maintain the peak bone mass until age 30 to 40 years. At this time, resorption begins to exceed formation, and the total mass slowly decreases.

The process of bone turnover in the adult is known as *remodeling,* which is also one of the major mechanisms for maintaining calcium homeostasis. The life span of a typical bone modeling unit is 6 to 9 months. About 10% of the total adult bone mass normally turns over each year in the remodeling process. Cortical bone turns over much more slowly than does trabecular bone (4% vs. 28%/year). Endocrine diseases that disrupt the coupling of formation and resorption have severe consequences on bone. The dysfunction is more pronounced if these diseases occur during the early

phase of growth and the late phase of senescence, when a natural disequilibrium already exists between bone formation and resorption. *Women experience severe consequences of such diseases more often than do men, because women have a 25% smaller peak bone mass and an accelerated rate of loss during the first 5 years after the menopause.*

Four major cell (**osteoblasts, osteocytes, lining cells,** and **osteoclasts**) types are recognized in histological sections of bone (Fig. 42-4). Osteoblasts arise from pluropotential primitive stem cells within the connective tissue of the mesenchyme. These cells can differentiate into adipocytes, myoblasts, and chondrocytes, as well as into osteoprogenitor cells. A variety of 15 bone morphogenetic proteins (BMPs) act through several transcription factors to direct the differentiation of precursors preferentially into osteoblasts and to stimulate their growth.

The BMPs appear to act synergistically with another class of proteins, which are products of the *hedgehog* genes. The latter regulate the very earliest steps in vertebrate skeletal development. About one-third of osteoblasts either become lining cells or osteocytes and two-thirds undergo apoptosis, as described in Chapter 39. The average life span of osteoblasts is 3 months, whereas osteocytes live 20 years. The osteoclasts, which are much fewer in number, originate from the same bone marrow stem cells as do tissue macrophages and circulating monocytes. Strong evidence indicates that a factor(s) secreted by differentiating osteoblasts

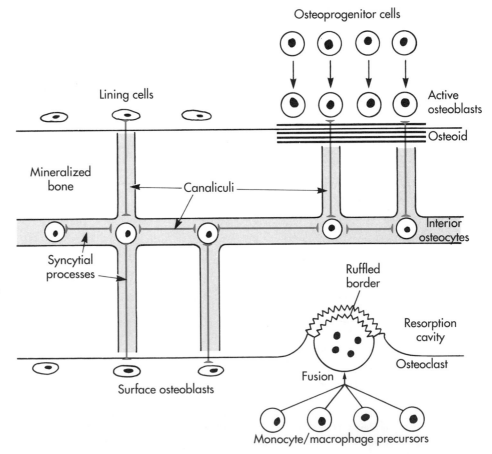

■ **Fig. 42-4** The relationships between bone cells and bone surfaces. The canaliculi provide a huge interface between the interior surfaces of mineralized bone and intercellular fluid. This permits efficient osteolysis with transfer of calcium and phosphate to the exterior via syncytial processes connecting interior osteocytes and surface lining cells. (Redrawn from Avioli LV et al: Bone metabolism and disease. In Bondy PK, Rosenberg LE, editors: *Metabolic control and disease,* Philadelphia, 1980, WB Saunders.)

is required for differentiation of mature osteoclasts from their precursors. Osteoclasts have a short life span of about 2 weeks.

Bone Formation

Bone formation is carried out by active osteoblasts, which synthesize and extrude the type 1 procollagen molecule into the adjacent extracellular space. There further processing results in three chained molecules that form fibrils spontaneously by interconnecting collagen molecules with pyridinoline cross-links that are unique to bone. The osteoblasts also secrete into the matrix other proteins, namely osteocalcin and osteonectin, which help regulate the quantity and quality of the final formed bone. The collagen fibrils line up in regular arrays and produce an organic matrix, known as **osteoid.** Calcium is then deposited as amorphous masses of calcium phosphate in an environment of calcium and phosphate concentrations that is regulated by the osteoblasts. About 10 days elapse between osteoid formation and mineralization, and a distance of 8 to 10 μm separates the leading edges of the two processes. Once mineralization is initiated, however, most of the calcium phosphate is deposited within 6 to 12 hours. Thereafter, hydroxide and bicarbonate ions are gradually added to the mineral mixture, and mature **hydroxyapatite** crystals are slowly formed. These crystals have a calcium/phosphate ratio of 2.2 by weight and of 1.7 by moles. As this completely mineralized bone accumulates and surrounds the osteoblast, this cell decreases its synthetic activity and it becomes an interior osteocyte (Fig. 42-4). Osteoblastic activity, therefore, is usually observed only along the surfaces of bone—the concentric **lamellae** of cortical bone or the linear lamellae of the interior bridging trabeculae (Fig. 42-3). Lining cells are arranged along these surfaces, and these cells may initiate the cycle of remodeling in each osteon, as described below.

The mineralization process requires adequate plasma concentrations of calcium and phosphate, and it is dependent on vitamin D. The enzyme, **alkaline phosphatase,** and other macromolecules from the osteoblast also participate in this process. **Osteonectin** binds to collagen, and the resultant complex in turn binds hydroxyapatite crystals. **Osteocalcin** is distinguished by the presence of γ-carboxyglutamate residues, which have an affinity for calcium and a strong avidity for uncrystallized hydroxyapatite. The plasma levels of alkaline phosphatase and of osteocalcin are standard markers of osteoblastic activity. Specific peptide derivatives of procollagen, are excreted in the urine, and they serve as indices of bone formation.

Within each bone unit, minute fluid-containing channels, called **canaliculi,** traverse the mineralized bone. Through these channels, the interior osteocytes remain connected with surface lining cells and with other osteocytes via syncytial cell processes (Fig. 42-4). This arrangement permits transfer of calcium from the enormous surface area of the interior to the exterior of the bone units, and then into the extracellular fluid. This transfer process, which is carried out by the osteocytes, is known as **osteocytic osteolysis.** It prob-

ably does not actually decrease bone mass, but it simply removes calcium from the most recently formed crystals.

Bone Resorption

In contrast to osteocytic osteolysis, the process of resorption of bone does not merely extract calcium; it destroys the entire matrix of bone and thereby diminishes the bone mass. The cell responsible for bone resorption is the osteoclast. This giant (50-100 μm) multinucleated (10-20 nuclei) cell is formed by fusion of several precursor cells (Fig. 42-4). Before osteoclastic resorption can begin, a thin 1- to 2-μm outer layer of unmineralized osteoid must be removed. This is achieved by collagenase released from lining cells. The latter also secrete molecules that attract osteoclasts to the site of the now denuded bone. The osteoclast contains large numbers of mitochondria and lysosomes. It attaches to the endosteal and periosteal surfaces of bone modeling units, a process mediated by integrins. At the point of attachment, a ruffled border is created by infolding of the osteoclast's plasma membrane. Within this sealed off zone, surrounded by a clear cytoplasmic space, the process of bone dissolution is carried out by type 4 collagenase, phosphatase, and lysosomal enzymes. An essential local acidic environment is created by operation of an ATP-driven proton pump.

Thus, osteoclasts literally tunnel their way into the mineralized bone at a rate of 25 μm per day. In this microenvironment, Ca^{2+} concentrations can rise as high as 40 mM. Calcium, phosphate, the amino acids, **hydroxyproline** and **hydroxylysine,** that are unique to collagen, and the fluorescent products of collagen cross-linkages, **pyridinolines,** are all released into the extracellular fluid during resorption. Urinary excretion rates of the organic products provide quantitative indices of bone resorption.

Coordination of Resorption and Formation in Remodeling

Remodeling occurs in areas of bone that have been structurally weakened by "fatigue," by having unusual mechanical stress placed on them, or by disuse. The osteocytes, imbedded deep within mineralized bone (Fig. 42-5), are the mechanosensors that pick up mechanical signals transmitted via interstitial fluid. The mechanical stress increases the flow of fluid and the fluid shear forces within the canaliculi. Osteocytes respond by increasing phospholipase C, Ca^{2+}, and protein kinase C activity. These lead to stimulation of phospholipase A_2 and production of prostaglandins (PGE_2). PGE_2 in turn reaches the lining cells via the syncytial processes (Fig. 42-4) or the canaliculi. The lining cells then initiate recruitment and differentiation of osteoclasts via communications with stromal precursors in the bone marrow, which in turn communicate with endothelial cells. Thus, remodeling ultimately requires a chain involving all the cells in bone and some of the cells in the bone marrow. As noted previously, resorption and formation are usually closely coordinated within each bone modeling unit.

Resorption is the initial process, but it is triggered by signals from osteoblasts and cells of its lineage. As osteoclasts

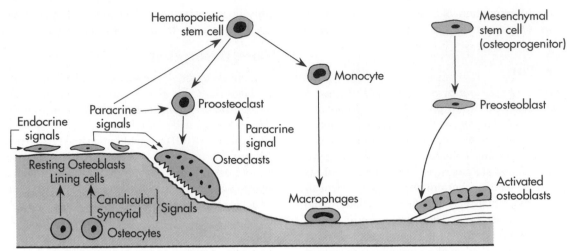

■ **Fig. 42-5**   Process of bone remodeling. Signals carried by canalicular and syncytial routes from interior osteocytes, and endocrine signals to resting osteoblasts and lining cells generate local paracrine cytokine signals to nearby osteoclasts and osteoclast precursors. Osteoclasts also recruit their own precursors by paracrine signals. The osteoclasts resorb an area of mineralized bone, and local macrophages complete the clean-up of dissolved elements. The process then reverses to formation as osteoblast precursors are recruited to the site and differentiate into active osteoblasts. These lay down new organic matrix and mineralize it. Thus, new bone replaces the previously resorbed mature bone. (Modified from Raisz LG: *N Engl J Med* 318:820, 1988.)

form, they secrete **annexins,** which are signaling molecules that recruit more osteoclasts from precursors. Moreover, as old bone is resorbed by osteoclasts and the products are cleaned up by macrophages, bone formation by osteoblasts follows at the same site and fills in the cavity with new and stronger bone. The resorption phase lasts about 10 days and the succeeding formation phase lasts 3 month. A single remodeling unit creates about 0.025 mm³ of bone and it has a life span of about 6 to 9 months.

All aspects of the remodeling cycle are influenced by a large array of hormones and growth factors, as well as by cytokines from immune cells (Table 42-1). These molecules can affect one or more of the various steps either positively or negatively, or even both, in different cells. The response depends on the concentration of each regulatory factor and on the duration of exposure. For example, transforming growth factor β stimulates apoptosis in osteoclasts, but it inhibits apoptosis in osteoblasts. The process of bone modeling is one example of coordinated function of the endocrine and immune systems.

Bone remodeling is ordinarily regulated to compensate for change. For example, if the primary effect of a hormone is to stimulate resorption, this effect will be at least partially balanced by a secondary increase in formation. This compensation occurs by the mechanism of coupling. Therefore, the net effect of any endocrine abnormality depends on the degree to which the total bone mass is defended by the compensatory process of coupling.

The total bone mass of humans, which may be individually determined genetically, peaks at 25 to 35 years of age. At this time, men have a larger bone mass than do women. A gradual decline occurs in both genders with

■ **Table 42-1**   Major effects of various hormones on bone

Bone formation	Bone resorption
Stimulated by	**Stimulated by**
Growth hormone (constant)	Parathyroid hormone (constant)
Insulin-like growth factors	Vitamin D
Insulin	Cortisol
Estrogen	Thyroid hormone
Androgen	Prostaglandins
Vitamin D (mineralization)	Interleukin-1
Transforming growth factor–β	Interleukin-6
Skeletal growth factor	Tumor necrosis factor α
Bone-derived growth factor	Tumor necrosis factor β
Calcitonin	
Parathyroid hormone (intermittent)	
Inhibited by	**Inhibited by**
Cortisol	Estrogen
	Androgen
	Calcitonin
	Transforming growth factor–β
	γ-Interferon
	Nitric oxide

aging, but women undergo an accelerated phase of bone loss, caused by increased resorption in the perimenopausal period. The turnover of bone decreases with age, but the osteoblasts do not refill resorptive cavities with normal speed; that is, bone resorption exceeds formation. The reduced bone density (Fig. 42-6) and mass, called **osteoporosis,** creates a susceptibility to wrist and vertebral fractures, particularly in women in the sixth and seventh decades of life.

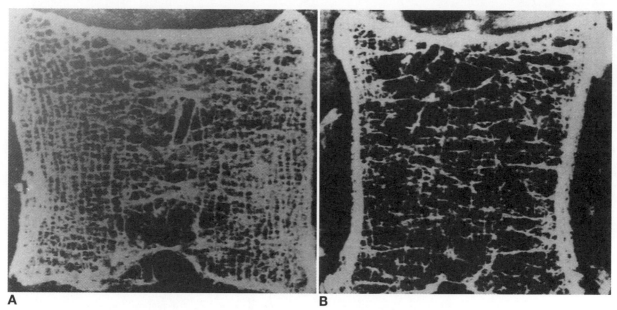

■ **Fig. 42-6** **A,** Radiograph of a normal vertebra from a 40-year-old woman. **B,** Radiograph of a vertebra from a 92-year-old woman. Note the marked loss of trabeculae with relative preservation of cortex in the aged woman. (From Atkinson P: *Calcif Tissue Res* 1:24, 1967.)

By the eighth and ninth decades, hip fractures become prevalent in both genders. A generous calcium intake, habitual exercise, and avoidance of smoking and excessive alcohol intake, throughout life, reduce the risk of osteoporosis.

VITAMIN D

Vitamin D, after its activation to the hormone $1,25\text{-}(OH)_2\text{-}D$, is one of the two major regulators of calcium metabolism. *$1,25\text{-}(OH)_2\text{-}D$ increases calcium absorption from the intestine and calcium resorption from bone.* Both actions raise or sustain the plasma calcium concentration. Vitamin $1,25\text{-}(OH)_2\text{-}D$ has similar effects on phosphate. $1,25\text{-}(OH)_2\text{-}D$ also plays an essential role in bone formation.

Vitamin D Production

Humans acquire vitamin D from two sources. Vitamin D is produced in the skin by ultraviolet irradiation (D_3) and it is also ingested in the diet (D_3 and D_2). In this sense, vitamin D itself is not a "classic hormone," because it is not produced by an endocrine gland. However, vitamin D undergoes molecular modification to yield a metabolite that then acts on distant target cells, and its mechanism of action is similar to that of thyroid and steroid hormones. These actions justify its classification as a hormone.

The structures of vitamin D_3, its precursors, and its metabolites are shown in Fig. 42-7. Vitamin D_2, which differs from vitamin D_3 only in an additional double bond at the 21 to 22 position, is derived from the plant sterol, ergosterol, by ultraviolet radiation. Vitamin D_2 is a major dietary source in many countries. Because vitamin D_2 has biological actions identical to those of vitamin D_3, the term *vitamin D* will generally be used to indicate both forms.

Vitamin D_3 synthesis occurs primarily in specialized skin cells, called **keratinocytes,** which are located in the epidermis. Under the influence of summer sunlight [ultraviolet (UV) radiation at 270 to 300 nm], **7-dehydrocholesterol** is photoconverted to **previtamin** D_3 (Fig. 42-7). A minimum of 20 mJ radiation energy per square centimeter of skin is required. The amount of previtamin D_3 formed is related in exponential fashion to the UV input. Previtamin D_3 is then converted spontaneously over 3 days to vitamin D_3, in a reaction that is driven by thermal energy from sunshine. Continuous exposure to sunlight also causes photodegradation of previtamin D_3 to inactive products in reactions that are catalyzed by UV radiation at 315 to 330 nm. *Thus, although sunlight stimulates vitamin D_3 production, it also restrains overproduction, so that excessive exposure to sunlight does not cause systemic vitamin D toxicity. Synthesis of vitamin D_3 is inhibited by $1,25\text{-}(OH)_2\text{-}D$ and it is stimulated by PTH.*

In winter or in sunlight-poor climates, dietary vitamin D may be essential for health. The most important sources are fish, liver, and irradiated milk. The minimal daily dietary requirement of vitamin D is approximately 2.5 μg, and the recommended daily intake is 10 μg (400 units). Because of its fat solubility, vitamin D absorption from the intestine is mediated by bile salts, and it occurs via the lymphatic glands. Excesses are efficiently stored in adipose tissue and liver, and it can take several months for these stores to be dissipated.

Vitamin D has very little, if any, intrinsic biological activity. It must undergo successive hydroxylations in order to act as a hormone (Fig. 42-7). In the liver, it is hydroxylated by a microsomal and mitochondrial enzyme to 25-OH-D. This reaction requires NADPH and O_2. From the liver, 25-OH-D is transported to the kidney (and possibly to other sites),

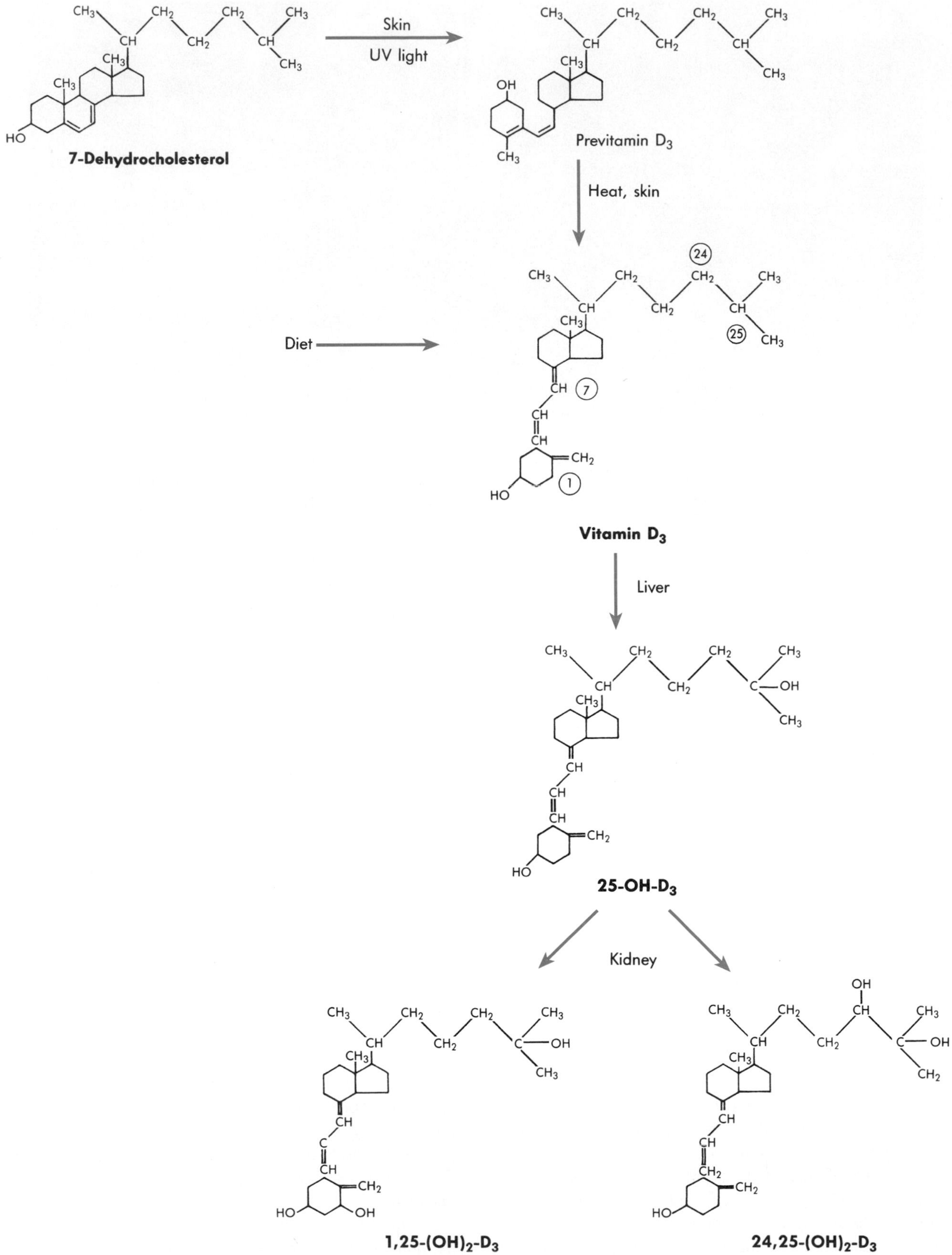

■ **Fig. 42-7** Structures of vitamin D_3, its precursor, and its metabolites.

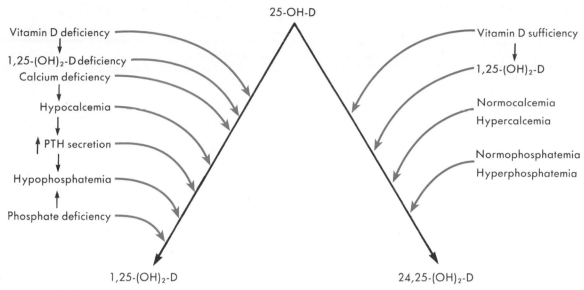

■ **Fig. 42-8** Factors that regulate conversion of 25-OH-D₃ to either 1,25-(OH)₂-D or 24,25-(OH)₂-D. The former is increased by either calcium or phosphate lack.

where it undergoes further alteration (Fig. 42-7). Although 25-OH-D does have intrinsic activity in vitro and in intact humans, it is essentially inactive in the absence of the kidneys. Its physiological function in calcium regulation appears to be that of a circulating plasma storage pool and a precursor to much more highly active metabolites.

The alteration that 25-(OH)-D undergoes in the kidneys yields two metabolites. Hydroxylation of 25-(OH)-D in the 1 position to 1,25-(OH)₂-D occurs in the mitochondria of the proximal convoluted and straight tubules of the kidneys. The 1α-hydroxylase enzyme is a mixed function P-450 steroid hydroxylase that requires NADPH, O₂, and a flavoprotein, known as **renoredoxin** or **ferredoxin.** Vitamin 1,25-(OH)₂-D is the most potent vitamin D metabolite in vivo, and it expresses all the known activities of vitamin D. Alternatively, 25-OH-D may be hydroxylated in the 24 position to 24,25-(OH)₂-D in a mitochondrial reaction that again requires NADPH and O₂. Whether 24,25-(OH)₂-D has significant biological activity remains controversial. However, it is far less potent than 1,25-(OH)₂-D in most assay systems. Preventing 24 hydroxylation by putting a fluorine atom at the 24 position does not reduce the activity of the hydroxylated derivative. Although 24 hydroxylation in the kidney probably represents only a means of inactivating excess vitamin D, 24,25-(OH)₂-D could still possibly play a separate role in expressing particular vitamin D actions.

Regulation of 1,25-(OH)₂-D production largely occurs in the kidney. (The rate of 25-OH-D synthesis in the liver is decreased by 1,25-(OH)₂-D via product inhibition.) Regulation primarily occurs at the alternative 1- or 24-hydroxylase step (Fig. 42-8). Vitamin 25-OH-D is preferentially directed toward the active metabolite, 1,25-(OH)₂-D when vitamin D, calcium, or phosphate is lacking. In vitamin D-deficient states, it is partly the lack of 1,25-(OH)₂-D itself that enhances

1-hydroxylation, because 1,25-(OH)₂-D suppresses 1-hydroxylase synthesis and activity.

Even when the amount of vitamin D is sufficient, the 1-hydroxylase enzyme is still subject to regulation by calcium and phosphate levels. Calcium deprivation leads to hypocalcemia, which in turn stimulates PTH hypersecretion. The decreased plasma calcium concentration and the increased PTH concentration both stimulate independently the synthesis and activity of 1-hydroxylase. Phosphate deprivation leads to hypophosphatemia and a lowered renal cortical phosphate content, which also directly increases 1-hydroxylase activity. *Thus, the supply of active 1,25-(OH)₂-D is augmented whenever the mobilization of calcium or phosphate from intestine and bone into the extracellular fluid is needed.* Conversely, the supply of inactive 24,25-(OH)₂-D is augmented when 1,25-(OH)₂-D and phosphate are plentiful, and bone formation can be sustained.

Vitamin D, 25-OH-D, 1,25-(OH)₂-D, and 24,25-(OH)₂-D all circulate bound to an α-globulin. This vitamin D–binding protein has a half-life of only 3 days. It binds 25-OH-D with high affinity, and binds D and 1,25-(OH)₂-D with much lower affinities. The concentrations, approximate half-lives, and estimated daily production rates for the three key vitamin D metabolites in humans are shown in Table 42-2. Vitamin 1,25-(OH)₂-D has the shortest half-life of the three and by far the lowest concentration, which befits its potency. Because of the difference in binding protein affinities, however, 0.4% of plasma 1,25-(OH)₂-D is free, compared to 0.04% of 25-(OH)-D.

Certain relationships among the plasma concentrations of the three metabolites are also physiologically significant. Vitamin 1,25-(OH)₂-D concentration is ordinarily independent of 25-OH-D concentration. Except in severe vitamin D deficiency or toxicity states, the regulatory factors previously described can maintain the appropriate concentration of

■ Table 42-2   Vitamin D metabolism in humans

	Plasma concentration (μ/L)	Plasma half-life (days)	Estimated production rate (μ/day)
1,25-(OH)$_2$-D$_3$	0.03	0.25	1
24,25-(OH)$_2$-D$_3$	2	15 to 40	1
25-OH- D$_3$	30	15	10

■ Table 42-3   Target genes of vitamin D

Gene	Transcription
Vitamin D receptor	Increased
Calcium-binding proteins (calbindins)	Increased
Calcium pump	Increased
Osteocalcin	Increased
Alkaline phosphatase	Increased
24-Hydroxylase	Increased
Parathyroid hormone	Decreased
1-Hydroxylase	Decreased
Collagen	Decreased
Interleukin-2	Decreased
γ-Interferon	Decreased

the active metabolite, irrespective of the supply of precursor. In contrast, 24,25-(OH)$_2$-D concentration is ordinarily directly proportional to 25-OH-D concentration. This proportional relationship reflects the role of 24-hydroxylation as a key sluicing mechanism for disposing of excess precursor. Vitamin 1,25-(OH)$_2$-D can be further hydroxylated to 1,24,25-(OH)$_3$-D, a compound that has little activity. Thus, if an excess of 1,25-(OH)$_2$-D should develop, it can still be inactivated by 24-hydroxylation. Many other hydroxylated vitamin D metabolites have been described, but their function is unknown.

In one respect, the orally absorbed vitamin D$_2$ may have a different metabolic fate than the endogenously produced D$_3$. Vitamin D$_2$ can first be 24-hydroxylated in the liver, followed by 1-hydroxylation. 24-(OH)-D$_2$ and 1,24-(OH)$_2$-D$_2$ may have specific biological actions, or they may serve as alternates to the 25-hydroxylated D$_3$ and D$_2$ metabolites. Both active and inactive vitamin D metabolites undergo biliary excretion and enterohepatic recycling.

Vitamin D deficiency results from inadequate access to sunlight and/or inadequate dietary sources. Preterm black infants who live in air-polluted cities (inadequate UV radiation) and who are breast fed (inadequate ingestion of the vitamin) are at increased risk for rickets, a disease characterized by bone deformation (e.g., bowlegs). Elderly institutionalized individuals are also at increased risk of suffering from vitamin D deficiency and from resulting fractures. Intestinal diseases that cause malabsorption of fats and decreased enterohepatic recycling of vitamin D and its critical metabolites also lead to deficiency states. Vitamin D can be used as replacement therapy for all of these vitamin D-deficient states. Hepatic disease, kidney failure, and defective genes that encode the 25-hydroxylase or 1-hydroxylase enzyme may prevent the normal conversion from vitamin D to 1,25-(OH)$_2$-D, and they can be treated with the specific deficient metabolite.

Vitamin D Actions

Vitamin 1,25-(OH)$_2$-D acts through the general nuclear mechanism outlined for steroid hormones (see Fig. 39-17). The vitamin D receptor is found in both the cytoplasm and nucleus. Binding of 1,25-(OH)$_2$-D induces receptor phosphorylation, and the resultant complex attaches to 1,25-(OH)$_2$-D regulatory elements in target DNA molecules. An accessory protein is required to facilitate this attachment. Heterodimers between the vitamin D receptor and the retinoid receptor

also play a role in the induction or suppression of target gene transcription.

Table 42-3 lists some of the important genes involved in vitamin D actions. Vitamin D may also downregulate the Ca^{2+} receptor in some target cells. This constitutes a positive feedback mechanism that augments the effect of vitamin D and raises the plasma Ca^{2+} concentration. The vitamin D receptor is upregulated by 1,25-(OH)$_2$-D. It is also upregulated by PTH, insulin-like growth factors, estrogen, and cortisol.

One major product of 1,25-(OH)$_2$-D action is a series of calcium binding proteins, called **calbindins** of various molecular weights. These proteins bind calcium ions in various stoichiometric proportions, and they exhibit significant homology with calmodulin and myosin light chain. In contrast to the slowly developing nuclear effects via its receptor (and not through a transcriptional mechanism), 1,25-(OH)$_2$-D also has rapid membrane effects that involve an increase in cGMP and in intracellular calcium levels.

The major action of 1,25-(OH)2-D is to stimulate absorption of calcium from the intestinal lumen against a concentration gradient. A rapid phase of action is evident within a few minutes to about 6 hours; a slower phase takes 24 to 96 hours. Vitamin 1,25-(OH)$_2$-D localizes to the nuclei of intestinal villus and crypt cells, but not to goblet or submucosa cells. There, it acts on the brush border and increases the number of calcium pump molecules in the basolateral membrane. Hours after calcium entry from the intestinal lumen to the capillaries has been rapidly stimulated, the calbindin concentration rises. These molecules may ferry calcium across the intestinal cell or they may buffer the high calcium concentrations that result from the initial entry of the ion. The rate of calcium absorption across the duodenum is proportional to the cell content of calbindin. Vitamin 1,25-(OH)$_2$-D is responsible for the adaptation, described previously, whereby intestinal calcium absorption can be adjusted to alterations in the amount of dietary calcium. A daily dose of only 0.5 μg of 1,25-(OH)$_2$-D produces a 25% increase above baseline in calcium absorption. Although 50 μg of 25-(OH)-D is required to produce the same increment, because of its much higher plasma concentration (Table 42-2), 25-(OH)-D contributes about 10% of the stimulated calcium absorption. In addition to calcium absorption, 1,25-(OH)$_2$-D stimulates the active absorption of phosphate and magnesium across the intestinal cell membrane. The mechanisms for the absorption of phosphate and magnesium are independent of and less well defined than those that regulate the absorption of calcium.

Another major target organ of $1,25\text{-}(OH)_2\text{-}D$ is bone, where it causes complex effects. Osteoblasts, but not osteoclasts, have $1,25\text{-}(OH)_2\text{-}D$ receptors. Nonetheless $1,25\text{-}(OH)_2\text{-}D$ stimulates bone resorption, probably by stimulating a cytokine signal that originates in the lining cell or osteoblast. In this way, $1,25\text{-}(OH)_2\text{-}D$ increases the recruitment, differentiation, and fusion of precursors into active osteoclasts, which carry out their resorptive missions. Vitamin $1,25\text{-}(OH)_2\text{-}D$ also increases osteocytic osteolysis. The concurrent presence of PTH is required for $1,25\text{-}(OH)_2\text{-}D$-stimulated bone resorption.

Vitamin D also plays a key role in bone formation. The normal mineralization of newly formed osteoid along a calcification front is critically dependent on vitamin D. In its absence, excess osteoid accumulates from lack of $1,25\text{-}(OH)_2\text{-}D$ repression of collagen synthesis by osteoblasts (Table 42-3). The bone formed in the absence of $1,25\text{-}(OH)_2\text{-}D$ is weak. It is still unclear whether this action of vitamin D is accounted for entirely by the augmentation of the supply of calcium and phosphate in the fluid bathing the osteoblast, or whether $1,25\text{-}(OH)_2\text{-}D$ also acts in a direct manner on the bone matrix or cells to hasten mineralization. A direct effect on bone formation is supported by the fact that $1,25\text{-}(OH)_2\text{-}D$ induces the synthesis of osteocalcin in osteoblasts. In any case, the first observable effect of vitamin D replacement on the bone in vitamin D-deficient animals and humans is the reappearance of a normal mineralized calcification front. The vitamin D receptor is also expressed by chondrocytes, and $1,25\text{-}(OH)_2\text{-}D$ may stimulate cartilage development in the epiphyseal growth plate.

Vitamin D–related abnormalities may play a role in the senescent bone loss described above. Aging changes in bone are associated with decreases in exposure to sunlight, synthesis of vitamin D from 7-dehydrocholesterol (Fig. 42-7), dietary intake of vitamin D, synthesis of $1,25\text{-}(OH)_2\text{-}D$, D receptors in the intestine, and therefore decreased calcium absorption. Lack of calcium impairs bone formation. Mild vitamin D deficiency in the aged leads to secondary hyperparathyroidism and increased bone turnover. Severe deficiency leads to **osteomalacia,** a condition analogous to rickets that is associated with an accumulation of an excess of unmineralized osteoid.

An important negative feedback action of $1,25\text{-}(OH)_2\text{-}D$ is to directly repress the gene responsible for the synthesis of PTH. This action is facilitated by $1,25\text{-}(OH)_2\text{-}D$ induction of its own receptor, as well as by a calbindin in parathyroid cells. $1,25\text{-}(OH)_2\text{-}D$ also inhibits expression of the PTH receptor in osteoblasts.

Vitamin $1,25\text{-}(OH)_2\text{-}D$ weakly stimulates renal calcium reabsorption by increasing the number of calcium pumps. It also stimulates calcium transport into skeletal and cardiac muscle; muscle weakness and cardiac dysfunction can result from vitamin D deficiency.

The same skin cells (keratinocytes) that synthesize vitamin D, and other epidermal cells, also produce $1,25\text{-}(OH)_2\text{-}D$ from $25\text{-}OH\text{-}D$. In a paracrine and autocrine manner, $1,25\text{-}(OH)_2\text{-}D$ stimulates differentiation and inhibits proliferation of these cells. Thus, formation of the outer cornified layer of the epidermis, with its appropriate content of enzymes and structural proteins, is regulated by vitamin D.

A new role for vitamin D in immunomodulation has also emerged. Macrophages, monocytes, and transformed lymphocytes can synthesize $1,25\text{-}(OH)_2\text{-}D$ from $25\text{-}OH\text{-}D$. Promyelocytes, monocytes, and activated T lymphocytes also express the $1,25\text{-}(OH)_2\text{-}D$ receptor. The hormone stimulates T-helper-2 cells to secrete interleukin-4 (IL-4) and TGF-β and T-helper-1 cells to decrease their production of interleukin-2, γ-interferon, and tumor necrosis factor α. The proliferation of T and B lymphocytes as well as immunoglobulin synthesis by B-lymphocytes are decreased by $1,25\text{-}(OH)_2\text{-}D$. Thus, vitamin D participates in autocrine and paracrine actions that are important in the regulation of immune responses, which are diminished in vitamin D-deficient states.

Macrophages and osteoclasts also have common ancestors. Therefore, $1,25\text{-}(OH)_2\text{-}D$ probably mediates an integrated endocrine, paracrine, and autocrine system, whereby osteoclasts and tissue macrophages are recruited sequentially when they are needed for bone resorption and for clean-up of the resultant waste products.

In diseases characterized by the formation of granulomas that contain mononuclear inflammatory cells (e.g., **sarcoidosis** and **tuberculosis**), these cells can synthesize excess $1,25\text{-}(OH)2\text{-}D$. Symptomatic hypercalcemia may result.

Finally, vitamin D receptors are found also in the pancreatic islets, anterior pituitary, hypothalamus, placenta, ovary, aortic endothelium, and skin fibroblasts. The presence of these receptors accounts for various other vitamin D actions that involve calcium, such as enhancement of insulin (see Chapter 41) and prolactin (see Chapter 43) secretion.

Vitamin D actions can be lost as a result of mutant receptors (e.g., in vitamin D-resistant **rickets**), hormone antagonists, and hormone deficiency. In children, the epiphyseal growth centers suffer defective mineralization of bone. This defect leads to the typical manifestations of rickets (Fig. 42-9), which include bowing of the extremities and collapse of the chest wall. In adults, pain, vertebral collapse, and fractures along stress lines characterize the condition known as **osteomalacia.** In children and adults, excess osteoid accumulates in the bone. Plasma calcium and phosphate levels are decreased, whereas alkaline phosphatase and PTH levels are increased. Therapy requires the appropriate form of vitamin D in amounts that range from physiological to pharmacological.

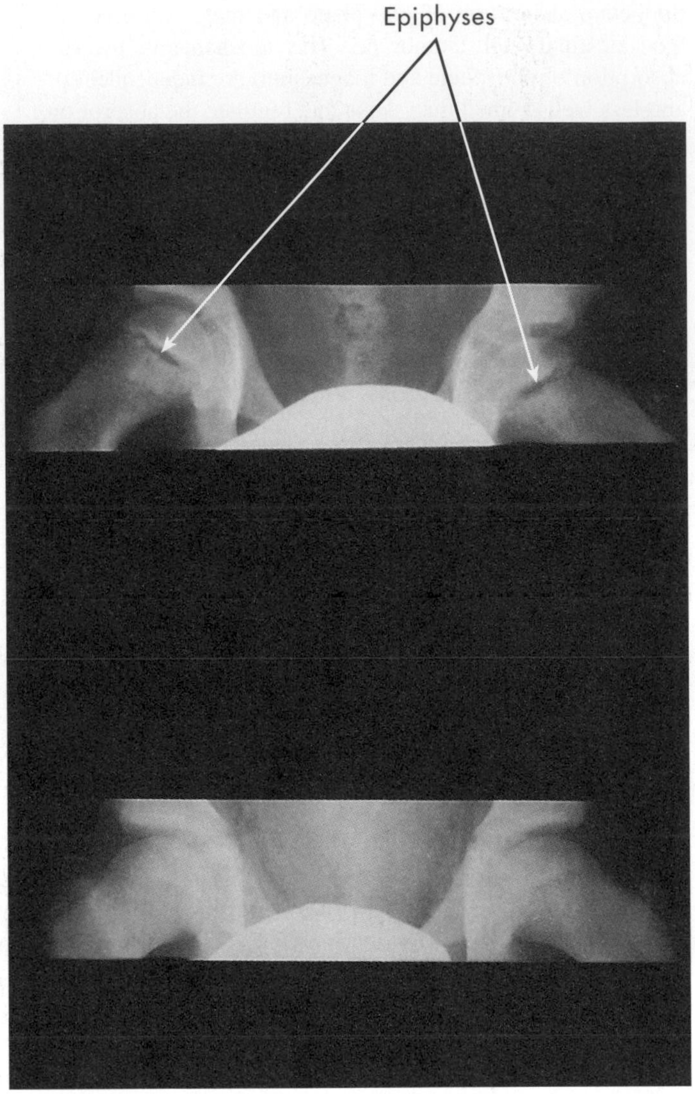

Epiphyses

■ **Fig. 42-9** **A,** Radiograph of the hips of a child with deficient 1,25-$(OH)_2$-D action because of renal failure and reduced production from 25-(OH)-D. Note the widened irregular epiphyseal growth areas. **B,** The same hips after treatment with vitamin D has mineralized the epiphyses.

Excessive vitamin D action causes overabsorption of calcium from the diet and increased bone resorption. Hypercalcemia, hypercalciuria, and kidney stones often result. Hyperphosphatemia is also present because of increased phosphate influx and suppression of PTH secretion (see below). The duration of toxicity is greatest with an excess of vitamin D, because of its large storage capacity, and is least in 1,25-$(OH)_2$-D excess, because of rapid removal of the active hormone. Treatment consists of blocking the effects of the vitamin D excess with calcitonin or with cortisol analogues.

PARATHYROID HORMONE

The parathyroid glands secrete **parathyroid hormone (PTH),** the other major regulator of calcium and phosphorus metabolism. *The paramount effect of PTH is to increase plasma calcium levels directly by stimulating bone resorption and renal tubular calcium reabsorption, and indirectly by stimulating renal 1,25-$(OH)_2$-D synthe-*

sis. At the same time, PTH decreases plasma phosphate concentration by inhibiting renal tubular phosphate reabsorption.

Four parathyroid glands develop at 5 to 14 weeks of gestation from the third and fourth branchial pouches. Normally, they descend to lie posterior to the thyroid gland, but ectopic locations in the neck and mediastinum can also occur. The total weight of adult parathyroid tissue is about 130 mg, and that of any one gland is 30 to 50 mg. The blood supply of the parathyroid glands, which is from the thyroid arteries, is easily interrupted during thyroid surgery. Samples drawn from the left and right thyroid veins can localize the site of unilateral parathyroid gland hyperfunction, when necessary.

The histological appearance of the parathyroid glands changes with age. The predominant cell, known as the **chief cell,** is present throughout life and is the normal source of PTH. Resting chief cells have abundant glycogen, an involuted Golgi apparatus, and a few clusters of secretory granules. Activated cells have little glycogen, a large convoluted Golgi apparatus with vacuoles and vesicles, and a granular endoplasmic reticulum. A second, less numerous cell type—

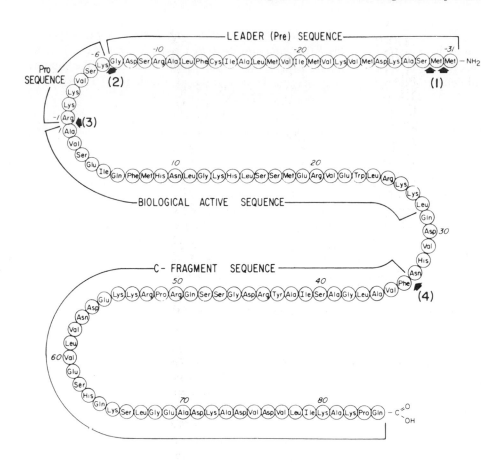

■ **Fig. 42-10** Structure and processing of preproparathyroid hormone (prepro-PTH). The N-terminal leader (signal) sequence is cleaved *(steps 1 and 2)* leaving pro-PTH. Removal of six more amino acids *(step 3)* yields the 1-84 PTH structure. Further cleavage within the gland as well as in peripheral tissues *(step 4)* yields as the major metabolic product of PTH a C-terminal fragment that is biologically inactive. (Redrawn from Habener J et al: *Physiol Rev* 64:985, 1984.)

the **oxyphil cell**—which first appears at puberty, is distinguished by an eosinophilic cytoplasm. Either of these cells may hypersecrete PTH pathologically.

Synthesis and Release of PTH

PTH is a single-chain protein of 9000 molecular weight. It contains 84 amino acids (Fig. 42-10). The biological activity of PTH resides in the N-terminal portion of the molecule within amino acids 1 to 27. The larger C-terminus portion may carry out other functions that are unrelated to calcium metabolism or are not mediated by the PTH receptor.

PTH is synthesized from a precursor molecule, called *prepro*-PTH (Fig. 42-10), which contains 115 amino acids. As the peptide chain of prepro-PTH grows to its complete length on the ribosomes, the N-terminal signal sequence is enzymatically removed in two steps, leaving pro-PTH. The prohormone is transported to the Golgi apparatus, within which the processing of pro-PTH to PTH is completed very efficiently. Consequently, the parathyroid glands normally contain much less pro-PTH than PTH. Some PTH is packaged for storage in mature secretory granules and is later released by exocytosis. In addition, some newly synthesized PTH may be transported, still in Golgi vesicles, directly through the cell for immediate constitutive release. Cleavage of PTH between amino acids 33 and 40 (Fig. 42-10) also occurs within the gland and prevents release of the intact hormone into the circulation.

The dominant regulator of parathyroid gland activity is the plasma calcium level. PTH and calcium form a nega-

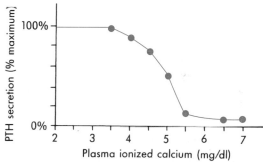

■ **Fig. 42-11** The inverse relationship between PTH and plasma ionized calcium concentration in humans. (Redrawn from Brent GA et al: *J Clin Endocrinol Metab* 67:944, 1988.)

tive feedback pair. Secretion of PTH is inversely related to the plasma calcium concentration in a sigmoidal fashion (Fig. 42-11). Maximal secretory rates of PTH are achieved below a total calcium concentration of 7 mg/dl (ionized calcium, 3.5 mg/dl). As total calcium concentration increases to 11 mg/dl (ionized calcium, 5.5 mg/dl), PTH secretion is progressively diminished to a persistent low basal rate that is not suppressible by further elevation of plasma calcium. It is actually the ionized fraction of plasma calcium that regulates PTH secretion. PTH secretion responds to small alterations in the concentration of ionized plasma calcium within seconds, even if total calcium concentration is kept constant. The dose-response curve is steep, with a set point for half-maximal secretion at an ionized calcium level of about 4.5 mg/dl (Fig. 42-11). The greater the *rate of fall* in the concentration of ionized calcium, the larger is the PTH secretion response. This relationship suggests that the parathyroid cells possess an "anticipatory" capability.

Suppression of PTH secretion by an increased concentration of ionized calcium represents one of the few exceptions to the usual rule that calcium influx into the cytoplasm of endocrine cells stimulates protein hormone secretion by exocytosis (see Fig. 39-3). However, *the calcium receptor (see above) within the plasma membrane of the parathyroid cell senses changes in the extracellular fluid concentration of ionized calcium* (Fig. 42-12). When the plasma calcium level exceeds normal, *an increase in binding of Ca^{2+} to the extracellular component of the receptor activates phospholipase C and inhibits adenylyl cyclase. The resultant rise (via generation of inositol trisphosphate) in the intracellular*

calcium level and the fall in cAMP levels stop exocytosis of the PTH-containing secretory granules (Fig. 42-12). When the binding of Ca^{2+} to the receptor decreases, the suppression of granule exocytosis is lifted and PTH secretion increases (Fig. 42-12).

When plasma calcium falls below normal, transduction of this signal by the calcium receptor also leads to an increase in PTH synthesis and secretion, and a decrease in PTH degradation within the parathyroid cells. Exposure to a high calcium concentration or to any noncalcium agonist of the calcium receptor for hours to days represses PTH gene transcription and eventually decreases the proliferation of parathyroid cells. Thus, hypercalcemia decreases PTH synthesis, stores, and release, as well as (ultimately) the parathyroid cell mass. Conversely, hypocalcemia increases PTH synthesis, stores, and secretory rates, and it ultimately stimulates growth of the glands.

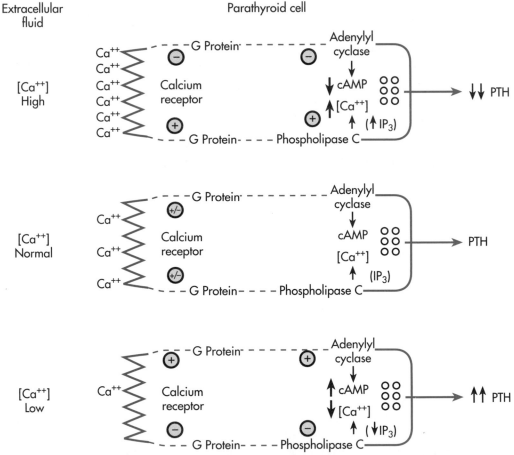

■ **Fig. 42-12**   Mechanism of regulation of PTH secretion by changes in extracellular fluid ionized calcium [Ca^{2+}] concentration. An increase in [Ca^{2+}] is sensed by a plasma membrane [Ca^{2+}] receptor in the parathyroid cell *(top tier)*. The activated receptor is linked to an inhibitory G-protein, which inhibits adenylyl cyclase. As a result, intracellular cAMP levels fall. The activated receptor is also linked to a stimulatory G-protein that stimulates phospholipase C. As a result, inositol trisphosphate (IP₃) levels increase and transduce a rise in intracellular [Ca^{2+}]. Exocytosis of PTH secretory granules and PTH release are *decreased*. The opposite sequence occurs when there is a decrease in extracellular fluid [Ca^{2+}]; in that case, exocytosis of PTH secretory granules and PTH release are increased. *IP₃*, Inositol trisphosphate; ⊕, disinhibited or stimulated; ⊖, inhibited or unstimulated; ⊕, balanced between inhibited and stimulated.

The divalent cation Mg^{2+} acutely modulates PTH secretion in a manner analogous to that of Ca^{2+}, that is, a decrease in magnesium levels stimulates PTH secretion. Because Mg^{2+} is less effective on a molar basis, it is much less important than is calcium in its normal physiological range (1.5-2.5 mEq/L). In contrast, *chronic hypomagnesemia strongly inhibits PTH synthesis,* and in severely magnesium-depleted individuals, the rate of PTH release is reduced. In addition, hypomagnesemia impairs the response of target tissues to PTH. Both of these effects lead to concurrent hypocalcemia.

A rise in plasma phosphate concentration causes an immediate fall in ionized calcium concentration, which in turn stimulates PTH secretion. In addition, high phosphate levels directly increase PTH secretion when ionized calcium concentration is kept constant. Phosphate shifts the PTH-calcium curve to the right (Fig. 42-11) raising the set point for calcium suppression of PTH secretion. This direct effect of phosphate on PTH may be mediated by "phosphatonin," the putative phosphate receptor, followed by a rise in arachidonic levels within the parathyroid cell.

Vitamin 1,25-$(OH)_2$-D inhibits transcription of the PTH gene and decreases PTH secretion. It also inhibits proliferation of parathyroid cells. 1,25-$(OH)_2$-D upregulates the Ca^{2+} receptor in parathyroid cells. All these actions, which decrease the plasma calcium level, coupled with the direct stimulatory effect of PTH on 1,25-$(OH)_2$-D synthesis, which increases the plasma calcium level, constitute yet another negative feedback loop that regulates calcium metabolism.

PTH secretion is also pulsatile and increases at night independent of the plasma calcium concentration. In response to diminished calcium absorption, aging leads to an increase in PTH secretion, and bone resorption is consequently increased.

Phosphodiesterase inhibitors (by increasing cAMP), epinephrine (via its β-adrenergic receptor), dopamine, and histamine (via H_2 receptors) all stimulate PTH secretion. α-Adrenergic agonists and prostaglandins inhibit PTH secretion by decreasing cAMP levels. Cosecreted chromogranin (Chapter 39) and related products feed back negatively on PTH secretion; this relationship may constitute an autocrine regulatory mechanism.

An excess of aluminum, commonly present in antacids, inhibits PTH secretion. Lithium, often used to treat **manic-depressive disorders,** shifts the PTH-calcium curve to the right (Fig. 42-11). Lithium as well as thiazide diuretic drugs stimulate PTH secretion modestly and can cause mild hypercalcemia.

Under normal circumstances, neither prepro-PTH nor pro-PTH is secreted from the parathyroid glands. One or more products of the intraglandular degradation of PTH, however, are released. In addition, PTH undergoes rapid metabolism in the peripheral tissues. The hormone is predominantly split in the liver. The major product is a circulating, 6000 molecular weight, carboxy-terminal fragment that is further acted upon in the kidney. Amino-terminal

fragments generated during cleavage of PTH also circulate, but they are not biologically active. The plasma concentration of intact PTH is about 30 pg/ml (approximately 3×10^{-12} M), and its plasma half-life is 5 to 8 minutes. The carboxy-terminal fragment has a much longer plasma half-life of 6 to 12 hours. This fragment is a valid index of chronic hypersecretion, but only so long as renal function is normal.

PTH Actions

PTH action is initiated by binding to a plasma cell membrane receptor (Fig. 39-11). The 14 to 34 region of PTH contains the receptor-binding sequence. Constant exposure of bone target cells to PTH downregulates the PTH receptor, whereas intermittent exposure upregulates the receptor. In all target cells, hormone binding to a cell membrane receptor leads to G-protein–mediated activation of adenylyl cyclase (see Fig. 39-9). The subsequent intracellular events mediated by the increased cAMP levels are not known in detail. Presumably, increased levels of cAMP trigger a protein kinase cascade that leads to phosphorylation of proteins necessary for enhanced transport of calcium and other ions. In some target cells, via phospholipase C, PTH generates phosphatidylinositol products that have second messenger roles by increasing protein kinase C activity. Activation of phospholipase C, however, requires a much higher concentration of PTH than does stimulation of adenylyl cyclase.

Independent of cAMP, PTH also stimulates the uptake of calcium into the cytosol of bone cells from the fluid that bathes them. Whether this calcium itself acts as another intracellular second messenger or whether it acts only to modulate the adenylyl cyclase response by counterregulatory inhibition remains unclear. The initial uptake of calcium by bone cells is reflected by a slight, transient hypocalcemia that follows PTH administration and precedes the classic hypercalcemic response. The presence of 1,25-$(OH)_2$-D is required for the exhibition of the full spectrum of PTH actions. A sufficient intracellular concentration of magnesium is also necessary for maximal PTH responsiveness.

The overall effect of PTH is to increase the plasma calcium concentration and decrease the plasma phosphate concentration by acting on three major target organs: directly on bone and kidney, and indirectly on the gastrointestinal tract. All three actions ultimately increase calcium influx into the plasma and raise the plasma calcium concentration. Although PTH acts on bone and intestine to increase phosphate influx, this effect is overwhelmed by the action on the kidney. This action increases phosphate efflux, and hence plasma phosphate concentration falls (Fig. 42-13).

Bone. PTH receptors are present in both osteoblasts and osteoclasts. PTH accelerates removal of calcium from bone by two processes. Its initial effect is to stimulate osteolysis. This process causes calcium to be transferred from the bone canalicular fluid into osteocytes and then into the extracellular fluid. The canalicular fluid is probably replenished with calcium from the surface of partially mineralized bone. Phosphate does not appear to be mobilized with calcium in this process.

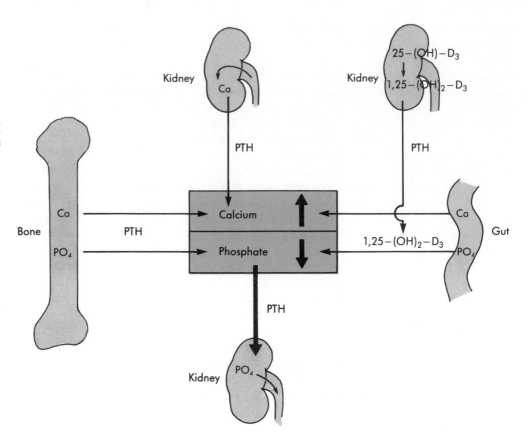

■ **Fig. 42-13**   The sites of PTH actions that lead to a net increase in serum calcium level and a net decrease in serum phosphate level. PTH stimulates calcium and phosphate resorption from bone. In contrast, PTH stimulates calcium reabsorption but inhibits phosphate reabsorption in the kidney. PTH stimulates renal formation of 1,25-(OH)$_2$-D, and the latter in turn increases absorption of both minerals from the intestine.

A second, more slowly developing effect of constant exposure to PTH is to stimulate the osteoclasts to resorb completely mineralized mature bone. In this process, both calcium and phosphate are released for transfer into the extracellular fluid. The organic bone matrix is hydrolyzed by the increased activity of collagenase (PTH increases expression of the collagenase gene) and of lysosomal enzymes. PTH initially increases the ruffled border of the osteoclast and the clear resorptive zone that develops between it and the mineralized bone. Increases in osteoclast size, RNA synthesis, and the number of osteoclast nuclei then follow. In a later phase of PTH action, differentiation of precursor cells to osteoclasts and their proliferation is stimulated. The giant osteoclasts create large resorption cavities in both cortical and trabecular bone, although the former is absorbed preferentially. PTH also induces increases in acid phosphatase and carbonic anhydrase and the accumulation of lactic acid and citric acid. The resultant increase in protons lowers the ambient pH and contributes to the resorptive process. Hence, various products of bone destruction are released into the plasma and then excreted in the urine.

Although PTH receptors are present on osteoclasts, the resorptive effects of PTH cannot be demonstrated in vitro unless osteoblasts are also present as intermediary cells. Osteoblasts, and particularly a precursor variety termed **proosteoblasts,** respond to the hormone in a number of ways. One response is an early alteration in cellular shape and cytoskeletal arrangement, probably by cAMP-induced phosphorylation of myosin light chains. PTH also inhibits the synthesis of collagen by osteoblasts, probably at the

level of transcription. The proosteoblast has long syncytial processes that extend through the bone matrix and intertwine with other cells and vascular structures. Thus, they may mediate the resorptive effects of PTH by stimulating the secretion of osteoblast products, such as interleukin-6 or macrophage colony-stimulating factor, which have paracrine effects on neighboring osteoclasts and their precursors. The resorptive effects of PTH on bone are achieved by the elevated concentrations of hormone that result from stimulation of the parathyroid glands by hypocalcemia. Thus, the resorption of boane completes a negative feedback loop that restores the plasma calcium level to normal. Bone resorptive effects seen on histological examination reflect continuous exposure to PTH.

However, PTH also has anabolic actions on bone. In culture, PTH via cAMP as second messenger, causes an increase in the number of osteoblasts, by inhibiting their rate of apoptosis by 80% to 90%, and an increase in collagen synthesis. *When given in low doses and intermittently, PTH stimulates bone formation in humans.* The plasma levels of alkaline phosphatase and osteocalcin, markers of bone formation, are often increased by PTH. These anabolic actions are mediated by PTH-induced increases in local insulin-like growth factors and transforming growth factors. The net effect of sustained increases in PTH may be either a decrease or an increase in total skeletal mass. Trabecular bone may be preserved by PTH at the expense of cortical bone. Whether total skeletal mass increases or decreases probably depends on concomitant factors that affect bone remodeling; these factors include mechanical stress, the level of exercise, and the availability of calcium, phosphate, vitamin D, and many other hormones with endocrine or paracrine actions (Table 42-1).

Primary hyperparathyroidism usually results from a benign parathyroid neoplasm (adenoma). Hypercalcemia, hypophosphatemia, hypercalcinuria, and renal calculi (stones) are typical manifestations. This condition seldom causes clinically evident bone disturbances, because the hallmark of hyperparathyroidism, hypercalcemia, is usually discovered early by health screening tests. However, long-term secondary massive overproduction of PTH, typical of slowly developing renal failure (which stimulates parathyroid gland hyperplasia by hyperphosphatemia, hypocalcemia, and decreased 1,25-(OH)$_2$-D levels), causes major effects on bone. Areas of osteoclastic hyperactivity and rampant bone resorption are present next to areas of excessive and disorganized trabecular bone formation. Pain, fractures, and deformity result. Alkaline phosphatase and osteocalcin levels are elevated. In **hypoparathyroidism,** bone mass is generally increased.

Parathyroid cells normally turn over at a rate of about 5% per year. However, overexpression of cyclin D1 in parathyroid cells increases their rate of mitosis and causes hyperplasia. At the same time there is a decrease in the expression of calcium receptor and the PTH-Ca^{2+} set point, which causes hypercalcemia. Benign parathyroid neoplasms (adenomas) may be monoclonal or polyclonal. Infrequently, the neoplasms result from mutations of known tumor suppressor genes, such as p53 and pRb (retinoblastoma). In familial cases, the MEN 1 tumor suppressor gene, whose product, **menin,** binds to the growth transcription factor Jun D, is mutated, and parathyroid cell growth is uncontrolled. A few parathyroid adenomas have cyclin D mutations.

Kidney. PTH increases the reabsorption of calcium from the ascending loop of Henle and the distal tubule of the kidney (see also Chapter 37). By this action, the PTH secreted in response to hypocalcemia immediately helps to raise the decreased plasma calcium concentration. Reabsorption of calcium is mediated by PTH stimulation of cAMP production at the capillary surface of the renal tubular cell. The cAMP is transported to the luminal surface of the cell, where it activates protein kinases that are located in the brush border and that are involved in calcium reabsorption. The previously described calcium-sensing receptor is also present, and it modulates calcium reabsorption by these cells. The relationship between urinary calcium excretion and plasma calcium concentration is shifted to the right by PTH (Fig. 42-14). *Therefore, acute stimulation of PTH secretion by calcium deficiency helps prevent hypocalcemia by causing the kidney to reabsorb a greater fraction of the filtered calcium.*

In **hyperparathyroidism,** the plasma calcium level can become high enough from the direct actions of PTH on

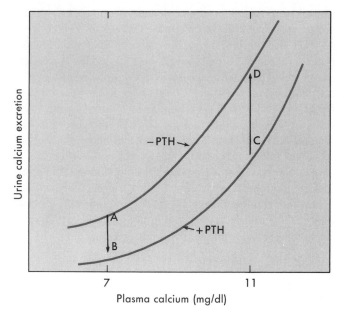

■ **Fig. 42-14**   Effect of PTH on the relationship between urine calcium excretion and plasma calcium level. At a low plasma calcium level, PTH secretion is stimulated, and the hormone shifts urine calcium excretion from point *A* to point *B,* thus conserving calcium. At a high plasma calcium level, PTH secretion is suppressed, and urine calcium excretion is shifted from point *C* to point *D,* thus disposing of excess calcium. (Redrawn from Nordin BEC et al: *Lancet* 2:1280, 1969.)

bone and the indirect actions on intestine for the hormone's primary renal tubular calcium reabsorbing action to be overwhelmed by the increased filtered load of calcium. The result is **hypercalciuria** and an increased frequency of renal calcium stone formation.

The most dramatic effect of PTH on the kidney is to inhibit the reabsorption of phosphate in the proximal tubule, and thereby to increase the urinary phosphate excretion (see also Chapter 37). PTH stimulates return of the Na-P$_i$ cotransporters from the brush border membrane of renal proximal tubule cells to the lysosomes, where they are presumably degraded. A transient activation of microtubule rearrangement is involved. cAMP excretion into the urine also increases, as expected, just before that of phosphate. The important phosphaturic effect of PTH allows disposition of the extra phosphate released by PTH-stimulated bone resorption. Without this effect, simultaneous plasma elevation of calcium and phosphate concentration could occur, with the potential danger of precipitating calcium-phosphate complexes in critical tissues. In contrast, under circumstances of primary phosphate deprivation, the plasma calcium concentration tends to rise and thus suppress PTH secretion. A lower level of PTH in turn allows more tubular phosphate reabsorption and conserves this essential mineral.

Although PTH stimulates phosphate entry into the plasma and phosphate elevation stimulates PTH secretion, PTH facilitates phosphate excretion in the urine. Thus, the phosphate-PTH pair constitutes another complex feedback loop, independent of the calcium-PTH loop.

PTH also inhibits the reabsorption of sodium and bicarbonate in the proximal tubule and stimulates a Na^+-H^+ exchanger. This acidification may prevent the occurrence of metabolic alkalosis, which could result from the release of bicarbonate during the dissolution of hydroxyapatite crystals in bone. In addition, PTH stimulates reabsorption of magnesium by the renal tubules, an action that helps to conserve this important cation.

A most important action of PTH in the kidney is to stimulate the synthesis of vitamin 1,25-$(OH)_2$-D. This activity occurs via increased levels of cAMP; protein kinase A phosphorylates and activates a protein phosphatase, which then dephosphorylates the ferroprotein renoredoxin. In its dephosphorylated active form, renoredoxin is essential to the activity of the renal 1-hydroxylase enzyme. In addition, the decrease in plasma and renal cortical phosphate caused by PTH enhances 1-hydroxylation of 25-OH-D_3. *Thus, PTH increases the level of available 1,25-$(OH)_2$-D, and in this indirect but critical way, it increases calcium absorption from the intestine.*

All the above renal effects explain why hyperparathyroidism is often accompanied by **hypophosphatemia,** a mild **hyperchloremic metabolic acidosis,** and elevated plasma 1,25-$(OH)_2$-D levels. The reverse findings are seen in hypoparathyroidism.

Overall action of PTH. The outcome of all the major biochemical effects of PTH is illustrated in Fig. 42-15, which demonstrates the results of administering the hormone

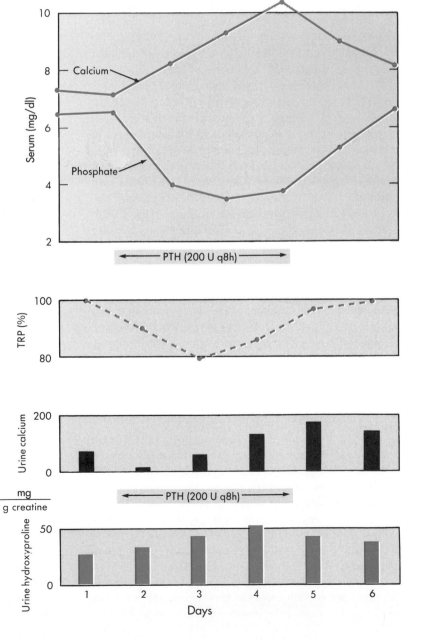

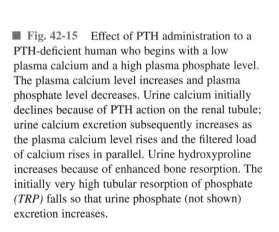

■ **Fig. 42-15** Effect of PTH administration to a PTH-deficient human who begins with a low plasma calcium and a high plasma phosphate level. The plasma calcium level increases and plasma phosphate level decreases. Urine calcium initially declines because of PTH action on the renal tubule; urine calcium excretion subsequently increases as the plasma calcium level rises and the filtered load of calcium rises in parallel. Urine hydroxyproline increases because of enhanced bone resorption. The initially very high tubular resorption of phosphate *(TRP)* falls so that urine phosphate (not shown) excretion increases.

to a hypoparathyroid patient. Figure 42-15 shows that there is a prompt increase in plasma calcium concentration and a decrease in plasma phosphate concentration. The renal tubular reabsorption of phosphate falls. Urinary excretion of calcium initially declines as its tubular reabsorption increases. However, as the plasma calcium concentration continues to increase, the filtered load increases and urinary calcium excretion then rises. Urinary excretion of hydroxyproline increases as a result of PTH-stimulated bone resorption.

Hypoparathyroidism is usually caused by inadvertent surgical removal of the glands; less often, the cause is autoimmune destruction. Both conditions are marked by hypocalcemia, hyperphosphatemia, and low plasma PTH concentrations. Rarely, patients have mutant G-proteins that cannot effectively transduce the PTH-receptor signal. Although plasma calcium concentration is low in this form of hypoparathyroidism, fractional calcium excretion in the urine is increased, and plasma PTH concentration is high (because of negative feedback). The clinical consequences of hypocalcemia were described above. Because PTH therapy, though experimentally effective, is still not available, oral calcium and 1,25-(OH)$_2$-D must be used to treat all forms of hypoparathyroidism in order to return plasma calcium concentration to normal. Because PTH stimulation of renal tubular calcium reabsorption is absent, the result can be hypercalciuria, with the threat of kidney stones.

PTH-Related Protein

PTH-related peptide or protein (PTH$_{rp}$) was originally discovered as a product of human cancers that were of squamous cell origin and that were associated with hypercalcemia. It is now known that normal tissues also express this molecule. These tissues include skin keratinocytes, lactating mammary epithelium, placenta, and fetal parathyroid glands.

The gene for PTH$_{rp}$ and the gene for PTH are on paired chromosomes, and they have evolved from a common ancestor. Three products of amino acid length 139 to 173 are expressed by alternate splicing of the PTH$_{rp}$ gene primary transcript. As a result of the striking homology between the N-terminal amino acids of PTH$_{rp}$ and of PTH, PTH$_{rp}$ exhibits most of the actions of PTH on bone and kidney. PTH$_{rp}$ exerts these actions by binding to the PTH receptor, although the amino acids in the receptor binding sequences of the two hormone molecules are not homologous. One action of PTH, stimulation of renal 1-hydroxylase, is not shared by PTH$_{rp}$. Hence, patients with hypercalcemia caused by PTH$_{rp}$ do not have elevated plasma levels of 1,25-(OH)$_2$-D.

The most likely and important physiological role for PTH$_{rp}$ is in the regulation of endochondral bone formation. The latter requires first the recruitment of chondrocytes from their precursors by BMPs and by *hedgehog* proteins. Then the proliferating chondrocytes progress in an orderly way through a transitional zone to become hypertrophic chondrocytes that lay down a matrix of type 2 collagen. After

they mineralize the matrix, the hypertrophic chondrocytes die off by apoptosis. The mineralized cartilage is subsequently changed to bone by invading osteoblasts.

Hedgehog proteins are secreted by strategically located chondrocytes in the transitional zone. These proteins induce secretion of PTH$_{rp}$ by other nearby cells. PTH$_{rp}$ reacts with the identical receptor as PTH on late proliferating chondrocytes, accelerating their growth but inhibiting their differentiation into hypertrophic chondrocytes. In this complex manner the chondrocytes committed to forming mineralized cartilage regulate the rate at which they will be replaced by proliferating and maturing new chondrocytes. Thus the bone lengthens by orderly progression of the growth plates at either end. Without PTH$_{rp}$ or a functional PTH$_{rp}$/PTH receptor, the process is severely disorganized, and the resulting bone becomes very abnormal. At puberty, sex steroids stop the operation of the hedgehog protein/PTH$_{rp}$ system and the epiphyseal growth plate permanently closes.

There are likely other physiological roles for PTH$_{rp}$ during intrauterine life and early infancy. These roles, like that in bone, are probably mostly carried out by paracrine actions. PTH$_{rp}$ in the placenta and the fetus is thought to function in maintaining the 30% to 40% increased ionized calcium concentration gradient that exists between the fetal and the maternal plasma.

PTH$_{rp}$ is also importantly involved in breast development and lactation, and it probably stimulates the presence of high concentrations of calcium in breast milk. The latter also contains PTH$_{rp}$ itself, in concentrations 10^4 times higher than in serum. PTH$_{rp}$ swallowed by the infant may thus react with its receptor, known to be present in intestinal epithelial cells, or it may be absorbed into the infant's bloodstream to fulfill a systemic role.

Other roles for PT$_{rp}$ include (1) resorbing alveolar bone, so as to allow normal tooth development and eruption; (2) regulating the rate of differentiation of skin keratinocytes and growth of hair follicles; and (3) protection of central nervous system neurons from toxic overstimulation by glutamate receptors that activate voltage-dependent calcium channels.

Not all the actions of PTH$_{rp}$ are carried out by the N-terminal sequence it shares with PTH. The midregion of the molecule appears responsible for placental calcium transport while the C-terminal region is active in alveolar bone resorption and in the brain. Processing of PTH$_{rp}$ within its various cells of origin leads to secretion of the fragments appropriate for the needed physiological function.

CALCITONIN

Synthesis and Release of Calcitonin

The parafollicular, or C, cells of the thyroid gland secrete another protein hormone, **calcitonin,** which can influence calcium metabolism. *Whereas PTH acts to increase the plasma calcium concentration, calcitonin acts to lower it.* The parafollicular cells are of neural crest origin. In humans, they are concentrated in the lateral lobes of the thyroid gland, where they constitute 0.1% of the epithelial cells. They are distinguished from ordinary thyroid hormone-producing cells (see Chapter 44) by their large size, pale cytoplasm, and small secretory granules.

Calcitonin is a straight-chain peptide composed of 32 amino acids. The hormone contains a seven-membered disulfide ring at the N-terminus that stabilizes the molecule and prolineamide at the C-terminus. Both fish and animal calcitonins are active in humans. The biologically active core of the molecule probably resides in its central region.

Calcitonin synthesis proceeds from a large preprohormone. The hormone is packaged in granules along with N-terminal and C-terminal copeptides. The gene for calcitonin again illustrates the significant relationship that exists between the endocrine and nervous systems. In some cells, the primary RNA transcript encodes preprocalcitonin and directs synthesis of calcitonin. However, in other cells (in both thyroid and nervous tissue), the same primary RNA transcript encodes the precursor for, and directs the synthesis of, a different peptide with 37 amino acids and a completely different C-terminal portion. This molecule, known as **calcitonin gene-related peptide (CGRP),** circulates in human plasma and probably arises from perivascular nerves. CGRP is a potent vasodilator and cardiac inotropic agent. The evolutionary path by which a hormone and a neuropeptide arose from alternate expression of the same gene and the functional significance of this relationship remain to be determined.

The major stimulus of calcitonin secretion is a rise in the plasma calcium concentration. This is sensed by the plasma membrane calcium receptor, previously described. A consequent increase in cAMP prompts exocytosis of calcitonin-containing granules. However, the degree of response seen in various species is related to their need to prevent hypercalcemia. Vertebrates that originated in fresh water (of low calcium concentration) but that migrated into the sea (with a calcium concentration of 40 mg/dl) were the first to require and develop a calcium-lowering hormone. When vertebrates moved to land, the emphasis in calcium economy shifted away from defense against hypercalcemia toward defense against hypocalcemia. PTH was developed, and the importance of calcitonin in regulating plasma calcium concentration probably declined.

Calcitonin circulates in humans at concentrations of 10 to 20 pg/ml (5×10^{-12}), and it increases 2-fold to 10-fold after an acute increase in the plasma calcium concentration of as little as 1 mg/dl. Much larger responses of the hormone to calcium infusion are elicited in patients with calcitonin-secreting tumors. Conversely, in such patients, a sharp reduction in the ionized calcium concentration lowers the plasma calcitonin concentration. $1,25\text{-}(OH)_2\text{-}D$ increases plasma calcitonin levels. Ingestion of food also stimulates calcitonin secretion without elevating the plasma calcium concentration. Food-stimulated calcitonin secretion is mediated by several gastrointestinal hormones, of which gastrin is the most potent. The rise in calcitonin could protect against too great a rapid influx of calcium from the diet. Excessive responses to gastrin provide a useful diagnostic test for

states of calcitonin hypersecretion. Circulating calcitonin is heterogeneous, and it is largely degraded and cleared by the kidney.

Calcitonin Actions

In bone, the target cell of calcitonin is the osteoclast. Binding of calcitonin to its plasma membrane receptor on the osteoclast (Fig. 39-11) is followed by an elevation of the intracellular concentration of cAMP, the second messenger for calcitonin in all target cells. The affected osteoclasts rapidly lose their ruffled borders, undergo cytoskeletal rearrangement, exhibit reduced motility, detach from bone surfaces, and are deactivated. Bone resorption is thus decreased.

The major effect of calcitonin administration is a rapid fall in the plasma calcium concentration, caused by inhibition of bone resorption. The magnitude of this decrease in humans is proportional to the baseline rate of bone turnover. In normal adults, the effect is minimal. However, in individuals with diseases that cause high rates of bone resorption, significant hypocalcemia can result. These individuals also display an escape from the calcitonin effect, caused by downregulation of calcitonin receptors. The mechanism of downregulation by calcitonin is not suppression of the receptor gene expression, but increased degradation of its mRNA. Nevertheless, continued provision of calcitonin eventually decreases the number of osteoclasts as well as their activity. More dense bone with fewer resorption cavities eventually results.

Calcitonin is clearly a physiological antagonist to PTH, with respect to calcium. However, with respect to phosphate, it has the same net effect as PTH; that is, it decreases the plasma phosphate level. This decrease is caused by inhibition of bone resorption, promotion of phosphate entry into bone, and a small increase in urinary phosphate excretion. This hypophosphatemic effect is independent of the hypocalcemic effect. Calcitonin also inhibits renal tubular calcium reabsorption, and thereby increases calcium excretion in the urine. This represents another mechanism for preventing or reducing hypercalcemia.

The importance of calcitonin to normal human calcium economy is still unclear. Ordinarily, the absorption of dietary calcium loads produces little, if any, elevation of the plasma calcium concentration. Calcitonin deficiency that results from complete removal of the thyroid gland does not lead to significant hypercalcemia. A chronic excess of calcitonin, generated either by a C-cell tumor of the thyroid gland or by exogenous administration, does not produce hypocalcemia. At present, it may be most reasonable to conclude that any effects of calcitonin deficiency or excess are easily offset by appropriate adjustments of PTH and vitamin D concentrations.

On the other hand, the possibility that calcitonin significantly regulates bone remodeling cannot be easily excluded. Calcitonin may protect bone from excessive resorption during periods when demand for calcium, to be used elsewhere, dramatically increases, such as in pregnancy, lactation, or growth. Calcitonin could participate in fetal skeletal development. The fact that plasma calcitonin is lower in women than in men and that it declines with aging may suggest a functional role for the hormone in the development of accelerated bone loss after the menopause.

Calcitonin is used in the acute treatment of hypercalcemia and in certain bone diseases, in which a sustained reduction in osteoclastic resorption is therapeutically beneficial. Finally, the discovery of calcitonin and CGRP in a number of locations throughout the body—in the pituitary gland and hypothalamus, and within cells of neural crest origin—has raised the possibility that calcitonin and CGRP may also have paracrine and neurotransmitter functions. In this regard, calcitonin does exhibit analgesic properties independent of the opioid system.

INTEGRATED HORMONAL REGULATION OF CALCIUM AND PHOSPHATE

The previous discussion indicates that a complex interplay of several hormones that act on a number of tissues, as well as the function of the calcium receptor itself, is responsible for maintenance of normal concentrations of calcium and phosphate in body fluids. This integrated system is best visualized by tracing the compensatory responses to deprivation of calcium and of phosphate (Figs. 42-16 and 42-17).

Calcium deprivation causes hypocalcemia, which acts as a signal via the calcium receptor for the stimulation of PTH

secretion (Fig. 42-16). PTH increases bone resorption and renal tubular calcium reabsorption, and thereby raises plasma calcium concentration. PTH also increases urinary phosphate excretion, and thereby decreases the plasma phosphate concentration and renal cortical phosphate content. All three factors—hypocalcemia, excess PTH, and hypophosphatemia—act to stimulate the production of 1,25-$(OH)_2$-D. The latter steroid hormone raises the plasma calcium concentration toward normal by increasing absorption of calcium from the gastrointestinal tract and, in concert with PTH, by increasing the rates of osteolysis and osteoclastic bone resorption. Thus, this beautifully integrated response to calcium deprivation increases the flux of calcium into the extracellular fluid. Simultaneously, the extra phosphate that enters with the calcium from the bone and intestine is eliminated by excretion in the urine. The recovery of plasma calcium concentration to normal shuts off PTH hypersecretion by negative feedback, augmented by a suppressive effect of 1,25-$(OH)_2$-D on PTH synthesis. 1,25-$(OH)_2$-D synthesis will then decline and 24,25-$(OH)_2$-D synthesis will increase; thus, the whole compensatory sequence will diminish. As a further safety valve, should the compensatory rise in the plasma calcium level greatly exceed the normal concentration, stimulation of calcitonin secretion would moderate it as well.

In a contrasting sequence, phosphate deprivation via hypophosphatemia directly stimulates 1,25-$(OH)_2$-D production (Fig. 42-16). The participation of a phosphate receptor is strongly suspected, but not yet proven. Vitamin

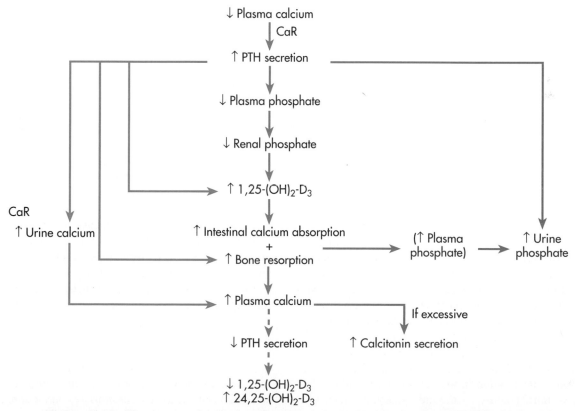

■ **Fig. 42-16**   The compensatory response to calcium deprivation. See text for explication. *CaR,* calcium receptor.

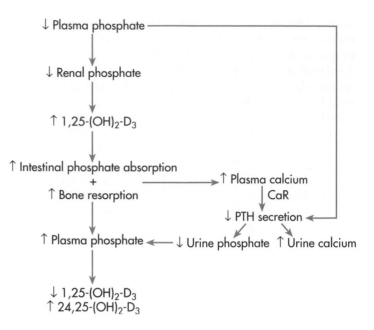

■ **Fig. 42-17** The compensatory response to phosphate deprivation. See text for explication. A putative phosphate receptor likely plays a fundamental role in organizing these responses.

1,25-$(OH)_2$-D increases the flux of phosphate into the extracellular fluid by stimulating its absorption from the intestine and by stimulating bone resorption. The extra calcium that simultaneously enters with phosphate raises the plasma calcium concentration, and this calcium increase, along with a direct effect of the low plasma phosphate, suppresses PTH secretion. The absence of PTH causes the kidney tubules to increase reabsorption of phosphate. Urinary phosphate is conserved, and thus aids in the restoration of plasma phosphate concentration to normal. At the same time, the lack of PTH permits easier disposal of the extra mobilized calcium. This process diminishes the renal tubular reabsorption of calcium and increases calcium excretion in the urine. As plasma phosphate returns to normal, 24,25-$(OH)_2$-D production is favored, 1,25-$(OH)_2$-D concentrations decline, and the whole process is reversed.

The combined arrangement of dual hormone regulation and dual hormone action permits selective defense of either the plasma calcium or plasma phosphate concentration, without creating a circulatory excess of the other. The same principles apply in reverse to the imposition of excess calcium or excess phosphate loads of either endogenous or exogenous origin.

Certain characteristics of these homeostatic systems for adjustment of body calcium and phosphate stores deserve emphasis. The renal responses to PTH provide the most rapid (within minutes) defense against perturbations in both calcium and phosphate stores. As PTH secretion ranges from very high to very low concentrations, the rate of urinary calcium excretion can rise 25-fold from approximately 0.05 to 1.2 mg/min, and that of phosphate can fall from 2 to 0 mg/min. A sudden 2- to 3-mg/dl increase in either calcium or phosphate concentration in the extracellular fluid can be corrected within 24 hours by the kidney, acting under the appropriate alteration in PTH concentration. In response to complete phosphate and calcium deprivation, the renal con-

servation of phosphate is complete, whereas that of calcium is not.

The gastrointestinal component of this homeostatic system is both slower and narrower in range than the renal component. As a result of variations in 1,25-$(OH)_2$-D, the absorption of dietary calcium increases from 20% to 70% as calcium intake decreases from 2000 to 200 mg/day. Thus, absorbed calcium can effectively range from 140 to 400 mg/day. Hormonal effects on phosphate absorption are even less striking, because the latter is virtually a linear function of dietary intake.

Bone responses to regulatory fluctuations in both PTH and 1,25-$(OH)_2$-D are rapid when produced by osteocytic osteolysis and relatively slow when caused by osteoclastic resorption. However, the capacity for compensatory calcium and phosphate uptake and release is enormous. In humans, 10-fold variations in calcium turnover have been observed.

Finally, an important difference between renal and gastrointestinal mechanisms on the one hand and bone mechanisms on the other hand must be considered. The compensatory responses of the kidney and the intestine are able to defend total body and bone stores of calcium and phosphate against erosion or inundation. In contrast, the skeletal mechanisms of defense against perturbations in plasma calcium and phosphate concentrations eventually sacrifice the chemical and structural integrity of the bone mass if they are employed for long periods.

SUMMARY

1. Calcium participates critically in a myriad of biological functions, including neurotransmission, hormone secretion and action, enzyme activities, muscle contraction, and blood clotting. Calcium is also the chief mineral that contributes to the structural integrity of the skeleton and teeth.

2. Extracellular Ca^{2+} concentration (approximately 10^{-3} M) is closely controlled in order to regulate the wide, transient swings in the much lower intracellular Ca^{2+} concentration (approximately 10^{-7} M). A specific G-protein–coupled calcium receptor in the plasma membrane of regulatory cells mediates the responses to changes in the extracellular ionized calcium concentration.

3. Phosphate is critical to all major enzymatic pathways involved in energy generation, substrate disposition, and synthesis of protein and other macromolecules. Phosphate is also the main anion partner of calcium in bone structure.

4. Calcium balance and plasma calcium homeostasis depend on dietary intake, fractional gastrointestinal absorption, regulation of renal excretion, and the internal movement of calcium into and out of skeletal reservoirs.

5. Phosphate balance and plasma phosphate homeostasis reflect dietary intake, renal excretion, and internal shifts among extracellular fluid, large soft tissue contents, and the skeletal reservoir.

6. Bone is a complex organ with cells specifically devoted to a continuous process of remodeling. In this process, mineralized bone is reabsorbed by osteoclasts (releasing calcium and phosphate) and is then reformed by osteoblasts (assimilating calcium and phosphate). This process is augmented during growth periods. With aging, resorption exceeds formation and bone mass declines.

7. Vitamin D is a steroid molecule that is either synthesized from cholesterol in the skin in the presence of ultraviolet light or is absorbed from the diet. The basic structure is modified successively in the liver and kidney to $1,25\text{-(OH)}_2$-D, the active metabolite.

8. $1,25\text{-(OH)}_2$-D acts via its nuclear receptor to increase calcium (and phosphate) absorption from the gastrointestinal tract. The hormone is therefore critical to maintaining the supply of calcium for bone formation and growth, as well as other calcium-dependent processes. Together with PTH, it also enhances bone resorption. Overall, $1,25\text{-(OH)}_2$-D increases plasma calcium and plasma phosphate concentrations.

9. Parathyroid hormone (PTH) is a straight-chain peptide synthesized from a prohormone in the four parathyroid glands. PTH is released by exocytosis in response to a decrease in plasma calcium concentration that is sensed by the calcium receptor in the parathyroid cell. PTH synthesis and secretion and parathyroid gland mass are suppressed by calcium and $1,25\text{-(OH)}_2$-D.

10. PTH acts via a plasma membrane receptor and cAMP (1) to increase osteoclastic bone resorption, (2) to increase renal tubular reabsorption of calcium, (3) to increase $1,25\text{-(OH)}_2$-D synthesis in the kidney, and (4) to decrease renal tubular phosphate reabsorption and increase urinary excretion of phosphate. Overall, PTH increases plasma calcium and decreases plasma phosphate concentrations.

11. Calcium deficiency evokes a synergistic sequence that increases PTH and $1,25\text{-(OH)}_2$-D secretion. The combined actions of these two hormones increase the inflow of calcium and restore plasma concentrations to normal. They simultaneously dispose of the inflow of extra phosphate by enhancing its renal excretion.

12. In contrast, phosphate deprivation evokes a synergistic sequence that increases $1,25\text{-(OH)}_2$-D secretion, but reduces PTH secretion. The result is to restore the plasma phosphate concentration toward normal while disposing of the inflow of extra calcium by increasing its renal excretion.

13. Calcitonin is a peptide hormone synthesized in C cells within the thyroid gland. It is a PTH antagonist in bone, and it is secreted in response to hypercalcemia. Thus, it acts to lower the plasma concentration of calcium.

BIBLIOGRAPHY

Journal articles

Allmaden Y et al: Direct effect of phosphorus on PTH secretion from whole rat parathyroid glands in vitro, *J Bone Miner Res* 11:970, 1996.

Amizuka N et al: Vitamin D_3 differentially regulates parathyroid hormone/parathyroid hormone-related peptide receptor expression in bone and cartilage, *J Clin Invest* 103:373, 1999.

Bell NH: Vitamin D metabolism, aging, and bone loss (editorial), *J Clin Endocrinol Metab* 80:1051, 1995.

Bikle DD, Pillai S: Vitamin D, calcium, and epidermal differentiation, *Endocr Rev* 14:3, 1993.

Blaustein MP, Lederer WJ: Sodium/calcium exchange: its physiological implications, *Am Physiol* 79:763, 1999.

Bouillon R, Okamura WH, Norman AW: Structure-function relationships in the vitamin D endocrine system, *Endocr Rev* 16:200, 1995.

Brown EM, MacLeod RJ: Extracellular calcium sensing and extracellular calcium signaling, *Physiol Rev* 81:240, 2001.

Burger EH, Klein-Nulend J: Mechanotransduction in bone: role of the lacuno-canalicular network, *FASEB J* 13:S101, 1999.

Dempster DW et al: Anabolic actions of parathyroid hormone on bone, *Endocr Rev* 14:690, 1993.

Epstein S: Serum and urinary markers of bone remodeling: assessment of bone turnover, *Endocr Rev* 9:437, 1988.

Gambacciani M et al: The relative contributions of menopause and aging to postmenopausal vertebral osteopenia, *J Clin Endocrinol Metab* 77:1148, 1993.

Gross M, Kumar R: Physiology and biochemistry of vitamin D-dependent calcium binding proteins, *Am J Physiol* 259:195, 1990.

Heaney RP et al: Calcium absorptive effects of vitamin D and its major metabolites, *J Clin Endocrinol Metab* 82:4111, 1997.

Holick MF: Skin: site of the synthesis of vitamin D and a target tissue for the active form, 1,25-dihydroxyvitamin D3, *Ann NY Acad Sci* 548:14, 1988.

Jilka RL et al: Increased bone formation by prevention of osteoblast apoptosis with parathyroid hormone, *J Clin Invest* 104:439, 1999.

Jones G et al: Current understanding of the molecular actions of vitamin D, *Physiol Rev* 78:1193, 1998.

Kumar R: Phosphatonin: a new phosphaturetic hormone? (Lessons from tumour-induced osteomalacia and X-linked hypophosphataemia), *Nephrol Dial Transplant* 12:11, 1997.

Lanske B et al: Ablation of the PTHrp gene or the PTH/PTHrp receptor gene leads to distinct abnormalities in bone development, *J Clin Invest* 104:399, 1999.

Lotscher M et al: Rapid downregulation of rat renal Na/P$_i$ cotransporter in response to parathyroid hormone involves microtubule rearrangement, *J Clin Invest* 104:483, 1999.

Mahonen A et al: Effect of 1,25-(OH)2-D3 on its receptor mRNA concentration and osteocalcin synthesis in human osteosarcoma cells, *Biochim Biophys Acta* 30:1048, 1990.

Manolagas SC: Birth and death of bone cells: basic regulatory mechanisms and implications for the pathogenesis and treatment of osteoporosis, *Endocr Rev* 21:115, 2000.

Marx SJ: Hyperparathryoid and hypoparathryoid disorders, *Med Progr* 343:1863, 2000.

Mawer EB et al: Unique 24-hydroxylated metabolites represent a significant pathway of metabolism of vitamin D$_2$ in humans: 24-hydroxyvitamin D$_2$ and 1,24-dihydroxyvitamin D$_{23}$ detectable in human serum, *J Clin Endocr Metab* 83:2156, 1998.

Munson PL, Hirsch PF: Importance of calcitonin in physiology, clinical pharmacology, and medicine, *Bone Miner* 16:162, 1992.

Murer H et al: Proximal tubular phosphate reabsorption: molecular mechanisms, *Am Physiol Soc* 80:1373, 2000.

Nemeth EF, Scarpa A: Are changes in intracellular free calcium necessary for regulating secretion in parathyroid cells? *Ann NY Acad Sci* 493:542, 1987.

Raisz LG: Local and systemic factors in the pathogenesis of osteoporosis, *N Engl J Med* 318:818, 1988.

Roodman GD: Advances in bone biology: the osteoclast, *Endocr Rev* 17:308, 1996.

Ross TK, Darwish HM, Deluca HF: Molecular biology of vitamin D action, *Vitam Horm* 49:281, 1994.

Rouleau MF et al: Characterization of the major parathyroid hormone target cell in the endosteal metaphysis of rat long bones, *J Bone Miner Res* 10:1043, 1990.

Schipani E et al: Constitutively activated receptors for parathyroid hormone and parathyroid hormone-related peptide in Jansen's metaphyseal chondrodysplasia, *N Engl J Med* 335:708, 1996.

Schmid C: IGFs: function and clinical importance to the regulation of osteoblast function by hormones and cytokines with special reference to insulin-like growth factors and their binding proteins, *J Intern Med* 234:535, 1993.

Silver J: Cycling with the parathyroid, *J Clin Invest* 107:1079, 2001.

Slatopolsky E et al: Phosphorus restriction prevents parathyroid gland growth: high phosphorus directly stimulates PTH secretion in vitro, *J Clin Invest* 97:2534, 1996.

Stern PH: Vitamin D and bone, *Kidney Int* 29:S17, 1990.

Strewler GJ: Mechanisms of disease, *N Engl J Med* 342:177, 2000.

Takasu H et al: Dual signaling and ligand selectivity of the human PTH/PTH$_{rp}$ receptor, *J Bone Miner Res* 14:11, 1999.

Webb AR et al: Sunlight regulates the cutaneous production of vitamin D$_3$ by causing its photodegradation, *J Clin Endocrinol Metab* 68:882, 1989.

Yamaguchi A et al: Regulation of osteoblast differentiation mediated by bone morphogenetic proteins, hedgehogs, and Cbfa1, *Endocr Rev* 21:393, 2000.

Books and monographs

Bouillon R: Vitamin D: from photosynthesis, metabolism, and action to clinical applications. In DeGroot LJ, Jameson JL, editors: *Endocrinology,* ed 4, Philadelphia, 2001, WB Saunders.

Bringhurst FR: Regulation of calcium and phosphate homeostasis. In DeGroot LJ, Jameson JL, editors: *Endocrinology,* ed 4, Philadelphia, 2001, WB Saunders.

Bringhurst FR, Demay MB, Kronenberg HM: Hormones and disorders of mineral metabolism. In Wilson JD et al, editors: *Williams textbook of endocrinology,* ed 9, Philadelphia, 1998, WB Saunders.

Coleman DT, Fitzpatrick LA, Bilezikian J: Biochemical mechanisms of parathyroid hormone action. In Bilezikian J, editor: *The parathyroids: basic and clinical concepts,* New York, 1994, Raven Press.

Juppner HW et al: Parathyroid hormone and parathyroid hormone-related peptide in the regulation of calcium homeostasis and bone development. In DeGroot LJ, Jameson JL, editors: *Endocrinology,* ed 4, Philadelphia, 2001, WB Saunders.

Kronenberg HM et al: Parathyroid hormone biosynthesis and metabolism. In Bilezikian J, editor: *The parathyroids: basic and clinical concepts,* New York, 1994, Raven Press.

Martin TJ, Moseley JM, Sexton PM: Calcitonin. In DeGroot LJ, Jameson JL, editors: *Endocrinology,* ed 4, Philadelphia, 2001, WB Saunders.

Rodan GA: Bone development and remodeling. In DeGroot LJ, Jameson JL, editors: *Endocrinology,* ed 4, Philadelphia, 2001, WB Saunders.

chapter forty-three

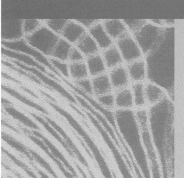

The Hypothalamus and Pituitary Gland

The hypothalamus-pituitary unit forms the most complex and, in some respects, the most dominant component of the entire endocrine system. Its internal anatomical and functional relationships are elaborate and subtle. *The output of the hypothalamus-pituitary unit regulates the function of the thyroid, adrenal, and reproductive glands and is directly responsible for somatic growth and lactation and milk secretion. It also helps maintain body fluid homeostasis.*

Numerous hormones are synthesized, stored, and released by the hypothalamus-pituitary unit. Two hormones, **antidiuretic hormone (ADH or arginine vasopressin)** and **oxytocin,** are synthesized by neurons in the hypothalamus, but they are stored and secreted by the posterior pituitary gland, or **neurohypophysis.** A group of tropic hormones—**adrenocorticotropic hormone (ACTH), thyroid-stimulating hormone (TSH), luteinizing hormone (LH), follicle-stimulating hormone (FSH), growth hormone (GH),** and **prolactin**—is synthesized, stored, and secreted mostly by hormone-specific endocrine cell types in the anterior pituitary gland, or adenohypophysis. A set of releasing and inhibiting hormones that are produced in the hypothalamus and travel to the adenohypophysis regulates the synthesis and secretion of these adenohypophyseal tropic hormones. All of these hormones emanate from a mass of only 500 mg of pituitary tissue in association with 10 g of adjacent hypothalamus.

ANATOMY

A knowledge of the embryological development of the pituitary gland is crucial to an understanding of its anatomy and function. *The fully developed gland is actually an amalgam of hormone-producing glandular cells (the adenohypophysis, or anterior pituitary), constituting 80%, and of neural cells with secretory function (the neurohypophysis, or posterior pituitary).* The anterior endocrine portion of the pituitary gland develops from an upward outpouching (Rathke's pouch) of ectodermal cells from the roof of the oral cavity. This pouch eventually pinches off and becomes separated from the oral cavity by the sphenoid bone of the skull. The lumen of the pouch is reduced to a small cleft. The posterior neural portion of the pituitary gland develops from a downward outpouching of ectoderm from the brain in the floor of the third ventricle. The lumen of this pouch is obliterated inferiorly as the sides fuse into the infundibular process. Superiorly, the lumen remains contiguous with, and forms a recess in, the adult third ventricle. The upper portion of this neural stalk expands to invest the lowest portion of the hypothalamus then called the **median eminence.** The cleftlike remnant of Rathke's pouch demarcates the interwoven anterior and posterior portions of the pituitary. In some animals, but not in humans, cells in the area of Rathke's pouch and adjacent to the neurohypophysis form a distinct intermediate lobe.

The entire pituitary gland sits in a socket of sphenoid bone, called the **sella turcica.** A reflection of the dura mater, called the **diaphragm,** extends across the top of the sella turcica and separates the bulk of the pituitary gland from the brain. However, the neural stalk penetrates the diaphragm, maintaining its continuity with the hypothalamus. These anatomical relationships are shown in Fig. 43-1, *B.* The human pituitary gland can be visualized (Fig. 43-1, *A*) by computed tomography (CT) and by nuclear magnetic resonance imaging (MRI). The volume of the pituitary gland decreases with aging and increases during pregnancy.

The blood supply to this amalgam of neural and endocrine tissue is complex. In the posterior pituitary gland, the neural tissue of the infundibular process is supplied with blood, mostly from the **inferior hypophyseal artery.** The fenestrated capillary plexus of this artery drains into the dural sinus. The neural tissue of the upper stalk and of the median eminence is supplied largely by the **superior hypophyseal artery.** After investing the axons in these areas, the capillary plexus that emanates from this artery forms a set of long portal veins that carry the blood downward into the anterior pituitary gland. There, these **portal veins** give rise to a second capillary plexus that supplies the anterior pituitary endocrine cells with most of their blood supply, which is then drained off into the dural sinus. The anterior pituitary gland also

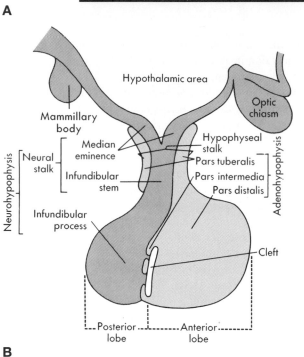

Fig. 43-1 **A,** Magnetic resonance image of the head shows the proximity of the hypothalamus and pituitary gland and their connection by a neurohypophyseal stalk. (Courtesy of Steven Wiener, MD.) **B,** Diagram of the pituitary gland shows its division into the adenohypophysis and neurohypophysis. (Adapted from an original painting by Frank H. Netter, MD, from The CIBA Collection of Medical Illustrations, Division of CIBA-Geigy Corporation.)

receives blood via a set of short portal veins that originate in the capillary plexus of the inferior hypophyseal artery within the neural stalk. Thus, very little direct arterial blood supply reaches the adenohypophyseal cells. Note also that the anterior pituitary gland lies outside the blood-brain barrier, and that it receives no direct innervation.

The implications of the anatomical arrangement of the hypothalamus-pituitary complex and its blood supply become apparent when the functional relationships are examined in Fig. 43-2. Aside from a small number of glial cells *(pituicytes)*, the neurohypophysis represents mainly a collection of axons whose cell bodies lie in the hypothalamus. Peptide hormones synthesized in the cell bodies of these hypothalamic neurons travel down their axons in neurosecretory granules to be stored in the nerve terminals lying in the posterior pituitary gland. These terminals consist of neurosecretory vesicles invested with modified astroglial cells, known as pituicytes. Upon stimulation of the cell bodies, the

granules are released from the axonal terminals by exocytosis. The peptide hormones then enter the peripheral circulation via the capillary plexuses of the inferior hypophyseal artery. Thus, a single neural cell performs the entire process of hormone synthesis, storage, and release.

In contrast, the adenohypophysis is a collection of endocrine cells regulated by blood-borne stimuli that originate in neural tissue. Cell bodies of particular hypothalamic neurons synthesize releasing and inhibiting hormones, which travel in packets down their axons only as far as the median eminence. Here, these hormones are stored within neurosecretory granules in the nerve terminals. After these hypothalamic neurons are stimulated by nerve impulses, the releasing or inhibiting hormones are discharged into the median eminence and enter the capillary plexus of the superior hypophyseal artery. From here, they are transported down the long portal veins and then exit from the secondary capillary plexus to reach their specific endocrine target cells in the adenohypophysis. A

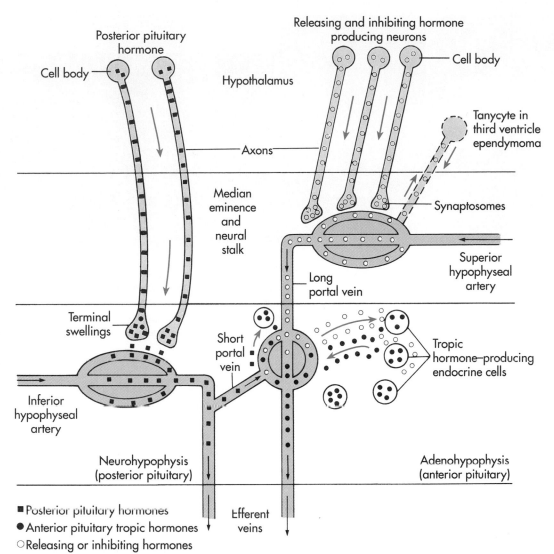

■ **Fig. 43-2** Anatomical and functional relationships between the hypothalamus, the pituitary gland, and their blood supply. Note that the adenohypophysis has no direct arterial supply but receives blood from the median eminence, which contains hypothalamic releasing and inhibiting hormones. *Arrows* indicate direction of movement of hormone molecules. Posterior pituitary hormones reach their storage and release area by axonal transport from the neuron cell bodies where they are synthesized. Anterior pituitary hormones are synthesized and stored in situ. They are secreted in response to hypothalamic peptides that reach the anterior pituitary by axonal transport followed by blood transport via portal veins.

similar arrangement can bring neurohormone signals from the neurohypophysis via the short portal veins. The endocrine cells respond to the releasing or inhibiting hormones by increasing or decreasing their output of tropic hormones that are stored in secretory granules. These hormones enter the same second capillary plexus through which they ultimately reach the peripheral circulation. Thus, two cells—one neural and one endocrine—participate in the processes that lead to synthesis and release (by exocytosis) of the anterior pituitary tropic hormones, a combination of neurocrine and endocrine function. Key evidence in support of this functional arrangement includes the following observations:

1. Neural tracts that contain hypothalamic peptides can be traced by immunohistochemical techniques down to the median eminence, where they end in proximity to capillaries (Fig. 43-3).
2. Direct measurement reveals that the concentrations of hypothalamic peptides are 10-fold to 20-fold higher in pituitary portal venous blood than in peripheral blood.
3. Exposure of anterior pituitary tissue to individual hypothalamic peptides in perfusion systems or in tissue culture causes specific patterns of stimulation or inhibition of the release of the corresponding tropic hormones.

The above description implies an entirely unidirectional arrangement. However, not all the venous drainage from the anterior pituitary gland necessarily empties directly into the systemic circulation. The short portal veins may act as

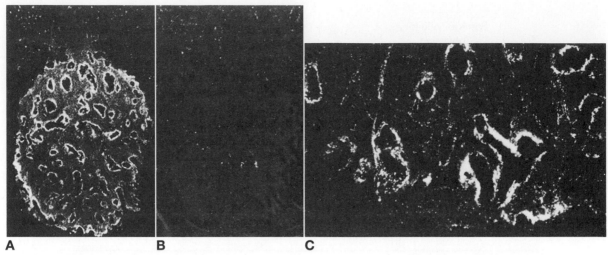

A   **B**   **C**

■ **Fig. 43-3**   Immunohistochemical localization of growth hormone-releasing hormone (GHRH) in the median eminence of the squirrel monkey. **A,** Section stained with fluorescent-labeled antibody to GHRH shows localization of GHRH around capillaries of the median eminence. **B,** Section stained with fluorescent-labeled control serum shows little reaction, demonstrating specificity of the antibody to GHRH. **C,** Higher power of **A** showing GHRH in axonal tracts ending in the vicinity of the capillaries. (From Bloch B et al: *Nature* 301:607, 1983.)

conduits for a reverse flow of blood from the anterior pituitary cells through the neurohypophyseal capillary plexus back up to the axons or cell bodies in the median eminence or in the hypothalamus. This direction of flow permits high concentrations of anterior pituitary tropic hormones to bathe these neurons without impedance from the blood-brain barrier, and thus it allows short-loop feedback from the endocrine to the neural cells.

Two-way traffic may also exist between the cerebrospinal fluid and the neurohypophysis and adenohypophysis. Specialized ependymal cells in the interior recess of the third ventricle send down long processes that interdigitate with the blood vessels in the median eminence and infundibular stalk (Fig. 43-2). These cells, known as pituitary tanycytes, may facilitate transfer of regulatory substances from the cerebrospinal fluid to the pituitary. They could also allow posterior pituitary peptide hormones, hypothalamic-releasing or -inhibiting hormones, or even anterior pituitary tropic hormones to have access to the brain via the cerebrospinal fluid.

HYPOTHALAMIC FUNCTION

The hypothalamus clearly plays a key role in regulating pituitary function. This structure can be considered a central relay station for collecting and integrating signals from diverse sources and funneling them to the pituitary (Fig. 43-4). The hypothalamus receives afferent nerve tracts from the thalamus, the reticular-activating substance, the limbic system (amygdala, olfactory bulb, hippocampus, and habenula), and the eyes and remotely from the neocortex. Some of the connections to the hypothalamus are multisynaptic. Through this input, pituitary function can be influenced by pain, sleep, wakefulness, emotion, fright, rage, olfactory sensa-

tions, light, and possibly even thought. These influences can coordinate pituitary function with patterned behavior and mating responses of neural origin. The proximity of other hypothalamic nuclei that govern thirst, appetite, energy stores, temperature regulation, and autonomic nervous system function also allows coordination between the output of pituitary hormones and a wide variety of basic functions.

The proximity of these various hypothalamic areas to each other has functional logic. For example, hormones of the thyroid gland increase energy expenditure, metabolic rate, and thermogenesis. The neurons that ultimately control output of the thyroid gland via secretion of its tropic hormone, TSH, are anatomically close to, and connect with, neurons that regulate energy intake via appetite control and temperature.

Other tracts within the hypothalamus can integrate multiple simultaneous pituitary responses with each other and regulate pituitary function in accordance with changes in temperature, energy needs, or fluid balance. The neurotransmitters involved in afferent impulses to the hypothalamus are largely norepinephrine, acetylcholine, and serotonin. Dopamine, acetylcholine, γ-aminobutyric acid (GABA), and the opioid peptide β-endorphin act as neurotransmitters for efferent impulses to the median eminence. These impulses regulate the discharge of releasing or inhibiting hormones into the adjacent capillaries (Fig. 43-2). In addition, neurotransmitters, such as dopamine from the hypothalamus may reach the portal vein blood. Via receptors in the endocrine cells, these transmitters may directly influence the output of anterior pituitary tropic hormones. Dopamine and β-endorphin also modulate efferent hypothalamic outflow by transmitting signals between different areas of the hypothalamus.

The hypothalamus-pituitary axis is also under the influence of blood-borne substances from the periphery. Virtually

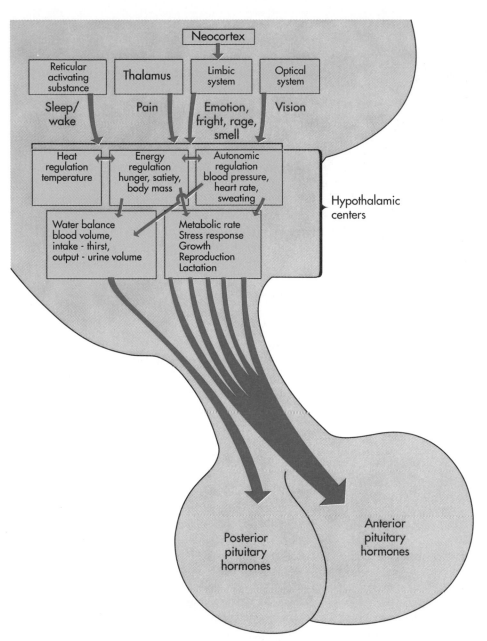

Fig. 43-4 The interrelationships among various hypothalamic centers and their inputs from various other areas of the brain and their outputs to the posterior and anterior pituitary gland. Using the hypothalamus as a relay station, a factor such as pain can influence secretion of hormones, modulating water balance or responses to stress.

all the tropic hormones from the adenohypophysis cause changes in the concentrations either of peripheral target gland hormones (thyroid, adrenal, gonadal) or of substrates, such as glucose or free fatty acids. Conditions exist for at least three levels of humoral feedback, as illustrated in Fig. 43-5. Peripheral gland hormones or substrates that arise from tissue metabolism can exert feedback control on both the hypothalamus and the anterior pituitary gland. This mechanism is known as **long-loop feedback,** and it is usually negative, although it can occasionally be positive. Negative feedback can also be exerted by the tropic hormones themselves through effects on the synthesis or discharge of the related hypothalamic-releasing or -inhibiting hormones. This mechanism is known as **short-loop feedback.** Because tropic hormones do not ordinarily cross the blood-brain barrier, short-loop feedback may occur either by specialized transport across fenestrated endothelial cells of the capillar-

ies that bathe hypothalamic neurons, or by reverse flow through the short portal veins, as previously described. Finally, hypothalamic-releasing hormones may even inhibit their own synthesis by stimulating the discharge of a paired hypothalamic inhibitory hormone that suppresses secretion by the releasing hormone neuron. This mechanism, called **ultra-short-loop feedback,** could occur in two ways: by neurotransmission between two hypothalamic cells, or by transport of the releasing hormone, via the pituitary tanycytes, to the cerebrospinal fluid and then back to the hypothalamus.

The anterior pituitary gland is the central point of the hypothalamic pituitary-peripheral gland axis. At this level, *hypothalamic-releasing hormones and peripheral target gland hormones are usually antagonists: one accelerates while the other brakes anterior pituitary hormone secretion.* The short- and ultra-short-loop feedback mechanisms help maintain the balance.

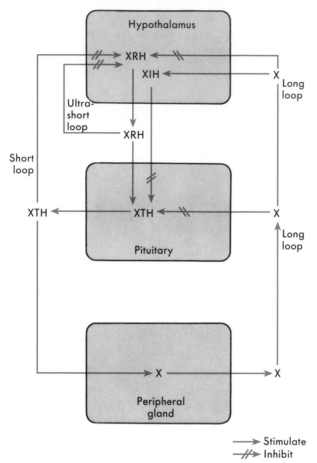

■ **Fig. 43-5** Negative feedback loops regulating hormone secretion in a typical hypothalamus-pituitary-peripheral gland axis. *X,* Peripheral gland hormone; *XTH,* pituitary tropic hormone; *XRH,* hypothalamic-releasing hormone; *XIH,* hypothalamic-inhibiting hormone.

Table 43-1 lists the currently known or suspected hypothalamic-releasing or -inhibiting hormones.

The hypothalamus can be subdivided into endocrinologically distinct functional areas. In general, the lateral hypothalamus receives afferent impulses, and it relays them to the neurosecretory nuclei of the anterior and medial basal portions of the hypothalamus. The anterior segment of the hypothalamus contains two well-defined collections of large (magnocellular) neurons, the supraoptic and paraventricular nuclei. These nuclei are responsible for the synthesis of the two posterior pituitary peptide hormones (oxytocin and ADH). Their axons project primarily to the posterior pituitary gland, although some fibers also project to the median eminence and to other neurons in the floor of the third ventricle and the brainstem. Clustered immediately beneath the third ventricle, in the arcuate nucleus and the periventricular nucleus of the medial basal hypothalamus, are small (parvicellular) neurons that are responsible for synthesis of the various hypothalamic-releasing and -inhibiting hormones. Some of these neurons are also located in the paraventricular nucleus. The axons of these small neurons project to the median eminence. However, cells that also contain hypotha-

lamic releasing hormones are scattered in numerous other areas of the hypothalamus. In these neurons, the hypothalamic peptide hormones may have particular neurotransmitter roles related to or distinct from their known endocrine functions. Immunohistochemical mapping has shown a substantial anatomical separation between the dense collections of hypothalamic peptides. This separation suggests that only one cell type produces each neurohormone. However, in at least one instance, two peptide hormones [corticotropin-releasing hormone (CRH) and ADH] are colocalized within certain hypothalamic neurons.

The names of all the hypothalamic peptides are based on the anterior pituitary hormone whose secretion they were originally discovered to influence. It was initially presumed that each tropic hormone was controlled by a unique hypothalamic-releasing or -inhibiting hormone. Also, each hypothalamic hormone was presumed to have only one target anterior pituitary cell. However, the actual physiology is more complex. **Thyrotropin-releasing hormone (TRH)** can also stimulate the secretion of prolactin. **Somatostatin,** discovered as a GH-inhibiting factor, can also inhibit the secretion of TSH. Growth hormone releasing peptide stimulates the secretion of ACTH and prolactin.

Hypothalamic peptide hormones have also been found outside the hypothalamus, in such diverse areas as the cerebral cortex, limbic area, spinal cord, autonomical ganglia, sensory neurons, pancreatic islets, and throughout the gastrointestinal tract. In such areas, these peptides serve neuromodulatory roles that may be related to or independent of their endocrine function. Especially noteworthy is the finding of numerous hypothalamic-releasing and -inhibiting hormones in the anterior pituitary gland itself, and the expression of their genes within their own normal target endocrine cells. This finding suggests that these hypothalamic peptides also have both paracrine and autocrine functions.

The hypothalamic peptides are synthesized via prepro-hormones, as described in Chapter 39. Many common features characterize their functional behavior.

Pathologically functioning adenohypophyseal cells in pituitary tumors may have receptors for unrelated hypothalamic regulatory peptides, whereas the normal adenohypophyseal cells generally do not. For example, **anterior pituitary adenomas** that secrete GH may have TRH receptors. These tumor cells respond to this hypothalamic peptide by the secretion of GH. This aberrant response is a useful diagnostic test for the presence of such adenomas. Tumor cells from types other than the GH-secreting line may have receptors for the peptide somatostatin, which inhibits GH. The presence of somatostatin receptors on the tumor cells makes possible the use of analogs of this peptide to treat such adenomas by reducing the size of these tumors and by stopping the hypersecretion of their hormone product.

The secretion of hypothalamic-releasing and -inhibiting hormones into the pituitary portal veins is pulsatile. This pul-

■ Table 43-1 Hypothalamic hormones and factors

Hormone	Predominant hypothalamic localization	Structure	Target pituitary hormones
Thyrotropin-releasing hormone (TRH)	Paraventricular	pGLU-HIS-PRO-NH$_2$	Thyrotropin Prolactin Growth hormone (pathological)
Gonadotropin-releasing hormone (GnRH)	Arcuate	pGLU-HIS-TRP-SER-TYR-GLY-LEU-ARG-PRO-GLY-NH$_2$	Luteinizing hormone Follicle-stimulating hormone Growth hormone (pathological)
Corticotropin-releasing hormone(CRH)	Paraventricular	SER-GLN-GLU-PRO-PRO-ILE-SER-LEU-ASP-LEU-THR-PHE-HIS-LEU-LEUARG-GLU-VAL-LEU-GLU-MET-THR-LYS-ALA-ASP-GLN-LEU-ALA-GLN-GLN-ALA-HIS-SER-ASN-ARG-LYS-LEU-LEU-ASP-ILE-ALA-NH$_2$	Adrenocorticotropin β- and γ-Lipotropin β-Endorphins
Growth hormone–releasing hormone (GHRH)	Arcuate	TYR-ALA-ASP-ALA-ILE-PHE-THR-ASN-SER-TYR-ARG-LYS-VAL-LEU-GLY-GLN-LEU-SER-ALA-ARG-LYS-LEU-LEU-GLN-ASP-ILE-MET-SER-ARG-GLN-GLN-GLY-GLU-SER-ASN-GLN-GLU-ARG-GLY-ALA-ARG-ALA-ARG-GLY-ALA-ARG-ALA-ARG-LEU-NH$_2$	Growth hormone
Growth hormone–inhibiting hormone (somatostatin)	Anterior periventricular	ALA-GLY-CYS-LYS-ASN-PHE-PHE-TRP-LYS-THR-PHE-THR-SER-CYS	Growth hormone Prolactin Thyrotropin Adrenocorticotropin (pathological)
Prolactin-inhibiting factor (PIF)	Arcuate	Dopamine	Prolactin, thyrotropin Growth hormone (pathological)
Prolactin-releasing factor (PRF)	Not known	Not established	Prolactin

satile pattern apparently depends on intrinsic neural oscillators within the cells that release these hormones. Pulsatile secretion of these hormones is critical for maintenance of the appropriate pattern and level of secretion of their target anterior pituitary hormones. Pulsatility may also determine whether the receptors for hypothalamic peptides are up- or downregulated.

To exert their effects, releasing and inhibiting hormones first bind to plasma membrane receptors in the anterior pituitary cells. The cytosolic calcium concentration, and then the cAMP concentration, is altered. In addition, diacylglycerols, inositol phosphates, and arachidonic acid from membrane phospholipids help mediate the intracellular effects that follow. Specific proteins are presumably phosphorylated by activated protein kinase A or C. Granule exocytosis is rapidly stimulated and stored tropic hormones are released. In addition, tropic hormone synthesis is stimulated or inhibited by increasing or decreasing the transcription of their genes. In some instances, the biological activity of the target pituitary hormones may also be increased after translation by modifying their content of carbohydrate or sialic acid or by phosphorylation.

Another factor of hypothalamic origin was identified in the anterior pituitary gland and was named the pituitary adenylyl cyclase–activating peptide (PACAP) (see Table 39-1).

Via a class 2 plasma membrane receptor and cAMP, this peptide hormone regulates both positively and negatively pituitary cell cycle and development, apoptosis, and release of ACTH, MSH, GH, LH, FSH, and from FS cells, interleukin-6 (IL-6). Subsequently PACAP has been found to have a much wider tissue distribution and to influence such diverse processes as insulin secretion, bone metabolism, melatonin synthesis, adrenocortical and adrenomedullary function, ovarian and testicular function, vascular dilation, and male erection.

The anterior pituitary contains at least five endocrine cell types (Table 43-2) that arise from a common precursor in the following order: corticotrophs, thyrotrophs, gonadotrophs, somatotrophs, and mammotrophs. A specific protein transcription factor, called **Pit-1,** is involved in the differentiation and proliferation of somatotrophs, mammotrophs, thyrotrophs, and gonadotrophs. The synthesis of Pit-1 in the precursor cells is induced by cAMP, the level of which is raised or lowered by the appropriate hypothalamic peptides. Other transcription factors also contribute to the specific differentiation of individual cell types.

Nonsense mutations in the Pit-1 gene result in **hypoplasia** of the anterior pituitary gland and in the deficient secretion

■ **Table 43-2**   Anterior pituitary cells and hormones

Cell	Pituitary population (%)	Products/molecular weight	Targets
Corticotroph	15-20	Adrenocorticotropin (ACTH), 4500 β-Lipotropin, 11,000	Adrenal gland Adipose tissue Melanocytes
Thyrotroph	3-5	Thyrotropin (TSH), 28,000	Thyroid gland
Gonadotroph	10-15	Luteinizing hormone (LH), 28,000 Follicle-stimulating hormone (FSH), 33,000	Gonads
Somatotroph	40-50	Somatotropin, growth hormone (GH), 22,000	All tissues
Mammotroph	10-25	Prolactin, 23,000	Breasts Gonads

of GH, prolactin, and TSH (Table 43-2). Mutations in another developmental gene, prophet of pituitary-1 (PROP-1), also cause combined deficiencies of anterior pituitary hormones.

Anterior pituitary cells cannot be completely distinguished from each other by conventional histological staining, and they are not localized to exclusive areas. However, immunohistochemical techniques that employ hormone-specific antisera have permitted each type to be identified. About 10% of anterior pituitary cells, known as folliculostellate (FS) cells, are devoid of protein hormone-containing granules. These cells are homologous to dendritic/macrophage cells, and they release immune cytokines such as IL-1, IL-6, and tumor necrosis factor-α (TNF-α), which can modulate endocrine function. FS cells send out long cytoplasmic processes that invest the hormone-secreting cells and affect hormone release. In at least one instance, certain FS cells express the receptor for an anterior pituitary tropic hormone (TSH); thus, a paracrine short-loop feedback with the pituitary thyrotrophic cell that secretes TSH can be visualized to operate in some physiological circumstances.

The distribution of endocrine cell types within the gland is not random. Certain endocrine cell types tend to associate with each other, intertwine, and even form junctional complexes. Growth factors are localized within certain anterior pituitary cells, and they may also express the receptor for the hormone that they secrete. Thus, paracrine interactions and autocrine effects are likely characteristics of anterior pituitary function. Leptin and leptin receptor, as well as interleukins (cytokines) and their receptors, are also expressed in the anterior pituitary cells. This gives leptin and interleukins a putative role in regulating anterior pituitary function. Similar observations have been made for endogenous cannabinoids (marihuana-like components) and to their receptors.

Mathematical modeling of the plasma profiles of human anterior pituitary hormones suggests that tonic secretion of these hormones is negligible. Rather, secretion is episodic, prompted by pulses of hypothalamic-releasing hormones. Secretion bursts probably last only a few minutes. The longer duration (90-140 minutes) of the resultant plasma peaks reflects the slow metabolic clearance rates of the anterior pituitary hormones.

ANTERIOR PITUITARY HORMONES

The anterior pituitary gland secretes three glycoprotein proteins with structural similarities. Each contains an almost identical α-subunit of 92 to 96 amino acids and a distinctive β-subunit. Each subunit is a product of a separate gene. Hence, synthesis of the whole hormone requires the coordinated expression of the α-subunit and the β-subunit genes. The α- and β-subunits are noncovalently linked, and the three-dimensional structures are determined by intramolecular S–S bonds.

Each hormone has different primary target cells and functions. However they bind to specific class 1 plasma membrane receptors, which also have some homology. These receptors are linked via stimulatory G-proteins to adenylyl cyclase, and thus generate cAMP as a second messenger. The extracellular portions of these receptors are also glycosylated. This modification is necessary for the proper folding and transport of these receptors to the cell membrane, but it is not necessary for hormone binding. Two amino acids in the α-subunit and seven amino acids in the β-subunit are essential for hormone binding to the receptor. Sequences 93 to 100 in the β-subunit interact with the α-subunit and determine the specificity of each hormone. Each glycoprotein hormone downregulates its respective receptor.

Each hormone has N-linked glycosylation sites (asparagine) and the oligosaccharide components are esterified to sulfuric acid and sialic acid. These hormones undergo hepatic and renal clearance after enzymatic removal of sialic acid moieties in the circulation. Specific hepatic receptors exist for the sulfated, desialylated hormone molecules. Small amounts of biologically active hormone are excreted in the urine. Variation in the degree of glycosylation during hormone synthesis in various physiological states determines the hormone clearance, modulates the plasma hormone concentration profiles, and therefore helps regulate the hormone action on target cells.

Thyrotropic Hormone (Thyroid-Stimulating Hormone; TSH)

TSH is a glycoprotein hormone whose function is to regulate the growth and metabolism of the thyroid gland and the secretion of its hormones, **thyroxine (T₄)** and **triiodothyronine (T₃)**. The TSH-producing cells normally form 5% of the adult human anterior pituitary population, and they are found predominantly in the anteromedial area of the gland. These cells develop at about 13 weeks of gestation, at the same time that the fetal thyroid gland begins to secrete thyroid hormone. Thyrotroph embryonic factor stimulates the synthesis of fetal TSH.

TSH has a molecular weight of 28,000, and it contains carbohydrate units that are bound covalently to the peptide chains. The β-subunit of 110 amino acids confers the specific biological activity on the TSH molecule. Nevertheless, both α- and β-subunits are required for receptor binding and subsequent hormone action.

TSH synthesis. Separate genes, located on different chromosomes, code for the individual α- and β-subunits. A signal N-terminal peptide is eliminated from each primary translation product (termed a prehormone). Subsequently, the N-glycoside–linked sugar moieties, which are rich in mannose and which protect the nascent molecule from premature intracellular proteolysis, are added. During transport of the carbohydrate units from the rough endoplasmic reticulum and packaging in the Golgi apparatus, these units are further modified, sialic acid and sulfate are added, and intramolecular disulfide bonds are formed. These changes ensure the proper conformation that permits the two individual subunits to combine in the mature TSH molecule, which is stored in secretory granules. In addition, the sialic acid and sulfate residues render the molecule more acidic and thereby prolong its plasma half-life. Expression of the α- and β-subunit genes is separately regulated, but in coordination with each other. Ordinarily, an excess of the nonspecific α-subunit is produced. However, the selective addition of an extra O-linked oligosaccharide renders the excess α-subunits incapable of combining with β-subunits. Transcription of both TSH subunit genes is stimulated by the hypothalamic TRH, and transcription is suppressed by thyroid hormone. In addition, TRH modulates the glycosylation process to increase biological activity, whereas thyroid hormone modulates this process to decrease biological activity. Transcription of the α-subunit gene is also regulated by cAMP.

TSH secretion. The secretion of TSH is reciprocally regulated by two major factors. TRH increases the rate of secretion, whereas thyroid hormone decreases the rate of secretion by negative feedback (Fig. 43-6). As a result of this balance, TSH is secreted in a relatively steady, but somewhat pulsatile, fashion. This pattern is congruent with that of its target gland, whose output is steady and whose hormones' actions slowly wax and wane.

TRH is a tripeptide, pyroglutamine-histidine-proline-amide. Its synthesis in the hypothalamus is directed by a gene that codes for a large precursor molecule that contains the small sequence of glutamine-histidine-proline-glycine. After translation, glutamine undergoes cyclization, and the terminal glycine is replaced with an amino group. TRH is stored in the median eminence and reaches its target cells via the pituitary portal vein. TRH then interacts with specific plasma membrane receptors on thyrotroph cells. This interaction

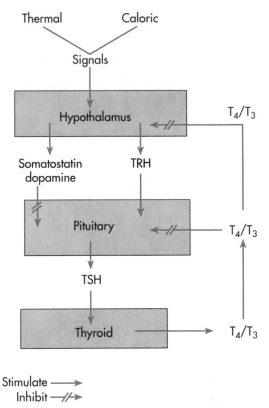

■ **Fig. 43-6** Regulation of thyroid-stimulating hormone (TSH) secretion. Thyroxine (T_4) and triiodothyronine (T_3) from the thyroid gland exert negative feedback on the pituitary by blocking the action of thyroid-releasing hormone (TRH). Negative feedback of T_4 and T_3 at the level of the hypothalamus also occurs. Somatostatin and dopamine each inhibits TSH secretion tonically.

triggers an influx of calcium and an increase in phosphatidyl-inositol products, which act as second messengers. TSH is then released by exocytosis. TRH eventually downregulates its own receptors, and the releasing hormone loses effectiveness. Another product of prepro-TRH processing, the 160 to 169 amino acid peptide, exhibits many of the actions of TRH itself.

After the intravenous administration of TRH, the plasma TSH levels rise as much as 10-fold, and they return toward baseline levels by 60 minutes (Fig. 43-7). With repeated TRH injections, the TSH response diminishes over time, mainly because the secondarily stimulated thyroid gland increases its output of T_4 and T_3 (Fig. 43-7). This clinical experiment demonstrates vividly the negative feedback regulation of TSH secretion depicted in Fig. 43-6. Small increases in thyroid hormone concentration suppress TSH secretion by blocking the stimulatory action of TRH; conversely, small decreases of thyroid hormone augment TSH responsivity to TRH. Significant modulation of TSH secretion is associated with variations in plasma thyroid hormone concentrations of only 10% to 30% above or below the individual's baseline level. The thyrotroph's response to continuous TRH stimulation is also limited by downregulation of the TRH receptor.

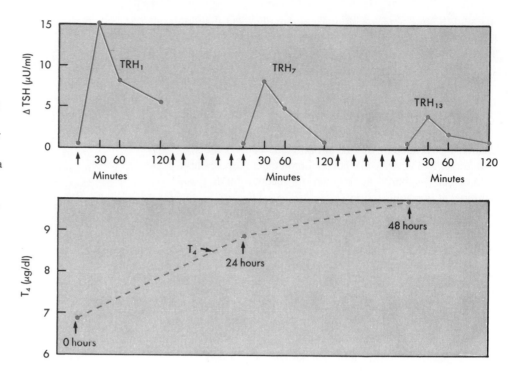

■ **Fig. 43-7** Pituitary and thyroid gland responses to repetitive injections of TRH every 4 hours for 48 hours in humans. Note that as plasma thyroxine (T_4) increases as a result of stimulation of the thyroid gland by TSH, the pituitary TSH responses to TRH are progressively blunted. *TRH₁*, First injection; *TRH₇*, seventh injection; *TRH₁₃*, thirteenth injection. (From Snyder PJ: *J Clin Invest* 52:2305, 1973.)

The intracellular mediator of thyroid hormone's effect on TSH is probably T_3. Furthermore, the T_3 that is generated within the pituitary cell from T_4 is more effective and important in this regard than is the T_3 that enters from the circulation. The suppressive effect of thyroid hormone on TSH release has a half-life of several days, and it may be mediated by the induction of a protein that suppresses TSH. In addition, T_3 decreases the number of TRH receptors. A negative feedback hypothalamic effect of T_3 in the hypothalamus reduces the synthesis or release of TRH; this feedback effect is mediated by one of the three thyroid hormone nuclear receptors (Chapter 44). In individuals who have thyroid diseases that result in deficiency of thyroid hormone **(hypothyroidism),** TRH actions are relatively unrestrained, because of negative feedback. As a result, these individuals have very high plasma TSH levels and hyperplasia of the thyrotrophs. Return of plasma TSH to normal is the most useful indicator that the dose of thyroid hormone replacement therapy is correct.

Physiological modulation of TSH secretion (and consequently of thyroid hormone output) occurs in at least two circumstances: fasting and exposure to cold. TSH responsiveness to TRH (and possibly TRH release itself) is diminished during fasting. This downward regulation coincides with a decrease in metabolic rate that helps the fasting individual adapt to the absence of energy intake. In animals, TSH secretion is augmented by exposure to cold, but this effect is difficult to demonstrate conclusively in adult humans. Because TSH increases thermogenesis via stimulation of the thyroid gland, this response to cold is logical.

Other hormonal and neural influences on TSH secretion have been noted. There is a slight diurnal variation, such that the highest TSH levels occur at night. A tonic inhibitory

effect on TSH secretion is exerted by the hypothalamic peptide, somatostatin, and by the hypothalamic neurotransmitter, dopamine. Cortisol (a hormone from the adrenal cortex) decreases both TRH and TSH secretion; GH also reduces TSH secretion. Plasma TSH fluctuates synchronously with the plasma leptin level, and leptin stimulates TRH release from the hypothalamus.

TSH normally circulates in plasma at a concentration of 0.3 to 5 µU/ml, which approximates a concentration of 10^{-11} M. Daily TSH production (about 165,000 µU) is approximately equivalent to the entire content of one normal pituitary gland. The metabolic clearance rate of TSH is 50 L/day, and this rate is inversely related to the degree of glycosylation of the TSH molecule. In normal individuals, the α-subunit is also secreted, and it circulates at low levels.

When TSH secretion is chronically hyperstimulated in response to deficient function of the thyroid gland, the circulating levels of both β- and α-subunits are elevated. Plasma levels of α units are also elevated in patients who appear to have nonfunctioning pituitary tumors. These tumors probably arise from less differentiated precursor cells or from dedifferentiated cells in the thyrotroph or gonadotroph lines.

TSH actions. TSH binds to a plasma membrane receptor, and cAMP is the second messenger for many of the hormone's effects. The only important TSH actions are those that are exerted on the thyroid gland, where it promotes growth and differentiation of the gland and stimulates all of the steps in thyroid hormone secretion. These steps include glandular uptake of iodide, its organification, the completion of thyroid hormone synthesis, and the subsequent release of

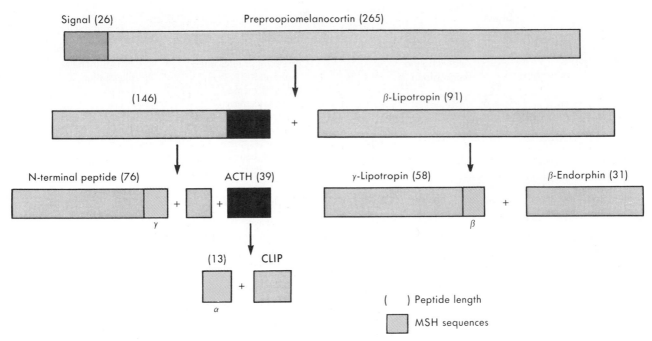

■ **Fig. 43-8** The processing of preproopiomelanocortin. In the anterior lobe of the human pituitary, adrenocorticotropic hormone (ACTH), β-lipotropin, γ-lipotropin, β-endorphin, and a 76-amino acid N-terminal fragment are end products that are released. In other species, ACTH is further cleaved to α-melanocyte-stimulating hormone (α-MSH) and corticotropin-like intermediate peptide *(CLIP)* in the neural intermediate lobe. In humans, MSH activity is provided by MSH sequences within larger molecules such as ACTH.

thyroid gland products (Fig. 43-6). These effects are described in detail in Chapter 44.

Adrenocorticotropic Hormone (ACTH)

ACTH is an anterior pituitary polypeptide hormone whose function is to regulate the growth of the adrenal cortex and the secretion of its steroid hormones. Its most important target gland hormone is cortisol. The corticotrophs form 20% of the anterior pituitary population. Although these cells are found mainly in the pars distalis of the anterior lobe (Fig. 43-1, *B*), ACTH-producing cells may also exist in vestigial intermediate lobes of humans under pathological conditions. In the human fetus, ACTH synthesis and secretion begin at 10 to 12 weeks of gestation, just before the adrenal cortex develops. Corticotroph upstream transcription-binding element (CUTE) and a neurotrophic factor (neuro D1/β2) stimulate corticotroph development and ACTH synthesis in the fetus.

ACTH is a straight-chain peptide with 39 amino acids and a molecular weight of 4500. The N-terminal 1 to 24 sequence contains full biological activity, and sequence 5 to 10 is critical for stimulating the adrenal cortex. The remaining C-terminal portion probably prolongs the hormone's action by protecting it from enzymatic degradation.

Synthesis of ACTH.   The synthesis of ACTH illustrates vividly the principle that the primary gene product in peptide hormone synthesis may yield several biologically active molecules by translational mechanisms. As shown in Fig. 43-8, the mature messenger RNA transcript of the gene directs the synthesis of a 31,000-molecular-weight protein known as **preproopiomelanocortin.** Sequential processing of this primary gene product in humans gives rise to ACTH, along with several other products that are cosecreted into the plasma. These products include β-lipotropin, γ-lipotropin, β-endorphin, and the N-terminal peptide. Some ACTH molecules may undergo posttranslational phosphorylation or glycosylation.

Melanocyte-stimulating hormone (MSH) activity resides within several of these peptides: α-MSH within ACTH, β-MSH within γ-lipoprotein, and γ-MSH within the N-terminal peptide. In extrapituitary sites (such as brain, hypothalamus, gastrointestinal tract, pancreatic islets, adrenal medulla, and skin), the various MSH molecules, their parent molecules, and ACTH are also produced from proopiomelanocortin, and they may subserve different signaling functions.

Finally, the N-terminal pentapeptide of β-endorphin is identical to metenkephalin, with which it shares the analgesic and mood-modifying effects of opioids. The brain enkephalins, however, do not arise by cleavage of β-endorphin, but are synthesized from an entirely different precursor that is expressed by a separate gene.

Secretion of ACTH.   *The regulation of ACTH secretion is among the most complex of all the pituitary hormone regulatory patterns* (Fig. 43-9). *ACTH exhibits circadian rhythms, cyclic bursts, and feedback control, and it responds to a wide variety of stimuli* (Table 43-3). Hypothalamic CRH is the important final mediator of the regulatory inputs. CRH is a peptide with 41 amino acids that originates in

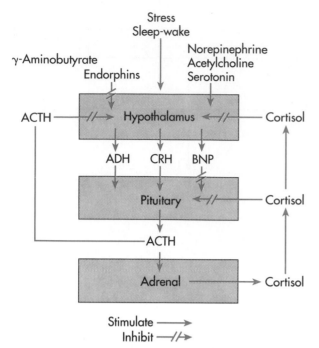

■ **Fig. 43-9** Regulation of ACTH secretion. Corticotropin-releasing hormone (CRH) and antidiuretic hormone (ADH) stimulate ACTH secretion. Brain natriuretic peptide (BNP) inhibits ACTH secretion. Cortisol from the adrenal glands exerts negative feedback (1) at the pituitary level by blocking CRH action and (2) at the hypothalamus level by inhibiting CRH release. Norepinephrine, acetylcholine, and serotonin are positive modulators, whereas endorphins, ACTH itself, and γ-aminobutyric acid are negative modulators of CRH release.

■ **Table 43-3**   Regulation of ACTH secretion

Stimulation	Inhibition
Corticotropin-releasing hormone	Cortisol increase
Cortisol decrease	Enkephalins
Adrenalectomy	Opioids
Metyrapone	ACTH
Sleep-wake transition	Somatostatin
Stress	γ-Aminobutyric acid (GABA)
Hypoglycemia	
Anesthesia	
Surgery	
Trauma	
Infection	
Pyrogens	
Psychiatric disturbance	
Anxiety	
Depression	
Antidiuretic hormone	
α-Adrenergic agonists	
β-Adrenergic antagonists	
Serotonin	
Acetylcholine	
Interleukins	
Gastrointestinal peptides	

small cells of the paraventricular nucleus (Table 43-1). It stimulates the synthesis and release by exocytosis of ACTH and of its proopiomelanocortin coproducts via calcium and cAMP as second messengers. A lack of CRH (as in a CRH gene knockout model) greatly impairs the ACTH diurnal rhythm and its response to stress. ADH also exhibits corticotropin-releasing activity. Under certain physiological circumstances, such as stress, ADH significantly augments the effect of CRH. The gene that directs the synthesis of prepro-CRH has considerable homology with the gene for prepro-ADH; this homology suggests a common evolutionary starting point for these molecules.

CRH receptors (Fig. 43-9) are also found throughout the brain and spinal cord, and CRH itself is synthesized in many peripheral cells, including immune cells and cells in the skin. The widespread distribution of CRH receptors in the central nervous system indicates that CRH has other important central functions related to or independent of stimulating ACTH release. CRH causes central arousal, increases sympathetic nervous system activity, and increases blood pressure. In contrast, CRH diminishes reproductive function by decreasing the synthesis of gonadotropin-releasing hormone (GnRH) and gonadotropins and by inhibiting sexual behavior. CRH also decreases feeding activity and growth. CRH may also regulate β-endorphin and its analgesic action. Finally, in immune cells, CRH stimulates the release of cytokines

and also augments their activity on target cells. CRH circulates at very low plasma levels and it is bound to a specific protein. A related peptide with 45% homology to CRH, called urocortin, is a very potent stimulator of ACTH secretion. Urocortin is present in the supraoptic and paraventricular nuclei and in the median eminence, and it is likely important physiologically.

ACTH secretion has a markedly diurnal pattern. As shown in Fig. 43-10, a large peak occurs 2 to 4 hours before awakening. Thereafter, the average level decreases to virtually zero, just before or after the subject falls asleep. A rise and fall in the major adrenocortical hormone, cortisol, is entrained in this ACTH secretion pattern. The timing of the diurnal pattern can be shifted by altering systematically the sleep-wake cycle for a number of days; however, the ACTH peak is not entrained with a specific stage of sleep. Quite the opposite, in fact, is true; slow-wave sleep decreases the ACTH and cortisol response to CRH, irrespective of the time of day. As individuals reach middle age, slow-wave sleep declines and CRH causes greater arousal. The circadian rhythm of ACTH is diminished or abolished by loss of consciousness, blindness, or constant exposure to either dark or light.

The nocturnal ACTH surge is primarily generated in the suprachiasmatic nucleus of the hypothalamus by CRH release. Although this peak is not directly caused by negative feedback from its target adrenal gland hormone, cortisol, the nocturnal peak is augmented by previous cortisol deficiency. Conversely, this peak can be completely suppressed by excess cortisol, which decreases expression of the CRH gene. The diurnal pattern is composed of pulses of ACTH release, with little or no tonic or constitutive secretion. Up to three pulses occur per hour, and each pulse lasts

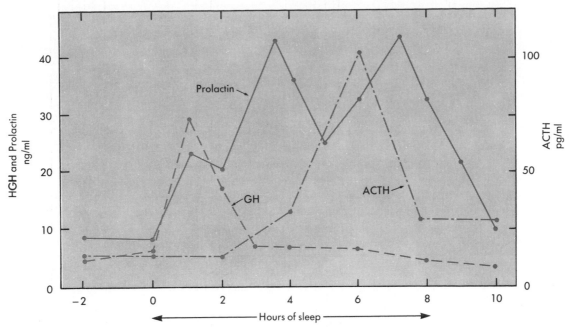

■ **Fig. 43-10** Nocturnal release of ACTH, growth hormone (GH), and prolactin. Note the distinctive pattern for each hormone. (From Takahashi Y et al: *J Clin Invest* 47:2079, 1968; Berson SA et al: *J Clin Invest* 47:2725, 1968; and Sassin JF et al: *Science* 177:1205, 1972.)

about 20 minutes. Major ACTH peaks appear to be caused by increased amplitude rather than by increased frequency of the secretory bursts. As would be expected, pulses of cosecreted β-endorphin occur simultaneously with those of ACTH, whereas cortisol pulses follow 10 minutes later. Men exhibit both a greater frequency and a greater amplitude of ACTH pulses than do women. Age has little effect on ACTH secretion.

Negative feedback inhibition of ACTH secretion is produced by cortisol, or by any synthetic analog with a potency that is proportional to its other cortisol-like activity (Fig. 43-9). The mass of ACTH secreted in each burst, the 24 hour rhythmicity, and the orderliness of ACTH secretion are all reduced by cortisol. The suppressive action of cortisol may outlive the duration of cortisol exposure. Conversely, when (1) cortisol action is blocked by an antagonist, (2) cortisol secretion is reduced by disease, or (3) cortisol release is inhibited pharmacologically (Fig. 43-11), ACTH secretion is stimulated. Cortisol suppresses ACTH secretion by the pituitary gland by blocking the stimulatory action of CRH (Fig. 43-12). Cortisol decreases the synthesis of ACTH by inhibiting the transcription of preproopiomelanocortin and by blocking hypothalamic release of CRH. Cortisol also induces a molecule called lipocortin-1 in FS cells, and this molecule mediates by paracrine action some of cortisol's inhibitory effects on the CRH-ACTH axis. Complete negative feedback requires the loss of cortisol's actions at the pituitary and hypothalamic sites.

The negative feedback effects of cortisol on diurnal and stress-induced ACTH release are also indirectly mediated by neural input from the hippocampus to the CRH neurons of the hypothalamus. Two distinct cortisol receptors in the hippocampus provide a range of affinities to accommodate the usual range of plasma cortisol levels. In the evening, when plasma cortisol is low the high-affinity type 1 glucocorticoid receptor in the hippocampus maintains a degree of negative feedback influence on ACTH secretion. When this receptor is blocked by a specific antagonist, plasma ACTH and cortisol levels, and their responses to CRH and ADH, are increased.

Overactivity of the hypothalamic-pituitary-adrenal axis is characteristic of some types of depressive illness. The pituitary corticotrophs are superresponsive to stimulation by CRH, and they are underresponsive to suppression by cortisol. Hence, cortisol is secreted in mild excess. These features suggest a primary overdrive of the system by CRH neurons in the hypothalamus.

ACTH may inhibit its own secretion by decreasing CRH release; this is an example of short-loop feedback. Chronic deficiency of cortisol leads to persistent elevation of the plasma ACTH concentration, but the diurnal and pulsatile patterns are preserved, indicating their basic nonfeedback origin.

Atrial natriuretic hormone (ANH), in the form of its brain analog, and its sister peptide products from the pro-ANH gene transcript (e.g., kaliuretic hormone) also inhibit basal CRH and ACTH release and the ACTH responses to CRH stimulation in humans. These peptides are synthesized in the hypothalamus and are found in the median eminence, so they may be the suspected corticotroph in release-inhibiting hormones. Because cortisol increases the expression of the pro-ANH gene, all the elements of still another negative feedback brake on ACTH secretion exist.

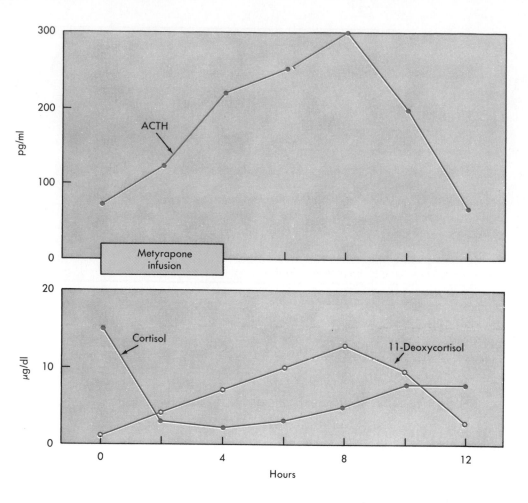

■ **Fig. 43-11** Negative feedback stimulation of ACTH release by metyrapone, a drug that blocks the conversion of 11-deoxycortisol to cortisol in the adrenal gland. Note that plasma ACTH increases as plasma cortisol decreases. The biologically inactive precursor 11-deoxycortisol increases as a result of ACTH action on the adrenal gland. (From Jubiz W et al: *Arch Intern Med* 125:468, 1970.)

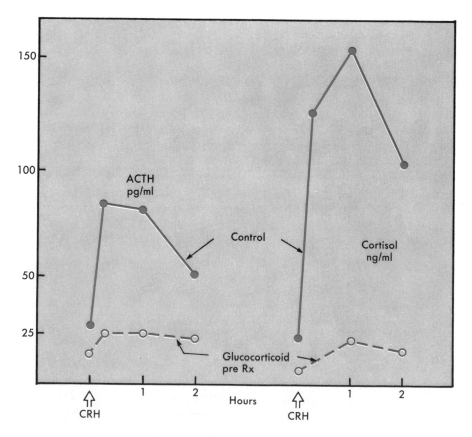

■ **Fig. 43-12** Plasma ACTH and cortisol responses to administration of CRH. Pretreatment with a synthetic glucocorticoid (an analog of cortisol) suppresses the action of CRH on the pituitary. The diminished ACTH response leads secondarily to a diminished secretion of cortisol by the adrenal glands. (From Copinschi G et al: *J Clin Endocrinol Metab* 57:1287, 1983.)

Chronic autonomous hypersecretion of cortisol or the long-term administration of cortisol analogs to treat various diseases leads to functional atrophy of the CRH-ACTH-adrenal axis. Complete recovery of this axis after the suppressive influence has been removed may take up to 1 year. During that time, the individual often requires exogenous cortisol if a stressful medical or surgical situation arises, because a normal adrenal gland response to the stress cannot be assured.

ACTH secretion responds most strikingly to stressful stimuli, a response that is critical to survival. Numerous factors that elicit the stress reaction in humans are noted in Table 43-3. The response to insulin-induced hypoglycemia is illustrated in Fig. 43-13. In some circumstances, such as major abdominal surgery or a severe psychiatric disturbance, the stress-induced hypersecretion of ACTH completely overrides the negative feedback. The hypersecretion cannot be suppressed even if the adrenal cortex secretes cortisol at its maximal level. Stress also may obliterate the diurnal variation of ACTH levels, although pulsatility persists. The pathways vary by which each particular stress signals, senses, and then stimulates CRH (and ADII) secretion. For example, hypothalamic sensitivity to glucose levels augmented by norepi-

nephrine (via α-adrenergic receptors) and by serotonin input induces the ACTH response to hypoglycemia. GABAergic influences dampen the ACTH responses to negative feedback. There are also gender-related influences. The ACTH and cortisol responses to the stress of exercise are modulated by the menstrual cycle in women. Greater responses are evoked during the midluteal phase than during the early follicular phase of the menstrual cycle (see Chapter 46).

However, in its most general sense, stress is a life-threatening situation that usually evokes CRH secretion and the activation of the sympathetic nervous system (see Fig. 45-27). As detailed in Chapter 45, CRH secretion and sympathetic nerve activation have mutually reinforcing actions.

ACTH circulates unbound in plasma, and its half-life is 15 minutes. Basal concentrations at 6 AM range from 20 to 100 pg/ml (average 50 pg/ml). Daily production is less than one third of the pituitary content in the average adult human. Because the bulk of the ACTH is secreted during a limited period in each day, there is sufficient time for ACTH stores to be replenished.

Action of ACTH. ACTH combines with its adrenal cell plasma membrane receptor to increase its principal second messenger, cAMP (see Fig. 45-8). *ACTH stimulates not*

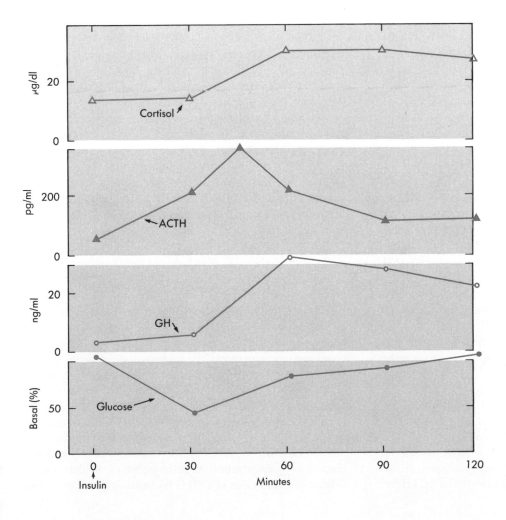

■ **Fig. 43-13**   Stimulation of ACTH, cortisol, and GH secretion by insulin-induced hypoglycemia in humans. (From Ichikawa Y et al: *J Clin Endocrinol Metab* 34:895, 1972.)

only the growth of specific zones of the adrenal cortex, but also the synthesis and secretion of cortisol and other steroid hormones. ACTH increases the size rather than the number of adrenal cells; in the absence of ACTH, the relevant adrenal zones atrophy. All steps in the synthesis of adrenal steroids, which are detailed in Chapter 45, are stimulated by ACTH. Adrenal responsiveness to ACTH is attenuated and delayed by chronic underexposure to the tropic hormone; conversely, responsiveness is accentuated by chronic overexposure.

ACTH synthesis and receptors for ACTH are located in the brain and gastrointestinal tract, where the peptide may have neuromodulatory or paracrine functions. An important relationship also exists between ACTH and the immune system. ACTH receptors and ACTH secretion occur in lymphocytes, and cytokines released by activated lymphocytes stimulate ACTH release by corticotrophs. Within the anterior pituitary, IL-6 from FS cells stimulates ACTH secretion and augments the corticotrophic cell response to CRH. Cytokines increase the expression of the POMC gene by two mechanisms. Binding of cytokines to their plasma membrane receptors leads to generation of STAT-3 (a signal-transducing and -activating transcription molecule), which binds to the promoter region of the POMC gene. STAT-3 also recruits expression of c-*jun* and c-*fos,* which combine to form AP-1 (see Chapter 45) and the latter also activates the POMC gene. Within the corticotrophic cell, the stimulatory effect of cytokines is reduced by subsequent cytokine recruitment of suppressor of cytokine signaling (SOCS) proteins, which inhibit the STAT-3 signaling cascade. This extraordinarily complex arrangement fine tunes ACTH and cortisol secretion and their responses to the degree and duration of stress. For example, obese subjects tend to have a subtle defect in negative feedback regulation. This defect leads to elevated plasma ACTH levels during the day and night and it increases the turnover of cortisol, but the plasma cortisol levels remain normal.

Because of its MSH sequences, ACTH increases skin pigmentation. MSH acts on melanocytes and causes the dispersal of melanin pigment granules within these cells and their dendrites. MSH also stimulates the key enzyme (tyrosinase) in melanin synthesis and the transfer of melanin from the melanocytes to epidermal cells (keratinocytes). These actions are mediated (1) by specific plasma membrane MSH receptors that differ from MC4R (Chapter 43), and (2) by cAMP, which causes the skin to darken. Skin keratinocytes express the proopiomelanocortin gene and its various translation products (see above); both CRH and urocortin are found in the skin. Therefore, under normal circumstances, these MSH actions may probably occur in paracrine rather than in endocrine fashion.

Hyperpigmentation of the skin characterizes diseases in which very large increases in ACTH secretion occur chronically. ACTH excess and MSH effects result (1) from negative feedback, when the adrenal cortex is destroyed (**Addison's disease,** or primary adrenocortical insufficiency) or (2) from ectopic production of ACTH by malignant neural crest cells. A mutant MSH receptor has been reported in association with fair skin and red hair.

Secretion and actions of other proopiomelanocortin peptides.   The remaining peptides in proopiomelanocortin are under the same transcriptional and translational control as is ACTH. The functional significance of this fact is still not well understood, although it could reflect a coordinated physiological response. The plasma level of each peptide rises and falls in parallel with the ACTH level in feedback and stress situations. The molar ratios of these levels differ from the expected 1.0 because of differences in metabolic clearance rates.

The proopiomelanocortin products were named **lipotropins** because of their lipolytic activity, but their role in mobilizing fatty acids from human adipose tissue is unknown. Similarly, the low plasma levels—or even all of the sources—of circulating β-endorphin are of uncertain endocrine significance. When administered to humans, β-endorphins (like opioids) inhibit the secretion of ACTH and of gonadotropins. These observations point to the neurocrine action of β-endorphin, which is generated in the hypothalamus.

Gonadotropic Hormones [Luteinizing Hormone (LH) and Follicle-Stimulating Hormone (FSH)]

LH and FSH are glycoproteins that regulate development, growth, pubertal maturation, reproductive processes, and sex steroid hormone secretion of the gonads of either sex. Both hormones are usually secreted by a single cell type, the gonadotroph. Gonadotrophs make up about 15% of the anterior pituitary cell population, and they are scattered throughout the gland. Small subclasses of gonadotrophs secrete only LH or only FSH. Gonadotrophs also appear to go through cycles in which differential expression of the two gonadotropins occurs at different times. Both hormones are present by 10 to 12 weeks of fetal life; however, neither is absolutely required for the initial intrauterine development of the gonads or for the initial steps in sexual differentiation. Steroidogenic factor-1 stimulates fetal gonadotrophic development and function.

LH, with a molecular weight of 28,000, and FSH, with a molecular weight of 33,000, have similar structures. Each is composed of the common pituitary hormone α-subunit (see above) and of a unique β-subunit (Fig. 43-14). The unique β-subunit differentiates the two hormones from each other, as well as from TSH and HCG. The α- and β-subunits are held together by noncovalent forces, and disulfide bridges create tertiary structures. The carbohydrate moieties (15%-25% by weight) contain oligosaccharides that are composed of mannose, galactose, fucose, galactosamine, acetylglucosamine, and sialic acid. The carbohydrate groups function in receptor binding and responses, and they increase the rate of LH degradation, whereas the sialic acid residues decrease the rate of FSH degradation. The α-subunit is required for binding of gonadotropins to their receptors; neither the β-subunit of LH nor that of FSH is biologically active by itself.

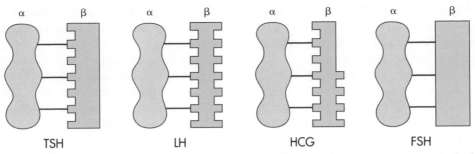

■ Fig. 43-14 Structural similarities among TSH, luteinizing hormone (LH), human chorionic gonadotropin (HCG), and follicle-stimulating hormone (FSH) are depicted schematically. Note that all share the same α-subunit.

The details of LH and FSH biosynthesis resemble those already described for glycoprotein hormones. Individual genes code for the α-subunit and two β-subunits; transcription of the β-subunit genes is rate limiting for gonadotropin synthesis. Also, FSH can be secreted in a nonglycosylated form. The more usual addition and later modification of the carbohydrate moieties by sulfation and sialylation allow considerable variation of the bioactivity of secreted LH and FSH molecules in different physiological circumstances. More basic, less acidic forms have increased potency but decreased half-lives, and they appear to be present at the mid-point of the menstrual cycle. More acidic forms are present after the menopause. In women, the pituitary stores of LH and FSH fluctuate, and they are highest just before ovulation. The patterns of release also suggest the existence of more than one intracellular pool of LH.

Secretion of LH and FSH. *The regulation of LH and FSH secretion is even more complex than that of ACTH. Regulation embodies pulsatile, periodic, diurnal, cyclic, and stage-of-life elements.* Regulation is also different in women and men. The main factors that control secretion of the gonadotropins are discussed in this chapter; their reproductive function is reviewed and discussed in detail in Chapter 46. The secretions of both LH and FSH are stimulated primarily by a single hypothalamic hormone, known either as **gonadotropin-releasing hormone (GnRH)** or as **luteinizing hormone-releasing hormone (LHRH).** As the latter alternate name implies, this hormone causes a much greater increase in LH than in FSH secretion. Whether a separate hypothalamic-releasing hormone exists with a greater specificity for FSH remains uncertain. GnRH is a decapeptide (Table 43-1) that is synthesized from a large prohormone that also yields other products. The cells of origin of GnRH are predominantly in the arcuate nucleus and in the preoptic area of the hypothalamus. These cells have migrated from olfactory epithelium anlage in the early embryo. After transport to the median eminence, GnRH is stored in small granules.

Various influences regulate the release of GnRH. GnRH neurons are under dopaminergic, serotonergic, noradrenergic, and endorphinergic influence (Fig. 43-15). In particular, GnRH neurons are closely associated with dopamine neurons within the arcuate nucleus of the hypothalamus. Dopamine inhibits LH secretion by decreasing GnRH release and also

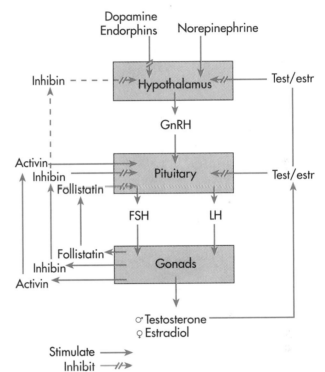

■ Fig. 43-15 Regulation of gonadotropin secretion. Gonadotropin-releasing hormone (GnRH) stimulates LH and FSH release. The gonadal steroids, estradiol in women and testosterone in men, exert negative feedback (1) at the pituitary level by blocking GnRH action and (2) at the hypothalamic level by inhibiting GnRH release. Negative modulation by endorphins and dopamine may mediate some of the steroid hormone feedback. Separate gonadal protein products selectively suppress (inhibin and follistatin) or stimulate (activin) FSH release. These protein products may be expressed locally in the pituitary gland and exert their effects by paracrine and autocrine actions.

by acting directly on the gonadotrophs. Endorphins also inhibit GnRH release and LH secretion. Neural input from the retina to the hypothalamus accounts for the influence of light-dark cycles on GnRH release. In some species, **melatonin** from the pineal gland mediates the seasonal variations in gonadotropin secretion and in reproductive activity that are related to daylight length. The production of melatonin, which inhibits gonadotropin release, is itself suppressed by light and stimulated by darkness. Although melatonin levels and gonadotropin secretion are inversely related in humans, the role of melatonin in the regulation of human reproduction has not yet been conclusively established.

Stress also has a substantial influence on reproductive functions. Menstrual function in women and sperm production in men are commonly lost during prolonged physical or psychic stress. These effects may be mediated by CRH, which inhibits GnRH release. GnRH is the dominant peptide regulator of the secretion of gonadotropins. However, numerous other peptides originate (1) in the hypothalamus, and gain access to the gonadotroph via the portal veins, or (2) in the pituitary cells themselves, and act in paracrine fashion. These peptides may influence the secretion of basal or GnRH-stimulated gonadotropin. The list of peptides includes galanin, PACAP, NPY, neurotensin, endorphins, endothelin, oxytocin, IL-6, and substance P. Their modulatory influences may be restricted to certain physiological circumstances, and they may be affected by changes in the sex steroid environment. Hence they may vary over time.

Another influence of interest are **pheromones,** which are airborne or waterborne chemical exciters or inhibitors. These neurons in the vomeronasal organ of the nose are distinct from those that detect odors, and specific pheromone receptor genes have been cloned. Transmission of impulses from the vomeronasal neurons to the olfactory bulb, and then to the hypothalamus, regulates the secretion of GnRH by signals from the environment and from other individuals.

GnRH-triggered release of LH and FSH begins with the binding of GnRH to its class 1 plasma membrane receptor on the gonadotroph. In response to this binding, calcium-calmodulin and phosphatidylinositol products are generated as principal second messengers. The exocytosis of gonadotropin secretory granules is rapidly stimulated. GnRH also stimulates transcription of the LH and FSH β-subunit genes. Intracellular signaling molecules are subsequently generated by protein kinase C activation, and they feed back on GnRH signal transduction to regulate the duration and amplitude of the response. GnRH both downregulates and upregulates its receptor.

Intravenous infusion of GnRH causes a biphasic response in plasma LH. An initial peak of LH concentration is reached at 30 minutes, followed by a secondary rise that begins at 90 minutes and continues for hours thereafter (Fig. 43-16). In contrast, GnRH causes only a uniphasic progressive rise in FSH (Fig. 43-16). In women, LH is secreted in pulses that are characterized by a 15-minute upsurge and a downslope with a half-life of 60 minutes. These peaks of plasma LH concentration have a periodicity that varies from 1 to 7 hours, depending on the phase of the menstrual cycle. The amplitude of the pulses can be equivalent to 100% changes in the plasma LH level, except at the time of ovulation, when the response is much greater. Men also exhibit 8 to 10 secretory bursts of LH per day (Fig. 43-17).

Pulsatile secretion of LH, which is due mainly to pulsatile secretion of GnRH (Fig. 43-18), does not depend on the presence of sex steroid hormones from target glands; agonadal

individuals and postmenopausal women exhibit even sharper spikes of the plasma LH level. Pulsatile secretion of LH is dampened in young children, but the pulse amplitude increases sharply as puberty approaches. At first, these higher amplitude pulses increase only at night, coincident with a modest reduction in melatonin levels from childhood to puberty. Thus, during the initial stages of puberty, LH peaks sharply at night. Although this diurnal pattern lasts only 1 or 2 years, and it disappears as puberty is completed, the heightened amplitude of LH pulses becomes fixed. The most striking feature of LH secretion in women, as opposed to secretion in men, is its monthly cyclicity. The menstrual cycle results from a complex interaction between the GnRH neuron-gonadotroph unit and feedback by sequential changes in secretion of ovarian steroid and protein products; these changes are detailed in Chapter 46.

Some women are infertile because disordered hypothalamic regulation fails to produce proper pituitary gonadotroph function and ovulation. Normal menstrual cycles and ovulation can be restored only if exogenous GnRH is administered to these women in pulses that mimic the timing, amplitude, and frequency of the normal hypothalamic generator. The same is true for spermatogenesis in infertile men. In contrast, continuous administration of GnRH to either gender ultimately downregulates the GnRH receptor and produces gonadotropin deficiency, with consequent loss of gonadal function. This technique is employed therapeutically, for example, to suppress painful menses in women with endometriosis or to inhibit the growth of prostate cancer in men.

FSH secretion also exhibits a pulsatile pattern that is generally synchronized with the pattern of LH secretion but is of lesser magnitude (Fig. 43-17). Because the ratio of FSH to LH levels in plasma can fluctuate considerably, the existence of a separate and specific hypothalamic-releasing hormone for FSH is postulated. Other explanations for changing plasma ratios of LH to FSH can be offered. Temporal differences in the hormonal, particularly the sex steroid, milieu of the gonadotrophic cell may cause differences between LH and FSH synthesis, glycosylation, and storage. Different subpopulations of gonadotrophs may have variable responsiveness to GnRH. The GnRH pulse pattern has variable affects on the release of the two gonadotropins. Greater pulsatility favors LH secretion, whereas longer interpulse intervals favors FSH secretion. Other modulators mentioned above may specifically stimulate expression of the LH or FSH β-subunit gene. An interesting difference between the two hormones is evident when hypothalamic connections to gonadotrophic cells are cut or when the cells are placed in tissue culture. LH secretion disappears rapidly in the absence of GnRH, whereas a basal constitutive level of FSH secretion persists. Finally, variability in metabolic clearance rates of the two gonadotropins could change their plasma concentration ratios, independent of any changes in their secretion patterns.

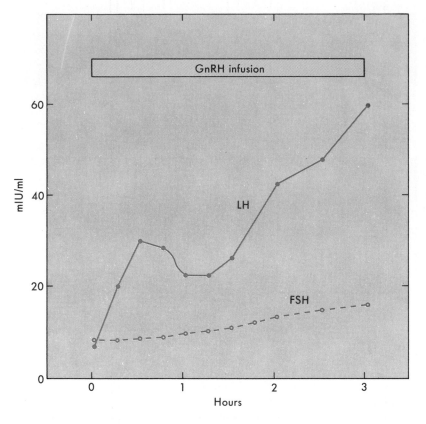

■ **Fig. 43-16** Stimulation of gonadotropin release by GnRH. Note the biphasic response of LH and uniphasic response of FSH. The initial LH response represents immediate release from a subset of secretory granules. The later response is from other secretory granules and augmented synthesis of LH. *LHRH,* Luteinizing hormone-releasing hormone. (From Wang CF et al: *J Clin Endocrinol Metab* 42:718, 1976.)

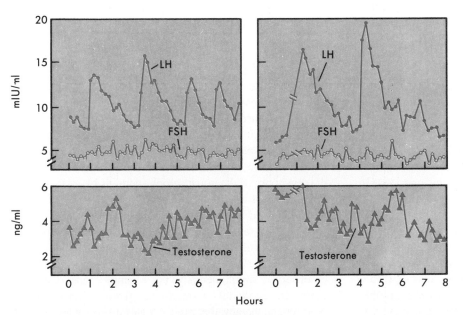

■ **Fig. 43-17** Pulsatile fluctuations in plasma LH levels are reflected in pulsatile fluctuations in its target hormone, testosterone, in men. Pulsatility of the lower FSH level is much less. (From Naftolin F et al: *J Clin Endocrinol Metab* 36:285, 1973.)

Notably, GnRH and its receptor are expressed in immune cells, and they may modulate lymphocyte function. The peptide and receptor are also present in the ovary, testis, and prostate gland, where they might subserve reproductive functions by paracrine and autocrine effects.

Feedback regulation of gonadotropins. The secretion of both LH and FSH is regulated by gonadal products. However, the patterns and mechanisms are more complex than are those that have already been described for TSH and ACTH. In general, the basic regulatory mechanism of LH

and FSH secretion is classic negative feedback. Thus, when the gonads are functionally inactive or surgically removed, the plasma levels of FSH and LH become elevated. FSH, however, usually increases proportionally more than does LH. In women, prominent increases in plasma FSH and LH occur after the menopause. In men, these increases are more subtle during the gradual male climacteric. A number of gonadal products from at least two gonadal cell types normally act to restrain the secretion of each gonadotropin by negative feedback. The basic schema is depicted in Fig. 43-15.

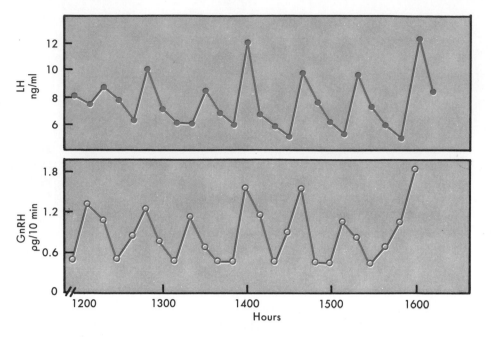

■ **Fig. 43-18** Fluctuation of peripheral vein plasma LH levels and portal vein plasma GnRH levels in unanesthetized, ovariectomized female sheep. Each pulse of LH is coordinated with a pulse of GnRH. This supports the view that pulsatility of LH release is dependent on pulsatile stimulation of the pituitary by GnRH. (From Levine J et al: *Endocrinology* 111:1449, 1982.)

The gonadal steroid hormones, **testosterone** in men and **estradiol** in women, are the most important of these negative feedback signals. The major androgen, testosterone, from the Leydig cells of the testis and the interstitial cells of the ovary, inhibits the release of LH. The major estrogen, estradiol, which arises from the granulosa cells of the ovary and from the Leydig and Sertoli cells of the testis (as well as by conversion from testosterone in peripheral tissues and in the hypothalamus), also inhibits the release of LH. Both the amplitude and the frequency of the LH pulses are affected; such changes indicate that both the pituitary gland and the hypothalamus are sites of feedback.

Both estradiol and testosterone administration blunt the response of the gonadotroph to a single pulse of GnRH. Conversely, in estradiol-deficient women and in testosterone-deficient men, LH responses to GnRH are exaggerated. In addition to inhibiting the release of LH (and FSH), estradiol decreases their synthesis by repressing transcription of their common α-subunit and their specific β-subunits. Estradiol may produce some of these effects by altering the number of GnRH receptors on the gonadotroph. In addition to these pituitary effects, estradiol and testosterone also decrease GnRH secretion, probably via interaction with endorphin neurons in the hypothalamus. The latter then complete this pathway of negative feedback by suppressing the discharge of GnRH from the median eminence into the portal blood (Fig. 43-2).

An additional feedback complexity occurs in men. Testosterone must first be converted to an estrogen product in the hypothalamus, where it decreases GnRH (and therefore LH) pulsatility, and in the pituitary gland, where it decreases the amplitude of LH pulses in response to GnRH. FSH secretion is also inhibited by estradiol and testosterone, which block the pituitary response to GnRH. However, feedback inhibition of FSH secretion is specifically carried out

by another gonadal product, a glycoprotein called **inhibin** (Chapter 46). Inhibin, which is secreted by ovarian granulosa cells and testicular Sertoli cells, suppresses FSH β-subunit synthesis, GnRH-stimulated FSH release, and possibly GnRH secretion. In contrast to its effects on FSH secretion, inhibin has much less effect on LH secretion.

In addition to exerting negative feedback on LH and FSH secretion in women, estradiol also exerts positive feedback effects. Regulation of LH and FSH secretion is thus very complex. When estradiol is administered to women in an appropriate dose range and for a sufficient number of days, the LH response to GnRH is *increased* rather than reduced. Furthermore, if GnRH is administered repetitively to properly estradiol-primed women, the cumulative increments in plasma LH are amplified. This response signifies that both the sensitivity of the gonadotroph (perhaps by an increase in the number of its GnRH receptors) and its LH stores have been enhanced by estradiol treatment. Moreover, in women so treated, a rapid further increase in estradiol raises the plasma levels of LH significantly.

Some aspects of this positive and negative feedback can be observed simultaneously. For example, when estradiol-deficient, agonadal women are given initial estradiol replacement therapy, the originally elevated basal levels of LH and FSH decline (negative feedback) after 7 days of treatment. However, the capacity to respond to subsequent repetitive doses of GnRH actually increases (positive feedback).

Progesterone, another major steroid product of the ovary, also modulates LH release. Administered acutely, progesterone can increase plasma LH levels 24 to 48 hours later. Progesterone can also either enhance or blunt the positive feedback effects of estradiol on the responsiveness of the gonadotroph to GnRH. The effect on feedback depends on the timing of the administration of the two hormones. However, continuous administration of progesterone (or analogs with mild androgenic effects, such as 19-nortestosterone) inhibits gonadotropin secretion by an action that does not involve the androgen receptor.

> Oral contraceptives use the negative feedback effects of estradiol (or its analogs) plus progesterone (or its suppressive analogs) to interfere with the normal timing and quantities of LH and FSH secretion. As a result, the delicately balanced stimulation of the ovaries by the two gonadotropins is lost, and ovulation is prevented.

Other protein products of the gonads influence FSH secretion. **Activin,** related structurally to inhibin, stimulates FSH synthesis and release. Activin is also synthesized within pituitary cells and its autocrine and paracrine actions may be more important than its endocrine action. **Follistatin** passively inhibits FSH secretion, by binding activin. **Prolactin,** a mammotropic hormone from the anterior pituitary, also inhibits GnRH release, and lowers basal secretion of LH and FSH. Finally, LH can inhibit the secretion of its own releasing hormone via short-loop negative feedback.

LH and FSH both circulate unbound to plasma proteins. The average concentrations of both hormones are in the range of 4 to 20 mIU/ml in men and in reproductive-age women. In the latter, the levels of both hormones are higher in the first half of the menstrual cycle than in the second half. Furthermore, both hormones show sharp, single-day peaks at the time of ovulation. Basal plasma concentrations of each hormone are of the order of 10^{-11} M. The metabolic clearance rates of LH and FSH are 36 and 20 L/day, respectively, and their half-lives in plasma are approximately 1 and 3 hours. The more rapid clearance of LH depends on prior desialylation of the molecule, followed by hepatic uptake through binding of its sulfated N-linked oligosaccharides to a specific plasma membrane receptor on hepatocytes. The receptor-hormone complex is internalized, transported to lysosomes, and degraded. The slower rate of degradation of FSH reflects its high sialic acid content. In contrast to the trivial excretion of other peptide hormones, 10% of the daily production of LH and FSH appears in the urine. This amount permits employment of urinary gonadotropin measurements as a reflection of integrated plasma concentrations. Such measurements are particularly useful when plasma levels of the hormones are low, as in children.

> Home measurements of urinary LH by women can help them anticipate ovulation and can assist in conception. Measurement of human chorionic gonadotropin (HCG), the pregnancy gonadotropin, can detect early pregnancy.

The common α-subunit is secreted to a small extent by normal gonadotrophs. Most plasma α-subunit molecules stem from thyrotropic cells. The individual β-subunits of LH and FSH are virtually undetectable, but they are cosecreted with LH and FSH, respectively, when GnRH stimulation increases (e.g., just before ovulation or after the menopause).

Actions of gonadotropins. LH and FSH reach their target cells by transcytosis through endothelial cells that possess receptors for the hormones. LH and FSH then bind to specific G-protein–linked class 1 plasma membrane receptors (see Fig. 39-11); in each case, cAMP is generated as the primary second messenger. The cAMP stimulates production of CREB-P and CREM-P (Chapter 46), transcription factors that initiate expression of target genes. FSH stimulates ovarian granulosa cells and testicular Sertoli cells to synthesize and secrete estradiol and inhibin, as well various protein products that are essential to oogenesis and spermatogenesis, respectively. LH stimulates ovarian interstitial (thecal) cells and testicular Leydig cells to secrete testosterone and other products that play roles in reproduction. Both gonadotropins downregulate their receptors.

Optimal LH action in target cells requires short pulses of the hormone's availability and rapid turnoff of its action. The latter effect is partly accomplished by a molecule known as β-arrestin, which binds to the activated LH receptor complex and uncouples it from adenylyl cyclase. The LH receptor complex is then internalized. Replenishment of free LH receptor within the plasma membrane occurs during the LH interpulse interval. The actions of gonadotropins are discussed in detail in Chapter 46.

> Activating mutations of the FSH receptor and the LH receptor cause precocious puberty. Inactivating mutations lead to infertility via (1) decreased or absent spermatogenesis, (2) disruption of the orderly process of producing an ovum, or (3) failure to sustain the zygote/embryo in its earliest phase of life.

Growth Hormone (Somatotropin, GH)

GH stimulates postnatal somatic growth and development, and it helps to maintain normal lean body mass and bone mass in adults. In addition, it has numerous actions on protein, carbohydrate, and fat metabolism. The hormone originates in anterior pituitary somatotrophs that make up 40% to 50% of the adult gland. GH is stored in large, dense granules. In humans, somatotrophs can form tumors that secrete excess GH and produce a highly distinctive disease called **acromegaly.**

GH is a single-chain polypeptide with a usual molecular weight of 22,000. It contains 191 amino acids and two disulfide bridges (Fig. 43-19). GH is a member of a large family of "helix bundle proteins." In the GH molecule, the amino acids form four helixes that are connected by thin loops. This structure is important for binding GH to its receptor. A 20,000-molecular-weight species lacking residues critical for binding the hormone to its receptor forms 10% of the pituitary content of GH, and it fluctuates in plasma coordinately with GH.

Synthesis of GH. The normal pituitary GH gene is one of a five-gene cluster from a gene family that also directs synthesis of structurally related hormones, such as prolactin, human placental lactogen, and a GH variant that is produced

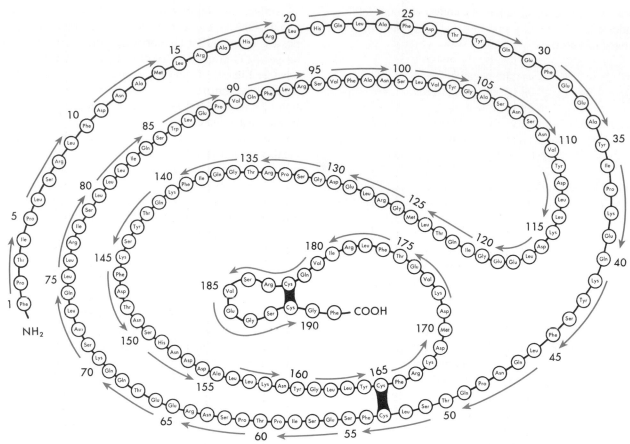

■ **Fig. 43-19** Structure of HGH. Although consisting of nearly 200 amino acids and containing two disulfide bridges, growth hormone (GH) is a single polypeptide chain. It does form a helical tertiary structure. The three-letter amino acid code is used. (From Li C et al: *Proc Natl Acad Sci USA* 74:1016, 1977.)

exclusively in the placenta. A tissue-specific constitutive protein transcription factor (Pit-1 or POUIFI) that binds to two sites in the promotor region of the GH gene is essential to that gene's selective expression in the pituitary gland. Four additional genes that are capable of directing synthesis of slightly larger GH molecules are present, but these genes are not normally expressed. The GH gene transcribes a messenger RNA that directs synthesis of a prehormone. Subsequently, a signal peptide is removed, and the final form of the hormone is stored in granules. The synthesis of GH is increased by its specific hypothalamic **growth hormone–releasing hormone (GHRH),** and it is decreased by **somatostatin,** its hypothalamic inhibitor (Table 43-1). GHRH (via cAMP) and Pit-1 act in concert to increase protein kinase A phosporylation of CREB (see Chapter 43 and Fig. 39-13), which then binds a CRE on the GH gene. Histone acetylase activity is increased, and thereby displaces the GH gene from nucleosomes and activates it.

Secretion of GH. GH release is stimulated by binding GHRH to its plasma membrane receptor. cAMP and Ca^{2+} are primary mediators of GH release, and phosphatidylinositol products are secondary mediators of GHRH action. Prostaglandins are also potent stimulators of GH release in vitro.

The hypothalamic peptide, somatostatin (Table 43-1), is a powerful inhibitor of GH release. Somatostatin blocks GHRH stimulation in a noncompetitive manner. It acts through its own plasma membrane receptor, in part by decreasing intracellular cAMP and calcium levels. GH is secreted in 10 to 20 pulses per day. This pulsatility arises from some combination of the pulsatile release of GHRH and of somatostatin into the portal blood. GHRH increases the amplitude of each pulse, whereas somatostatin diminishes the degree to which the somatotroph can respond to GHRH.

As seen in Table 43-4, GH secretion is under many different influences. An acute fall in the plasma levels of either of the major energy-yielding substrates, glucose or free fatty acids (FFAs), produces an increase in GH secretion. For example, when insulin is administered intravenously, the plasma level of GH increases up to 10-fold within 30 to 60 minutes after the plasma glucose level has fallen to below 50 mg/dl (Fig. 43-13). Conversely, a carbohydrate-rich meal or a pure glucose load causes a prompt decrease in plasma GH level by at least 50%. Responses to similar alterations in FFA levels are slower and smaller. Both glucose and FFAs mainly suppress GH secretion by increasing somatostatin release.

A high-protein meal or the infusion of a mixture of amino acids raises the plasma GH level; arginine is the most con-

■ Table 43-4 Regulation of growth hormone secretion

Stimulation	*Inhibition*
Growth hormone-releasing hormone	Somatostatin
Glucose decrease	Glucose increase
Free fatty acid decrease	Free fatty acid increase
Amino acid increase (arginine)	
Fasting	Somatomedins
Prolonged caloric deprivation	Growth hormone
Stage IV sleep	β-Adrenergic agonists
Exercise	
Stress (Table 43-3)	Cortisol
Puberty	Senescence
Estrogens	Obesity
Androgens	Pregnancy
Dopamine	
Acetylcholine	
Serotonin	
α-Adrenergic agonists	
γ-Aminobutyric acid	
Enkephalins	
Growth hormone releasing peptide (ghrelin)	

sistent amino acid stimulator, and it acts by inhibiting somatostatin release. However, prolonged protein-calorie deprivation or total fasting also stimulates GH secretion. This occurs because of (1) decreasing negative feedback from a peripheral product of GH action, and (2) decreased glucose and insulin levels. Furthermore, it occurs despite elevation of suppressive free fatty acid levels and enhanced NPY expression. Exercise and various acute stresses, including blood drawing, anesthesia, fever, trauma, and major surgery, rapidly stimulate GH secretion. Chronic stress, such as a protracted illness, decreases GH levels through an inhibitory affect of CRH. GH is secreted episodically at 2-hour intervals, and a regular nocturnal GH peak occurs 1 hour after the onset of deep, stage 3 or 4, sleep (Fig. 43-10). Although this GH peak is preceded by a nocturnal plasma GHRH peak, somatotroph responsiveness to GHRH is also increased by sleep.

The recent search for therapeutically useful, orally administered enhancers of growth hormone secretion has led to the discovery of another endogenous regulator of growth hormone secretion. This regulator is called the growth hormone secretogogue, or growth hormone–releasing peptide (GHRP). A natural receptor for this secretogogue is present both in the pituitary gland and in the hypothalamic neurons that secrete GHRH and NPY. The receptor is G-protein linked to phospholipase C and Ca^{2+} is its second messenger. GHRP synergizes with GHRH to increase basal GH secretion and the mass of GH in each pulsatile secretory burst, but GHRP does not alter pulse frequency. A natural ligand for the GHRP receptor, and likely GHRP itself, is a 28-amino acid peptide with an octanoyl group linked to one of its serine residues. This GHRP is named ghrelin and is synthesized in the oxyntic glands of the stomach. Ghrelin circulates at a low plasma level of about 10^{-13} M, and it is an orexigen (see Chapter 43). The widespread tissue distribution of the ghrelin receptor suggests that this peptide has other functions as well.

The neurotransmitters dopamine, norepinephrine, acetylcholine, serotonin, GABA, and histamine all increase GH secretion by stimulating the release of GHRH or by blocking the release of somatostatin. The GH responses to exercise, stress, hypoglycemia, and arginine administration are augmented by α-adrenergic stimulation, and they are reduced by β-adrenergic stimulation of the receptors in neurons that release GHRH and somatostatin. The sleep-induced rise in GH and the response to hypoglycemia are enhanced by serotonergic pathways from the brainstem. Cholinergic pathways augment GH response to GHRH and to other stimuli by inhibiting somatostatin release. NPY inhibits GH secretion, whereas leptin stimulates it.

GH secretion is greater in premenopausal women than in men, and it is greatest just before ovulation. Although the pattern and frequency of pulses are the same, women secrete more GH in each secretory burst. The gender difference is explained by the stimulating effect of estradiol on GH secretion. However, testosterone also increases GH secretion.

GH levels reach a peak in midgestation after the initial appearance of GHRH in the fetal hypothalamus by 18 weeks of gestational age. Daily GH production remains slightly increased in children, it rises further during the period of puberty, and it then decreases in young adults (Fig. 43-20) after puberty is completed. A further reduction in GH secretion in response to GHRH and to other stimuli occurs in aging individuals. This decline in GH secretion is partly responsible for the decline in lean body mass, physical fitness, protein synthesis, and metabolic rate, as well as the increase in adipose mass that characterizes elderly humans.

GH secretion begins to rise before puberty and it increases over 2-fold by late adolescence. Pulse amplitude and duration increase, but not the pulse number. However, greater intrinsic fluctuation in GH secretion over weeks correlates with short-term gains in height and with eventual tall stature. Furthermore, especially tall adults demonstrate greater GH responses to GHRH than do adults of average height. Thus, the final height of humans may be partly determined by their inherent GH secretory capacity. In some otherwise normal children of short stature, a subtle deficiency in integrated 24-hour GH secretion has been observed.

Like the regulation of other anterior pituitary hormones, feedback regulation of GH is also complex (Fig. 43-21). For example, GH inhibits its own secretion. Administration of exogenous GH dampens subsequent endogenous GH responsiveness to a number of stimuli, including hypoglycemia and stage 4 sleep. The mechanisms for this self-regulation may involve short-loop feedback, because GH stimulates the synthesis and release of its inhibitor, somatostatin (Fig. 43-21). However, GHRH release is also decreased, and somatostatin synthesis and release are also increased, by **somatomedins,** which are circulating **insulin-like growth factor** peptides (IGF-1 and IGF-2) that are generated outside the pituitary gland, and mediate many of the actions of GH. Somatomedins

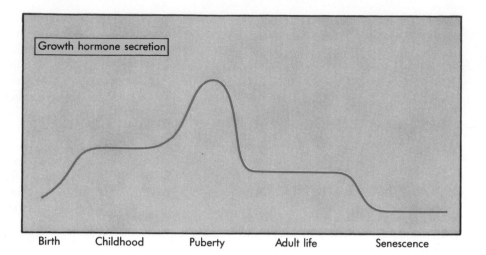

Growth hormone secretion

Birth   Childhood   Puberty   Adult life   Senescence

■ **Fig. 43-20**   Lifetime pattern of GH secretion. GH levels are higher in children than in adults, with a peak period during puberty. GH secretion declines with aging.

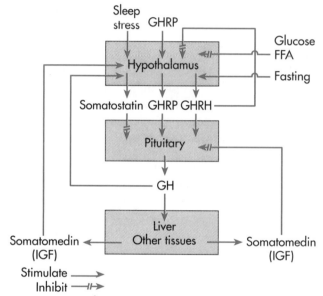

■ **Fig. 43-21**   Regulation of GH secretion. The hypothalamic peptide *(GHRH)* stimulates growth hormone release, whereas the hypothalamic peptide somatostatin inhibits it. Negative feedback is by the peripheral mediators of GH action: somatomedins, also known as insulin-like growth factors. Negative feedback occurs both via somatomedin inhibition of GHRH action and by somatomedin stimulation of somatostatin release. Another factor, GHRP, stimulates both GHRH and GH release. GH inhibits its own secretion by short-loop feedback. In addition, GHRH inhibits its own release via ultra-short-loop feedback. In both these cases, the negative feedback is probably affected by increasing the release of inhibitory somatostatin. Likewise, glucose and free fatty acids *(FFA)* inhibit GH secretion at the hypothalamic level.

also act at the pituitary level to decrease responsiveness to GHRH (Fig. 43-21). Finally, GHRH itself, in doses too small to stimulate the somatotrophs, but administered in a manner that allows access to the hypothalamus, may decrease, rather than increase, GH secretion. This ultra-short-loop paradoxical effect probably results from a stimulation of somatostatin release, and it may reflect the existence of axonal connections between GHRH neurons and somatostatin neurons.

Other negative regulatory influences have also been noted. Although basal cortisol and thyroid hormone levels synergistically stimulate GH gene expression, an excess of either hormone decreases the GH responses to GHRH by enhancing somatostatin release. Insulin also represses GH gene expression. A decline in pituitary GH secretion occurs during the latter part of pregnancy, perhaps in response to production of placental GH and placental lactogen. Obese individuals exhibit dampened GH responses to all stimuli, including GHRH itself, even though leptin levels are elevated. These responses are restored to normal by weight reduction.

The basal plasma GH concentration is 0.5 to 5 ng/ml (about 10^{-10} M). This concentration may increase up to 50-fold in response to various stimuli. Circulating GH is bound to a plasma protein whose structure is identical to the extracellular portion of the hepatic plasma membrane GH receptor. This GH-binding protein arises by cleavage of the receptor at the cell's surface. One molecule of GH binds two of the circulating binding protein molecules. The plasma half-life of GH is 20 minutes, and the metabolic clearance rate is 350 L/day. Daily secretion in prepubertal children and in normal young adults is 200 to 600 µg, which is only a small fraction of the large pituitary store. Although only a trivial portion of secreted GH is excreted unchanged by the kidneys, daily urinary GH excretion correlates well with the integrated 24-hour plasma GH profile.

Actions of GH.   *GH is a hormone with profound anabolic action. In its absence, growth is stunted in humans. When the hormone is administered to unequivocally GH-deficient individuals, it causes prompt nitrogen retention and hypoaminoacidemia. Decreased urea production also results, because the amino acids are diverted from oxidation to protein synthesis as growth ensues.* Many GH actions are carried out by the peripherally generated mediators, somatomedins IGF-1 and IGF-2.

The various major GH targets and effects are indicated in Fig. 43-22. The most striking and specific effect of GH is the stimulation of linear growth (gain in height) that results from GH action on the epiphyseal cartilage or growth plates of long bones (see Chapter 42). All aspects of the metabolism

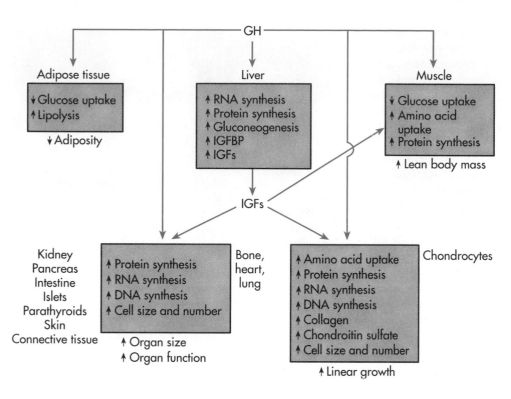

■ **Fig. 43-22** Biological actions of GH. The effects on linear growth, organ size, and lean body mass are at least partly mediated by insulin-like growth factors (IGFs) (somatomedins) produced in the liver and in the GH target tissues as well. *IGFBP*, Insulin-like growth factor-binding protein.

of the cartilage-forming cells, the chondrocytes, are stimulated. These metabolic effects include (1) the incorporation of the amino acid, proline, into collagen and its conversion to hydroxyproline, and (2) the incorporation of sulfate into the proteoglycan chondroitin. Together, chondroitin and collagen form the resilient extracellular matrix of cartilage. GH also stimulates the differentiation of prechondrocytes into chondrocytes and the proliferation and hypertrophy of the chondrocytes, as well as their synthesis of DNA, RNA, and proteins. GH further supports protein synthesis by stimulating cellular uptake of certain amino acids.

Other tissues participate in the anabolic response to GH. This hormone increases the activity and probably the number of bone modeling units (Chapter 42). After GH administration, urinary hydroxyproline and calcium excretions initially increase. This response indicates the activation of osteoclastic bone resorption (see Chapter 42). However, plasma osteocalcin levels subsequently rise, and this osteoblastic response reflects bone formation (see Chapter 42). Ultimately, total bone mass and mineral content are increased by GH.

Visceral organs (liver, kidney, pancreas, and intestines), endocrine glands (adrenals, parathyroids, and pancreatic islets), skeletal muscle, heart, skin, and connective tissue all undergo hypertrophy and hyperplasia in response to GH. In most instances, the functional capacity of the enlarged organ is enhanced. For example, GH increases renal plasma flow, glomerular filtration, cardiac output, and hepatic clearance of test substances. GH also increases cardiac muscle size and contractility (see also Chapter 16), and it induces muscle enzymes involved in contraction. The net result is an increase in cardiac output. In addition to stimulating height increase during puberty, GH sensitizes the gonads to LH and FSH and thereby promotes pubertal sexual maturation.

GH exerts several actions on carbohydrate and lipid metabolism. Normal levels of GH are required to sustain normal pancreatic islet function; in the absence of GH, insulin secretion declines. However, an excess of GH decreases glucose uptake by insulin-sensitive tissues, such as muscle and adipose tissue, and it increases hepatic glucose output. Insulin secretion then rises to compensate for the GH-induced insulin resistance. GH inhibits insulin action in the phosphatidylinositol 3-kinase pathway, and thus prevents activation of protein kinase B (see Fig. 41-10). Moreover the clearance of insulin from the plasma increases, which diminishes its availability to target tissues. GH decreases adipose tissue mass and is also lipolytic; this characteristic leads to increases in plasma FFAs and ketoacids, especially when the increased insulin secretion cannot compensate adequately. The increased FFA levels may themselves contribute to GH-induced insulin resistance. Increased oxidation of fat and decreased oxidation of glucose are reflected in a decreased respiratory quotient; total metabolic rate is also usually increased. On balance, *GH is a diabetogenic hormone.*

GH increases the volume of extracellular fluid by stimulating the renin-angiotensin-aldosterone axis (see Chapter 36), by suppressing atrial natriuretic peptide (ANP), and by the action of its mediator, somatomedin, on the renal tubules. Proximal tubular phosphate reabsorption, and thus the plasma phosphate concentration, are increased by GH. Calcium absorption from the intestine is enhanced, probably by GH stimulation of $1,25\text{-}(OH)_2$-vitamin D_3 production.

Deficiency of GH in children can result from hypothalamic dysfunction, pituitary destruction, a defective GHRH receptor, a biologically incompetent GH or GH receptor molecule, failure to generate somatomedins normally, or

GH receptor deficiency. Short stature and correspondingly delayed bone and sexual maturation are the consequences of GH deficiency. Mild obesity is common, and puberty is usually delayed. In adults, decreased muscle and total lean body mass, decreased muscle strength and exercise performance, decreased cardiac function and mass, and decreased bone density occur. The diagnosis of GH deficiency is established by demonstrating low levels of somatomedins, and low plasma GH levels, which fail to rise during the night or after various stimuli. Replacement treatment with GH causes nitrogen retention, increased lean body mass, increased cardiac and skeletal muscle performance, increased bone density and calcium content, decreased adipose mass, decreased insulin sensitivity and insulin secretion, and a greater sense of well-being. In children, growth rate increases, pubescence occurs, and fertility is established.

Sustained hypersecretion of GH results from pituitary tumors and produces a unique syndrome called **acromegaly.** If hypersecretion of GH begins before puberty is completed, the individual grows very tall and has long arms and legs. If hypersecretion occurs after puberty, only periosteal bone growth can be increased by GH. This bone growth causes widened fingers, toes, hands, and feet; prominent bony ridges above the eyes; and a prominent lower jaw (Fig. 43-23). Facial features are coarsened by accumulation of excess soft tissue resulting in a bulbous nose (Fig. 43-23). The tongue is enlarged and the skin is thick, whereas subcutaneous fat is sparse. Virtually all organ sizes are increased. Enlargement of the heart, hypertension, and accelerated atherosclerosis often lead to a shortened lifespan. The antagonistic effect of GH on insulin produces an abnormal tolerance to carbohydrate, or even frank diabetes mellitus that requires treatment with insulin. The diagnosis of acromegaly is confirmed by demonstrating elevated plasma GH levels, which are not suppressed when glucose is administered. Plasma levels of somatomedins are also high. Definitive treatment requires surgical removal of the tumor. Somatostatin analogs that diminish GH hypersecretion are also useful.

Mechanisms of GH action.   Plasma membrane GH receptors of various sizes are present in the target cells found in many tissues, including the liver and adipose tissue. GH receptors belong to the cytokine family of receptors composed of glycoprotein disulfide–linked subunits that span the plasma membrane once (Fig. 39-16). The length of the intracellular cytoplasmic receptor tail varies from tissue to tissue and among the hormone ligands. The latter include prolactin, erythropoietin, interleukins, and granulocyte-macrophage colony-stimulating factors. Of GH receptors 90% are full length; alternate splicing of the GH receptor gene yields receptors that are missing almost all of the intracellular portion. As shown in Fig. 43-24, one GH molecule binds two GH receptor molecules; the receptor dimer then initiates GH actions by attracting a set of intracytoplasmic tyrosine kinases (Janus kinases), docking them, and activating signal

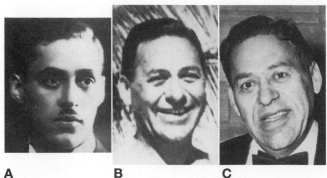

A   **B**   **C**

■ **Fig. 43-23   A** to **C,** A patient with acromegaly, a GH excess syndrome. Note the gradual coarsening of the face and increasing prominence of the jaw over many years before diagnosis.

transducer and activator of transcription (STAT) proteins by phosphorylating them.

Two different amino acid sequences in GH bind the identical amino acid sequence in each of the two receptor molecules. For this reason, an excess of GH may inhibit the hormone's actions, because two receptor monomers may each bind a GH molecule at the same GH site. This binding prevents formation of the active receptor dimer, and it nullifies hormone action. Synthesis of GH receptors requires the presence of GH itself, but an excess of GH downregulates synthesis of its receptors. The GH receptor is also induced by insulin and estrogens, and it is repressed by fasting.

Many hours must elapse after administration of GH before its anabolic, growth-promoting effects become evident. Most, if not all, of these effects require the GH-induced generation of a family of peptide hormone intermediaries, the somatomedins or IGFs.

These compounds have a molecular weight of about 7000, and they are structurally related to proinsulin. IGF-1 is a 70-amino acid straight-chain peptide with 50% homology to the A-chain and B-chain domains of proinsulin (see Fig. 43-3). IGF-2 has 70% homology with IGF-1 in these same domains. Both somatomedins, however, have distinctive C-chain domains. Circulating somatomedins originate as a result of GH-stimulated expression of the IGF genes, primarily but not solely in the liver. In contrast to the sharp and rapid fluctuations of plasma GH, the IGF-1 and IGF-2 concentrations are relatively stable. For example, neither IGF increases after hypoglycemia, as GH does. In general, the plasma concentration of IGF-2 is 3-fold to 4-fold higher than that of IGF-1.

The plasma half-life of the IGF molecules is much longer than that of GH, because they circulate bound to at least six carrier proteins. Circulating **insulin growth factor-binding proteins (IGFBP$_{1-6}$)** are primarily synthesized in the liver, and they are secreted as phosphoproteins, but local synthesis also occurs in other tissues. IGFBP$_1$ is a major regulator of the plasma-free IGF-1 and IGF-2 concentrations. Insulin, IGF-1, and IGF-2 suppress IGPBP$_1$ gene expression, whereas cortisol, glucagon, and cAMP increase it. Thus during fasting, when the insulin level declines, IGFBP$_1$ levels rise;

Mechanism of GH Action

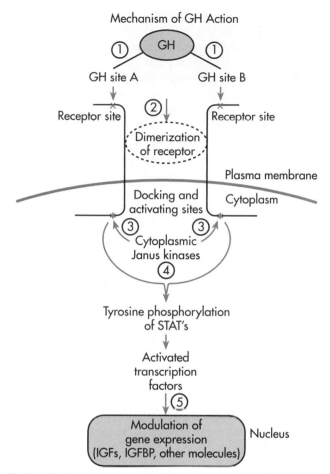

■ **Fig. 43-24** Transduction of GH signals. *1,* One GH molecule binds two plasma membrane GH receptor molecules to different sites on the hormone. *2,* This causes dimerization of the two receptor molecules, which activates them. *3,* The intracytoplasmic portions of the receptors attract, dock, and activate Janus kinases. *4,* These phosphorylate signal transducer and activator of transcription factors (STATs) that *(5)* induce or repress expression of GH target genes such as IGFs.

related to IGFBP$_1$ levels. In addition, paracrine hormonal actions of its own may be conferred on IGFBP$_1$ by its binding to an integrin, which serves as a cell surface receptor for fibronectin. Local IGFBP proteases regulate tissue IGFBP concentrations and modulate their independent and IGF binding functions. IGFBP$_1$ probably plays a complex role in implantation of the human embryo within the uterus.

The growth-promoting effects of GH can be accounted for largely by the IGFs. These factors stimulate typical GH responses in cartilage, muscle, adipose tissue, fibroblasts, and tumor cells in vitro. IGF molecules also stimulate nitrogen retention and enhance renal function in vivo. IGF molecules that are generated locally within clones of GH target cells (e.g., osteoblasts) and that act in an autocrine or paracrine fashion may even be more important than the IGF molecules that are derived from the plasma.

Somatomedins bind to specific plasma membrane receptors of their own. The receptor for IGF-1 is a dimer that is structurally similar to the insulin receptor (see Figs. 43-12 and 41-10), and that has intrinsic tyrosine kinase activity that phosphorylates the insulin receptor substrates (Chapter 41). IGF-1 also binds both the insulin and the IGF-2 receptor, although with lower affinities. The receptor for IGF-2 is a monomer that does not resemble the IGF-1 and the insulin receptors. It binds IGF-1 with lower affinity, but it does not bind insulin at all. IGF-2 acts largely through the IGF-1 receptor and through the insulin receptor A, to which it binds with high affinity. The IGF receptor tyrosine kinases phosphorylate various cytoplasmic protein substrates. These in turn set up mitogenic signals probably in the same manner as has been described for insulin (see Chapter 41). Indeed, an important proliferative action of IGF-1 is to inhibit apoptosis in target cells, by tyrosine phosphorylation of insulin receptor substrate-1 (IRS-1). In turn, phosphorylated IRS-1 activates PI$_3$ kinase and protein kinase B, as well as the mitogen-activated kinase. All of these kinases mediate the inactivating phosphorylations of molecules that are essential to the apoptosis process.

therefore, free IGF-1 and IGF-2 levels fall, thereby reinforcing the withdrawal of the insulin effects on substrate flow (Chapter 40 and 41). IGFBP$_1$ may also serve to transfer IGF molecules out of the plasma, so that they can act on certain target cells.

IGFBP$_3$ (the most prevalent IGFBP) forms a large ternary complex with IGF-1 or IGF-2 and an acid-labile protein. This complex serves as a reservoir that keeps the IGF molecules from leaving plasma and protects them from degradation. The hepatic synthesis of IGFBP$_3$ and of the acid-labile protein are both increased by GH.

The presence of the binding proteins and the expression of their genes in many tissues suggest that these proteins also have important modulating effects on the actions of IGF molecules produced in those tissues. Thus IGFBP$_1$ administration decreases linear growth and weight gain in experimental animals. Whereas human birth and fetal weight correlate positively with fetal IGF levels, they are inversely

The cross-reactivities among insulin, IGF-1, and IGF-2 may assume biological importance when the concentrations of either IGF or of insulin are very high. For example, some patients with tumors that secrete IGF-2 develop spontaneous hypoglycemia, because the IGF-2 activates the insulin and IGF-1 receptors in the liver and elsewhere. In other patients who have insulin receptor deficiency and who have (in compensation) extremely high plasma insulin levels, the soft tissues grow excessively. This growth is mediated by the activation of the IGF receptors and their downstream mitogenic pathways by insulin. Mutations in the IGF-1 receptor also retard intrauterine growth. Activating mutations of the IGF-2 gene or failure to inactivate that gene by methylation produce large size individuals. The IGF-2 gene normally shows "genetic imprinting," with only the paternal allele being active in most tissues. If both parental alleles are active, tissue and somatic overgrowth occur.

Plasma somatomedins are increased by administration of GH, with a time lag of 12 to 18 hours, and they are absent in GH-deficient individuals. IGF-1 synthesis is GH dependent, and its plasma levels are very sensitive to changes in GH availability. In contrast, IGF-2 levels do not reflect GH status nearly as well. During adolescence, the augmented secretion of GHRH and of GH increases the plasma levels of IGF-1. The levels of IGF-1 correlate well with the progression of pubertal growth.

Although GH itself is not essential for fetal growth, one or more of the somatomedins produced in the embryo or placenta likely is. IGF-2 and its receptor are expressed very early in fetal development (at the two-cell stage in mice). IGF-2 stimulates placental growth and is found in trophoblast cells (see Chapter 46). IGF-2 also stimulates growth of both the preimplantation and postimplantation embryo. In contrast, IGF-1 and its receptor are expressed later in life. Both IGF-1 and IGF-2 stimulate progression through the G_1 phase of the cell cycle that leads to the phase of DNA synthesis. In newborns, plasma IGF-2 levels decline, whereas those of IGF-1 increase. IGF-1 stimulates neuronal development during early postnatal life.

GH and IGF-1 are also important for normal development and function of the immune system. Both molecules are produced by monocytes and macrophages. In addition, IGF-1 stimulates the functioning of neutrophils.

Somatomedin production is reduced by factors that can override GH. Fasting, low energy or low protein intake, and insulin deficiency all diminish the liver production of IGFs and decrease their plasma levels, despite increases in GH secretion. In fact, in these pathophysiological states, the lack of somatomedin is the likely cause of the elevated GH levels through negative feedback. Estrogens and cortisol also decrease somatomedin production. This response may account for their antagonism to GH action, despite their stimulation of GH secretion.

It is difficult to explain and integrate the various roles and interactions of GH, its circulating and locally produced IGF products, and its circulating and locally produced IGFBPs. Gene knockout experiments suggest that GH and IGFs have some independent actions on growth processes that nonetheless correlate. For example, GH may stimulate differentiation of precursor cells into chondroblasts and osteoblasts, whereas IGF-2 may subsequently stimulate proliferation of the differentiated cells. IGF-1 may then stimulate hypertrophy of these cells by antiapoptotic and anabolic effects. Both GH and IGF-1 stimulate production of bone morphogenetic proteins (see Chapter 42), but the GH effect can also occur independent of functioning IGF-1. By contrast, infertility results from lack of the ovarian actions of IGF-1, but not from the lack of GH. The relative roles and importance to growth of circulating IGF and IGFBP versus IGF and IGFBP produced in tissues also require clarification. For example, circulating IGF produced by the liver may serve, by negative feedback, primarily to prevent GH overproduction.

Overall role of GH in substrate flow. Some of the interactions between GH and insulin are presented in Fig. 43-25. When protein and energy intake are both ample, the absorbed amino acids are used for protein synthesis and to stimulate growth. Hence, both GH and insulin secretion are stimulated by amino acids, and together they augment the production of somatomedins. The latter in turn, with GH, stimulate the accretion of lean body mass. (These actions are probably directly enhanced by insulin also.) The insulin antagonistic effect of the GH molecule on carbohydrate metabolism helps to prevent hypoglycemia, which might result from insulin stimulation in the absence of carbohydrate.

On the other hand, when a carbohydrate load is ingested and insulin secretion is correspondingly increased, GH secretion is decreased. In this circumstance, the actions of free circulating somatomedins are not needed, because protein anabolism is not advantageous in the absence of amino acid inflow. Neither is insulin antagonism necessary. On the contrary, the unrestrained expression of insulin action permits efficient storage of the excess carbohydrate calories.

Finally, when an individual is fasting, insulin secretion falls, partly because the plasma glucose levels diminish. Although this decline in insulin secretion increases GH secretion (and IGFBP$_3$), the calorie deficit and the significant deficiency of insulin decrease the production of somatomedin. Again, these effects are appropriate when an increase in protein anabolism is disadvantageous and when protein catabolism is essential. However, the increase in GH may still be beneficial during fasting, because it enhances lipolysis, decreases peripheral glucose use, and increases glucose production.

Prolactin

In humans, prolactin is a protein hormone that is principally concerned with stimulating breast development and milk production. In addition, it influences reproductive function and immune responses. Prolactin originates in specific anterior pituitary cells called mammotrophs or lactotrophs, which make up 10% to 25% of the pituitary population. These cells increase in number during pregnancy and lactation, and in response to estrogen treatment. The estrogen receptor also contributes to mammotroph development in the fetus. Some cells, somatomammotrophs, have both growth hormone and prolactin secretion capabilities. These cells may differentiate further into unifunctional cells under certain physiological circumstances, such as pregnancy when mammotrophs emerge.

Prolactin is a single-chain protein of molecular weight 23,000. The molecule contains 199 amino acids and three intramolecular disulfide bridges (Fig. 43-26). Its gene and structure are homologous to those of GH (Fig. 43-19), but the molecule has a major midportion loop. Synthesis of prolactin proceeds from a prehormone. The N-terminal signal peptide is cleaved, and transient N-glycosylation takes place before the compound arrives in the Golgi apparatus. There, the hormone molecules that are subsequently destined to be stored in granules and released by acute stimuli (or secreted during pregnancy) are deglycosylated. However, some of the N-glycosylated molecules escape complete processing, and they are secreted constitutively. These molecules form a major

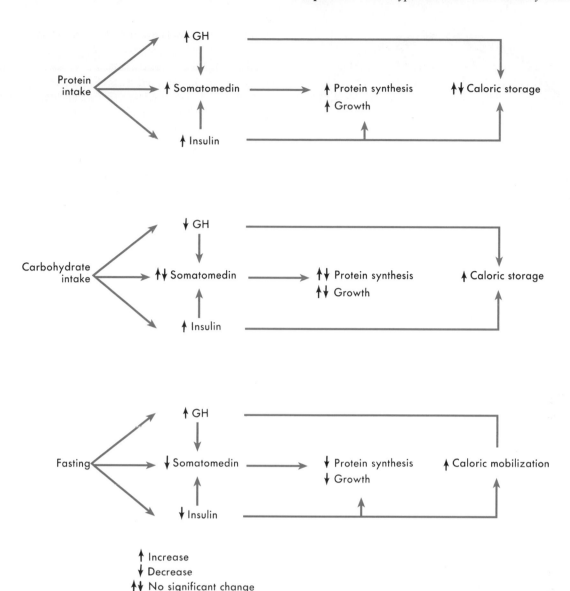

↑ Increase
↓ Decrease
↑↓ No significant change

■ **Fig. 43-25** Complementary regulation of GH and insulin secretion coordinate nutrient availability with anabolism and either caloric storage or mobilization. Note that both hormones are increased by protein, and both stimulate protein synthesis.

part of the circulating prolactin in nonpregnant women, and they have a lower biological activity. Phosphorylated prolactin and the products of proteolytic cleavage have been found but their functional significance is unknown. Transcription of the prolactin gene is regulated by factors that also regulate secretion of the hormone. Thus, TRH increases prolactin messenger RNA, whereas dopamine decreases it.

Prolactin is also synthesized in the brain including the hypothalamus, and in specialized cells of the uterus, placenta, and breast, and in lymphocytes. In these areas it has paracrine and autocrine functions. It is also secreted into breast milk, and it has functions in the neonate.

Secretion of prolactin. Table 43-5 lists the most important influences on prolactin secretion. Consistent with its essential role in lactation, prolactin secretion increases steadily during pregnancy. This increase is probably mediated by the large increase in estrogen, which stimulates hyperplasia of

prolactin-producing cells and synthesis of the hormone by inducing transcription of the gene. Although estrogen does not itself stimulate the release of prolactin, it enhances responsiveness to other stimuli. If a new mother does not nurse her child, the plasma level of prolactin declines to the normal (nonpregnant) range 3 to 6 weeks after delivery. However, suckling (or any other form of nipple stimulation) maintains elevated levels of prolactin secretion, especially for the first 8 to 12 weeks after birth (Fig. 43-27).

Prolactin secretion from mammotrophs is stimulated in paracrine fashion by the presence of neighboring gonadotrophs, which are themselves responding to GnRH. These gonadotrophs, which also release **angiotensin II,** increase prolactin release by nearby mammotrophs.

There is a circadian pattern of prolactin secretion, which rises at night (Fig. 43-10). The first peak appears 60 to 90 minutes after the onset of slow-wave sleep, and subsequent

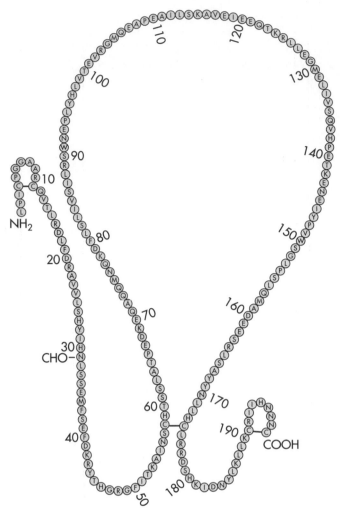

■ **Fig. 43-26** Structure of prolactin. This molecule is a single polypeptide chain with a major midportion loop and three intramolecular disulfide bridges. Residue 31 is an asparagine that is N-glycosylated (CHO). The single-letter amino acid code is used. (From Cooke NE: In DeGroot LJ, editor: *Prolactin: basic physiology in endocrinology,* ed 3, Philadelphia, 1995, WB Saunders.)

■ **Table 43-5**   Regulation of prolactin secretion

Stimulation	Inhibition
Pregnancy	Dopamine
Estrogen	Dopaminergic agonists
Nursing—breast manipulation	Somatostatin
Sleep	GnRH-associated peptide
Stress (Table 43-3)	Prolactin
TRH	γ-Aminobutyric acid (GABA)
Dopaminergic antagonists	
Opioids	
Serotonin	
Histamine antagonists (H_2)	
Adrenergic antagonists	
Candidate prolactin-releasing factors	
Vasoactive intestinal peptide	
Peptide histidine-isoleucine	
Oxytocin	
Angiotensin II	
Neurotensin	
Galanin	
Neurophysin II	
Intermediate lobe product	

pituitary tissue in vitro. After dopamine is bound to its receptors on the mammotrophs, its inhibiting action is mediated by G-proteins and by the consequent lowering of the levels of calcium and cAMP.

A dopaminergic tract runs from the arcuate nucleus of the hypothalamus to the median eminence. The dopamine concentrations in the long portal veins of the pituitary gland are elevated to levels that can inhibit prolactin release in vitro. In addition, a dopaminergic tract from the periventricular nucleus of the hypothalamus to the posterior pituitary gland provides dopamine via the short portal veins. Dopamine generated or concentrated in adjacent anterior pituitary cells also inhibits prolactin secretion by paracrine or autocrine action. Somatostatin, GABA, and a peptide derived from the processing of the gene transcript of GnRH are other hypothalamic inhibitors of prolactin secretion.

The inhibitory effect of dopamine on prolactin secretion is useful therapeutically. Pathological prolactin hypersecretion from tumors, for example, is readily suppressed by dopamine agonists. They may even shrink such tumors. In contrast, numerous dopaminergic analogs, used to treat psychiatric disorders, elevate prolactin levels and increase the biological effects of the hormone.

Prolactin inhibits its own secretion via a short-loop feedback. It does so by directly increasing the synthesis and release of dopamine, its hypothalamic inhibitor. The hypothalamus has positive as well as negative effects on prolactin secretion. Several candidates exist for the role of prolactin-releasing hormone (PRH) (Table 43-5). TRH, for example, stimulates prolactin synthesis and release; it acts through specific membrane receptors in the mammotroph, and phosphatidylinositol products are generated as second messen-

peaks occur later, after cycles of rapid eye movement (REM) sleep. Stresses, including anesthesia, surgery, insulin-induced hypoglycemia, fear, and mental tension, all cause prolactin release. The purpose of sleep- or stress-induced prolactin release is unknown.

The details of the pathways for regulating prolactin release in each physiological circumstance are not completely known. *However, uniquely among the pituitary hormones, prolactin secretion is tonically inhibited by the hypothalamus* (Fig. 43-28). Disruption of the hypothalamic-pituitary connection induces prompt and enduring increases in plasma prolactin levels. **Dopamine** has many characteristics that qualify it for the role of primary **prolactin-inhibiting factor (PIF),** although it is not a hypothalamic peptide. This catecholamine strongly inhibits prolactin release, either when it is generated within the brain in vivo or when it is applied to

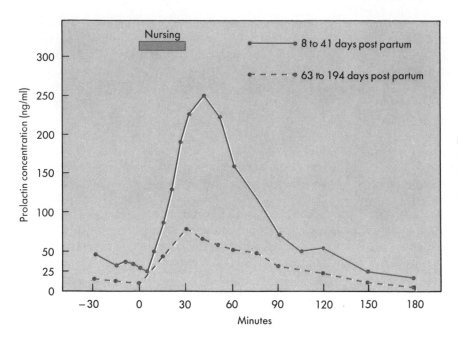

■ **Fig. 43-27** Stimulation of prolactin secretion by nursing. Note the decreased responses as the interval of time from delivery increases. (From Noel GL et al: *J Clin Endocrinol Metab* 38:413, 1974.)

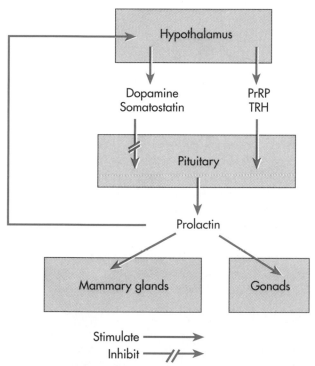

■ **Fig. 43-28** Regulation of prolactin secretion. The predominant mode of hypothalamic regulation is tonic inhibition by dopamine with a contribution from somatostatin. TRH and a number of prolactin-releasing factor *(PRF)* candidates stimulate prolactin release, but their relative roles are uncertain. Prolactin itself exerts negative feedback by stimulating secretion of its inhibitor dopamine.

Suckling, for example, does not produce a simultaneous, acute rise in plasma levels of TSH, as would be expected if TRH mediated the plasma prolactin increase. Some evidence links oxytocin, transmitted to mammotrophs via the short portal veins, to this particular prolactin-stimulating function.

A number of other peptides that are found in the hypothalamus or median eminence and that have receptors in the anterior pituitary gland have prolactin-releasing activity (Table 43-5), but their functional roles are unclear. Most recently, a 31-amino acid peptide called prolactin-releasing peptide (PrRP), has been described. This peptide stimulates prolactin release from human pituitary glands in vitro, in a manner that is augmented by pretreatment with estrogen. PrRP-positive neurons are found in the dorsomedial and ventromedial nuclei of the hypothalamus, and axons that contain PrRP contact oxytocin neurons in the latter nucleus and are also present in the posterior pituitary gland. Thus, oxytocin, arriving from short portal veins, may mediate some PrRP action. PrRP may also increase prolactin secretion indirectly, by stimulating the release of other putative prolactin secretogogues, galanin and VIP.

Normal basal plasma concentrations of prolactin are about 10 ng/ml (5×10^{-10}), and they are similar in women and men. The half-life of the hormone is 20 minutes, and the daily production is around 350 µg. The kidney is a likely organ of prolactin degradation, because patients with renal failure often have high plasma prolactin levels. Prolactin is also present in amniotic fluid; its source is pregnancy-modified cells of the uterus stimulated by a placental prolactin-releasing factor.

Biological effects of prolactin. *Prolactin participates in stimulating the original development of breast tissue and its further hyperplasia during pregnancy. It is the principal hormone responsible for lactogenesis.* Before and after puberty, prolactin, together with estrogens, progesterone,

gers. When TSH secretion is chronically increased as a result of negative feedback from the thyroid gland, prolactin tends to increase modestly, probably because of increased endogenous TRH release. However, TRH is probably not the sole or most important stimulator of prolactin release.

cortisol, and GH, stimulates the proliferation and branching of ducts in the female breast. During pregnancy, prolactin, along with estrogen, progesterone, and cortisol, causes the development of lobules of alveoli within which milk is produced. Finally, after parturition, prolactin, together with insulin and cortisol, stimulates milk synthesis and prolactin with oxytocin maintains milk secretion during the nursing period.

To exert these effects, prolactin binds to plasma membrane receptors (Fig. 43-29) homologous to those of GH in their extracellular binding domains. The intracytoplasmic tails of the prolactin receptors are different from and shorter than those of the GH receptors. As in the case of growth hormone, one prolactin molecule binds two prolactin receptors into a dimer (Fig. 43-24). Signal transduction is effected via activation of cytoplasmic tyrosine kinases, and regulation of target genes by phosphorylated STAT proteins as described for GH (Fig. 43-25). The intracellular tail of the prolactin receptor is also phosphorylated in this process by Janus kinase.

Prolactin stimulates the uptake of some amino acids and it induces transcription of genes for the milk proteins casein, lactalbumin, and β-lactoglobulin, whose messenger RNAs it also stabilizes. Galactosyltransferase and *N*-acetyllactosamine synthetase are also induced. These enzymes are necessary for synthesis of lactose, which is the major sugar in milk. The synthesis of fatty acids and phospholipids is also stimulated by prolactin, specifically in breast tissue. Prolactin upregulates the number of its own receptors. Estrogen also increases the number of prolactin receptors. However, estrogen and progesterone directly antagonize the stimulatory effects of prolactin on milk synthesis.

Additional prolactin action pathways include MAP kinase, inositol phosphate second messengers, and calcium channels. Downregulation of the JAK-STAT pathway occurs by acute and transient induction of inhibitory proteins.

Prolactin has both stimulating and inhibiting effects on reproduction. The effects depend in part on the phase of the reproductive process during which it acts. Excess prolactin blocks the synthesis and release of GnRH; this action causes the loss of normal GnRH pulses, and it prevents ovulation in females and normal sperm production in males. Prolactin can both induce and repress gene transcription for certain enzymes that are essential to production of gonadal steroid hormones, particularly progesterone. Whether induction or repression occurs depends on the species, which cell type is affected, and, in females, on the stage of the menstrual cycle. In addition, certain reproductive behavioral effects of prolactin have been described, such as inhibition of libido in humans and stimulation of parental protective behavior toward the newborn in animals. Prolactin receptors are present in those areas of the hypothalamus that are associated with sexual behavior and prolactin levels are elevated in women with pseudopregnancy.

Certain effects of prolactin on cell growth and proliferation are under investigation. Although the effects resemble GH effects, they are expressed through prolactin receptors. In addition, prolactin, like GH, may induce an intermediary growth molecule, **synlactin,** which is synthesized and released by the liver, in analogy to the somatomedins. Extrapituitary production of prolactin suggests a role for this hormone in the immunological balance required for the acceptance of fetal tissues by the mother, and the protection of maternal tissues from fetal invasion. During pregnancy, locally produced prolactin may participate in the osmoregulatory function of amniotic fluid.

In women, prolactin deficiency, caused by destruction of the anterior pituitary gland, results in the inability to lactate. Prolactin excess results from hypothalamic dysfunction or from pituitary tumors. In women, prolactin

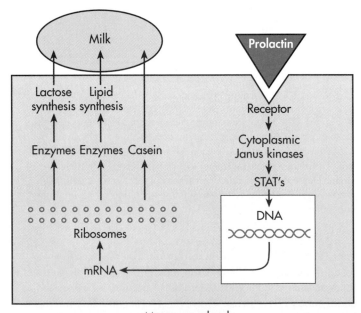

■ **Fig. 43-29** Mechanism of prolactin action. After binding to a plasma membrane receptor, cytoplasmic Janus kinases phosphorylate signal transducer and activation of transcription (STATs) factors that stimulate expression of genes. These genes direct synthesis of the milk protein casein and of enzymes essential for production of other milk components: lactose and lipids.

Mammary gland

hypersecretion causes infertility, and even a complete loss of menses. Less often, lactation unassociated with pregnancy (**galactorrhea**) occurs. In men, decreased testosterone secretion and sperm production result from prolactin excess. Stimulation of breast development is uncommon, and lactation is rare. In both sexes, libido is decreased. The diagnosis of excess prolactin is established by demonstrating a high plasma prolactin level. If surgical removal of a mammotrophic tumor is not required, dopaminergic drugs reduce prolactin secretion to normal levels and restore fertility.

POSTERIOR PITUITARY HORMONES

Two nonapeptides of homologous structure (Fig. 43-30), **antidiuretic hormone (ADH),** also known as **arginine vasopressin (AVP),** and **oxytocin (OTC),** are secreted from the posterior pituitary gland. In humans, *the primary role of ADH is to conserve body water and to regulate the osmolality of body fluids; the primary role of OTC is to eject milk from the lactating mammary gland and to facilitate uterine contractions during labor.* In subprimate species, some actions of ADH and OTC overlap. Although their primary human functions are different, the synthesis, storage, and mode of secretion of the two hormones are similar, and they will be discussed together.

Both hormones are synthesized in the cell bodies of hypothalamic neurons. ADH originates largely in the supraoptic nucleus, and OTC originates largely in the paraventricular nucleus of the hypothalamus. However, each hormone is also synthesized in the alternate site. The genes that direct the synthesis of the respective preprohormones are remarkably similar, and they are located on the same chromosome, only a few kilobases apart (Fig. 43-31). Enhancer elements lie next to each other between the genes and are transcribed in opposite directions (Fig. 43-32). The hormone sequences are contained within exon-1 (Fig. 43-31).

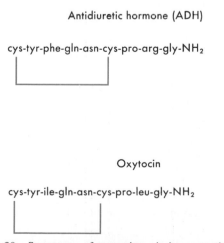

Antidiuretic hormone (ADH)

cys-tyr-phe-gln-asn-cys-pro-arg-gly-NH$_2$

Oxytocin

cys-tyr-ile-gln-asn-cys-pro-leu-gly-NH$_2$

■ **Fig. 43-30** Structures of posterior pituitary peptides. The alternative term for ADH is arginine vasopressin (AVP).

In addition to ADH or OTC, the products from these genes include certain distinctive proteins, known as **neurophysins,** of molecular weight 10,000. Neurophysin I (for OTC) and neurophysin II (for ADH) are virtually identical in their large central cores (corresponding to exon-2 in each gene). The two neurophysins differ in their N-terminal portions, which are coded for by exon-1 (Fig. 43-31), and in their C-terminal portions, which are coded for by exon-3. In the case of ADH, an additional glycopeptide is coded for by exon-3. After processing of the preprohormones, ADH and OTC are bound to their respective neurophysins and packaged together in the acidic environment of the neurosecretory granules. The neurophysins serve as carrier proteins in the process of transport of the neurohormones down the axons. Mutations of the ADH gene, which express functionally inactive neurophysin-2, are associated with peripheral signs of ADH deficiency. These changes are accompanied by retention of ADH in the endoplasmic reticulum of the hypothalamic neurons, decreased processing of ADH, and loss of these neurons.

The axons of ADH and OCT neurons end in the posterior pituitary gland as terminal swellings, known as **Herring bodies.** ADH and OTC are released when a nerve impulse is transmitted from the cell body in the hypothalamus down the axon, where it depolarizes the neurosecretory vesicles within the terminal Herring body (Fig. 43-2). An influx of calcium into the neurosecretory vesicle then results in hormone secretion by exocytosis. After the hormone is released from the granule, it dissociates from its neurophysin in the neutral environment, and each separately enters the closely adjacent capillary. Subsequent passage of the hormone into the bloodstream is accomplished by endocytosis into the endothelial cell, and then by diffusion through pores in the fenestrated capillary endothelium.

Mechanical disruption of the neurohypophyseal tract by trauma, tumor, or surgery temporarily causes ADH (and OTC) deficiency, which can disappear with regeneration of the axons. However, if disruption occurs at a high enough level, the cell bodies in the hypothalamus die and ADH deficiency is permanent.

Secretion of ADH

ADH is detectable in the fetal hypothalamus by 10 weeks of gestation. It is synthesized as described above from a preprohormone containing 145 amino acids. Consistent with its role in water metabolism, *secretion of ADH is primarily regulated by osmotic and volume stimuli* (Table 43-6). Water deprivation increases the osmolality of plasma, and hence of the fluids bathing the brain. This hyperosmolality induces a loss of intracellular water from osmoreceptor neurons in the hypothalamus. Although these neurons could be identical with the magnocellular neurons that secrete ADH, evidence favors the existence of a distinct population of osmoreceptor neurons in the anterior circumventricular region that connects with the ADH neurons. In either case, the shrinkage of

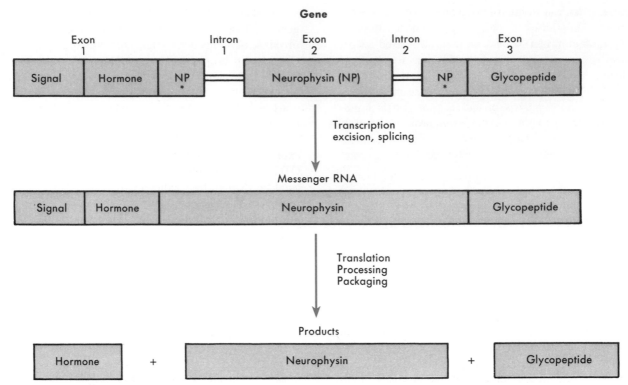

Fig. 43-31 Schematic representation of the synthesis of the two posterior pituitary peptides, ADH and oxytocin. The two gene structures are similar. In each case, exon 1 codes for the signal peptide, the hormone, and a variable portion of its corresponding neurophysin. Exon 2 is virtually identical in the two genes and codes for the homologous large central core of each neurophysin. In the case of ADH only, exon 3 contains a base sequence extension that codes for a C-terminal glycopeptide, which is coreleased with ADH. (From Richter D, Ivell R: Gene organization, biosynthesis, and chemistry of neurohypophyseal hormones. In Imura H: *The pituitary gland,* New York, 1985, Raven Press.)

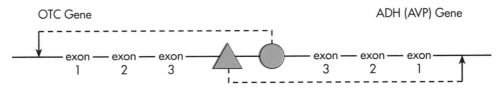

Fig. 43-32 Relationship between ADH (AVP) and OTC genes. The two genes lie on the same chromosome in tandem arrangement and in reverse order. The enhancer unit for ADH transcription *(triangle)* lies closer to the OTC gene and the enhancer unit for OTC transcription *(circle)* lies closer to the ADH gene. (From Gimpl G, Farenholz F: *Physiol Rev* 8:629, 2001.)

neuronal cell volume or increase in intracellular osmolality may cause ADH to be released. Conversely, water ingestion suppresses osmoreceptor firing, and consequently shuts off ADH release to a low constitutive level. ADH is initially suppressed by reflex neural stimulation shortly after water is swallowed, but before plasma osmolality declines. The plasma ADH level then declines further, after the water is absorbed from the intestine and plasma osmolality falls.

If plasma osmolality is increased directly by administration of solutes, only those solutes, such as sodium, that do not freely or rapidly penetrate cell membranes cause release of ADH. Substances, such as urea, that enter cells rapidly do

not stimulate ADH secretion, because they do not produce an osmotic disequilibrium between the extracellular and neuronal intracellular fluids. A selective increase in sodium concentration of the cerebrospinal fluid also increases ADH secretion. The hypothalamic osmoreceptors are extraordinarily sensitive and respond to changes in osmolality of only 1% to 2% (Fig. 43-33). An increase in plasma osmolality of 1 mOsm/kg increases the ADH level by 0.2 to 0.3 pg/ml. If water deprivation is prolonged, ADH synthesis is also increased.

In response to plasma hyperosmolality, osmoreceptor neurons also stimulate thirst. These neurons are probably

■ **Table 43-6**   Regulation of ADH secretion

Stimulation	*Inhibition*
Extracellular fluid osmolality increase	Extracellular fluid osmolality decrease
Volume decrease	Volume increase
Pressure decrease	Temperature decrease
Cerebrospinal fluid sodium increase	α-Adrenergic agonists
	γ-Aminobutyric acid (GABA)
Angiotensin II	Ethanol
Pain	Cortisol
Nausea and vomiting	Thyroid hormone
Stress (see Table 43-3)	Atrial natriuretic peptide
Hypoglycemia	
Cytokines	
Temperature increase	
Senescence	
Drugs	
Nicotine	
Opiates	
Barbiturates	
Sulfonylureas	
Antineoplastic agents	

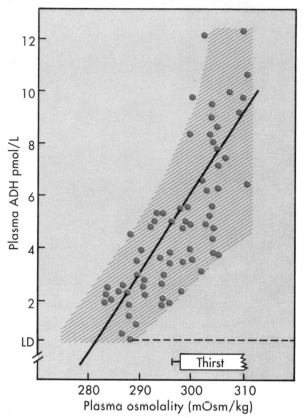

■ **Fig. 43-33**   Correlation between plasma ADH and plasma osmolality in humans. As plasma osmolality is increased by infusing hypertonic sodium chloride, ADH secretion is stimulated, and plasma ADH rises over a linear concentration range. This response to hyperosmolality just precedes the response of thirst. Both ADH release and thirst lead to increases in body water that limit further increments in the osmolality of body fluids. (From Baylis P: *Clin Endocrinol Metab* 12:747, 1983.)

separate from those that stimulate ADH secretion, and they are located elsewhere in the hypothalamus. In humans, the threshold for this action is close to, or slightly higher than, the threshold for ADH release of around 284 mOsm/kg. These relationships take linear forms: plasma AVP = 0.43 (plasma osmolality – 284) and thirst = 0.39 (plasma osmolality – 285). Therefore, ADH secretion is at least as important as thirst in maintaining normal body water content. The slopes and intercepts of these equations are quite similar in monozygotic twins, which strongly suggest that they have a genetic determinant.

ADH release is also stimulated by a decrease of 5% to 10% in total circulating blood volume, central blood volume, cardiac output, or blood pressure (Fig. 43-34). Hemorrhage is a potent stimulus of ADH release (see also Chapter 24). Quiet standing, tilting, or positive-pressure breathing also reduce central blood volume; therefore, they increase ADH secretion, particularly if blood pressure falls. Conversely, administration of blood or isotonic saline solution, which increases total circulating blood volume, or immersion up to the neck in water, which increases central blood volume, suppresses ADH release.

Hypovolemia is perceived by a number of pressure sensors in the body (see Chapters 17 and 21). These sensors include carotid and aortic baroreceptors, stretch receptors in the walls of the left atrium and pulmonary veins, and possibly the juxtaglomerular apparatus of the kidney. The afferent impulses of this neurohumoral arc are carried by the ninth and tenth cranial nerves to their respective nuclei in the medulla. From the medulla, the impulses are carried by way of the midbrain via adrenergic neurotransmitters to the supraoptic nuclei of the hypothalamus. Normally, the pressure receptors *tonically inhibit* ADH release by modulating an inhibitory flow of adrenergic impulses from the medulla to the hypothalamus. A decrease in pressure increases ADH

secretion by reducing the flow of neural impulses from the baroreceptors to the brainstem. The reduced neural input from the baroreceptors relieves the source of tonic inhibition on the hypothalamic cells that secrete ADH.

Hypovolemia also stimulates the generation of renin and angiotensin directly within the brain. This local angiotensin II enhances the release of ADH, in addition to stimulating thirst. Furthermore, volume regulation of ADH is partly mediated or reinforced by **atrial natriuretic peptide (ANP).** When circulating volume is increased, ANP is released by cardiac myocytes; this ANP, along with a homologous natriuretic peptide generated locally in supraoptic hypothalamic neurons (brain ANP), acts to inhibit ADH release (see also Chapter 24). Plasma ADH rises to much higher levels in response to hypotension than in response to hyperosmolarity (compare Fig. 43-34 with Fig. 43-33). This exaggerated response indicates that the vascular system is less sensitive to ADH than is the kidney.

The two major stimuli of ADH secretion interact. Increases or decreases in circulating volume reinforce the osmolar responses by raising or lowering, respectively, the threshold for osmotic release of ADH. Thus, hypovolemia sensitizes

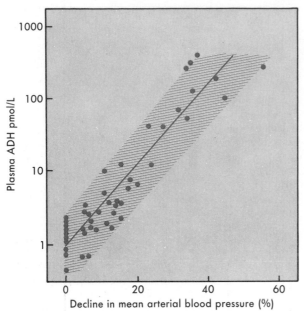

■ **Fig. 43-34** Correlation between plasma ADH and declining blood pressure in humans. As blood pressure is decreased by infusing an agent that blocks sympathetic ganglion function, ADH secretion is stimulated. Note that in this response, plasma ADH rises over an exponential concentration range (compare Fig. 43-33). (From Baylis P: *Clin Endocrinol Metab* 12:747, 1983.)

the ADH response to hyperosmolarity. However, if hypovolemia is severe, baroregulation overrides osmotic regulation, and ADH secretion is stimulated, even though plasma osmolality may be below 270 mOsm/kg (see also Chapter 24).

Secretion of ADH is also influenced by various other conditions (Table 43-6). Pain, emotional stress, heat, and various drugs are stimulators; nausea and vomiting are especially potent. Inflammatory cytokines, such as interleukin-6, also stimulate ADH release. The size of ADH neurons, the rate of ADH secretion, and the plasma levels of ADH are all greater in men than women. Elderly individuals secrete more ADH then do younger individuals, probably in compensation for a diminished ability of their kidneys to concentrate urine. The threshold for ADH release is lower in women during the luteal phase of the menstrual cycle and during pregnancy. Ethanol is a commonly encountered inhibitor of ADH secretion. As little as 30 to 90 ml of whiskey is sufficient to suppress ADH secretion. Cortisol and thyroid hormones restrain ADH release; in their absence, ADH may be secreted, even though plasma osmolality is low.

ADH circulates unbound to protein at an average basal concentration of 1 pg/ml (10^{-12} M). ADH does bind to platelets. The plasma half-life is 5 to 15 minutes, although the half-life of biological action may be as long as 20 minutes. Metabolic clearance of ADH increases with its plasma level, and it averages 600 ml/min when plasma concentrations are about 10 pg/ml. Urinary clearance of ADH consistently averages 5% of total metabolic clearance. Therefore, urinary excretion rates are usually a valid index of ADH secretion. The latter is normally about 1 mg/day.

During water deprivation, the secretion of ADH increases 3-fold to 5-fold. Maximum antidiuresis is reached at a plasma level of 4 to 5 pg/ml. Transient 50-fold increases can occur in response to hemorrhage (see Chapter 24), severe pain, or nausea. Neurophysin II also circulates in plasma, and its levels rise and fall parallel with ADH. The C-terminal glycopeptide of prepro-ADH origin is also present in plasma. No functional role for these peptides in peripheral tissues has yet been identified.

Actions of ADH

ADH binds to a class 1 G-protein–linked plasma membrane receptor (see Fig. 44-11) of three types. cAMP, phosphoinositol, and Ca^{2+} are second messengers. *The major action of ADH is on renal cells that are responsible for reabsorbing free (i.e., osmotically unencumbered) water from the glomerular filtrate* (Chapter 36). These ADH-responsive cells line the distal convoluted tubules and collecting ducts of the renal medulla. *ADH increases the permeability of these cells to water.* ADH binds to a specific plasma membrane receptor (known as the V_2 receptor) on the capillary (basal) side of the cell, where it activates adenylyl cyclase. The increase in intracellular cAMP activates a protein kinase on the opposite, luminal (apical) side of the cell. The activated protein kinase phosphorylates a water channel protein, aquaporin-2, at a serine site in its C-terminus. As a result, aquaporin-2 vesicles are transported to the luminal plasma membrane. The vesicles fuse with the plasma membrane and insert aquaporin-2 water channels, through which water rapidly moves from the tubular lumen into the collecting duct cell. By a separate mechanism, urea is also reabsorbed.

The increase in membrane permeability to water permits back diffusion of water along an osmotic gradient, from the hypotonic tubular urine that emerges from the loop of Henle to the hypertonic interstitial fluid of the renal medulla. The mechanisms for establishing this gradient are discussed in Chapter 36. ADH also acts on the ascending limb of the loop of Henle to enhance sodium transport into the medullary interstitium. The resultant increase in the osmolality of the interstitium helps create the osmotic gradient for water reabsorption. The net result of ADH action is to increase the osmolality of urine to a maximum value that is 4-fold greater than that of the glomerular filtrate or plasma (Fig. 43-35). In other words, ADH significantly reduces free-water clearance by the kidney.

Water deprivation stimulates ADH secretion, and it thereby decreases free-water clearance and enhances water conservation. A water load decreases ADH secretion, and thus increases free-water clearance and the efficiency of water excretion. Thus, ADH and water form a negative feedback loop. The sigmoidal dose-response relationship between plasma levels of ADH and urine osmolality is shown in Fig. 43-35. Most of the renal effect occurs at plasma ADH levels between 2 and 5 pg/ml. In this range, urine osmolality correlates directly with plasma ADH concentrations. An increase in plasma ADH concentration of only 0.3 pg/ml increases urine osmolality from 60 to 300 mOsm/kg

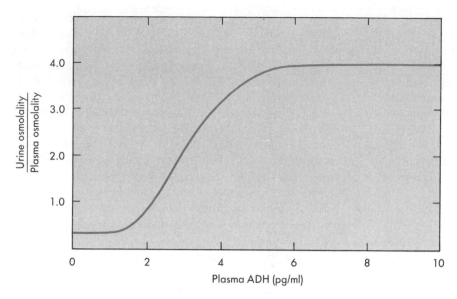

Fig. 43-35 Dose-response curve for the effect of ADH in increasing renal tubular reabsorption of free water, expressed as the ratio of urine to plasma osmolality. A maximal ratio of 4.0 is reached. (Data from Moore WW: *Fed Proc* 30:1387, 1971.)

in water-loaded humans. At an ADH level of 5 pg/ml, a maximal urine osmolality is achieved.

ADH deficiency is caused by destruction or dysfunction of the supraoptic and paraventricular nuclei of the hypothalamus. The inability to produce concentrated urine is the hallmark of ADH deficiency; the condition is called **diabetes insipidus.** In normal individuals, water deprivation can be compensated for by an increase in urine osmolality to 1000 to 1400 mOsm/kg. Individuals who lack ADH cannot achieve osmolalities higher than that of plasma (290 mOsm/kg), and in severe cases, it cannot exceed 50 mOsm/kg. Because a typical diet generates up to 900 mOsm of solute per day, which must be excreted by the kidney, urine volumes may be as high as 18 L/day in patients with diabetes insipidus, in contrast to the usual 1 to 3 L. Patients therefore urinate frequently both day and night, and they must also drink excess fluids to replace the loss of water. Despite this water intake, chronic elevation of serum osmolality (>290 mOsm/kg) and of serum sodium concentration (>145 mEq/L) can occur. Replacement with ADH or with long-acting analogs relieves the frequent urination and thirst, and prevents disastrous dehydration.

Many factors blunt the action of ADH on the tubular cell: solute diuresis, chronic water loading (which reduces medullary hyperosmolarity), prostaglandin E (which interferes with ADH activation of adenylyl cyclase), ANP, cortisol, potassium deficiency, calcium excess, and lithium (which is used in the treatment of psychiatric disorders). Certain sulfonylurea drugs, formerly used in the treatment of diabetes mellitus, and a tetracycline antibiotic can enhance ADH action.

ADH subserves other functions in addition to its primary role in water metabolism. In response to hemorrhage, ADH contributes to increasing vascular tone by binding to arteri-

olar smooth muscles via the V_{1a} receptor and causing the smooth muscles to constrict. This action is mediated by Ca^{2+} and phospholipase C-generated second messengers. In contrast, a V_2 receptor-mediated vasodilator effect of ADH may prevent blood pressure from changing too much when ADH secretion is in the physiological range. However, when ADH is administered systemically in large doses, it elevates the blood pressure and constricts the coronary and splanchnic vascular beds. The latter effect has been exploited therapeutically in controlling serious gastrointestinal bleeding.

ADH excess, inappropriate to either the osmolarity or volume of the body fluids, can result from (1) increased secretion caused by central nervous system disease, trauma, or psychosis; (2) increased secretion, mediated by cytokines that are released during infections or other medical or surgical stress; (3) ectopic production of the hormone by tumors; or (4) potentiation of hormone secretion or action by drugs. The reduction in free-water clearance caused by ADH, combined with voluntary or involuntary water intake, leads to water retention. Plasma sodium concentration and osmolality are significantly lowered, whereas urine osmolality is increased.

Characteristically, sodium excretion in the urine is also increased, despite the hyponatremia, as a result of a compensatory increase in ANP secretion. Both intracellular and extracellular fluid volumes are expanded. The swelling of brain cells and hypoosmolality can cause headache, nausea, lethargy, somnolence, convulsions, and coma, when plasma osmolality declines to below 250 mOsm/kg and plasma sodium levels fall below 125 mEq/L. Water restriction is a logical and effective acute treatment. Occasionally, this treatment must be supplemented with drugs that induce a hypotonic diuresis or with hypertonic sodium chloride solutions to raise osmolality more rapidly.

ADH also functions as a corticotropin-releasing factor via axons that transmit the peptide to the median eminence. From there, it travels via the portal veins to the anterior pituitary gland, where it interacts with a V_{1b} receptor, which generates phospholipase C-released second messengers. ADH also serves as a neurotransmitter in the brain, where it is involved in memory, regulation of temperature and blood pressure, circadian rhythms, and brain development. Finally, ADH, present locally in high concentrations and acting via a V_1 receptor in a paracrine manner, stimulates smooth muscle contraction in the human spermatic cord. This effect may facilitate the ejaculation of sperm.

Oxytocin Secretion

Oxytocin (OTC) is known as the milk letdown factor. *Suckling is an immediate and major stimulus for OTC release.* Afferent neural impulses are carried from sensory receptors in the nipple to the spinal cord, where they ascend in the spinothalamic tract. From relays in the brainstem and midbrain, they reach the paraventricular nuclei of the hypothalamus. From there, they trigger OTC release from the neurosecretory vesicles in the posterior pituitary. As suckling is continued, OTC synthesis and its transfer down the hypothalamic axon are also stimulated. As shown in Fig. 43-36, the stimulus of suckling is specific for OTC, because little release of ADH is noted. Likewise, the various stimuli for ADH secretion stimulate little or no OTC release in humans. Opioid (endorphinergic) input to the hypothalamus inhibits the OTC responses to various stimuli. OTC circulates unbound, and it exhibits a plasma half-life of 3 to 5 minutes. It is degraded by the kidneys and liver.

Oxytocin Actions

OTC binds to plasma membrane receptors distinct from, but with 50% homology to, those of ADH. Binding takes place mostly in the extracellular and transmembrane loops. Binding affinity is greatly increased by Mg^{2+} and cholesterol, and it is inhibited by progesterone. Increases in calcium levels and in phosphatidylinositol products then mediate actions of OTC. *The unique effect of OCT is to cause contraction of the myoepithelial cells of the alveoli of the mammary glands,* in response to cries of the infant and the stimulus of sucking the nipple. As a result, milk is forced from the alveoli into the ducts, from where it is evacuated by the infant. The response is very rapid and milk flows within 1 minute. Repeated high-frequency bursts of OTC secretion lead to huge increases in plasma OTC and to sustained stimulation of milk release. Estrogens augment and catecholamines block the action of OTC.

OTC also has a powerful action on smooth muscle in the uterus. Formation of Ca^{2+}-calmodulin complexes leads to activation of myosin light chains and to contraction of smooth muscle cells. Rhythmic contractions of the myometrium are stimulated by very small doses of OTC, which act by lowering slightly the threshold for membrane depolarization. Large doses lower the threshold still further, prevent repolarization and spiking discharges, and induce a sustained tetanic contraction. Neither maternal plasma OTC levels nor fetal OTC availability bears a consistent relationship to the progress of labor during childbirth. Therefore, despite the ability to stimulate rhythmic uterine contractions, secreted OTC seems to be more a contributing factor than an essential hormone of human parturition (see Chapter 46). However, after delivery, it may play an important role in the sustained contractions that help to maintain hemostasis after the placenta is evacuated. OTC is used to induce labor in women who are physiologically ready, and it is also used therapeutically to decrease immediate postpartum bleeding. OTC and its receptor are also present in the ovary, where OTC may have a

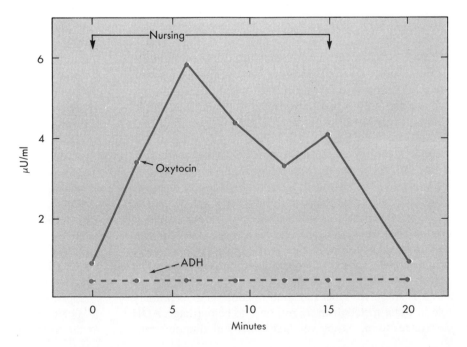

■ **Fig. 43-36**   Stimulation of oxytocin secretion by nursing in humans. Note the specificity of response as no release of ADH is observed. (From Weitzman RE et al: *J Clin Endocrinol Metab* 41:836, 1980.)

paracrine role in terminating the corpus luteum at the end of the menstrual cycle (see Chapter 46).

OTC has other functions in the reproductive activity of both genders. OTC and its receptor are found in the testis, epididimus, and prostate gland of men and thus may assist in the movement of sperm, in ejaculation, and in the addition of seminal fluid to the sperm (Chapter 46). OTC plasma levels rise during male sexual activity, and they peak at ejaculation.

OTC plasma levels also rise during female sexual activity. The hormone and its receptor are found in the ovary, and OTC assists in ovulation and in the termination of the corpus luteum (Chapter 46).

SUMMARY

1. The hypothalamic-pituitary unit regulates growth, lactation, fluid homeostasis, and the functions of the thyroid gland, adrenal glands, and gonads. This unit receives input from the thalamus, the reticular activating substance, the limbic system, and from olfactory and visual stimuli. These signals are then relayed to various parts of the endocrine system.

2. Peptide hormones that are synthesized in the cell bodies of certain hypothalamic neurons pass down their axons to be stored in and released into the circulation from the posterior pituitary gland.

3. Other hypothalamic peptides travel down axons to the median eminence, from which they are released into a portal venous circulation that carries them to the anterior pituitary gland. There, they stimulate or inhibit release of target hormones.

4. Hypothalamic-releasing and -inhibiting peptides are secreted in pulses, and they induce effects via cAMP, Ca^{2+}, and phosphatidylinositol products as second messengers. They stimulate or inhibit transcription, modulate translation, and stimulate or inhibit secretion of the target anterior pituitary hormones.

5. The anterior pituitary gland contains five functional cell types that are in close proximity, and thus they are capable of paracrine interactions. These cell types are thyrotrophs, adrenocorticotrophs, gonadotrophs, somatotrophs, and mammotrophs. Each cell type secretes a hormone or hormones in response to hypothalamic stimulation. Peripheral target gland hormones or other peripheral products of hormonal action feed back negatively to inhibit their respective anterior pituitary hormones.

6. Thyrotropin (TSH) is a glycoprotein that contains an α- and β-subunit. TSH stimulates secretion and growth of the thyroid gland. It is released in response to thyrotropin-releasing hormone (TRH) and to thyroid hormone deficiency.

7. Adrenocorticotrophin (ACTH) is a peptide that stimulates the secretion and growth of the adrenal cortex. It is synthesized from a multifunctional precursor, and it is secreted in bursts in response to corticotropin-releasing hormone,

antidiuretic hormone, cortisol deficiency, and various stresses, such as trauma and hypoglycemia.

8. Follicle-stimulating hormone (FSH) and luteinizing hormone (LH) are both made primarily by a single gonadotrophic cell type. These glycoprotein hormones share common α-subunits with each other and with TSH, but they have distinctive β-subunits.

9. In women, FSH stimulates the development of ovarian follicles and estradiol secretion, and in men spermatogenesis. LH stimulates steroid hormone secretion in both genders, primarily estradiol and its precursors in women, and testosterone in men. LH also stimulates ovulation. Estradiol and testosterone, as well as the gonadal protein hormone inhibin, feed back on FSH and LH secretion in complex ways.

10. Growth hormone (GH) is a large protein that stimulates cartilage development and growth, bone growth, and accretion of lean body mass. It acts primarily via peptide mediators (insulin-like growth factors, or somatomedins) that are produced in the liver and in many GH target cells.

11. GH also acts to antagonize insulin, stimulate lipolysis, and increase the metabolic rate. GH is secreted in response to growth hormone–releasing hormone (GHRH), hypoglycemia, amino acids, and stress. Its secretion is inhibited by somatostatin from the hypothalamus, somatomedin, and glucose.

12. Prolactin is structurally similar to GH, but it specifically stimulates growth of the mammary glands and production of milk. Prolactin is tonically inhibited by dopamine from the hypothalamus. Its synthesis is markedly increased during pregnancy and it is augmented by estrogens. Its release is stimulated by suckling.

13. Antidiuretic hormone (ADH) is a small peptide that acts on the renal tubules via cAMP as messenger. ADH increases the reabsorption of free water and the final urine osmolality. ADH also acts as a vasoconstrictor via a separate plasma membrane receptor and raises blood pressure. ADH is secreted from the posterior pituitary gland in response to an increase in plasma osmolality or to a decrease in plasma volume or blood pressure.

14. Oxytocin (OTC) is structurally very similar to ADH, but it acts specifically on the mammary gland to release milk. It is secreted in response to suckling. OCT also contracts the uterus, and it plays a role in the overall process of parturition.

BIBLIOGRAPHY

Journal articles

Amato G et al: Body composition, bone metabolism, and heart structure and function in growth hormone (GH)-deficient adults before and after GH replacement therapy at low doses, *J Clin Endocrinol Metab* 77:1671, 1993.

Argetsinger LS et al: Identification of JAK2 as a growth hormone receptor-associated tyrosine kinase, *Cell* 74:237, 1993.

Arvat E et al: Mineralocorticoid receptor blockade by canrenoate increses both spontaneous and stimulated adrenal function in humans, *J Clin Endocrinol Metab* 86:3176, 2001.

Barni T et al: Sex steroids and odorants modulate gonadotropin-releasing hormone secretion in primary cultures of human olfactory cells, *J Clin Endocrinol Metab* 84:4266, 1999.

Bousquet C et al: Direct regulation of pituitary proopiomelanocortin by STAT3 provides a novel mechanism for immuno-neuroendocrine interfacing, *J Clin Invest* 106:1417, 2000.

Brixen K et al: A short course of recombinant human growth hormone treatment stimulates osteoblasts and activates bone remodeling in normal human volunteers, *J Bone Miner Res* 5:609, 1990.

Conn PM, Crowley WF Jr: Gonadotropin-releasing hormone and its analogues, *N Engl J Med* 324:93, 1991.

Cooke NE, Liebhaber SA: Molecular biology of the growth hormone–prolactin gene system, *Vitam Horm* 50:385, 1995.

Corpas E, Harman SM, Blackman MR: Human growth hormone and human aging, *Endocr Rev* 14:20, 1993.

Date Y et al: Ghrelin, a novel growth hormone-releasing acylated peptide, is synthesized in a distinct endocrine cell type in the gastrointestinal tracts of rats and humans, *Endocrinology* 141:4255, 2000.

deBoer H, Blok G-J, Van der Veen EA: Clinical aspects of growth hormone deficiency in adults, *Endocr Rev* 16:63, 1995.

Engler D, Redei E, Kola I: The corticotropin-release inhibitory factor hypothesis: a review of the evidence for the existence of inhibitory as well as stimulatory hypophysiotropic regulation of adrenocorticotropin secretion and biosynthesis, *Endocr Rev* 20:460, 1999.

Evans JJ: Modulation of gonadotropin levels by peptides acting at the anterior pituitary gland, *Endocr Rev* 20:46, 1999.

Freeman ME et al: Prolactin: structure, function, and regulation of secretion, *Physiol Rev* 80:1523, 2000.

Gharib SD et al: Molecular biology of the pituitary gonadotropins, *Endocr Rev* 11:177, 1990.

Gill MS et al: Patterns of GH output and their synchrony with short-term height increments influence stature and growth performance in normal children, *J Clin Endocrinol Metab* 86:5860, 2001.

Gimpl G, Fahrenholz F: The oxytocin receptor system: structure, function, and regulation, *Physiol Rev* 81:629, 2001.

Giudice LC et al: Insulin-like growth factors and their binding proteins in the term and preterm human fetus and neonate with normal and extremes of intrauterine growth, *J Clin Endocrinol Metab* 80:1548, 1995.

Giustina A, Veldhuis JD: Pathophysiology of the neuroregulation of growth hormone secretion in experimental animals and the human, *Endocr Rev* 19:717, 1998.

Horseman ND, Yu-Lee L-Y: Transcriptional regulation by the helix bundle peptide hormones: growth hormone, prolactin, and hematopoietic cytokines, *Endocr Rev* 15:627, 1994.

Hulthen L et al: GH is needed for the maturation of muscle mass and strength in adolescents, *J Clin Endocrinol Metab* 86:4765, 2001.

Hunt G: Melanocyte-stimulating hormone: a regulator of human melanocyte physiology, *Pathobiology* 63:12, 1995.

Lee PDK et al: Insulin-like growth factor binding protein-1: recent findings and new directions, *Proc Soc Exp Biol Med.* 216(3):319, 1997.

Le Roith D et al: The somatomedin hypothesis: 2001, *Endocr Rev* 22:53, 2001.

Lofqvist C et al: Reference values for IGF-1 throughout childhood and adolescence: a model that accounts simultaneously for the effect of gender, age, and puberty, *J Clin Endocrinol Metab* 86:5870, 2001.

Magner JA: Thyroid stimulating hormone: biosynthesis, cell biology and bioactivity, *Endocr Rev* 11:354, 1990.

Miller N et al: Short-term effects of growth hormone on fuel oxidation and regional substrate metabolism in normal man, *J Clin Endocrinol Metab* 70:1179, 1990.

Muller EE, Locatelli V, Cocchi D: Neuroendocrine control of growth hormone secretion, *Physiol Rev* 79:511, 1999.

Prummel MF et al: Expression of the thyroid-stimulating hormone receptor in the folliculo-stellate cells of the human anterior pituitary, *J Clin Endocrinol Metab* 85:4347, 2000.

Rubinek T et al: Prolactin (PRL)-releasing peptide stimulates PRL secretion from human fetal pituitary cultures and growth hormone release from cultured pituitary adenomas, *J Clin Endocrinol Metab* 86:2826, 2001.

Samuels MH et al: Pathophysiology of pulsatile and copulsatile release of thyroid-stimulating hormone, luteinizing hormone, follicle-stimulating hormone, and alpha-subunit, *J Clin Endocrinol Metab* 71:425, 1990.

Seeman TE, Robbins RJ: Aging and hypothalamic-pituitary-adrenal response to challenge in humans, *Endocr Rev* 15:233, 1994.

Southworth MB et al: The importance of signal pattern in the transmission of endocrine information: pituitary gonadotropin responses to continuous and pulsatile gonadotropin-releasing hormone, *J Clin Endocrinol Metab* 72:1286, 1991.

Spencer SA et al: Growth hormone receptor and binding protein, *Recent Prog Horm Res* 46:165, 1990.

Suter KJ, Pohl CR, Wilson ME: Circulating concentrations of nocturnal leptin, growth hormone, and insulin-like growth factor-I increase before the onset of puberty in agonadal male monkeys: potential signals for the initiation of puberty, *J Clin Endocrinol Metab* 85:808, 817, 2000.

Takano A et al: Growth hormone induces cellular insulin resistance by uncoupling phosphatidylinositol 3-kinase and its downstream signals in 3T3-L1 adipocytes, *Diabetes* 50:1891, 2001.

Theill LE, Karin M: Transcriptional control of growth hormone expression and anterior pituitary development, *Endocr Rev* 14:670, 1993.

Thissen JP, Ketelslegers JM, Underwood LE: Nutritional regulation of the insulin-like growth factors, *Endocr Rev* 15:80, 1994.

Thompson CJ et al: Reproducibility of osmotic and nonosmotic tests of vasopressin secretion in men, *Am J Physiol* 260:R533, 1991.

Turnbull AV, Rivier CL: Regulation of the hypothalamic-pituitary-adrenal axis by cytokines: actions and mechanisms of action, *Physiol Rev* 79:1, 1999.

Veldhuis JD: Nature of altered pulsatile hormone release and neuroendocrine network signaling in human aging: clinical studies of the somatotropic, gonadotropic, corticotropic and insulin axes, *Novartis Found Symp* 227:163, 2000.

Veldhuis JD, Roemmich JN, Rogol AD: Gender and sexual maturation-dependent contrasts in the neuroregulation of growth hormone secretion in prepubertal and late adolescent males and females—a general clinical research center-based study, *J Clin Endocrinol Metab* 85:2385, 2000.

Veldhuis JD et al: Corticotropin secretory dynamics in humans under low glucocorticoid feedback, *J Clin Endocrinol Metab* 86:5554, 2001.

Vesely DL et al: Atrial natriuretic hormone, vessel dilator, long-acting natriuretic hormone, and kaliuretic hormone decrease the circulating concentrations of CRH, corticotropin, and cortisol, *J Clin Endocrinol Metab* 86:4244, 2001.

Wells JA et al: The molecular basis for growth hormone-receptor interactions, *Recent Prog Horm Res* 48:253, 1993.

Wennink JM et al: Growth hormone secretion patterns in relation to LH and testosterone secretion throughout normal male puberty, *Acta Endocrinol (Copenh)* 123:263, 1990.

Werner H et al: Molecular and cellular aspects of insulin-like growth factor action, *Vitam Horm* 48:1, 1994.

Books and monographs

Asa SL, Horvath E, Kovasc KT: Functional pituitary anatomy and histology. In DeGroot LJ, Jameson JL, editors: *Endocrinology,* ed 4, Philadelphia, 2001, WB Saunders.

Baylis PH: Vasopressin, diabetes insipidus and syndrome of inappropriate antidiuresis. In DeGroot LJ, Jameson JL, editors: *Endocrinology,* ed 4, Philadelphia, 2001, WB Saunders.

Horseman ND: Prolactin. In DeGroot LJ, Jameson JL, editors: *Endocrinology,* ed 4, Philadelphia, 2001, WB Saunders.

Patel YC: Neurotransmitters and hypothalamus in the control of anterior pituitary function. In DeGroot LJ, Jameson JL, editors: *Endocrinology,* ed 4, Philadelphia, 2001, WB Saunders.

Reeves WB, Bichet DG, Anderoli TE: The posterior pituitary and water metabolism. In Foster D et al, editors: *Williams textbook of endocrinology,* ed 9, Philadelphia, 1998, WB Saunders.

Reichlin S: *Neuroendocrinology.* In Foster D et al, editors: *Williams textbook of endocrinology,* ed 9, Philadelphia, 1998, WB Saunders.

Thorner MO et al: The anterior pituitary. In Foster DF et al, editors: *Williams textbook of endocrinology,* ed 9, Philadelphia, 1998, WB Saunders.

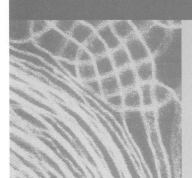

chapter forty-four

The Thyroid Gland

The thyroid gland was the first endocrine gland to be recognized as such on the basis of the symptoms associated with excess or deficient function. Physicians had previously speculated that deficiency of an internal secretion caused the clinical state associated with atrophy of the gland. This speculation was borne out when crude thyroid extracts successfully reversed the symptoms associated with thyroid atrophy; these extracts were the first example of successful hormonal therapy. Soon *thereafter, the most important mission of the thyroid gland was discovered to be regulation of the overall rate of body metabolism, including its most fundamental component—oxygen utilization. In addition, the gland was found to be critical for normal growth and development.*

The thyroid gland develops from endoderm associated with the pharyngeal gut. The gland descends to the anterior part of the neck, where it divides into two halves that lie on either side of the trachea (Fig. 44-1, *A*). Abnormal descent may locate the thyroid anywhere from the base of the tongue to the anterior mediastinum. By 11 to 12 weeks of gestational age, the gland is capable of synthesizing and secreting thyroid hormones under the stimulus of fetal thyroid-stimulating hormone (TSH). Both fetal TSH and thyroid hormone are required for the normal intrauterine development of the central nervous system and skeleton (although not for body growth), because only small amounts of this needed thyroid hormone reach the fetus from the maternal circulation.

Together, the two lobes of the adult thyroid gland weigh approximately 20 g. They receive a rich blood supply from the thyrocervical arteries and innervation from the autonomic nervous system. The basic histological structure of the thyroid gland is shown in Fig. 44-1, *B*. A single layer of hormone-producing, cuboidal epithelial cells forms a circular follicle 200 to 300 µm in diameter. Within the lumen of the follicle, newly synthesized hormone is stored in the form of a **colloid** material. The base of each epithelial cell (follicular cell) is covered by a basement membrane, and tight junctions connect adjacent cells at both their basal and apical (luminal) portions. When the gland is intensely stimulated, the endocrine cells enlarge and assume a more columnar shape, and their nuclei move toward the base of the cell (Fig. 44-1, *C*). The lumens of the follicles then appear scalloped because of endocytic resorption of the hormone-containing colloid (Fig. 44-1, *C*). Evidence suggests that the follicular cells are polyclonal and that their capacity to perform various steps in hormone synthesis in response to stimulation differs from cell to cell.

The growth and differentiation of thyroid follicular cells and their expression of genes of unique proteins required for thyroid hormone synthesis are stimulated and regulated by three nuclear transcription factors: thyroid transcription factors 1 and 2 (TTF-1 and TTF-2) and PAX 8. Thyroid volume increases during puberty in both genders, and thyroid size increases further after the onset of menses in girls.

The thyroid gland contains another type of cell in addition to follicular cells. Scattered within the gland, in close association with the epithelial cells, are parafollicular cells, called **C cells.** These cells are the source of the polypeptide hormone **calcitonin,** which is discussed in Chapter 42.

SYNTHESIS AND RELEASE OF THYROID HORMONES

The secretory products of the thyroid gland are **iodothyronines** (Fig. 44-2), a series of compounds resulting from the coupling of two iodinated tyrosine molecules. Approximately 90% of the thyroid output is **3,5,3′,5′-tetraiodothyronine (thyroxine, or T_4); 10% is 3,5,3′-triiodothyronine (T_3); and less than 1% is 3,3′,5′-triiodothyronine (reverse T_3, or rT_3).** Normally, these three compounds are secreted in the same proportions as they are stored in the gland. *However, T3 is the molecule responsible for most of the tissue actions of thyroid hormone.*

Because of the unique role of iodide in thyroid physiology, a description of thyroid hormone synthesis properly begins with a consideration of iodide turnover (Fig. 44-3). An average of 400 µg of iodide per person is ingested daily in the United States, versus a minimum daily requirement of

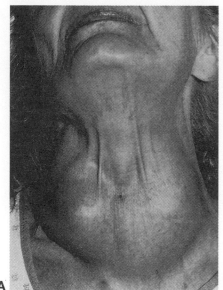

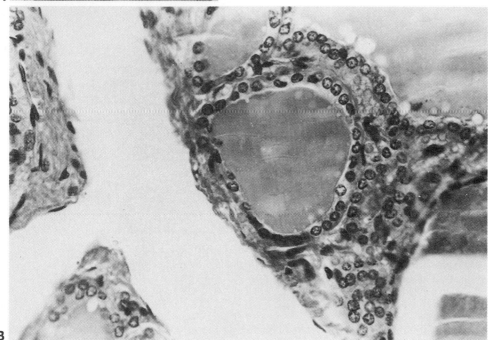

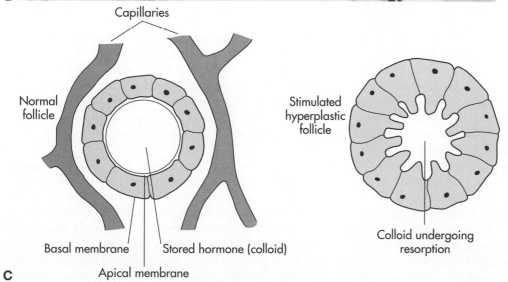

■ Fig. 44-1   **A,** The thyroid gland is located in the anterior neck, where it is easily visualized and palpated when it is enlarged (goiter). **B,** Photomicrograph of a thyroid gland follicle. **C,** Schematic drawing of a normal thyroid gland follicle and a follicle stimulated by thyrotropin (TSH). Note the change in cellular shapes from cuboidal to columnar, the relocation of the nuclei to the base of the cells, and the scalloped appearance of the follicle lumen.

Capillaries

Normal follicle

Stimulated hyperplastic follicle

Basal membrane

Apical membrane

Stored hormone (colloid)

Colloid undergoing resorption

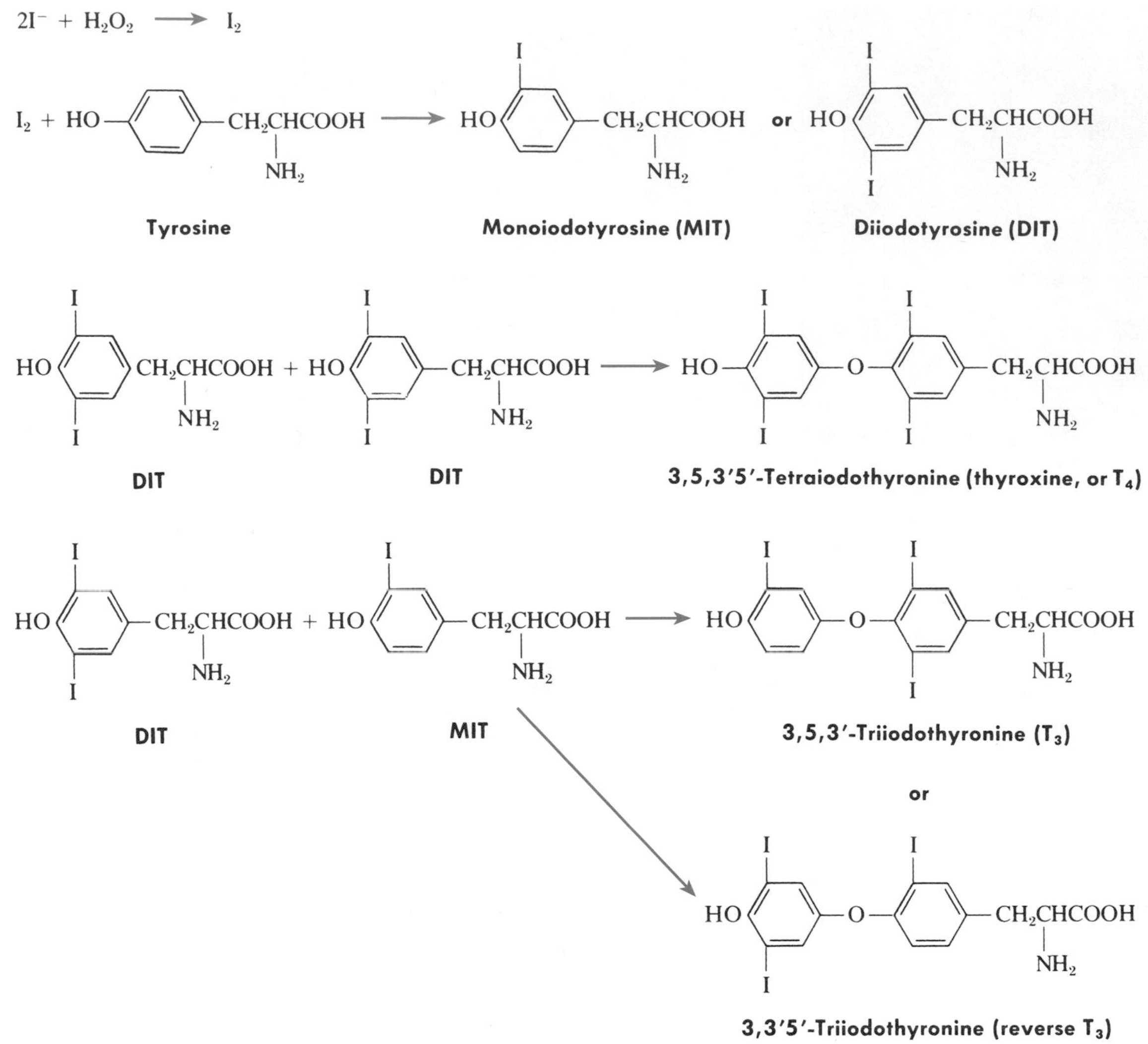

■ Fig. 44-2 Overall chemical pathway of thyroid hormone synthesis. All these reactions occur with tyrosine molecules that are incorporated into the protein thyroglobulin by peptide linkages. T_4 and T_3 are the biologically active hormone molecules.

150 µg. In a steady state, virtually the same amount, 400 µg, is excreted in the urine. Iodide is actively concentrated in the thyroid gland, salivary glands, gastric glands, lacrimal glands, mammary glands, and choroid plexus. About 70 to 80 µg of iodide is taken up daily by the thyroid gland from a circulating pool that contains approximately 250 to 750 µg of iodide. If this extrathyroidal iodide pool is labeled with a small dose of radioactive iodine (^{123}I or ^{131}I), the percentage of thyroid uptake of this tracer in 24 hours (8% to 35%) gives a dynamic index of thyroid gland activity. The total iodide content of the thyroid gland averages 7500 µg, virtually all of which is in the form of iodothyronines. In a steady-state condition, 70 to 80 µg of iodide, or about 1% of the total, is released from the gland daily. Of this amount, 75% is secreted as thyroid hormone and the remainder is free iodide. The large ratio (100:1) of iodide stored in the form of hormone to the amount turned over daily protects the individual from the effects of iodide deficiency for about 2 months. Iodide is further conserved by a marked reduction in the renal excre-

tion of iodide as the circulating concentration and filtered load fall.

Iodide is not plentiful in the environment, and deficiency of iodide is a major cause of **hypothyroidism** in such varied areas of the world as China and the Peruvian Andes. This tragic form of endemic **cretinism** (see below) can be easily prevented by public health programs that add iodide to table salt or that provide yearly injections of a slowly absorbed iodide preparation.

Iodide is actively transported into the gland against chemical and electrical gradients by a Na$^+$-I$^-$cotransport (symport) system (see Chapter 1) that is located in the basal membrane of the thyroid epithelial cells. Normally, a thyroid/ plasma-free iodide ratio of 30 is maintained. This so-called **iodide trap** requires energy generation by oxidative phosphorylation and displays saturation kinetics. The sodium-iodide symporter (NIS) is a plasma membrane

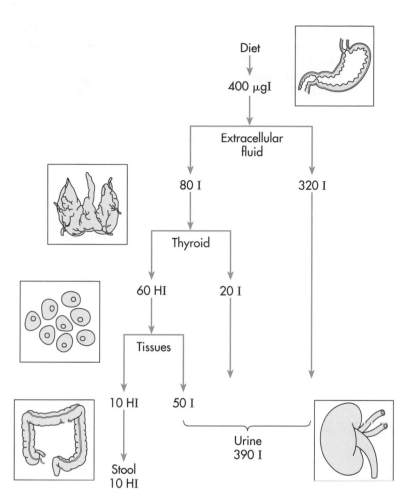

Diet

400 μgI

Extracellular fluid

80 I   320 I

Thyroid

60 HI   20 I

Tissues

10 HI   50 I

Urine
390 I

Stool
10 HI

■ **Fig. 44-3** Average daily iodide turnover in humans in the United States. Note that 20% of the intake is taken up by the thyroid gland and 15% turns over in hormone synthesis and disposal. The unneeded excess is excreted in the urine. *I,* Iodide; *HI,* hormonal iodide.

protein with 643 amino acids and 13 transmembrane loops. One iodide anion is contransported uphill against an iodide gradient, while two sodium ions move down a natural sodium gradient from the extracellular fluid into the thyroid cell. The energy source for this transfer is provided by a Na^+,K^+-ATPase in the plasma membrane, which is ouabain inhibited (Chapter 1). Expression of the NIS gene is inhibited by iodide and stimulated by TSH. Numerous inflammatory cytokines also suppress NIS gene transcription. A primary reduction in dietary iodide intake depletes the circulating iodide pool and greatly enhances the activity of the iodide trap. Under these circumstances, the percentage of thyroid uptake of iodide can reach 80% to 90%.

A number of anions, such as thiocyanate (CNS^-), perchlorate ($HClO_4^-$), and pertechnetate (TcO_4^-) act as competitive or noncompetitive inhibitors of iodide transport via NIS. If iodide cannot be rapidly incorporated into tyrosine after its uptake by the cell, administration of one of these anions will, by blocking further iodide uptake, cause a rapid discharge of the iodide from the gland. This discharge occurs as a result of the high thyroid/plasma concentration gradient.

Rapid iodide discharge can be demonstrated by monitoring the thyroid gland in vivo after the iodide pool is labeled with radioactive iodine. This procedure assists in the diagnosis of biosynthetic defects in hormone synthesis. In its radioactive form as $^{99m}TcO_4$, pertechnetate is a useful substitute for radioactive iodine in the measurement of the trapping function and in the visualization of thyroid gland anatomy by external isotope scanning with a photon detector.

The steps in thyroid hormone synthesis subsequent to entry of iodide into the gland are shown in Fig. 44-2 and depicted in Fig. 44-4. Once within the gland, iodide rapidly moves to the apical surface of the epithelial cells. From there, it is transported into the lumen of the follicles by a sodium-independent iodide/chloride transporter, named **pendrin**. Iodide (I^-) is immediately oxidized to iodine (I^0) and incorporated into tyrosine molecules (Fig. 44-2). The latter are not free in solution, but they are incorporated by peptide linkages within **thyroglobulin.** Thyroglobulin is a large glycoprotein that also contains covalently bound phosphate and sulfate residues. Thyroglobulin is synthesized on the rough endoplasmic reticulum of thyroid epithelial cells as peptide units of molecular weight 330,000 (the primary translation product of its messenger RNA). These units combine into a dimer, after which carbohydrate moieties are added as the molecule moves to the Golgi apparatus. The completed protein is contained in small vesicles, which move to the apical plasma membrane and into the adjacent lumen of the follicle (Fig. 44-4).

Immediately within the follicle, at the apical membrane-colloid interface, thyroglobulin is iodinated to form both **monoiodotyrosine (MIT)** and **diiodotyrosine (DIT)** (Fig. 44-2). After iodination, two DIT molecules are coupled to form T_4, or one MIT and one DIT molecule are coupled to form T_3. Very little reverse T_3 (rT_3) is synthesized. This entire sequence of reactions is catalyzed by **thyroid peroxidase (TPO),** an enzyme complex largely localized to the apical membrane. TPO is a glycosylated heme-containing protein that spans the follicular apical membrane. The immediate oxidant (electron acceptor) for the reaction iodide $\rightarrow$ iodine is hydrogen peroxide (H_2O_2). The mechanism whereby H_2O_2 is itself generated in the thyroid gland likely involves reduction of oxygen by NADPH via a calcium-stimulated NADPH oxidase that is also localized to the apical membrane. A mechanism also exists for disposing of excess H_2O_2 and other peroxides that may be generated as intermediates in the complex reactions leading to T_4 and T_3. Several selenium-containing enzymes, including 5-monodeiodinases and thioredoxin reductase, catalyze the reduction of potentially toxic concentrations to the thyroid cell of H_2O_2 and other peroxides.

A closer look at the formation of MIT and DIT reveals that a single tyrosine, located at the fifth position from the N terminus of both MIT and DIT (site A), is a preferential but not an exclusive site of synthesis of T_4 or T_3. About 10% of all tyrosines in thyroglobulin are iodinated. Both iodide and tyrosines are complexed to sites on the peroxidase enzyme; they undergo oxidation by H_2O_2 and are then combined to form MIT or DIT. The next step, coupling, may be facilitated by the three-dimensional structure of thyroglobulin. This structure brings an MIT or DIT molecule at site A next to a second MIT or DIT molecule at site B, which is buried deeper within thyroglobulin. The second MIT or DIT at site B donates its iodinated phenolic ring to the first MIT or DIT at site A. Depending on the pairing, this process produces T_4 or T_3 at site A, and it leaves dehydroalanine at site B in peptide linkage within thyroglobulin.

Thyroglobulin iodination occurs rapidly; labeled iodide appears in hormone molecules 1 minute after in vivo administration. After 1 hour, 90% to 95% of iodide is organically bound, with each thyroglobulin molecule containing 5 to 50 iodine atoms. The usual distribution of iodoamino acids, as residues per molecule of thyroglobulin, is MIT, 7; DIT, 6; T_4, 2; and T_3, 0.2. Approximately one third of the iodine in thyroglobulin is in the form of calorigenic hormone (T_4 and T_3). Certain factors regulate the ratio of T_3 synthesis to T_4 synthesis. When iodide availability is restricted, the formation of T_3 is favored. Because T_3 is three times as potent as T_4, this response provides more active hormone per molecule of organified iodide. The proportion of T_3 is also increased when the gland is hyperstimulated by TSH or other activators.

Once thyroglobulin has been iodinated, it is stored in the lumen of the follicle as colloid (Fig. 44-4). Release of the peptide-linked T_4 and T_3 into the bloodstream requires pro-

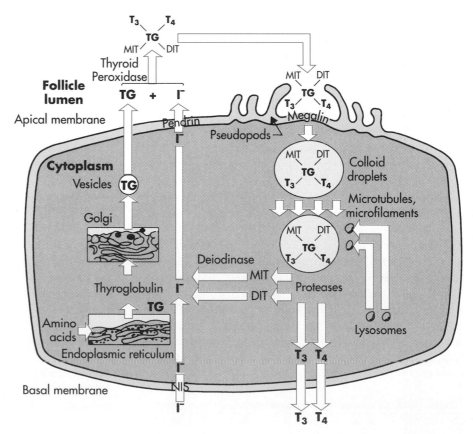

■ **Fig. 44-4** Overall schema of thyroid hormone synthesis and release. (1) Iodide is taken up by a sodium-iodide-symporter (NIS) in the basal membrane and crosses to the apical membrane where it is transferred into the follicular lumen. (2) T_4 and T_3 synthesis, catalyzed by thyroid peroxidase (TPO), occurs within the protein molecule thyroglobulin *(TG)* at the membrane between the cytoplasm and the follicle lumen. (3) Retrieval of stored hormone requires endocytosis of the colloid, facilitated by the TG receptor "megalin," followed by intracytoplasmic proteolysis by lysosomes. Iodide in the precursor molecules monoiodotyrosine *(MIT)* and diiodotyrosine *(DIT)* is recovered by the action of the enzyme deiodinase.

teolysis of the thyroglobulin. Histochemical and radiographic studies have demonstrated that the colloid is retrieved from the lumen of the follicle by the epithelial cell through endocytosis. An apical membrane molecule, similar to the low-density lipoprotein (LDL) cholesterol receptor, called **megalin,** mediates the uptake of thyroglobulin from the follicle. Endocytosis starts when the plasma cell membrane forms pseudopods that engulf a pocket of colloid. After this portion of the luminal content has been pinched off by the plasma cell membrane, it appears as a colloid droplet within the cytoplasm (Fig. 44-5). The droplet consists of thy-

roglobulin in small vesicles, which moves through the cytoplasm toward the basal membrane, probably as a result of microtubule and microfilament function. At the same time, lysosomes move from the base toward the apex of the cell and fuse with the colloid droplets. The action of the lysosomal proteases (cathepsins common to many tissues) then releases free T_4 and T_3, which leave the cell through the plasma membrane at the basal end and enter the bloodstream via the adjacent rich capillary plexus.

The MIT and DIT molecules, which also are released during proteolysis of thyroglobulin, are rapidly deiodinated

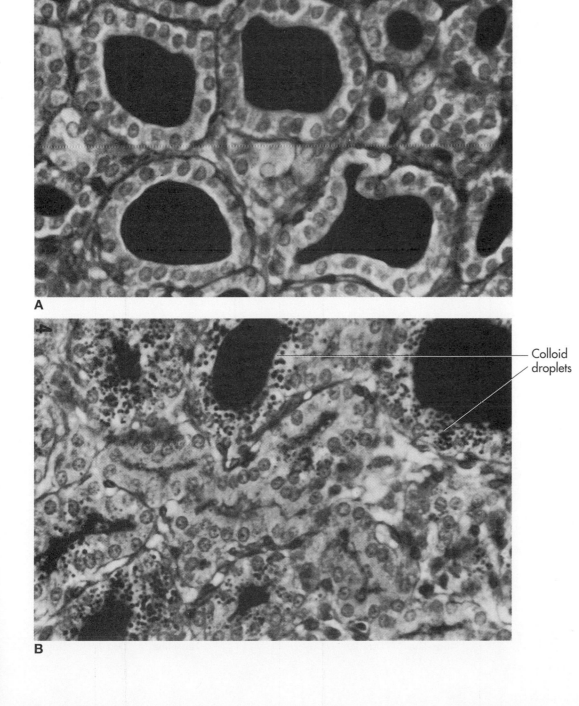

■ Fig. 44-5
Histological demonstration of the process of resorption of colloid.
A, Unstimulated follicles. **B,** Within minutes of TSH administration, colloid droplets are seen inside the follicular cells. (From Wollman SH et al: *J Cell Biol* 21:191, 1964.)

Colloid droplets

within the follicular cell by the enzyme **deiodinase** (Fig. 44-4). Because MIT and DIT are metabolically useless and would be lost in the urine if secreted, their deiodination retrieves the iodide for recycling into T_4 and T_3 synthesis. Only minor amounts of intact thyroglobulin leave the follicular cell under normal circumstances.

In acute and subacute inflammations of the thyroid gland, disruption of thyroid follicles leads to leakage of thyroglobulin into the circulation. The elevated plasma levels of thyroglobulin can be diagnostic of such diseases. In cases of thyroid cancer, total surgical removal of the gland and subsequent ablation of any gland remnants by radioactive iodine are usually performed. After such treatment, the presence of significant levels of thyroglobulin in the plasma indicates that persistent or recurrent cancer cells exist somewhere in the body.

REGULATION OF THYROID GLAND ACTIVITY

The most important regulator of thyroid gland function and growth is the hypothalamic-pituitary Thyroid-releasing hormone (TRH)-TSH axis (see Chapter 43 and Fig. 43-6).

Because the diurnal variation of TSH secretion is small, thyroid hormone secretion and plasma concentrations are relatively constant. Only small nocturnal increases in secretion of TSH and release of T_4 occur. *TSH stimulates the synthesis of thyroglobulin, the process of iodide trapping, and each of the subsequent steps in T_4 and T_3 synthesis. It also stimulates the endocytosis of colloid, the proteolysis of thyroglobulin, and the release of T_4 and T_3 from the gland.*

TSH increases expression of the genes for NIS, thyroglobulin, TPO, and megalin. In response to human TSH administration, serum T_4 and T_3 levels and radioactive iodine uptake approximately double, whereas serum thyroglobulin level increases 10-fold (Fig. 44-6). Sustained TSH stimulation leads to hypertrophy and hyperplasia of the follicular cells. The enlarged cells show an increased volume of endoplasmic reticulum, increased numbers of ribosomes, a larger and more complex Golgi apparatus, and an increase in DNA synthesis. Capillaries also proliferate, and thyroid blood flow increases. In the absence of TSH, marked atrophy of the gland occurs. However, in humans, a low basal level of thyroid hormone production and release can continue seemingly independent of TSH.

The regulatory effects of TSH are exerted through multiple actions (Fig. 44-7). The initial step is binding of TSH to a plasma transmembrane receptor of 764 amino acids. The

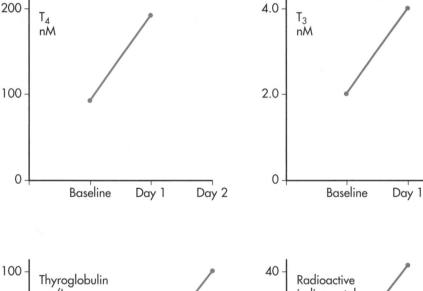
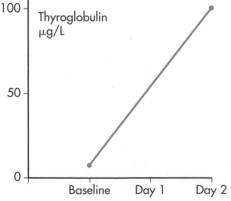
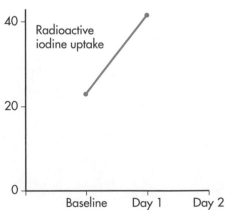

■ **Fig. 44-6**   Effect of administering a single dose of human TSH to normal individuals. Uptake of radioactive iodine by the thyroid gland, plasma thyroglobulin, and plasma T4 and T3 all rise. This shows that TSH stimulates all aspects of thyroid hormone synthesis and release by the gland. (From Torres et al: *J Clin Endocrinol Metab* 86:1660, 2001.)

extracellular α-subunit of the receptor binds the α- and β-subunits of TSH. The β-subunit of the receptor probably winds through the plasma membrane seven times and is functionally linked to adenylyl cyclase by a G-protein. The β-subunit ends in a short intracellular tail of about 80 amino acids. Although the β-subunit of TSH confers its specificity for the TSH receptor, it is the α-subunit of TSH (common to luteinizing hormone and follicle-stimulating hormone) that initiates the messenger cascade. This subunit of the TSH molecule binds to the N-terminus of the extracellular domain of the receptor. The binding triggers a conformational change in the receptor and causes the C-terminus of its extracellular domain to contact the transmembrane sites in the receptor. The latter then interact with neighboring G-proteins that activate adenylyl cyclase. The resultant increases in cAMP levels mediate TSH stimulation of iodide uptake by the cell, as well as many of its other actions on T_4 and T_3 synthesis. The phosphatidylinositol second messenger system helps to mediate some TSH effects.

Within minutes of thyroid cell exposure to TSH, thyroglobulin, which is stored within the follicular lumen, undergoes endocytosis, and colloid droplets appear in the cytoplasm (Fig. 44-5). Shortly thereafter, iodide uptake and TPO activity increase. Concurrently, TSH also stimulates glucose oxidation, especially via the hexose monophosphate shunt. This

reaction may be the means for generating the NADPH that is needed for the peroxidase reaction.

Further effects of TSH on the thyroid gland occur after a delay of hours to days. TSH stimulates transcription of the thyroglobulin and TPO genes, an action mediated by a specific protein transcription factor. Both insulin and insulin-like growth factors (IGFs) are also required for thyroglobulin synthesis to proceed. Nucleic acid and protein synthesis are also generally increased, via effects on both transcription and translation. These actions, which underlie the growth-promoting effects of TSH on the gland, are supported by local production of IGFs and epidermal growth factor in response to TSH.

The regulation of thyroid hormone secretion by TSH is under exquisite negative feedback control (see Fig. 43-6). Circulating T_4 and T_3 act on the pituitary gland to decrease TSH secretion; if the levels of T_4 and T_3 fall, TSH secretion increases. It is free T_4 and T_3, not the protein-bound portions, that regulate pituitary TSH output. The pituitary gland is capable of deiodinating T_4 to T_3, and the latter acts as the final effector molecule in turning off TSH.

Mutant TSH receptors or their G-proteins that are constitutively activated without hormone binding are one cause of thyroid adenomas and **hyperthyroidism.** These

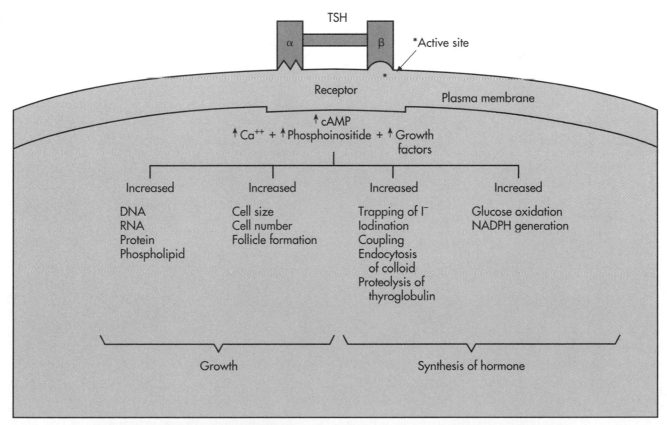

■ **Fig. 44-7** TSH actions on the thyroid cell. Cyclic adenosine monophosphate (cAMP) along with calcium ions (Ca^{2+}) and phosphoinositol products act as second messengers generated by TSH binding to its receptor. All steps in thyroid hormone production, as well as many aspects of thyroid cell metabolism and growth, are stimulated by TSH. Growth factors are important intermediaries in cell proliferation and in synthesis of some proteins such as thyroglobulin.

adenomas secrete T_4 and T_3 autonomously, that is, independent of TSH. The excessive production of T_4 and T_3 suppresses TSH secretion by negative feedback. The lack of TSH then leaves the remaining normal thyroid tissue atrophied and functionless. In another form of hyperthyroidism, **Graves' disease,** autoantibodies to the TSH receptor are produced. These immunoglobulins react with the TSH receptor and activate adenylyl cyclase, just as TSH does. The results are again a stimulated, TSH-independent gland and very low plasma TSH levels. Only rarely is hyperthyroidism caused by excess TSH from an adenoma of the pituitary thyrotrophs.

Another important regulator of thyroid gland function is iodide itself, which has a biphasic action. At relatively low levels of iodide intake, the rate of thyroid hormone synthesis is directly related to iodide availability. However, if the intake of iodide exceeds 2 mg/day, the intraglandular concentration of iodide reaches a level that suppresses NADPH oxidase activity and the NIS and TPO genes, and thereby the mechanism of hormone biosynthesis. This autoregulatory phenomenon is known as the **Wolff-Chaikoff effect.** As the intrathyroidal iodide level subsequently falls, NIS and TPO genes are derepressed and the production of thyroid hormone returns to normal. In unusual instances, the inhibition of hormone synthesis by iodide can be great enough to induce thyroid hormone deficiency. The temporary reduction in hormone synthesis by excess iodide can also be used therapeutically in hyperthyroidism.

Other modes of autoregulation may help prevent excessive responses to TSH stimulation. Thyroglobulin inhibits binding of TSH to its receptors, as well as the response of adenylyl cyclase to the tropic hormone. On the other hand, thyroglobulin and iodide both upregulate pendrin levels. The thyroid also receives adrenergic, VIPergic, and cholinergic innervation. Epinephrine and vasoactive intestinal polypeptide (VIP) stimulate T_4 release via increased cAMP, and acetylcholine inhibits it via increased cGMP. Prostaglandins also mimic some of the effects of TSH. The physiological roles of the above influences are not clear.

Thyroid hormones increase oxygen utilization, energy expenditure, and heat production. Therefore, it is logical to expect that the availability of active thyroid hormone correlates with changes in the body's caloric and thermal status. In fact, ingestion of excess calories, particularly in the form of carbohydrate, increases the production and plasma concentration of T_3 as well as the individual's metabolic rate, whereas prolonged fasting leads to corresponding decreases. Because most T_3 arises from circulating T_4 (Table 44-1), peripheral mechanisms are important in mediating these changes. However, starvation also lowers T_4 levels, rapidly in small animals and more gradually in humans.

Regulation of T_4 levels by energy intake and adipose tissue stores occurs through leptin effects in the central nervous system (CNS). Leptin directly stimulates TRH neurons, which leads to increased TSH and T_4. In addition, leptin-regulated neurons in the paraventricular nucleus (see Fig.

■ Table 44-1 Average thyroid hormone turnover

	T_4	T_3	rT_3
Daily production (μg)	90	35	35
From thyroid (%)	100	25	5
From T_4 (%)	—	75	95
Extracellular pool (μg)	850	40	40
Plasma concentration			
Total (μg/dl)	8.0	0.12	0.04
Free (ng/dl)	2.0	0.28	0.20
Half-life (days)	7	1	0.8
Metabolic clearance (L/day)	1	26	77
Fractional turnover per day (%)	10	75	90

40-14) reinforce the direct effects. Thus, leptin-stimulated proopiomelanocortin (POMC) neurons release *more α-melanocyte–stimulating hormone (MSH)*, which increases satiety (decreases energy intake) and also stimulates TRH neurons. Leptin-inhibited AgRP neurons release *less AgRP.* This increases α-MSH action and relieves the inhibition of TRH secretion by AgRP. Not surprisingly a negative feedback relationship also exists between leptin and thyroid hormones. High leptin levels increase thyroid hormone levels and thyroid hormone deficiency engenders high leptin levels. Thus when excess T_4 causes too much energy expenditure and loss of adipose tissue energy stores, leptin levels fall (see Fig. 44-8) and food intake is increased in compensation. When a deficiency of T_4 causes too little energy expenditure and a gain in adipose tissue stores, leptin levels rise (see Fig. 44-8) and food intake is decreased in compensation.

In animals, exposure to cold increases thyroid gland activity. Humans living in very cold regions also increase T_3 production and modestly increase TSH responsiveness to TRH. In the neonatal period, when the infant suddenly becomes responsible for maintenance of its own body temperature, facultative thermogenesis in its brown adipose tissue is required (see below). An acute rise in TSH secretion after birth is followed by a rise in plasma T_4 to levels well above those of adults. Over the ensuing weeks or months, plasma T_4 then subsides to a range that remains stable in adult life, until a small decline occurs with senescence.

Pharmacological inhibition of thyroid gland activity is of major therapeutic importance. A class of drugs, known as **thiouracils,** suppresses the synthesis of T_4 and T_3 by inhibiting peroxidase activity. Because organification is blocked, iodide taken up by the activity of the iodide trap is rapidly discharged again, as can be shown by studies with radioactive iodine (see above). After administration of thiouracils has continued for weeks, the stores of thyroid hormone (and of iodide) become depleted. These drugs are effective in the treatment of **hyperthyroidism.**

Lithium, frequently used to treat manic-depressive illness, inhibits the release of thyroid hormones and, secondarily, their synthesis, probably by blocking adenylyl cyclase and cAMP accumulation. Thus, lithium can cause **hypothyroidism.** Finally, a large excess of iodide, in

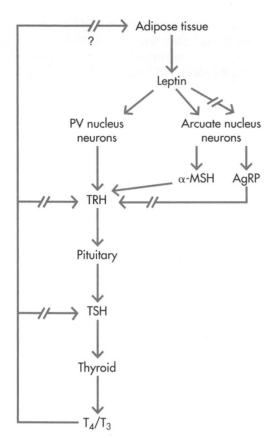

■ **Fig. 44-8** Relationship between regulation of energy turnover and of thyroid hormone production and action. An increase in leptin signaling from expanded adipose tissue energy stores leads, via connections with hypothalamic TRH neurons in the paraventricular nucleus and anorexigenic neurons in the arcuate nucleus, to increased TRH release and consequent TSH release. In turn, T_4/T_3 levels increase and energy expenditure therefore increases. The inhibitory effect of T_4/T_3 on TRH and TSH release, along with a likely downregulating effect on leptin production, prevents an overshoot by stimulating release of hypothalamic orexigenic signals. The latter part of the pathway may account for the increased appetite that characterizes hyperthyroidism.

addition to the effects previously noted, can also promptly inhibit thyroid hormone release. Although this action is transient, the administration of iodide for several weeks may benefit individuals with severe hyperthyroidism.

METABOLISM OF THYROID HORMONES

Table 44-1 shows the average daily production rates, pool sizes, plasma concentrations, half-lives, metabolic clearances, and fractional turnovers of T_4, T_3, and rT_3. *T_4 is clearly the dominant secreted and circulating form of thyroid hormone.* In contrast, the major portion of T_3 and virtually all of rT_3 are derived secondarily from circulating T_4, rather than primarily from thyroid gland secretion. *Thus, T_4 serves primarily as a prohormone for T_3; probably in addition, T_4 provides some intracellular action of its own.* The "storage" function of plasma T_4 is also reflected in its much lower

metabolic clearance and fractional turnover rates, compared with those of T_3 or rT_3. The small amount of intact thyroglobulin that is secreted circulates at an average plasma concentration of 5 ng/ml.

Most conversion of T_4 to T_3 occurs in tissues with high blood flows and rapid exchanges with plasma; such tissues include the liver and the kidneys. This process supplies circulating T_3 for uptake by other tissues in which local T_3 generation is too restricted to provide sufficient thyroid hormone action. Aging is associated with a decrease in TSH secretion, which in turn leads to a decrease in T4 production. Because this decrease in the T_4 level is balanced by a reduction in T_4 degradation, plasma T_4 levels are essentially unchanged. However, plasma T_3 levels decline slightly.

Secreted T_4 and T_3 circulate in the bloodstream almost entirely bound to proteins. Normally, only about 0.03% of total plasma T4 and 0.3% of total plasma T_3 exist in the free state (Table 44-1). However, free T_4 and T_3 are the critical fractions that are *biologically active,* not only in exerting thyroid hormone effects on peripheral tissues, but in pituitary feedback as well. The major binding protein is **thyroxine-binding globulin (TBG).** TBG is a glycoprotein α-globulin that is synthesized in the liver. Each TBG molecule binds one molecule of T_4; at the normal TBG concentration of 1.5 ng/dl, 20 μg of T_4 can be bound per deciliter of plasma.

About 70% of circulating T_4 and T_3 is bound to TBG; 10% to 15% is bound to another specific thyroid-binding protein, called **transthyretin (TTR).** Albumin binds 15% to 20%, and 3% is bound to lipoproteins. Compared with TBG, TTR and albumin have much lower affinities but much higher capacities for binding T_4 and T_3. Ordinarily, however, only alterations in TBG concentration significantly affect total plasma T_4 and T_3 levels.

Two important biological functions have been ascribed to TBG. First, it maintains a large circulating reservoir of T_4, which buffers any acute changes in thyroid gland function. Even the instantaneous addition to the plasma of the amount of calorigenic hormone needed for an entire day would cause only a barely perceptible increase in the total T_4 concentration. Conversely, after removal of the thyroid gland, it would take 1 week for the plasma T_4 concentration to fall as much as 50%. Second, the binding of plasma T_4 and T_3 to large proteins prevents the loss of these relatively small hormone molecules into the urine, and thereby helps conserve iodide. The roles of TTR and perhaps also of albumin are to deliver T_4 and T_3 to cells; TTR, in particular, may provide thyroid hormones to the central nervous system.

Recently a third function for TBG has been proposed, based on its identification as a member of a large family of proteins, most of which have serine protease *inhibitor* properties. Their most distinctive characteristic is that when a certain peptide bond is cleaved by a serine protease, the remaining molecule is transformed in its three-dimensional structure. In the case of TBG, this change results in a much lower affinity for T_4 and release of the free hormone. This occurs on contact of TBG with polymorphonuclear leukocytes that have been activated, for example, by a bacterial infection. Production of a very high local concentration of free T_4, followed by rapid deiodination of the T_4, would generate a high local iodine concentration. This iodine would create an antibacterial environment and the local T_4 might also serve unknown physiological or pathophysiological functions.

The reservoir function of TBG is best understood by examining the chemical equilibrium between T_4 and TBG. This equilibrium governs the distribution of the hormone between the free (T_4) and bound ($T_4 \cdot$ TBG) forms.

$$T_4 + TBG \leftrightarrows T_4 \cdot TBG \qquad (44.1)$$

$$Keq = \frac{[T_4 \cdot TBG]}{[T_4][TBG]} \qquad (44.2)$$

$$\frac{[T_4]}{[T_4] \cdot [TBG]} = \frac{Free\ T_4}{Bound\ T_4} = \frac{1}{Keq\ [TBG]} \qquad (44.3)$$

$$[T_4] = [T_4 \cdot TBG] \times \frac{1}{Keq\ [TBG]} \qquad (44.4)$$

A temporary decrease in free T_4, caused either by a decrease in thyroid gland output or by an accelerated uptake by target cells, can be rapidly compensated for by the dissociation of bound T_4 ($T_4 \cdot$ TBG), until the new ratio of T_4/($T_4 \cdot$ TBG) returns to that required by Keq (equation 44-3). A temporary increase in free T_4, caused by endogenous secretion or exogenous administration, can be rapidly compensated for by association of the excess T_4 with TBG, because normally only 30% of the available T_4-binding sites on TBG are occupied. Of course, *sustained decreases or increases in T_4 supply, which are caused by thyroid disease, eventually lead to sustained decreases or increases in free T_4, because the latter is directly proportional to $T_4 \cdot$ TBG* (equation 44-4).

Note also that a primary change in TBG concentration will also disturb the ratio of free to bound T_4 (equation 44-3). In this situation, the normal thyroid gland must increase or decrease its rate of hormone secretion appropriately, until the new equilibrium state restores the free T_4 level to normal.

TBG concentration can decrease because of reduced hepatic synthesis (liver disease) or excessive loss in the urine (kidney disease). The free T_4 concentration will then increase temporarily. In compensation, pituitary TSH secretion will be suppressed by negative feedback. T_4 output by the thyroid gland will then decrease until the new, lower steady-state level of bound $T_4 \cdot$ TBG yields a normal level of free T_4 (equation 44-4). TBG levels can also increase, most commonly because of estrogen administration or pregnancy. In this situation, free T_4 will decrease temporarily; this decrease will stimulate pituitary secretion of TSH. Consequently, T_4 output by the thyroid gland will increase. T_4 output will continue until the elevated level of bound $T_4 \cdot$ TBG is sufficient to restore the free T_4 level to normal in a new steady-state condition.

Although major alterations in TBG are not usually caused by thyroid gland disease, TBG levels must be considered when the total thyroid hormone concentrations in the plasma are measured for diagnostic purposes.

Identical considerations govern the circulating levels of free and bound T_3. However, the buffering action of TBG is less effective for T_3, because the Keq for T_3 is an order of magnitude lower than that for T_4 (2×10^9 versus 2×10^{10}, respectively), and because the total extrathyroidal pool of T_3 is much smaller than that of T_4 (Table 44-1). Thus, rapid addition of T_3, in an amount equivalent to the calorigenic hormone needed for an entire day, produces greater swings in the concentrations of total and free T_3.

The major pathways of peripheral metabolism of circulating thyroid hormones are outlined in Fig. 44-9. Most of the T_4 that is released by the gland daily undergoes deiodination. However, approximately 15% is irreversibly excreted in the bile, as the various iodothyronines in hydrophilic glucuronide or sulfate conjugates. Tetraiodoacetic acid and triiodoacetic acid are less important metabolites. The liver, kidneys, and skeletal muscles are the major sites of T_4 degradation. The overall rate of disposal of T_4 is directly related to the free T_4 concentration in the plasma. Thus, T_4 increases its own degradative metabolism. The entire cascade of products—T_3, T_2, and T_1—of the sequential deiodination steps is regularly increased in the plasma in hyperthyroidism (T_4 excess) and is usually decreased in hypothyroidism (T_4 deficiency).

RELATIONSHIP BETWEEN HORMONE METABOLISM AND HORMONE ACTION

The initial step in T_4 metabolism—the intracellular conversion of T_4 to either T_3 or rT_3—is of critical importance to thyroid hormone action. T_3 is the hormone of greatest biological activity, whereas rT_3 has no significant calorigenic action. Therefore, factors that regulate the relative rates of outer ring versus inner ring monodeiodination (Fig. 44-9) also determine the quantitative biological effect of secreted T.

At least three types of deiodinases have been identified, distinguished by the presence of a rare amino acid in which the trace element selenium is substituted for sulfur in cysteine (selenocysteine). The function of these enzymes depends critically on the presence of selenium at the active catalytic sites. For type 1 5'-deiodinase (D1), rT_3 is the preferred substrate yielding *3,3-T_2* (Fig. 44-9). Type 2 5'-deiodinase (D2) efficiently converts T_4 to T_3 (Fig. 44-9). Both types are present in the pituitary gland, whereas D1 is also expressed in the thyroid gland, liver, and kidney, and D2 in skeletal muscle, brain, and brown fat. Type 3 5-deiodinase converts T_4 to rT_3 (Fig. 44-9) and is found in the brain, skin, and placenta. The T_3-generating activity, **5'-monodeiodination,** is supplied by D1 and D2. In the pituitary gland and certain areas of the brain, D2 strongly favors local T_3 generation. In the liver and kidney D1 5'-monodeiodinase activity has a lower affinity but a higher capacity for T_4 than does D2. D1 5'-

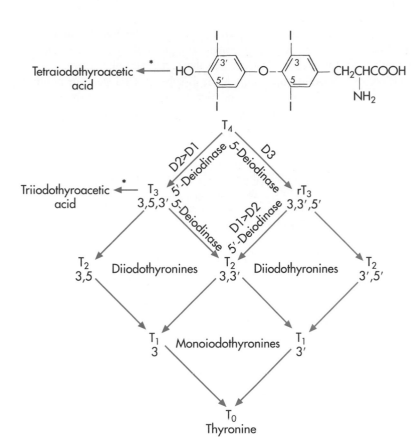

Fig. 44-9 Peripheral metabolism of thyroxine *(T₄)* is largely by successive deiodinations. A key regulatory step is the proportion of T_4 undergoing the initial deiodination to metabolically active T_3 versus metabolically inactive rT_3. Asterisks signify oxidative deamination and decarboxylation. T_4 and T_3 sulfates and glucuronides are also formed in small amounts.

monodeiodinase activity has both a high affinity and a high capacity for rT_3. Thus D1 regulates the circulating T_3 supply by augmenting T_3 production and disposing of rT_3 generated from excess T_4. Prior sulfation of iodothyronine molecules greatly increases their rate of deiodination by D1 in the liver.

In humans, the normal distribution of T_4 products is approximately 45% T_3 and 55% rT_3. An increase in T_4 concentration leads to a decrease in its conversion to T_3. Thus, the biological effects of T_4 excess or deficiency are automatically mitigated slightly by accelerated or retarded metabolic inactivation, respectively.

Certain clinical states and factors are associated with a reduced conversion of T_4 to T_3, and often with a reciprocally enhanced conversion of T_4 to rT_3. These conditions include the gestational period, fasting, major medical and surgical stress, catabolic diseases, hepatic disease, renal failure, thiouracil drugs, and β-adrenergic blockade. In many cases, inhibition of hepatic D1 activity appears to explain this switch. As seen in Fig. 44-9, inhibition of 5′-monodeiodinase decreases the production of T_3 from T_4 (reducing plasma T_3), and it simultaneously decreases the degradation of rT_3 to $3,3′-T_2$ (increasing plasma rT_3). The reduction of 5′-monodeiodinase activity may also result from decreased glucose metabolism, increased free fatty acid (FFA) metabolism, and excess secretion of the stress hormone cortisol. When 5′-monodeiodinase activity is reduced, sulfation of T_4 and T_3 increases, and the addition

of sulfate greatly diminishes the biological activity of whatever T_3 is produced.

The biological effects of T_4 are largely a result of its intracellular conversion to T_3. T_3 has 10 times the affinity for the thyroid receptor (TR) than does T_4 (and 100 times the affinity for rT_3). When administered exogenously, T_3 is three to four times more potent than T_4 in humans. However, evidence continues to favor some intrinsic biological activity of T_4 itself. For example, in hypothyroid individuals, a low plasma T_4 level (and high TSH level) can be accompanied by a state of biological thyroid deficiency, despite a normal plasma T_3. Conversely, a clinically normal state can exist with a normal plasma T_4 concentration, despite a low plasma T3. In the absence of endogenous thyroid gland function, the maintenance of a euthyroid (normal) state requires exogenous doses of T_3 that sustain supranormal plasma T_3 levels, whereas only doses of T_4 that sustain normal plasma T_4 levels are required. An alternative possible explanation for these phenomena is that the T_3 that has been generated from T_4 *intracellularly* might be more effective than the T_3 that reaches its intracellular sites of action from the circulation.

INTRACELLULAR ACTIONS OF THYROID HORMONE

Free T_4 and T_3 both enter cells by a carrier-mediated, energy-dependent process. The plasma membrane carriers for T_4

and T_3 resemble organic anion transporters and T and L-type amino acid transporters. The transport of T_4 is rate limiting for the intracellular production of T_3. T_4 transport is inhibited by aromatic amino acids, free fatty acids, and carnitine. Within the cell, most, if not all, of the T_4 is converted to T_3 (or rT3). T_3 and T_4 bind to a nuclear receptor of the steroid hormone, vitamin D, retinoid family (Fig. 44-10) (see also Chapter 39 and Fig. 39-13), which acts as a transcription factor.

Two main TRs are expressed by different genes on separate chromosomes, and are designated α and β. Each gene is alternatively spliced, yielding $TR_{\alpha-1}$ and $TR_{\alpha-2}$ and $TR_{\beta-1}$ and $TR_{\beta-2}$. These receptor subtypes range from 410 to 514 amino acids in length, and they have strong homologies in their ligand-binding and DNA-binding domains. $TR_{\alpha-2}$ is noteworthy for being homologous to a viral oncogene, c-erbA. $TR_{c-erbA-\alpha 2}$ cannot bind T_3, and its weak binding to TREs cannot transactivate the T_3 target genes; $TR_{c-erb-\alpha 2}$ may actually inhibit transcription by other T_3-liganded TRs. The tissue distribution of $TR_{\alpha-1}$ and $TR_{\beta-1}$ is widespread. The former is especially expressed in cardiac and skeletal muscle, and $TR_{\alpha-1}$ is the dominant TR that transduces thyroid hormone actions on the heart. By contrast, $TR_{\beta-1}$ is expressed more in the brain, liver, and kidney. $TR_{\beta-2}$ expression is restricted to the pituitary and critical areas of the hypothalamus. T_3-bound $TR_{\beta-2}$ is responsible for inhibiting the expression of the prepro-TRH gene in the paraventricular neurons of the hypothalamus and of the β-subunit TSH gene in pituitary thyrotropes. Thus negative feedback effects of thyroid hormone on both TRH and TSH secretion are largely mediated by $TR_{\beta-2}$. T_3 also downregulates $TR_{\beta-2}$ gene expression in the pituitary gland.

An understanding of TR subtypes and tissue expression is of more than academic interest because inactivating mutant genes have been found increasingly to be causes of clinical syndromes manifest by resistance to thyroid hormone. The most common mutations occur in the $TR_{\beta-2}$ subtype; therefore there is incomplete negative thyroid hormone feedback at the hypothalamic-pituitary level. Typically, plasma TSH is elevated and the excessive stimulation of the thyroid gland in turn causes high plasma levels of T_4 and T_3. When the resistance is purely at the hypothalamic-pituitary level, the patient may exhibit signs of hyperthyroidism due to excess effects of high thyroid hormone levels on peripheral tissue, particularly on the heart through $TR_{\alpha-1}$. In other patients with more global resistance to thyroid hormone, hypothyroid

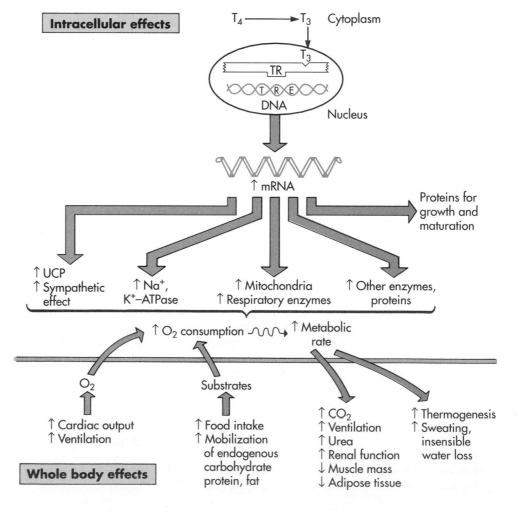

Fig. 44-10 Overall schema of thyroid hormone effects. The upper portion represents intracellular actions resulting from T_3 binding to its nuclear receptor *(TR)*, which is linked to thyroid regulatory elements (TREs) in target DNA molecules. The lower portion catalogs all the various whole body effects of thyroid hormone that sustain increased oxygen consumption and permit disposal of the excess CO_2, heat, and metabolic products.

manifestations may predominate. A mutant TR allele that cannot be expressed causes no discernible abnormality, because a single normal TR allele can sustain normal thyroid function. An expressed allele with a point mutation may bind to TREs and thereby inhibit binding of the T_3-liganded normal TR allele, thus causing loss of thyroid function.

Detailed knowledge of TR subtypes and the actions they mediate holds great pharmacological promise. Specific subtype agonists and antagonists will make it possible to selectively invoke desirable thyroid hormone actions and to inhibit others, depending on the circumstances. Examples may include ameliorating obesity, decreasing tachycardia, increasing cardiac inotropic effects, and decreasing chronic anxiety.

Usually, *TR constitutively represses target gene expression, although certain genes may be constitutively activated.* Binding of T_3 (or possibly T_4, see below) to TR relieves the repression exerted through the TRE, and thus gene expression is induced. Several corepressors, including histone deacetylase (see Chapter 39), are involved in TR inhibition of basal transcription. Coactivators of TR have also been described, and phosphorylation of TR by mitogen-activated protein (MAP) kinase may also enhance its transcriptional activity.

TREs have two half-sites, with the nucleotide base sequence AGGTCA. Two TRs can form a homodimer that binds to both TRE half-sites. More often, however, one TR molecule and one retinoid receptor molecule form a heterodimer that, when bound to T_3, activates the target gene. A TR-retinoid receptor (RXRα) dimer mediates thyroid hormone suppression of the TSH β-subunit gene. The two TRE half-sites can function as direct repeats of each other, as palindromes, as reverse palindromes, or even as single sites themselves. Additional cell-specific, constitutive basal factors are necessary to permit T_3-receptor complex action on certain genes in some cells and at certain stages of development. Subsequent to T_3-TR-TRE interactions, a large number of messenger RNA levels are increased or decreased, and the synthesis of the related proteins is altered accordingly. Examples of the many T_3 target genes include those for growth hormone, osteocalcin, myosin chains, malic enzyme, enzymes of lipogenesis, TSH, and the T_3 receptor itself.

In addition to nuclear receptors, thyroid hormone-binding sites have been identified in ribosomes, mitochondria, and the plasma membrane. Binding of thyroid hormone to these sites may mediate either posttranscriptional and pretranslational events, such as association of messenger RNA with ribosomes, or posttranslational processes, such as membrane transport. These mechanisms may explain some thyroid hormone actions that are not presently accounted for by modulation of gene expression.

The responsiveness of tissues to T_3 correlates with their nuclear receptor number and with the degree of receptor saturation, although the correlation is not always linear. In humans, about half the available T_3 receptor sites are usually occupied. In some tissues, T_3 downregulates its own receptors by inhibiting their synthesis at the level of gene expression; this action provides still another means for receptor modulation of T_3 action. Because thyroid hormone appears to act largely through influencing transcription, many of its effects can be blocked by inhibitors of protein synthesis. Usually, there is a 12- to 48-hour delay before most of the hormone's effects become evident in vivo. Indeed, several weeks of T_4 replacement are required in humans before all the consequences of the hypothyroid state are eliminated.

The multitude of thyroid hormone actions is still difficult to explain exactly on an intracellular basis. A large catalog of changes in enzymes, structural and functional proteins, and substrates—all induced by thyroid hormone—can be listed (Table 44-2). However, a single final common pathway that serves as a unifying mechanism of the hormone's actions, particularly on oxygen utilization, has not yet been established incontrovertibly. The hormone acts at multiple loci, which vary in different tissues. General effects in the nucleus include stimulation of RNA polymerase and phosphoprotein kinases and the synthesis of other nuclear proteins. These nuclear effects are followed or paralleled by an increase in the biogenesis of mitochondria and in their rate of respiration. The number and size of the inner membrane components and the areas of mitochondria, as well as protein synthesis and RNA synthesis of these organelles, are all increased by thyroid hormone. These effects may also involve mitochondrial DNA. Key respiratory chain enzyme activities, such as NADPH cytochrome c reductase and cytochrome oxidase, are increased by thyroid hormone. α-Glycerophosphate dehydrogenase and pyridine nucleotide transhydrogenases, which are important in regulating the levels of pyridine nucleotide cofactors, are likewise

■ **Table 44-2** Selected molecules whose concentration, activity, and/or gene expression is modulated by thyroid hormone

Increased	*Decreased*
Na$^+$,K$^+$-ATPase (in some tissues)	TSH (thyrotropin)
Cytochrome oxidase	Thyroid hormone receptor
α-Glycerophosphate dehydrogenase	Myosin heavy chain-β
Pyridine nucleotide transhydrogenases	Creatine kinase
Urea	Inhibitory G-protein
Malic enzyme	Total and LDL cholesterol
Ca-ATPase	
Myosin heavy chain-α	
Glucose transporters	
β-Adrenergic receptor	
Stimulatory G-protein	
cAMP	
Erythropoietin	
Tyrosine	
Osteocalcin	
Alkaline phosphatase	
Hydroxyproline	
Growth hormone	
Antidiuretic hormone	
Sex steroid-binding globulin	
Metabolites of cortisol	

increased. Clearly, these stimulatory actions of thyroid hormone on mitochondrial metabolism and size increase oxygen uptake and CO_2 production.

The experimental observation that excess thyroid hormone increases the rate of oxygen use and of heat production disproportionately to any particular amount of muscle work suggested that the hormone decreases the efficiency with which high-energy phosphate bonds are formed during aerobic respiration. However, this attractive hypothesis has not yet been completely proven. For instance, the normal P/O ratios of approximately 3 (fixation of phosphate/O_2 uptake) reported in muscle from a relatively small number of hyperthyroid humans controverts this hypothesis.

However, further insight into the regulation of O_2 utilization and thermogenesis by thyroid hormone has been gained by studies of facultative thermogenesis in brown adipose tissue (BAT) in rodents (Fig. 44-11). Humans and other mammals maintain a constant body temperature (homeothermy), irrespective of fluctuations in the environmental temperature. When challenged by a cold environment, temperature sensors in the hypothamus stimulate increased activity by the nearby sympathetic nervous system (SNS) center. Increased SNS output releases norepinephrine at nerve terminals in BAT, where the norepinephrine reacts with adrenergic receptors in the plasma membrane. Coupling via a G-protein and adenylyl cyclase results in an increased concentration of cAMP. This entire sequence, starting with the number of adrenergic receptors in BAT, is increased by thyroid hormone. Among its many other effects, cAMP increases the activity of D2 5′-monodeiodinase, and thereby generates

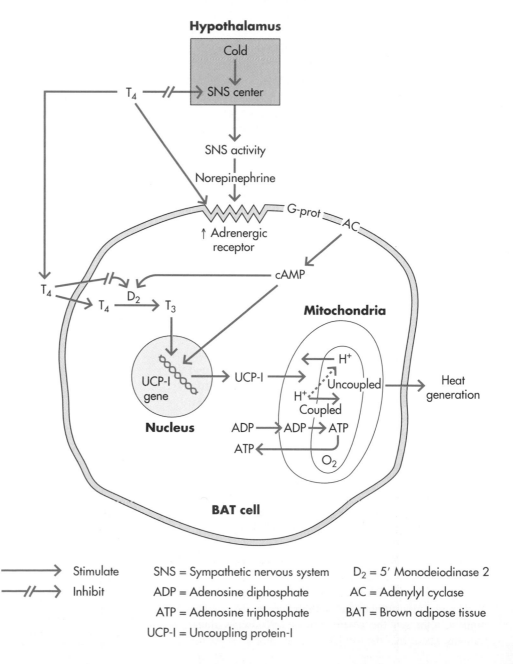

■ **Fig. 44-11** Interaction between thyroid hormones and the sympathetic nervous system in regulating facultative thermogenesis in brown adipose tissue. In response to cold, hypothalamic thermal sensors increase sympathetic outflow to adipose cells. Via β-adrenergic receptors, norepinephrine stimulates adenylyl cyclase activity and increased cAMP levels. T_4 enters the BAT cell where it is converted to T_3 and T_3 increases the norepinephrine receptor. Together T_3 and cAMP increase expression of the gene for uncoupling protein-1. UCP-1 uncouples synthesis of ATP from O_2 utilization by creating *a leak* of protons back into the mitochondria. The effect of an excessive amount of T4 can be partially offset by two other actions of T_4: (1) an inhibition of hypothalamic sympathetic outflow and (2) an inhibition of the 5′-deiodinase (D2) that converts T_4 to the more active T_3.

Stimulate   SNS = Sympathetic nervous system D_2 = 5′ Monodeiodinase 2

Inhibit   ADP = Adenosine diphosphate   AC = Adenylyl cyclase

ATP = Adenosine triphosphate   BAT = Brown adipose tissue

UCP-I = Uncoupling protein-I

more T_3 from the available intracellular T_4. Together the cAMP interaction with the CRE, and the T_3 interaction with the TRE, stimulate the promoter area of the gene for uncoupling protein-1 (UCP-1). UCP-1 levels increase and create a larger leak of protons across the mitochondrial membranes, thereby reducing the amount of adenosine triphosphate (ATP) that is generated from the passage of electrons up the respiratory chain (Chapter 40). Effectively, the oxidation of substrates and the utilization of O_2 has resulted in more of the available energy being used to maintain body temperature by the "wasteful" production of heat. This co-stimulatory effect of thyroid hormone and cAMP on facultative thermogenesis is moderated at two other levels. T_4 inhibits D2 activity in BAT, which limits T3 generation when T_4 levels become too high. T_4 also limits SNS output from the hypothalamus, and thus SNS stimulation of BAT is reduced (Fig. 44-11). The increase in cAMP (SNS effect) induced by T_3 occurs via interaction of T_3 with TRa-1. T_3 interacts with TR_β to increase the expression of UCP-1.

The above paradigm has been applied to explain the increase in obligatory thermogenesis, which is largely the consequence of an increase in the resting/basal metabolic rate that results from thyroid hormone action. Certain elements of the system are present in human skeletal muscle, which is the largest contributor to the BMR. The expression of D2 5′-monodeiodinase is stimulated by β-adrenergy via cAMP, and it is inhibited by high T_4 levels. T_3 upregulates the UCP-2 and UCP-3 genes in human muscle, independently of increasing mitochondrial respiratory chain enzymes, but associated with a significant increase in BMR. Skeletal muscle in mice, over- or underexpressing UCP-3 coordinately increases or decreases the coupling of ATP generation to O_2 utilization. Conversely, in a study of humans with variable levels of BMR induced by a various energy intake regimens, the BMR did not correlate with the level of skeletal muscle UCP-2 or UCP-3 gene expression. Moreover, with fasting, as the BMR falls UCP-2 and UCP-3 gene expression rises. Although these discrepant observations may have other explanations, they appear to counter the theory that thyroid hormone raises BMR by inducing UCP-2 and UCP-3 in muscle.

Another explanation for thyroid hormone's ability to increase oxygen consumption arose from the observation that the hormone increases the activity and amount of plasma membrane Na^+,K^+-ATPase, an enzyme essential for membrane cation transport (see also Chapter 1). Ouabain, an inhibitor of this enzyme, also blocks the action of thyroid hormone on respiration. Because the sodium pump is responsible for up to 80% of the energy turnover in some tissues, large amounts of adenosine diphosphate (ADP) would be generated by augmenting its activity. The extra ADP that results from the increased Na^+,K^+-ATPase activity would then stimulate oxygen utilization in the mitochondria.

In keeping with this mechanism is a report that T_3 binds to the inner mitochondrial membrane enzyme, adenine nucleotide translocase, which is responsible for transporting ADP into and ATP out of the mitochondria. However, in some thyroid-sensitive tissues, Na^+,K^+-ATPase accounts for only 15% of total oxygen utilization. Hence, it is doubtful that this mechanism unifies thyroid hormone action on oxygen utilization. Another suggestion is that thyroid hormone simultaneously stimulates fatty acid synthesis and fatty acid oxidation, and it thereby operates a futile thermogenic energy cycle in order to produce heat for temperature regulation.

In tissues such as brain, in which oxygen consumption is not stimulated at all, thyroid hormones still increase the synthesis of specific structural or functional proteins. In brain and other tissues, thyroid hormones also stimulate the transport of amino acids across the cell membrane and thereby facilitate protein synthesis. On the other hand, proteolytic and lysosomal enzyme activities in muscle are also increased by thyroid hormone. T_4 and T_3 augment leucine flux and protein turnover (Fig. 40-7), and yet they also increase the ability of insulin to inhibit proteolysis.

WHOLE BODY ACTIONS OF THYROID HORMONE ON METABOLISM

General Effects

The most obvious in vivo effect of thyroid hormone is to increase the basal rate of oxygen consumption and heat production (Fig. 44-10). This action is demonstrated in all tissues except the brain, gonads, and spleen. Resting oxygen use in humans ranges from about 150 ml/min in the hypothyroid state to about 400 ml/min in the hyperthyroid state (normal, 225 to 250 ml/min). When standardized to body surface area, the basal metabolic rate ranges from −40% to +80% of normal at the clinical extremes of thyroid function. The respiratory quotient (RQ) is slightly decreased by thyroid hormone, suggesting a relative increased use of fatty acid substrates (Chapter 40). Glucose and fatty acid uptake and oxidation are both overall increased, as are lactate-glucose recycling and fatty acid-triglyceride recycling. Thyroid hormone does not specifically augment diet-induced oxygen utilization, and it may not change the efficiency of energy use during exercise.

Thermogenesis must also increase concomitantly with oxygen use (see above). Thus, changes in body temperature parallel fluctuations in thyroid hormone availability. The potential increase in body temperature, however, is moderated by a compensatory increase in heat loss through appropriate thyroid hormone-mediated increases in blood flow, sweating, and ventilation.

Respiratory Effects

Thyroid hormone could not stimulate oxygen utilization for long without also enhancing oxygen supply. Thus, T_4 and T_3 increase the resting respiratory rate, minute ventilation, and the ventilatory responses to hypercapnia and hypoxia (see Chapters 27 and 28). These actions maintain a normal arterial P_{O_2} when O_2 utilization is increased, and a normal P_{CO_2} when CO_2 production is increased. Additionally, the red blood cell mass increases slightly and thereby enhances the oxygen-carrying capacity. This increase in red blood cell mass results from stimulation of erythropoietin production, which arises directly by alteration of its gene expression and indirectly by way of the renal tissue hypoxia that results from increased O_2 use.

Cardiovascular Effects

Most important, thyroid hormone increases cardiac output, ensuring sufficient oxygen delivery to the tissues (Fig. 44-12). The resting heart rate and the stroke volume are both increased. The speed and force of myocardial contractions are enhanced, and the diastolic relaxation time is shortened. Systolic blood pressure is modestly augmented and diastolic blood pressure is decreased. The resultant widened pulse pressure reflects the combined effects of the increased stroke volume and the reduction in total peripheral vascular resistance that results from blood vessel dilation in skin, muscle, and heart. These effects in turn are partly secondary to the increase in tissue production of heat and CO_2 (see Chapter 17) that thyroid hormone induces. In addition, however, thyroid hormone directly decreases systemic vascular resistance by dilating resistance arterioles in the peripheral circulation. Total blood volume is increased also by activating the renin-angiotensin-aldosterone axis and thereby increasing renal tubular sodium reabsorption (see Chapter 36). Offsetting this latter, there is a negative feedback relationship between thyroid hormone and atrial natriuretic hormone (ANH). T_4/T_3 stimulate expression of the proANH gene by myocytes, and raise plasma ANH, thereby promoting sodium excretion. Conversely, ANH, which is present in thyroid follicular cell granules, decreases plasma T_4/T_3 by inhibiting TSH action on the thyroid gland.

The cardiac inotropic effects are partly indirect, via adrenergic stimulation, and partly direct (Fig. 44-12). Myocardial calcium uptake and adenylyl cyclase activity are increased and enhance contractile force. Thyroid hormone induces the myosin heavy-chain α gene and represses the β gene, thereby increasing the velocity of myocardial contraction. The calcium-ATPase of the sarcolemmal reticulum and its protein stimulator, phospholamban (see Chapter 16), are increased by T_3, which facilitates sequestration of calcium during diastole and shortens the relaxation time. Many of the cardiac muscle effects of thyroid hormone are mediated by $TR_{\alpha-1}$. Moreover, conversion of T_4 to T_3 is negligible in myocytes, so cardiac effects are dependent on T_3 transported in from the plasma.

Thyroid hormone levels in the normal range are necessary for optimum cardiac performance. A deficiency of thyroid hormone in humans reduces stroke volume, left ventricular ejection fraction, cardiac output, and the efficiency of cardiac function. The latter defect is shown by the fact that the stroke work index [(stroke volume/left ventricular mass) × peak systolic blood pressure] is decreased even more than is myocardial oxidative metabolism. The rise in systemic vascular resistance may contribute to this cardiac debility. On the other hand, though an excessive amount of thyroid hormone increases cardiac output, it also increases UCP-2 and UCP-3 in cardiac muscle. These increases uncouple energy generation from oxygen utilization during the β-oxidation of free fatty acids such as palmitate. Ultimately a form of high output cardiac failure can result.

> The cardiac effects of thyroid hormone are particularly important when aging individuals develop hyperthyroidism. The only clinical manifestation may be the development of rapid **atrial arrhythmias,** such as **flutter** or **fibrillation** (see Chapter 15). Alternatively, unexplained heart failure may occur or symptoms of coronary insufficiency may develop if the aging heart cannot meet its own increased oxygen need or the increased tissue oxygen demands.

■ **Fig. 44-12**   Mechanisms by which thyroid hormone increases cardiac output. The indirect mechanisms are probably quantitatively more important.

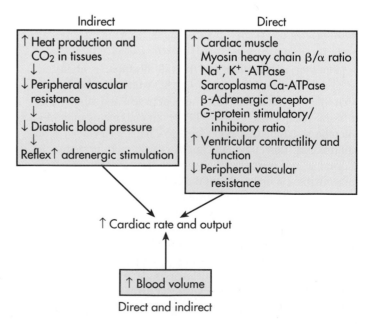

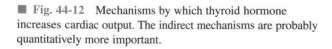

Normal function of skeletal muscles also requires optimal amounts of thyroid hormone. This requirement may also be related to the regulation of energy production and storage in this tissue. Glycolysis and glycogenolysis are increased and concentrations of glycogen and creatine phosphate are reduced by an excess of T_4 and T_3; the inability of muscle to take up and phosphorylate creatine leads to its increased urinary excretion. The role of increased expression of UCP-2 and UCP-3 and the uncoupling in skeletal muscle may mirror that in cardiac muscle.

Metabolic Effects

Increased oxygen use ultimately depends on an increased supply of necessary substrates for oxidation. Thyroid hormone stimulates the provision of these substrates. T_4 and T_3 augment glucose absorption from the gastrointestinal tract and they increase glucose turnover (glucose uptake, oxidation, and synthesis). In adipose tissue, thyroid hormone induces enzymes of fatty acid synthesis, acetyl-CoA carboxylase, and fatty acid synthase and enhances lipolysis by increasing the number of β-adrenergic receptors. Thyroid hormone also enhances clearance of chylomicrons. Thus, lipid turnover (FFA release from adipose tissue and oxidation) is augmented.

Protein turnover (release of muscle amino acids, protein degradation, and, to a lesser extent, protein synthesis and urea formation) is also increased. Multiple enzymes in these protein pathways are also increased by thyroid hormone. T_4 and T_3 potentiate the respective stimulatory effects of epinephrine, norepinephrine, glucagon, cortisol, and growth hormone on gluconeogenesis, lipolysis, ketogenesis, and proteolysis of the labile protein pool. *The overall metabolic effect of thyroid hormone has therefore been aptly described as accelerating the response to starvation.* In addition, thyroid hormone stimulates the synthesis of cholesterol, but more so its oxidation and biliary secretion. The net effect is a decrease in the body pool and in the plasma levels of total and low-density lipoprotein cholesterol. The synthesis of bile acids is decreased.

The metabolic disposal of adrenal and gonadal steroid hormones, some B vitamins, and some administered drugs is increased by thyroid hormone. Therefore, the endogenous secretion rates of such hormones as cortisol, the dietary requirements of such vitamins as riboflavin, and the doses of such drugs as digoxin that are necessary to maintain normal or effective plasma levels of these substances are all increased by thyroid hormone.

THYROID HORMONE AND THE SYMPATHETIC NERVOUS SYSTEM

One of the prominent but incompletely understood features of thyroid hormone is its interaction with the sympathetic nervous system. Certain effects of thyroid hormone, such as the increases in metabolic rate, heat production, heart rate, motor activity, and central nervous system excitation, are also produced by the adrenergic catecholamines, epinephrine and norepinephrine. An indisputable explanation for this striking similarity remains to be found. Most studies show that thyroid hormone does not increase the levels of catecholamine hormones or their metabolites in blood, urine, or tissues. Indeed, norepinephrine levels—a marker of sympathetic nervous system activity—are reduced by thyroid hormone. However, increased levels of cAMP, a β-adrenergic second messenger, are found in plasma, urine, and muscle. Furthermore, the cAMP response to epinephrine in cultured myocardial cells is augmented by T_3. At least one mechanism for this important effect is that T_3 increases the number of β-adrenergic receptors in heart muscle. Synergism between catecholamines and thyroid hormones is also required for maximal thermogenesis (Fig. 44-11), lipolysis, glycogenolysis, and gluconeogenesis to occur.

Studies of heart rate variability in humans exposed to excess thyroid hormone show evidence of both increased sympathetic activity and decreased parasympathetic tone. By contrast, hypothyroid animals show blunted baroreflex responses (increase in heart rate) to lowering of blood pressure.

Hyperthyroidism has a number of causes. Most commonly, the entire gland undergoes hyperplasia as a result of autoimmune stimulation (**Graves' disease**). In this condition, antibodies formed against the TSH receptor bind to it and mimic TSH actions on thyroid growth and hormone synthesis. The next most common cause of hyperthyroidism is the formation of benign neoplasms in one or more areas of the thyroid. These neoplasms have activating mutations of the TSH receptor or its related stimulatory G-protein and having escaped from normal hypothalamic-pituitary regulation, they secrete thyroid hormone autonomously. The least common causes are inflammation of the thyroid, excessive pituitary secretion of TSH, ingestion of exogenous T_4 or T_3, and activating mutations of TRs.

The patient with an excess of thyroid hormone presents one of the most striking pictures in clinical medicine. *The large increase in metabolic rate is accompanied by the highly characteristic combination of weight loss, despite an increased intake of food.* The increased heat production causes discomfort in warm environments, excessive sweating, and a greater intake of water. The increase in adrenergic activity is manifested by a rapid heart rate, hyperkinesis, tremor, nervousness, and a wide-eyed stare. Weakness is caused by a loss of muscle mass, as well as by an impairment of muscle function. Other symptoms include a labile emotional state, breathlessness during exercise, and difficulty in swallowing or breathing, due to compression of the esophagus or trachea by the enlarged thyroid gland (**goiter**).

The diagnosis of hyperthyroidism is established by demonstrating an elevated serum T_4 or T_3 level (appropriately corrected for any abnormalities in TBG concentrations). In most cases, the thyroid uptake of iodine (labeled with ^{123}I) is excessive. Serum TSH levels are low, because the hypothalamus and the pituitary gland are inhibited by the high levels of T_4 and T_3. In rare cases an adenoma of the pituitary thyrotrophs causes hyperthyroidism, and plasma TSH levels are high. The most definitive treatment of hyperthyroidism is ablation of thyroid tissue, either by radiation effects of ^{131}I or by surgery. Alternatively, thiouracil drugs are administered.

EFFECTS ON GROWTH AND TISSUE DEVELOPMENT

Another major effect of thyroid hormone is on growth and maturation. The most spectacular example is the process of metamorphosis in nonhuman vertebrates. Endogenous thyroid hormone levels are very low in amphibians, until just before the major stage of metamorphosis. At this point, the hormone levels increase sharply and parallel the rapid change from the larval to the adult form, after which the levels again decline. Thyroid hormone accelerates all aspects of tadpole metamorphosis, including limb growth, tail resorption, shortening of the gastrointestinal tract, and induction of hepatic ureagenesis. These effects are accomplished by thyroid hormone-induced increases in protein and nucleic acid synthesis in the limb buds, by proteolytic and hydrolytic enzyme activities in the tail, and by the hepatic content of carbamyl phosphate synthase, which is the rate-limiting enzyme in the urea cycle.

EFFECTS ON BONE

In humans, thyroid hormone stimulates endochondral ossification, linear growth of bone, and maturation of the epiphyseal bone centers (see Chapter 42). T_3 enhances the maturation and activity of chondrocytes in the cartilage growth plate, in part by increasing local somatomedin production and action (see Chapter 43). Although thyroid hormone is not required for linear growth until after birth, it is essential for normal maturation of growth centers in the bones of the developing fetus. T_3 also stimulates adult bone remodeling. T_3 receptors, TRα more than TRβ, are present in osteoblasts and in bone marrow stromal cell osteoblast precursors. Increased osteoid and bone formation, stimulated by T_3 induction of insulin growth factor-1, are manifested by increases in the production and plasma levels of alkaline phosphatase and osteocalcin. Increased bone resorption, possibly stimulated by the T_3-induced release of interleukin 6 and 8 from osteoblasts, is apparent from increases in the urinary excretion of hydroxyproline and pyridinium cross-link compounds (see Chapter 42).

A reduction in bone mass (**osteoporosis**) is recognized as one of the potential consequences of long-term exposure to excess thyroid hormones. Therefore, to prevent this initially silent complication, thyroid hormone replacement therapy for hypothyroid individuals must be carefully titrated.

The regular progression of tooth development and eruption depends on thyroid hormone, as does the normal cycle of growth and maturation of the epidermis, its hair follicles, and nails. The normal degradative processes in these structural and integumentary tissues are also stimulated by thyroid hormone. Thus, either too much or too little thyroid hormone can lead to hair loss and abnormal nail formation.

Thyroid hormone alters the characteristics of subcutaneous tissue by inhibiting the synthesis and increasing the degradation of mucopolysaccharides (glycosoaminoglycans) in the intercellular ground substance; thyroid hormone has similar effects on **fibronectin,** a fibroblast product that causes adherence.

EFFECTS ON THE NERVOUS SYSTEM

Thyroid hormone performs a critical set of actions on the timing and pace of development of the central nervous system. *If thyroid hormone is deficient in utero and in early infancy, growth of the cerebral and cerebellar cortex, proliferation of axons, and branching of dendrites, synaptogenesis, myelinization, and cell migration are all decreased. Irreversible brain damage can result when the deficiency of thyroid hormone is not recognized and treated promptly after birth.* The above structural defects are paralleled by biochemical abnormalities. In various areas of the brain of hypothyroid embryos, the cell size, RNA and protein content, the amount of tubulin- and microtubule-associated protein, the protein and lipid content of myelin, the local production of critical growth factors, and the rates of protein synthesis are reduced. Enzymes such as succinic dehydrogenase (which is essential for energy generation), galactosyl sialyl transferase (which is essential for myelin formation), and various biosynthetic enzymes and receptors for neurotransmitters are also diminished.

The crucial role of thyroid hormone in central nervous system development is underscored by a number of adaptive phenomena that occur specifically in the neonatal brain that increase the biological effectiveness of thyroid hormone at this critical time. In the cortex and other areas of the brain, $TR_{\alpha-1}$ is expressed throughout fetal life, whereas a dramatic increase in $TR_{\beta-1}$ occurs shortly after birth. *The activity of D2 5'-monodeiodinase is augmented, and it enhances the local conversion of T_4 to T_3. Conversely, the activity of brain D1 5'-monodeiodinase is diminished,* and this reduces the local degradation of T3 to 3,3′ T2 (see Fig. 44-9). Because only T_4—and not T_3—is effectively taken up by immature brain tissue, the two deiodinase activities work in concert to maintain sufficient T_3 concentrations in the developing brain. An increase in D3 5-deiodinase protects the brain from excess T_4.

Thyroid hormone induces the expression of important brain genes that direct the synthesis of myelin basic protein, neurotropic factor, neural cell adhesion molecules, and proteins involved in neuronal migration.

In adults lacking thyroid hormone, positron emission tomography demonstrates a generalized reduction in cerebral blood flow and glucose metabolism. This abnormality may explain the psychomotor retardation and depressed affect of hypothyroid individuals.

Thyroid hormone also enhances wakefulness, alertness, responsiveness to various stimuli, auditory sense, awareness of hunger, memory, and learning capacity. Normal emotional tone also depends on proper thyroid hormone availability. Furthermore, the speed and amplitude of peripheral nerve reflexes are increased by thyroid hormone, as is the motility of the gastrointestinal tract.

In both women and men, thyroid hormone plays an important permissive role in the regulation of reproductive function. The normal ovarian cycle of follicular development, maturation, and ovulation; the homologous testicular process of spermatogenesis; and the maintenance of the healthy pregnant state are all disrupted by significant deviations of thyroid hormone levels from the normal range. In part, these deleterious effects may be caused by alterations in the metabolism or availability of steroid hormones. For example, thyroid hormone stimulates hepatic synthesis and release of sex steroid-binding globulin. T_3 also promotes differentiation of prepubertal testicular *Sertoli cells* (see Chapter 46).

Thyroid hormone also has significant effects on other parts of the endocrine system. Pituitary production of growth hormone is increased by thyroid hormone, whereas that of prolactin is decreased. Adrenocortical secretion of cortisol, as well as the metabolic clearance of this hormone, is stimulated, but plasma free cortisol levels remain normal. The ratio of estrogens to androgens (see Chapter 46) is increased in men (in whom breast enlargement may occur with hyperthyroidism). Decreases in both parathyroid hormone and in $1,25\text{-}(OH)_2$-vitamin D production are compensatory consequences of the effects of thyroid hormone on bone resorption, as described above.

Kidney size, renal tubular epithelium, renal plasma flow, glomerular filtration rate, and tubular transport maximums for a number of substances are also increased by thyroid hormone.

Hypothyroidism in adults most often results from idiopathic atrophy of the gland, which is thought to be preceded by a chronic autoimmune inflammatory reaction. In this form of **lymphocytic thyroiditis,** the antibodies that are produced may block hormone synthesis or thyroid gland growth, or they may have cytotoxic properties. Other causes of hypothyroidism include radiation damage, surgical removal, nodular goiters, and hypothalamic or pituitary destruction. In children, iodide deficiency, mutant genes for NIS, TPO, thyroglobulin, and pendrin, and resistance to the action of thyroid hormones caused by mutant thyroid hormone receptors (usually TR_β) can also cause hypothyroidism.

The clinical picture of hypothyroidism is in many respects the exact opposite of that seen in hyperthyroidism. *The lower-than-normal metabolic rate leads to weight gain without an appreciable increase in caloric intake.* The decreased thermogenesis lowers body temperature and causes intolerance to cold, decreased sweating, and dry skin. Adrenergic activity is decreased, and therefore bradycardia may occur. Movement, speech, and thought are all slowed, and lethargy, sleepiness, and a lowering of the upper eyelids (ptosis) occur. An accumulation of mucopolysaccharides—ground substance—in the tissues also causes an accumulation of fluid. This **myxedema** produces puffy features; an enlarged tongue; hoarseness; joint stiffness; effusions in the pleural, pericardial, and peritoneal spaces; and pressure on peripheral and cranial nerves, entrapped by excess ground substance, with consequent thyroid dysfunction. Constipation, loss of hair, menstrual dysfunction, and anemia are other signs.

Notably, hypothyroidism in infancy or childhood causes marked retardation of growth (Fig. 44-13, *A*) and even greater slowing in the maturation of the epiphyseal growth centers of the bone (Fig. 44-13, *B* and *C*). If hypothyroidism is present at birth and remains untreated for only 2 to 4 weeks, the central nervous system will not normally mature in the first year of life. Developmental milestones, such as sitting, standing, and walking, will be late, and severe irreversible mental retardation can result. Such individuals are known as **cretins** (Fig. 44-13, *A*).

Hypothyroidism is diagnosed by finding a low serum T_4 level. (The exception would be in cases caused by thyroid hormone receptor abnormalities.) Serum TSH is elevated because of negative feedback, unless the hypothyroidism is caused by hypothalamic or pituitary disease. If the pituitary gland is at fault, TSH levels will be low and will respond inadequately to administration of TRH. Replacement therapy with T_4 is curative. T_3 is not needed, because it will be generated intracellularly from the administered T_4. Furthermore, giving T_3 raises plasma T_3 to unphysiological levels.

The stepwise nature of thyroid hormone synthesis offers many possible causes of congenital hypothyroidism that result from specific enzyme deficiencies. These syndromes are characterized by the symptoms of hypothyroidism noted previously, plus thyroid gland enlargement (congenital goiter) (Fig. 44-1) that results from persistent hypersecretion of TSH. Table 44-3 lists the best understood of these rare syndromes, with the biochemical findings that point to the lesion. Replacement therapy with T4 corrects the hormone deficiency in each instance and reduces the size of the goiter. Large amounts of iodine alone can be used successfully if the NIS (iodide trap) is defective.

SUMMARY

1. The thyroid gland is the source of tetraiodothyronine (thyroxine, T_4) and triiodothyronine (T_3).

2. The basic endocrine unit in the gland is a follicle that consists of a single circular layer of epithelial cells surrounding a central lumen that contains colloid or stored hormone.

■ **Fig. 44-13** **A,** A normal 6-year-old child (left) and a congenitally hypothyroid 17-year-old child (right) from the same village in an area of endemic cretinism. Note especially the short stature, obesity, malformed legs, and dull expression of the mentally retarded hypothyroid child. Other features are a prominent abdomen, a flat broad nose, a hypoplastic mandible, dry scaly skin, delayed puberty, and muscle weakness. (From Delange FM: Endemic cretinism. In Braverman LE, Utiger RD, editors: *Werner and Ingbar's the thyroid,* ed 7, Philadelphia, 1996, Lippincott-Raven.) Hand x-ray films of a 13-year-old normal child **(B)** and a 13-year-old hypothyroid child **(C).** Note that the hypothyroid child has a marked delay in development of the small bones of the hands, in growth centers at either end of the fingers, and in the growth center of the distal end of the radius. **(B** from Tanner JM et al: *Assessment of skeletal maturity and prediction of adult height (TW2 method),* New York, 1975, Academic Press. C from Andersen HJ: Nongoitrous hypothyroidism. In Gardner LI, editor: *Endocrine and genetic diseases of childhood and adolescence,* Philadelphia, 1975, WB Saunders.)

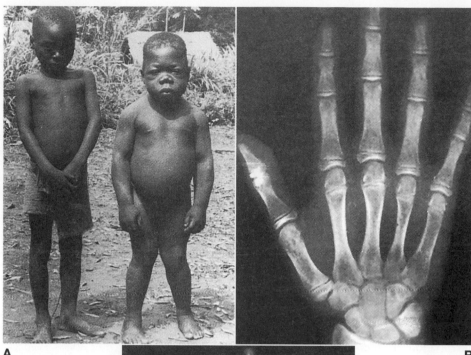

A

B

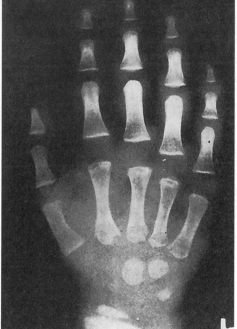

C

3. Iodide is taken up into thyroid cells by a sodium iodide symporter in the basal plasma membrane.

4. T_4 and T_3 are synthesized from tyrosine and iodide by the enzyme complex, peroxidase. Tyrosine is incorporated in peptide linkages within the protein thyroglobulin. After iodination, two iodotyrosine molecules are coupled to yield the iodothyronines.

5. Secretion of stored T_4 and T_3 requires retrieval of thyroglobulin from the follicle lumen by endocytosis. To sup-

port hormone synthesis, iodide is conserved by recycling the iodotyrosine molecules that escape coupling within thyroglobulin.

6. Thyrotropin (TSH) acts on the thyroid gland via its plasma membrane receptor and cAMP to stimulate all steps in the production of T_4 and T_3. These steps include iodide uptake, iodination and coupling, and retrieval from thyroglobulin.

7. TSH also stimulates glucose oxidation, protein synthesis, and growth of the epithelial cells.

■ Table 44-3 Some congenital defects in thyroid hormone synthesis

Defect	Diagnostic pattern
Iodide trap	Decreased uptake of radioactive iodine; decreased salivary/blood ratio of radioactive iodine
Peroxidase	Increased early uptake of radioactive iodine*; rapid discharge by perchlorate
Deiodinase	Increased uptake of radioactive iodine*; increased MIT and DIT in urine
Coupling	Increased uptake of radioactive iodine*; increased MIT and DIT and decreased T_4 and T_3 in thyroid tissue

*Radioactive iodine uptake is increased because of increased TSH secretion, which stimulates the iodine trap.

8. More than 99.5% of the T4 and T3 circulates bound to the following proteins: thyroid-binding globulin (TBG), transthyretin, and albumin. Only the free fractions of T_4 and T_3 are biologically active.

9. T_4 functions largely as a prohormone whose disposition is regulated by three types of deiodinases. Monodeiodination of the outer ring yields 75% of the daily production of T_3, which is the principal active hormone. Alternatively, monodeiodination of the inner ring yields reverse T_3, which is biologically inactive. Proportioning of T_4 between T_3 and reverse T_3 regulates the availability of active thyroid hormone.

10. T_3 and, to a much lesser extent, T_4 binds to three thyroid hormone receptor (TR) subtypes that exist linked to thyroid regulatory elements (TREs) in target DNA molecules. As a result, induction or repression of gene expression increases or decreases a large number of enzymes, as well as structural and functional proteins.

11. Thyroid hormone increases and is a major regulator of the basal metabolic rate. Oxygen utilization, CO_2 production, and thermogenesis are stimulated by mechanisms that include uncoupling of ATP synthesis from substrate oxidation, increases in the size and number of mitochondria, increased Na^+,K^+-ATPase activity, and increased rates of glucose and fatty acid oxidation and synthesis.

12. Additional important actions of thyroid hormone are to increase heart rate, cardiac output, and ventilation and to decrease peripheral resistance. The corresponding increase in heat production leads to increased sweating. Substrate mobilization and disposal of metabolic products are enhanced.

13. Other thyroid hormone effects on the central nervous system and skeleton are crucial to normal growth and development. In the absence of the hormone, brain development is retarded and cretinism results. The stature shortens and the bones fail to mature. In adults, thyroid hormone increases the rates of bone resorption and degradation of skin and hair.

BIBLIOGRAPHY

Journal articles

Abel E et al: Critical role for thyroid hormone receptor β2 in the regulation of paraventricular thyrotropin-releasing hormone neurons, *J Clin Invest* 107:1017, 2001.

Acheson K et al: Thyroid hormones and thermogenesis: the metabolic cost of food and exercise, *Metabolism* 33:262, 1984.

Barbe P et al: Triiodothyronine-mediated up-regulation of UCP2 and UCP3 mRNA expression in human skeletal muscle without coordinated induction of mitochondrial respiratory chain genes, *FASEB* 15:13, 2001.

Bengel F et al: Effect of thyroid hormones on cardiac function, geometry, and oxidative metabolism assessed noninvasively by positron emission tomography and magnetic resonance imaging, *J Clin Endocrinol Metab* 85:1822, 2000.

Boehm E et al: Increased uncoupling proteins and decreased efficiency in palmitate-perfused hyperthyroid rat heart, *Am J Physiol Heart Circ Physiol* 280:H977, 2001.

Brown D et al: Amphibian metamorphosis: a complex program of gene expression changes controlled by the thyroid hormone, *Recent Prog Horm Res* 50:309, 1995.

Burggraaf J et al: Sympathovagal imbalance in hyperthyroidism, *Am J Physiol Endocrinol Metab* 281:E190, 2001.

Constant EL: Cerebral blood flow and glucose metabolism in hypothyroidism: a positron emission tomography study, *J Clin Endocrinol Metab* 86:3864, 2001.

Contempre B et al: Detection of thyroid hormones in human embryonic cavities during the first trimester of pregnancy, *J Clin Endocrinol Metab* 77:1719, 1993.

de Jesus L et al: The type 2 iodothyronine deiodinase is essential for adaptive thermogenesis in brown adipose tissue, *J Clin Invest* 108:1379, 2001.

de La Vieja A et al: Molecular analysis of the sodium/iodide symporter: impact on thyroid and extrathyroid pathophysiology, *Physiol Rev* 80:1083, 2000.

Flier J et al: Leptin, nutrition, and the thyroid: the why, the wherefore, and the wiring, *J Clin Invest* 105:859, 2000.

Foley C et al: Thyroid status influences baroreflex function and autonomic contributions to arterial pressure and heart rate, *Am Physiol Soc* 280:H2061, 2001.

Hennemann G et al: Plasma membrane transport of thyroid hormones and its role in thyroid hormone metabolism and bioavailability, *Endocr Rev* 22:451, 2001.

Howie AF et al: Identification of a 57-kilodalton selenoprotein in human thyrocytes as thioredoxin reductase and evidence that its expression is regulated through the calcium-phosphoinositol signaling pathway, *J Clin Endocrinol Metab* 83:2052, 1998.

Kim MS et al: The central melanocortin system affects the hypothalamo-pituitary thyroid axis and may mediate the effect of leptin, *J Clin Invest* 105:1005, 2000.

Klein I: Thyroid hormone and the cardiovascular system, *Am J Med* 88:631, 1988.

Klein I et al: Thyroid hormone and the cardiovascular system, *N Engl J Med* 344:501, 2001.

Kohn LD et al: The thyrotropin receptor, *Vitam Horm* 50:287, 1995.

Kohrle J: The deiodinase family: selenoenzymes regulating thyroid hormone availability and action, *Cell Mol Life Sci* 57:1853, 2000.

Larsen PR et al: Relationships between circulating and intracellular thyroid hormones: physiological and clinical implications, *Endocr Rev* 2:87, 1981.

Lazar MA: Thyroid hormone receptors: multiple forms, multiple possibilities, *Endocr Rev* 14:184, 1993.

Lebon V et al: Effect of triiodothyronine on mitochondrial energy coupling in human skeletal muscle, *J Clin Invest,* 108:733, 2001.

Mariotti S et al: The aging thyroid, *Endocr Rev* 16:686, 1995.

Mihaly E et al: Hypophysiotropic thyrotropin-releasing hormone-synthesizing neurons in the human hypothalamus are innervated by neuropeptide Y, agouti-related protein, and α-melanocyte-stimulating hormone, *J Clin Endocrinol Metab* 85:2596, 2000.

Misrahi M et al: Cloning, sequencing and expression of human TSH receptor, *Biochem Biophys Res Commun* 166:394, 1990.

Mutvei A et al: Thyroid hormone and not growth hormone is the principal regulator of mammalian mitochondrial biogenesis, *Acta Endocrinol (Copenh)* 121:223, 1989.

Nelson BD: Thyroid hormone regulation of mitochondrial function: comments on the mechanism of signal transduction, *Biochim Biophys Acta* 1018:275, 1990.

Pinkney JH et al: Thyroid and sympathetic influences on plasma leptin in hypothyroidism and hyperthyroidism, *Int J Obes Relat Metab Disord* 24:S165, 2000

Porterfield SP, Hendrich CE: The role of thyroid hormones in prenatal and neonatal neurological development: current perspectives, *Endocr Rev* 14:94, 1993.

Reed HL et al: Changes in serum triiodothyronine (T3) kinetics after prolonged Antarctic residence: the polar T3 syndrome, *J Clin Endocrinol Metab* 70:965, 1990.

Ribeiro MO et al: Thyroid hormone-sympathetic interaction and adaptive thermogenesis are thyroid hormone receptor isoform-specific, *J Clin Invest* 108:97, 2001.

Robbins J: Editorial: new ideas in thyroxine-binding globulin biology, *J Clin Endocrinol Metab* 85:3994, 2000.

Rochon C et al: Response of leucine metabolism to hyperinsulinemia in hypothyroid patients before and after thyroxine replacement, *J Clin Endocrinol Metab* 85:697, 2000.

Silva JE: The multiple contributions of thyroid hormone to heat production, *J Clin Invest* 108:35, 2001.

Spitzweg C et al: Review: thyroid iodine treatment, *Thyroid* 10:321, 2000.

Sterling K: Direct thyroid hormone activation of mitochondria: identification of adenine nucleotide translocase (AdNT) as the hormone receptor, *Trans Assoc Am Physicians* 100:284, 1987.

Taylor T, Weintraub B: Thyrotropin (TSH)-releasing hormone regulation of TSH subunit biosynthesis and glycosylation in normal and hypothyroid rat pituitaries, *Endocrinology* 116:1968, 1985.

Viguerie N et al: Regulation of human adipocytes gene expression by thyroid hormone, *J Clin Endocrinol Metab* 87:630, 2002.

Vulsma T et al: Maternal-fetal transfer of thyroxine in congenital hypothyroidism due to a total organification defect or thyroid agenesis, *N Engl J Med* 321:13, 1989.

Yen PM: Physiological and molecular basis of thyroid hormone action, *Physiol Rev,* 81:1097-1128, 2001.

Books and monographs

Anderson, GW, Mariash, CN, Oppenheimer JH: The molecular actions of thyroid hormone. In Braverman LE, Utiger RD, editors: *Werner and Ingbar's the thyroid,* ed 8, Philadelphia, 2000, Lippincott-Raven.

Delange FM: Endemic cretinism. In Braverman LE, Utiger RD, editors: *Werner and Ingbar's the thyroid,* ed 8, Philadelphia, 2000, Lippincott-Raven.

Dunn JT: Thyroglobulin: chemistry, biosynthesis and proteolysis. In Braverman LE, Utiger RD, editors: *Werner and Ingbar's the thyroid,* ed 8, Philadelphia, 2000, Lippincott-Raven.

Klein I, Ojamaa, K: The cardiovascular system in thyrotoxicosis. In Braverman LE, Utiger RD, editors: *Werner and Ingbar's the thyroid,* ed 8, Philadelphia, 2000, Lippincott-Raven.

Scanlon MF, Toft AD: Regulation of thyrotropin secretion. In Braverman LE, Utiger RD, editors: *Werner and Ingbar's the thyroid,* ed 7, Philadelphia, 1996, Lippincott-Raven.

Smallridge RD: Metabolic, physiologic and clinical indexes of thyroid function. In Braverman LE, Utiger RD, editors: *Werner and Ingbar's the thyroid,* ed 8, Philadelphia, 2000, Lippincott-Raven.

Taurog A: Hormone synthesis: thyroid iodine metabolism. In Braverman LE, Utiger RD, editors: *Werner and Ingbar's the thyroid,* ed 8, Philadelphia, 2000, Lippincott-Raven.

chapter forty-five

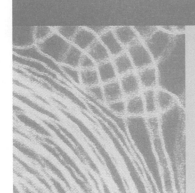

The Adrenal Glands

The adrenal glands are complex, multifunctional endocrine organs that are essential for life. Severe illness results from their atrophy, and death follows their complete removal, unless life-essential hormones are replaced.

Each adrenal gland consists of two distinct functional parts (Fig. 45-1). The outer zone, or **cortex**, makes up 80% to 90% of the gland and is derived from mesodermal tissue. The cortex is the source of corticosteroid hormones. The inner zone, or **medulla,** makes up the other 10% to 20% of the adrenal gland, and it is derived from neuroectodermal cells of the sympathetic ganglia. The medulla is the source of catecholamine hormones. In actuality this division is far from absolute. Cortical cells are present as single cells, as rays from the cortex, or as islets within the medulla. Similarly medullary (chromaffin) cells are scattered throughout all three zones of the cortex. This intimate relationship between the endocrine cells of the cortex and the neuroendocrine cells of the medulla makes possible paracrine influence of each cell type's secretory products on the release of secretory products from the other cell type.

The adrenal glands are located in the retroperitoneum, just above each kidney. Their total weight is 6 to 10 g. The adrenal glands have one of the body's highest rates of blood flow per gram of tissue. They receive arterial blood from branches of the aorta, the renal arteries, and the phrenic arteries. Arterial blood enters sinusoidal capillaries in the cortex and then drains into medullary venules. This arrangement exposes the medulla to relatively high concentrations of corticosteroids from the cortex. The right adrenal vein drains directly into the inferior vena cava, whereas the left adrenal vein drains into the renal vein on that side. The human adrenals can be visualized radiographically by computed tomography (CT) or by magnetic resonance imaging (MRI), and each adrenal vein can be catheterized for blood sampling to help localize which adrenal gland (or both) is the source of excessive hormone secretion.

THE ADRENAL CORTEX

The major hormones secreted by the adrenal cortex are (1) the **glucocorticoids, cortisol** and **corticosterone,** which are critical to life because of their effects on carbohydrate and protein metabolism; (2) a **mineralocorticoid, aldosterone,** which is vital to maintaining sodium and potassium balance and extracellular fluid volume; and (3) precursors to the **sex steroids, androgens** and **estrogens,** which contribute to establishing and maintaining secondary sexual characteristics. The discovery of the potent antiinflammatory effects of glucocorticoids generated intense medical interest in cortisol and its glucocorticoid analogs, which have wide therapeutic usefulness.

The cortical portion of the adrenal gland differentiates by 8 weeks of gestation and is initially much larger than the adjacent kidney. At this time, the cortex contains two zones. The **peripheral neocortex,** making up 15% of the cortex, is undifferentiated and relatively inactive. The inner 85%, known as the **fetal cortex,** is highly active, and it produces fetal adrenal steroids throughout almost all intrauterine life. Shortly after birth, the fetal cortex begins to involute, and it disappears completely in 3 to 12 months. At the same time, the thin outer zone of the fetal cortex enlarges and differentiates into the permanent three-layered adrenal cortex of the mature human. Each layer or zone secretes mainly one of the three types of corticosteroids (Fig. 45-1). A nuclear receptor with a currently uncertain ligand, steroidogenic factor-1 (SF-1), is essential for development of the adrenal cortex and expression of the enzymes of steroid hormone biosynthesis.

The three mature cortical zones differ in their histological appearances. The outermost **zona glomerulosa** is very thin, and it consists of small cells that have numerous elongated mitochondria with lamellar cristae. The middle **zona fasciculata** is the widest zone, and it consists of columnar cells that form long cords. The cytoplasm is highly vacuolated, and it contains lipid droplets. The mitochondria of the zona fasciculata cells are distinguished by their large size and numerous vesicular cristae within their membranes. The innermost **zona reticularis** contains networks of interconnecting cells. These cells contain fewer lipid droplets than fasciculata cells, but they have similar mitochondria. When stimulated by **adrenocorticotropic hormone (ACTH),** the

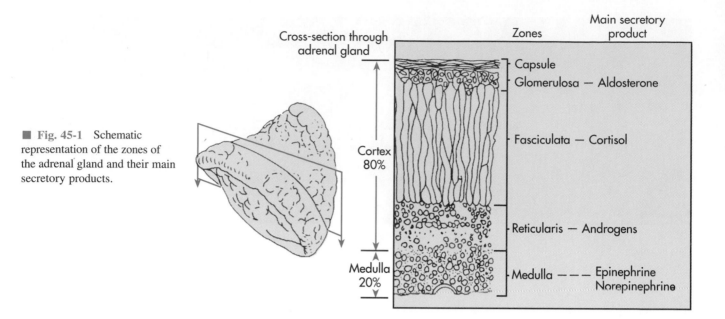

■ **Fig. 45-1**   Schematic representation of the zones of the adrenal gland and their main secretory products.

size and number of cells in the fasciculata and reticularis increase. In addition, their mitochondria become larger and more numerous, and they develop central ribosomes and vesicular cristae. The mitochondria also develop polylamellar membranes that extend to nearby cholesterol-containing vacuoles. The endoplasmic reticulum also increases. These changes relate to ACTH effects on steroid hormone synthesis, as detailed later.

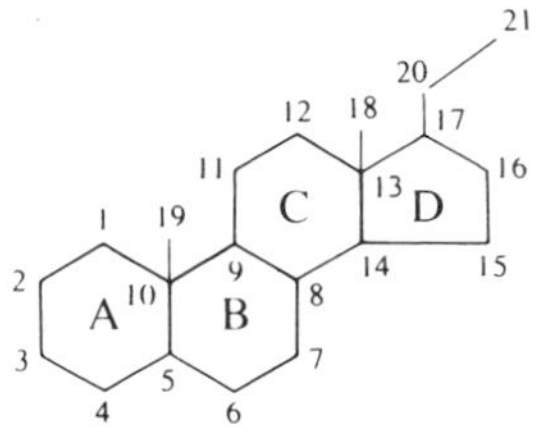

Synthesis of Adrenocortical Hormones

All hormones of the adrenal cortex represent chemical modifications of the steroid nucleus shown in Fig. 45-2. Potent glucocorticoids require the presence of a ketone at the 3 position and hydroxyl groups at the 11 and 21 positions. Potent mineralocorticoids require an oxygenated carbon at the 18 position. Potent androgens are characterized by the elimination of the C_{20-21} side chain and the presence of an oxygenated carbon at the 17 position. Estrogens are characterized by aromatization of the A ring in androgens. In the course of adrenal development, adrenocortical cells migrate inward from the outermost layer; during this migration, they increase the 17-hydroxylating activity and decrease the 18-hydroxylating activity. Those cells that migrate farthest inward also lose 11-hydroxylating activity.

The precursor for all adrenocortical hormones is cholesterol, which is actively taken up from the plasma by adrenal cells. Specific adrenal plasma membrane receptors bind both circulating low-density (LDL) and high-density (HDL) lipoproteins, which are rich sources of cholesterol. After transfer into the cell by endocytosis, microtubules move the cholesterol to cytoplasmic vacuoles, within which most of the cholesterol is esterified and then stored. A small amount of cholesterol is also synthesized in adrenal cells from acetyl-coenzyme A (acetyl-CoA) by the usual biochemical pathway. Under basal conditions, free cholesterol from plasma is the major source used for adrenocortical hormone synthe-

■ **Fig. 45-2**   The adrenocorticosteroid nucleus.

sis. When production of corticosteroids is stimulated by ACTH, however, the stored esterified cholesterol becomes the most important precursor.

Most of the synthetic reactions from cholesterol to active hormones involve **cytochrome P-450** enzymes, which are **mixed oxygenases** that catalyze steroid hydroxylations. These hydrophobic hemoproteins are located in the lipophilic membranes of the endoplasmic reticulum and mitochondrial cristae. Molecular oxygen is split so that one of its oxygen atoms is inserted between the carbon and hydrogen of the steroid site, whereas the other oxygen atom is reduced by hydrogen to H_2O. NADPH and, to some extent, NADH, which are generated by oxidation of a variety of substrates, are the ultimate donors of the hydrogen. A flavoprotein enzyme, **adrenoxin reductase,** and an iron-containing protein, **adrenoxin,** are intermediates in the transfer of hydrogen from NADPH to the P-450 enzymes.

Glucocorticoids. The synthesis of glucocorticoids occurs largely in the zona fasciculata, with a smaller contribution from adjoining cells in the zona reticularis. **Cortisol** is the dominant glucocorticoid in humans. However, if cortisol synthesis is blocked, but the pathway to **corticosterone** is open, increased synthesis of corticosterone can provide the glucocorticoid activity necessary for maintaining health.

The sequence of reactions in glucocorticoid synthesis is shown in Fig. 45-3. The intracellular localization and

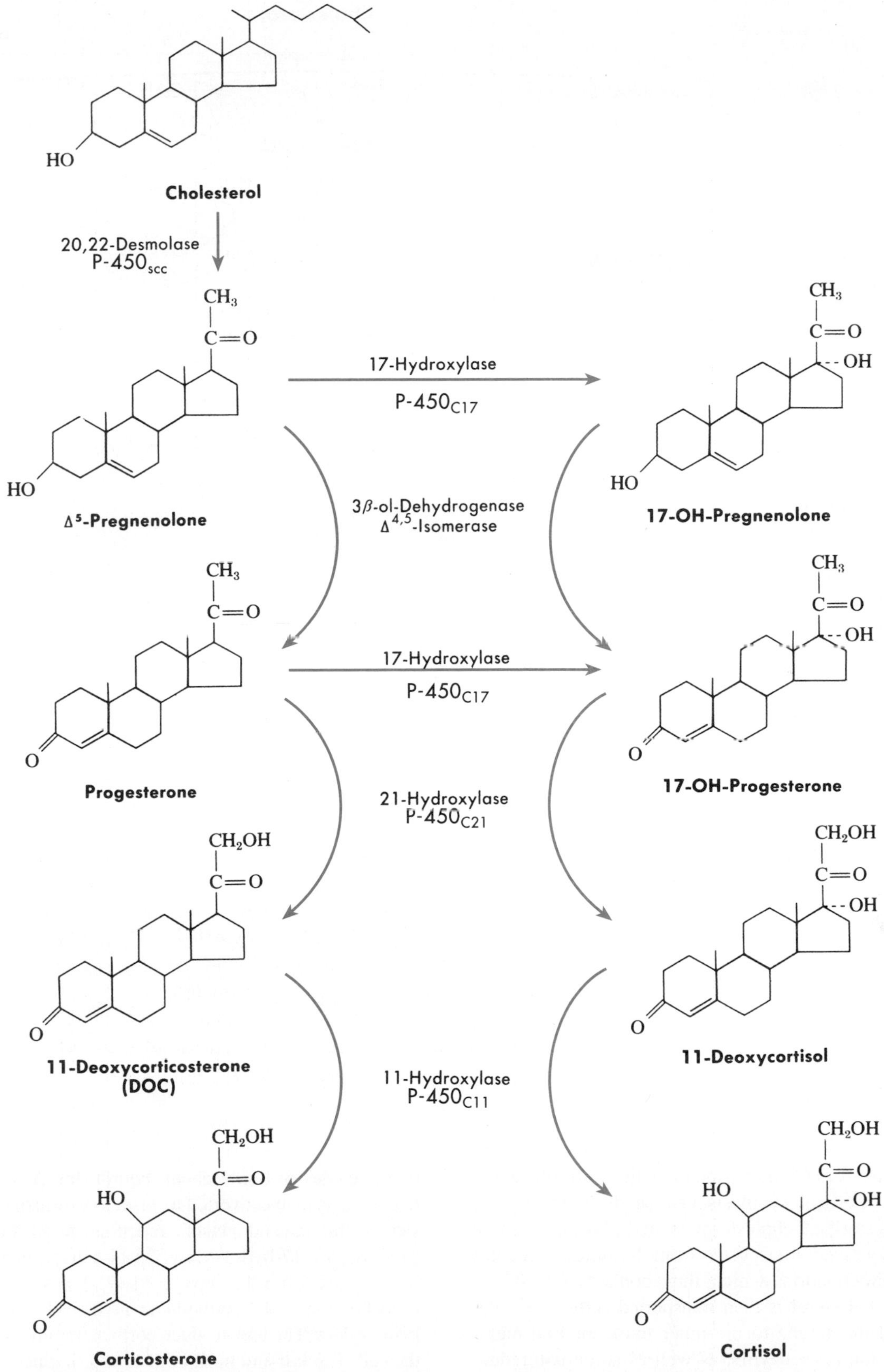

Fig. 45-3 Synthesis of glucocorticoids in the zona fasciculata. Cortisol is the major glucocorticoid in humans. When cortisol cannot be synthesized, corticosterone is an adequate endogenous alternative.

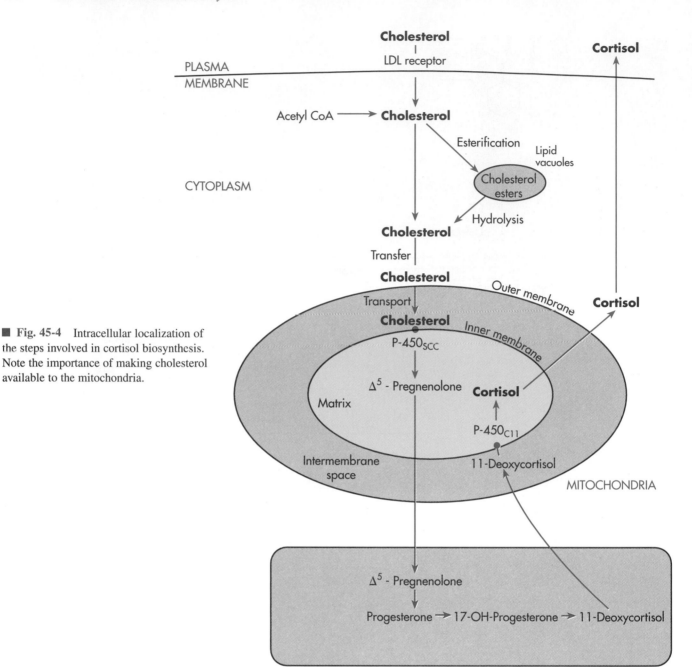

Fig. 45-4   Intracellular localization of the steps involved in cortisol biosynthesis. Note the importance of making cholesterol available to the mitochondria.

mediating activators of the various reactions are illustrated in Fig. 45-4. Cortisol synthesis can be described in five steps. First, esterified cholesterol is hydrolyzed, and free cholesterol is actively transported from the storage vacuoles to nearby mitochondria, which they contact (Fig. 45-5). Second, the cholesterol is then transported across the outer mitochondrial membrane to the inner mitochondrial membrane, where the first enzyme, as well as adrenoxin reductase and adrenoxin, is localized. Third, the initial reaction that converts cholesterol to Δ^5-pregnenolone is catalyzed by a side chain cleavage enzyme P-450$_{scc}$, also known as 20,22-desmolase. This inner mitochondrial membrane complex carries out successive hydroxylations, followed by cleavage

of the cholesterol side chain. Fourth, the Δ^5-product, pregnenolone, is then converted to 11-deoxycortisol by successive steps within the endoplasmic reticulum (Figs. 45-3 and 45-4) catalyzed by 17-hydroxylase, 3β-ol-dehydrogenase, and 21-hydroxylase. Fifth, 11-deoxycortisol is transferred back to the mitochondria and hydroxylated in the 11 position by 11-hydroxylase. The end product, cortisol, rapidly diffuses out of the cell. The last and most critical step in glucocorticoid synthesis, 11-hydroxylation, is very efficient in humans; 95% of the 11-deoxycortisol formed is converted to cortisol.

The order of hydroxylations, from Δ^5-pregnenolone to 11-deoxycortisol, can vary. Even the 3β-ol-dehydrogenase and $\Delta^{4,5}$-isomerase reactions can occur after all the hydroxy-

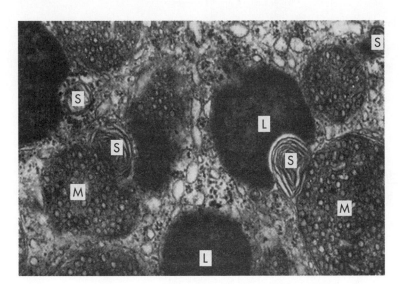

■ **Fig. 45-5**   Electron micrograph of rat cell from adrenal cortex. Note how lipid vacuoles *(L)* containing cholesterol attach to mitochondria *(M)* via syncytial membranes *(S)* to accomplish transfer of the cholesterol into the mitochondria for the first step in steroid hormone synthesis. (From Merry BJ: *J Anat* 119:611, 1975.)

lations, rather than before. However, the sequences presented in Fig. 45-3 (17-21-11) show the usual pattern of precursor accumulation that occurs when the various hydroxylases are either chemically blocked or congenitally deficient. A limited degree of 18-hydroxylation in the zona fasciculata also produces small amounts of 18-OH-cortisol, 18-OH-deoxycorticosterone (18-OH-DOC), and 18-OH-corticosterone. Some 19-OH-cortisol is also produced.

Cortisol is not stored appreciably in the adrenocortical cell. Hence, an acute need for increased amounts of circulating cortisol requires rapid activation by ACTH (Chapter 43) of the entire synthetic sequence from cholesterol.

Androgens and estrogens.   The synthesis of sex steroid precursors occurs largely in the zona reticularis. The 17-hydroxylated derivatives of Δ^5-pregnenolone and progesterone (Fig. 45-3) are the starting points for androgen and estrogen synthesis. Removal of the C_{20-21} side chain by a microsomal desmolase-like reaction is the key step, yielding dehydroepiandrosterone (DHEA) and androstenedione, respectively, as shown in Fig. 45-6. This reaction is catalyzed by the same enzyme, $P-450_{c17}$, that catalyzes the previous 17-hydroxylation step. DHEA is then largely sulfated by a specific enzyme; the sulfate donor is 3'-phosphoadenosine 5'-phosphosulfate. Dehydroepiandrosterone sulfate (DHEA-S), DHEA, and androstenedione are the major androgen precursor products of the adrenal glands. Although they are weak androgens themselves, they are converted to the more potent androgen, **testosterone** (see Chapter 46) in peripheral tissues. Only tiny amounts of testosterone itself are secreted by the zona reticularis. The same is true for the potent estrogen, **estradiol** (see Chapter 46), which is derived from testosterone.

In women, the adrenal glands ultimately supply 50% to 60% of the androgenic hormone requirements. In contrast, adrenal androgen precursors are of little biological importance to men, because the testes produce a large quantity of

testosterone. The further conversion of androgen precursors to estrogens within the adrenal cortex is not significant in women until the ovaries cease to function. After the menopause, estrogens secreted directly by the adrenal glands or arising in peripheral tissues from adrenal androgen precursors become important sources of estrogenic activity. Note that 17-hydroxylation is the last reaction common to the synthesis of cortisol and the adrenal androgens (compare Fig. 45-3 with Fig. 45-6). When cortisol synthesis is impaired at any point beyond this step, the accumulation of 17-hydroxypregnenolone and 17-hydroxyprogesterone leads to greatly increased androgen synthesis.

Mineralocorticoids.   The synthesis of **aldosterone,** the major mineralocorticoid, is carried out exclusively by the zona glomerulosa (Fig. 45-7). The initial sequence of synthesis from cholesterol to corticosterone is identical to that in the zona fasciculata (Fig. 45-3, left side). The C18 methyl group of corticosterone is then hydroxylated and converted to an aldehyde by aldosterone synthase, a mitochondrial P-450 mixed oxygenase, to yield aldosterone, which is rapidly released. 18-OH corticosterone is not a direct intermediate but a by-product of this enzymatic reaction. The fasciculata 11-hydroxylase and glomerulosa aldosterone synthase enzymes are 95% homologous in their amino acid sequences. They are coded for by separate genes, situated in tandem on chromosome 8. The former is expressed in both the zonae fasciculata and glomerulosa, and the latter is expressed exclusively in the glomerulosa. Their differing activity is determined by amino acid differences at two sites. Aldosterone synthase has a glycine at position 288 and an alanine at position 320. 11-Hydroxylase has serine and valine, respectively, at these positions. The two genes are also regulated independently (see below).

DOC and 18-OH DOC have some mineralocorticoid activity. However, only rarely are they secreted in physiologically significant amounts by the zona fasciculata under ACTH stimulation.

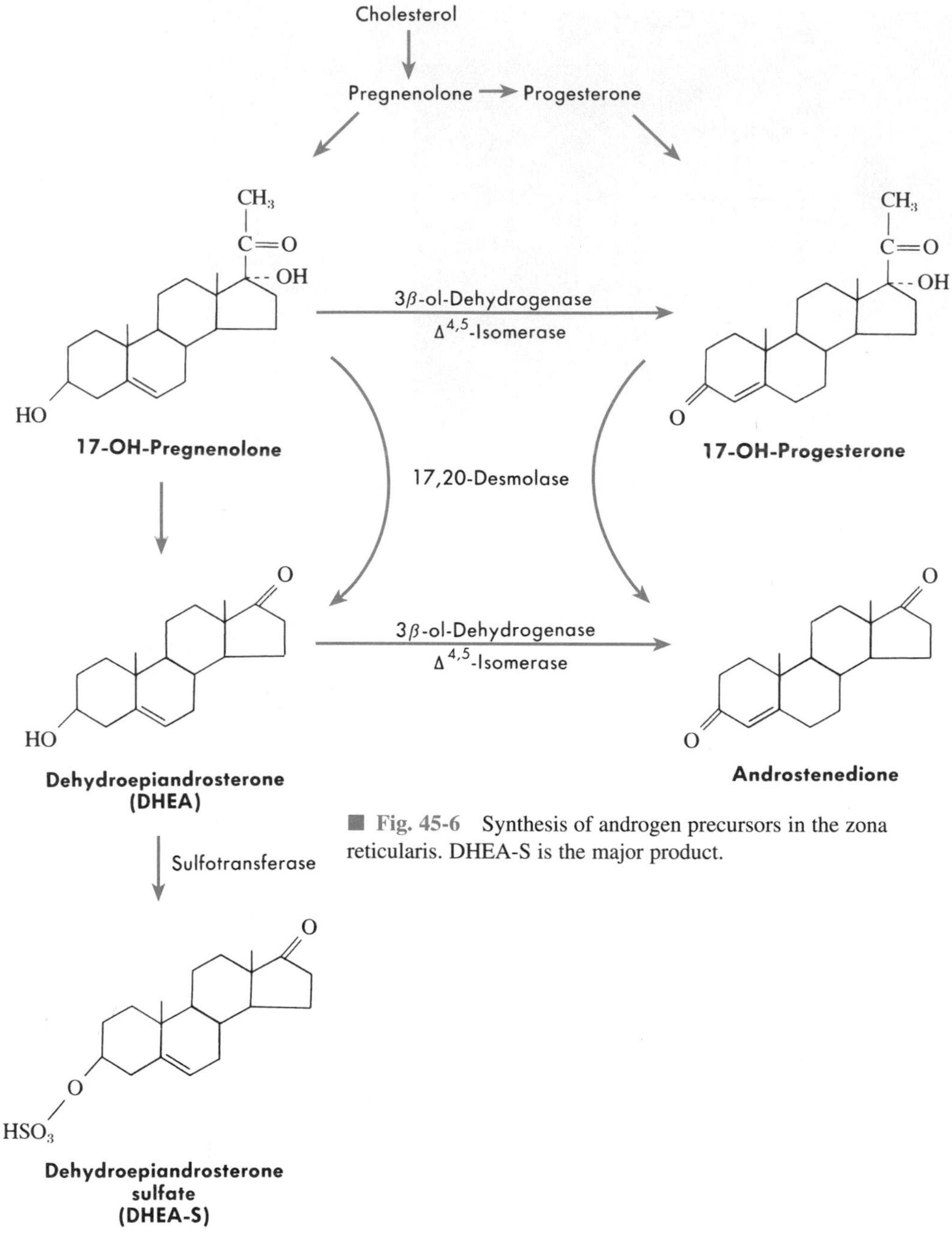

Fig. 45-6   Synthesis of androgen precursors in the zona reticularis. DHEA-S is the major product.

Genetic defects in cortisol biosynthesis have important and varied consequences. A defect in either the 21- or 11-hydroxylase enzyme gene leads to overproduction of androgenic steroids from the accumulated precursors, 17-OH progesterone and 17-OH pregnenolone (Fig. 45-3). Excess androgens cause masculinization of female fetuses in utero and early secondary sexual changes in male infants and young boys. Severe deficiency of 21-hydroxylase activity may also cause manifestations of cortisol (glucocorticoid) and aldosterone (mineralocorticoid) deficiency. Deficiency of 11-hydroxylase leads to overproduction of 11-deoxycorticosterone (Fig. 45-3), large amounts of which cause excess mineralocorticoid activity. Chimeric genes, composed of one

element from 11-hydroxylase and one from aldosterone synthase, cause abnormal regulation of cortisol or aldosterone secretion, depending on which promoter region and which exons are expressed by the chimera. Deficiency of 17-hydroxylase/17,20-desmolase activity leads to absent androgens and estrogens. Men and women who lack androgens and estrogens have absent secondary sexual characteristics, and women are without menses. Corticosterone provides normal glucocorticoid activity, but overproduction of 11-deoxycorticosterone causes excess mineralocorticoid activity. Each specific enzyme defect is diagnosed by demonstrating low plasma levels of the missing hormone product and elevated levels of the hormone precursors. Plasma ACTH

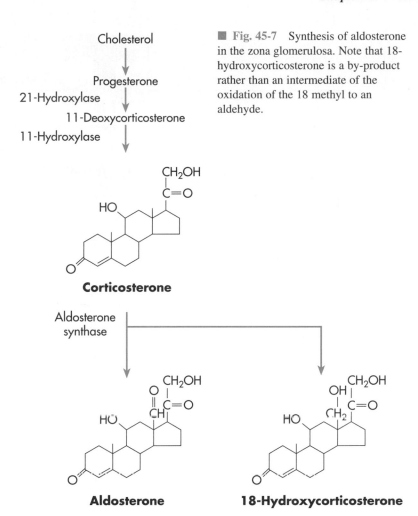

Cholesterol

↓

Progesterone

21-Hydroxylase ↓

11-Deoxycorticosterone

11-Hydroxylase ↓

Corticosterone

Aldosterone synthase

Aldosterone　　　**18-Hydroxycorticosterone**

■ **Fig. 45-7** Synthesis of aldosterone in the zona glomerulosa. Note that 18-hydroxycorticosterone is a by-product rather than an intermediate of the oxidation of the 18 methyl to an aldehyde.

levels are also elevated by negative feedback (see Fig. 43-9 and below).

Inhibitors of adrenocortical hormone synthesis. Several drugs that block steroid synthesis at various steps have diagnostic and therapeutic usefulness. **Metyrapone** inhibits 11-hydroxylation, the last and critical step in cortisol synthesis. Administration of this drug creates acute cortisol deficiency and thereby stimulates ACTH secretion via negative feedback. As a result of the increase in ACTH, adrenal production of the immediate precursor to cortisol, 11-deoxycortisol (Fig. 45-3), markedly increases. This adrenal response demonstrates the reserve capacity of the normal hypothalamic-pituitary-ACTH axis (see Fig. 43-11). Failure to respond to this drug indicates a hypothalamic-pituitary disease that has abolished this function.

Aminoglutethimide is a potent inhibitor of the desmolase reaction, and it thereby decreases all adrenal steroid synthesis. This drug has been used to treat women with breast cancer to diminish estrogen production. **Ketoconazole,** an antifungal agent, also inhibits several steps in adrenocorticosteroid synthesis, and thus it is effective in treating states of cortisol excess.

Regulation of Zona Fasciculata and Zona Reticularis Functions

The secretion of cortisol by the zona fasciculata is primarily controlled by the hypothalamic-pituitary corticotropin-releasing hormone (CRH)-ACTH axis (see Chapter 43 and Figs. 43-9 to 43-13). The secretion of adrenal androgens is likewise regulated by ACTH, but some evidence suggests that a separate, still not definitely characterized, pituitary tropic hormone may act specifically on the zona reticularis. In the absence of ACTH, adrenocortical secretion virtually ceases, except for aldosterone from the zona glomerulosa.

ACTH initiates its regulatory action by binding to its plasma transmembrane receptor, a step that requires calcium (Fig. 45-8). This binding is followed by G-protein activation of adenylyl cyclase and a rise in cAMP levels as the principal second messenger. Phosphatidylinositol products play adjunctive second messenger roles. Protein kinases A and C probably phosphorylate various protein mediators of ACTH action. A **steroidogenesis activator protein** mediates immediate hydrolysis of stored cholesterol esters. A **sterol transfer protein** transports the released cholesterol to the outer mitochondrial membrane (Fig. 45-5). The ACTH-activated **steroidogenic acute regulatory protein** (StAR), a 30-kDa phosphoprotein, mediates transfer of the cholesterol

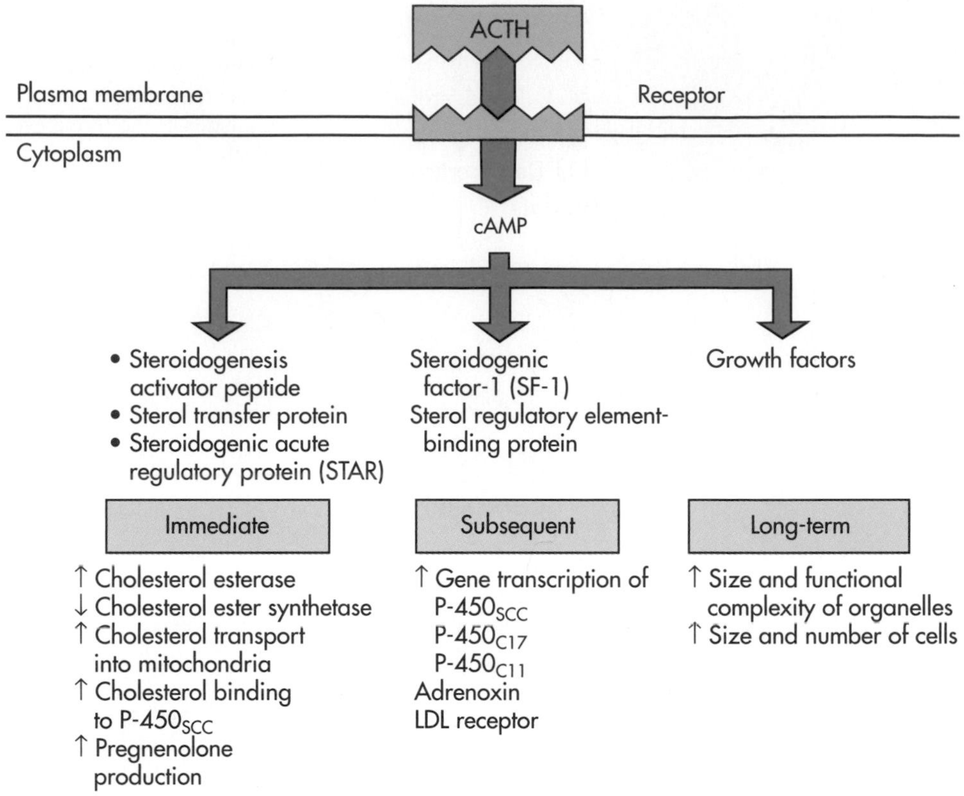

■ **Fig. 45-8** Overview of adrenocorticotropic hormone *(ACTH)* actions on target adrenocortical cells. Note that the major second messenger, cyclic adenosine monophosphate *(cAMP),* activates immediate protein mediators and also induces production of later protein mediators. *LDL,* Low-density lipoprotein.

to the inner mitochondrial membrane, where it can react with the P-450$_{scc}$, adrenoxin reductase-adrenoxin complex. An arachidonic acid metabolite, released by phospholipase A$_2$, is essential for maximum StAR function. Later, steroidogenic factor-1 (SF-1) and sterol regulatory element-binding protein, which are transcription factors activated by ACTH, increase transcription of the genes for P-450$_{scc}$, P-450$_{c17}$, P-450$_{c11}$, adrenoxin, and the LDL receptor. *Thus, all steps in corticosteroid hormone synthesis, from cholesterol entry into the mitochondria to the generation of final products, are increased by ACTH in two phases, acute activation followed by induction of the enzyme genes.*

In addition, ACTH acts on the cytoskeleton to bring cholesterol-containing vacuoles into intimate association with the mitochondria. The role of StAR is crucial, because it mediates the rate-limiting step in the entire sequence, which is the transfer of cholesterol to the first inner mitochondrial membrane enzyme. SF-1 also increases expression of the StAR gene, further amplifying the effects of a subsequent ACTH pulse. ACTH administered chronically increases the size and number of adrenal cells and their mitochondria. This trophic effect is enhanced, because ACTH initially upregulates its own receptor, and both ACTH and insulin-like growth factor (IGF) upregulate each other's receptors.

An inactivating mutation of the StAR gene has been discovered. Affected individuals cannot make steroid hormones, and they have enlarged adrenal glands filled with cholesterol and cholesterol esters. The condition is lethal.

As seen in Fig. 45-9, plasma levels of cortisol, adrenal androgens, and their precursors rise within minutes of intravenous ACTH administration to humans. ACTH induces a sustained, 2-fold to 5-fold increase in cortisol secretion. An intravenous bolus of as little as 0.01 to 0.03 μg of ACTH is enough to produce an adrenocortical response. Plasma ACTH concentrations of about 300 pg/ml, or six times the basal level, are maximally effective in stimulating cortisol secretion in the short term. However, when the adrenal gland is chronically hyperstimulated by ACTH, the gland undergoes hyperplasia, and its capacity for cortisol secretion rises up to 20-fold.

All the factors that influence ACTH secretion, as detailed in Chapter 43, likewise affect cortisol secretion; plasma levels of the latter generally follow those of the former by 15 to 30 minutes. Thus, cortisol secretion, like that of ACTH, exhibits distinct diurnal variation; the peak occurs just before the subject awakens in the morning, and the nadir occurs from the late afternoon on. The lowest level of cortisol secretion (near zero) occurs just after the subject falls into slow-wave sleep (Fig. 45-10), which independently blunts the response of corticotrophs to CRH. The diurnal curve of total and free plasma cortisol includes 7 to 13 pulses or episodes of cortisol secretion per day. Half of the total daily cortisol is secreted within the major predawn burst.

The plasma peaks of cortisol are determined by the frequency and duration of secretory bursts, rather than by gradual changes within a range of cortisol secretion rates. Thus, the basal unstimulated rate of secretion is actually near zero, and acute ACTH pulses produce essentially all-or-none

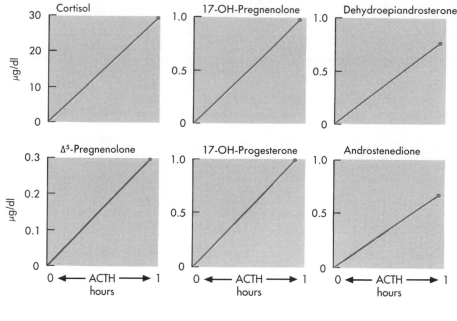

■ **Fig. 45-9** Increments in plasma adrenocortical hormones in response to a 1-hour infusion of ACTH in humans. Note the increase of both precursors and hormonally active products. These changes indicate that ACTH activates the entire biosynthetic sequence. (From Lachelin GCL et al: *J Clin Endocrinol Metab* 49:892, 1979.)

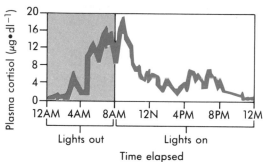

■ **Fig. 45-10** Pulsatile and diurnal nature of cortisol secretion. (From Weitzman ED et al: *J Clin Endocrinol Metab* 33:14, 1971.)

adrenal responses. The reason for each of the daytime bursts of cortisol is unknown. However, exposure to bright light, after a long period of wakefulness, from 5 AM to 8 AM, causes a prompt rise in cortisol secretion, and a reduction in the loss of alertness that accompanies sleep deprivation. A consistent burst after lunch suggests that cortisol secretion may be entrained with feeding patterns. The entrainment is not necessarily in response to plasma substrate fluctuations, but it is more likely coordinated with appetite and satiety regulation. For example, Orexin A, a hypothalamic appetite stimulant, its prohormone precursors, and its receptor, are all present in the adrenal cortex. Orexin A stimulates cortisol release, likely by paracrine action. The plasma profiles of other adrenal steroids, such as DHEA, parallel that of cortisol; any disparities reflect differences in their metabolic clearance rates.

Plasma cortisol levels are increased by the stress of surgery, burns, infection, fever, psychosis, electroconvulsive therapy, acute anxiety, prolonged and strenuous exercise, and hypoglycemia. Injection of a dose of endotoxin that causes a one degree rise in rectal temperature [and concomitant increases in the plasma levels of the inflammatory cytokines interleukin-6 (IL-6) and tumor necrosis factor-α

(TNF-α)] evokes significant increases in plasma ACTH and cortisol and much smaller increases in DHEA or DHEA-S. If stress-related pain is prevented by disruption of the sensory input to the hypothalamus or by opioid analgesia, the cortisol response is blocked or diminished, because CRH and ACTH secretion are less. Plasma cortisol levels are decreased promptly by the administration of synthetic glucocorticoids, such as dexamethasone (Table 45-1), which suppresses ACTH secretion by negative feedback (see Fig. 43-12). A single dose of dexamethasone that is biologically equivalent to twice the daily secretion rate of cortisol is sufficient to completely eliminate the nocturnal ACTH peak and the subsequent morning rise in plasma cortisol level. However, major stress often overrides feedback suppression and eliminates the diurnal pattern of cortisol secretion. Atrial natriuretic peptide is an endogenous inhibitor of corticosteroid hormone synthesis that acts by repressing the StAR gene (see above).

Responses of the hypothalamic-pituitary-adrenal axis to stress are variable, yet quite individualistic. For example, among people there are differences in response to exercise and to psychological stress. Low responders to one are low responders to the other; there is also concordance among high responses to each stimulus. Moreover high responders during exercise also show a tendency to escape earlier from suppression with dexamethasone. These differences have clinical importance. In a severe pediatric illness, such as meningococcal sepsis, nonsurvivors maintain very high plasma levels of ACTH, but inexplicably only marginally increased levels of cortisol, compared to survivors. There is also some evidence for familial, even genetic, influences on cortisol secretion and metabolism.

Some of this variability in adrenal responsiveness to stress may occur because of the operation of an *intraadrenal* CRH-ACTH system and other regulatory neuropeptides that emanate from the adrenal medulla. Intraadrenal cytokine and lymphokine production by resident immune cells and

■ **Table 45-1** Relative glucocorticoid and mineralocorticoid potency of natural corticosteroids and some synthetic analogs in clinical use*

	Glucocorticoid	Mineralocorticoid
Cortisol	1.0	1.0
Cortisone (11-keto)	0.8	0.8
Corticosterone	0.5	1.5
Prednisone (1.2 double bond)	4	<0.1
6α-Methylprednisone (Medrol)	5	<0.1
9α-Fluoro-16α-hydroxyprednisolone (triamcinolone)	5	<0.1
9α-Fluoro-16α-methylprednisolone (dexamethasone)	30	<0.1
Aldosterone	0.25	500
Deoxycorticosterone	0.01	30
9α-Fluorocortisol	10	500

*All values are relative to the glucocorticoid and mineralocorticoid potencies of cortisol, which have each been set at 1.0 arbitrarily. Cortisol actually has only 1/500 the potency of the natural mineralocorticoid aldosterone.

by medullary and cortical cells can likewise influence adrenocortical output during individual stresses.

The average normal 8 AM plasma levels of cortisol and of other adrenal steroids in humans, as well as their estimated secretion rates, are given in Table 45-2. The dominance of cortisol over corticosterone as a glucocorticoid is evident. Under severe stress, the maximal rate of cortisol secretion is 300 to 400 mg/day. Therefore, this amount is usually provided to patients who lack adrenal function and who are either acutely ill or must undergo surgery; without the steroid, they may not survive. Plasma cortisol concentration varies little from childhood to senescence, but negative feedback control of ACTH by cortisol is somewhat delayed and lessened in the elderly. Cortisol secretion rates are correlated with lean body mass.

In contrast, DHEA and DHEA-S increase to adult levels during late childhood and puberty. These adrenal steroids then decline significantly, along with androstenedione and its peripheral product testosterone, as women and men age. Because ACTH secretion does not vary appreciably throughout life, the selective change in DHEA versus cortisol with age suggests that intraadrenal factors may be responsible for these differences. Epidemiological evidence suggests that low plasma levels of DHEA are correlated with a tendency to weight gain and an increased risk of cardiovascular disease later in life. In individuals with adrenocortical insufficiency, addition of DHEA to cortisol replacement is reported to improve psychological well-being. However, the physiological importance of DHEA remains debatable.

Metabolism of Adrenocorticosteroids

Most of the cortisol (75%-80%) that circulates in plasma is bound to a specific corticosteroid-binding α_2-globulin (CBG), called **transcortin.** Each molecule of this glycoprotein binds a single molecule of cortisol. The normal plasma concentration of transcortin is 3 mg/dl, and its binding capacity is 20 μg cortisol/dl. An additional 15% of plasma cortisol is bound to albumin, and only 5% to 10% is free. The concentration of transcortin, and therefore of total cortisol, is increased during pregnancy and by estrogen administration. The physiological effects of increased cortisol

■ **Table 45-2** Average 8 AM plasma concentrations and secretion rates of adrenocortical steroids in adult humans

	Plasma concentration (μg/dl)	Secretion rate (mg/dl)
Cortisol	13	15
Corticosterone	1	3
11-Deoxycortisol	0.16	0.40
Deoxycorticosterone	0.07	0.20
Aldosterone	0.009	0.15
18-OH corticosterone	0.009	0.10
Dehydroepiandrosterone sulfate	115	15

binding are determined by principles similar to those that characterize thyroxine binding (see Chapter 44).

Transcortin may have functions of its own when bound to cortisol, because cellular receptors for the transcortin-cortisol complex that activate adenylyl cyclase have been found. Transcortin is also cleaved by a leukocyte enzyme, a process that could increase free cortisol concentration at sites of inflammation. The plasma half-life of cortisol is about 70 minutes, and the metabolic clearance rate averages 200 L/day. The cortisol circulating free in plasma is filtered by the kidney, but only about 0.3% of the total daily secretion, or approximately 50 μg, is excreted in the urine.

Measurements of 24-hour urinary free cortisol excretion or the cortisol/creatinine ratio in urine collected from midnight to morning reflect cortisol secretion rates reasonably well. Sufficient cortisol is present in saliva to make salivary concentrations useful.

Cortisol is in equilibrium with its biologically inactive 11-keto analog, **cortisone,** via the enzyme 11β-hydroxysteroid dehydrogenase (HSD) (Fig. 45-11). The plasma ratio of total cortisone to total cortisol is 0.1 to 0.2, but because cortisone binds only weakly to CBG, the plasma ratio of free cortisone to free cortisol is close to 1.0. Moreover there is little diurnal variation in plasma total cortisone levels. Therefore, in effect circulating cortisone is something of a prohormone for cortisol, and exogenous cortisone is an effective, though not ideal, replacement in cortisol deficient individuals.

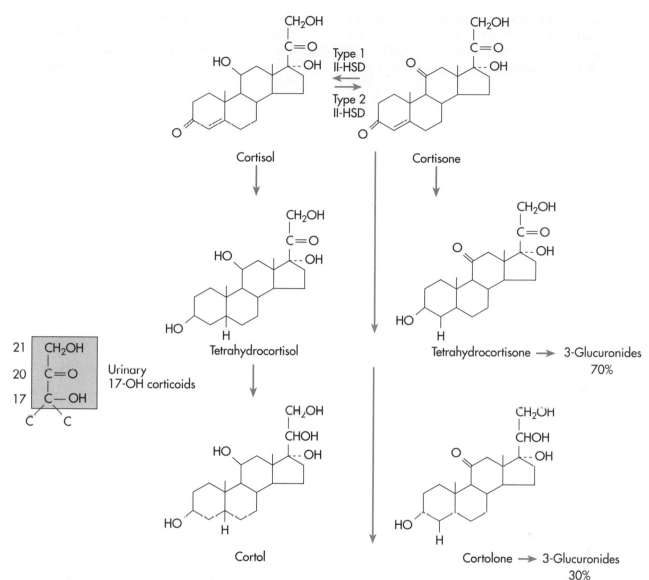

■ Fig. 45-11 Major pathways of cortisol metabolism. The analogous metabolites are formed from cortisol and cortisone. The ratio of cortisol to cortisone metabolites is normally about 1:1. Cortisol is converted to cortisone in the kidney by type 2 11-HSD (11-hydroxysteroid dehydrogenase); the cortisone is returned to the plasma from which it enters cortisol target cells. There cortisone is reconverted to cortisol by type 1 11-HSD.

There are at least two types of 11-hydroxysteroid dehydrogenases. Type 1 11-HSD is present in liver, bone, muscle, adipose tissue, and gonads. It is a bidirectional enzyme that uses NADPH to reduce cortisone to cortisol, as the latter is needed in cortisol target tissues. Type 2 11-HSD is present in the kidney and in other aldosterone target tissues, where it unidirectionally oxidizes cortisol to cortisone by using NAD. This reaction removes cortisol from competition with aldosterone for a common nuclear receptor. Only type 1 variant of 11-HSD is found in the pituitary gland. The two forms of 11-HSD are expressed by different genes, and they are only 14% homologous in structure.

Most cortisol and cortisone is metabolized in the liver; the reduced metabolites, cortols and cortolones are conjugated and excreted in the urine as glucuronides. About half

of these excretory products are normally derived from cortisol and half from cortisone (Fig. 45-11).

The measurement of urinary metabolites of cortisol provides a reliable index of cortisol secretion as long as hepatic and renal functions are normal. Particularly useful has been the 17,21-dihydroxy-20-ketone configuration of tetrahydrocortisol and tetrahydrocortisone (Fig. 45-11). The excretion of these so-called "17-hydroxycorticoids" represents up to 50% of total daily cortisol secretion. Normal excretion rates of 17-hydroxycorticoids range from 2 to 12 mg/day, and they are slightly higher in men than in women, as are cortisol secretion rates. Adrenocortical responsiveness to ACTH (or metyrapone), or suppressibility by exogenous synthetic glucocorticoids, can be assessed by daily measurements of urinary 17-hydroxycorticoids.

The cortisol precursors, progesterone and 17-hydroxyprogesterone, are metabolized to the respective, cortols, which are known as **pregnanediol** and **pregnanetriol,** respectively. In adult females, these urinary metabolites reflect both adrenal and ovarian secretion. In prepubertal children, however, elevation of urinary pregnanetriol specifically indicates increased secretion of adrenal 17-hydroxyprogesterone. Therefore, it is a valuable marker for particular congenital defects in cortisol secretion caused by abnormalities in the genes that express 21- and 11-hydroxylases.

The metabolism of androgens, in general, involves reduction of the 3-ketone group and the A ring in the liver. The two isomers that are formed, androsterone and etiocholanolone, are then excreted in the urine. However, these metabolites are not specific for the adrenal gland, because they also arise from gonadal androgens. DHEA-S is entirely excreted directly in the urine, and it is virtually adrenal specific.

Androsterone, etiocholanolone, and DHEA-S together constitute the major part of a urinary fraction, traditionally called **17-ketosteroids.** Normal 17-ketosteroid values range from 5 to 14 mg/day in women and 8 to 20 mg/day in men. Two thirds of this fraction is normally derived from adrenal secretions and one third from gonadal androgen secretions. In virilized children or adult women, a large increase in urinary 17-ketosteroid excretion almost always indicates an adrenal abnormality. Similar information can now be more readily obtained by measurement of plasma or urinary DHEA-S.

General Actions of Glucocorticoids

Cortisol is essential for life. Although provision of carbohydrate and of a pure mineralocorticoid or sodium chloride can postpone death, human beings cannot survive removal of both adrenal glands for long without glucocorticoid replacement. Cortisol maintains glucose production from protein, facilitates fat metabolism, supports responsiveness of the vascular tree, modulates central nervous system function, and profoundly affects the immune system and inflammatory responses. In addition, cortisol affects skeletal turnover, muscle function, and renal function. The net effect of its metabolic actions is either catabolic or antianabolic and diabetogenic. The term *permissive* has been used to describe many of cortisol's actions. This term implies that the hormone may not directly *initiate,* so much as *allow,* certain processes to occur. Several examples may serve to better define this permissive role:

1. Cortisol may amplify the effect of another hormone on a process that it does not affect directly. For example, cortisol does not itself stimulate glycogenolysis, but it augments the stimulation of glycogenolysis by glucagon.
2. Cortisol and glucagon individually increase the activity of the enzyme, phosphoenolpyruvate carboxykinase (see Fig. 41-14). However, their combined effect on this important regulatory step of gluconeogenesis is synergistic rather than additive.
3. The enzyme, tyrosine transaminase, is inducible by cortisol. It is not normally inducible by its substrate, tyrosine. However, in the presence of small doses of cortisol, tyrosine administration will now induce the enzyme.

Intracellular actions of glucocorticoids. In vitro and in vivo, the effects of cortisol (e.g., inhibition of ACTH release) may be evident within 10 to 30 minutes. However, cortisol effects usually require hours (increase in plasma glucose) or days (induction of glucose-6-phosphatase) to be expressed. Cortisol enters target cells freely by simple or facilitated diffusion, and it is then bound to one of two types of glucocorticoid receptors (GR). Most cortisol effects in peripheral tissues are exerted through the type II GR. Without its ligand, this receptor may shuttle back and forth between the cytoplasm and the nucleus. GR belongs to the superfamily of steroid, thyroid, vitamin D, and retinoid receptors (see Chapter 39) and consists of four identical subunits. The GR is found in many tissues, including numerous areas of the brain, where it is mainly expressed as the type I GR. Although each GR appears to be the same molecule in all cells, GR concentration varies with the cell type, the degree of cellular differentiation, and the phase of the cell cycle (lowest in G-I and M, highest in S and G-II). GR_α and GR_β result from alternate splicing of the initial GR gene product. Differences in the carboxyl terminus make GR_α active and GR_β inactive, because the latter cannot bind its ligand cortisol. Moreover, GR_β can combine with GR_α to form a heterodimer, which is also inactive. Thus regulation of the splicing pattern of the GR gene is another component in regulating cortisol action.

In the cytoplasm, cortisol combines noncovalently, but strongly, with its receptor. Binding of cortisol dissociates GR from chaperone molecules such as heat shock proteins, and allows it to be hyperphosphorylated. Hyperphosphorylation of the receptor exposes C-terminus sites that facilitate the translocation of the hormone-receptor complex into the nucleus and the binding to glucocorticoid regulatory elements (GREs) on target DNA molecules (Fig. 45-12). Two liganded GRs combine to form a *homodimer unit,* which latches on with zinc fingers to two palindromic GRE half-sites (5′ TGTTCT 3′), which are separated by 3 base pairs.

GREs are usually located upstream from the gene promotor, but they may be downstream or may even exist within the gene. A single gene may have more than one type of paired GRE half-sites. To free genes for transcription, cortisol-bound GR interacts with histone acetylators (Chapter 39) and with the ATP-dependent chromatin remodeling process. Constitutive protein transcription factors may also be required to facilitate binding of a cortisol-GR complex to a GRE. Still other transcription factors (even induced by other hormones) may block the interaction of the GR with the GRE.

Once the cortisol-GR complex has bound to a GRE, initiation or repression of gene transcription takes place. Repression may sometimes occur by displacement of activating factors from the DNA molecule, as is the case when cortisol inhibits certain inflammation-related genes that lack

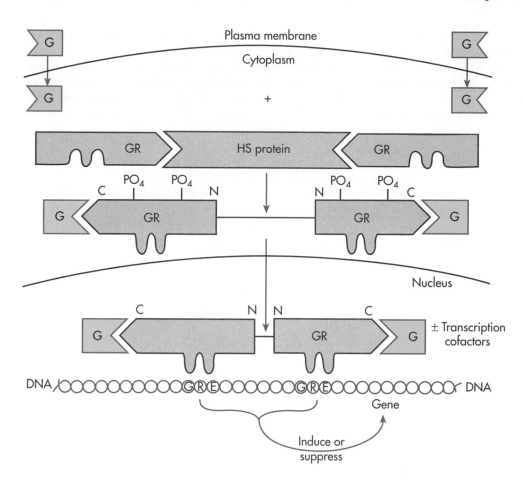

■ **Fig. 45-12** Mechanism of glucocorticoid (cortisol) action. The hormone *(G)* enters the cytoplasm and displaces a heat shock *(HS)* protein or other chaperone from the ligand-binding portion of the glucocorticoid receptor *(GR)*. This leads to hyperphosphorylation of GR and changes its conformation, so that it can readily enter the nucleus. There, complexed to G in the form of homodimers, GR then interacts with glucocorticoid regulatory elements *(GRE)* in target DNA molecules. Transcription cofactors may enhance or repress gene expression. *G,* Glucocorticoid; *GR,* glucocorticoid receptor; *GRE,* glucocorticoid-regulating element; *HS,* heat shock.

GREs. In other instances, a negative GRE exists within the gene, as is the case when cortisol suppresses transcription of the proopiomelanocortin gene (see Chapter 43).

In any one target cell type, only certain genes are affected. For example, in the anterior pituitary gland, the growth hormone gene is induced by cortisol, but the gene for the enzyme tyrosine aminotransferase is not. The opposite is true in the liver. GR can also bind other steroids, such as progesterone, and GREs can bind other steroid receptors, such as the progesterone receptor. However, only the simultaneous combination of glucocorticoid plus GR plus GRE produces the conformation necessary to induce the unique glucocorticoid effect on the expression of a gene.

Mutant GRs with deficient activity have been found in families that are resistant to cortisol action. Such individuals have compensatory increases in plasma cortisol levels, because of inadequate negative feedback on CRH and ACTH secretion. Some AIDS patients appear to have acquired altered GRs with a markedly reduced affinity for cortisol. As a result, the number of GRs per cell is increased, owing to the inadequate repression of the GR gene itself by cortisol. When the GR is severely defective, cortisol action may be so impaired that the patient is clinically deficient in cortisol (see below).

Cortisol downregulates its receptor by repressing expression of GR_α, by decreasing stability of GR_α mRNA, and by inducing expression of GR_β. This important mechanism limits cortisol actions.

The mineralocorticoid receptor (MR) shows strong homology to GR in its C terminus and DNA-binding domains; therefore, it is also known as the type I GR. Although this receptor exerts its physiological function mainly by binding mineralocorticoids, it actually binds cortisol 10 times more strongly than does the type II GR. Thus, MR or type I GR may mediate some cortisol actions when the basal concentrations of cortisol are low, whereas type II GR may mediate actions when stimulated cortisol concentrations are high. The selective central nervous system distribution of MR also suggests that it specifically mediates certain actions of cortisol in the brain.

Other intracellular mechanisms of cortisol action also probably exist. Cortisol does not generally alter intracellular cAMP levels. It does, however, synergize with the nucleotide in many situations, and cAMP can mimic some actions of cortisol. Cortisol may also act by altering cGMP levels and the phospholipid component of various intracellular membranes. Even within a single cell type, various enzyme changes produced by cortisol are not necessarily simultaneous or proportional in magnitude. This observation suggests the existence of multiple mechanisms of action.

Effects on metabolism. *Cortisol acts permissively to facilitate the mobilization of fuels. The nocturnal surge in cortisol supports the enhancement of gluconeogenesis, lipolysis, and ketogenesis, which are necessary for overnight* *metabolic stability. The most important overall action of cortisol is to facilitate the conversion of protein to glycogen* (Fig. 45-13). Cortisol enhances the mobilization of muscle protein for gluconeogenesis by accelerating protein degradation and inhibiting protein synthesis. In fasted humans, the rates of entry of essential and nonessential amino acids into the blood are increased by cortisol levels that are raised to those seen in trauma or acute illness. This change indicates that proteins are being broken down (Fig. 45-14). The plasma concentrations of the branched-chain amino acids increase; however, alanine levels do not rise, because the conversion of alanine to glucose is increased simultaneously by cortisol (Fig. 45-14). Branched-chain amino acids directly stimulate muscle protein synthesis, and this effect is blunted by glucocorticoids. Nonetheless the increased availability of amino acids produced by cortisol does itself increase protein synthesis. Therefore, the overall effect of cortisol is to increase protein *turnover,* with net loss of protein from the whole body.

The combined catabolic and antianabolic action of cortisol in normal amounts is physiologically beneficial.

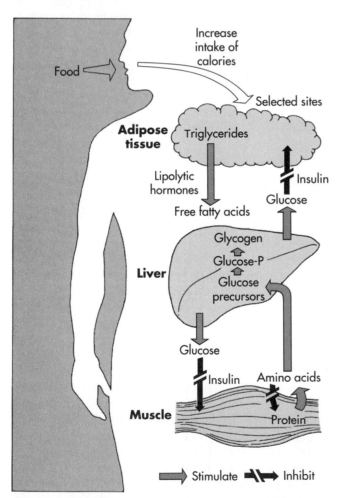

■ **Fig. 45-13** Effect of cortisol on the overall flow of fuels facilitates release of amino acids from muscle, their use for gluconeogenesis, storage and release of glucose, and acute release of free fatty acids from adipose tissue. Appetite is increased as are adipose tissue fat stores.

However, a continuous excess of glucocorticoid action can drain the body's protein stores remarkably, in muscle, bone, connective tissue, and skin. Dietary protein cannot make up for this drain, because protein synthesis is partially inhibited. Cortisol further stimulates the transformation of proteolytically derived amino acids into glucose precursors, and then into glucose (Fig. 45-13). Table 45-3 lists enzymes that are induced by cortisol, and that are important to glucose production and to the disposition of ammonia released from gluconeogenic amino acids.

Glucocorticoids are critical for the survival of a fasting animal or human. Without glucocorticoids, proteolysis does not increase much, as evidenced by the lack of increase in urinary nitrogen excretion (see Chapter 40). Therefore, when liver glycogen stores are depleted, deficient gluconeogenesis from protein may lead to death from hypoglycemia. The secretion of cortisol is modestly increased by fasting, but it is the previous exposure to normal levels of cortisol that permits the initial augmentation of amino acid mobilization.

Cortisol plays a similar role in the defense against hypoglycemia that is evoked by insulin. The rapid release of the glycogenolytic hormones glucagon and epinephrine is mainly responsible for the rapid recovery of plasma glucose levels. However, the *previous* action of cortisol leads to the build-up of sufficient gluconeogenic enzyme levels and glycogen stores, on which the other hormones can act. The critical enzyme glucose-6-phosphatase, which catalyzes glucose release from the liver, is also cortisol dependent. During the late phase of recovery from hypoglycemia, cortisol also decreases peripheral glucose utilization.

Although the major impact of cortisol is on liver glycogen, an excess of the hormone eventually increases plasma glucose levels. *This increase occurs because cortisol powerfully antagonizes the actions of insulin on glucose metabolism. Hence, cortisol inhibits insulin-stimulated glucose uptake in muscle and adipose tissue, and it reverses the insulin suppression of hepatic glucose production.* As shown in Fig. 44-15, cortisol decreases tissue sensitivity, but not maximal responsiveness, to insulin. This antagonism takes place largely at postreceptor steps; for example, insulin represses, whereas cortisol induces, transcription of the gluconeogenic phosphoenolpyruvate carboxykinase gene. Cortisol also demobilizes glucose transporters from the plasma membrane back to intracellular sites, and thus directly reduces glucose uptake. As is the case with another insulin antagonist, growth hormone (see Chapter 43), cortisol eventually enhances the increase in insulin secretion that compensates for the insulin resistance produced by cortisol.

Cortisol also plays a somewhat analogous and permissive role in fat metabolism (Fig. 45-13). Although cortisol itself has only a slight lipolytic activity, its presence is necessary for epinephrine, growth hormone, and other lipolytic substances to stimulate hydrolysis of stored triglycerides at maximal rates. Thus, during fasting, cortisol permits the accelerated release of stored energy in the form of fatty acids and of glycerol for gluconeogenesis. Fatty acid oxidation and basal metabolic rate (BMR) are sustained, and RQ is decreased.

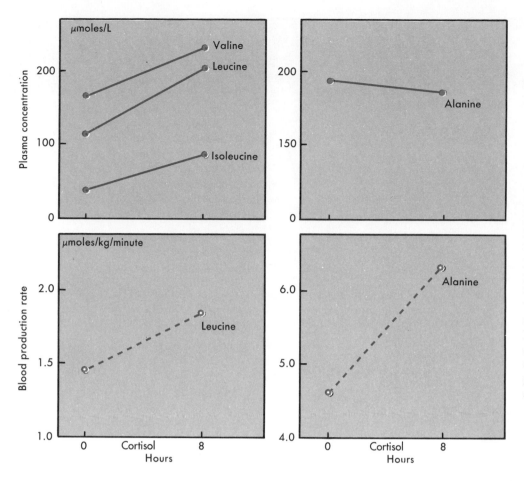

■ **Fig. 45-14**   Effect of cortisol infusion for 8 hours in normal humans on the plasma concentrations and blood production rates of several amino acids. The plasma concentrations of leucine and two other essential branched-chain amino acids increase. The increase of leucine is accomplished by an increase in its production rate and therefore indicates that cortisol stimulates proteolysis. Although the blood production rate of alanine also increases, its plasma concentration does not, because (in contrast to the nongluconeogenic leucine) cortisol simultaneously stimulates alanine use by augmenting its conversion to glucose. (From Simmons PS et al: *J Clin Invest* 73:412, 1984.)

■ **Table 45-3**   Enzymes whose activities are increased by cortisol

Provide carbon precursors	Convert pyruvate to glycogen	Release glucose	Dispose of ammonia liberated from amino acids in urea cycle
Alanine transaminase	Pyruvate carboxylase	Glucose-6-phosphatase	Arginine synthetase
Tyrosine transaminase	Phosphoenolpyruvate carboxykinase		Argininosuccinase
Tryptophan pyrrolase	Phosphoglyceraldehyde dehydrogenase		Arginasenase
Threonine dehydrase	Aldolase		
Serine dehydrase	Fructose 1,6-biphosphatase		
	6-Phosphofructo-2-kinase/fructose 2,6-biphosphatase		
	Phosphohexoisomerase		
	Glycogen synthase		

Cortisols actions on body fat are complex. The hormone increases appetite and caloric intake, by inducing neuropeptide Y (NPY) synthesis and NPY receptors in the hypothalamus, and by suppressing CRH release (see Chapter 40). It also increases differentiation of adipose tissue cells from preadipocytes to adipocytes, and stimulates lipogenesis by increasing adipocyte lipoprotein lipase and glucose-6-phosphate dehydrogenase activity. These actions vary in different regions of the body. *Therefore, an excess of cortisol finally results in obesity, with a peculiar distribution of fat that favors the abdomen, trunk, and face, but spares the extremities* (Fig. 45-16). Because cortisol also induces **leptin**

synthesis in adipocytes, the gain in fat mass is eventually limited by the negative feedback action that leptin exerts on the appetite center in the hypothalamus (see Chapter 40).

In short, cortisol is an important diabetogenic, antiinsulin hormone. Its primary hyperglycemic and lipolytic and secondary ketogenic actions are usually exhibited only when its secretion is greatly stimulated by stress. Cortisol then potentiates and extends the duration of the hyperglycemia evoked by glucagon, epinephrine, and growth hormone, and it accentuates the loss of body protein. These diabetogenic and catabolic actions are markedly amplified when insulin secretion is deficient. Cortisol also affects numerous

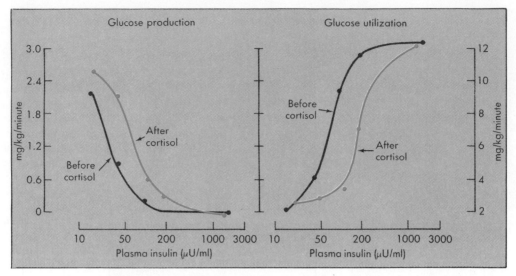

■ **Fig. 45-15** Effect of cortisol on glucose turnover in response to increasing levels of insulin in a human. Cortisol decreases the sensitivity to insulin (the dose-response curve is shifted to the right) with regard to both insulin inhibition of glucose production and insulin stimulation of glucose use. (From Rizza RA et al: *Am J Med* 70:169, 1981.)

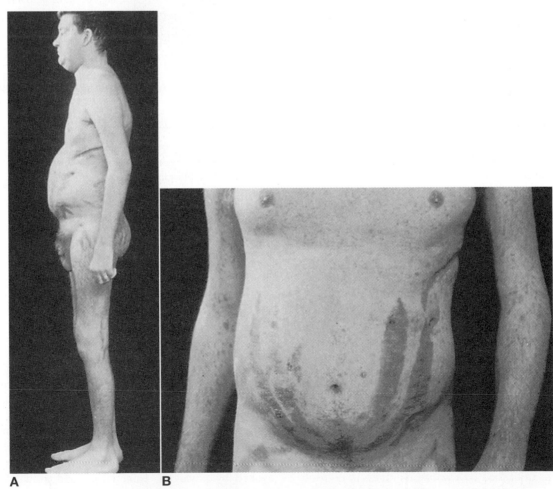

A   **B**

■ **Fig. 45-16** An individual suffering from cortisol excess (Cushing's syndrome). **A,** Note the loss of muscle mass in extremities and selective accumulation of fat in the abdomen and above the clavicles. **B,** The extremely thin skin reveals blood flowing through vessels just below.

organs and systems throughout the body, as depicted in Fig. 45-17.

Effects on muscle. Cortisol maintains the contractility and work performance of skeletal and cardiac muscle. This inotropic action of cortisol on skeletal muscle may be exerted at the myoneural junction via an increase in acetylcholine synthesis. In addition, cortisol increases myocardial Na$^+$,K$^+$-ATPase and β-adrenergic receptors. However, an excess of cortisol decreases muscle protein synthesis, increases muscle catabolism, and consequently reduces muscle mass and muscle strength. The ratio of the insulin-sensitive, slow oxidative type I muscle fibers to the fast glycolytic type II-B muscle fibers is decreased by cortisol. This effect adds to the insulin resistance.

Effects on bone. *Glucocorticoids increase bone resorption in a transient manner by several actions.* Cortisol reduces the expression of a family of transcription factors, known as NF-κB, which regulate immune and inflammatory cytokines that stimulate osteoclast formation and bone resorption by the osteoclasts (Chapter 42). In addition, cortisol increases mRNA of collagenase, the enzyme essential for destroying the organic matrix of bone.

However, the most profound effect of glucocorticoids is to inhibit bone formation. Osteoblasts and osteocytes (but not osteoclasts) contain GR$_\alpha$. Cortisol decreases collagen synthesis and formation of mature osteoblasts from their undifferentiated precursors, while at the same cortisol increases the rate of apoptosis of osteoblasts and osteocytes, which are the functional cells in bone formation (Chapter 42). The shrinkage of these cell masses comes about partly because cortisol decreases the systemic and local generation of anabolic IGF-1 molecules (Chapter 43). Cortisol also impedes calcium absorption from the intestinal tract by antagonizing the action of 1,25-(OH)$_2$-vitamin D and inhibiting its synthesis. This causes mild secondary hyperparathyroidism (Chapter 42), which adds to the bone-resorbing effect of cortisol.

Osteoporosis is a feared and sometimes devastating complication of glucocorticoid therapy that lasts more than a few weeks. Because therapy to restore lost bone mass is not fully effective, preventive treatment with calcium, vitamin D, and a drug class (diphosphonates) that inhibits bone resorption is advisable.

Effects on connective tissue. Inhibition of collagen synthesis by cortisol produces thinning of the skin and the walls of capillaries. The resultant fragility of the capillaries leads

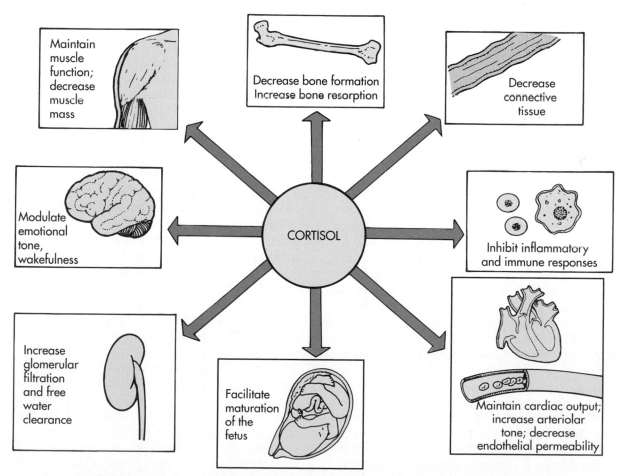

■ **Fig. 45-17** Overview of cortisol effects on various tissues, organs, and systems other than its effects on general metabolism as noted in Fig. 45-13.

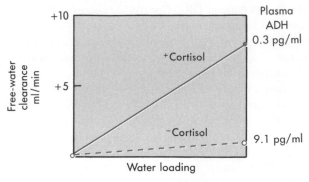

■ **Fig. 45-18** Effect of cortisol on the response of adrenalectomized dogs to water loading. In the absence of the hormone, there is little increase in free-water clearance, and antidiuretic hormone *(ADH)* levels remain high (because of negative feedback on ADH neurons). Cortisol replacement allows a normal suppression of ADH levels and a sharp increase in free-water clearance. (From Boykin J et al: *J Clin Invest* 62:738, 1978.)

to their easy rupture and to intracutaneous hemorrhage (Fig. 45-16).

Effects on the vascular system. *Cortisol is required for the maintenance of normal blood pressure.* In addition to sustaining myocardial performance, the hormone permits normal responsiveness of arterioles to the constrictive action of catecholamines and angiotensin II. The mechanism for this effect may be inhibition of the membrane sodium-calcium exchanger, which would prolong the transient calcium increases produced by the vasoconstrictors. Cortisol decreases production of vasodilator prostaglandins and helps to maintain blood volume by decreasing the permeability of the vascular endothelium.

Effects on the kidney. *Cortisol increases the rate of glomerular filtration* by decreasing preglomerular resistance and increasing glomerular plasma flow. *The hormone is also essential for the rapid excretion of a water load.* In the absence of cortisol, the synthesis and secretion of antidiuretic hormone (ADH) are increased (by negative feedback on hypothalamic neurons), and its action on renal tubules is enhanced. Therefore, free-water clearance is diminished and dilution of the urine is limited (Fig. 45-18). Cortisol is also required for generation of the ammonium ion from glutamate in response to acid loads. The hormone increases calcium excretion and phosphate excretion by decreasing their reabsorption in the proximal tubules.

Effects on the central nervous system. Cortisol modulates excitability, behavior, and mood of individuals; the electrical activity of neurons is influenced. Both type I and type II GRs are present in various areas of the brain, particularly in the limbic system and the hippocampus. In normal subjects, exogenous glucocorticoids decrease rapid eye movement (REM) sleep, but they increase both slow-wave sleep and the time spent awake. However, studies in subjects with cortisol deficiency suggest that permissive amounts of cortisol are needed to facilitate initiation and maintenance of REM sleep and the accompanying easy arousability. The

early morning rise in ACTH and cortisol generally precedes S_1, or light, sleep. Some of these apparent cortisol effects may be caused secondarily by changes in CRH release. In excess, cortisol can cause insomnia, can strikingly elevate or depress moods, can decrease memory function, and can lower the threshold for seizure activity. Atrophy of the brain, with particular loss of hippocampus volume, has been noted. Cortisol also specifically decreases the ability to detect a salty taste and it dampens the acuity to gustatory, olfactory, auditory, and visual stimuli. On the other hand, cortisol improves the ability to integrate those sensations that are perceived and to organize appropriate responses.

Effects on the fetus. *Cortisol facilitates in utero maturation of the central nervous system, retina, skin, gastrointestinal tract, and lungs.* The latter two effects have been best studied. The digestive enzyme capacity of the intestinal mucosa changes from a fetal pattern to a mature adult pattern under the influence of cortisol. This maturation process permits the newborn child to use disaccharides present in milk. Timely preparation of the fetal lung to permit satisfactory breathing immediately after birth is facilitated by cortisol, which increases the rate of development of the alveoli, the flattening of the lining cells, and the thinning of the lung septa. Most important, during the last weeks of gestation, the synthesis of surfactant, a phospholipid vital for maintaining alveolar surface tension, is increased (see Chapter 26). This last effect is mediated by increasing the activity of key enzymes, such as phosphatidyl acid phosphatase and choline phosphotransferase, which are involved in the biosynthetic pathway of surfactant.

Effects on inflammatory and immune responses. *Cortisol has a profound influence on the complex set of reactions that are revoked by tissue trauma, chemical irritants, infection, or foreign proteins* (Fig. 45-19). The immediate local reaction to injury consists of dilation of capillaries and endothelial cell membrane changes that increase microvascular permeability and enhance the trapping of circulating leukocytes at the site of injury. These reactions, mediated by **prostaglandins, thromboxanes, leukotrienes, nitric oxide,** and **platelet-activating factor,** are profoundly inhibited by cortisol, and all of the currently available synthetic glucocorticoids that are used therapeutically. The inhibition of these reactions by cortisol stems initially from the hormone's suppression of the synthesis and release of **arachidonic acid,** which is a precursor of many of the lipid immune mediators. Cortisol decreases the availability of arachidonic acid by inducing **lipocortin,** a phosphoprotein that inhibits the activity of the enzyme phospholipase A_2. This phospholipase releases arachidonic acid from its linkage to phosphatidylcholine. Arachidonic acid is the immediate precursor of the proinflammatory prostaglandins, thromboxanes, and leukotrienes, and its production is the rate-limiting step in their synthesis. In addition, cortisol decreases the expression of the gene that codes for cyclooxygenase 2, an enzyme that directs prostaglandin synthesis toward inflammatory products. Cortisol also decreases the expression of the gene that encodes nitric oxide synthase.

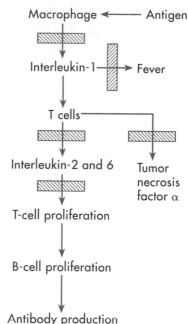

Inflammatory response

Production of

Platelet-activating factor   Nitric oxide

Phosphatidyl choline

Phospholipase

Arachidonic acid

Cyclooxygenase   Lipooxygenase

Prostaglandins
Thromboxanes

Leukotrienes

Neutrophil function

Phagocytosis

Vasodilation

Bacterial killing

Permeability
Leukocyte trapping

Immune response

Macrophage ←— Antigen

Interleukin-1 →→ Fever

T cells

Interleukin-2 and 6   Tumor necrosis factor α

T-cell proliferation

B-cell proliferation

Antibody production

▨▨▨ **Inhibition by Cortisol**

■ **Fig. 45-19** Mechanisms whereby cortisol inhibits many steps in the processes involved in inflammation and immune system responses. Inhibition of the enzymes phospholipase and cyclooxygenase and the synthesis of nitric oxide and platelet-activating factor impairs the vascular component of inflammation. Inhibition of leukotriene actions impairs neutrophil phagocytosis and bactericidal abilities. Inhibition of antigen presentation and macrophage cytokine release impairs proliferation and cytokine release of T cells. Ultimately, B cell function is reduced so that both cellular and humeral immunity are decreased.

In addition, glucocorticoids stabilize lysosomes and thereby reduce the local release of proteolytic enzymes and hyaluronidase, which contribute to tissue swelling. The differentiation and proliferation of local inflammatory mast cells (but not their release of histamine) are also inhibited by cortisol.

Cortisol inhibits the recruitment of circulating leukocytes to the site of trauma or infection. The hormone also decreases margination of leukocytes from blood vessels and their adherence to capillary endothelium. This process requires interaction between various **chemotactic peptides** that attract the leukocytes and specific endothelial cell surface receptors. Cortisol inhibits the production and binding of these peptides to their receptors. Cortisol also decreases the phagocytic and bactericidal activity of neutrophils and the leukotriene-stimulated respiratory burst that accompanies these activities. *Because cortisol increases the release of neutrophils from bone marrow, the circulating number of these cells actually increases* (Fig. 45-20), *although their effectiveness decreases. In contrast, cortisol decreases the number of circulating eosinophils by stimulating* **apoptosis.**

Cortisol also decreases the proliferation of fibroblasts and their synthesis and deposition of fibrils. This process forms the basis for the chronic inflammatory response to injury. *The net result of inhibiting fibroblast function is to impede the local responses to irritants or invading microorganisms, and thus to prevent the walling off of an infection.*

Cortisol also profoundly suppresses the immune system responses to foreign substances. The hormone decreases the number of circulating thymus-derived lymphocytes (T cells), especially the proportion of type 1 T helper lymphocytes, by stimulating apoptosis (Fig. 45-20). In addition, their transport to the site of antigenic stimulation and their functions are decreased. *Thus, cell-mediated immunity, as typified by the rejection of transplanted tissue of nonself origin, is markedly inhibited by the hormone.*

The mechanism of this inhibition by cortisol is multifactorial (Fig. 45-19). When a foreign protein, or antigen, enters the body, it is engulfed by a monocyte/macrophage. This cell "presents" the antigen to T cells and simultaneously elaborates **interleukin-1 (IL-1),** a peptide lymphokine that activates a subset of T cells with helper or inducer function. In turn, the helper T cells secrete various interleukins that produce a cascade of still more T cells and cytokines of various functions. Cortisol inhibits the initial presentation of antigen and the production of IL-1, IL-2, IL-6, interferon gamma (INF-γ), TNF-α, and other macrophage and lymphocyte products. Cortisol affects resting immune cells more than those that are already activated by antigens, and lymphocyte proliferation is arrested in cell stages G_0 and G_1. Even the differentiation of monocytes to macrophages is inhibited by cortisol.

The antiinflammatory action of glucocorticoids also includes the suppression of the febrile response to infections

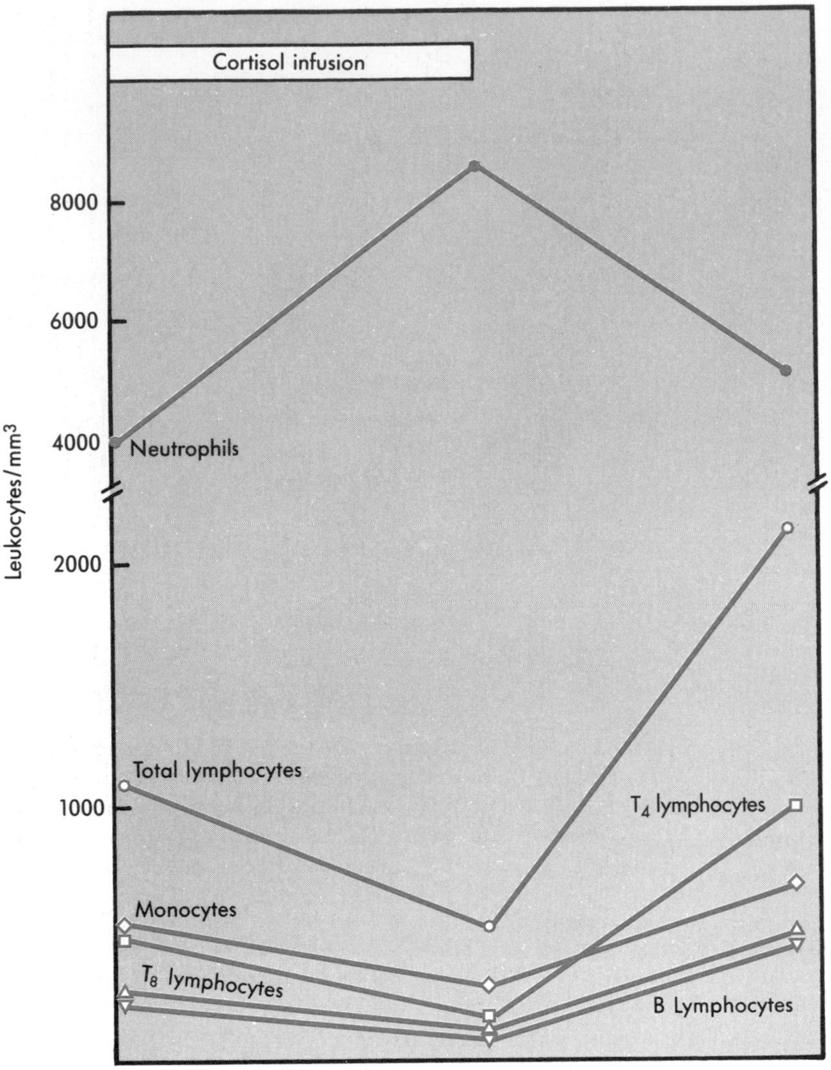

■ **Fig. 45-20**   Effects of cortisol on circulating leukocytes. Note the increase in neutrophils and decrease in monocytes and lymphocytes of all types. T_4 helper lymphocytes were disproportionately reduced. Eosinophils (not shown) also decrease. (From Calvano SE et al: *Surg Gynecol Obstet* 164:509, 1987.)

or tissue injury. This action occurs from decreased production of IL-1, which acts as an endogenous pyrogen.

One of the results of T cell activation is the recruitment and activation of B lymphocytes, which produce neutralizing **antibodies** that are directed against specific antigens. Thus, the proliferation and differentiation of B lymphocytes and their production of antibodies are influenced at least indirectly by cortisol. However, the specific reaction of antibodies with antigen molecules is not affected by glucocorticoids, nor is the degradation of the antibodies.

In patients with asthma (who are often sensitized to allergens), cortisol increases immunoglobulin E (IgE) antibody production by increasing the stimulating lymphokine IL-4 from T helper cells. The action of IL-4 is aided by the costimulatory molecule CD-40, which is expressed on the surface of activated T cells. CD-40 ligand production is also increased by cortisol. The beneficial effect of cortisol on allergic reactions, however, is mediated by suppression of T-cell responses.

A negative feedback relationship between the hypothalamic-pituitary-adrenal axis and the immune system also exists. Immune reactivity varies in a diurnal pattern that is opposite to that of cortisol secretion. *Whereas cortisol inhibits immune responses as described above, inflammatory cytokines stimulate cortisol release.* IL-1, IL-6, and TNF-α all stimulate CRH and then ACTH secretion; this in turn stimulates the adrenal zona fasciculata to synthesize and secrete cortisol. A complex relationship also exists between cortisol and an interesting cytokine that was originally associated with macrophages; this cytokine is called the migration inhibitory factor (MIF). Cortisol at relatively low levels induces expression of MIF, whose release is stimulated during a stress by INF-α and TNF-α. As stress continues and becomes severe, for example, septic shock, the antiinflammatory and immunosuppressive actions of cortisol, which may have detrimental effects, are overridden by MIF. Yet MIF is also expressed in the pituitary gland, where it likely regulates ACTH (and hence cortisol) secretion by a paracrine effect. Finally, CRH and ACTH genes are expressed by some immune cells, and therefore these two peptides may also exert autocrine or paracrine effects on the immune response.

It has been repeatedly emphasized that cortisol is essential to the survival of the severely stressed, traumatized, or infected individual. However, many of the defense mechanisms incorporated in the response to injury are inhibited by elevated levels of glucocorticoids. To explain this paradox, it has been suggested that permissive basal levels or modestly elevated levels of cortisol are required for the initial, beneficial, metabolic responses to stress (and possibly also for some of the immunological, e.g., MIF) However, if a local inflammatory reaction becomes too intense or spreads to adjacent uninjured tissue, the reaction may create local pressure or ischemia. Furthermore, if the initially selective immune system reaction broadens to include responses to nonspecific antigens or even to self-antigens, these defensive processes could become more damaging than the original injury. Thus, the later and more greatly elevated cortisol levels produced by cytokine feedback on the hypothalamus-pituitary-adrenal axis serve to limit cellular and tissue responses, so that they do not destroy normal structure and function, for example, by autoimmune reactions. A proper balance between inflammatory/immune responses to invasion and modulation of those responses by cortisol is necessary to an ultimately successful defense.

The antiinflammatory and immunosuppressive actions of glucocorticoids are used in treating nonendocrine diseases. Administered in high doses, they represent a double-edged sword. When the symptoms of tissue injury that result from disease are functionally disabling or life threatening or when the rejection of transplanted vital organs (kidney, heart, liver) must be prevented, glucocorticoids are dramatically beneficial. However, if glucocorticoids are administered therapeutically for very long, they may increase the susceptibility to bacterial, fungal, and viral infections or allow their dissemination. They may also prevent or delay normal wound healing after injury or surgery. These serious adverse effects, along with diabetes, osteoporosis, and psychiatric disorders, enjoin physicians to prescribe glucocorticoids only when no safer form of treatment can succeed. This injunction obviously does not apply to the use of cortisol as replacement therapy in individuals who have lost adrenocortical function.

Action of Adrenal Androgens

The adrenal steroids, DHEA-S, DHEA, and androstenedione, are relatively weak androgens. Their physiological function is largely expressed by their peripheral conversion to the potent androgen, testosterone (see Chapter 46). However, the adrenal androgens as well as some cortisol precursors, may serve as neurosteroids, which are synthesized in certain areas of the brain. In females, testosterone derived from adrenal androgen precursors sustains normal pubic and axillary hair. It may also contribute to the maintenance of red blood cell production. In males, the amount of testosterone produced in the testicle far exceeds that produced in the adrenal glands, and thus the latter is an unimportant source of androgen. Estradiol, of direct or indirect adrenal origin, is an important source of estrogen activity after the menopause.

The most common cause of endogenous cortisol excess is bilateral hyperplasia of the adrenal cortex, which results from hypersecretion of ACTH. Tumors that autonomously secrete cortisol also occur. The major manifestations of endogenous hypercortisolism include (1) obesity, with a peculiar distribution of fat in the cheeks, the supraclavicular areas, the posterior cervicothoracic junction, the trunk, and the abdomen (the extremities and gluteal area are spared) (Fig. 45-16); (2) loss of bone mass (osteoporosis), vertebral fractures, and necrosis of the hips; (3) loss of connective tissue integrity, associated with fragile capillaries, easy bruisability, and thin skin through which the underlying blood vessels may be seen (purple **striae**) (Fig. 45-16); (4) increased protein catabolism, which results in atrophy and weakness of the muscles of the trunk and extremities, poor wound healing, and stunted growth in children; (5) abnormal carbohydrate metabolism, or even overt diabetes; (6) increased VLDL and LDL cholesterol; (7) hypertension; (8) cardiovascular disease, if Cushing's syndrome is prolonged; (9) insomnia, euphoria, or depression; and (10) impaired wound healing and response to infections. All these pathological consequences can also be produced by large therapeutic doses of synthetic glucocorticoids.

Endogenous glucocorticoid excess is diagnosed by demonstrating elevated plasma cortisol levels or urinary free cortisol levels, loss of normal cortisol diurnal variation, and loss of normal suppressibility of cortisol secretion by potent exogenous glucocorticoids, such as **dexamethasone** (Table 45-1). If the pituitary gland causes cortisol hypersecretion, plasma ACTH is elevated. If autonomous adrenal tissue has developed, negative feedback decreases the levels of plasma ACTH, and inhibits the normal rise in plasma ACTH produced by CRH administration (see Fig. 43-12).

Cortisol concentrations inside target cells are maintained at appropriate levels, partly by the operation of a subtle intracellular negative feedback system (Fig. 45-21) involving the activity of the type 1 11β-hydroxysteroid dehydrogenase (11-HSD). Cortisol induces 11-HSD, by combining with GR_α. However, cortisol also downregulates GR_α, by repressing its synthesis. Hence, when intracellular cortisol levels become too high, GR_α falls, 11-HSD declines, less cortisone entering from the plasma is converted to cortisol, and the level of cortisol decreases. The reverse sequence can raise intracellular cortisol from suboptimal levels.

Interest is currently high in mechanisms that might influence intracellular cortisol levels, and hence might affect cortisol actions. This is because the phenotype of excess

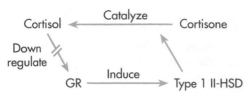

Fig. 45-21 Regulation of intracellular cortisol. Cortisol is produced from cortisone that enters the cell from plasma in a reaction catalyzed by type 1 11-hydroxysteroid dehydrogenase *(11-HSD)*. This enzyme is induced by ligand-bound glucocorticoid receptor *(GR)*. By downregulating GR, less 11-HSD is produced, hence less cortisol is made from cortisone.

cortisol effect (Cushing's syndrome, Fig. 45-16) has many similarities to that of the increasingly prevalent prediabetic and precardiovascular disease, "metabolic syndrome." The latter consists of insulin resistance, hyperinsulinemia, hypertension, dyslipidemia, and accumulation of excess abdominal (especially visceral) fat. Type 1 11-HSD is plentiful in visceral fat, in both stromal cells and adipocytes, and is present in liver and muscle. By maintaining high intracellular cortisol levels derived from plasma cortisone, cortisol's adipose tissue-generating effect and cortisol's insulin-inhibiting effect could contribute to the metabolic syndrome, even though plasma cortisol levels are not elevated. Obese individuals have normal plasma cortisol levels, but increased cortisol turnover to cortisone apparently secondary to an altered set point of type 1 11-HSD.

Adrenal androgen hypersecretion is clinically silent in adult males, but it is detectable in females by their signs of masculinization. This includes loss of regular menses, regression of breast tissue, increased body hair, acne, deepening of the voice, enlargement of the clitoris, increased muscularity, and heightened libido. In such women, plasma and urinary DHEA-S and plasma testosterone levels are elevated.

Regulation of Zona Glomerulosa Function

The principal function of aldosterone, the major mineralocorticoid, is to sustain extracellular fluid volume by conserving body sodium. Hence, aldosterone is largely secreted in response to signals that arise from the kidney when a reduction in circulating fluid volume is sensed. As shown in Fig. 45-22, when body sodium is depleted (e.g., by dietary restriction), the fall in extracellular fluid and plasma volume decreases renal arterial blood flow and pressure. The juxtaglomerular cells of the kidney respond to this change by secreting the enzyme **renin** into the peripheral circulation. As detailed in Chapter 36, renin acts on its substrate, **angiotensinogen** (an α_2-globulin of hepatic origin), to form the decapeptide **angiotensin I.** This decapeptide is then further cleaved by an angiotensin-converting enzyme to the octapeptide **angiotensin II.** This potent vasoconstrictor binds to specific plasma membrane receptors in the adrenal zona glomerulosa cells. Through G-protein linkages, cal-

cium and phosphatidylinositol products are generated as second messengers. Protein kinase C is translocated to the plasma membrane and is activated. Subsequently, the transfer of cholesterol to the mitochondria and P450$_{scc}$ and aldosterone synthase steps in the synthesis of aldosterone are stimulated (Fig. 45-7). Minute increases in plasma angiotensin II are sufficient to stimulate maximal aldosterone release. Angiotensin II also stimulates expression of the aldosterone synthase gene and proliferation of the zona glomerulosa cells.

During several days of an intake of only 10 mEq of sodium, the aldosterone secretion rates increase 4-fold to 8-fold. The renin and aldosterone responses to hypovolemia are also rapidly evoked by hemorrhage, by assuming an upright posture for several hours, or by an acute diuresis (see also Chapters 24 and 36). Such maneuvers increase plasma aldosterone levels 2-fold to 4-fold. Conversely, when excess sodium is ingested and extracellular fluid volume expands, rcnin release, angiotensin II generation, and aldosterone secretion all are suppressed. *Thus, the juxtaglomerular cells and the zona glomerulosa form a negative feedback system. Sodium deprivation induces aldosterone hypersecretion via renin and angiotensin. When the additional aldosterone has caused sufficient sodium retention and the extracellular fluid and plasma volume are restored to normal, the extra renin release is shut off and aldosterone hypersecretion ceases.* In this manner, daily aldosterone secretion ranges from 50 µg (with a dietary sodium intake of 150 mEq) to 250 µg (with a dietary sodium intake of 10 mEq).

The release of renin, which is induced by hypovolemia, is enhanced by increased sympathetic neural activity, via norepinephrine and β-adrenergic receptors in the kidney. The release of renin is also stimulated by certain local prostaglandins; therefore, prostaglandin synthesis inhibitors (e.g., nonsteroidal antiinflammatory agents) can reduce aldosterone responses. Short-loop feedback inhibition of renin release is exerted by angiotensin II, but there is no direct feedback on the juxtaglomerular cells by aldosterone.

The actions described above form part of the physiological basis for the therapy of **hypertension.** β-Adrenergic antagonists lower blood pressure, in part by reducing the sodium retention caused by renin-aldosterone activity. In a similar way, inhibitors of angiotensin-converting enzyme or angiotensin II receptor blockers also lower blood pressure. Antagonists of aldosterone at the renal tubule cell level directly prevent sodium reabsorption and reduce hypertension.

Atrial natriuretic peptide (ANP) reinforces the effects of the renin-angiotensin system on aldosterone secretion. In response to volume expansion, atrial myocytes release ANP, which binds to specific receptors in the zona glomerulosa and inhibits the synthesis and release of aldosterone. This direct inhibitory effect is mediated by decreased cAMP and increased cGMP levels. ANP also reduces aldosterone secretion indirectly by decreasing renin release. B-type ANP

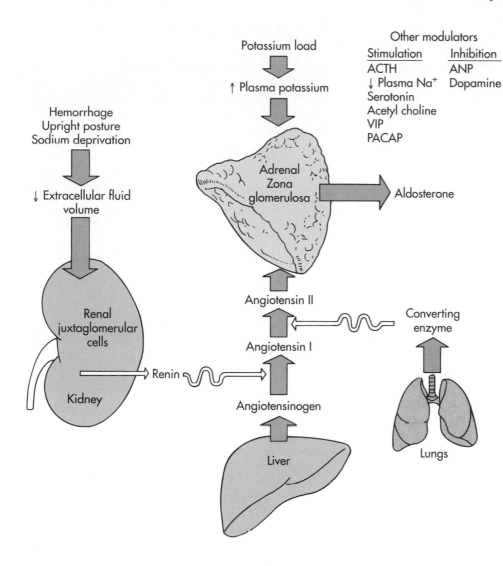

Potassium load

↑ Plasma potassium

Other modulators

Stimulation	Inhibition
ACTH	ANP
↓ Plasma Na⁺	Dopamine
Serotonin	
Acetyl choline	
VIP	
PACAP	

Hemorrhage
Upright posture
Sodium deprivation

↓ Extracellular fluid volume

Adrenal
Zona
glomerulosa

Aldosterone

Renal
juxtaglomerular
cells

Angiotensin II

Converting
enzyme

Angiotensin I

Renin

Kidney

Angiotensinogen

Liver

Lungs

■ **Fig. 45-22** Regulation of aldosterone secretion. Activation of the renin-angiotensin system in response to hypovolemia is the predominant stimulus to aldosterone production. Elevation of plasma potassium is the other major stimulus. ACTH has a minor tonic stimulatory role. *ANP,* Atrial natriuretic hormone is inhibitory. Neurotransmitters and neuropeptides, probably produced in the adrenal gland, modulate aldosterone secretion.

released by ventricular myocytes in response to increased end-diastolic pressure and volume and C-type ANP released by endothelial cells in response to shear stress also decease aldosterone secretion.

Finally, a local renin-angiotensinogen-angiotensin-converting enzyme system, expressing all the necessary genes, exists within the adrenal gland. It is activated by sodium depletion and potassium excess. The additional contribution of the local angiotensin II-generating system to systemically derived angiotensin II production of the adrenal aldosterone response, needed in various physiological circumstances, is currently unknown.

Aldosterone also participates in a vital negative feedback relationship with potassium (Fig. 45-20). *The hormone facilitates the clearance of potassium from the extracellular fluid, and in physiological concordance, potassium acts to stimulate aldosterone secretion.* In humans, an increase of plasma potassium of only 0.5 mEq/L immediately raises plasma aldosterone levels 3-fold, and an increase in dietary potassium from 40 to 200 mEq/day increases plasma aldosterone levels 6-fold. Conversely, potassium depletion lowers aldosterone secretion. Potassium stimulates aldosterone release by depolarizing the adrenal cell membrane.

As a result, voltage-dependent calcium channels open, and the intracellular calcium concentration increases. Accordingly, calcium channel blockers may inhibit aldosterone release.

ACTH, in doses similar to those that increase cortisol secretion, also acutely stimulates aldosterone secretion as effectively as that of cortisol (Fig. 45-7). However, the response to ACTH is blunted if angiotensin II levels are decreased by inhibitors of the angiotensin-converting enzyme. The stimulatory effect of ACTH on aldosterone secretion in vivo wanes after several days. Because of the increased action of aldosterone, sodium is retained and extracellular fluid volume rises above normal; therefore, the release of renin and angiotensin is suppressed, and ANP release is stimulated. Together, these compensatory responses to overhydration return aldosterone levels to baseline and prevent further fluid retention.

The physiological role of ACTH in maintaining aldosterone output is a tonic one; that is, when ACTH is deficient, the zona glomerulosa is less able to respond to its primary stimulus of angiotensin II. This debility is seldom critical in patients with **hypopituitarism.** ACTH also stimulates the secretion of deoxycorticosterone (DOC) and 18-OH-DOC from the zona fasciculata. Rarely these steroids can generate clinical syndromes of mineralocorticoid excess.

The major factors that stimulate aldosterone secretion act in an interrelated way. A low sodium intake or a low plasma sodium level potentiates aldosterone responsiveness to angiotensin, potassium, and ACTH. The increased sensitivity to angiotensin is explained by increased binding of angiotensin II to its receptors, and by enhanced activity of the biosynthetic pathway. Conversely, if the potassium content of the adrenal cell is depleted, the responses to angiotensin and ACTH are diminished. The neural transmitters, acetylcholine and serotonin, also stimulate aldosterone secretion; serotonin is produced by intraadrenal perivascular mast cells. Dopamine released locally decreases aldosterone secretion via an inhibitory G-protein and lowered levels of cAMP. The neuropeptides VIP and PACAP (Table 40-1), synthesized in adrenomedullary cells, interact with their receptors in zona glomerulosa cells to stimulate aldosterone secretion.

In humans, the plasma aldosterone level fluctuates diurnally; the highest concentration occurs at 8 AM and the lowest at 11 PM. Although this profile correlates with similar directional changes in plasma renin and plasma cortisol levels, the diurnal pattern of aldosterone seems to arise independently of these levels. It is not affected by variations in sodium intake, posture, ACTH suppression by exogenous glucocorticoids, or plasma potassium levels.

Aldosterone circulates in plasma bound to a specific aldosterone-binding globulin, to transcortin, and to albumin. Overall binding to these proteins is weaker than it is for cortisol. Hence, the plasma half-life is only 20 minutes, and the metabolic clearance rate is 1600 L/day. Ninety percent of aldosterone is cleared by the liver in a single passage. There, aldosterone is reduced to tetrahydroaldosterone, the major metabolite that is excreted in the urine as its 3-glucuronide conjugate. A smaller portion of aldosterone is excreted simply as its own 18-glucuronide conjugate. The latter metabolite, however, is most commonly measured in the urine for diagnostic purposes. The values of aldosterone 18-glucuronide in subjects with a normal sodium diet range from 5 to 20 µg/day.

Actions of Aldosterone and Other Mineralocorticoids

Aldosterone binds to the mineralocorticoid receptor (type 1 glucocorticoid receptor) in target cells, and the hormone-receptor complex affects gene transcriptional changes in a manner similar to that described for cortisol. Various proteins (described below) that mediate the hormone's effects are induced or suppressed. A lag of 1 to 2 hours is required between exposure to aldosterone and the onset of its action, in most cases. However, considerable evidence of a rapid nongenomic effect, via phosphatidylinositol products and Ca^{2+}, has been adduced. The effects of this nongenomic action on blood pressure, systemic vascular resistance, and rapid sodium exchange are not blocked by inhibitors of protein synthesis or of gene transcription.

The kidney is the major site of mineralocorticoid activity (Fig. 45-23). Aldosterone stimulates the active reabsorption

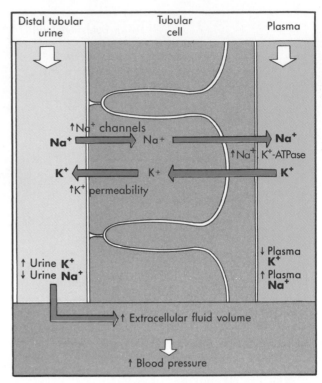

■ **Fig. 45-23**   Action of aldosterone on the renal tubule. Sodium reabsorption from tubular urine into the tubular cell is stimulated by increasing sodium channels in the apical membrane of the cell. Simultaneously, potassium secretion from the tubular cell into the tubular urine is increased. At the capillary surface, Na^+,K^+-ATPase activity is increased so that sodium exits the cell into the capillary and potassium enters the cell from the capillary.

of sodium from the tubular urine back into the nearby capillaries by collecting duct cells and by late distal convoluted tubule cells (see also Chapter 36). Thus, net urinary sodium excretion is diminished and this vital extracellular cation is conserved. Because water is passively reabsorbed with the sodium, there is little increase in the plasma sodium concentration. Hence, extracellular fluid volume expands in a virtually isotonic fashion. Although only 3% of total sodium reabsorption is regulated by aldosterone, its deficiency produces a significant negative sodium balance.

Aldosterone acts via the following mechanisms: (1) Aldosterone stimulates expression of the gene for the α-subunit of the α, β, γ trimeric epithelial Na channel in the principal cells of the collecting duct. The hormone also increases the expression of a serine protease that cleaves the original inactive 85-kDa γ-subunit of this Na channel to a 70-kDa active γ-subunit. Aldosterone then increases the number of these fully functional Na channels in the apical membrane of the principal cells. (2) Aldosterone also increases the number of thiazide-sensitive Na-Cl cotransporters in the apical membrane of the distal convoluted tubule cells. Together these actions increase inflow of Na from the tubular urine to the renal cell. (3) At the basal (capillary) surface of the cell, aldosterone increases the content of Na^+,K^+-ATPase, which pumps the sodium out and then back into the

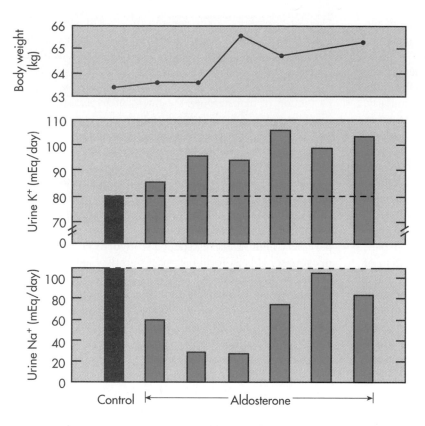

■ **Fig. 45-24** Effects of aldosterone administration in a normal human. Note the eventual escape from sodium retention with stabilization of body weight after a small gain. However, potassium continues to be lost in the urine. Dashed lines represent levels of sodium and potassium intake. (From August JT et al: *J Clin Invest* 37:1549, 1958.)

plasma. (4) In the mitochondria, aldosterone stimulates Krebs cycle enzyme activity, such as citrate synthase, that helps generate the needed energy for extrusion of sodium into the interstitial fluid and capillary blood. (5) In the cytosol, aldosterone increases phospholipase activity and the synthesis of fatty acids, possibly for use in membrane generation.

Aldosterone also stimulates the active secretion of potassium out of the tubular cell and into the urine (Fig. 45-21) *concurrently with sodium reabsorption.* However, this coincidence of effects does not constitute a direct and stoichiometric exchange of potassium for sodium. Stimulation of Na⁺,K⁺-ATPase brings potassium from the plasma into the renal cell; the active reabsorption of sodium at the apical membrane makes the tubular lumen electronegative, which stimulates the transfer of potassium from the cell into the tubular urine. The ability of the tubules to excrete a potassium load depends on distal nephron flow and sodium delivery. Aldosterone allows a small secretion of potassium, even when sodium intake is restricted. However, the extent of kaliuresis increases in parallel with the rate of delivery of sodium to the distal tubule. Thus, a high sodium intake will greatly exacerbate urinary potassium losses caused by aldosterone.

Most of the potassium that is excreted daily results from distal tubular secretion. *Hence, aldosterone is critical for disposal of the daily dietary potassium load at a normal plasma potassium concentration.* However, unlike what occurs with sodium flux, potassium flux does not cause an osmotically balancing movement of water. Therefore, in the absence of aldosterone, potassium retention can cause a dan-

gerous rise in the plasma potassium concentration. An excess of the hormone decreases the plasma potassium level. The control of plasma potassium by aldosterone is relatively slow, compared to the lowering of plasma potassium by insulin and epinephrine, which induce the rapid uptake of potassium by muscle cells.

Continued administration of aldosterone when sodium intake is normal (ad libitum) produces sodium retention, weight gain (Fig. 45-24), and an increase in blood pressure as a result of the expanded extracellular fluid volume. However, after several days and an accumulation of 200 to 300 mEq of sodium, retention ceases, balance is achieved, and body weight stabilizes. This eventual escape from sodium retention is partly caused by a decrease in proximal tubule sodium reabsorption, which in turn results from expansion of the extracellular fluid volume, and the subsequent release of ANP. In addition, the increased renal vascular perfusion pressure decreases the sodium channels in the principal cells of the collecting ducts. Nonetheless, aldosterone-induced potassium loss continues because a high rate of sodium delivery to the distal tubule is maintained and hypokalemia can result.

In addition to its effects on potassium secretion, aldosterone enhances the tubular secretion of hydrogen ions as sodium is reabsorbed. Therefore, aldosterone excess leads to the development of mild systemic metabolic alkalosis, which can be further aggravated by the depletion of potassium (see Chapters 37 and 38). Ammonium excretion is also increased. The final urine pH is usually alkaline, however, because the expansion of extracellular fluid volume inhibits bicarbonate reabsorption. In contrast, a deficiency of aldosterone produces a hyperchloremic non-anion gap metabolic acidosis. Finally, aldosterone also stimulates the excretion of magnesium.

Aldosterone also affects mineral transport in other organs. The hormone stimulates sodium reabsorption from the colon while enhancing potassium excretion in the feces. Similarly, the hormone decreases the ratio of sodium to potassium in fluids from the salivary and sweat glands. These actions, however, have little importance in overall cation balance. Aldosterone significantly affects sodium and potassium exchange between the extracellular fluid and intracellular fluid. The net result is to increase the potassium content of the intracellular space.

A clinically important effect is the increased blood pressure that results from an excess of aldosterone. In part, hypertension is an indirect consequence of the retention of sodium, expansion of the extracellular fluid volume, and a slight increase in cardiac output. However, infusion of small doses of aldosterone into the cerebral ventricles raises blood pressure without altering plasma aldosterone. This response indicates a central action of the hormone on the blood pressure-regulating centers. Moreover, recent evidence demonstrates that endothelial cells and vascular smooth muscle cells can *synthesize* angiotensin II and aldosterone itself. The gene for aldosterone synthase is expressed and aldosterone production by endothelial cells is stimulated by angiotensin II and potassium, just as zona glomerulosa cells are. In addition, smooth muscle cells express the mineralocorticoid receptor and have Na channels. Thus, an entire local system exists for the regulated synthesis and release of aldosterone, and for a paracrine action by aldosterone to increase Na uptake by the vascular smooth muscle cells. Aldosterone is also synthesized at low levels in the human heart, where it may play a paracrine role in sustaining normal cardiac output and tissue remodeling. Finally, aldosterone antagonists can lower peripheral resistance rapidly, even before Na excretion has been enhanced significantly.

The above effects of aldosterone, when it is released excessively for long periods of time, can lead to sustained hypertension and to myocardial necrosis and fibrosis, with impairment of cardiac output. For these reasons, angiotensin-converting enzyme inhibitors (ACEI) and angiotensin receptor antagonists have become first line drugs in the treatment of hypertension. In addition, ACEIs and aldosterone antagonists such as spironolactone, in doses that do not lower blood pressure, have been shown to reduce morbidity and mortality from congestive heart failure.

An excess of aldosterone **(hyperaldosteronism),** or of any other mineralocorticoid, produces a clinical syndrome characterized by hypertension, a slightly expanded extracellular fluid volume, hypokalemia with metabolic alkalosis, and slight hypernatremia. The diagnosis of hyperaldosteronism is established by demonstrating that plasma Sand urinary aldosterone (or rarely, DOC or 18-OH-DOC) are elevated even when the patient has a high sodium intake. If the secretion of aldosterone is autonomous, plasma renin levels are low, because of the expanded extracellular volume. Obstructive lesions of the renal arteries, which reduce renal perfusion pressure, stimulate excess renin secretion and, secondarily, hypersecretion of aldosterone. Treatment of hyperaldosteronism caused by zona glomerulosa tumors is accomplished by removal of the neoplasm or by treatment with drugs that antagonize aldosterone action (see below).

Although cortisol binds well to the mineralocorticoid receptor, it is normally prevented from contributing significantly to renal mineralocorticoid action, because the kidneys (and other aldosterone target tissues, such as sweat glands) have very high levels of type 2 **11β-hydroxysteroid dehydrogenase.** This isoform inactivates cortisol locally by converting it to cortisone (Fig. 45-11). Aldosterone actions in the kidney are blocked by high concentrations of progesterone and 17-hydroxyprogesterone. An important inhibitor, which is used clinically as a diuretic and antihypertensive agent, is **spironolactone.** This drug is a competitive antagonist that binds to the mineralocorticoid receptor.

Complete destruction of the adrenal cortex, or **Addison's disease,** results from autoimmune, infectious, and malignant processes. Addison's disease usually progresses slowly as cortisol, aldosterone, and adrenal androgen deficiencies develop. A lack of cortisol leads to anorexia, weight loss, malaise, lethargy, fatigue, muscle weakness, nausea, vomiting, abdominal pain, fever, poor tolerance of minor medical or surgical stress, fasting hypoglycemia, an increase in circulating lymphocytes and eosinophils, and a reduction in neutrophils. A loss of adrenal androgens may contribute to anemia and, in females, to a loss of pubic and axillary hair. Because of negative feedback, the secretion of ACTH and all proopiomelanocortin products increases as cortisol levels decline. The melanocyte-stimulating activity of ACTH and its MSH coproducts (Chapter 43) produces striking hyperpigmentation of the skin. The diagnosis of Addison's disease is confirmed by demonstrating low plasma cortisol levels, decreased urinary excretion of 17-hydroxycorticoids, and elevated plasma ACTH. If exogenous ACTH is administered, the levels of cortisol and its urinary metabolites fail to increase normally.

Deficiency of aldosterone is marked by polyuria, which is caused by natriuresis. Dehydration, hypotension, hyperkalemia, hyponatremia, and metabolic acidosis are characteristic. Plasma and urinary aldosterone levels are low, whereas plasma renin and angiotensin levels are elevated consequent to the depletion of sodium.

When adrenal insufficiency is caused by ACTH deficiency (resulting from disease of the hypothalamus or pituitary), the clinical picture is the same as that described for loss of cortisol and adrenal androgen. However, plasma aldosterone and potassium levels remain normal, because renin-angiotensin II stimulation is intact. Hyperpigmentation does not occur, because ACTH and MSH are not present in excess.

Treatment of acute adrenal insufficiency (adrenal crisis) requires doses of intravenous cortisol that produce plasma cortisol levels typical of stress, and sufficient isotonic sodium chloride must be infused to restore normal extracellular fluid volume and to lower plasma potassium levels. For maintenance, patients require oral cortisol (or cortisone) and a synthetic mineralocorticoid, such as 9α-fluorocortisol (Table 45-1).

THE ADRENAL MEDULLA

The adrenal medulla is the source of the circulating catecholamine hormone **epinephrine.** The medulla also secretes small amounts of **norepinephrine,** nominally a neurotransmitter, which in select circumstances may also function as a hormone. These compounds have diverse effects on metabolism, as well as on virtually all organ systems in the body. *The adrenal medulla essentially represents an enlarged and specialized sympathetic ganglion. However, the neuronal cell bodies of the medulla do not have axons; instead, they discharge their catecholamine hormones directly into the bloodstream, and thus function as endocrine cells rather than as nerve cells.* The adrenal medulla is formed in parallel with the peripheral sympathetic nervous system. At about 7 weeks of gestation, neuroectodermal cells from the neural crest invade the anlage of the primitive adrenal cortex. There, these cells develop into the adrenal medulla, which begins to secrete catecholamines during gestation, and by birth the medulla is completely functional. The development of sympathetic nervous tissue and induction of neural hormone synthesis are stimulated by **nerve growth factor.**

Adrenomedullary tissue in the adult weighs about 1 g and consists of **chromaffin cells** (so named for their affinity for chromium stains). These cells are organized in cords and clumps, in intimate relationship with venules that drain the adrenal cortex and with nerve endings from *cholinergic preganglionic fibers* of the sympathetic nervous system. Within the chromaffin cells are numerous granules that are 100 to 300 nm in diameter, similar to those found in postganglionic sympathetic nerve terminals. These granules contain the catecholamine hormones, epinephrine and norepinephrine (20% by weight), adenosine triphosphate and other nucleotides (15%), proteins (35%), and lipids (20%). They also contain enkephalins, β-endorphin, other proopiomelanocortin peptides, neuropeptide Y, and chromogranin.

The adrenal medulla is often activated in association with the rest of the sympathetic nervous system and acts in concert with this system. Some actions of the neurotransmitter norepinephrine (which is released locally at the effector site of the postganglionic sympathetic nerve endings) are duplicated and amplified by the hormone, epinephrine, which reaches similar sites via the circulation. However, epinephrine has unique effects of its own, some of which modulate those of norepinephrine. Furthermore, under certain circumstances (e.g., during hypoglycemia), the adrenal medulla is probably activated selectively, with less involvement of the sympathetic nervous system.

Synthesis and Storage of Catecholamine Hormones

The catecholamine hormones are synthesized within the chromaffin cells by the series of reactions shown in Fig. 45-25. The first reaction, catalyzed by the enzyme **tyrosine hydroxylase,** is the rate-limiting step in the sequence, and it occurs in the chromaffin cell cytoplasm. The conversion of tyrosine to dihydroxyphenylalanine (DOPA) requires molecular oxygen, the cofactor tetrahydrobiopterin, and NADPH. The subsequent catecholamine products through norepinephrine all inhibit this initial reaction. The conversion of DOPA to dopamine is catalyzed by a nonspecific aromatic L-amino acid decarboxylase that uses pyridoxal phosphate as a cofactor. The dopamine thus formed in the cytoplasm must be taken up by the chromaffin granules before it can be acted on further.

The next enzyme in the sequence, **dopamine β-hydroxylase,** is found only in the granules. In the presence of molecular oxygen and a hydrogen donor, it catalyzes the formation of norepinephrine from dopamine. In approximately 15% of the granules, the sequence ends here and the norepinephrine is stored. In the rest of the granules, norepinephrine diffuses back into the cytoplasm. There, it is *N*-methylated by **phenylethanolamine *N*-methyltransferase,** which uses *S*-**adenosylmethionine** as the methyl donor. The resultant epinephrine is then taken back up by the chromaffin granules, in which it is stored as the predominant adrenomedullary hormone. The uptake of dopamine, norepinephrine, and epinephrine by the secretory granules is an active process that requires adenosine triphosphate (ATP) and magnesium. The storage of the catecholamine hormones at such high intragranular concentrations also requires energy in the form of ATP. In the granules, ATP is stored in a complex consisting of 1 mole of ATP with 4 moles of catecholamine and chromogranin.

Several factors regulate the synthesis of epinephrine and norepinephrine. Acute sympathetic stimulation activates tyrosine hydroxylase, possibly by decreasing cytoplasmic catecholamine levels and relieving product inhibition. Chronic stimulation of the preganglionic fibers increases the concentrations of both tyrosine hydroxylase and dopamine β-hydroxylase, and thus helps to ensure maintenance of the output of both catecholamines when the demand is continuous. The mechanism of induction may involve a cAMP-dependent protein kinase. ACTH acts directly and helps to sustain the levels of the same two enzymes under stressful conditions. By contrast, cortisol specifically induces the *N*-methyltransferase, and therefore selectively stimulates epinephrine synthesis. The anatomical relationship between the medulla and the cortex subserves this action, because blood from the cortex has a high concentration of cortisol, and it directly perfuses the chromaffin cells. In turn, epinephrine diffuses into the cortex, and it can stimulate adrenocortical

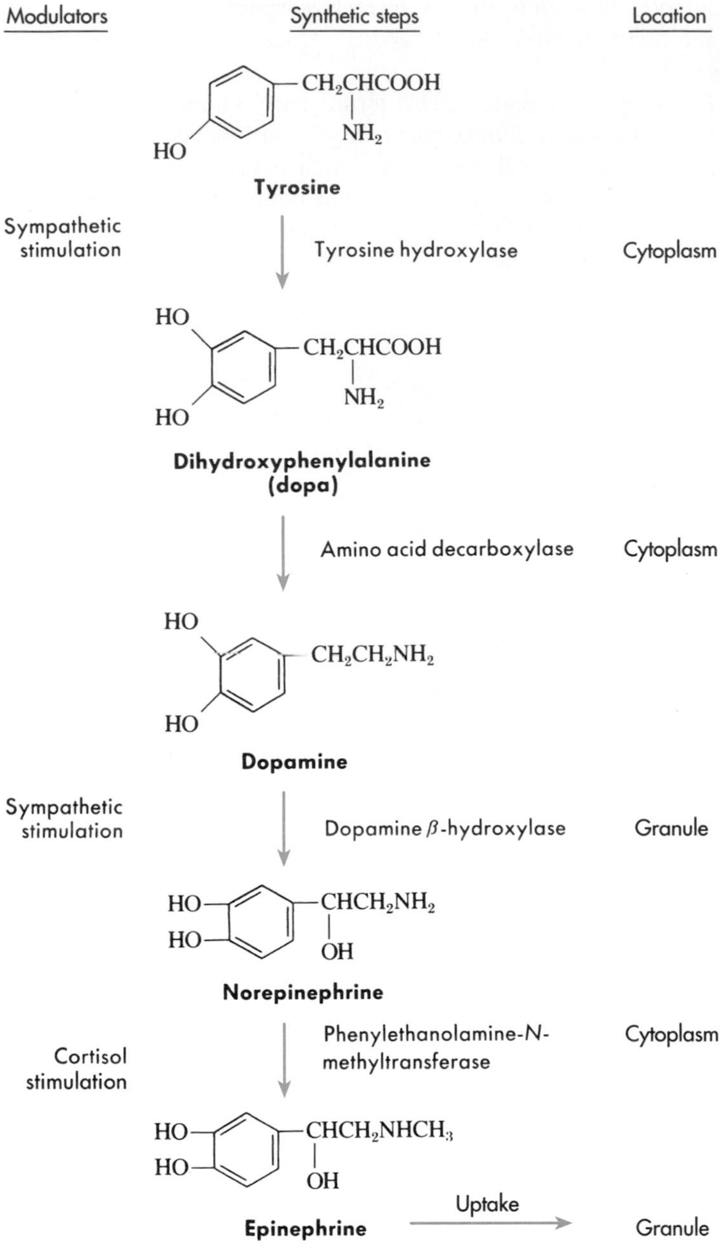

Modulators   Synthetic steps   Location

CH₂CHCOOH
NH₂

Tyrosine

Sympathetic
stimulation   Tyrosine hydroxylase   Cytoplasm

CH₂CHCOOH
NH₂

**Dihydroxyphenylalanine
(dopa)**

Amino acid decarboxylase   Cytoplasm

CH₂CH₂NH₂

Dopamine

Sympathetic
stimulation   Dopamine β-hydroxylase   Granule

CHCH₂NH₂
OH

Norepinephrine

Cortisol
stimulation   Phenylethanolamine-N-
methyltransferase   Cytoplasm

CHCH₂NHCH₃
OH

Uptake

Epinephrine ————————→   Granule

■ Fig. 45-25 Pathway of catecholamine hormone
synthesis in the adrenal medulla. Note that the dopamine
β-hydroxylase reaction occurs within the secretory granule in
which norepinephrine and epinephrine finally reside. Note
also the stimulatory effects of sympathetic nerve impulses
and of cortisol to which the adrenal medulla has preferred
vascular access (see text).

steroid synthesis by activating the expression of the StAR
gene (see above).

Regulation of Adrenomedullary Secretion

*Secretion from the adrenal medulla is an integral part of the
"fight-or-flight" reaction that is evoked by stimulation of the
sympathetic nervous system (Fig. 45-26). Thus, perception
or even anticipation of danger or harm (anxiety), trauma,
pain, hypovolemia from hemorrhage or fluid loss, hypotension, anoxia, extremes of temperature, hypoglycemia, and
severe exercise cause the rapid secretion of epinephrine
(and probably norepinephrine) from the adrenal medulla.*
These stimuli are sensed at various higher levels in the sympathetic nervous system, and responses are initiated in the
hypothalamus and brainstem (see Chapter 11). Usually, activation of the adrenal medulla follows activation of the sym-

pathetic nervous system, and the adrenomedullary responses
are activated by more intense stimuli.

The final common effector pathway that activates the adrenal medulla consists of cholinergic preganglionic fibers in the
greater splanchnic nerve. When these fibers are stimulated,
acetylcholine is released from the nerve terminals. This neurotransmitter depolarizes the chromaffin cell membrane by
increasing its permeability to sodium. Depolarization in turn
induces an influx of calcium ions, which stimulate exocytosis
of the secretory granules. Epinephrine, norepinephrine, ATP,
the enzyme dopamine β-hydroxylase, and chromogranin are
released into the circulation. The membranous material of the
granule is retained in the chromaffin cell and probably recycled.

Adrenomedullary cells bind plasminogen and tissue plasminogen activator to their plasma membranes. Locally
released chromogranin undergoes proteolysis by plasmin

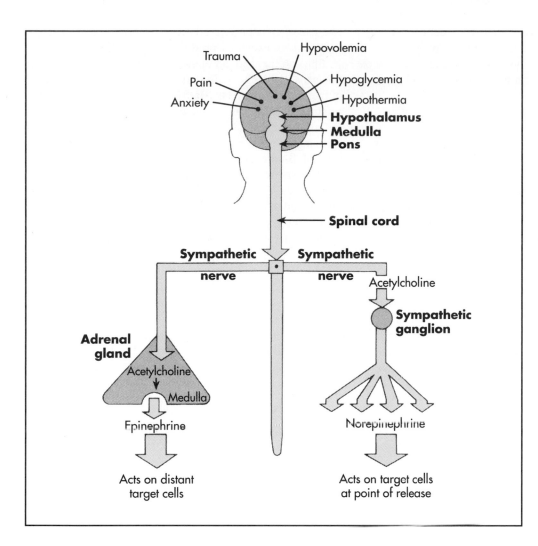

■ **Fig. 45-26** Stimuli to activation of catecholamine effects and their pathways. The adrenal medulla is homologous to a sympathetic ganglion. The latter releases norepinephrine into synaptic clefts. The adrenal medulla releases primarily epinephrine into the bloodstream, where it acts on distant targets.

■ **Table 45-4**   Comparison of circulating concentrations of catecholamine hormones with biologically effective concentrations

		Plasma Epinephrine (pg/ml)		Plasma Norepinephrine (pg/ml)	
Physiological state	*Relevant biological action*	*Observed*	*Effective range for relevant biological action*	*Observed*	*Effective range for relevant biological action*
Basal	—	34	—	228	—
Upright position	↑ Heart rate and blood pressure	73	50–125	526	1800
↓ Plasma glucose	↑ Plasma glucose	230	150–200	262	1800
Severe hypoglycemia	—	1500	—	770	—
Diabetic ketoacidosis	↑ Lipolysis and ketosis ↓ Insulin	510	100–400	1270	1800

Based on data from Clutter WE et al: *J Clin Invest* 66:94, 1980; Silverberg AB et al: *Am J Physiol* 234:E252, 1978; and Christensen NJ: *Diabetes* 23:1, 1974.

(whose usual substrate is fibrin formed by the clotting system). The chromogranin split products then feed back to inhibit release of the catecholamines.

Basal plasma epinephrine levels are 25 to 50 pg/ml (6 × 10^{-10} M). The estimated daily basal delivery rate of epinephrine is 150 μg. The rate of epinephrine release can increase greatly in response to physiological stimuli (Table 45-4). For example, with a modest fall in plasma glucose concentration to 55 to 60 mg/dl, epinephrine concentrations rise to approximately 250 pg/ml. If epinephrine is infused exogenously at a rate sufficient to achieve this epinephrine concentration, the plasma glucose level rises. Hence, the adrenal medulla secretes enough epinephrine to contribute to glucose homeostasis.

The same relationship between epinephrine secretion and its effects characterizes the cardiovascular responses. An increase in heart rate and systolic blood pressure can be produced by the concentrations of epinephrine that are generated endogenously when an individual assumes an upright position (Table 45-4). In addition, the high concentrations of epinephrine that occur in illnesses such as diabetic ketoaci-dosis (see Chapter 41) can contribute to the pathological state by stimulating glycogenolysis, lipolysis, and ketosis. Thus, epinephrine functions as a true hormone in all these situations.

In contrast, circulating norepinephrine levels do not gen-erally increase to levels sufficient to produce relevant bio-logical actions (Table 45-4). Therefore, norepinephrine does not usually function in an endocrine fashion, although it may do so in severe, stressful illnesses, such as myocardial infarction. Instead, the effects of norepinephrine on metab-olic processes, such as glucose production or lipolysis, result from its role as a neurotransmitter. The necessary high concentrations of norepinephrine are thus generated locally at the effector site.

Metabolism of Catecholamines

Essentially all the epinephrine that circulates in the body is derived from the adrenal medulla. In contrast, most of the circulating norepinephrine is derived from sympathetic nerve terminals and from the brain, having escaped immedi-ate local reuptake from synaptic clefts. However, the metab-olic fate of epinephrine and norepinephrine merges into one or two major excretory products (Fig. 45-25).

Epinephrine and norepinephrine have extremely short lifespans in the circulation; this feature allows rapid turnoff of their dramatic effects. Half-lives are in the range of 1 to 3 minutes, and their metabolic clearance rates range from 2.0 to 6.0 L/min. The clearance rates of both hormones can be further increased by the hormones themselves by activa-tion of β-adrenergic receptors. This constitutes another mechanism that helps to limit the actions of these hor-mones. Only 2% to 3% of catecholamines is excreted unchanged in the urine. The normal total daily excretion is about 50 µg, of which 20% is epinephrine and 80% is nor-epinephrine. Another 100 µg is excreted as sulfate or glu-curonide conjugates. Most epinephrine is metabolized within the adrenomedullary chromaffin cell when synthe-sis exceeds the capacity for storage. Circulating epineph-rine and norepinephrine are metabolized predominantly in the liver and kidney.

The catecholamine hormones are metabolized by the reac-tion sequences shown in Fig. 45-27. The key enzymes are **catecholamine *O*-methyltransferase** and the combination of

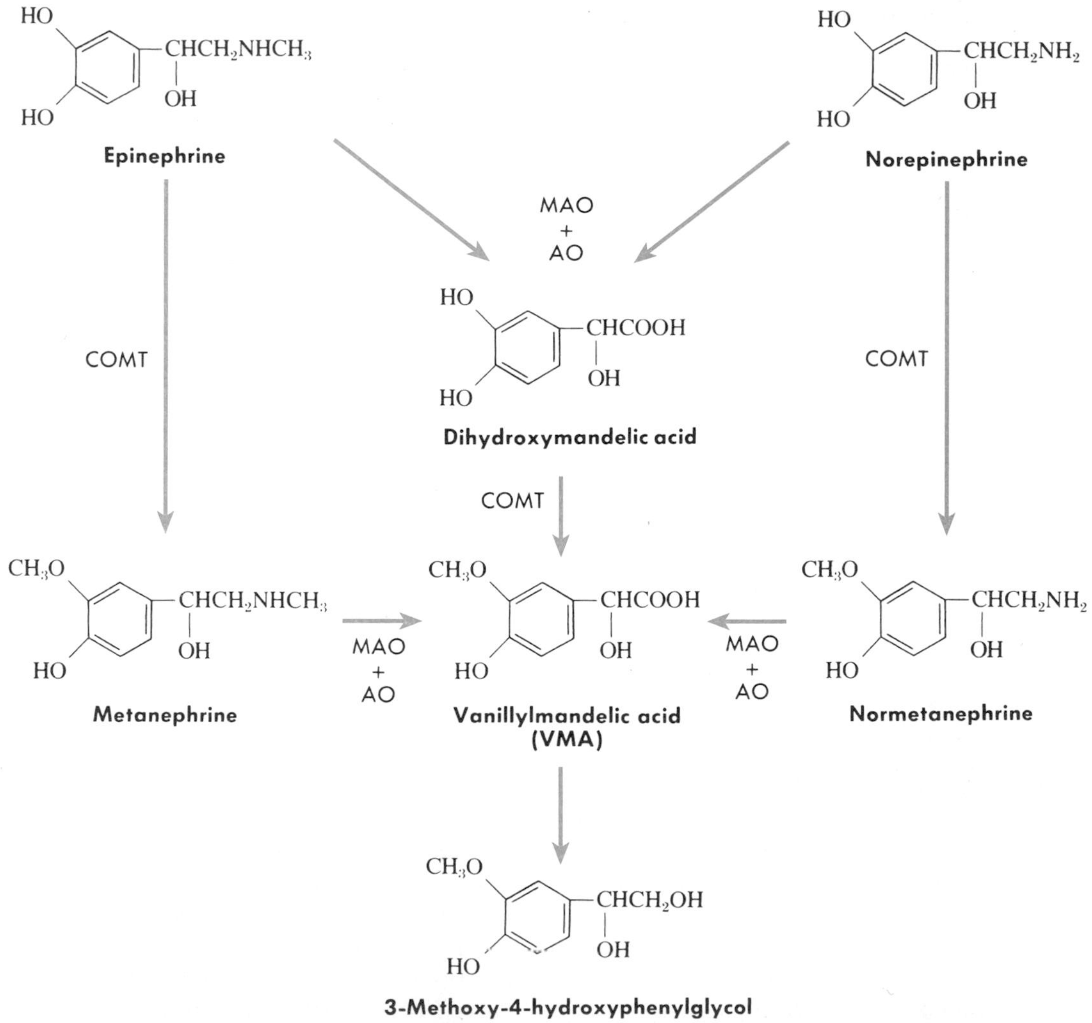

■ Fig. 45-27   Metabolism of catecholamine hormones. VMA is quantitatively the main product.
MAO, Monoamine oxidase; *AO,* aldehyde oxidase; *COMT,* catecholamine-*O*-methyltransferase.

monoamine oxidase and **aldehyde oxidase.** *O*-Methylation and oxidative deamination can be carried out in either order; these reactions give rise to several products that are then excreted in the urine. *O*-Methylation alone yields an average daily excretion of metanephrine (from epinephrine) plus normetanephrine (from norepinephrine) of 300 μg. In contrast, the excretion of the common deaminated products, vanillylmandelic acid (VMA) and methoxyhydroxyphenylglycol (MOPG), averages 4.0 mg and 2.0 mg, respectively. Normally, epinephrine accounts for only a minor fraction of urinary VMA and MOPG; the majority is derived from norepinephrine, and it mainly reflects the activity of the sympathetic nervous system. *Activity of the adrenal medulla can be assessed specifically only by measurement of plasma epinephrine levels or of urinary free epinephrine excretion.*

Actions of Catecholamines

Intracellular actions. Epinephrine and norepinephrine exert their effects on a group of plasma membrane receptors that are designated β_1, β_2, β_3, α_1, and α_2. The relative potency of the two catecholamines varies with each receptor type. Epinephrine tends to react more strongly with β receptors, and norepinephrine with α receptors, but overlap is considerable. Specific agonists and antagonists have been developed for each receptor type.

The β_1, β_2, and α_2 receptors are structurally similar. All three of these receptors are single-unit transmembrane glycoproteins (see Fig. 39-11). α_1 Receptors differ from these receptors and have higher molecular weights. β_1, β_2, and β_3 receptors are coupled to and stimulate adenylyl cyclase; thus, cAMP is the second messenger for these biological effects. Protein kinase A is then activated, and a cascade of changes in enzyme activities follows. The α_2 receptor, in contrast, is coupled to an inhibitory G-protein; thus, hormone binding decreases cAMP levels and protein kinase A activity. The α_1 receptor is coupled to the phosphatidylinositol membrane system; calcium, along with protein kinase C, mediates the hormone effects.

Continuous stimulation of catecholamine release or exposure to catecholamine agonists downregulates the number of adrenergic receptors and induces partial refractoriness to hormone action. Conversely, sympathectomy increases the number of receptors and enhances sensitivity to catecholamines. Acute exposure to catecholamine hormones produces rapid desensitization to subsequent doses. This effect is caused by phosphorylation of the various receptors by the hormone-activated protein kinase A or C. Phosphorylation renders the receptors inaccessible to further hormone binding. Receptor desensitization is a form of rapid intracellular negative feedback, which limits hormone actions.

β-Agonists are used clinically to relieve bronchial constriction in patients with asthma. However, overuse leads to a state of refractoriness to such therapy by the mechanisms detailed above.

Effects on metabolism. A list of epinephrine and norepinephrine actions is presented in Table 45-5. The overall effects on metabolism are depicted in Fig. 45-28. Both catecholamine hormones increase glucose production. They stimulate glycogenolysis in the liver by binding to β receptors and by activating phosphorylase through the same cAMP-initiated cascade that is produced by glucagon. Glycogen synthase activity is concurrently restrained. The adrenomedullary epinephrine response to hypoglycemia is not needed, as long as glucagon secretion is intact. However, in the absence of glucagon, epinephrine becomes essential for recovery from hypoglycemia.

Epinephrine and norepinephrine also stimulate gluconeogenesis by activation of α and β receptors on the liver cells. In addition, they stimulate muscle glycogenolysis, and the released lactate increases plasma lactate levels and provides additional gluconeogenic substrates to the liver. Simultaneously, epinephrine inhibits insulin-mediated glucose uptake by muscle and adipose tissue. By activating α receptors, the catecholamines also stimulate glucagon secretion and inhibit insulin secretion. *All these catecholamine actions help to prevent hypoglycemia, or to restore plasma glucose levels and glucose delivery to the central nervous system, if hypoglycemia does occur.* At the same time, epinephrine activates adipose tissue lipase, and thereby increases the plasma free fatty acid levels, their β-oxidation in muscle and liver, and ketogenesis.

When the catecholamine hormones are secreted during exercise, they promote (1) use of muscle glycogen stores by stimulating phosphorylase, (2) efficient hepatic reutilization for gluconeogenesis of the lactate that is released by the exercising muscle, and (3) provision of free fatty acids as alternative fuels. When epinephrine secretion is stimulated by "stress," such as during illness or surgery, its actions on

■ **Table 45-5** Some actions of catecholamine hormones

β *Epinephrine > norepinephrine*	α *Norepinephrine > epinephrine*
↑ Glycogenolysis	↑ Gluconeogenesis (α_1)
↑ Gluconeogenesis (β_2)	↑ Glycogenolysis (α_1)
↑ Lipolysis (β_3) (β_2)	
↑ Calorigenesis (β_1)	
↓ Glucose utilization	
↑ Insulin secretion (β_2)	↓ Insulin secretion (α_2)
↑ Glucagon secretion (β_2)	
↑ Muscle K$^+$ uptake (β_2)	↑ Cardiac contractility (α_1)
↑ Cardiac contractility (β_1)	
↑ Heart rate (β_1)	
↑ Conduction velocity (β_1)	
↑ Arteriolar dilation: ↓ BP	↑ Arteriolar vasoconstriction;
(β_2) (muscle)	↑ BP (α_1) (splanchnic, renal, cutaneous, genital)
↑ Muscle relaxation (β_2)	↑ Sphincter contraction (α_1)
Gastrointestinal	Gastrointestinal
Urinary	Urinary
Bronchial	Platelet aggregation (α_2)
	Sweating ("adrenergic")
	Dilation of pupils (α_1)

BP, Blood pressure.

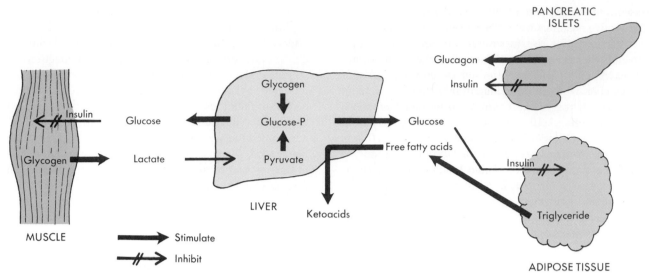

■ Fig. 45-28   Metabolic actions of epinephrine. The hormone stimulates glucose production and inhibits glucose use. It also stimulates lipolysis and ketogenesis. Insulin secretion is inhibited. The net effect is a rise in plasma glucose, free fatty acids, and ketoacids.

fuel turnover contribute significantly to the induction of hyperglycemia and ketosis, that is, epinephrine is a diabetogenic hormone.

Epinephrine increases the basal metabolic rate by 7% to 15%, and it also increases nonshivering thermogenesis and diet-induced thermogenesis. The increase in BMR is less in old than in young people, in women than in men, and in sedentary than in physically fit people. Therefore, epinephrine is an important part of the response to cold exposure, and it helps to regulate overall energy balance and energy stores. In neonates of many species, brown adipose tissue* is an important site in which catecholamines increase heat production (see Chapter 40). Here, they stimulate proton conductance into the mitochondria and thereby uncouple ATP synthesis from oxygen utilization.

In most metabolic effects, epinephrine is more potent than norepinephrine. The latter nonetheless contributes to the regulation of metabolism via the activity of the sympathetic nervous system. For example, sympathetic nervous system activity, with norepinephrine as the mediator, decreases with fasting and increases after feeding. By modulating thermogenesis, norepinephrine thus helps to adapt total energy utilization to energy availability. In contrast, epinephrine secretion increases modestly during prolonged fasting, and also 4 to 5 hours after a meal, in both cases in response to a declining plasma glucose level. This increase in epinephrine levels helps to sustain glucose production for use by the central nervous system.

Effects on the cardiovascular system.   The cardiovascular effects of epinephrine reinforce its metabolic actions. Heart rate, contractile force, and cardiac output increase; on

the other hand, arteriolar constriction is selectively produced in the renal, splanchnic, and cutaneous vascular beds. Systolic blood pressure increases, whereas diastolic blood pressure remains unchanged or decreases slightly. During exercise, the net effect of these changes is to shunt blood toward the active muscles while maintaining coronary and cerebral blood flow (see Chapters 23 and 24). These changes guarantee delivery of substrate for energy production to the critical organs in the fight-or-flight situation. During exposure to cold, constriction of cutaneous vessels helps to conserve heat, and thereby reinforces the thermogenic action of epinephrine.

The cardiovascular responses to catecholamines also initially benefit an individual who has suffered major trauma, circulatory failure, or hypoxia. Without catecholamine release, death might rapidly ensue. However, prolonged secretion of catecholamines eventually becomes deleterious. Reduced blood flow to the kidneys leads to renal failure; reduced blood flow to the splanchnic bed leads to hepatic failure, as well as to intestinal paralysis and necrosis; and reduced blood flow to many other tissues leads to decreased oxygenation and increased lactate production. In the face of decreased lactate utilization in the liver, increased lactate production produces metabolic (lactate) acidosis (see Chapter 38).

Effects on other systems.   Catecholamines exert other diverse effects. Inhibition of gastrointestinal and genitourinary motor activity, relaxation of bronchioles to prevent expiratory airway obstruction and to improve gas exchange, and dilation of the pupils to permit better distant vision benefit the endangered individual. Catecholamines modulate ADH release (β receptors stimulate and α receptors inhibit). They

---

* The role of this specialized adipose tissue in human physiology is controversial.

increase renin release by stimulation of β receptors in the kidney. The increase in renin increases aldosterone secretion, which in turn enhances sodium retention. This action is augmented by the local catecholamine effects in the kidney on the distribution of blood flow and on renal tubular function. Epinephrine stimulates influx of potassium into muscle cells via β_2 receptors. The movement of potassium into the intracellular space helps to prevent hyperkalemia. The important interaction between catecholamine and thyroid hormone function is reviewed in Chapter 44. Thyroid hormone secretion is enhanced by catecholamines under some circumstances, and the peripheral conversion of T_4 to T_3 is stimulated via β_2 receptors.

Catecholamine agonists and antagonists are used widely in medicine. A group of agonists, called **amphetamines,** is used as nasal decongestants, appetite suppressants, and general stimulants. Amphetamines may be prescribed or sold over the counter, but their illicit availability has also become a public health problem. They may cause hypertension; exacerbate tachycardia, palpitations, and nervousness in hyperthyroid patients; or increase plasma glucose levels in diabetic patients. In large doses, they can produce life-threatening "highs." Certain β-agonists are used to quiet premature uterine contractions in pregnancy. β Adrenergic antagonists, α_1-antagonists, and α_2-agonists are used to treat hypertension. β-Antagonists relieve symptoms and extend life in coronary artery disease. They also counteract the hyperactive adrenergic state in hyperthyroid patients.

A recently discovered peptide product of the adrenal medulla, named **adrenomedullin** (AM), has also been shown to be widely produced by vascular endothelial and smooth muscle cells. AM is structurally homologous to the calcitonin gene-related peptide (CGRP) (see Chapter 42). AM is synthesized from a large preprohormone, along with a copeptide named prohormone adrenomedullin peptide (PAMP). Release of AM is stimulated by the cytokines IL-1 and INF-α, and by various growth factors, mineralocorticoids, and glucocorticoids.

AM binds to its own G-protein receptor, as well as to the CGRP receptor. An increase in nitric oxide is followed by vasodilation and a fall in blood pressure. Renal blood flow and sodium excretion are increased. Angiotensin II and potassium-stimulated aldosterone release are inhibited, as is the release of ACTH and cortisol. PAMP decreases catecholamine release by a paracrine effect within the adrenal medulla. Both AM and PAMP decrease sodium and water intake and ADH release.

Pathological Secretion of Catecholamines

Spontaneous deficiency of epinephrine is unknown as an adult disease, and adrenalectomized patients do not require epinephrine replacement. Hypersecretion of epinephrine and norepinephrine from tumors of the chromaffin cells (**pheochromocytoma**) results in a well-defined syndrome. Dramatic clinical episodes are caused by bursts of catecholamine release. These bursts can result from stress or from a rapid change in posture. Sudden severe headache, palpitations, chest pain, extreme anxiety with a sense of impending death, and cold perspiration may occur. Blood pressure may rise to levels as high as 250/150. If epinephrine is mainly being secreted, the heart rate will be increased; if norepinephrine is the predominant hormone, the heart rate will decrease in a reflex response to the marked hypertension. In addition to these episodes, chronic catecholamine excess may produce weight loss, as a result of an increased metabolic rate and decreased appetite. Hyperglycemia can result from inhibition of insulin secretion. The roles of AM and PAMP in the syndrome of septic shock are being explored.

The diagnosis of a pheochromocytoma is established by detecting high plasma levels of epinephrine or norepinephrine when the patient is recumbent and at rest. In addition, urinary excretion of free catecholamines, metanephrines, and VMA is usually increased. The tumor is usually visualized by CT or MRI scan.

Definitive treatment requires removal of the adrenomedullary tumor. Symptomatic treatment is provided by α-adrenergic antagonists, which lower the elevated blood pressure, and β-adrenergic antagonists, which reduce a dangerous tachycardia.

INTEGRATION OF THE RESPONSE TO STRESS

The intimate anatomical relationship between the adrenal medulla and the adrenal cortex mirrors a fundamental functional relationship between the adrenergic nervous system and the CRH-ACTH-cortisol axis. Both the adrenal cortex and the adrenal medulla are major participants in the adaptation to stress. In addition, interactions between these two physiological entities and the immune system add further complexity to this adaptive response, particularly when stress is produced by foreign substances or invading organisms. Thus, it is useful to present an integrated overview of the adaptation to stress (Fig. 45-29).

Stress is perceived by many areas of the brain, from the cortex down to the brainstem. Major stresses activate the CRH and ADH neurons in the paraventricular nucleus and adrenergic neurons elsewhere in the hypothalamus. The activation is mutually reinforcing, because norepinephrine increases CRH release and CRH increases adrenergic discharge, particularly from the locus coeruleus (Fig. 45-29). CRH and ADH release stimulates ACTH release and ultimately elevates plasma cortisol levels; adrenergic stimulation elevates plasma levels of epinephrine and norepinephrine. Together, these hormones increase glucose production. Catecholamines do so rapidly by activating glycogenolysis, and cortisol acts more slowly by providing amino acid substrate for gluconeogenesis. Together, they shift glucose

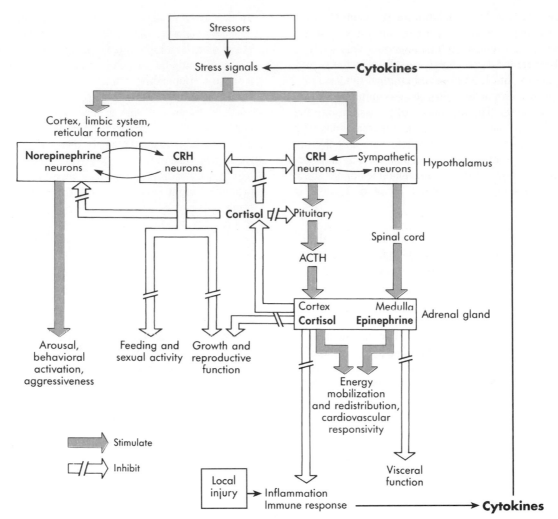

Fig. 45-29   Integrated responses to stress. Responses mediated by the sympathetic nervous system (SNS) and the hypothalamic-pituitary-adrenocortical axis (HPA) are mutually reinforcing, at both the central and peripheral levels. Negative feedback by cortisol can also limit an overresponse that might be harmful to the individual. A feedback relationship between local immune responses to injury and the HPA-SNS consortium also exists. Cytokines from the periphery stimulate the central responses, and cortisol inhibits excessive cytokine production. Cytokines are also produced within the pituitary, stimulated by CRH, and these contribute to the increased ACTH secretion. *Colored arrows,* Stimulation; *open arrows,* inhibition; *CRH,* corticotropin-releasing hormone; *ACTH,* adrenocorticotropic hormone.

utilization toward the central nervous system and away from peripheral tissues. Epinephrine also rapidly augments the supply of free fatty acid to the heart and to the muscles, and cortisol facilitates this lipolytic response. Both hormones raise blood pressure and cardiac output, and they improve the delivery of substrates to tissues that are critical to the immediate defense of the organism.

The neurotransmitter, norepinephrine, and the neuropeptide, CRH, can produce other adaptive responses to stress. A general state of arousal and vigilance, focused attention, an activation of defensively useful behavior, and appropriate aggressiveness result from adrenergic stimuli to the pertinent brain centers. At the same time, CRH input to other hypothalamic neurons inhibits growth hormone and gonadotropin

release. CRH also inhibits sexual activity. These CRH effects presumably occur because growth and reproduction are not useful functions during stress. These actions are reinforced by the excess of cortisol, which also suppresses growth and ovulation. In addition, CRH inhibits appetite and feeding behavior, which again are inappropriate when the organism perceives itself to be in immediate danger. CRH input into the arcuate nucleus of the hypothalamus, hindbrain, and spinal cord increases awareness of pain; in contrast, proopiomelanocortin peptide products related to ACTH (see Chapter 43) produce analgesia and feedback to dampen the excessive CRH and norepinephrine release caused by stress.

At the same time, a variety of cytokines are released at local sites of injury. These immune system "hormones" stimulate cellular and humoral defenses that repel, neutralize, or eliminate harmful organisms or foreign molecules. However, a balance is needed between these useful local responses and their possibly counterproductive systemic spread. If plasma concentrations of cytokines (such as IL-1, IL-6, and TNF-α) become greatly elevated, they stimulate CRH release, which increases ACTH secretion and ultimately raises plasma cortisol levels (Fig. 45-29). Cytokines produced locally within the pituitary gland (Chapter 43) augment ACTH secretion. As the level of plasma cortisol becomes progressively elevated, the production of these same cytokines is inhibited by the glucocorticoid.

Individuals who respond strongly to stress with CRH release, and therefore with cortisol release, have less chance of activating any underlying autoimmune disease process, but they may increase their risk of disseminating an infection. The reverse is true in individuals who are unable to mount even a "normal" stress response.

In short, the hypothalamic CRF-pituitary ACTH-adrenal cortisol axis and the sympathetic nervous system operate jointly in the adaptation to stress. These responses reinforce each other's actions to promote life-saving behavior and to inhibit activities that divert individuals and their resources from defensive responses to danger. They also interact with the immune system to produce a balance between useful local cytokine production at threatened or imperiled sites and potentially dangerous systemic effects of these immune system products.

SUMMARY

1. The two adrenal glands consist of an outer three-layered cortex and an inner medulla. The cortex secretes three types of steroid hormones: cortisol, a glucocorticoid; aldosterone, a mineralocorticoid; and androgen precursors. The medulla secretes the catecholamine hormones, epinephrine and norepinephrine. The adrenal glands are richly vascularized and are essential to survival, because of the cortisol they produce.

2. All adrenocorticosteroids are synthesized from cholesterol by sequential enzymatic steps, which consist of side-chain cleavage and hydroxylation of key sites in the steroid nucleus. Cortisol specifically requires an 11-hydroxyl group; aldosterone, an 18-hydroxyl group; and androgens, a 17-hydroxyl group for their respective activities. The mitochondrial and microsomal enzymes involved are P-450 mixed oxygenases.

3. Steroid hormones are not stored directly. Rather, increased secretory demands require rapid synthesis from stored cholesterol.

4. Cortisol and androgen secretion are regulated by adrenocorticotropic hormone (ACTH). The pituitary hormone acts through a plasma membrane receptor, with cAMP as the main second messenger. ACTH stimulates cellular uptake of cholesterol, its movement from storage vacuoles into mitochondria, and all subsequent biosynthetic steps.

5. Cortisol has major effects on protein, glucose, and fat metabolism. The hormone binds to its receptor, and the complex links to a glucocorticoid regulatory element on target DNA molecules. Modulation of gene expression of numerous enzymes and proteins follows.

6. Cortisol increases muscle proteolysis and stimulates hepatic conversion of the liberated amino acids into glucose, which is then released into the circulation or stored in the liver as glycogen. Cortisol also inhibits insulin-stimulated glucose uptake by muscle. Cortisol stimulates caloric intake and favors deposition of fat in selected sites. By inhibiting collagen synthesis, cortisol reduces bone formation and impairs the integrity of capillaries and skin.

7. Cortisol strongly inhibits the entire process of inflammation, including the recruitment of neutrophils and the release of numerous inflammatory mediators. It also inhibits the immune system and prevents proliferation of thymus-derived lymphocytes and production of lymphokines. These actions underlie the broad therapeutic use of synthetic analogs of cortisol as antiinflammatory and immune suppressant agents.

8. Aldosterone is a major regulator of sodium, potassium, and fluid balance. Aldosterone secretion is regulated mainly by the renin-angiotensin system. In response to sodium deprivation, production of angiotensin II is increased. This hormone stimulates aldosterone secretion via Ca^{2+} and phosphatidylinositol second messengers. Aldosterone secretion is also directly stimulated by potassium.

9. Aldosterone acts on the renal tubule via a specific nuclear receptor and gene expression. Sodium channels are recruited to the apical membrane and sodium reabsorption is increased, with the concomitant expansion of extracellular fluid. Potassium excretion is simultaneously increased, and plasma potassium concentration is lowered.

10. The adrenal medulla is an enlarged, specialized sympathetic ganglion. It synthesizes epinephrine and norepinephrine from tyrosine, and it stores these catecholamine hormones in granules. They are released in response to stimulation of preganglionic cholinergic sympathetic nervous system fibers. Hypoglycemia, hypovolemia, hypotension, stress, and pain are major stimuli.

11. Epinephrine, and to a lesser extent norepinephrine, act as true hormones to increase glycogenolysis in liver and muscle, and lipolysis in adipose tissue. Epinephrine also decreases insulin-stimulated glucose uptake and increases the metabolic rate. cAMP and Ca^{2+} are second messengers. Epinephrine increases the plasma levels of glucose, free fatty acids, and ketoacids. Numerous vascular and visceral actions of the sympathetic nervous system are also reinforced by circulating epinephrine.

BIBLIOGRAPHY

Journal articles

Allison AC, Lee SW: The mode of action of anti-rheumatic drugs. I. Anti-inflammatory and immunosuppressive effects of glucocorticoids, *Prog Drug Res* 33:63, 1989.

Auernhammer C, Melmed S: The central role of SOCS-3 in integrating the neuro-immunoendocrine interface, *J Clin Invest* 108:1735, 2001.

Bamberger CM, Schulte HM, Chrousos GP: Molecular determinants of glucocorticoid receptor function and tissue sensitivity to glucocorticoids, *Endocr Rev* 17:245, 1996.

Barbarino A et al: Corticotropin-releasing hormone inhibition of gonadotropin release and the effect of opioid blockade, *J Clin Endocrinol Metab* 68:523, 1989.

Barrett PQ et al: Role of calcium in angiotensin II-mediated aldosterone secretion, *Endocr Rev* 10:496, 1989.

Bergendahl M et al: Fasting as a metabolic stress paradigm selectively amplifies cortisol secretory burst mass and delays the time of maximal nyctohemeral cortisol concentrations in healthy men, *J Clin Endocrinol Metab* 81:692, 1996.

Born J et al: Influences of cortisol on auditory evoked potentials (AEPs) and mood in humans, *Neuropsychobiology* 20:145, 1989.

Brillon DJ et al: Effect of cortisol on energy expenditure and amino acid metabolism in humans, *Am J Physiol* 268:E501, 1995.

Burnstein KC, Cidlowski JA: Regulation of gene expression by glucocorticoids, *Annu Rev Physiol* 51:603, 1989.

Canalis E, Giustina A: Glucocorticoid-induced osteoporosis: summary of a workshop, *J Clin Endocrinol Metab* 86(12):5681, 2001.

Cato ACB, Wade E: Molecular mechanisms of anti-inflammatory action of glucocorticoids, *BioEssays* 18:371, 1996.

Christ M et al: Nongenomic steroid actions: fact or fantasy? *Vitam Horm* 57:325, 1999.

Chrousos GP: The hypothalamic-pituitary-adrenal axis and immune-mediated inflammation, *Semin Med Beth Israel Hosp Boston* 332:1351, 1995.

Chrousos GP, Gold PW: The concepts of stress and stress system disorders, *JAMA* 267:1244, 1992.

Cidlowski JA et al: The biochemistry and molecular biology of glucocorticoid-induced apoptosis in the immune system, *Recent Prog Horm Res* 51:457, 1996.

Darmaun D et al: Physiological hypercortisolemia increases proteolysis, glutamine, and alanine production, *Am J Physiol* 255:E366, 1988.

DeFeo P et al: Contribution of cortisol to glucose counterregulation in humans, *Am J Physiol* 257:E35, 1989.

Ehrhart-Borntein M et al: Intraadrenal interactions in the regulation of adrenocortical steroidogenesis, *Endocr Rev* 19(2):101, 1998.

Estaban NV et al: Daily cortisol production rate in man determined by stable isotope dilution/mass spectrometry, *J Clin Endocrinol Metab* 72:39, 1991.

Garcia-Borreguero D et al: Glucocorticoid replacement is permissive for rapid eye movement sleep and sleep consolidation in patients with adrenal insufficiency, *J Clin Endocrinol Metab* 85(11):2002.

Goodfriend TL, Elliott ME, Catt KJ: Angiotensin receptors and their antagonists, *N Engl J Med* 334:1649, 1996.

Gustafsson J et al: Biochemistry, molecular biology and physiology of the glucocorticoid receptor, *Endocr Rev* 8:185, 1987.

Hauner H et al: Glucocorticoids and insulin promote the differentiation of human adipocyte precursor cells into fat cells, *J Clin Endocrinol Metab* 64:832, 1987.

Herndon DN et al: Reversal of catabolism by beta-blockade after severe burns, *N Engl J Med* 345(17):1223, 2001.

Horber FF et al: Differential effects of prednisone and growth hormone on fuel metabolism and insulin antagonism in humans, *Diabetes* 40:141, 1991.

Horrocks PM et al: Patterns of ACTH and cortisol pulsatility over twenty-four hours in normal males and females, *Clin Endocrinol (Oxf)* 32:127, 1990.

Hunt PJ et al: Improvement in mood and fatigue after dehydroepiandrosterone replacement in Addison's disease in a randomized, double blind trial, *J Clin Endocrinol Metab* 85:4650, 2000.

Kayes-Wandover KM, White PC: Steroidogenic enzyme gene expression in the human heart, *J Clin Endocrinol Metab* 85:2519, 2000.

Kim GH et al: The thiazide-sensitive Na-Cl cotransporter is an aldosterone-induced protein, *Proc Natl Acad Sci USA* 95:14552, 1998.

Kirkham BW, Panayi GS: Diurnal periodicity of cortisol secretion, immune reactivity and disease activity in rheumatoid arthritis: implications for steroid treatment, *Br J Rheumatol* 28:154, 1989.

Kotelevtsev Y et al: 11β-Hydroxysteroid dehydrogenase type 1 knockout mice show attenuated glucocorticoid-inducible responses and resist hyperglycemia on obesity or stress, *Proc Natl Acad Sci USA* 94:14924, 1997.

Lainchbury JG et al: Hemodynamic, hormonal, and renal effects of short-term adrenomedullin infusion in healthy volunteers, *J Clin Endocrinol Metab* 85:1016, 2000.

Lundgren JD et al: Mechanisms by which glucocorticosteroids inhibit secretion of mucus in asthmatic airways, *Am Rev Respir Dis* 141:S52, 1990.

Masilamani S et al: Aldosterone-mediated regulation of ENaC α, β, and γ subunit proteins in rat kidney, *J Clin Invest* 104:R19, 1999.

Mastorakos G, Chrousos GP, Weber JS: Recombinant interleukin-6 activates the hypothalamic-pituitary-adrenal axis in humans, *J Clin Endocrinol Metab* 77:1690, 1993.

Matthews DE et al: Effect of epinephrine on amino acid and energy metabolism in humans, *Am J Physiol* 258:E948, 1990.

Muglia LJ et al: Corticotropin-releasing hormone links pituitary adrenocorticotrophin gene expression and release during adrenal insufficiency, *J Clin Invest* 105:1269, 2000.

Miller WL: Molecular biology of steroid hormone synthesis, *Endocr Rev* 9:295, 1988.

Napolitano A et al: 11 β-Hydroxysteroid dehydrogenase 1 in adipocytes: expression is differentiation-dependent and hormonally regulated, *J Steroid Biochem Mol Biol* 64:251, 1998.

Norbiato G et al: Cortisol resistance in acquired immunodeficiency syndrome, *J Clin Endocrinol Metab* 74:608, 1992.

Pacak K, Palkovits M: Stressor specificity of central neuroendocrine responses: implications for stress-related disorders, *Endocr Rev* 22:502, 2001.

Parmer RJ et al: Processing of chromogranin A by plasmin provides a novel mechanism for regulating catecholamine secretion, *J Clin Invest* 106:907, 2000.

Peers SH, Flower RJ: The role of lipocortin in corticosteroid actions, *Am Rev Respir Dis* 141:S18, 1990.

Penhoat A et al: Synergistic effects of corticotropin and insulin-like growth factor I on corticotropin receptors and corticotropin responsiveness in cultured bovine adrenocortical cells, *Biochem Biophys Res Commun* 165:355, 1989.

Prummel MF et al: The course of biochemical parameters of bone turnover during treatment with corticosteroids, *J Clin Endocrinol Metab* 72:382, 1991.

Pushkala K, Gupta PD: Steroid hormones regulate programmed cell death: a review, *Cytobios* 106:201, 2001.

Rebuffe-Scrive M et al: Muscle and adipose tissue morphology and metabolism in Cushing's syndrome, *J Clin Endocrinol Metab* 67:1122, 1988.

Rosner W: The functions of corticosteroid-binding globulin and sex hormone-binding globulin: recent advances, *Endocr Rev* 11:80, 1990.

Samson WK: Adrenomedullin and the control of fluid and electrolyte homeostasis, *Annu Rev Physiol* 61:363, 1999.

Schenker Y: Atrial natriuretic hormone and aldosterone regulation in salt-depleted state, *Am J Physiol* 257:E583, 1989.

Schleimer RP: Effects of glucocorticosteroids on inflammatory cells relevant to their therapeutic applications in asthma, *Am Rev Respir Dis* 141:S59, 1990.

Simpson ER, Waterman MR: Regulation of the synthesis of steroidogenic enzymes in adrenal cortical cells by ACTH, *Annu Rev Physiol* 50:427, 1988.

Smith JB, Lee H-W, Smith L: Regulation of expression of sodium-calcium exchanger and plasma membrane calcium ATPase by protein kinases, glucocorticoids, and growth factors, *Ann NY Acad Sci* 779:258, 1996.

Stewart PM, Krozowski ZS: 11β-Hydroxysteroid dehydrogenase, *Vitam Horm* 57:249, 1999.

Stocco DM: StAR protein and the regulation of steroid hormone biosynthesis, *Annu Rev Physiol* 63:193, 2001.

Stocco DM, Clark BJ: Regulation of the acute production of steroids in steroidogenic cells, *Endocr Rev* 17:221, 1996.

Takeda R et al: Aldosterone biosynthesis and action in vascular cells, *Steroids* 60:120, 1995.

Taupenot L et al: Peptidergic activation of transcription and secretion in chromaffin cells cis and trans signaling determinants of pituitary adenylyl cyclase-activating polypeptide (PACAP), *J Clin Invest* 101:863, 1998.

Taylor AL, Fishman LM: Corticotropin-releasing hormone, *N Engl J Med* 319:213, 1988.

Umeki S, Soejima R: Hydrocortisone inhibits the respiratory burst oxidase from human neutrophils in whole-cell and cell-free systems, *Biochim Biophys Acta* 1052:211, 1990.

Vamvakopoulos NC, Chrousos GP: Hormonal regulation of human corticotropin-releasing hormone gene expression: implications for the stress response and immune/inflammatory reaction, *Endocr Rev* 15:409, 1994.

Veldhuis JD et al: Amplitude modulation of a burstlike mode of cortisol secretion subserves the circadian glucocorticoid rhythm, *Am J Physiol* 257:E6, 1989.

Wallberg AE, Wright A, Gustafsson JA: Chromatin-remodeling complexes involved in gene activation by the glucocorticoid receptor, *Vitam Horm* 60:75, 2000.

Wick G et al: Immunoendocrine communication via the hypothalamo-pituitary-adrenal axis in auto-immune diseases, *Endocr Rev* 14:539, 1993.

Wisialowski T et al: Adrenalectomy reduces neuropeptide Y-induced insulin release and NPY receptor expression in the rat ventromedial hypothalamus, *J Clin Invest* 105:1253, 2000.

Wong MM et al: Long-term effects of physiologic concentrations of dexamethasone on human bone-derived cells, *J Bone Miner Res* 5:803, 1990.

Young DB: Quantitative analysis of aldosterone's role in potassium regulation, *Am J Physiol* 255:F811, 1988.

Zuckerman-Levin N et al: The importance of adrenocortical glucocorticoids for adrenomedullary and physiological response to stress: a study in isolated glucocorticoid deficiency, *J Clin Endocrinol Metab* 86:5920, 2001.

Books and monographs

Keiser HR: Pheochromocytoma and related tumors. In DeGroot LJ, editor: *Endocrinology,* ed 3, Philadelphia, 1995, WB Saunders.

Lansberg L, Young JB: Catecholamines and the adrenal medulla. In Wilson JD, Foster DW, editors: *Williams textbook of endocrinology,* Philadelphia, 1992, WB Saunders.

Meikle AW: Secretion and metabolism of the corticosteroids and adrenal function and testing. In DeGroot LJ, editor: *Endocrinology,* Philadelphia, 1989, WB Saunders.

Mortensen RM, Williams GH: Aldosterone action. Physiology. In DeGroot LJ, editor: *Endocrinology,* ed 3, Philadelphia, 1995, WB Saunders.

Munck A, Náray-Fejes-Tóth A: Glucocorticoid action. Physiology. In DeGroot LJ, editor: *Endocrinology,* ed 3, Philadelphia, 1995, WB Saunders.

Orth DN, Kovacs WJ, Debold CR: The adrenal cortex. In Wilson JD, Foster DW, editors: *Williams textbook of endocrinology,* Philadelphia, 1992, WB Saunders.

chapter forty-six

The Reproductive Glands

The endocrine glands that have been discussed in previous chapters are essential to the maintenance of the life and the well-being of the individual. The endocrine function of the reproductive glands, or gonads, is primarily concerned with the preservation and the well-being of the species. The evolution of sexual reproduction has required the development of highly complex patterns of gonadal function. The gonads govern the development, maturation, and nutritional support of the individual male and female germ cells and their successful union in reproduction. They also assist in the early growth and development of the offspring within the body of the mother.

Although the classic endocrine principle that hormones are carried through the bloodstream to act on distant target cells does operate in the reproductive system, paracrine signaling is especially prominent. Thus, cross-talk between different cells within each gonad, between endocrine and germ cells that are close to each other, and between cells of maternal and fetal origin is characteristic. Autocrine functioning generates positive feedback loops. In addition, peptides that are synthesized in the hypothalamus and that initiate functioning of the hypothalamic-pituitary-gonadal axis may also be produced locally within the gonads and placenta, where they may have additional functions.

Despite the many obvious differences that exist between the functioning of the testes and the ovaries, there are also important basic conceptual similarities and operational homologies. Therefore, this chapter presents human gonadal endocrinology as a single unit in the following sequence: (1) sexual differentiation, (2) homologous aspects of gonadal structure and function, (3) testicular function, (4) ovarian function, and (5) endocrine aspects of pregnancy.

SEXUAL DIFFERENTIATION

The process of sexual differentiation (i.e., the pattern of development of the gonads, genital ducts, and external genitalia) produces the most fundamental and obvious differences between the genders. However, during the first 5 weeks of gestation, the gonads of males and females are indistin-

guishable and their genital tracts are unformed. Between this stage of the "indifferent gonad" and that of the mature individual of either gender, the process of sexual differentiation (Figs. 46-1 to 46-3) takes place. Before this process is described, it is useful to consider the gonadal cell lines and functions that are common to both genders (Fig. 46-1).

Primordial germ cells generate the oogonia and spermatogonia, which undergo eventual reductional division and maturation into large numbers of ova and sperm, respectively. Only a few of each eventually unite with each other to reproduce the species, in a manner that guarantees an almost infinite variety of individual characteristics.

One cell line of the indifferent gonad becomes the **granulosa cells** of the **ovarian follicle** and the **Sertoli cells** of the **testicular seminiferous tubules.** The function of these cells is homologous: to sustain or "nurse" the germ cells, to foster their maturation, and to guide their movement into the genital duct system. This cell line is also the main source of estrogenic hormones in females. Another cell line of the indifferent gonad, the **interstitial cells,** gives rise to **theca cells** in the ovary and to **Leydig cells** in the testis. The primary function of this cell line is to secrete androgenic hormones. These hormones are essential to the development of masculine sex characteristics and of sperm production and, in females, as precursors for estrogen synthesis.

The final maleness or femaleness of individuals is best characterized in terms of differences in genetic sex (genotype), gonadal sex, and genital sex (phenotype).

Genetic Sex

Human sexuality is genetically determined by two sex chromosomes with very different characteristics. The X chromosome is much larger, constitutes 5% of the total length of one set of chromosomes, and contains 3000 to 4000 genes, of which about 1000 have been cloned. Only 30 genes have thus far been cloned from the Y chromosome, despite considerable screening. Much of the Y chromosome consists of functionless repetitive sequences. One genetic theory holds that the Y chromosome is an evolutionary descendent of the X

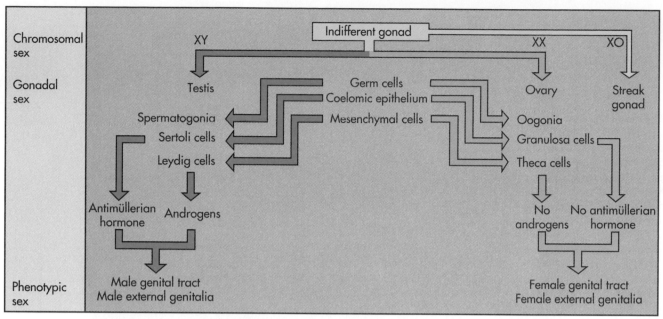

■ **Fig. 46-1** Overview of the development of the cells of the ovary and testis from the primitive indifferent gonad. The hormonal products from the testis and the absence of these products from the ovary determine the gender differences in the internal genital tracts and the external genitalia.

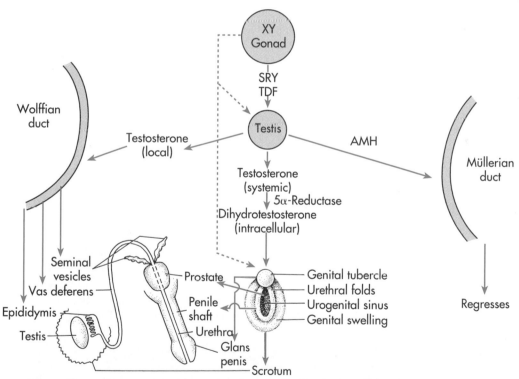

■ **Fig. 46-2** Development of the human male reproductive organs and tract. Note the *dependence on SRY*, a gene on the Y chromosome that expresses the testis-determing factor, and on hormone products of the gonad (testosterone, dihydrotestosterone, and anti-Müllerian hormone [AMH]).

chromosome, and that the Y chromosome is disintegrating over evolutionary time. Each of the sex chromosomes has a pseudoautosomal region (PAR) at the tip of the short arm. These PARs facilitate the crossing over and exchange of genes during meiosis.

The normal male chromosome complement is 44 autosomes and two sex chromosomes, X and Y. *The presence of the Y chromosome is a positive and the single most constant determinant of maleness.* Without a Y chromosome (or critical material translocated from a Y to an X

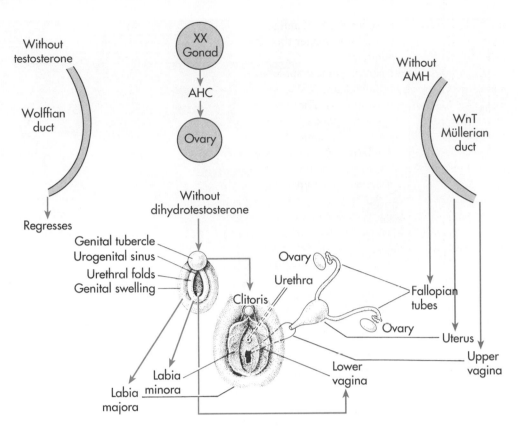

■ **Fig. 46-3** Development of the human female reproductive organs and tract. Note the *independence* from hormonal products of the gonad. Nonetheless, a gene on the X chromosome, AHC, helps determine development of an ovary and the Wnt gene stimulates Müllerian duct development in the absence of AMH. In the absence of any gonads, the female format results. *AMH,* Anti-Müllerian hormone.

chromosome), neither testes nor a masculine genital pattern can develop.

The Y chromosome contains the 14-kilobase segment known as the SRY gene (it is the sex determining region of the Y chromosome). This gene is located on the short arm of the human Y chromosome (Y_p), just below the PAR. SRY encodes the **testis-determining factor (TDF),** a transcription factor protein with a "zinc finger" configuration that binds to DNA molecules. The TDF is a member of a superfamily of nuclear transcription factors that all contain a homologous high mobility group (MHG) protein, which consists of 77 amino acids in the case of the SRY gene product. The rest of this family of over 20 transcription factors is known as SOX (SrybOX) proteins. These orphan nuclear receptors bind to the minor groove of target DNA molecules, where they cause the DNA molecule to bend. This alteration presumably brings specific nucleotide base regions or other DNA-bound transcriptional protein complexes into proper architectural alignment for expression.

SRY interacts with other SOX proteins. Acting briefly in the indifferent gonad on the genital ridge, SRY (TDF) appears to initiate differentiation of the gonad into a testis by relieving the repression that is exerted by SOX-9 on the programmed development of Sertoli and Leydig cells (Fig. 46-1). SRY and SOX-9 also appear to act on pre-mRNA to facilitate splicing. Either SRY or SOX-9 can induce testis development when transferred into XX mice.

Although the SRY gene is essential for masculinization, it is not sufficient for complete maleness. Autosomal and X-chromosomal genes also play roles. The SOX-9 gene, for

example, is on chromosome 17. As already mentioned in Chapter 45, steroidogenic factor-1 (SF-1) acts as an essential component in the development of the adrenal cortex and its synthesis of steroid hormones. SF-1 has an analogous critical role in gonadal development of both sexes. Located on chromosome 9, SF-1 is an orphan nuclear receptor, which is first expressed in the urogenital ridge, then in the adrenal primordium. In the gonad, SF-1 binds to target DNA molecules as a monomer and interacts with SRY, SOX-9, WT-1 (Wilms tumor gene), and DAX-1 (see below). In Leydig cells, SF-1 induces the enzymes of testosterone synthesis; in granulosa cells it induces the key enzyme, aromatase, of estradiol synthesis. SF-1 also regulates the transcription of other molecules involved in reproduction. These molecules include the β-subunit of luteinizing hormone (LH), oxytocin, the α-subunit of inhibin, and the receptors for gonadotropin-releasing hormone (GnRH), follicle-stimulating hormone (FSH), and prolactin. Virilization of the genital ducts and external genitalia requires the presence of an androgen hormone receptor, which is encoded by genes on the X chromosome. In addition, a gene that is called SOX-3, homologous to TDF, is present on the X chromosome. Hence, a dose effect of TDF + SOX-3 (X and Y genes), rather than simply a Y-gene qualitative effect, may help to determine maleness.

Male haploid cells carry a histocompatibility antigen, known as the H-Y antigen (and male plasma contains related heterogeneous H-Y antigens). These antigens are involved in the rejections of male tissue by female recipients. At least one of these molecules is coded by a gene on the Y chromosome. However, the H-Y antigen has now been found in XX males, and it is no longer thought to play any role in sexual differentiation.

The normal female chromosome complement is 44 autosomes and two sex chromosomes, XX. *Both of the X chromosomes are active in germ cells. The genesis of a normal ovary is dependent on the presence of two X chromosomes and on the absence of a Y chromosome* (Fig. 46-1).

Adrenocortical hypoplasia congenital (AHC), formerly called DAX-1, is a gene located on the short arm of the X-chromosome (X_p) that codes for another nuclear transcription factor. AHC is thought to play a positive role in ovarian development, because duplication of the X_p in an XY individual causes female development. This effect might, however, result from the double dose of AHC, which suppresses testicular development. In addition, autosomes participate in ovarian development, because individuals with a normal complement of XX sex chromosomes can still inherit defective gonads as an autosomal recessive trait.

The second X chromosome of an XX female is normally inactivated early in all extragonadal tissues. However, differentiation of feminine genital ducts and external genitalia requires only that the remaining single X chromosome be active in directing transcription within the cell. *Therefore, if an abnormality of meiosis or mitosis produces an individual with only a single X chromosome and no Y chromosome (XO karotype), the phenotype will still be female, although the gonads will be defective* (Fig. 46-1).

Gonadal Sex

Before any gonad appears, primordial germ cells differentiate in the 5-day-old blastocyst. At 22 to 24 days of gestation, the germ cells are present within the yolk sac endoderm. They then migrate to the genital ridge, where they associate with mesonephric tissue to form an indifferent gonad that is present for only 7 to 10 days. The primitive gonad consists of coelomic epithelium, which is the precursor of granulosa (female) and Sertoli (male) cells; of the mesenchymal stromal cells, which are the precursors of theca (female) and Leydig (male) cells; and of the germ cells (Fig. 46-1). A specific transcription factor that binds to a GATA motif in *cis*-acting promoter elements of many gonadal genes is important to the development of Leydig and Sertoli cells in the testis, and of granulosa and thecal cells in the ovary. The entire assembly of the primitive gonad is organized as an outer **cortex** and an inner **medulla.**

In a normal genetic male at 6 to 7 weeks of gestational age, the **seminiferous tubules** begin to form as the Sertoli cells differentiate under SOX-9 influence and they enclose the germ cells. The Leydig cells appear at 8 to 9 weeks. At that time, there is a recognizable testis that initiates secretion of **testosterone,** which is the hormone critical for further male development. The synthesis of estrogen may be prevented by another SRY gene product that inhibits expression of the crucial enzyme, **aromatase** (see later). The medulla of the testis dominates anatomically, whereas the cortex regresses.

In the normal genetic female, differentiation of the indifferent gonad into an ovary does not start until 9 weeks of age. At this time, *both X chromosomes* within the germ cells become activated (Fig. 46-1). Activation of both X chromosomes is an absolute requirement for the further development and survival of the germ cells. These germ cells begin to undergo mitosis, giving rise to oogonia, which continue to proliferate. Shortly thereafter, meiosis is initiated in some of the oogonia, and they become surrounded by granulosa cells and stroma; interstitial cells subsequently appear from the stroma. The germ cells, now known as **primary oocytes,** remain in the diplotene, or late prophase, stage of meiosis, until possible ovulation many years later. In contrast to the male gonad, the cortex predominates in the developed ovary, while the medulla regresses. The ability of the primitive ovary to synthesize estrogenic hormones develops at about the same time that testosterone synthesis begins in the testis. The estrogens may contribute to further female development by blocking the masculinizing actions of any available androgens (see below).

Genital (Phenotypic) Sex

Up to this point in fetal development, sexual differentiation does not require any known hormonal products. However, differentiation of the genital ducts and of the external genitalia does require hormones. *The guiding principle is that positive hormonal influences, normally arising from the gonad, are required to produce male genitals. In the absence of any gonadal hormonal input, female genitals will develop.*

During the sexually indifferent stage, from 3 to 7 weeks of gestational age, two genital ducts develop on each side of the embryo. In the male, at about 9 to 10 weeks, the **wolffian,** or **mesonephric, ducts** begin to grow and eventually give rise to the epididymis, the vas deferens, the seminal vesicles, and the ejaculatory duct (Fig. 46-2). This system is responsible for delivering sperm from the testis into the vagina for reproduction. The differentiation of the wolffian ducts is preceded by the appearance of the testosterone-secreting Leydig cells in the testis. Testosterone stimulates the growth and differentiation of the wolffian ducts in the male. Furthermore, *the testosterone produced by each testis acts unilaterally on its own wolffian duct* (Fig. 46-2), as shown by gonadal transplantation experiments or testosterone implantations. Testosterone need not be converted to its hormonally active product, **dihydrotestosterone (DHT),** to act within the wolffian duct cells, as it does in some other tissues (described later). Indeed, these cells do not develop the 5α-reductase activity necessary for this conversion, until after they have fully differentiated. In the female, the wolffian ducts begin to regress at 10 to 11 weeks, because the ovary does not secrete testosterone.

The Müllerian ducts arise parallel to and in part from the wolffian ducts on each side. A gene, known as Wnt, induces Müllerian ducts in both genders; the expression of Wnt ceases soon after in males, but persists in females. In the male, these ducts begin to regress at 7 to 8 weeks of gestational age, about the same time that the Sertoli cells of the testis appear. These cells produce a glycoprotein hormone, which is a disulfide-linked homodimer, called **Müllerian-inhibiting factor (MIF).** This hormone is also called **anti-Müllerian hormone (AMH),** because it causes the **Müllerian ducts** to atrophy. AMH is encoded by a gene from a superfamily of growth-regulating factors, including **transforming growth factors** α and β, **epidermal growth factor, inhibin,** and **activin.** SOX-9 and SF-1 both activate early AMH production in males. AMH acts through a sequential pair of single transmembrane receptors that leads to phosphorylation of a nuclear transcription factor. This action results in accentuated apoptosis of Müllerian duct cells in a cranial to caudad direction that reflects a similar wave of AMH receptor expression. A product of the Wnt gene mediates this apoptotic action of the liganded AMH receptor in males, even though it stimulates growth of Müllerian duct tissue in females. AMH may also participate in organizing the testis into seminiferous tubules, in restraining overdevelopment of Leydig cells, and in initiating descent of the testis into the inguinal area. Although AMH is found in the postnatal testis and in the plasma of male infants and children, its function after birth remains unclear.

AMH is not produced constitutively by granulosa cells until late in gestation or after birth, and it is present at much lower levels in female than in male infants and children. Therefore, in females, who lack early substantial amounts of AMH, the Müllerian ducts continue to grow. They differentiate into fallopian tubes at the upper ends, whereas at the lower ends they join to form the uterus, cervix, and upper vagina (Fig. 46-3). This *differentiation* is completed at 18 to 20 weeks of gestational age, and it does not require any known ovarian hormone or even the presence of ovaries. However, if estradial is lacking, hypoplasia (e.g., of the uterus) can result.

The external genitalia of both sexes begin to differentiate at 9 to 10 weeks of gestation. They are derived from the same anlage: the genital tubercle; the genital swelling; the urethral, or genital, folds; and the urogenital sinus. In males, testosterone must be secreted into the fetal circulation and then be converted to dihydrotestosterone within the cells of the anlage tissues for the external genitalia to differentiate normally. As a result of dihydrotestosterone stimulation, the genital tubercle grows into the glans penis, the genital swellings fold and fuse into the scrotum, the urethral folds enlarge and enclose the penile urethra and corpora spongiosa, and the urogenital sinus gives rise to the prostate gland (Fig. 46-2). In addition to an androgenic hormone, the presence of a functional androgen receptor is required in these target tissues.

In normal females or in the absence of any gonads, the anlage tissues develop into the clitoris, labia majora, labia minora, and lower vagina, respectively (Fig. 46-3). Hormones may not be essential for this development to occur, although the presence of estradiol may oppose the effect of any androgen secretion in the female. Growth to normal size (e.g., of the labia) requires estrogen. *However, if the normal female fetus is exposed to an excess of testosterone or of other androgens (e.g., from the adrenal glands) during the period of differentiation of the external genitalia, a male pattern can result.* Once the female pattern of differentiation has been achieved, androgen exposure cannot change it to the male pattern, although it can cause enlargement of the clitoris.

The androgen production necessary for early sexual differentiation does not depend on fetal pituitary gonadotropins (see Chapter 43). A luteinizing hormone, called **chorionic gonadotropin,** from the placenta, stimulates testosterone production by the fetal Leydig cells. However, placental steroid hormone precursors, such as pregnenolone, might serve as a source of fetal androgens. Such placental precursors might obviate the necessity for gonadotropin stimulation (analogous to ACTH stimulation) of the reactions from cholesterol to pregnenolone (see later discussion). The growth of the male external genitalia in the last 6 months of gestation does require fetal pituitary LH to stimulate the necessary quantity of androgen. Similarly, the final molding and size of the female external genitalia in utero may be affected by estrogens whose secretion depends on pituitary LH stimulation of the ovaries.

Other aspects of phenotypic sexual differentiation are not evident until well after birth. Such differences include the relatively constant pattern of gonadotropin secretion in the male versus the monthly cyclic pattern in the female, the different degree of breast development, and the psychological identification with a unique gender. The factors that imprint or regulate these traits in humans have not been established conclusively. In rodents, circulating androgens induce the fetal hypothalamus to set a constant pattern of gonadotropin secretion in the postpubertal male. To do so, androgens (paradoxically) require metabolism to estrogens within the target neurons. In the absence of androgens, the cyclic pattern of the female rodent ultimately results. This is yet another instance in which the female pattern is the "neutral pattern," whereas the male pattern requires an action ultimately derived from the Y chromosome. Exposure to androgens in the prenatal or early postnatal period also establishes rodent male sexual behavior, such as mounting. Whether the same mechanism operates in humans is not certain.

Mammary gland development in the rodent embryo also is clearly regulated by hormones. In the absence of testosterone, a normal female breast develops; in the presence of testosterone, the breast ductal system is suppressed. However, in humans, male or female differences in breast development are not apparent before puberty. At that time, the estrogenic milieu in the female induces growth and differentiation of breast tissue, whereas the androgenic milieu in the male suppresses it.

Psychological gender identity, and its expression as gender role behavior, is probably the result of a complex interaction of numerous factors. Genetic sex is not an absolute determinant: a Y chromosome does not guarantee male gender identity, nor does its absence guarantee a female gender identity. Sex assignment at birth almost always accords with the predominant anatomy of the external genitalia. The latter reflects early embryonic exposure to androgens, prenatal testosterone and dihydrotestosterone, and the essential mediation of the androgen receptor. Therefore, androgens can be said to influence gender identity. Individuals with complete androgen insensitivity have high testosterone levels throughout life but remain female in identity. Parental rearing cues and social recognition in accord with sex assignment then establish and reinforce the initial gender identity. A possible later endocrine influence on gender identity is revealed by the natural history of individuals with defective synthesis of testosterone or dihydrotestosterone. Because of incomplete virilization at birth, these XY individuals are raised with female gender identities (or at least expectations). During puberty, compensatory mechanisms lead to normal testosterone or dihydrotestosterone production, growth of the penis, erections, and fertility. Most such individuals then change to male gender identity and male role behavior. However, this reversal, though occurring during a period of increasing androgen action, could also partly result from a change in the way such individuals are viewed by family and friends.

Abnormalities of Sexual Differentiation

Anatomical aberrations that result from certain genetic errors are listed in Table 46-1. Sexual differentiation can be distorted by abnormalities in either sex chromosomes or autosomes.

Individuals with the XO chromosomal karyotype have a vestigial gonadal streak, because they lack the ovarian organizational input of two active X chromosomes or the testicular organizational input of the Y chromosome. The absence of AMH and of testosterone secretion in turn leads to Müllerian duct development, female external genitalia, and wolffian duct regression.

XY individuals who cannot respond to androgenic hormones because of severe androgen receptor deficiency (as in the X-linked **testicular feminization syndrome**) still develop testes, because of the presence of the Y chromosome. These individuals demonstrate Müllerian duct regression, caused by the presence of AMH. However, they show no growth or development of the wolffian ducts nor masculinization of the external genitalia, because the lack of androgen receptors prevents effective testosterone or dihydrotestosterone action. The external genitalia are feminine and breast development is marked because of unopposed estrogen action.

XY individuals who have genetic defects in testosterone biosynthesis develop testes, because of the presence of the Y chromosome, and the Müllerian ducts regress, because of the presence of AMH. Depending on the degree of testosterone deficiency, however, the wolffian duct structures are variably underdeveloped, and the external genitalia may show effects ranging from a failure of complete fusion of the urethral folds to an entirely female pattern.

XY individuals who cannot adequately convert testosterone to dihydrotestosterone because of a deficiency of the 5α-reductase-2 enzyme have a normal testis because of the presence of the Y chromosome. Their Müllerian ducts regress because of the presence of AMH. The development of the epididymis, vas deferens, and seminal vesicles is normal because of the presence of testosterone. However, the external genitalia vary from a partial to a complete female pattern, depending on the degree of deficiency of dihydrotestosterone.

XX individuals who overproduce adrenal androgens in utero (see Chapter 45) have ovaries, because of the presence of two X chromosomes and absence of a Y chromosome. The Müllerian ducts develop normally, because of the absence of AMH. The wolffian structures regress, because of the absence of local gonadal testosterone and the relatively late exposure to excess adrenal androgen. However, depending on the severity of androgen hypersecretion, the external genitalia show variable degrees of the male pattern, ranging from mild enlargement of the clitoris to complete scrotal fusion of the labia and a persistent urogenital sinus.

Individuals with more than two X chromosomes develop testes if a Y chromosome is also present, and they develop ovaries if a Y chromosome is absent. Their genital ducts and

■ **Table 46-1** Examples of abnormal development of the reproductive system

Genetic state	Gonad	Müllerian duct	Wolffian duct	External genitalia
XY, normal ♂	Testis	Regressed	Developed	♂
XX, normal ♀	Ovary	Developed	Regressed	♀
XO, Turner's syndrome	Streak*	Developed	Regressed	♀
XY, loss of X-linked gene for androgen receptor	Testis	Regressed	Regressed	♀
XY, deficient testosterone synthesis	Testis	Regressed	Regressed to variably developed	♀/♂
XY, deficient 5α-reductase	Testis	Regressed	Developed	♀/♂
XXY, Klinefelter's syndrome	Dysgenetic testis	Regressed	Developed	♂
XX, adrenal 21- or 11-hydroxylase deficiency	Ovary	Developed	Regressed	♀/♂
XY, SRY mutation	Dysgenetic	Developed	Regressed	♀
XY, SF-1 deletion	Agenesis	Developed	Regressed	♀
XY, SOX-9 haplo insufficient	Dysgenetic	Developed	Regressed	♀
XX, SOX-9 duplication	Testis	Regressed	Developed	♂
XY, AHC duplication	Ovary	Developed	Regressed	♀
XY, AMH/AMH receptor mutation	Testis	Developed	Developed	♂

*A fibrous streak essentially devoid of germ cells.

external genitalia develop normally. However, spermatogenesis and seminiferous tubule development are markedly deficient in XXY males **(Klinefelter's syndrome)**. XXX females may have shortened reproductive lives. The mechanisms by which extra X chromosomes damage germ cell function are unknown.

Other abnormal patterns of sexual differentiation are caused by mutations of autosomal genes (SF-1, SOX-9, AMH). Their phenotypes are predictable from the actions of the products they express (Table 46-1). Of note, duplication of a gene on the X chromosome, AHC, leads to development of ovaries, even in an XY individual.

COMMON ASPECTS OF GONADAL FUNCTION

Pathway of Gonadal Steroid Synthesis

Both genders use the same pathway of steroid hormone biosynthesis in gonadal tissue (Fig. 46-4). The biosynthetic pathway of steroid hormone in the gonads starts with cholesterol, and it is essentially identical to that of the adrenal cortex. The enzyme genes and characteristics, cofactor requirements, stimulators such as StAR, and localizations are also the same as those described in Chapter 45 for the adrenal glands. More in situ cholesterol may be synthesized from acetyl-CoA in the gonads than in the adrenal glands. As noted, the key enzymes are upregulated by SF-1.

Although two parallel synthetic pathways lead to testosterone, the Δ^5 pathway from pregnenolone is favored (Fig. 46-4). Oxidation of the A ring by the 3β-ol-dehydrogenase-isomerase complex can take place at any point, from pregnenolone to androstenediol. A small quantity of testosterone undergoes 5α-reduction to dihydrotestosterone, and a further α-reduction of the 3-ketone position to 5α-androstenediol also takes place within the testis (Fig. 46-4).

Androgens are the obligate precursors of estrogens. The key step in conversion to estrogen is aromatization of the A ring; this reaction is heavily favored in the ovary and placenta. The aromatase enzyme complex is a cytochrome P-450, localized in the endoplasmic reticulum. It sequentially hydroxylates the 19-methyl group, oxidizes it to the aldehyde, hydroxylates the 2 position, and then creates a 1-2 double bond by reduction. Following these steps, the 19-carbon is removed by decarboxylation, and the characteristic benzene ring is formed. Estradiol and estrogen are formed from testosterone and androstenedione, respectively. The two estrogens may also be interconverted by 17-hydroxysteroid dehydrogenase.

Other Gonadal Products

Testicular Sertoli and Leydig cells and ovarian granulosa cells synthesize and secrete numerous peptide and protein products that act in endocrine, paracrine, and even autocrine fashion to modulate the process of gametogenesis. Inhibins and activins are members of the same superfamily of such growth-regulating factors as AMH. These factors are constructed by combining three basic subunits in various combinations, as shown in Fig. 46-5. **Inhibin** is a glycoprotein that circulates in plasma and inhibits GnRH-stimulated FSH secretion by the pituitary gland. Activin has the opposite action and stimulates FSH secretion. Each factor also has intragonadal actions (described later). **Activin** also stimulates development of some embryonic tissues. **Follistatin** is another FSH-suppressing protein, but its structure is entirely unrelated to that of inhibin. It acts by binding and neutralizing activin. (Inhibin, activin, and follistatin are all also synthesized in the pituitary gland, and this locally produced combination helps regulate FSH secretion.) Insulin-like growth factor-1 (IGF-1 or somatomedin C) and transforming growth factors α and β are also synthesized by Sertoli, Leydig, and granulosa cells, and they modulate cell growth and hormonal responses by paracrine effects within the gonads.

Leydig cells synthesize and secrete proopiomelanocortin products (see Chapter 43) and oxytocin. A peptide that functionally resembles GnRH, but that is structurally dissimilar to it, is also present in the gonads. A variety of trace metal-binding proteins (transferrin for iron, ceruloplasmin for copper), steroid-binding proteins, IGF-binding proteins (see Chapter 43), proteases, prostaglandins, immune cytokines, and extracellular matrix molecules, such as laminin, integrins, collagen types I and IV, and proteoglycans, are also produced by gonads. These substances have local functions in the nurture and development of the germ cells and in the later exodus of ova and sperm from the gonads.

Gonadotropin Actions in the Gonads

The general framework for the hypothalamic-pituitary-gonadal axis is presented in Chapter 43 (see Fig. 43-15). *LH and FSH are the coordinate pituitary regulators of gonadal function. Through negative feedback, their synthesis and secretion are increased by decreases in gonadal steroids.* LH stimulates the interstitial cell line of male and female gonads (Leydig and thecal cells), mainly to secrete androgens. LH also acts on female granulosa cells.

The term gonadotropin implies a "trophic" (i.e., a growth-promoting) effect of FSH and LH on their target cells. In this regard, both gonadotropins share sequence homology and three-dimensional structural features with a variety of growth factors, such as platelet-derived growth factor, AMH, and several bone morphogenetic proteins (Chapter 42). A "cysteine knot" motif, consisting of a cluster of three cysteine bridges, is a characteristic feature of this ligand family.

LH binds to a plasma membrane receptor, a single polypeptide that associates in oligomers. The receptor has a large extracellular portion, spans the plasma membrane seven times, and terminates in an intracellular carboxy tail. LH acts primarily by means of a stimulatory G-protein, adenylyl cyclase, and cAMP as a second messenger. At very high LH concentrations, phosphatidylinositol second messengers, Ca^{2+}, and mitogen-activated protein kinase (MAP) kinase also transduce LH actions.

The interaction of LH with its receptor is exquisitely sensitive. As little as 1% receptor occupancy by LH molecules

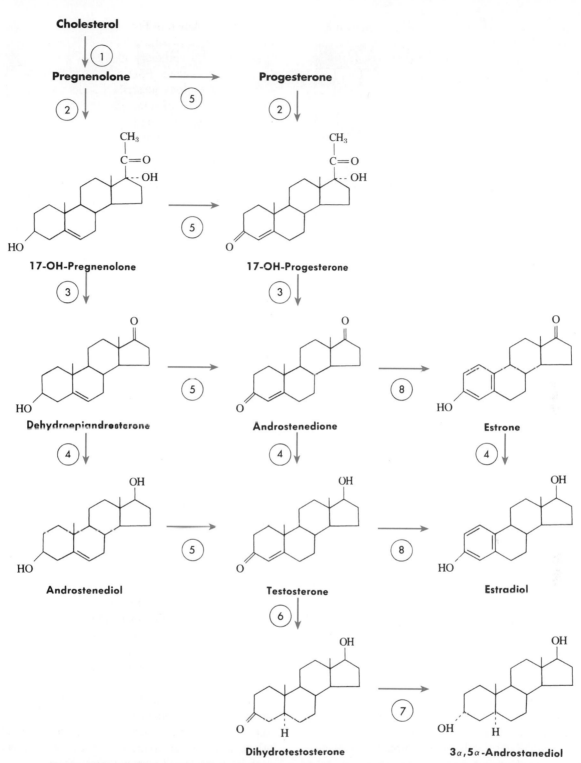

■ **Fig. 46-4** Pathways of synthesis of gonadal steroid hormones. Testosterone is the major secretory product of the testis. Estradiol and progesterone are the major secretory products of the ovary. Enzymes are 20,22-desmolase *(1)*, 17-hydroxylase *(2)*, 17,20-desmolase *(3)*, 17β-OH-steroid dehydrogenase *(4)*, 3β-ol-dehydrogenase and $\Delta^{4,5}$-isomerase *(5)*, 5α-reductase *(6)*, 3α-reductase *(7)*, and aromatase *(8)*.

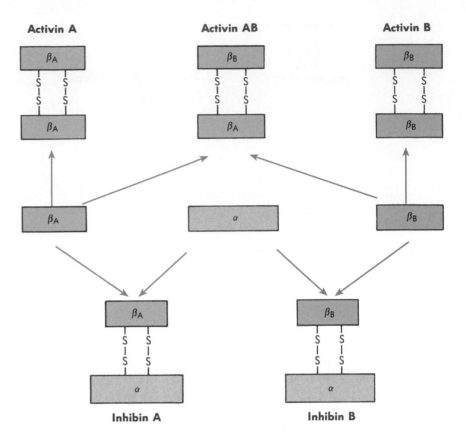

Activin A — Activin AB — Activin B

■ **Fig. 46-5** Synthesis of inhibin A and B from a common α-subunit and two distinct β-subunits. Activins are synthesized by combining the β-subunits into two homodimers (A-A and B-B) and one heterodimer (A-B).

Inhibin A — Inhibin B

can be sufficient for stimulation of some responses, and 5% to 10% occupancy can produce maximal cellular responses. Continued stimulation of gonadal cells by LH reduces the responsivity to the hormone by uncoupling of the LH receptor from its transducing G-protein and by internalization of the receptor. Prostaglandins are additional intermediaries in LH action, and they may potentiate the cAMP effects. LH increases the uptake and mobilization of cholesterol and its conversion to pregnenolone by stimulating the P-450 reaction. It also stimulates transcription of the genes for the enzyme 17-hydroxylase-17,20-desmolase (Fig. 46-4) and the cofactor, adrenoxin.

FSH acts on ovarian granulosa cells and testicular Sertoli cells by binding to a plasma membrane receptor. The FSH receptor shares partial homology with the LH receptor. The increase in cAMP concentration that follows FSH-receptor binding increases the transcription of the aromatase gene and markedly stimulates estrogen synthesis. FSH also stimulates synthesis of inhibin and numerous other protein products of Sertoli and granulosa cells. Another important effect of FSH is to increase the number of LH receptors in granulosa cells, thereby amplifying their sensitivity to LH.

In addition to their actions on steroidogenesis, LH and FSH produce diverse metabolic effects on their target gonadal cells. Glucose oxidation and lactic acid production are increased, effects that may lead to local vasodilation. The long-term tropic effects of the two hormones entail stimulation of amino acid transport, RNA synthesis, and general protein synthesis.

AGE-RELATED CHANGES IN GONADOTROPIN SECRETION

The hypothalamic-pituitary-gonadal axis is unique in that it changes throughout the human life span. Although the patterns of change in females and males differ, there are certain common aspects.

Intrauterine and Childhood Patterns

In humans, GnRH is present in the hypothalamus by 4 weeks of gestation, and FSH and LH are present in the pituitary gland by 10 to 12 weeks. A broad peak of gonadotropin concentrations occurs in fetal plasma at midgestation (Fig. 46-6). After the concentrations drop to low levels before birth, they increase transiently again at about 2 months of age (this increase is more prolonged in females). For the rest of childhood, both gonadotropins are secreted at very low, but detectable, levels. These changes are mirrored by fluctuations of plasma testosterone in males and of plasma estradiol in females. Plasma inhibin also rises and falls in temporal concert with plasma gonadotropins.

Puberty

The transition from a childhood nonreproductive state to a reproductive state during puberty requires maturation of the entire hypothalamic-pituitary-gonadal axis. *Before this maturation occurs, plasma LH and FSH levels are diminished despite low concentrations of gonadal steroids and inhibin. Therefore, either the negative feedback system is inoperative or restrained by other central nervous system input to the*

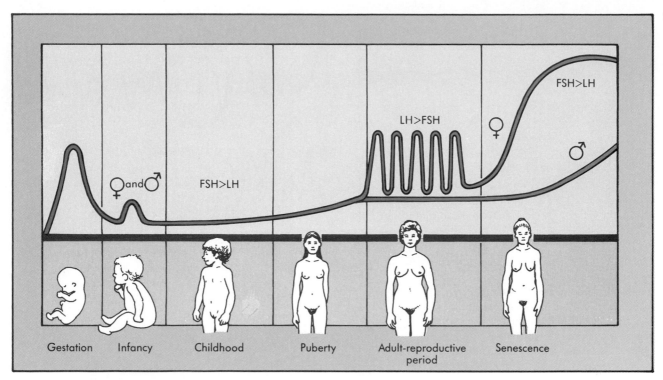

Fig. 46-6   Pattern of gonadotropin secretion throughout life. Note transient peaks during gestation and early infancy and low levels thereafter in childhood. Women subsequently develop monthly cyclic bursts, with luteinizing hormone *(LH)* exceeding follicle-stimulating hormone *(FSH)*; men do not. Both genders show increased gonadotropin production after age 50 years, with FSH exceeding LH.

GnRH neurons, or the hypothalamus and pituitary gland are exquisitely sensitive to testosterone, estradiol, and inhibin.

The gradual maturing of hypothalamic neurons during puberty leads to an increased synthesis and release of GnRH. As puberty approaches, the low-level pulsatile pattern of LH and FSH secretion becomes more pronounced. The ratio of plasma LH to FSH rises as the pulse frequency increases. During early and middle puberty, a barely detectable childhood nocturnal peak in LH secretion is greatly amplified. The nocturnal LH peak then disappears when adult status is reached (Fig. 46-7).

During early puberty, LH exceeds FSH output. More LH is synthesized and stored in the pituitary gland in response to amplified pulsatile GnRH secretion, perhaps because the pulsatility allows better maintenance of GnRH receptors. Although the gonadal target cells respond to LH in childhood, their responsiveness is greatly augmented by puberty. Therefore, testosterone levels in males and estradiol levels in females increase sharply. In addition, FSH stimulates a pubertal rise of inhibin levels in both genders. Thus, early puberty can be viewed as a cascade of increasing maturation from the hypothalamic to the pituitary to the gonadal level.

It is still not certain what sets the gradual process of puberty into motion, but there is no clinically evident precipitating event. More likely there is a preprogrammed schedule of expression of genes, possibly even controlled by an unknown master gene. The time of onset of puberty in sons and daughters correlates with that of their mother, and

50% to 80% of the variation in onset of puberty is likely genetic. There is also gender and ethnic variation. Of African-American girls 27% have some evidence of secondary sexual characteristics by age 7, whereas only 7% of white girls display these changes. Boys are more likely than girls to have delayed onset of puberty, whereas girls are more likely than boys to have precocious puberty.

The current concept of what determines the transition from little or no activity of GnRH neurons to full pubertal and then adult activity is shown in Fig. 46-8. After the gonadotropin burst in early infancy, a dominant negative GABAergic tone restrains the GnRH neurons, both directly and indirectly, by reducing the stimulation of these neurons from glutaminergic neurons. During the transition to puberty, the positive glutaminergic tone is strengthened as the negative GABAergic tone is diminished.

Additional inhibition of GnRH release during childhood comes from neuropeptide Y (NPY), endorphins, and nocturnal melatonin secretion. The very low levels of testosterone and estradiol from the gonads add little, if any, negative feedback. Indeed, the pubertal change in GnRH release occurs in humans who lack functioning gonads and in gonadectomized experimental animals. Endorphin inhibition is also not essential, because opioid antagonists do not increase LH or FSH levels during childhood before puberty. Although nocturnal plasma levels of melatonin are elevated in childhood (and in children with delayed puberty), the subsequent decrease in melatonin does not coordinate well with

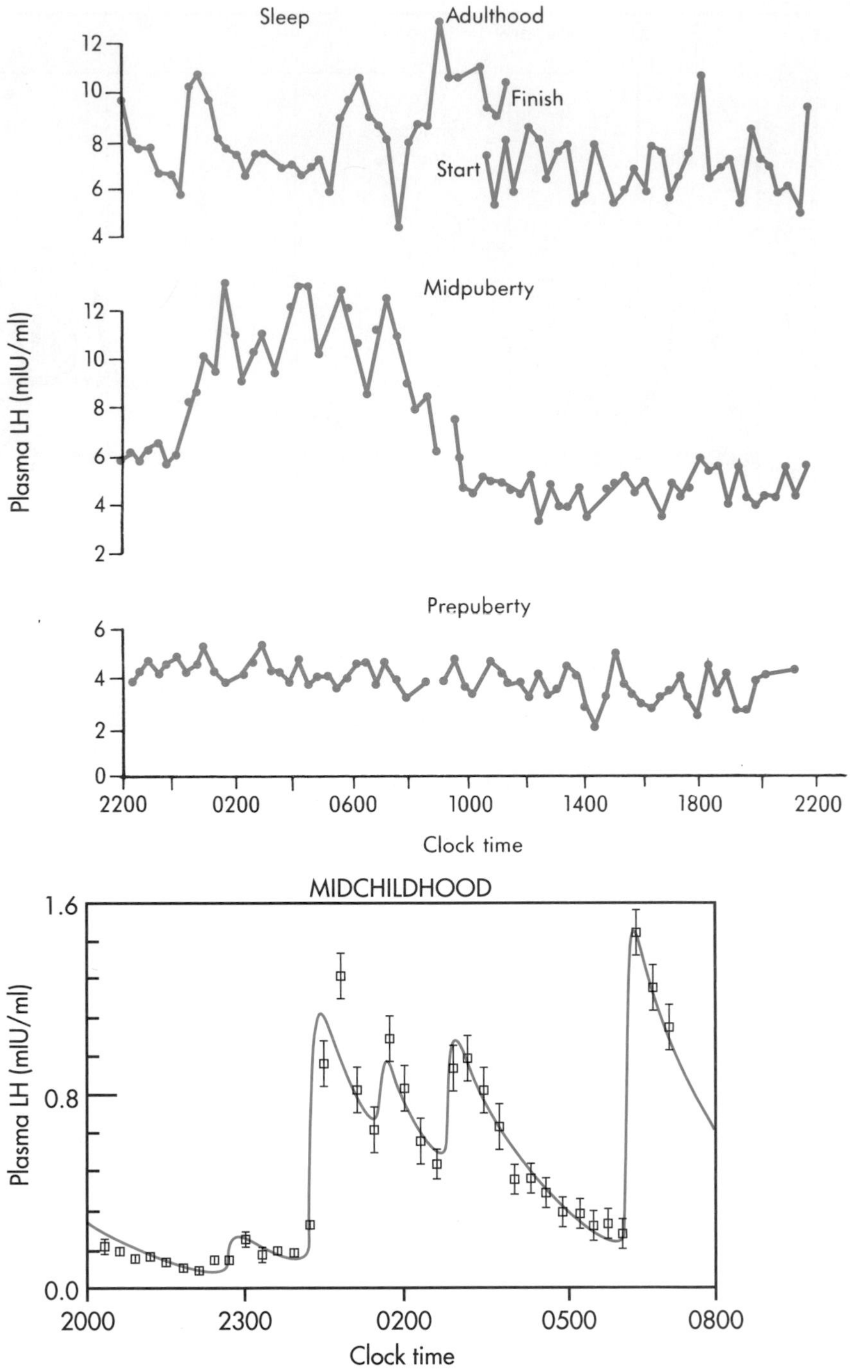

■ **Fig. 46-7**   LH secretion in childhood, puberty, and adult life. During puberty, the pattern of LH secretion becomes much more pulsatile. In addition, a nocturnal peak in LH is greatly amplified in early and middle puberty. This peak disappears when puberty is completed. Males and females both show these changes. As seen in the inset, nocturnal peaking is demonstrable even in childhood when a very sensitive LH assay is used. (From Boyar RM et al: *N Engl J Med* 287:582, 1972. Inset redrawn from Wu FC et al: *J Clin Endocrinol Metab* 81:1798, 1996.)

pubertal onset in primates. Moreover, blind girls with no light perception to suppress melatonin secretion (Chapter 39) actually have early, rather than delayed, menarche.

Individuals with low body weight have delayed puberty and obese individuals tend to pubesce early. It has long been proposed that attainment of a critical fat mass may be an essential condition to trigger puberty. The discovery of leptin (Chapter 40) provides a physiological link between adipose energy stores and reproductive functioning. Thus leptin has been found to increase GnRH release by stimulating GnRH neurons directly and, indirectly, by repressing NPY expression and release (see Chapter 40). At present, however,

most evidence suggests that leptin does not trigger puberty, but rather has an important permissive regulatory function.

Note that puberty entails a marked acceleration of growth, as well as sexual maturation (Chapter 43). Bone mass approximately doubles. Important mechanisms mutually reinforce these two processes that act in concert (Fig. 46-9). As testosterone and estradiol levels rise during puberty, they act on the pituitary gland to help produce a 2- to 3-fold increment in growth hormone (GH) pulse amplitude, without change in pulse frequency or duration. The effect of testosterone is likely mediated by prior aromatization to estradiol. Both steroids also directly increase bone mass,

Prepuberty

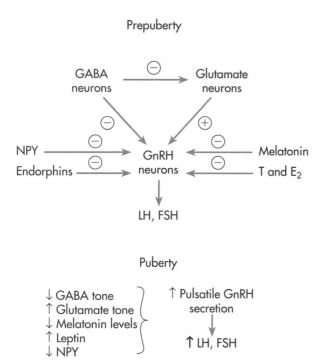

Puberty

■ **Fig. 46-8** Development of pubertal gonadotropin secretion. In childhood a dominant negative tone is exerted on GnRH neurons by GABA (γ-aminobutyric acid) neurons, supplemented by negative input from NPY (neuropeptide Y) neurons. During puberty, GABA tone diminishes permitting a dominant positive tone from glutamate neurons. A decrease in nocturnal melatonin and a decrease in NPY tone wrought by an increase in leptin also help relieve the prepubertal suppression of GnRH. Negative input by endorphins and negative feedback by T (testosterone) and E_2 (estradiol) are barely present before puberty but are greatly augmented by puberty. (From Delemarre-van de Waal HA. *Clin Endocrinol Metab* 16:1, 2002.)

and testosterone directly increases muscle mass in synergy with GH. Although estradiol produces higher GH levels in girls than those present in boys, the estrogen also decreases, rather than increases, the whole body response to GH. The synergy of GH with testosterone, and the lack of estradiol, accounts for the greater pubertal gain in muscle mass in boys than in girls. Conversely, IGF-1 and GH potentiate gonadal development and secretion of the sex steroid hormones. In addition, IGF-1 and other growth factors produced by glial cells in the brain can increase GnRH release.

About 2 years before puberty, adrenal androgen production increases, which is marked by a rise in plasma dehydroepiandrosterone-sulfate (DHEA-S) levels (Chapter 45). This stimulates the epiphyseal growth centers (Chapter 42), which generally must reach a certain level of maturation before puberty can begin. Although the increased adrenal androgens do not initiate puberty, the two developments— adrenarche and pubarche—are normally coordinated.

In both genders, a late onset of what will eventually be normal puberty may be difficult to distinguish from a disease of the hypothalamus or of the pituitary gland that

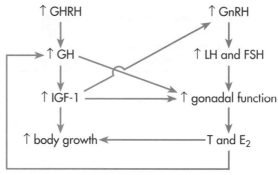

■ **Fig. 46-9** Interaction between growth and reproduction. The products of the GH (growth hormone)-IGF-1 (insulin growth factor-1) axis stimulate reproductive function in the GnRH (gonadotropin-releasing hormone)-LH (luteinizing hormone), FSH (follicle-stimulating hormone)-T (testosterone) and E_2 (estradiol) axis. Lkewise T and E_2 stimulate GH secretion and growth. (From Hull KL: *J Endocrinol* 172:1, 2002.)

prevents the expected increase in gonadotropins. Failure to show any physical signs of puberty by age 13 in girls, or by age 14 in boys, raises suspicion of hypothalamic-pituitary disease and is psychologically distressing. Treatment with sufficient testosterone or estradiol to induce pubertal changes and a growth spurt may be warranted. Such hormonal support does not cause fertility, and it can be withdrawn after an appropriate period to determine whether normal puberty has finally begun.

Once the adult pattern of gonadotropin secretion is established, the basal plasma concentrations of LH and FSH (approximately 10^{-11} M) are similar in men and women. However, an important distinguishing feature between the genders is the establishment of a dramatic monthly gonadotropin cycle in females, only, in which the LH bursts greatly exceed the FSH bursts (Fig. 46-6).

Climacteric

In both genders, a decline in gonadal responsiveness to gonadotropin stimulation occurs after the fifth decade of life. In males, this decline is gradual, and some reproductive capacity usually persists into the eighth decade. In females, full reproductive capacity is lost completely over a period of several years, and menopause occurs. In both genders, however, sex steroid and inhibin secretion decreases so that enhanced negative feedback leads to elevated plasma gonadotropin levels. The FSH level rises more than the LH level, and the increase is more distinct in females (Fig. 46-6). The decline in estradiol and testosterone levels is also accompanied by a decrease in GH secretion and in IGF-1 level, as well as a loss of bone and muscle mass and a gain in fat mass.

Germ Cell Development

Before discussing the gender-specific aspects of reproductive endocrine function, it is useful to examine the analogies

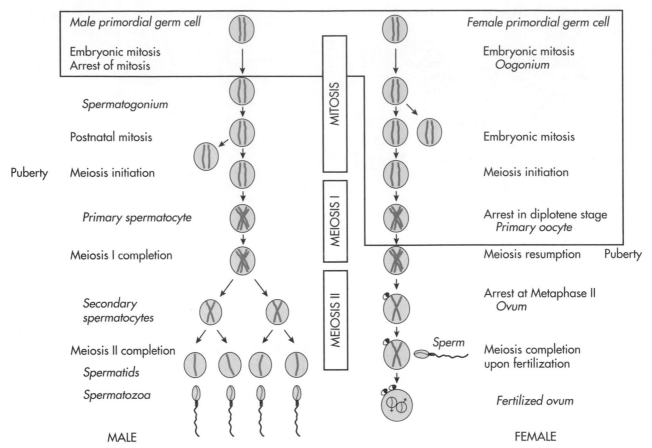

■ **Fig. 46-10** Comparison of male gamete and female gamete production from primitive germ cells. Whereas female germ cells enter meiosis in embryonic life and remain suspended in that state for many years before resuming development after puberty, male germ cells start into meiosis only after puberty. Each female germ cell yields a single ovum, whereas each male germ cell yields many sperm. Approximately 70 days elapse in each case, once meiosis is resumed or started, respectively, until an ovum or sperm is finally formed. (From Wohlgemuth DJ et al: *Recent Prog Horm Res* 57:75, 2002.)

and differences in male and female gamete production (Fig. 46-10). In the embryonic state, primordial germ cells in the male undergo only mitosis to primitive spermatogonia, but development stops there. Meiosis (cell division with chromosomal reduction to the haploid state) does not begin until puberty, but once it does, the process continues through two meiotic divisions to the final emergence of spermatozoa within 2 months. In females in the embryonic state, primordial germ cells not only undergo mitosis to oogonia, but the latter already begin meiosis, which stops in the diplotene stage of prophase. The first meiosis does not resume until many years later, following puberty, but after its completion, the second meiosis again arrests in the metaphase II stage, with extrusion of one polar body. The second meiosis of the ovum is completed only after entry of a sperm, and then the second polar body is extruded. Finally, after fertilization the two haploid pronuclei—one from the sperm and one from the ovum—begin DNA synthesis separately and then they fuse into the final diploid nucleus of the zygote.

THE TESTES

Anatomy

The human testes are normally situated in the scrotum, where they are maintained at a temperature 1° to 2° C below that of the body core temperature. *This lower temperature is essential for normal sperm production.* A lower temperature is partly maintained by the intertwined coiling of arteries and veins to facilitate heat exchange between them. Each testis weighs about 40 g and has a long diameter of 4.5 cm in adults. The testes receive blood from the spermatic arteries, which arise directly from the aorta.

Eighty percent of the adult testis is made up of the **seminiferous tubules;** the remaining 20% is composed of supportive connective tissue, throughout which Leydig cells are scattered (Fig. 46-11). The seminiferous tubules are a coiled mass of loops; each loop begins and ends in a single duct, the tubulus rectus. The tubuli recti, in turn, anastomose in the rete testis, and they eventually drain via the ductuli

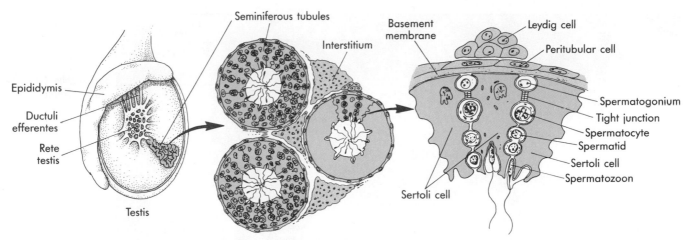

■ **Fig. 46-11** Schematic representation of the architecture of the testis. Note that the Leydig cells and peritubular cells are separated from the spermatogenic tubules by a basement membrane. Within the tubules, the germ cell line is completely invested by cytoplasm of the surrounding Sertoli cells. Tight junctions between adjacent Sertoli cells separate the ancestral spermatogonia from their descendent spermatocytes, spermatids, and spermatozoa. Thus, a blood-testis barrier effectively filters plasma, permitting only selected substances to reach the developing germ cells from Sertoli cell cytoplasm. (From Skinner MK: *Endocr Rev* 12:45, 1991.)

efferentes into the **epididymis.** The epididymis serves as a storage and maturation depot for spermatozoa. From the epididymis, the spermatozoa are carried via the vas deferens and ejaculatory duct into the penis, to be emitted during copulation.

The structure of the adult seminiferous tubule is complex (Fig. 46-11). Each tubule is bounded by a basement membrane that separates it from the Leydig cells, the peritubular (myoid) cells, and the surrounding connective tissue. Gap junctions connect adjacent Leydig cells. Located immediately beneath the basement membrane are spermatogonia and Sertoli cells. As the **spermatogonia** divide and develop successively into **spermatocytes** and **spermatids,** a column of germ cells is formed that reaches from the basement membrane to the lumen of the tubule, where it culminates in the spermatozoa.

In contrast, the cytoplasm of each Sertoli cell extends all the way from the basement membrane to the lumen of the tubule. This cytoplasm invests the spermatogonia and its germ cell line successors (Fig. 46-11). *Special processes of the Sertoli cell cytoplasm fuse into tight junctions, which create two compartments of intercellular space between the basement membrane and the lumen of the tubule.* The spermatogonia and early primary spermatocytes lie within the proximal **basal compartment,** whereas the later spermatocytes and their gradually maturing descendents, which lead to spermatozoa, lie in the distal **adluminal compartment.** This separation maintains a barrier between the blood and these compartments, a barrier that is begun by the basement membrane and the overlapping peritubular cells (Fig. 46-11). In even more discriminating fashion, the cytoplasm of the adjacent Sertoli cells excludes various circulating substances from the intercellular fluid that bathes the maturing germ cells, and from the seminiferous tubular fluid that bathes the

spermatozoa. This barrier also prevents late spermatogenic products from reaching the bloodstream, where, if recognized as foreign substances, they could evoke immune rejection mechanisms.

In short, the testis consists of separate, but interacting, functional elements (Figs. 46-11 and 46-12). The Leydig cells (the first element) are pure steroid-secreting cells. Their major product, testosterone, has important local effects on both germ cell replication and distant target cells. Peritubular myoid cells (the second element) secrete paracrine regulatory products and may produce contractile effects on the tubules and the vasculature (Fig. 46-11). The seminiferous tubules (the third element) are the site where spermatogenesis takes place. These tubules are bathed in Sertoli cell products and are exposed to locally generated testosterone.

The Biology of Spermatogenesis

The production of sperm takes place continuously throughout the reproductive life of the male. Approximately 100 to 200 million sperm are produced daily. Generating this large number of sperm requires the spermatogonia to renew themselves by cell division. This situation differs fundamentally from that in the female, who at birth has a fixed number of oocytes that decreases throughout her life.

Spermatogenesis consists of three distinct phases: (1) stem cell renewal and production of spermatogonia, (2) germ cell proliferation, and (3) spermiogenesis. The first phase is mitotic, with some cells being lost by apoptosis. Apoptosis at early stages of spermatogenesis may adjust the number of diploid spermatogenic cells to the number of Sertoli cells, thereby ensuring quality of the final sperm that are produced. The second phase is meiotic, occurring in the G_2 phase of primary spermatocytes; and the third phase is postmeiotic, as haploid spermatids develop into spermatozoa.

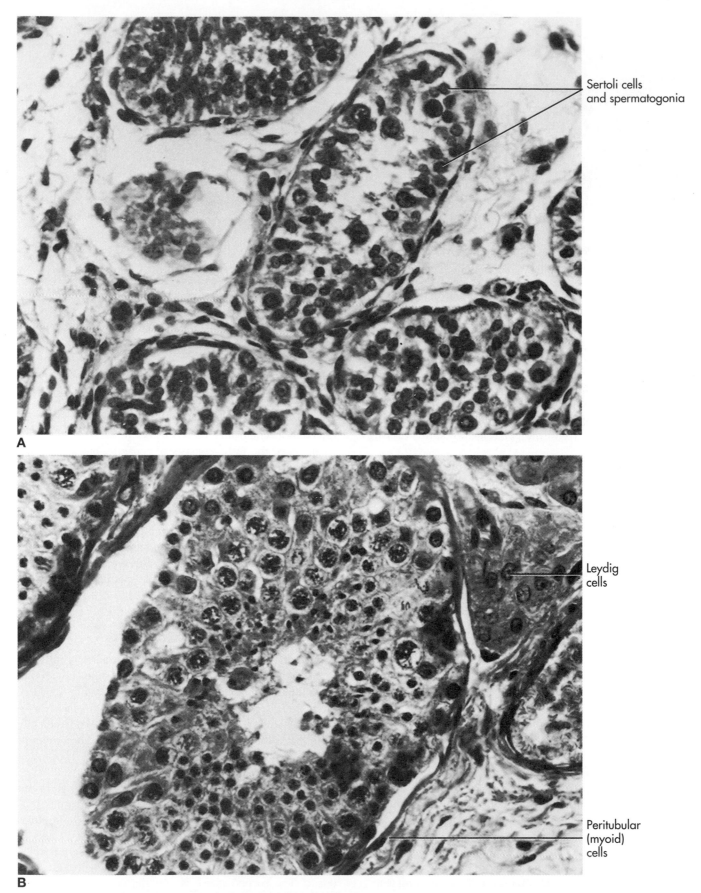

Sertoli cells
and spermatogonia

A

Leydig
cells

Peritubular
(myoid)
cells

B

■ Fig. 46-12   Histological sections of the testis from prepubertal **(A)** and postpubertal **(B)** males. Note the absence of Leydig cells and active spermatogenesis before puberty. (Courtesy of Dr. Howard Levin.)

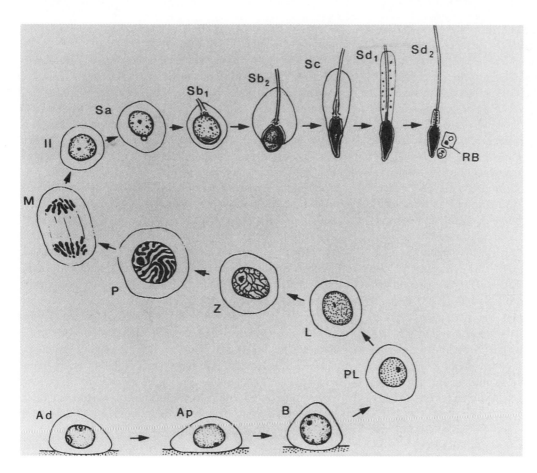

■ Fig. 46-13 Development of spermatozoa from spermatogonia in the human. *Ad,* Dark spermatogonium; *Ap,* pale spermatogonium; *B,* type B spermatogonium; *PL,* preleptotene primary spermatocyte; *L,* leptotene spermatocyte; *Z,* zygotene spermatocyte; *P,* pachytene spermatocyte; *M,* meiotic division; *II,* secondary spermatocyte; *Sa, Sb, Sc, Sd,* spermatids; *RB,* residual body. (Redrawn from DeKretser DM et al: In DeGroot LJ, editor: *Endocrinology,* ed 3, vol 3, Philadelphia, 1995, WB Saunders, p 2309.)

The latter two phases occur in the adluminal compartment, where the consecutive processes of meiosis, genetic recombination, haploid gene expression, formation of the sperm acrosome and flagellum, remodeling and condensing of chromatin, and finally extrusion of cytoplasm take place. Cyclins and cyclin-dependent kinases are essential mediators of mitosis and meiosis.

The whole sequence of spermatogenesis is under *intrinsic regulation* by a preprogrammed temporal pattern of germ cell expression that directs differentiation and morphogenesis. Some of the gene transcripts are unique to germ cells, and they are highly conserved in evolution, being shared among mammals, round worms, fruit flies, and budding yeast. Some of these unique genes are expressed by germ cells only at certain stages of their development. Other genes, such as those for glycolytic enzymes, have homologues in somatic cells. Some gene transcripts also result from alternate splicing of homologous genes. Another form of regulation is *interactive;* that is, products from cells in one stage of spermatogenesis may influence cells in earlier or later stages, directly through intercellular bridges or via Sertoli cell intermediates. Either the knockout or the overexpression of genes in germ cells of one stage can affect the numbers or functions of germ cells in another stage. An example of such interactive effects is seen with bone morphogenetic protein (BMP) (Chapter 42), which is initially produced by spermatogonia. Subsequently, when this production stops, spermatids produce BMP, and this molecule then feeds back to regulate

survival of spermatogonia. *Extrinsic* or hormonal regulation is engrafted on the intrinsic and interactive modes of regulation.

Changes in metabolism and structure occur during spermatogenesis. Glycolysis is ineffective in spermatids, whereas glucose utilization by sperm is an absolute requirement for fertilization to take place. In the last phase, nuclear histones are replaced by protamine, a basic molecule that allows packaging of the DNA into one-twentieth the volume that is required in somatic cells.

Each spermatogonium can give rise to 64 spermatozoa. The extraordinary metamorphosis from human spermatogonium to spermatozoon is depicted in Fig. 46-13. The first two mitotic divisions of a spermatogonium give rise to four cells: a single resting dark cell *(Ad),* that will eventually serve as the ancestor of a later generation of sperm, and three active pale cells *(Ap).* The Ap cells divide by further mitoses to yield type B spermatogonia, which then give rise to many primary spermatocytes. Some Ap cells may also transdifferentiate to Ad cells and form a reservoir. Primary spermatocytes enter the prophase of meiosis, the first reduction division, in which they remain for about 20 days. This process occurs within the basal compartment of the seminiferous tubule.

Meiosis is a complex process of chromosomal reduplication, synapsis, crossover, division, and cell separation. Genes unique to meiosis facilitate these operations, and this process is reflected histologically in the changing appearance of the **primary spermatocytes,** up through the pachytene stage (Fig. 46-13). Their daughter cells, the **secondary spermatocytes,** immediately divide again by mitosis in the adluminal compartment. These daughter cells, now called *spermatids,* each contains 22 autosomes and either an X or a Y sex chromosome. The spermatids lie near the lumen of the seminiferous tubule. *They are attached to the abutting Sertoli cells by specialized junctions. The spermatocytes and spermatids of each generation are connected with each other through intercellular bridges.*

The next process in spermatogenesis is called **spermiogenesis.** In this process, spermatids undergo nuclear condensation, shrinkage of cytoplasm, formation of an **acrosome,** and development of a tail, to emerge as flagellated spermatozoa (Figs. 46-13 and 46-14). The spermatozoa are then extruded into the lumen of the tubule by a process called spermiation, during which most of the cytoplasm of the spermatozoa is ejected as the residual body and remains embedded in the cytoplasm of a Sertoli cell.

Once in the seminiferous tubules, the spermatozoa appear as linear structures with several components (Fig. 46-14). The **head** contains the nucleus, with its haploid chromosome content. No new DNA can be synthesized nor can genes be expressed to enable new protein synthesis. An acrosomal cap, in which hydrolytic and proteolytic enzymes are concentrated, is also at the tip of the head. These enzymes facilitate penetration of the ovum and possibly also of the mucous plug of the female cervix. The **middle piece,** or body, contains mitochondria, which generate the motile energy of the spermatozoon. The chief piece of the tail contains stored adenosine triphosphate (ATP) and pairs of contractile microtubules down its entire length; one pair lies in the center, and nine pairs are located around the circumference. Cross-bridging arms contain **dynein,** a magnesium-dependent ATPase, which catalyzes the conversion of ATP energy into a sliding movement between the microtubules. *This sliding movement imparts flagellar motion to the spermatozoa.* Both cAMP and Ca^{2+} regulate sperm motility.

In a human, the entire sequence of development from spermatogonia to spermatozoa takes about 70 days. *However, individual resting spermatogonia do not enter the process of spermatogenesis randomly. Cycles of spermatogenesis exist with distinct cycle times.* Groups of adjacent resting spermatogonia initiate a new cycle about every 16 days, which thus constitutes one "generation." At about the same time that the primary spermatocytes of one cycle enter the prophase, a second cycle of spermatogonia is activated. A third cycle begins at approximately the same time that spermatids appear from the first cycle. By the time these spermatids are completely transformed into spermatozoa, a fourth cycle of spermatogonia development has been started.

The seminiferous tubules extend distally, coiled in a helical or spiral fashion. Therefore a cross section through the lumen usually reveals that several spermatogenic cycles are in process simultaneously, around the circumference. Within each cycle, specific stages of cellular development can be identified histologically. Thus, several cellular constellations can exist side by side. In some mammals, but possibly not in humans, spermatogenic cycles are repeated in a defined topographic relationship to each other along the length of each seminiferous tubule. This phenomenon has been termed "the **wave of spermatogenesis.**"

As previously noted, the individual germ cells that make up the successive descendants of type B spermatogonia and that lie within the adluminal compartment of the tubule are not totally separated. Continuity of cytoplasm and cell-to-cell intercommunication exists. Because of these possibilities and because of the regular topographic association of particular stages of spermatogenesis in neighboring cycles, products of germ cells in one stage of spermatogenesis initiate or regulate events in other stages.

After spermiation, the spermatozoa reach the epididymis, which they traverse in a period of 2 to 4 weeks. During this time, the spermatozoa undergo further maturation, gaining motility and losing all their cytoplasm.

Spermatozoa are initially transported into the epididymis by seminiferous tubular fluid currents that are generated by the peritubular myoid cells or by the contraction of the testicular capsule. The epididymis is lined by specialized epithelial cells, and it is surrounded by contractile muscle cells. The growth and differentiation of the epididymis, as well as the motility and fertility of the sperm that migrate through it, depend on androgens. Marked changes in fluid osmolality, electrolytes, and the concentrations of many small molecules occur progressively within the length of the epididymis. These changes suggest homologies with the function of the renal tubules.

Proteins provided by epididymal and seminiferous tubular fluid bind to the membranes of sperm, and they enhance their motility and fertilizing ability. These proteins include a forward-mobility protein, an acrosomal stabilizing or inhibiting factor, and a protein that binds to the outer membrane of the ovum. The amount of sperm contained in the epididymis is

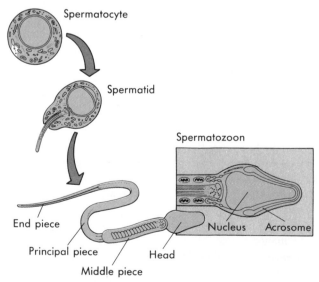

■ **Fig. 46-14** Schematic representation of the morphological alterations in the development of the spermatozoon from the spermatocyte.

about the equivalent of a single ejaculate or a single day's production. After reaching the vas deferens, sperm may be stored viably for several months between ejaculations.

Sexual Functioning

Delivery of spermatozoa into the female genital tract for reproductive purposes occurs by ejaculation from the vas deferens. To this initial ejaculate, successive fluids are added by various structures. The first secretions are added from the prostate gland, and they contain citrate, calcium, zinc, and acid phosphatase. The alkalinity of prostatic fluid helps neutralize the acid pH of the semen and of the vaginal and cervical secretions. The later secretions are from the seminal vesicles. These secretions contain fructose, another important oxidative substrate for the spermatozoa, and prostaglandins, which may stimulate contractions of the uterus and fallopian tubes and thereby help propel the spermatozoa toward the ovum.

Seminal fluid also contains LH, FSH, prolactin, testosterone, estradiol, inhibins, endorphins, oxytocin, kallikreins, relaxin (see later discussion), proteases, plasminogen activator, and sperm-coating proteins. Because the concentrations of these substances are usually higher than those in plasma, they have probably entered from cells of the genital tract (e.g., epididymal cells).

Ejaculation requires preceding penile erection, which is caused by blood filling the venous sinuses of the corpora cavernosa and spongiosa. An 8-fold increase in blood content converts the flaccid penis into a firm organ for penetration. This process may be initiated in the brain (mammillary body in the posterior hypothalamus), or it may begin with afferent sensory impulses that originate from the penis and are carried by the **pudendal nerve.** The process is further mediated by impulses in the pelvic nerves, which contain both parasympathetic and sympathetic fibers. During the **flaccid phase,** sympathetic neural tone dominates and the cavernosa are kept empty by constriction of smooth muscle and of the supplying arterioles. During the initial filling phase, parasympathetic stimuli dominate, arteriolar constriction diminishes, and the penis elongates without a change in cavernosa pressure. During the next **tumescence phase,** release of nitric oxide and prostaglandin E_1, and increase in intracellular cyclic GMP, causes relaxation of the cavernosa smooth muscle and an increase in its compliance, which allows easy entry of blood and engorgement of the penis. In the **full erection phase,** output of blood from the penis is markedly decreased by pressure on the veins from the engorged cavernosa. In this phase, the pressure of the engorged cavernosa rises to just below that of the systolic blood pressure. In the final **rigid phase,** cavernosa pressure exceeds systolic blood pressure. Ejaculation, which occurs during this phase, results from sympathetic stimuli that cause contraction of the ischiocavernosa and bulbocavernosa muscles.

Inability to ejaculate, or impotence, is a common problem. It may be caused by structural and functional disorders, including neuropathies and spinal cord lesions, or by psy-chogenic complications. New detailed knowledge about the physiology of erection has led to improved pharmacological therapy. Direct self-injection of α-adrenergic antagonists or appropriate prostaglandins into the cavernosa at the base of the penis generates erections that last 1 to 3 hours, and thereby permit satisfactory intercourse. In other instances, a simple mechanical pump creates a vacuum in an airbag placed around the penis; transmission of the negative pressure to the cavernosa results in their engorgement and in an adequate erection. A drug that inhibits cyclic GMP phosphodiesterase, sildenafil, increases cyclic GMP and facilitates erection under conditions of sexual stimulation.

A typical ejaculate contains 200 to 400 million spermatozoa in a volume of 2 to 4 ml. The first 1 ml has the highest concentration of sperm. Once within the vagina, the spermatozoa's rate of flagellated movement is up to 44 mm/min. However, to reach the ovum, sperm require assistance by smooth muscle contractions in the female genital tract. The lifespan of the spermatozoa within the female genital tract is approximately 2 days.

Ejaculated sperm cannot immediately fertilize an ovum. In vivo fertilization can take place only after the sperm have been within the milieu of the female reproductive tract for 4 to 6 hours. This process is termed **capacitation.** In vitro, human fertilization can take place after the spermatozoa have been washed free of seminal fluid. This suggests that seminal fluid contains substances that coat the sperm surface and that prevent union of a sperm with an ovum. Materials in the female genital tract might either remove or neutralize these substances. However, capacitation itself has proven to be a regulated process. A fertilization-promoting peptide (FPP) originates in the prostate gland and in other male reproductive tissues. FPP is a tripeptide pGlu-Glu-Pro-NH_2 that is very similar to TRH (Chapter 44). A receptor for FPP is expressed by a gene on an autosomal chromosome that is transcribed during late spermatogenesis and translated during spermiation. FPP interacts with its receptor to increase cAMP in uncapacitated sperm and to stimulate capacitation. However, FPP also actually works to halt capacitation in capacitated sperm, before the **acrosomal reaction** can occur prematurely during the transit of a sperm toward an ovum, and renders the sperm incapable of fertilization. Other peptide hormones, such as calcitonin and angiotensin, are found in semen, and they can also stimulate capacitation. In the course of capacitation, cholesterol is withdrawn from the sperm membrane, and the surface proteins of the membrane redistribute. In addition, calcium influx occurs and motility becomes more whiplike. This increases the forward velocity of sperm and enhances its ability to penetrate the ovum. Most importantly, capacitation permits the acrosomal reaction. In this reaction, the acrosomal membrane fuses with that of the outer sperm membrane (Fig. 46-14). Pores are created through which the acrosomal hydrolytic and proteolytic enzymes can escape. These enzymes then create a path through the protective membranes of the ovum for penetration of the sperm.

Hormonal Regulation of Spermatogenesis

The endocrine mechanisms that govern human spermatogenesis are not completely understood. Demonstrating with certainty at what particular stage and precisely how each reproductive hormone influences human spermatogenesis remains difficult for many reasons. Normal testicular tissue is seldom available for study in the basal state or after experimental manipulation. Ethical constraints prevent administering to men radioactive tracers that can quantiate cell turnover, differentiation, and function of germ cells at various stages in vivo. Wide species differences make direct extrapolation of experimental results from subprimates, e.g., rodents, to humans tentative or questionable. Even subhuman primates, like monkeys, have lesser cycle times (48 vs. 70 days), have more mitoses between type B spermatogonia and primary spermatocytes, and have more stages demarcated (13 vs. 6). However, they have only a single stage rather than multiple stages of spermatogenesis visible in any one cross section of a semniferous tubule.

Clearly, adult functioning of the GnRH-LH/FSH-testicular axis, as illustrated in Fig. 43-15, is essential for substantial spermatogenesis to occur in adults. *Of critical importance is the pulsatile release of GnRH and the resultant arrival of LH and FSH at their target cells.* Men with congenital GnRH deficiency can be made fertile only if exogenous GnRH is given in appropriately sized pulses and timed intervals, but not if it is given continuously.

LH, FSH, testosterone, and quite possibly its metabolites, DHT and estradiol, are essential. The role of LH is mainly limited to stimulating the Leydig cells to produce testosterone. The presence of high local concentrations of testosterone in the vicinity of the seminiferous tubules is an absolute requirement. FSH is no longer held to be absolutely necessary, but it is clearly very facilitory. Since the entire process of spermatogenesis is genetically programmed to occur in germ cells, the role of the endocrine system is best thought of as optimizing the rate and total quantity of sperm production, as well as enhancing the function—to fertilize an ovum—of the final product.

The prepubertal testis contains only resting spermatogonia and quiescent Sertoli cells. These cells do not exhibit cyclic alterations in structure or in biochemical functioning. Neither Leydig cells nor peritubular cells of the adult myoid character are present (Fig. 46-12A). Pubertal activation of gonadotropin secretion leads to dramatic and complex changes. The proximity of several stimulated endocrine cell types (with multiple secretory products) to each other and to the germinal cell line creates many potential and observed paracrine effects, and possibly also autocrine effects. These effects are in addition to central feedback actions. The specific or critical nature of each effect and the exact point in spermatogenesis at which it operates are still difficult to determine.

During fetal life, the transient midgestation surge of pituitary FSH, LH, and testosterone release may stimulate the transformation of some primordial germ cells into resting spermatogonia. Withdrawal of fetal gonadotropins then leaves the spermatogonia in suspended development throughout childhood, possibly through operation of a local meiosis inhibitor. Both AMH and inhibin have been proposed for this role. Shortly after FSH and LH secretion begins to rise at the onset of puberty, the spermatogonia are activated. The maximum rate of sperm production may be set by the number of Ap spermatogonia present at the end of puberty.

Although the most immature germ cells have been reported to have FSH receptors, evidence is lacking that FSH acts directly on germ cells. Although FSH alone cannot initiate and complete spermatogenesis, in its absence the process is arrested. Men with inactivating mutations of the FSH-β subunit gene have had azospermia (complete absence of sperm from the ejaculate). Men with inactivating mutations of the FSH receptor have quantitatively and qualitatively abnormal spermatogenesis, but they can still be fertile in some instances. FSH may act to promote transformation of Ap to type B spermatogonia, rather than to Ad spermatogonia. Downstream, FSH appears to facilitate the normal structural changes during spermiogenesis, and ultimately to ensure adequate acrosomal activity and motility of sperm. An important transcription factor for the genes expressed in the later postmeiosis stages of spermiogenesis is cAMP regulatory element modulator (CREM, Chapter 39). FSH stabilizes CREM transcripts in spermatocytes, leading to an increased number in the haploid spermatids. FSH certainly stimulates the Sertoli cells, whose functions are in turn required for initial germ cell mitotic and early meiotic activity. These cells are described in detail later.

LH stimulates the Leydig cells to secrete testosterone, which presumably diffuses across the basement membrane and can enter the Sertoli cells. The latter contain a high density of androgen receptors. The high local concentration of testosterone (50- to 100-fold greater than in plasma) is essential for completion of the later stages of spermatogenesis, at least by acting on the Sertoli cells. Testosterone prevents premature separation of the next to last stage spermatids from the Sertoli cell, thus promoting normal separation of the last stage of spermatids at the proper time (spermiation). This effect of testosterone may be explained by its ability to stimulate Sertoli cell synthesis and secretion of adhesion molecules, such as *N*-cadherins. In men who lack LH, testosterone administration to attain normal systemic plasma levels, even if given with FSH, cannot sustain spermatogenesis. It is possible that dihydrotestosterone may also enter and act within the germ cells; rodent germ cells contain both dihydrotestosterone and the 5α-reductase enzyme necessary for its production from testosterone (Fig. 46-4). When LH deficiency lowers intratesticular testosterone levels in men, their DHT levels remain normal. Because DHT has a higher affinity for the androgen receptor than does testosterone, preservation of DHT may preserve some androgen action. Conversion of small amounts of testosterone to estradiol within the Leydig and Sertoli cells makes this estrogen available as another local spermatogenesis modulator that is ultimately derived from LH and FSH action. Men with inactivating mutations of either estrogen receptors or the aromatase enzyme (necessary for estradiol synthesis) have diminished fertility and abnormal spermatogenesis. *The trophic effect of LH on Leydig cells is also essential to spermatogenesis, and FSH may contribute to a full Leydig cell response.*

Once regular spermatogenesis has been established during puberty, it can continue to a small extent in adults who have very low levels of FSH and LH (Fig. 46-15), provided that testosterone is present in high amounts. Under these circumstances type B spermatogonia were decreased 80% to 90%, spermiation was impaired, and the number of sperm was markedly reduced, but the sperm were normal in appearance. Moreover, in gonadotropin-deficient men, different degrees of suppression of spermatogenesis occur, even in adjacent tubules. Selective restoration of either FSH alone or LH alone can increase sperm numbers (Fig. 46-15), but both are required for normal levels to be reached. In some men, after a suitable period of exposure to FSH, LH alone can sustain sufficient sperm production (15 to 60 million per ejaculate) to permit fertility. LH receptors have been found on sperm.

Other pituitary hormones are also involved in spermatogenesis. Prolactin receptors are present on Leydig cells; prolactin increases the number of LH receptors and synergizes with LH to stimulate androgen production. Growth hormone is essential for the normally timed onset of reproductive function. A GH-variant gene (Chapter 43) and the GH receptor gene are expressed in the testis. GH stimulates growth of the wolffian duct structures, penis, and prostate gland. GH also increases the Leydig cell response to LH (i.e., it raises testosterone levels), probably by inducing the LH receptor. Via the local production of IGF-1, GH enhances testosterone

synthesis, possibly by increasing StAR and the 3β-OH-steroid dehydrogenase enzyme.

Despite the variability of spermatogenesis within each seminiferous tubule, the normal testis continuously releases spermatozoa. Furthermore, although gonadotropin release is pulsatile, the daily *mean* plasma levels of FSH and LH vary little in adult men. However, temporal or topographic differences may exist in the density of gonadotropin receptors or in the peritubular myoid cell control of capillary blood flow. Such variations could modulate gonadotropin availability and thereby be responsible for the cyclic and topographic nature of the spermatogenic process. In general, spermatogenesis obviously differs from that of oogenesis, in which a clear phasic pattern of gonadotropin secretion, highlighted by a single distinct burst, produces the monthly release of a single ovum.

Sertoli Cell Function and Its Regulation

The Sertoli cells and their responses to FSH and testosterone are crucial to spermatogenesis. Sertoli cells proliferate in two phases, during the infancy peak of FSH secretion (Fig. 46-6) and again during puberty. Between the fetal state and puberty, Sertoli cell function is unknown. The normal cell complement at birth increases 10-fold after puberty, but thereafter the Sertoli cells do not undergo any further cell divisions. Each cell remains in contact with up to five other Sertoli cells and with an estimated 47 germ cells in different stages of development. Because each Sertoli cell can support only a limited number of germ cells, the number of functioning Sertoli cells is a major determinant of the maximum rate of sperm production in each man. Ectoplasmic processes from Sertoli and germ cells invaginate into each

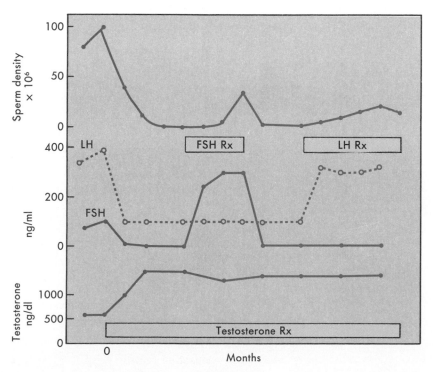

■ Fig. 46-15 Individual effects of FSH and LH on human sperm production. Normal men were given sufficient testosterone to suppress endogenous FSH and LH secretion by negative feedback. As a result, sperm density declined to very low but detectable levels. Selective restoration of either FSH or LH individually raised sperm levels. However, neither gonadotropin alone could return sperm production to normal. (Redrawn from Matsumoto AM et al: *J Clin Invest* 72:1005, 1983; and Matsumoto AM et al: *J Clin Endocrinol Metab* 59:882, 1984.)

other's plasma membranes. In close association with the cycle of spermatogenesis, Sertoli cells undergo regular changes in (1) the activity and shape of the nucleus; (2) the size, shape, and branching of the cytoplasmic processes; (3) the concentrations of lipid and glycogen; (4) mitochondrial function; and (5) enzyme content. These changes relate to the processing of the germ cells in an intimate and regular manner, which suggests that the Sertoli cells are responding in part to signals from the germ cells. One candidate germ cell signal is the cytokine, **tumor necrosis factor-α (TNF-α),** which is secreted by spermatids. Sertoli and Leydig cells have TNF-α receptors, and Sertoli cells secrete inhibin in response to TNF-α.

The cytoplasmic processes of the Sertoli cells extend from the basement membrane to the lumen of the seminiferous tubule. These processes act as conduits, between which the various stages of germ cells move in their passage to the lumen (Fig. 46-11). As spermatocytes mature, new tight junctions between the investing Sertoli cells develop behind them while the old tight junctions ahead of them "unzip." In this way, spermatocytes pass from the basal to the adluminal compartment without breaking the integrity of the blood-testis barrier that is formed by Sertoli cell cytoplasm. This cytoplasm acts as a filter, permitting only certain substances to reach the spermatocytes.

FSH receptors are present on Sertoli cells by 8 to 16 weeks of gestation. Over 100 proteins are synthesized and secreted by the Sertoli cells in response to FSH. Some of these secretions are directed into the lumen of the seminiferous tubule (Fig. 46-11). FSH induces the enzyme, aromatase, and stimulates estradiol production by Sertoli cells from androgen precursors of Leydig cell origin. FSH upregulates the androgen receptor, and makes the Sertoli cell more responsive to testosterone. In response to FSH and testosterone, which act synergistically, an **androgen-binding glycoprotein (ABP),** with an amino acid sequence identical to that of the circulating sex steroid-binding globulin is synthesized (see below). ABP binds testosterone, dihydrotestosterone, and estradiol with high affinity. In this way, ABP regulates the availability of these hormones to germ cells in the seminiferous tubular fluid (Figs. 46-11 and 46-16). ABP is also secreted into epididymal fluid, where it prevents reabsorption of sex steroids and ensures their continued presence for sperm needs. ABP may also regulate the inhibitory effect of estradiol on Leydig cell testosterone synthesis (Fig. 46-16).

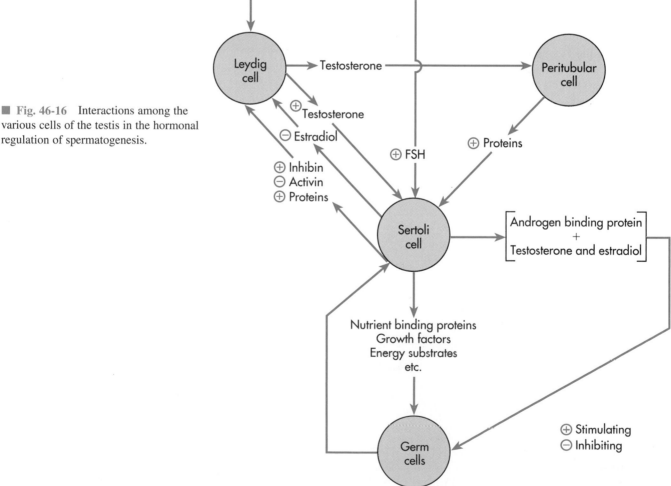

■ **Fig. 46-16** Interactions among the various cells of the testis in the hormonal regulation of spermatogenesis.

Inhibin B, activin, and various growth factors are also synthesized under the influence of FSH and testosterone. Inhibin A is not produced in detectable amount in males. Destruction or spontaneous loss of the spermatogenic cells suppresses inhibin secretion. This influence suggests that a signal from spermatogenic cells stimulates the synthesis of inhibin by the Sertoli cells (Fig. 46-16). In addition to their central feedback roles of inhibiting and stimulating FSH secretion, respectively, inhibin and activin may also have reciprocal local actions on the neighboring cells (Fig. 46-16). For example, inhibin increases testosterone secretion by the Leydig cells, whereas activin decreases testosterone secretion. Thus, FSH can also influence Leydig cell function indirectly by modulating the production of inhibin and activin. FSH promotes the availability of iron, copper, vitamin A, and crucial sphingolipids to the germ cells by stimulating synthesis of their binding proteins. Binding proteins then extract their respective ligands from plasma and transfer them to the germ cells. FSH also increases the glucose metabolism of Sertoli cells, and the resultant production of pyruvate and lactate provides available energy substrates for the spermatogenic cells.

A nerve cell factor is among the Sertoli cell signals to the germ cells. Of particular importance, Sertoli cells secrete IGF-2 and transforming growth factor-β (TGF-β), both of which interact with IGF-2 receptors on germ cells. In the latter, the mRNA level of *c-fos,* a mitogenic gene, is also increased by Sertoli cell products.

FSH-stimulated proteases and plasminogen activator are probably involved in the process of spermiation. Either by mechanical or chemical means, the Sertoli cell facilitates entry of the spermatozoa into the tubular lumen. In this process, the nucleus of the spermatozoon is oriented toward the base of the tubule. The bulk of the cytoplasm is then squeezed out past the nucleus and shed as the residual body (Fig. 46-13), while the spermatozoon is cast free. The residual body and other fragments are then phagocytosed by the Sertoli cells and subsequently degraded.

Other paracrine interactions may be important in maintaining the proper testicular environment to support spermatogenesis (Fig. 46-16). Thus, testosterone from the Leydig cells stimulates differentiation and proliferation of the peritubular myoid cells. These cells secrete a protein that stimulates some functions of Sertoli cells. A positive feedback loop exists between Leydig and Sertoli cells in that testosterone stimulates inhibin secretion and inhibin stimulates testosterone secretion. However, activin and estradiol from Sertoli cells reduce testosterone synthesis by Leydig cells. Each of these interactions may vary in functional significance at different points in the cycle of spermatogenesis.

One conceptual way to summarize and integrate the relationship between spermatogenesis and its major hormonal regulators is illustrated in Fig. 46-17. This figure shows that serum FSH and serum inhibin B have a reciprocal relationship with each other, as expected from a negative feedback pair (see Chapter 39). Figure 46-18 further shows that sperm count is **directly** related to serum inhibin but **inversely** related to serum FSH. These findings suggest that the germ cells

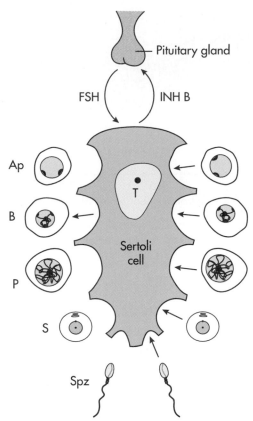

■ **Fig. 46-17** Endocrine and paracrine regulation of spermatogenesis. The preprogrammed development of sperm from spermatogonia is facilitated and maintained at a basal rate by T (testosterone) effects on Sertoli cells that are transmitted to and elicited by germ cells at various stages. The basal rate of production is augmented by FSH (follicle-stimulating hormone). When the rate is too low, signals from various stages of sperm development (B, spermatogonium B; P, primary spermatocyte; S, spermatid; Spz, spermatozoa) decrease output of inhibin B from the Sertoli cell. This results in increased FSH secretion from the pituitary gland. Likewise, when spermatogenesis is too brisk, Sertoli cells release more inhibin B, which suppresses FSH secretion and turns down the rate of spermatogenesis. (From Plant TM et al: *Endocr Rev* 22:764, 2001.)

themselves may control their own pace of development by signals to the Sertoli cells at various stages of spermatogenesis (Fig. 46-18). When sperm production is too brisk, Sertoli cells are caused to increase inhibin secretion, which then inhibits FSH secretion. As FSH levels fall, sperm production decreases to a more desirable rate. Conversely, when sperm production is inadequate, germ cells signal Sertoli cells to reduce inhibin secretion. This lessens the brake on FSH secretion. As FSH levels increase, sperm production increases to a more desirable rate. All of the above takes place in and depends on a high supportive concentration of testosterone around and within the Sertoli cell.

The clinical importance of understanding the extrinsic and interactive regulation of spermatogenesis is increasing. First, about 10% of otherwise normal men are infer-

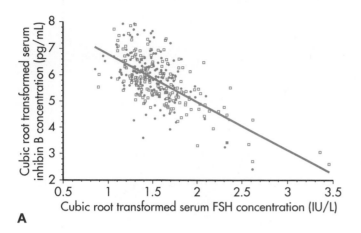

A

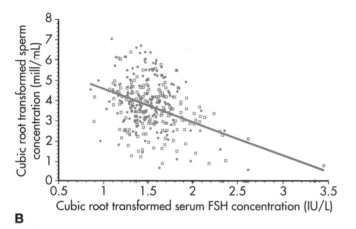

B

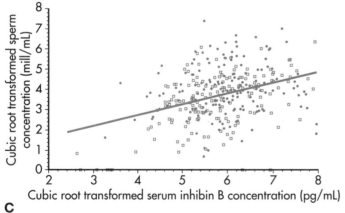

C

■ **Fig. 46-18**   Relationships between FSH (follicle-stimulating hormone), inhibin B, and sperm count in men. **A,** An inverse relationship between plasma FSH and inhibin B. **B,** An inverse relationship between sperm count and FSH. **C,** A direct relationship between sperm count and inhibin B. Open and closed circles represent two different populations of men. (From Jensen TK et al: *J Clin Endocrinol Metab* 82:4059, 1997.)

tile because of oligospermia, azospermia, or poor sperm quality. Therapy is presently ineffective for many such men. Second, a convenient, reliable, safe, and acceptable systemic form of male contraception is still unavailable, but it is clearly desirable.

Secretion and Metabolism of Androgens

Testosterone, the major androgenic hormone, is synthesized as described previously (Fig. 46-4). Its synthesis and release by the Leydig cells are regulated by LH; therefore, plasma testosterone levels undergo small coordinate pulses throughout the day (see Fig. 43-17). In addition, the plasma testosterone level follows a superimposed diurnal trend; plasma testosterone is about 25% lower at 8:00 PM than at 8:00 AM. When exogenous LH is supplied for a prolonged period, the plasma testosterone level initially rises, then briefly declines, and then rises again. The temporary decrease may be caused by downregulation of LH receptors by the peak concentrations of gonadotropin; the later upswing may reflect stimulation of the expression of enzyme genes that are involved in testosterone synthesis and in Leydig cell growth.

Testosterone gives rise to two other potent androgens: **dihydrotestosterone (DHT)** and **5α-androstenediol** (Fig. 46-4). The major portion of each of these two androgens is formed from the reduction of testosterone in peripheral tissues. The key enzyme, 5α-reductase, exists in two types. Type 2 is present in genital tissues, and it is essential to differentiation of these tissues in the male pattern in utero. This enzyme isotype is greatly downregulated at puberty, and the type 1 5α-reductase is responsible for DHT and androstenediol production thereafter in target tissues, such as the prostate gland. These two isoenzymes are located in microsomes and they use NADPH as the reductant. The plasma levels, blood production rates, and metabolic clearances of these androgens are shown in Table 46-2. The testosterone precursor, androstenedione, is also secreted in major amounts by the Leydig cells (Fig. 46-4), but it contributes little per se to androgen action.

The two estrogens—estradiol and estrone—are produced in significant amounts in men. However, only a trivial fraction of the daily production is provided directly by testicular secretion. Most is derived from circulating testosterone and androstenedione by aromatization, which takes place largely in the adipose tissue and liver.

Leydig cell function varies distinctively during the lifespan of males. As shown in Fig. 46-19, plasma testosterone concentration rises to levels of 400 ng/dl in the fetus when the external genitalia are undergoing differentiation to the masculine pattern. By birth, however, these levels have declined to less than 50 ng/dl. Soon thereafter, plasma testosterone again begins to rise, reaching a peak of 150 to 200 ng/dl at 4 to 8 weeks of age. The physiological significance of this elevation in testosterone concentration is not known. Plasma testosterone again falls to low levels and remains so throughout childhood; these low plasma levels correspond to the absence of Leydig cells (Fig. 46-12).

At about age 11 years, the plasma testosterone level begins to rise steeply, and it reaches the adult plateau of about 600 ng/dl at about age 17 (Fig. 46-19). After the third decade of life, total and free testosterone begin to decline at a rate of 0.5% to 1.0% a year. This decline results both from a reduction in GnRH release and from a loss of Leydig cell responsiveness to LH stimulation. Decreasing testosterone levels

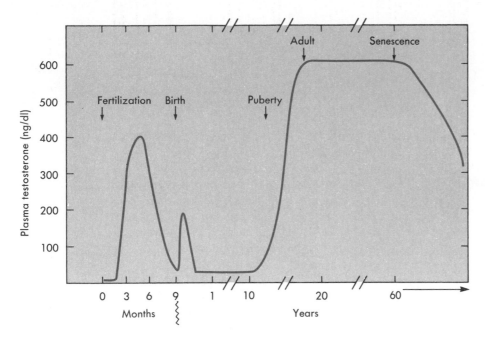

■ **Fig. 46-19** Plasma testosterone profile during the lifespan of a normal male. (Data from Griffin JE et al: In Bondy PK, Rosenberg LE, editors: *Metabolic control and disease,* Philadelphia, 1980, WB Saunders; and Winter JSD et al: *J Clin Endocrinol Metab* 42:679, 1976.)

■ **Table 46-2** Turnover of gonadal steroids in adult men

Steroid	Plasma concentration (ng/dl)	Blood production rate (µg/day)	Metabolic clearance rate (L/day)
Testosterone	650	7000	1100
Dihydrotestosterone	45	300*	600
5α-Androstenediol	12	200*	1800
Androstenedione	120	2400	2000
Estradiol	3.0	50†	1700
Estrone	2.5	60†	2500

*About 60% to 80% produced peripherally from testosterone.
†About 80% to 90% produced peripherally from testosterone and androstenedione, respectively.

may be associated with a decline in libido, a decrease in bone mass, an increased risk of fractures, a decrease in muscle mass, and a greater risk of falls. However, spermatogenesis itself is remarkably well preserved, even in octogenarians.

Only 1% to 2% of circulating testosterone is in the free form; 65% of testosterone is bound to a liver-derived glycoprotein, called **sex steroid-binding globulin (SSBG),** also known as **testosterone-estradiol–binding globulin.** SSBG differs from ABP only in its carbohydrate content. Most of the remaining testosterone is bound to albumin and other proteins. SSBG also binds dihydrotestosterone and 5α-androstenediol. The SSBG-bound fractions serve as circulating reservoirs of androgens, which are similar to those of thyroid hormone and cortisol. In general, only the free and the loosely bound albumin fractions of testosterone and of the other androgens diffuse into cells and are biologically active. However, receptors exist for SSBG itself in target tissues; therefore, SSBG may have actions of its own, or it may serve as a delivery molecule for androgens in certain cases. The concentration of SSBG is increased by thyroid hormone and estrogens, and it is decreased by androgens. Reciprocally, then, estrogen reduces the percentage of free testosterone, whereas androgen increases it.

The metabolism of testosterone to hormonally active intermediates (DHT, androstenediol, estradiol, and probably

testosterone glucuronide) and to inactive products (testosterone sulfate) is depicted in Fig. 46-20. It is especially noteworthy that a hormone, namely estradiol, that is usually thought of as feminine, is an important mediator of certain actions of the quintessentially masculine hormone, testosterone. About 1% of the daily production of testosterone (70 µg) is excreted daily in the urine as a glucuronide. Most of the remainder is excreted in the urine as 17-ketosteroids (see Chapter 45). Because most of the 17-ketosteroids arise from adrenal androgen precursors, measurement of plasma total and free testosterone (and occasionally urine testosterone) is the mainstay for assessing Leydig cell function.

Inhibin B (Fig. 46-5) circulates in the plasma of males and its level correlates inversely with FSH levels (Fig. 46-15). This inverse relationship supports the idea that inhibin B functions to suppress FSH secretion. Inhibin A (Fig. 46-5) is not detectable in males.

Androgen Actions

The extratesticular effects of testosterone and related androgens can be divided into two major categories: (1) effects that pertain specifically to reproductive function and to secondary sexual characteristics and (2) effects that pertain more generally to stimulation of nonreproductive tissue growth and maturation. Similar intracellular mechanisms

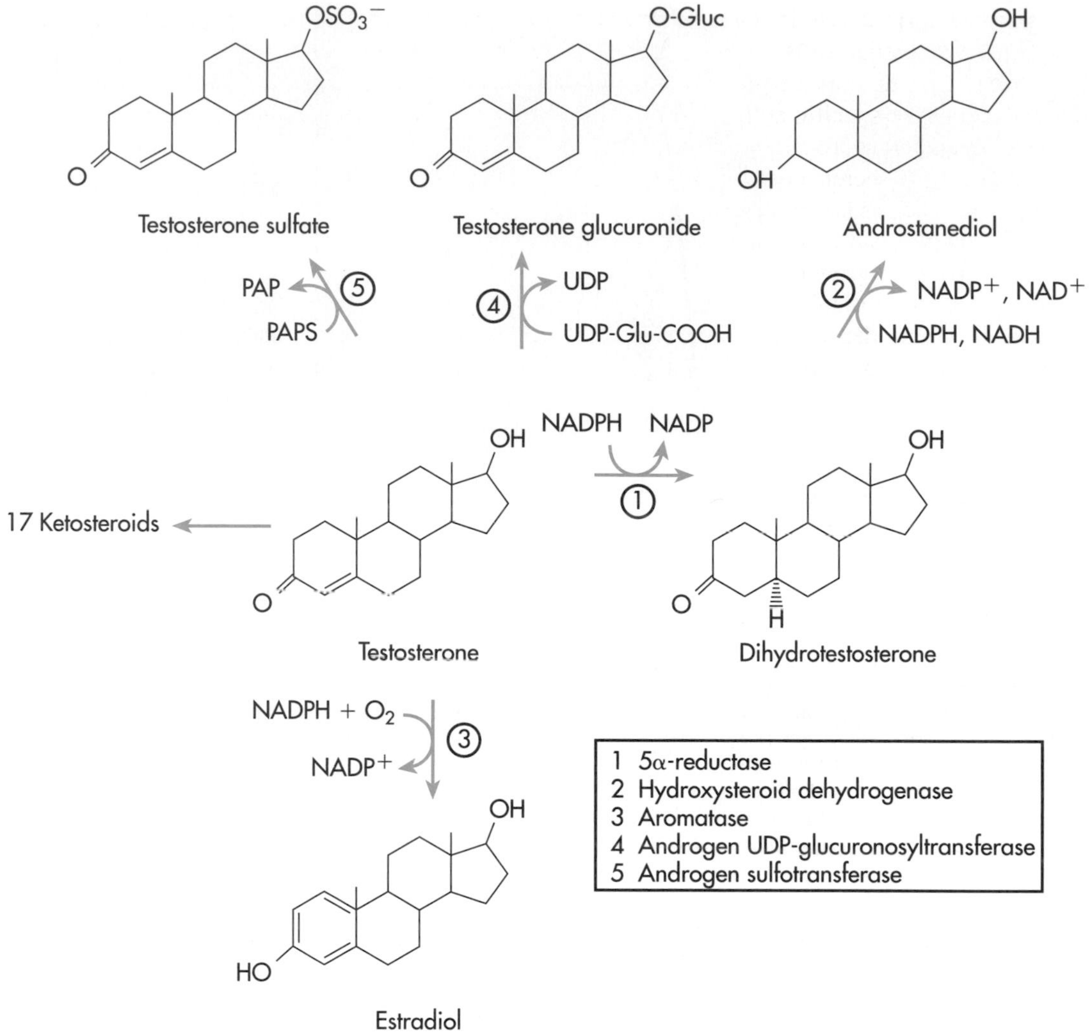

■ **Fig. 46-20**   The metabolism of testosterone. Testosterone is metabolized by enzymes 1 to 4 to intermediates that are hormonally active via the androgen receptor, except for estradiol, which acts through the estrogen receptor. Testosterone sulfate is inactive and the 17-ketosteroids (see Chapter 45) are very weakly active as androgens. (Modified from Roy AK et al: *Vitam Horm* 55:309, 1999.)

are involved in both categories of effects. In general, the model for steroid hormone effects is applicable (see Fig. 39-17).

Testosterone diffuses freely into cells. In many, but not all, target cells, it rapidly undergoes reduction to DHT and, in some cells, to 5α-androstenediol (Fig. 46-4). DHT is much more potent than testosterone in some biological actions, and it has a 3-fold greater affinity for the androgen receptor.

The androgen receptor, which is a member of the steroid receptor superfamily, is composed of approximately 900 amino acids (see Fig. 39-17). The DNA-binding domain is 56% homologous with that of the estrogen receptor. The androgen hormone-receptor complex is phosphorylated, disassociates from a chaperone heat shock protein, dimerizes, and then interacts with target DNA molecules. It is sometimes assisted by nuclear transcription factors. Binding of androgen to the receptor may relieve a constitutive repressing action of the receptor on target genes. As a result of this interaction, RNA polymerase, various messenger RNAs, and the synthesis of proteins are stimulated. In addition, the activities of enzymes, such as thymidine kinase and DNA polymerase, that play roles in DNA synthesis, are increased. Virtually all androgen actions can be blocked by inhibitors of RNA or of protein synthesis. Therefore, these actions require the induction of new enzyme molecules, as opposed to the allosteric or the covalent activation of existing enzyme molecules. The unliganded androgen receptor can also be activated by IGF-1, which acts through MAP kinase to phosphorylate the transactivating N terminus of the receptor. This action may contribute to the growth-promoting activity of the receptor.

The androgen receptor gene can be downregulated by androgen in some target cells, but it can be upregulated in others. The receptor can itself increase the translation of its own mRNA. In androgen target tissues, such as the prostate gland and seminal vesicles, polyamine (e.g., spermine and putrescine) synthesis is stimulated by testosterone, and these compounds in turn increase RNA synthesis. Androgens also stimulate the remarkable growth of these accessory organs of reproduction. This growth is characterized by hypertrophy and hyperplasia of the epithelial cells, stromal components, and blood vessels. In the prostate gland, a steroid-binding protein and a prostate-specific antigen (PSA) are induced. The DHT liganded androgen receptor causes prostate mesenchymal cells to secrete positive growth regulators of epithelial cells, such as keratinocyte growth factor and fibroblast growth factor; on the other hand, TGF-β, a repressor of prostate growth, is downregulated by DHT. Proliferation of the prostate epithelium is mediated by an increase in cyclin-dependent kinases. In the absence of androgen action, apoptosis of prostate cells is accelerated.

The mitogenic effects of androgens (and specifically of DHT) on the prostate gland are of great clinical importance. The conditions known as **benign prostatic hypertrophy (BPH)** and **prostate cancer** are common after age 50. BPH interferes with bladder function, and it can even cause renal failure by obstruction. Treatment with an inhibitor **(finasteride)** of the enzyme 5α-reductase reduces DHT concentrations in the prostate, and causes the gland to shrink. Prostate cancer can be detected early by screening; its presence is suggested by an elevated serum level of PSA (see above). Growth of prostate cancer is at least partly androgen dependent, and therefore complete removal of androgen action is a mainstay of treatment. Methods include (1) excision of the testes; (2) markedly reducing LH and hence testosterone secretion with long-acting continuous GnRH agonists that downregulate their receptors; and (3) inhibiting testosterone and DHT actions with a receptor blocker **(flutamide)** or with estrogens. Escape from the abolition of androgen actions occurs, possibly by the upregulation of the androgen receptor, and its activation by the above-mentioned growth factors.

The major circulating androgen by far is testosterone (Table 46-2). This hormone can be considered in part a prohormone for DHT and 5α-androstenediol, much as thyroxine is a prohormone for triiodothyronine. However, testosterone also has a definite intrinsic hormonal activity of its own in fetal and adult tissues that lack the enzyme 5α-reductase. For example, males who have congenital 5α-reductase deficiency cannot produce DHT. Although these individuals have feminized external genitalia at birth, during puberty they undergo selective masculinization in response to the rising testosterone secretion, and they produce sperm.

The effects of androgens are classified according to the probable actual effector molecule (Fig. 46-21). DHT is specifically required in the fetus for differentiation of the genital tubercle, genital swellings, genital folds, and urogenital sinus into the penis, scrotum, penile urethra, and prostate, respectively. During puberty, DHT is required again for growth of the scrotum and prostate and for stimulation of prostatic secretions.

DHT or 5α-androstenediol stimulates the hair follicles and produces the typical male pattern of hair growth characterized by beard growth, a diamond-shaped pubic escutcheon, relatively large amounts of body hair, and the recession of the temporal hairline. In some men this last response culminates in baldness. DHT or 5α-androstenediol is also responsible for increased production of sebum by the sebaceous glands, and the consequent development of acne, especially during puberty.

Testosterone, on the other hand, specifically stimulates the differentiation of the wolffian ducts into the epididymis, vas deferens, and seminal vesicles. During puberty, testosterone, with or without DHT, causes enlargement of the penis and the seminal vesicles. It also causes enlargement of the larynx and thickening of the vocal cords, which result in a deeper voice. Also, as noted, testosterone is the major local hormone required for initiation and maintenance of spermatogenesis.

Testosterone itself first stimulates the pubertal growth spurt. It then terminates linear growth by closing the epiphyseal growth centers. Androgen receptors in osteoblasts transduce testosterone-stimulated increases in the levels of transforming growth factors. Estradiol is an essential partner of testosterone and a mediator of testosterone's action on bone maturation in males.

Estradiol has also emerged as an important active testosterone metabolite, which mediates effects of testosterone, particularly in the hypothalamus, bone, and reproductive tract. Figure 46-22 demonstrates that selectively decreasing serum estradiol, and probably the hypothalamic conversion of testosterone to estradiol, causes an increase in the serum FSH and LH levels—even in the face of an LH-induced increase in the serum testosterone level. When the testosterone level is also decreased with estradiol, the serum LH level rises even further, whereas the same increase in the serum FSH level is seen. This suggests that estradiol may mediate all the negative feedback effect of testosterone on FSH, but may mediate only partly the feedback effect on LH.

In the male reproductive tract, estradiol regulates the reabsorption of luminal fluid by cells of the efferent ductules (Fig. 46-11). These cells function like those of the proximal tubule in the kidney, and contain Na^+,K^+-ATPase, Cl^- channels, and aquaporin (Chapter 43). Normally, 90% of the fluid in the rete testes is reabsorbed. This process concentrates the sperm in the final ejaculate and improves their maturation and survival. Without estradiol action via the estradiol receptor α, fluid resorption is defective and infertility results.

Recently, XY males have been discovered who either lack estrogen receptors or who have mutant genes for the enzyme aromatase and are therefore estradiol deficient. In both instances, the adult individuals are tall and their epiphyses are unfused. Plasma LH levels are elevated, despite normal or increased testosterone levels. These findings support a normal role for estradiol in epiphyseal function in males, and in gonadal feedback on the male hypothalamus.

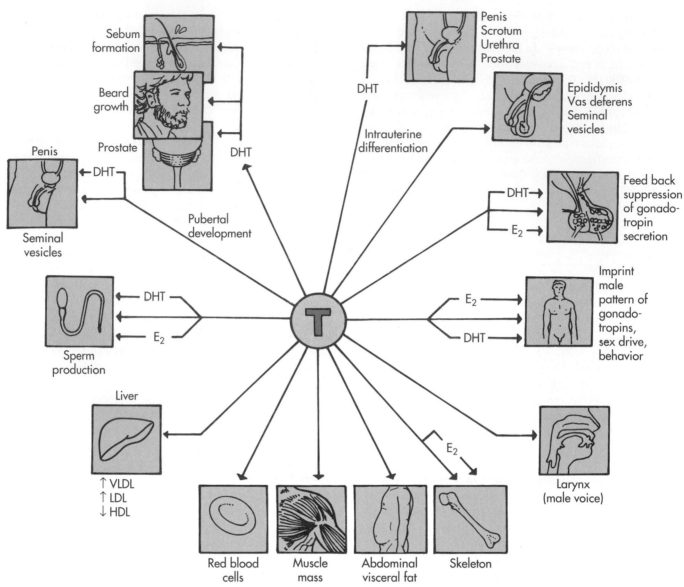

■ **Fig. 46-21** The spectrum of testosterone *(T)* effects. Note that some effects result from the action of T itself, whereas others are mediated by dihydrotestosterone *(DHT)* and estradiol *(E₂)* after they are produced from testosterone. *VLDL, LDL, HDL:* Very-low-density, low-density, and high-density lipoproteins, respectively.

Testosterone causes enlargement of the muscle mass in boys during puberty. In subsequent adult life, administration of testosterone to either sex causes nitrogen retention, which reflects protein anabolism. Note that the hypothalamus lacks significant 5α-reductase activity. Thus, androgen suppression of gonadotropin secretion by negative feedback is largely a function of testosterone, with a possible small additional effect from circulating DHT. As noted, estradiol, produced by aromatase action in the hypothalamus, mediates feedback by testosterone.

Testosterone has important actions on lipid metabolism. It increases levels of circulating low-density lipoprotein (LDL) cholesterol and decreases levels of circulating high-density lipoprotein (HDL) cholesterol (see Chapter 40). It also favors accumulation of upper body, abdominal, and visceral fat.

These lipid effects are associated with a greater risk of cardiovascular disease in men than in premenopausal women.

Certain other diverse androgenic actions can be ascribed to testosterone. These include (1) stimulation of erythropoietin synthesis and maturation of erythroid precursors, which help maintain a normal red blood cell mass; (2) stimulation of renal sodium reabsorption; (3) suppression of hepatic synthesis of SSBG, cortisol-binding globulin, and thyroxine-binding globulin; (4) suppression of mammary gland growth; (5) initiation of sexual drive (libido) and the ability to achieve a physiologically complete erection (potency); and (6) stimulation of aggressive behavior. The importance of testosterone to erectile function is supported by the high density of androgen receptors in that area of the primate brain, where electrical stimulation produces an erection.

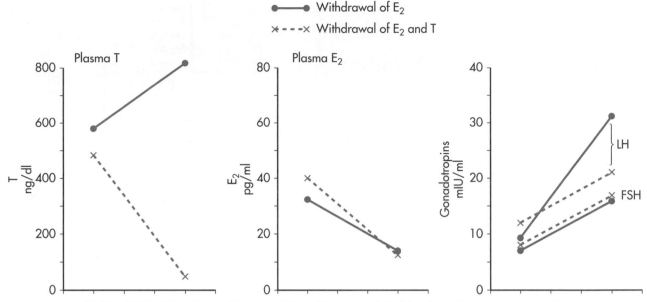

■ **Fig. 46-22**   The effects of 7 days withdrawal from estradiol (E_2) or from E_2 and testosterone (T) in normal men. E_2 withdrawal, by inhibiting aromatase, lowered plasma E_2, causing increases in plasma FSH (follicle-stimulating hormone) and LH (luteinizing hormone). Plasma T rose as a consequence of the increase in LH. Withdrawal of both T and E_2, by inhibiting all gonadal steroid synthesis with ketoconazole, caused a marked decrease in plasma T, along with E_2. There was no further increase in FSH, whereas LH did increase futher. This suggests that all FSH inhibition is via aromatization to E_2, whereas LH inhibition is also accomplished by T itself. (Data from Hayes FJ et al: *J Clin Endocrinol Metab* 86:53, 2001.)

Male Puberty

Beginning at an average age of 10 to 11 years, and ending at an average age of 15 to 17 years, males develop full reproductive function, Leydig cell proliferation, and adult levels of androgenic hormones (Figs. 46-12 and 46-19). They achieve adult size and function of the accessory organs of reproduction, complete secondary sexual characteristics, and adult musculature. They undergo a linear growth spurt, and the epiphyses close when they attain adult height. A composite picture of the measurable and visible portions of this sequence is shown in Fig. 46-23. Note that this process can start as early as age 8 and as late as age 20, without any evidence of disease. The mechanisms of pubertal onset were described previously (Figs. 46-7 and 46-8).

Enlargement of the testis is the first and most important clinical sign of puberty. This enlargement signals an increase in the volume of the seminiferous tubules, and it is preceded by small increases in plasma FSH levels. Testicular volume increases from childhood levels of less than 4 cm^3 to adult levels of 20 to 30 cm^3. As plasma LH levels increase, Leydig cells appear, and testosterone secretion is stimulated. The plasma testosterone level then climbs rapidly over a 2-year period, during which time pubic hair appears, the penis enlarges, and linear growth achieves peak velocity (Fig. 46-23). Males achieve a 10% greater average height and a 25% greater peak bone mass than do females. Sometime during this interval, at a median age of 13 years, sperm production begins. In about one third of boys, breast growth and tenderness appear transiently. These signs probably reflect

increased production of estradiol secondary to LH stimulation. As testosterone levels continue to climb, the breast tissue regresses. One to 2 years after adult testosterone levels are reached, closure of the epiphyseal growth centers ends puberty. The plasma AMH level decreases from childhood levels, in response to an inhibiting effect of pubertal testosterone on this Sertoli cell product. Testosterone, via conversion to estradiol as an intermediate active molecule, also promotes increases in growth hormone secretion during puberty (Fig. 46-9).

THE OVARIES

The **ovaries, fallopian tubes,** and **uterus** make up the internal reproductive organs of the female, and they are situated in the pelvis. Each adult ovary weighs approximately 15 g, and is attached to the lateral pelvic wall and to the uterus by ligaments, through which run the ipsilateral ovarian artery, vein, lymphatic vessels, and nerve supply.

The ovary consists of three zones (Fig. 46-24). The dominant zone is the **cortex,** which is lined by germinal epithelium and contains the **oocytes.** Each oocyte is enclosed within a *follicle.* Follicles in various stages of development and regression are present throughout the cortex during the reproductive years (Fig. 46-24). Interposed between the follicles is the stroma, which is composed of supporting connective tissue elements and interstitial cells. The other two zones of the ovary are the **medulla,** which consists of a heterogeneous group of cells, and the **hilum,** at which the

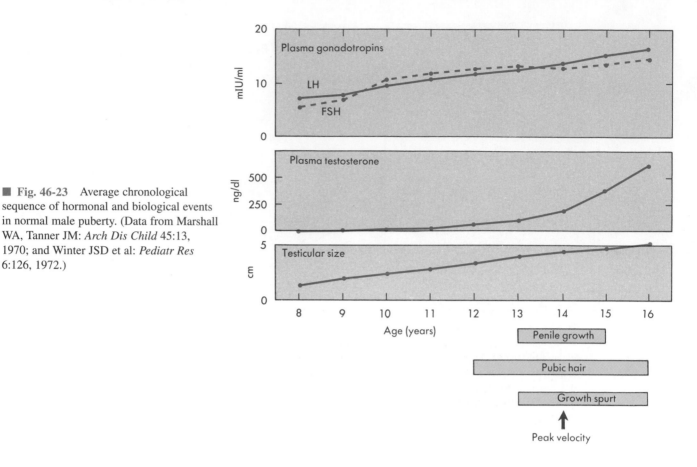

■ **Fig. 46-23**   Average chronological sequence of hormonal and biological events in normal male puberty. (Data from Marshall WA, Tanner JM: *Arch Dis Child* 45:13, 1970; and Winter JSD et al: *Pediatr Res* 6:126, 1972.)

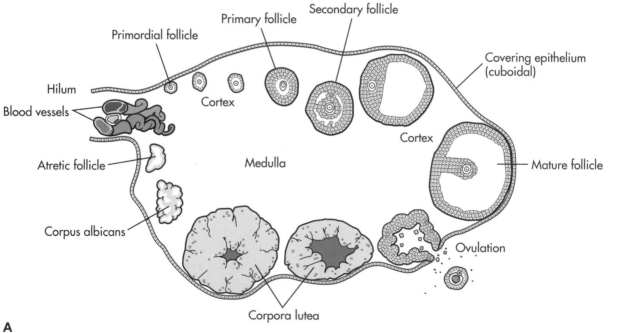

■ **Fig. 46-24**   **A,** Schematic representation (not to scale) of the ovary showing the various stages in the development of the follicle and its successor, the corpus luteum.

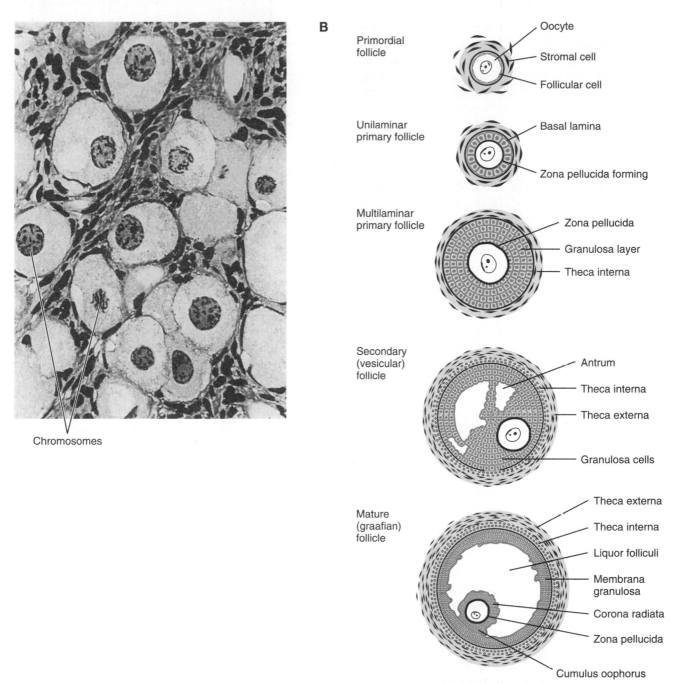

Chromosomes

B

Primordial follicle — Oocyte — Stromal cell — Follicular cell

Unilaminar primary follicle — Basal lamina — Zona pellucida forming

Multilaminar primary follicle — Zona pellucida — Granulosa layer — Theca interna

Secondary (vesicular) follicle — Antrum — Theca interna — Theca externa — Granulosa cells

Mature (graafian) follicle — Theca externa — Theca interna — Liquor folliculi — Membrana granulosa — Corona radiata — Zona pellucida — Cumulus oophorus

■ **Fig. 46-24, cont'd   B,** Details of each stage showing how the oocyte draws successive layers of nutritive, supportive, and protective cells around it as it reaches its maximum size in the secondary follicle. Note the chromosomes that are visible in the photomicrograph because the oocytes are suspended in meiosis. Hormones and other consitutents in the follicular fluid regulate this process. (Modified from Junquiera LC et al: In *Basic histology,* ed 9, Norwalk, Conn., 1998, Appleton & Lange.)

blood vessels enter. The hilum contains Leydig-like androgen-producing cells. During physical examination, the ovaries can be felt through the abdominal wall, and they can also be well visualized by ultrasonography and computed tomography (CT).

As a hormone-secreting organ, the ovary functions in two ways. First, the ovarian sex steroids and protein hormones function locally to modulate the complex events in the development and extrusion of the ova (the process is called

ovulation). Second, ovarian hormones are secreted into the circulation and they act on diverse target organs, including the uterus, fallopian tubes, vagina, breasts, hypothalamus, pituitary gland, adipose tissue, bones, kidney, liver, and vascular system. Many, but not all, of these distant effects are closely related to the reproductive sequence.

The fundamental reproductive unit in the female is the single ovarian follicle, which is composed of one germ cell completely surrounded by a cluster of endocrine cells. When fully developed and functional, the follicle (1) maintains and nurtures the resident oocyte, (2) matures the oocyte and releases it at the right time, (3) prepares the vagina and fallopian tubes to assist in fertilization, (4) prepares the lining of the uterus to accept and implant a zygote, and (5) maintains hormonal support for the fetus until the placenta can take over this function.

The Biology of Oogenesis

The primordial germ cells migrate from the yolk sac of the embryo to the genital ridge at 5 to 6 weeks of gestation. There, in the developing ovary, they produce oogonia by mitotic division until 20 to 24 weeks of gestation, when the total number of oogonia has reached a maximum of 7 million. Beginning at 8 to 9 weeks of gestation, some oogonia start into the prophase of meiosis and become primary oocytes. By 20 weeks, two thirds of the germ cells have entered into meiosis. This process continues until 6 months after birth, when all available oogonia have been converted to oocytes. At this time, oocytes are 10 to 25 μm in diameter. They grow to 50 to 120 μm at maturity; the sizes of the nucleus and cytoplasm increase proportionately. The first meiotic division is not completed until the time of ovulation; thus, primary oocytes have lifespans of up to 50 years. The lengthy suspension of the oocyte in prophase apparently depends on the hormonal milieu provided by its surrounding sustaining cells. Both X chromosomes are required in the ovary for oocyte meiosis and survival.

From the start of oogenesis, however, a process of oocyte attrition also occurs. Initially, the oogonia themselves undergo apoptosis. Once follicles begin to form, many of them undergo atresia by apoptosis. By birth, only 1 to 2 million primary oocytes remain, and by the onset of puberty the number falls to 400,000. Thus, in contrast to the male, who continuously produces spermatogonia and primary spermatocytes, the adult female cannot produce new oogonia. Hence, the woman must function with a continuously declining number of primary oocytes, from which ova can mature. At or soon after menopause, few, if any, oocytes are left, and reproductive capacity ends.

The process of oocyte attrition occurs by apoptosis (see Chapter 39). TGF-β and FAS ligand and their receptors stimulate oocyte apoptosis, whereas various survival factors, including fibroblast growth factor, LIF, and KIT-KIT LIGAND, oppose apoptosis. These vary in their influence on the early ovary, compared to the mature ovary.

The development of ovarian follicles from their primordial state to the point at which an ovum is launched can be divided into three stages.

Stage 1. Follicles begin to form in the fetal ovary at 12 to 16 weeks of gestation. The first stage of development of the ovarian follicle parallels the prophase of the oocyte. This stage progresses slowly, over a period that is usually not less than 13 years but may be as long as 50 years. As an oocyte enters meiosis, it induces a single layer of spindle cells from the stroma to surround it completely. These cells are the precursors of the **granulosa cells.** Cytoplasmic processes from

these cells attach to the plasma membrane of the oocyte. In addition, a membrane called the **basal lamina** forms outside the spindle cells, delimiting the complex from the surrounding stroma. The resultant structure constitutes the **primordial follicle,** which is about 25 μm in diameter (Fig. 46-24).

Beginning at 21 to 31 weeks of gestation, some of these follicles enter the next phase of development. The spindle-shaped cells around the oocyte change to a cuboidal shape and become a single layer of granulosa cells, and thus a unilaminar **primary follicle** is formed. As the granulosa cells divide and form several layers around the oocyte, a multilaminar primary follicle is created. Gap junctions, composed of proteins called **connexins,** lie between granulosa cells and create a syncytium. This allows the flow of nutrients and signaling molecules from cell to cell. The granulosa cells secrete mucopolysaccharides, which form a protective halo, the **zona pellucida,** around the oocyte (Fig. 46-24). The cytoplasmic processes of the granulosa cells, however, continue to penetrate the zona pellucida. This arrangement creates conduits through which these cells can selectively provide nutrients for the maturing primary oocyte within. Thus, the cytoplasm of the granulosa cells, like that of the male Sertoli cells, forms a filter through which plasma substances must pass before reaching the germ cell. Of note, neither the granulosa cells nor the oocyte have a direct blood supply. Exchange with plasma must take place by diffusion across the basal lamina. The penetration of the zona pellucida by cytoplasmic processes of the granulosa cells permits chemical signals to pass between the granulosa cells and their oocyte.

The multilaminar primary follicle continues to grow as granulosa cells proliferate and it reaches a diameter of 150 μm. At this point, the oocyte has reached its maximal size, on average 80 μm in diameter. Two other developments take place concurrently: (1) another layer of spindle interstitial cells is recruited outside the basal lamina and forms the **theca interna** and (2) the granulosa cells begin to extrude small amounts of fluid that form collections between them. Thus a **secondary follicle,** or vescicular follicle, with about 600 granulosa cells, is formed. The first stage of follicular development is now complete. With some exceptions, this first stage is the maximal degree of development found in the prepubertal ovary.

Stage 2. In contrast to the first stage, the second stage of follicular development is much more rapid, requiring only 70 to 85 days. This stage takes place mainly after menarche (i.e., after the onset of menses). Past the midpoint of each menstrual cycle, a small cohort of secondary follicles is recruited to enter the next sequence, which spans 2½ menstrual cycles. The small collections of follicular fluid coalesce into a single central area, called the **antrum** (Fig. 46-24). The fluid in the antrum contains mucopolysaccharides, plasma proteins, electrolytes, glycosoaminoglycans, proteoglycans, gonadal steroid hormones, FSH, LH, inhibin, activin, follistatin, several growth factors [IGF-1, IGF-2, IGFBP1-5, TGF-β, and epidermal growth factor (EGF)], oxytocin, arginine vasopressin, corticotropin-releasing hormone (CRH) and proopiomelanocortin products, the renin-angiotensin system, and various cytokines (interleukin-1 [IL-1], TNF-α). The steroid hormones reach the antrum by direct secretion from granulosa cells and by diffusion from the theca cells outside the basal lamina. A nonsteroidal substance, made by granulosa cells that can inhibit oocyte meiosis, is also secreted into the antral fluid. AMH, inhibin, or a related molecule may be this factor.

The granulosa cells continue to proliferate, and they displace the oocyte into an eccentric position on a stalk. Here the oocyte is surrounded by a distinctive granulosa cell layer, called the **cumulus oophorus,** which is two to three cells thick. These granulosa cells appear not to be engaged in steroid hormone production. The theca cells also proliferate, and those nearest the basal lamina are transformed into cuboidal, steroid-secreting cells of the theca interna. Additional peripheral layers of spindle cells from the stroma form around the theca interna and, together with an ingrowth of blood vessels, make up the theca externa. The new vessels give the follicle direct access to blood-borne molecules such as gonadotropins. By the end of this second stage, the entire complex, called a **graafian follicle** or **antral follicle** (Fig. 46-24), has reached an average diameter of 2 to 5 mm. Although graafian follicles are found in prepubertal ovaries, particularly during the postnatal period of high FSH and LH levels (Fig. 46-6), they are relatively small and in an early phase of development.

Stage 3. The third and final stage of follicular development is the most rapid, and it occurs only in the postpubertal reproductive ovary. *Five to 7 days after the onset of menses, a single graafian follicle is selected from its small cohort of about 20 sister follicles, and it becomes the dominant follicle* of that cycle. With rare exceptions, this process occurs in only a single ovary each month. A high mitotic index of its granulosa cells is a key characteristic of this selected dominant follicle. In addition to further cellular growth, the production of antral fluid is significantly increased. The colloid osmotic pressure of the fluid also increases because of depolymerization of the mucopolysaccharides, but the total intrafollicular pressure remains at 16 to 20 mm Hg. The granulosa cells spread apart and the cumulus oophorus loosens. At the same time, the vascularity of the theca increases greatly. With exponential growth, the total size of this follicle reaches 20 mm in the final 48 hours before ovulation, which takes place at the midpoint of the menstrual cycle. The portion of the basal lamina adjacent to the surface of the ovary then undergoes proteolysis. The follicle gently ruptures and releases the oocyte with its adherent cumulus oophorus into the peritoneal cavity. At this time, the first meiotic division is completed. The resultant secondary oocyte is drawn into the closely approximated fallopian tube. The other daughter cell, called the **first polar body,** is discarded. In the fallopian tube, penetration by a sperm stimulates the completion of the second meiotic division and yields the haploid (23 chromosome) ovum and the **second polar body.**

Corpus luteum formation. After ovulation, the remaining elements of the ruptured follicle next form a new endocrine structure, the **corpus luteum** (Fig. 46-24). *This new endocrine unit provides the necessary balance of gonadal steroids that optimizes conditions for implantation of a fertilized ovum, and for subsequent maintenance of the zygote until the placenta can assume this function.* The corpus luteum is made up of granulosa cells, theca cells, thecal capillaries, and fibroblasts. Vascular endothelial growth factor and fibroblast growth factor drive the rapid vascularization of the corpus luteum. The granulosa cells comprise 80% of the corpus luteum. They undergo hypertrophy to a diameter of 30 μm and become arranged in rows. The mitochondria develop dense matrices with tubular cristae, numerous lipid droplets form within the cytoplasm, and the smooth endoplasmic reticulum proliferates. These changes reflect the marked increase in the capacity of the cells to produce steroid hormones, as described in Chapter 45. This process, called **luteinization,** is precipitated by the exit of the oocyte from the follicle.

The remaining 20% of the corpus luteum consists of theca cells arranged in folds along its outer surface. The theca cells exhibit similar, although less dramatic, luteinization changes. The basal lamina between the theca and granulosa cells disappears, which allows direct vascularization of the granulosa cells. Gap junctions form between the luteal cells. Intake of LDL cholesterol from plasma provides the substrate for a new wave of steroid hormone production by the new entity.

The antrum may become engorged temporarily with blood from hemorrhaging thecal vessels, but a clot quickly forms and is subsequently lysed. If fertilization and pregnancy do not ensue, the corpus luteum begins to regress after a 14-day lifespan. In this process, known as **luteolysis,** the endocrine cells undergo apoptosis and necrosis, and the structure is invaded by leukocytes, macrophages, and fibroblasts. Gradually, the former corpus luteum is replaced by an avascular scar, known as the **corpus albicans** (Fig. 46-24).

Atresia of follicles. During the reproductive lifespan of the average woman, only 400 to 500 oocytes (one per month) undergo the complete sequence of events that culminate in ovulation. The remaining millions of oocytes disappear. A few are lost each month because they enter into a growth phase with other follicles, but they do not become dominant follicles. Most, however, undergo the process called **atresia,** which begins almost as soon as the first primordial follicles appear in the fetal ovary.

Atresia is caused by **apoptosis,** or programmed cell death (Chapter 39). In first-stage follicles, atresia appears to be a relatively simple process, precipitated by oocyte degeneration. The oocyte becomes necrotic, its nucleus becomes pyknotic, and the granulosa cells also degenerate. This simple type of atresia accounts for the disappearance of most follicles. In more advanced follicles, atresia is more complex. In some of these follicles, the granulosa cells furthest from the oocyte first undergo necrotic changes. Loss of their function may actually cause the oocyte to resume meiosis, to the point of extrusion of the first polar body. Eventually, however, the granulosa cells in the cumulus oophorus also die, the protective zona pellucida disappears, and the oocyte degenerates. Fibroblasts then invade the follicle, and everything inside the basal lamina collapses into an avascular scar. Outside the basal lamina, the theca cells dedifferentiate and return to the pool of interstitial cells from which they came.

Hormonal Patterns during the Menstrual Cycle

The menstrual cycle is divided physiologically into three sequential phases. The **follicular phase** begins with the onset of menstrual bleeding, and it averages 15 days (range, 9 to 23 days). The **ovulatory phase** lasts 1 to 3 days and culminates in ovulation. The **luteal phase** has a more constant length of 13 to 14 days, and it ends with the onset of menstrual bleeding. The overall duration of a normal menstrual cycle averages 28 days, but it can vary from 21 to 35 days, depending mostly on the length of the follicular phase.

A series of cyclic changes in gonadal steroid and protein hormone production characterizes adult ovarian function (Fig. 46-25, Table 46-3). This monthly hormone profile results from cyclic changes in pituitary gonadotropins (Fig. 46-25), coupled with paracrine and autocrine effects on the follicle. Critical changes in FSH and LH secretion largely reflect changes in pituitary sensitivity to GnRH (Fig. 46-26, *A*) but they also reflect changes in the pulsatility of the hypothalamic GnRH generator. However, the pattern of gonadotropin secretion is also critically regulated by both negative and positive feedback from gonadal steroids, and it is influenced by inhibin and activin. These interactions are described in detail in Chapter 43 and presented in Fig. 43-15.

Toward the end of the luteal phase (a few days before the onset of menstrual bleeding), plasma FSH and LH are at their lowest levels (Fig. 46-25). The LH/FSH ratio is slightly greater than 1. One or 2 days before the onset of menses, FSH levels begin to rise, followed somewhat later by a rise in LH levels. *The estrogen (estradiol and estrone) levels increase gradually, stimulated by the gradual rise in the FSH level in this first half of the follicular phase.* Progesterone, 17-hydroxyprogesterone, and the androgens, androstenedione and testosterone, remain at relatively low, constant levels.

During the second half of the follicular phase, FSH levels fall modestly, whereas LH levels continue to rise very slowly. The LH/FSH ratio therefore increases to about 2. *Concurrently, estradiol and estrone production and plasma levels rise sharply, and just before the ovulatory phase, they reach peaks that are 5-fold to 9-fold higher.* The estradiol is secreted directly by the dominant follicle. In contrast, estrone is produced largely by peripheral conversion from estradiol and androstenedione. Progesterone, largely secreted by the adrenal cortex, and 17-hydroxyprogesterone remain at low levels until just before the ovulatory phase, when the progesterone level begins to increase as a consequence of ovarian secretion. Androstenedione and testosterone also rise modestly in parallel with 17-hydroxyprogesterone. About half the androgenic steroids are derived from ovarian secretion, and half are derived from adrenal secretion. The ovarian contribution results from LH stimulation of the theca cells in the dominant follicle.

The succeeding ovulatory phase is characterized by a very sharp spike in plasma gonadotropin levels. The LH level increases much more than does the FSH level (Fig. 46-25), and hence the LH/FSH ratio rises to about 5. It takes an average of 14 hours for this surge to be achieved, and the doubling time is 5 hours. The plateau lasts 14 hours, and LH and FSH levels then decline over 20 hours. Plasma estradiol levels plummet from their peak at the same time that LH

■ **Table 46-3**   Turnover of gonadal steroids in adult women

Steroids	*Plasma concentration (ng/dl)*	*Production rate (μg/day)*	*Metabolic clearance rate (L/day)*
Estradiol			
Early follicular	6	80	1400
Late follicular	50	700	
Middle luteal	20	300	
Estrone			
Eary follicular	5	100	2200
Late follicular	20	500	
Middle luteal	10	250	
17-Hydroxyprogesterone			
Early follicular	30	600	2000
Late follicular	200	4000	
Middle follicular	200	4000	
Progesterone			
Follicular	100	2000	
Luteal	1000	25,000	
Testosterone	40	250	700
Dihydrotestosterone	20	50	400
Androstenedione	150	3000	2000
DHEA*	500	8000	1600

Modified from Lipsett MB: In Yen SSC, Jaffe RB, editors: *Reproductive endocrinology,* Philadelphia, 1978, WB Saunders.
DHEA, Dehydroepiandrosterone.

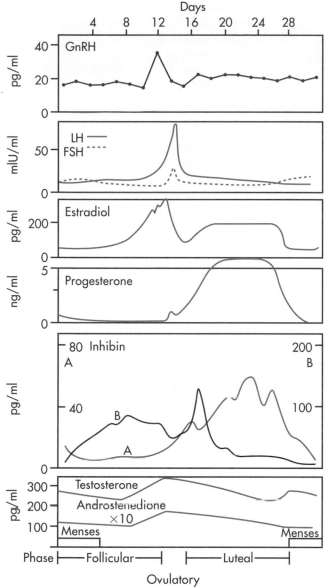

■ **Fig. 46-25** Plasma hormone levels throughout the menstrual cycle. Note the increases of estradiol from the dominant follicle and gonadotropin-releasing hormone *(GnRH)* preceding ovulatory surges of LH and FSH. The later broad peaks of progesterone and estradiol are produced by corpus luteum secretion. The earlier inhibin B peak results from follicle production; the later inhibin A peak results from corpus luteal production.

and FSH are on their ovulatory upswing. Estrone, 17-hydroxyprogesterone, androstenedione, and testosterone also now decrease, but much more gradually than does estradiol. In contrast, a small but significant rise in progesterone begins during the ovulatory phase.

After ovulation, LH and FSH both continue to decline during the luteal phase, and they reach their lowest points toward the end of the cycle, before the onset of menses. *The most distinctive and important feature of the luteal phase is a 10-fold increase in the progesterone level, which emanates from the corpus luteum.* Levels of estradiol, estrone, and 17-hydroxyprogesterone also increase, and broad second peaks

of each occur through the middle of the luteal phase. Levels of androstenedione and testosterone, however, continue to decline during the luteal phase.

Inhibin levels also fluctuate systematically throughout the cycle (Fig. 46-25). Inhibin B (Fig. 46-5) levels rise during the follicular phase as a result of follicle production, in parallel with FSH levels, and inhibin B displays a periovulatory phase peak. The levels become very low during the luteal phase. In contrast, inhibin A (Fig. 46-5) levels are low during the follicular phase, but they increase markedly in parallel with the progesterone level during the luteal phase, which reflects corpus luteum production. Thus, inhibin B comes from the dominant follicle, whereas inhibin A comes predominantly from the corpus luteum. Inhibin B plus estradiol feed back on the pituitary gland, to reduce FSH secretion during the latter part of the follicular phase. Inhibin A plus estradiol and progesterone feed back on the pituitary to suppress FSH and LH secretion throughout the luteal phase. If pregnancy does not occur, the menstrual cycle ends as estrogen and progesterone levels decrease dramatically to their lowest values. FSH levels again begin to rise, and bleeding signals the start of a new cycle.

Hormonal Regulation of Oogenesis and the Stages of Follicular Development

Stage 1. The initial growth of the primordial follicle appears to be a local phenomenon. It is independent of gonadotropins, but factors from the oocyte stimulate early granulosa cell development. In mouse oocytes several genes, including those coding for zona pellucida proteins, are essential to normal follicle development. In turn, granulosa cell products initiate formation of the theca, and then they stop maturation of the oocyte once the latter reaches 80 μm in diameter. Some of the cross-signaling between the oocyte and its surrounding granalosa cells may be mediated by TGF-α and EGF. Both of these growth factors, as well as the EGF and activin receptors, are present in oocytes. In addition, a growth differentiation factor, called GDF-9, is secreted by oocytes and affects granulosa cells.

In mouse studies, the protooncogene c-*kit* encodes a receptor of the tyrosine kinase growth factor type (Chapter 39). This receptor is termed KIT and it is activated by a signaling molecule called KIT LIGAND. KIT is present in oocytes and theca cells. KIT and KIT LIGAND are expressed at various stages of folliculogenesis, and their interaction inhibits apoptosis of oocytes, oogonia, and primordial germ cells. In mature ovaries, formation of an antral cavity and maximal androgen production by theca cells are partly facilitated by paracrine interactions that use this signaling system.

The transient surge of FSH and LH release that occurs midway through gestation, and even the normally low levels of gonadotropins that are secreted during childhood, are necessary for an adequate rate of follicular growth throughout the rest of life. Without any gonadotropin stimulation, follicular growth is greatly impaired. Nonetheless, the first stage, from primordial to primary follicle, continues until menopause; its occurrence does not appear to depend on the

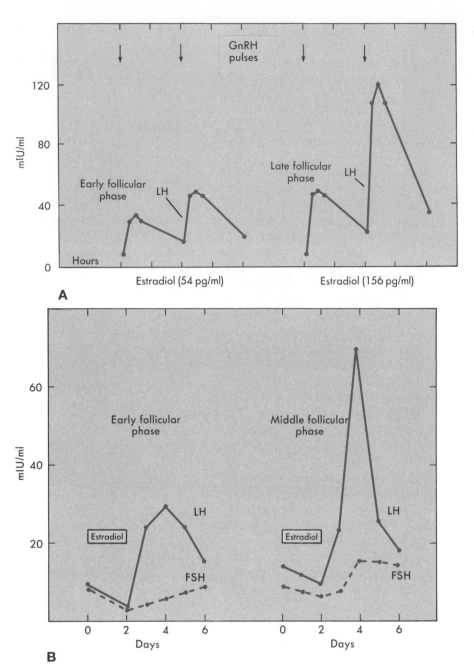

■ **Fig. 46-26** **A,** Increased responsiveness of pituitary gonadotrophs to GnRH in the late follicular phase of the menstrual cycle when endogenous estradiol levels are increased. **B,** Plasma LH and FSH after exogenous estradiol administration. After the initial decrease caused by negative feedback, plasma LH rebounds well above the baseline when estradiol is discontinued. This positive effect of estradiol is also accentuated as the follicular phase of the menstrual cycle progresses. (**A** redrawn from Wang CF et al: *J Clin Endocrinol Metab* 42:718, 1976. **B** redrawn from Yen SSC et al: In Ferin M et al, editors: *Biorhythms and human reproduction,* New York, 1974, John Wiley.)

presence or the state of reproductive cycling or, in particular, on FSH or FSH receptor functioning.

The exact mechanism by which a particular group of resting primordial follicles is recruited to descend from the cortex into the interstitium toward the medulla and to initiate development into primary follicles is unknown. However, the most "selectable" follicles are those whose theca interna begins to develop during the periovulatory phase of that cycle, when the surge of gonadotropin release increases the vascularity of the follicles and helps protect them from atresia.

Stage 2. After the menarche, recruitment of a cohort of primary follicles for second-stage development occurs in the early luteal phase of the menstrual cycle, and is dependent on the relatively low levels of FSH and LH during the luteal phase. Each cohort gradually develops further over a period of 60 to 70 days, until the late luteal phase two cycles later. At this point, a total of about 20 follicles in both ovaries, which have reached a size of 2 to 4 mm, is capable of responding further to the FSH increase in the follicular phase of the next cycle.

Before their selection, primary follicles show evidence of only the faint presence of steroid hormone–producing enzymes. *The initial action of FSH on primary follicles is to stimulate growth of the granulosa cells* (Fig. 46-27) with a 600-fold increase in granulosa cell numbers and a 15-fold increase in follicle diameter. Aromatase activity is also progressively increased by FSH, and hence estrogen synthesis from androgen precursors is enhanced. The increasing local estradiol concentration causes proliferation of its own receptors and of endocrine, paracrine, and autocrine growth fac-

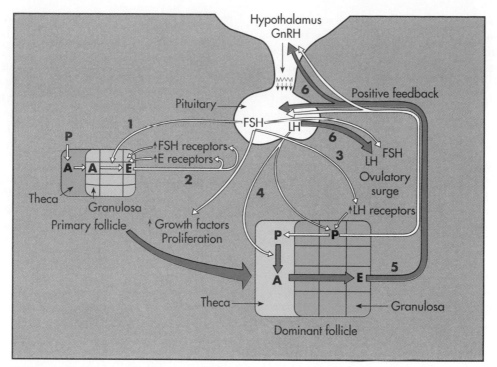

■ **Fig. 46-27** Hormonal regulation of follicular development. *1,* FSH stimulates granulosa cell growth and estradiol *(E)* synthesis in certain more receptive primary follicles. *2,* The local estradiol increases its own receptors and FSH receptors, amplifying both hormones' effects. Thus, a self-propelling mechanism is set into motion. *3,* FSH also stimulates growth factor production and granulosa cell proliferation. FSH later increases LH receptors, augmenting granulosa and theca cell responsiveness to LH. *4,* LH stimulates theca cell growth and androgen *(A)* production. Androgen is then converted to estradiol in the granulosa cells. LH also stimulates progesterone *(P)* production in the granulosa cells. *5,* As a result of two-way steroid traffic, the dominant follicle emerges as a very efficient secretor of estradiol. *6,* Rising estradiol, with late potentiation by progesterone, acts on the pituitary gland and hypothalamus to evoke the preovulatory surge of LH and FSH by positive feedback.

tors. It also reinforces FSH actions by increasing FSH receptors and by synergizing with FSH, along with locally produced activin, to stimulate further granulosa cell hyperplasia and hypertrophy (Fig. 46-27). These effects in turn further boost estradiol production. Local synthesis of IGF-1 and IGF-2, in response to FSH, further amplifies the primary FSH signals for proliferation and steroidogenesis. In contrast, EGF and TGF-α decrease FSH-induced estradiol synthesis, but reinforce granulosa cell proliferation. Thus, the initiation of second-stage follicular development may be viewed as a self-propelling mechanism that involves fine coordination between the pituitary gland and ovary, and that yields successively increasing rates of follicular growth and estradiol production. FSH is absolutely required for this advance in development beyond preantral follicles.

Three other important actions, which develop somewhat later in the second stage, contribute to this autocatalytic process. First, FSH, along with estradiol, induces LH receptors on the granulosa cells. Both FSH and LH receptors act via cAMP as a second messenger. However, as a follicle approaches ovulation, the increased production of cAMP in the granulosa cells becomes more influenced by LH than by FSH. The increased density of LH receptors also prepares

the granulosa cells for their later LH-regulated functioning as luteal cells in the corpus luteum. Second, the slowly rising plasma estradiol levels condition the hypothalamic gonadotropin axis, which maintains or slightly increases plasma LH, while plasma FSH is decreasing. Furthermore, pituitary LH stores are enhanced by estradiol. This enhancement is reflected by the fact that administration of exogenous pulses of GnRH increases the LH responses more in the second half of the follicular phase than in the first half (Fig. 46-26, *A*). Thus, pituitary stores of LH are built up for the coming essential ovulatory surge. Third, estradiol increases the number of LH receptors in theca cells, receptors that are essential to full androgen production.

The rising LH level stimulates the theca cells to synthesize increasing amounts of androgens, with androstenedione production predominating over testosterone production. These steroids diffuse across the basal lamina, where they serve as substrates for granulosa cell aromatase and sustain the augmented estradiol production (Figs. 46-4 and 46-27). In addition, LH stimulates the granulosa cells to produce progesterone, some of which can diffuse back into the theca cells to serve as substrate for androgen synthesis (Fig. 46-27). Thus, although granulosa cells and theca cells can individually synthesize both androgens and estrogens to some extent, their proximity and the two-way traffic of steroids between them greatly increase the overall efficiency of the follicle. Androgens and the androgen receptor also have important functions in the granulosa cells. They amplify the FSH-induced increase in cAMP and thereby contribute at an early stage to the growth of the dominant follicle. Androgens also upregulate aromatase activity. These actions are not carried out by dihydrotestosterone, which in the ovarian milieu may actually have a negative effect through the androgen receptor, and oppose those actions.

The local gonadal protein hormones also contribute paracrine effects to the two-cell process of estradiol production. Inhibin B from granulosa cells, together with IGF-1 stimulated by growth hormone action and locally produced IGF-2, augments androgen production by theca cells. Insulin itself also stimulates androgen synthesis. Although activin inhibits this synthesis, the inhibition may be offset by activin enhancement of FSH and LH receptors. Follistatin also inhibits activin actions and directly stimulates progesterone synthesis. As the follicle matures, inhibin and follistatin increase and activin declines. The influence of both IGFs is modulated by local production of their binding proteins.

Growth hormone (GH) also has a role in the development of the follicle and of its resident oocyte. In animal studies, the FSH-independent first stage in folliculogenesis may be stimulated by GH. Later, GH contributes to the hyperplasia of the granulosa cells and their accretion of steroids. In turn, GH facilitates growth and maturation of the oocyte, but does so indirectly because oocytes lack GH receptors. IGF-1 and IGF-2 mediate some, but not all, GH effects. Indeed, GH and IGF-1 may actually have synergistic actions.

All components of the hypothalamic-pituitary GH axis are present in the ovary, where the appropriate mRNAs indicate they are locally produced. This includes GHRH, somatostatin, GH, and their respective receptors. The relative roles, timing, and importance of endocrine actions of GH originating in the pituitary, versus paracrine and autocrine actions of GH originating in the ovary, remain to be deter-mined. Because not all women with partial pituitary GH deficiency are infertile, the ovarian GH axis may function in some instances as a back-up.

FSH stimulates the production of various other molecules by the granulosa cells, which probably have paracrine effects. The situation is analogous to that of the Sertoli cell and spermatogenesis. Thus, transferrin and ceruloplasmin pick up iron and copper, respectively, from their plasma-binding analogs and transfer these vital elements to the oocyte. FSH also stimulates granulosa cell metabolism and provides lactic acid and 2-ketoisocaproic acid as energy sources for the oocyte. IGFs and transforming growth factors may modulate oocyte development. Locally produced plasminogen activator and cytokines are involved in ovulation. Concentrations of renin, angiotensin, oxytocin, and GnRH-like peptides are all elevated in the follicular fluid, but their functions are obscure.

Stage 3. By days 5 to 7 of the follicular phase, only one follicle has reached a size greater than 11 mm. This **dominant follicle** selects itself by outstripping the others. Its key characteristic is increased aromatase activity, and therefore synthesis of estradiol is more efficient. The increased aromatase activity may result from greater vascularity, and therefore from greater accessibility to FSH. Because FSH is more available to this follicle, and it has an increased number of FSH receptors, the dominant follicle is not as dependent on the waning FSH supply in the middle to late follicular phase. A greater production of inhibin, a lesser production of activin, and a more favorable array of growth factors at this crucial time may increase LH receptors and cAMP. Hence, the supply of precursor androgens from the theca cells for estradiol synthesis tends to increase. *Whatever the mechanism, its greater production of estradiol permits the dominant follicle (1) to inhibit further substantive growth of its sister follicles, (2) to prime the GnRH-gonadotropin axis for generating the ovulatory LH surge, and (3) to alter the tissues of the genital tract to favor conception* (Fig. 46-28).

The remaining follicles undergo atresia, the largest of them in the midluteal phase when the FSH level is low. These

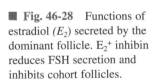

■ **Fig. 46-28** Functions of estradiol *(E₂)* secreted by the dominant follicle. E₂⁺ inhibin reduces FSH secretion and inhibits cohort follicles.

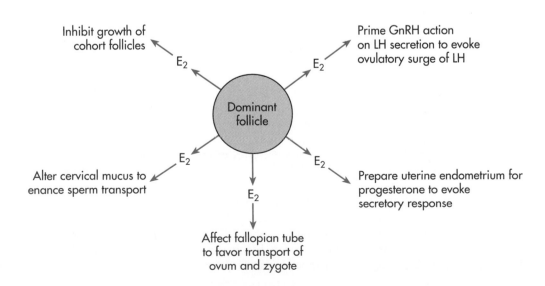

Inhibit growth of cohort follicles

E_2

Prime GnRH action on LH secretion to evoke ovulatory surge of LH

E_2

Dominant follicle

Alter cervical mucus to enance sperm transport

E_2

E_2

Prepare uterine endometrium for progesterone to evoke secretory response

E_2

Affect fallopian tube to favor transport of ovum and zygote

follicles have fewer FSH receptors, as well as a low FSH concentration, and a high androgen/estrogen ratio in the follicular fluid. Also, the fact that cohort follicles are stunted more severely in the ovary that contains the dominant follicle than in the contralateral ovary suggests that the dominant follicle increases the secretion of a specific paracrine inhibitor of steroidogenesis, such as activin.

The sharply increasing estradiol release from the dominant follicle triggers the ovulatory surge of gonadotropins (Figs. 46-26, *B,* and 46-29). A critical plasma estradiol level of at least 200 pg/ml, sustained for at least 2 days, is required to elicit this **positive feedback** effect on LH; this effect is more pronounced later than earlier in the follicular phase (Fig. 46-26, *B*). Although the much smaller periovulatory increase in progesterone is not absolutely required for ovulation, it does synergize with estradiol by amplifying and prolonging the gonadotropin surge. The loci of this positive feedback on gonadotropin secretion are both the pituitary gland and the hypothalamus. The mechanism involves decreasing the inhibitory activity of dopaminergic and endorphinergic neurons on GnRH neurons (Fig. 43-15). The pituitary gonadotrophs, appropriately primed by the preceding pattern of gonadal steroid exposure, respond to GnRH with heightened sensitivity at this time (Fig. 46-26, *A*). The LH molecules released are more bioactive, probably because of posttranslational modulation of their sialic acid content by estradiol. Also, a peak of peripheral plasma GnRH levels may precede the LH/FSH peak (Fig. 46-25). This peak likely indicates an augmented flow of GnRH from the hypothalamus to the pituitary, an effect that is also attributable to gonadal estrogens (Fig. 46-29).

The surge of LH with FSH then triggers ovulation by a multicomponent mechanism. LH stimulation of the granulosa cell neutralizes the action of an oocyte maturation inhibitor. Release from inhibition allows meiosis to be completed. Stimulation of progesterone levels enhances proteolytic enzyme activity and increases the distensibility of the follicle. As a result, follicular fluid volume rapidly increases. The LH surge, possibly via increasing progesterone and its receptor, also induces the enzyme, **prostaglandin endoperoxidase synthase,** in granulosa cells. This enzyme increases the synthesis of prostaglandins, thromboxanes, and leukotrienes, and thereby causes a pseudoinflammatory response that leads to follicular rupture. Mucification of the cumulus oophorus, and possibly contraction of the follicular wall stimulated by oxytocin, contribute to extrusion of the oocyte. Plasminogen activator, stimulated by FSH, generates the proteolytic enzyme, plasmin, which catalyzes breakdown of the follicular wall. Increases in the concentrations of histamine, bradykinins, platelet-activating factor, and blood flow then follow. FSH also stimulates the process whereby the oocyte-cumulus complex becomes detached and free-floating just before extrusion. Finally, immediately after the LH surge, the numbers of LH receptors are temporarily downregulated. This reduction in LH receptors desensitizes the granulosa and thecal cells to LH. The resultant rapid fall in androgen and estradiol production contributes to loss of integrity of the follicle. The LH surge also neutralizes the activity of the luteinization-inhibiting factor found in preovulatory fluid, and thereby stimulates luteinization of the granulosa cells.

Although the inflammatory reaction is essential to ovulation, its continuation after discharge of the ovary would not likely favor the establishment of the corpus luteum on that site. Thus, it is of interest that the LH surge induces type 1 11-hydroxysteroid dehydrogenase and downregulates the

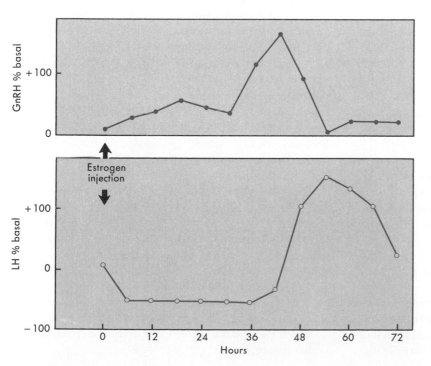

■ **Fig. 46-29** Effect of exogenous administration of estrogen on plasma GnRH and LH levels. After an initial phase of suppression, the positive feedback action of estrogen on LH secretion is seen at 48 hours. This delayed rise in LH levels is preceded by an increase in GnRH levels, suggesting a hypothalamic locus of estrogen action. (Redrawn from Miyake A et al: *J Clin Endocrinol Metab* 56:1100, 1983.)

type 2 enzyme isomer (Chapter 45). This increases the synthesis of cortisol from cortisone, and thereby provides the postovulation-suppressing effect of the active glucocorticoid, cortisol, on inflammation.

Corpus luteum function. Once the oocyte leaves the ovary, it is not under any other immediate hormonal influence. However, the organization and growth of the corpus luteum and its secretory pattern are under hormonal control. In humans, LH is essential for luteinization of the granulosa cells. Their subsequent high rate of progesterone production is facilitated by increased expression of StAR and increased activity of the enzymes 3β-hydrogenase and $\Delta^{4,5}$-isomerase (Fig. 46-4). Luteinization requires restoration and maintenance of LH receptors, which in turn depends on proper exposure to FSH and LH pulses in the preceding follicular phase. Prolactin may help sustain progesterone output by increasing the LH receptors. However, plasma prolactin levels vary only slightly throughout the menstrual cycle, and corpus luteum function has been observed in prolactin-deficient women. Estradiol also may play an autocrine role in maintaining the corpus luteum, possibly by facilitating vascular ingrowth. Vascular endothelial growth factor increases angiogenesis and vascular permeability thereby enhancing nutrition to the corpus luteum.

During the luteal phase, low-frequency/high-amplitude LH pulses replace the high-frequency/low-amplitude pulses of the follicular phase. This change in pulse characteristics may result from conditioning of the GnRH generator by the high progesterone concentrations. Also, the steadily increasing output of progesterone, estradiol, and inhibin A from the corpus luteum exerts negative feedback on the pituitary gland. As a result, the levels of LH and FSH (Fig. 46-25) gradually decline. If the declining LH levels of the late luteal phase are not replaced by the equivalent placental hormone, **human chorionic gonadotropin (HCG),** the corpus luteum regresses. Apoptosis of luteal cells is stimulated by interactions between essential transcription products of the tumor suppressor genes, p53 and Wilms tumor-1. LH and HCG inhibit expression of the oncogenic p53 gene. Secretion of progesterone and estradiol ceases completely in 14 days. In addition to LH, GH, IGF-1, prostaglandin (PG) E_2, and PGI_2 (Fig. 39-19) all participate in regulating corpus luteum function by increasing progesterone secretion. Prolactin also has a modulating role.

In the nonpregnant female who lacks HCG, the corpus luteum begins to regress by the eighth day after ovulation. The breakdown of the corpus luteum **(luteolysis)** is associated with decreasing LH receptors, steroidogenic enzymes, and vascularity. This process is also marked by increasing concentrations of cholesterol in the corpus luteum as progesterone synthesis declines. Luteolysis is itself a complexly regulated endocrine/paracrine process. Estradiol, by preovulatory follicles from the developing next cycle—if conception has not occurred—and estradiol from the corpus luteum itself stimulates oxytocin secretion from the posterior pituitary gland. Added to this is oxytocin, which is produced in the corpus luteum. Oxytocin stimulates production of $PGF_{2\alpha}$

(Fig. 39-19), which in turn inhibits the actions of LH on luteal cells. This inhibition leads to loss of steroid production and apoptosis. As macrophages and T lymphocytes are drawn to the site of luteolysis, they secrete TNF-α and interferon-γ (IFN-γ) which augment $PGF_{2\alpha}$ synthesis and accelerate the lutolytic process. Prolactin also stimulates particular lymphocytes to increase expression of fas-ligand, which mediates luteal cell death by apoptosis. By the twelfth postovulatory day, plasma progesterone, estradiol, and inhibin A have fallen to levels low enough to release the pituitary gland from negative feedback inhibition. FSH then begins to rise in the next cycle.

> Extraordinary coordination between the various elements of the female hypothalamic-pituitary-ovarian axis is clearly required for ovulation and conception. This creates numerous possibilities for failure, and infertility often arises from dysfunction of this system. Disease or conditions that disrupt GnRH release or impair the gonadotroph responsiveness prevent the necessary initial FSH pattern from recruiting a dominant follicle. Hence, complete loss of menses **(amenorrhea)** may result. A dominant follicle may produce enough estrogen for uterine bleeding to occur (see below), but not enough to induce a midcycle peak of the LH level. **Anovulatory cycles** result. An elevated ratio of LH to FSH levels in the follicular phase is associated with excessive theca cell production of androgens, which results in the formation of numerous atretic and cystic follicles. This condition is known as the **polycystic ovary syndrome.** Even if ovulation occurs, inadequate progesterone production by the corpus luteum may lead to poor preparation of the reproductive tract for either fertilization or implantation.

Various medical therapies are available for female infertility. For example, the drug clomiphene is an estrogen receptor antagonist that acts in the hypothalamus. By simulating estrogen deficiency and producing negative feedback, clomiphene increases GnRH and gonadotropin secretion in women who have a hypothalamic origin of infertility. Alternatively, endogenous pituitary function can be suppressed with a long-acting GnRH superagonist, and ovulation can then be induced by carefully timed doses of exogenous FSH and LH. LH is usually provided in the form of HCG.

The hormonal regulation of the female reproductive cycle, as just described, raises an important question: *What ultimately determines the monthly cyclicity of the LH/FSH surge and the resultant ovulation?* Although the concept of a primary central nervous system clock was initially favored, considerable evidence suggests that it is the ovary that principally determines the basic rhythm. Five observations support this point:

1. Cyclic release of gonadotropins is not observed in women whose ovaries never functioned or whose ovaries were removed during the reproductive years, or in postmenopausal women after follicular development has ceased.

2. During the reproductive years, the ovulatory gonadotropin surge does not occur until the dominant follicle has reached the appropriate stage of development, however long that may take.

3. When the antiestrogen, hypothalamic stimulator clomiphene, is given for 5 to 7 days to treat infertility, a *spontaneous* LH/FSH surge and ovulation can occur several days after the drug is stopped, provided that a dominant follicle has emerged and grown.

4. Administration of estrogen with or without progesterone in a format that resembles the normal preovulatory estradiol rise can induce an LH surge (Fig. 46-29), even in postmenopausal women.

5. In monkeys whose pituitary glands have been completely severed from the hypothalamus, central nervous system regulation of gonadotropin secretion is disrupted. However, if GnRH is replaced intravenously in a physiological pulsatile pattern to reinstitute and sustain basal FSH and LH secretion, subsequent cyclic ovarian function occurs with an LH/FSH surge that does not require any change in the rate or pattern of the GnRH infusion.

Such observations suggest that a GnRH pulse generator in the central nervous system is required to initiate and sustain follicular development. However, it is the subsequent developing pattern of ovarian events and secretions, most critically in the dominant follicle, that conditions this pulse generator and the pituitary gonadotrophs to respond later with an ovulatory LH/FSH surge. Perhaps no other phenomenon so clearly illustrates the intricate nature of the interactions among endocrine, paracrine, autocrine, and neural mechanisms of regulation. (Moreover, the suppression of competing follicles by the dominant follicle in an ovary may be analogous to the inhibition of growth in the earlier stages of spermatogenesis by products of the later stages.)

The close coordination between the emergence of a single dominant follicle and the ovulatory signal it recruits makes multiple pregnancies unlikely in humans. For example, the natural rate of occurrence of **dizygotic twins** is less than 1% of live births. By contrast, a much higher rate (15%) results from the multiple ova produced by cycles in which follicular development and ovulation are stimulated artificially "from above" by administration of exogenous FSH and LH in superimposed profiles.

Ovarian signals can be either overridden or reinforced by other influences on and from the hypothalamus. Loss of cyclic gonadotropin secretion can occur in situations that suggest that the hypothalamus is responding to a caloric signal or adipose mass, or to thermal, photic, olfactory, emotional, or inflammatory signals. Cyclic gonadotropin secretion can cease in women who are calorically deprived and who therefore lose considerable amounts of adipose tissue and lean body mass, and also in women who exercise excessively. This also occurs in women who undergo physical translocation, climatic change, or emotional deprivation or

who suffer from chronic inflammatory diseases. Such inhibitory influences may be mediated by hypothalamic endorphins, corticotropin-releasing hormone (CRH), or even leptin.

Well-known examples of anovulation or even complete amenorrhea occur in women with **anorexia nervosa,** in ballet dancers, or in marathon runners. The ovarian dysfunction can be so serious that it causes profound estrogen deficiency, with consequent **osteoporosis.**

Alterations in the levels of adrenal androgen, cortisol, or thyroid hormone can also inhibit ovulation. Seasonal variation in reproductive activity suggests modulation by melatonin, because human conception rates are lowest in the winter months (when darkness is most prevalent, and the secretion of inhibitory melatonin is highest). It has also been observed that women who live close to one another can adopt a common timing of their menstrual cycles, possibly because of chemical signals (**pheromones**) emitted by one individual that affect a nearby individual. In humans, no evidence exists that ovulation is directly stimulated by sexual behavior, as it is in other animals. However, female-initiated sexual activity is reportedly increased around the time of ovulation; this increase in libido is possibly caused by increased androgen levels at that time (Fig. 46-25).

Gonadal Steroid Hormone Effects

Intracellular actions. Estradiol, estrone, other estrogens, and progesterone all enter cells freely and bind to cytoplasmic receptors of the steroid-thyroid, vitamin D superfamily (see Figs. 43-17 and 43-18). The **estrogen receptor,** which is the oldest member of this family in vertebrates, preceded the androgen receptor. Two distinct estrogen receptors of 500 to 600 amino acids exist. They are coded for by different genes located on separate chromosomes, and they are termed ER_α and ER_β. Although the DNA-binding domains are very similar, the ligand-binding domains of ER_α and ER_β are only 55% homologous in amino acid sequence. Although they have equal affinity for estradiol, their affinities for estrone and numerous synthetic agonists and antagonists vary widely. Splice variants for ER_α and ER_β are also found. Their tissue distributions overlap somewhat but some distinct localizations have been noted. For example, uterine endometrium and breast cancer contain mostly ER_α, whereas granulosa cells and osteoblasts contain ER_β. After ligand binding, by the receptor, heat shock proteins are displaced and phosphorylation and dimerization occur. After transfer to the nucleus, binding of the hormone receptor complex to estrogen response elements on DNA molecules occurs. Although a consensus ERE has been defined (5′GGT-CAXXXTGACC3′), variant EREs are very common. Growth factors, acting through serine-threonine kinases, like MAP kinase (Chapter 39), can also activate nonliganded ERs by phosphorylating them. Likewise, cyclins (Chapter 39) can activate ER in the absence of estradiol. Numerous coactivators and corepressors of the activated liganded ER have also been discovered. Moreover, estradiol-ER$_\alpha$ complexes activate transcription, whereas estradiol-ER$_\beta$ complexes repress transcription at ERE sites.

> The importance of understanding the ERs has been greatly hightened by the discovery of **selective estrogen-receptor modulators (SERMs),** such as raloxifene and tamoxifen. These pharmaceutically produced non-steroidal ER ligands have varied ER profiles. Tamoxifen anatagonizes the action of estrogens on the breast, but mimics the action of estrogens on the uterine endometrium. It is an excellent chemotherapeutic agent for breast cancer, but it can also rarely produce endometrial cancer of the uterus. Raloxifene has beneficial agonist effects on bone and serum lipids, but not on breast or endometrium. It is therefore a safe treatment for osteoporosis, but its antagonist effects on the brain produce, as a side effect, the hot flashes associated with estrogen deficiency.

Nongenomic actions of estradiol that are evident within minutes also occur. These are mediated by ERs contained in plasma membrane invaginations, known as **caveolae.** These liganded receptors are linked to MAP kinases, which phosphorylate other proteins that yield such rapid effects of estradiol as dilating coronary arteries.

Some other relatively early and relatively rapid target cell responses to estrogen are likely due to protooncogenes, such as c-*jun* and c-*fos,* whose expression is induced by liganded ERs. These transcription factors, singly or combined as AP-1 (Chapter 39), may then facilitate later actions of ER via its EREs within more specific target DNA molecules. Numerous genes are regulated in various tissues. Examples include ovalbumin, ovomucoid, growth factors, the LDL receptor, type 1 collagen, the 1,25-(OH)$_2$-vitamin D receptor, and IGFBP-4. In addition, estradiol can stabilize mRNA levels of certain gene products, such as vitellogenin.

The **progesterone receptor (PR)** contains 934 amino acids. Its interaction with progesterone and progesterone regulatory elements (PREs) on DNA molecules resembles the cortisol format (see Fig. 45-12). Indeed, these interactions overlap in such a manner that a progesterone inhibitor that binds to PR (mifepristone, an abortifacient drug) also inhibits the binding of cortisol to its receptor. Not surprisingly, mifepristone is used to treat endogenous hypercortisolism.

One of estradiol's important actions is to increase the synthesis of ER and PR. In this way, estradiol amplifies its own effects on growth of the follicle and on proliferation of the endometrium. This action also prepares target tissues for subsequent, efficient progesterone action. Conversely, progesterone decreases the synthesis of ER. This action accounts for the inhibition by progesterone of further endometrial proliferation during the luteal phase.

The cyclic changes in estradiol and progesterone secretion produce effects on the uterus, fallopian tubes, vagina, and breasts (Fig. 46-30). These effects coordinate precisely with the expectation of conception and the institution of a pregnancy.

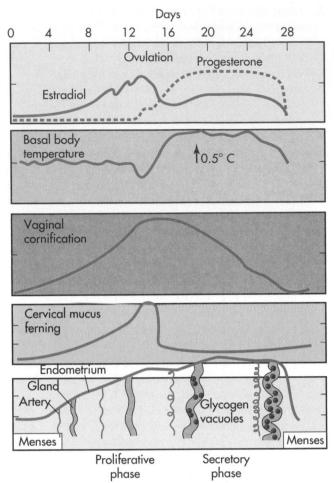

■ **Fig. 46-30**   Correlation of biological changes throughout the menstrual cycle with the profiles of plasma estradiol and progesterone levels. (Redrawn from Odell WD: In DeGroot LJ et al, editors: *Endocrinology,* vol 3, New York, 1979, Grune & Stratton.)

Uterus. The function of the uterus is to house and nurture the developing fetus until birth. The uterus is a muscular organ that encloses a cavity lined with stromal cells and a special mucous membrane, called the **endometrium.** At the beginning of the follicular phase of each menstrual cycle, the uterus is shedding its lining (menstruation) and is therefore incapable of receiving a conceptus. The endometrium is only 1 to 2 mm thick, and its glands are sparse and straight. The lumen of the glands is narrow and the glands themselves exhibit few mitoses (Fig. 46-30). After the menstrual endometrial slough ceases, the increase in estradiol secretion during the follicular phase causes a 3-fold to 5-fold increase in endometrial thickness to a maximum of 8 to 10 mm just before ovulation. Mitoses appear in the glands and stroma, the glands become tortuous, and the spiral arteries that supply the endometrium elongate. This stage is termed the **proliferative phase** of the endometrium. During the proliferative phase, the telomeres at the end of each chromosome, which are shortened during each mitosis leading to apoptosis of the cells, are repaired by the enzyme telomerase. Estradiol induces high levels of telomerase during the proliferative phase, and thereby prevents apoptosis in the endometrium. The mucus elaborated by the cervix also changes dramatically during the proliferative phase from a scant, thick, viscous material, to a copious, more watery, but more elastic substance that can be stretched into a long, fine thread. The mucus also produces a characteristic fernlike pattern when it is dried on a glass slide. In this estrogen-stimulated condition, the cervical mucus creates a myriad of channels in the opening of the cervix. These channels facilitate the entrance of the sperm and direct their motion forward into the uterine cavity.

Shortly after ovulation, the rise in the plasma progesterone level produces marked alterations (Fig. 46-30) in the endometrium. Its rapid proliferation slows, mitotic activity is reduced, and the endometrial thickness decreases to about 5 mm. In contrast to estradiol, progesterone suppresses telomerase, telomeres are lost, and apoptosis of endometrial cells is facilitated. The uterine glands become much more tortuous, and they begin to accumulate glycogen in large vacuoles at the base of each cell. As the luteal phase of the cycle progresses, these vacuoles move toward the lumen of the glands, and the mucus secretion of these glands greatly increases as a result of progesterone action. These secretions contain glycogen, glycoproteins, and glycolipids, which sustain and facilitate attachment of a conceptus. The stroma of the endometrium becomes edematous, and the originally straight spiral arteries elongate further and become coiled. These changes constitute the **secretory phase** of the endometrium. During this phase, progesterone decreases the quantity of the cervical mucus and causes it to return to its original thick, nonelastic state; the ferning pattern is not seen. Progesterone downregulates genes that direct the synthesis of voltage-dependent calcium channels, and thereby decreases the uptake of calcium by the myometrium. This prevents myometrial contractions and early expulsion of a newly implanted conceptus.

If pregnancy does not occur and the corpus luteum regresses, lymphocytes and neutrophils appear. The abrupt loss of estradiol and progesterone causes spasmodic contractions of the spiral arteries and uterine muscles. These effects are probably mediated by local production of leukotrienes and prostaglandins. The resultant ischemia produces necrosis, the stroma condenses and degenerates, and the superficial endometrial cells are sloughed, along with sludged blood. These changes constitute the **menstrual period.**

Fallopian tubes. The fallopian tubes (oviducts) are the normal site of fertilization and of the early development of the zygote. Pregnancy rates are highest when fertilization takes place in the tube, next highest when a zygote just created in vitro is placed in the tube, and lowest when a zygote, created in vitro, is implanted directly in the uterus. The bilateral tubes, 10 cm long, emerge from the uterus. Each tube ends in finger-like projections called **fimbriae,** which lie close to the ipsilateral ovary. The fallopian tube consists of a muscular layer that surrounds a mucosa that is lined by an epithelium that contains both ciliated and secretory cells. The cilia beat toward the uterus. During the follicular phase, estradiol increases the number of cilia and their rate of beating, as well as the number of actively secreting epithelial cells. Estradiol also stimulates tubal secretions that provide a mucoid medium in which the sperm may move upstream efficiently against the ciliary beat. In addition, the fimbria become more vascularized. These effects are antagonized by progesterone.

As ovulation approaches, tubal contractions increase, and the fimbria undulate so as to draw the shed ovum into the tube. During the luteal phase, progesterone acts to maximize the ciliary beat and to enhance the movement of any fertilized ovum toward the uterus. Progesterone also increases the secretion of materials that are nutritious to the ovum, to any incoming sperm, and to the zygote, should fertilization occur.

Vagina. The vaginal canal is lined with a stratified squamous epithelium that is highly sensitive to estradiol. In the absence of estradiol, only a thin layer of basal and parabasal cells is present. For the first few days of the follicular phase of the menstrual cycle, the vaginal epithelium is thin. Smears taken from the surface show cells, identified by their vesicular nuclei, that arise from the layer beneath the epithelium.

As the cycle progresses to the ovulatory phase, more layers of epithelium are added, and the maturing cells accumulate glycogen. Vaginal smears at this time show many large, eosinophilic-staining, cornified cells with small pyknotic or absent nuclei. The percentage of these cells on a vaginal smear is a sensitive index of estrogenic activity (Fig. 46-30). Progesterone, on the other hand, reduces the percentage of cornified cells. Vaginal secretions are increased by estradiol, and they too form an important element in the events that lead to fertilization.

Breasts. The mammary glands consist of a large series of lobular ducts lined by an epithelium that is capable of secreting milk. These ducts empty into larger milk-conveying ducts that converge at the nipple. These glandular structures are embedded in supporting adipose tissue, and the breasts are separated into lobules by connective tissue.

The development of adult-sized mammary glands depends absolutely on estrogens. Before puberty, the breasts grow only in proportion to the rest of the body. After estrogen secretion increases during puberty, the growth and differentiation of ductal epithelium, and the growth of connective tissue and of the lobular ducts accelerate, and the area around the nipple (the areola) enlarges. These effects of estrogen on the glandular cells may be mediated by its action on adjacent stromal cells. Moreover, estradiol, which is produced locally in the breast by the action of breast tissue aromatase on testosterone, contributes to these effects.

Estrogens also selectively increase the adipose tissue of the breast, and they give it its distinctive female shape. The lobular ducts are capable of outpouching to form numerous secretory alveoli. This process is stimulated by progesterone. In various ways, cortisol, growth hormone, prolactin, epidermal growth factor, insulin, IGF-1, and transferrin all contribute to the growth and differentiation of breast tissue. During each menstrual cycle, the lobules further proliferate, mainly in parallel with plasma estradiol levels and with the ER content of the breast tissue, but progesterone may also contribute to this process. This proliferation causes swelling of the breasts; however, by the end of the luteal phase, breast size and tenderness diminish.

Effects on other tissues. During puberty, estradiol action is to the female what testosterone action is to the male. Estradiol causes almost all the changes that result in the normal adult female phenotype. In addition to stimulating growth of the internal reproductive organs and breasts, estrogens cause pubertal enlargement of the labia majora and labia minora. Linear growth is accelerated by estradiol. However, because the epiphyseal growth centers are more sensitive to estradiol than to testosterone, they close sooner. For this reason, the average height of women is less than that of men. The hips enlarge and the pelvic inlet widens; these changes facilitate future pregnancy. The specific deposition of fat about the hips is another effect of estradiol. Because in women, estradiol predominates over testosterone, total body adipose mass is twice as large as that of men, whereas their muscle and bone mass is only two thirds that of men.

The skeleton, the kidney, the liver, and the vasculature are also important target tissues of estrogens. Estradiol restrains bone turnover in adults and keeps bone formation equal to bone resorption. Osteoclast formation and activity are decreased, and osteoclast apoptosis is increased. Osteoclast recruitment is reduced by estradiol's inhibition of the production of IL-1, TNF-α, and granulocyte-macrophage colony-stimulating factor, all of which are lymphokines that stimulate proliferation of osteoclasts (Chapter 42). Estradiol may also increase the formation, differentiation, and activity of osteoblasts. These skeletal effects are achieved through ER_α in cortical bone and ER_β in trabecular bone. Loss of estrogen action after the menopause shifts the balance markedly toward bone resorption. Reabsorption of sodium from the renal tubules is stimulated by estradiol; this response may contribute to the cyclic fluid retention noted by some women. The hepatic synthesis of a number of circulating proteins is increased by estrogens; these proteins include thyroxine-binding globulin, cortisol-binding globulin, SSBG, the renin substrate, angiotensinogen, very-low-density lipoproteins (VLDLs), and HDLs. LDL levels are decreased by estradiol, which increases the number of LDL receptors.

The effects of estrogen on the vasculature are important. In general, estradiol is vasodilatory and antivasoconstrictive. Estradiol increases the local release of vasodilators, such as nitric oxide, prostaglandin E_2, and prostacyclin, and it decreases production or activity of endothelin-1, a potent local vasoconstrictor. The marked fall in estradiol secretion at the end of the luteal phase alters the endometrial balance from vasodilator to vasoconstrictor, and it helps to initiate the ischemic necrosis of the endometrium.

The presence of ER_α and ER_β in areas of the brain outside the hypothalamus, plus other evidence, supports the existence of significant estrogen effects on central nervous system functioning. Interactions γ-aminobutyric acid with

(GABA), acetylcholine, and serotonin signaling have been identified. Of special note, E_α interacts with *N*-methyl-D-aspartate receptors in the hippocampus to induce formation of new synapses between axons and dendrites. Estradiol improves memory and learning in rats. Estradiol deficiency in women is associated with deficits in declarative memory and with subtle motor incoordination, and it may increase the risk of developing Alzheimer's disease. The A ring of estradiol may provide neuroprotection from damage by free radicals that are generated in response to brain injury.

Only a few systemic actions of progesterone are known. Progesterone accounts for the 0.5° C rise in body temperature that occurs shortly after ovulation (Fig. 46-30). Progesterone also acts on the central nervous system to increase appetite, to produce somnolence and anesthetic effects, and to increase the sensitivity of the respiratory center to stimulation by carbon dioxide. Because progesterone is an aldosterone antagonist, it can induce natriuresis (see Chapter 45). Progesterone decreases the expression of the genes for the GnRH receptor and for the β-subunits of LH and FSH. This negative feedback effect of progesterone on gonadotropin secretion requires the presence of adequate estrogen. The combination of hormonal actions is the basis for the use of oral contraceptives by women.

Metabolism of Gonadal Steroids

Estradiol and estrone bind to SSBG, but their affinities are much lower than that of testosterone. Therefore, the circulating estrogens are bound loosely to albumin, and their metabolic clearance rates are relatively high (Table 46-3). In menstruating women, most of the circulating estradiol is derived from ovarian secretion; a minor fraction is formed from testosterone in adipose tissue, liver, and other sites. Most of the circulating estrone is derived from estradiol by peripheral 17-hydroxysteroid dehydrogenases. Estrone can also be 16-hydroxylated and then reduced to estriol (Fig. 46-31).

Sulfated and glucuronidated derivatives of all three estrogens are excreted in the urine. Values range from 20 µg during the early follicular phase to 65 µg at the preovulatory peak. An additional pathway of estrogen metabolism involves 2-hydroxylation, and it produces the so-called *catechol estrogens* (Fig. 46-31). These compounds resemble the catecholamine neurotransmitters norepinephrine and dopamine, in their hydroxylated benzene rings. Because 2-hydroxylase activity is present in the hypothalamus, the catechol estrogens generated within the brain may modulate the estradiol effects on GnRH release. The catechol estrogens bind to estradiol receptors, but they do not have estradiol actions; in effect, they are natural antiestrogen agents that could increase GnRH by negative feedback.

Progesterone can bind to cortisol-binding globulin, but this binding is largely prevented by competition from the much higher plasma cortisol concentration. Therefore, progesterone circulates loosely bound to albumin. It is reduced to the urinary metabolite, pregnanediol. During the follicular phase of the cycle, about half of the circulating progesterone

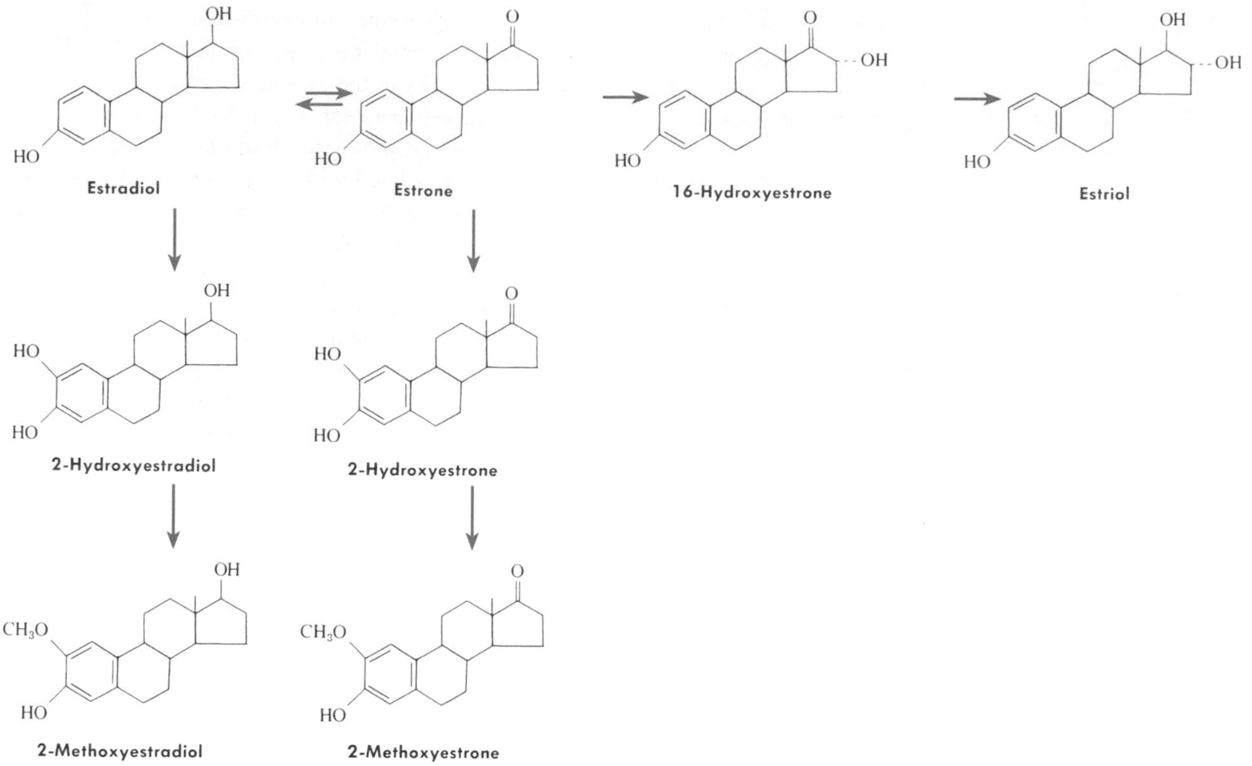

■ **Fig. 46-31** Metabolism of estradiol and estrone to catechol estrogens and estriol.

is secreted by the ovary and about half by the adrenal glands. During the luteal phase, however, most of the progesterone originates in the ovary.

In women, 70% to 80% of circulating testosterone is derived from peripheral conversion of DHEA and androstenedione. About half the daily production of testosterone comes from adrenal precursors, and about half from ovarian precursors. In some disorders, ovarian cells can secrete sufficient testosterone to cause virilizing effects.

Female Puberty

The general process by which puberty is initiated has already been described (Fig. 46-8). Reproductive function begins after an increase in gonadotropin secretion from the low levels of childhood (Fig. 46-32). However, FSH increases before LH more distinctly in females than in males (compare Figs. 46-23 and 46-32). Budding of the breasts is the first observable physical sign of female puberty, and it coincides with the first detectable increase in plasma estradiol, as ovarian secretion commences. The onset of menses (menarche) occurs approximately 2 years later, after LH levels have risen more sharply. Menarche correlates with both body height and bone maturation. Menarche can be delayed by undernutrition or strenuous exercise, and it occurs later in large sibships. Menarche is accelerated by obesity and blindness.

Development of the positive feedback effect of estradiol necessary to provoke a preovulatory LH burst is the last step in the maturation of the hypothalamic pituitary ovarian unit. Therefore, ovulation usually does not occur in the first few menstrual cycles. The initial menstrual cycles are usually irregular, as the menstrual bleeding is induced by withdrawal of estrogen from graafian follicles that are undergoing atresia.

The growth spurt and the peak velocity of growth characteristically occur earlier in girls than in boys, and they do not last as long. These differences help to account for the average lower height of girls. Further increase in height usually ceases 1 to 2 years after the onset of menses. The development of pubic hair precedes menses, and it correlates most closely with the rising levels of adrenal androgens, especially dehydroepiandrosterone sulfate (DHEA-S).

Sexual Functioning

The desire for sexual activity is increased by androgens. During sexual intercourse, vascular erectile tissue beneath the clitoris is activated by parasympathetic impulses. This causes the vaginal opening to be tightened around the penis. Simultaneously, these impulses stimulate copious secretion of mucus by glands located beneath the labia minora and in the vagina. The secretions lubricate the vagina and help it produce a massaging effect on the penis. Estrogen actions maintain these glands and their secretions.

Female orgasm results from spinal cord reflexes that are similar to those involved in male ejaculation. The skeletal muscle of the perineum and the musculature of the vagina, uterus, fallopian tubes, and the rectal sphincter contract reflexly. The clitoris retracts against the symphysis pubis. After orgasm, the cervix remains widely patent for 20 to 30 minutes, and thereby permits sperm to enter the uterus. The first wave of sperm may reach an ovum in the fallopian tube

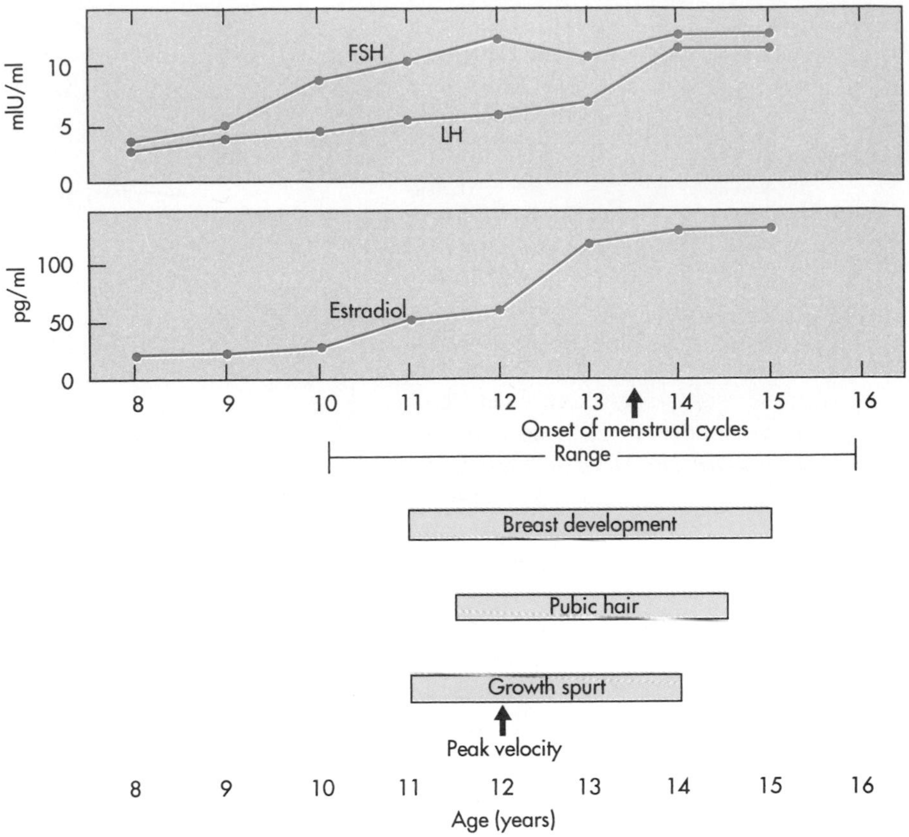

■ **Fig. 46-32**   Average chronological sequence of hormonal and biological events in normal female puberty. Note that the peak velocity of growth precedes the onset of menses, and the growth spurt ends shortly after menarche. (Redrawn from Lee PA et al: *J Clin Endocrinol Metab* 43:775, 1976; and Marshall WA, Tanner JM: *Arch Dis Child* 45:13, 1970.)

within 10 minutes. However, these sperm, lacking capacitation, are unlikely to fertilize an ovum.

Many spermatozoa are trapped and eventually destroyed in the vagina within a few hours. The remaining spermatozoa reach the cervix, where they dwell in storage sites formed by the convoluted mucosa (cervical crypts) and its mucus. Here, they undergo capacitation. From this reservoir, spermatozoa migrate into the uterine cavity and fallopian tubes over a 24- to 48-hour period. A tremendous number of sperm are lost along the way; fewer than one in every 100,000 eventually reaches an ovum.

Menopause

The reproductive capacity of women begins to wane in the fifth decade of life, and menses completely terminate at an average age of 50. For several years before menopause, the frequency of ovulation decreases. The menses occur at variable intervals and with decreased flow. These changes are caused by irregular peaks of estradiol secretion without adequate secretion of progesterone during the luteal phase. With the disappearance of virtually all the follicles, ovarian secretion of estrogens—and inhibins—essentially ceases. From then on, low plasma estradiol, inhibin A, and inhibin B concentrations (characteristic of menopause) are maintained. Most of this estradiol comes from peripheral conversion of androgen precursors that are secreted predominantly by the adrenal glands. However, some precursors come from ovarian stromal cells that remain responsive to high levels of LH. The dominant estrogen in plasma becomes estrone rather than estradiol; the ratio is maintained at 3:1.

During the last few years of reproductive life, follicular sensitivity to gonadotropin stimulation diminishes. The plasma FSH and LH levels gradually increase in compensation, along with inhibin B, 2 years before the final menstrual period. Once menopause occurs, inhibin levels decrease and the loss of negative feedback from ovarian estradiol and inhibin causes gonadotropin levels to average four to ten times those of the normal follicular phase; a plateau is reached 2 years after the last menstrual period. The LH/FSH ratio falls to less than 1. Although the monthly cyclicity of gonadotropin secretion is lost, pulsatile secretion persists.

The programmed decline in available estrogenic biological activity causes thinning of the vaginal epithelium and loss of its secretions. Breast mass decreases also. Vascular flushing is entrained with LH pulses, and emotional lability is also related to estrogen deficiency. Because adipose tissue contains aromatase activity, this tissue is an important site of production of estrogen from adrenal and ovarian stromal androgens. Obese women may therefore have fewer symptoms of estrogen deprivation. Ovarian secretion of androgens may mildly stimulate hair growth in a male pattern.

The hormonal characteristics of the postmenopausal period are of major health importance. Loss of estrogens produces a period of increased bone resorption, and bone loss is accelerated for approximately 5 years (**postmenopausal osteoporosis**). Fractures of the wrist and vertebrae increase in frequency. Postmenopausal osteoporosis also sets the stage for the later, but slower, senescent phase of bone loss. During this phase, women are at a greater risk of hip and vertebral fractures than are men, until age 80.

The loss of estrogens after the menopause increases the risk of coronary artery disease. By age 60, death from **coronary heart disease** becomes increasingly prevalent in women. This change is partly explained by loss of the beneficial effect of estrogen on the serum lipid pattern. In addition, loss of estrogen's vasodilator effect on the endothelium of the coronary circulation may add to the increasing risk of coronary events. Once coronary disease is established, however, estrogen replacement does not retard its progression. Because estrogen replacement is associated with small increases in breast cancer risk and, without accompanying progesterone, in uterine cancer risk, its routine long-term use in women is controversial at best.

Estrogen replacement therapy after the menopause is prescribed to relieve such symptoms as hot flashes. Progesterone is usually added to protect women from estrogen-induced endometrial hyperplasia and cancer.

PREGNANCY

Fertilization

After ovulation, the ovum is captured by the widened proximal portion (the ampulla) of the fallopian tube (ampulla). Retention of the ovum within the fallopian tube is aided by adherence of the "sticky" cumulus oophorus to the cilia in the fimbria. Muscle contractions produce a to-and-fro motion, which mixes the contents of the fallopian tube and increases the chance of a random encounter between the ovum and sperm, and thereby facilitates fertilization. GnRH, produced locally by the tube, increases binding of sperm to the zona pellucida of the ovum. The ovum is viable for only 12 to 24 hours. The sperm must reach the ovum within about 48 hours of ejaculation.

The conjunction of ovum with sufficient sperm is not an entirely random process. Chemotactants, secreted by the ovary, attract sperm and interact with receptors in the sperm membrane. cGMP, formed by such activators of guanylyl cyclase as **atrial natriuretic peptide (ANP)** and nitric oxide, mediates an increase in the velocity and directionality of sperm movement, and it stimulates the acrosome reaction. ANP is present in follicular fluid, and its receptors are present on sperm membrane. Nitric oxide synthase is present in sperm and ova.

Once sperm are very close to the zona pellucida of the ovum, they undergo the acrosomal reaction, which has been described previously. As a result of Ca^{2+} stimulation, as well as protein kinase C (PKC) and protein kinase A (PKA) activation, the acrosomal cap releases a corona-dispersing enzyme, a trypsin-like enzyme (known as acrosin), a neuraminidase, and hyaluronidases. Together, these enzymes

disperse and digest the granulosa cells of the cumulus oophorus, and they permit attachment of sperm to the zona pellucida. The acrosomal reaction is stimulated by, and penetration of the zona is facilitated by, species-specific zona receptors. These receptors have oligosaccharide-binding sites for sperm membrane proteins, in particular one receptor that is termed ZP_3. Many sperm bind to the zona, first reversibly and then tightly. The single successful sperm penetrates this barrier by the release of the proteolytic enzyme, **acrosin.** *Penetration of the zona pellucida by the first sperm creates a block to the entry of the other sperm.* This barrier is generated by the uptake of Ca^{2+} into the ovum, depolarization of its plasma membrane, and release of proteases and glycosidases that are contained in the granules within the ovum. This process alters zona surface glycoproteins, such as ZP_3, so that they reject, instead of attract, additional sperm. Hence, they prevent complete entrance of those spermatozoa that had partially penetrated. This important step prevents **polyploidy,** the production of an organism with more than two sets of homologous chromosomes. The polar body that results from the second reduction-division of meiosis is then released, and it leaves the ovum in a haploid state, that is, with 23 chromosomes. After fusion of their respective membranes, the chromatin material of the sperm head is engulfed by the ovum, and it forms the haploid male pronucleus. The two pronuclei generate a spindle on which the chromosomes are arranged, and a new diploid individual with 46 chromosomes is created. The mitochondria from the sperm are eliminated or diluted out by those of the ovum, so that mitochondrial DNA is essentially all inherited from the mother.

The zygote, now in the blastocyst stage, traverses the fallopian tube in about 3 days. Most of this time is spent in the ampulla of the tube, where a delay at the junction with the isthmus may allow time for the endometrium to become better prepared to accept the zygote. With the early rise in the luteal phase progesterone levels, the transit time through the tube rapidly increases. *After another 2 to 3 days in the uterus, the zygote initiates implantation, which consists of three successive processes: adhesion, penetration, and invasion.*

Implantation is a complex process that requires subtle interactions between maternal cells and signals and the cells and signals from the early embryo. Moreover, at least one segment of the endometrium must be in a state of receptivity that is optimal during only a narrow window of time. This window begins several days after fertilization, which allows for transit of the zygote through the tube and for differentiation of certain invasive cells of the blastocyst. The blastocyst must appose itself to a receptive area of endometrium, after it descends into the uterine cavity. For adhesion to take place, the requisite dissolution of the zona pellucida is brought about by alternate contraction and expansion of the blastocyst, as well as by lytic factors in the uterine secretions. These and other substances (e.g., epidermal growth factor) that facilitate implantation depend on adequate maternal progesterone levels during the luteal phase and on early paracrine signals (e.g., GnRH) from the zygote. Such signals induce further receptive endometrial responses at the site.

Attachment of the embryo to the endometrium is brought about by cell surface receptors for extracellular matrix on both the embryo and the endometrium. Initially, these receptors, called integrins, fix and bond endometrial cells to each other, and they bond blastocyst cells to each other. IL-1, from the blastocyst cells, upregulates integrin expression by the endometrial cells. In addition, the glandular epithelium of the uterus also expresses and secretes *osteopontin,* an adhesion molecule that interacts with *integrins.* Progesterone increases osteopontin secretion. Osteopontin (and perhaps other bridging molecules) then may bind to integrins both on the endometrial cells and on the embryo (Fig. 46-33), and causes them to adhere to each other.

From the initial solid mass of blastocyst cells, a layer of **trophoblasts** separates. Microvilli of these cells interdigitate with those of endometrial cells, and junctional complexes form between the respective cell membranes. Integrins, and other endometrial molecules, such as **laminin** and **fibronectin,** also facilitate this adhesion. Once firmly attached, trophoblast cells intrude between and burrow beneath endometrial cells, lysing the intercellular matrix with a variety of enzymes. Also, the trophoblasts phagocytize and digest dead endometrial cells. As the decidua (see below) forms, the trophoblasts invade and remodel the blood vessels at the junction of the endometrium and the decidua. The trophoblasts disrupt the tunica media of the uterine arteries and replace their endothelium.

Penetration by the trophoblasts is limited by concurrent changes in the stroma of the uterus. Late in the normal luteal phase, fibroblast-type stromal cells near uterine blood vessels enlarge and accumulate glycogen and lipid. These **decidual** cells disappear unless pregnancy occurs, and the corpus luteum is maintained. If pregnancy occurs, however, continuing estrogen, and especially progesterone, stimulation causes widespread decidualization, which rapidly changes the entire stroma into a sheet of compact decidual cells. At the same time, the endometrial glands progressively atrophy. The **decidua** functions initially as a source of essential nutrients for the embryo, until implantation of the embryo produces vascular connections between the mother and the embryo, and a single central circulation is established. Thereafter, the decidua provides a mechanical and an immunological barrier to further invasion of the uterine wall by the embryo. The decidua also functions as an endocrine organ; it releases prolactin, relaxin, prostaglandins, and other molecules that have paracrine actions on the muscles of the uterus and on the two fetal membranes: the **chorion** and **amnion.**

Numerous locally produced factors, such as IGFs, transforming growth factors, epidermal growth factor, and cytokines, contribute to implantation, the growth and differentiation of trophoblast cells, the growth and development of the embryo and fetus, and the process of decidua formation. Matrix metalloproteinases (MMPs), from the trophoblasts, degrade the extracellular matrix between decidual cells and they facilitate further trophoblast migration. Decidual cells, on the other hand, secrete inhibitors of MMPs. IGF-2, secreted by trophoblasts, and IGFBPs (Chapter 43), secreted by decidual cells, help regulate this balance between invasion and defense of the decidua. A further layer of complexity to this balancing results from secretion of a specific pregnancy-associated protein into the maternal plasma. This protease acts on the ternary complex of IGF-acid labile subunit-IGFBP to release free IGF. In addition to modulating implantation, the IGF stimulates the growth of fetal and maternal tissues.

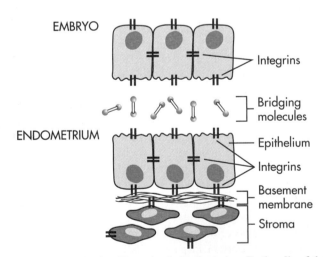

■ Fig. 46-33 Role of integrins in implantation. Both cells of the embryo and the endometrium have plasma membrane receptors with external extensions called integrins. These interact with each other to bind embryonic cells together and endometrial cells together and the latter to basement membrane and stromal cells as well. After the embryo apposes itself to a fixed receptive endometrial site, integrins from the embryo and integrins from the endometrial cells bind to each other via bridging molecules such as osteopontin, which is secreted by the embryo. (Modified from Lessey BA et al: *J Reprod Immunol* 39:105, 1998.)

> Implantation is more susceptible to mishap than is conception. Approximately 70% of all conceptions result in miscarriage; half are attributable to maternal uterine deficits and half to fetal abnormalities. Most miscarriages occur within 14 days of conception, and they are unrecognized by the woman, who may have only a slightly delayed menstrual period. Miscarriages later in the first trimester may still reflect suboptimal maternal-fetal attachment, but they are increasingly likely to be caused by fetal anomalies.

Functions of the Placenta

Pregnancy is marked by the development of a unique organ, the placenta, which has a limited lifespan. This organ has diverse functions. It serves (1) as the fetal gut in supplying nutrients, (2) as the fetal lung in exchanging oxygen and carbon dioxide, (3) as the fetal kidney in regulating fluid volumes and disposing of waste metabolites, and (4) as a versatile endocrine gland that synthesizes many steroid and protein hormones that affect both maternal and fetal metabolism. Some of these hormones can be found in maternal plasma, where they exhibit typical temporal profiles during pregnancy (Fig. 46-34), and some can also be found in fetal plasma and amniotic fluid.

Fetal trophoblasts differentiate very early into two cell types: an inner layer of **cytotrophoblasts,** and an outer layer of fused **syncytiocytotrophoblasts,** which are under the influence of epidermal growth factor and other stimuli. Both cell types synthesize peptide and protein hormones, many of which are very similar to hypothalamic, pituitary, and gonadal products. The syncytiocytotrophoblasts also synthesize increasingly large amounts of steroid hormones from precursors of various sources as pregnancy proceeds (Fig. 46-35). The adjacent arrangement of cytotrophoblast and syncytiocytotrophoblast layers forms a placental hypothalamus-pituitary-like unit. The cytotrophoblasts secrete mainly stimulatory [e.g., CRH and thyrotropin-releasing hormone (TRH)] and inhibitory (somatostatin) hypothalamic-like

peptides and gonadal growth factors. These substances regulate in a paracrine manner the output of pituitary-like hormones [e.g., adrenocorticotropic hormone (ACTH) and thyroid-stimulating hormone (TSH)] from the syncytiocytotrophoblast layer. However, the products of the two trophoblast layers overlap.

Hormones of Pregnancy

Human chorionic gonadotropin. *Human chorionic gonadotropin (HCG) is the first key hormone of pregnancy. It is secreted by the syncytiocytotrophoblast cells, stimulated by GnRH from cytotrophoblasts, and regulated by the inhibin-activin pair in an autocrine manner. HCG can be detected in maternal plasma and urine within 9 days of conception.* HCG is a glycoprotein with a molecular weight of 39,000, and it is composed of two subunits, an α-subunit and a β-subunit. The α-subunit is identical to that of TSH, LH, and FSH, whereas the β-subunit has 80% homology with the β-subunit of LH. Detection of HCG is the most commonly used and most specific test for pregnancy. The urine may be

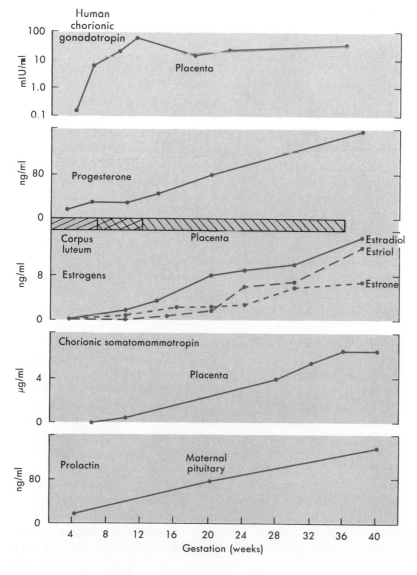

■ **Fig. 46-34** Profile of plasma hormone changes during normal human pregnancy. Note the logarithmic scale for human chorionic gonadotropin. Also note the shift from corpus luteum to placenta as the source of estrogens and progesterone between 6 and 12 weeks of gestation. Relaxin and inhibin A levels also rise, whereas inhibin B remains low. (Redrawn from Goldstein DP et al: *Am J Obstet Gynecol* 102:110, 1968; Rigg LA et al: *Am J Obstet Gynecol* 129:454, 1977; Selenkow HA et al: In Pecile A, Finzi C, editors: *The foetoplacental unit,* Amsterdam, 1969, Excerpta Medica; and Tulchinsky D et al: *Am J Obstet Gynecol* 112:1095, 1972.)

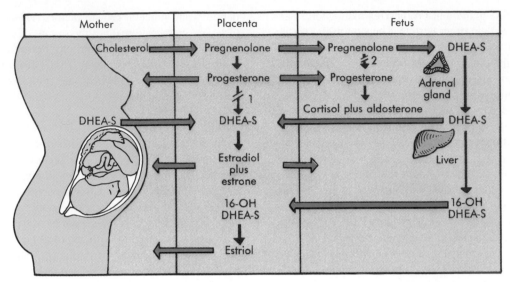

■ **Fig. 46-35** Maternal-fetal-placental unit in steroid hormone synthesis. Progesterone is synthesized in the placenta from maternal cholesterol. In turn, this progesterone acts on the mother. Placental progesterone is transferred to the fetus, where it serves as the precursor to cortisol and aldosterone synthesis by the fetal adrenal glands. Placental pregnenolone serves as the precursor to fetal DHEA-S and 16-OH-DHEA-S. Estradiol and estrone are synthesized in the placenta from maternal and fetal dehydroepiandrosterone sulfate *(DHEA-S)*, and estriol is synthesized from fetal 16α-hydroxydehydroepiandrosterone sulfate *(16-OH-DHEA-S)*. *1,* 17-hydroxylase/17,20-desmolase; *2,* 3β-ol-dehydrogenase-$\Delta^{4,5}$-isomerase.

tested at home. Maternal plasma levels of HCG increase at an exponential rate, reach a peak at 9 to 12 weeks, and then decline to a stable plateau for the remainder of pregnancy (Fig. 46-34). After the fetus is delivered, HCG disappears with a half-life of 12 to 24 hours from maternal plasma.

HCG maintains the function of the corpus luteum beyond its usual lifespan of 14 days (when conception does not occur). The placental gonadotropin stimulates ovarian secretion of progesterone and estrogens by mechanisms that are essentially identical to those previously described for LH; cAMP is the second messenger. When the placenta takes over the synthesis of these steroids, thereby relieving the fetus of its dependence on the corpus luteum, HCG secretion declines. HCG that reaches the fetus stimulates essential DHEA-S production by the fetal zone of the adrenal gland and testosterone production by the Leydig cells of the testis. Fetal pituitary LH is not needed to stimulate testosterone synthesis because of the availability of HCG. HCG may also stimulate the production of **relaxin** (see later discussion). In addition, HCG inhibits the maternal secretion of LH by the pituitary. Because of the structural overlap of HCG with TSH, the very high plasma concentrations of HCG that are maintained in early pregnancy can increase the maternal thyroid gland activity. In some women, this effect of HCG can even induce hyperthyroidism. HCG receptors are found in the endometrium and myometrium, and the gonadotropin can inhibit the contractions produced by oxytocin. Thus, HCG may also contribute to uterine quiescence, especially in the early phase of pregnancy.

Progesterone. *Progesterone is the hormone most directly responsible for the establishment and sustenance of the fetus*

in the uterine cavity. Even prior to this stage of the conceptus, progesterone facilitates sperm capacitation and motility, and the ZP_3-induced acrosomal reaction. During the first 2 weeks of pregnancy, progesterone stimulates the fallopian tubal and endometrial glands to secrete the nutrients on which the zygote depends. Thereafter, it maintains the decidual lining of the uterus. Progesterone, produced by the placenta, is the principal substrate for synthesis of cortisol and aldosterone by the fetal adrenal gland (Fig. 46-35), which lacks the 3β-ol-dehydrogenase-$\Delta^{4,5}$-isomerase enzyme complex necessary for progesterone synthesis. Progesterone may also modulate the secretion of HCG and human chorionic somatomammotropin (HCS) (see below).

Other actions of progesterone are important during pregnancy. *Progesterone inhibits uterine contractions, in part by inhibiting production of prostaglandins, and in part by decreasing sensitivity to oxytocin.* Progesterone thus prevents premature expulsion of the fetus. It also stimulates the development of the alveolar pouches of the mammary glands, and it greatly increases their eventual capacity to secrete milk. Progesterone may participate in the inhibition of maternal immune responses to antigens from the fetus, and thereby help prevent its rejection. Finally, progesterone stimulates the maternal respiratory center to increase ventilation, which helps to dispose of the increased carbon dioxide produced by the pregnant woman and her fetus.

The placenta begins to synthesize progesterone at about 6 weeks of gestation, and by 12 weeks it produces enough of this hormone to replace the corpus luteum for this purpose. During this transition period, the plasma progesterone level reaches a temporary plateau (Fig. 46-34). Cholesterol is extracted from maternal plasma, and it serves as the major precursor for placental progesterone. The synthetic pathway resembles that of the adrenal gland and the ovary. By term, progesterone production reaches a level of 250 mg/day, which is 10 times greater than the peak rates that prevail during the luteal phase of the menstrual cycle. About 90% of the progesterone goes to the mother and 10% goes to the fetus. Maternal urinary pregnanediol excretion also rises markedly; this metabolite reflects the enormous increase in production of progesterone.

Estrogens. The augmented production of estrogens (estradiol, estrone, and estriol) that occurs throughout pregnancy (Fig. 46-34) results in several important actions. *Estrogens stimulate the continuous growth of the uterine myometrium, and thereby prepares it for its role in labor. Estrogens stimulate the further growth of the ductal system of the breast, from which the alveoli will develop.* In addition, estrogen, along with relaxin, causes relaxation and softens the mother's pelvic ligaments and the symphysis pubis of her pelvic bones, and thus allows better accommodation of the expanding uterus.

Estrogens also play a paracrine role in placental function. They augment progesterone synthesis by increasing LDL cholesterol uptake and the activity of the P-450 enzyme. They also enhance placental conversion of cortisol to inactive cortisone (see Fig. 45-11). This inactivation may relieve the inhibition of fetal pituitary corticotropin by maternal cortisol that would otherwise cross the placenta; fetal ACTH could then stimulate production of essential adrenal androgen, and later of cortisol, by the fetus. Although estriol is in other respects a weak estrogen, it does increase uterine and placental blood flow.

Like progesterone, estrogens are initially produced by the corpus luteum under stimulation by HCG. The placenta then assumes this role, but it requires steroid hormone precursors from both the mother and the fetus to complete the synthesis of estrogens. This unique example of coordinated maternal-placental-fetal function is depicted in Fig. 46-35. The placenta lacks significant 17-hydroxylase and 17,20-desmolase activity, and therefore it cannot generate the androgens that serve as substrates for aromatization (Fig. 46-4). Instead, the placenta extracts DHEA-S produced by the maternal and fetal adrenal glands, removes the sulfate, and synthesizes estradiol and estrone. The fetus becomes the main source of DHEA-S as pregnancy progresses. Placental synthesis of estriol, a 16-hydroxylated estrogen (Fig. 46-31), almost entirely depends on precursors from the fetus. In this process, the fetal adrenal gland synthesizes DHEA-S from placental pregnenolone, the fetal liver hydroxylates it in the 16 position, and the placenta then desulfates it and aromatizes it to estriol.

One third of the unconjugated estrogens that circulate in maternal plasma at term are accounted for by estriol. Estriol, in the form of sulfate and glucuronic acid conjugates, represents 90% of the total estrogen excreted in maternal urine. Because estriol is derived almost entirely from the fetal placental unit, maternal plasma or urine estriol levels provide one index of the well-being of the fetus.

Human chorionic somatomammotropin. Another protein hormone unique to pregnancy is **human chorionic somatomammotropin (HCS),** also called **human placental lactogen (HPL).** The synthesis of HCS by the syncytiocytotrophoblasts can be detected at about 4 weeks of gestation. The maternal plasma concentration of HCS rises steadily to a peak of 6 μg/ml at term (Fig. 46-34). The HCS production rate of 1 to 2 g/day far exceeds that of any other human protein hormone. Maternal plasma HCS levels provide another indicator of placental function. After delivery of the fetus, the hormone rapidly disappears from maternal plasma; the half-life is 20 minutes.

HCS synthesis is directed by a gene in the growth hormone family. GHRH and somatostatin, produced in neighboring cytotrophoblasts, probably stimulate and inhibit, respectively, HCS synthesis by syncytiocytotrophoblasts. Although HCS has 96% structural homology with growth hormone, it has only 3% of the latter's growth-promoting activity. Nonetheless, its very high plasma concentrations contribute to anabolism in the pregnant woman. HCS also has lactogenic activity, but this action may not be needed, because of the high concentration of prolactin itself during pregnancy.

HCS stimulates maternal lipolysis and, like growth hormone, it antagonizes insulin actions on carbohydrate metabolism. These actions tend to raise the maternal plasma glucose concentration. Maternal fasting and hypoglycemia raise plasma HCS levels. As detailed later, HCS may direct maternal metabolism to maintain a continuous flow of substrates, especially glucose, to the fetus. HCS levels in fetal plasma are far below those in maternal plasma; however, somatomedins (IGF-2), produced in the placenta as the result of HCS action, may help to stimulate fetal growth.

A **placental human growth hormone variant,** closely related to, but distinct from, both growth hormone and HCS, has been characterized. This variant represents the major form of growth hormone in maternal plasma, and it reaches elevated levels of 15 ng/ml by term. It is probably regulated by placental GHRH and somatostatin, and because of its high concentrations, it may be as important to maternal metabolism as is HCS.

Prolactin. Another hormone secreted in excess during normal pregnancy is maternal pituitary prolactin. Plasma levels of prolactin rise linearly throughout pregnancy, and by term they reach values 8 to 10 times higher than those of nonpregnant women (Fig. 46-34). The prolactin synthesized during pregnancy is largely in the more bioactive, nonglycosylated form (see Chapter 43). Prolactin is essential for expression of the mammotropic effects of estrogen and progesterone, and it stimulates the lactogenic apparatus (see Fig. 43-29). A small amount of milk begins to be produced at about 5 months of gestation, but progressive increase in lactation is inhibited by the high levels of estrogen and progesterone.

Prolactin is also synthesized by the decidual cells of the uterus, where it helps to depress the immune responses to the fetus. The decidua is the source of amniotic fluid prolactin, which may help to regulate osmolarity in fetal fluids.

Relaxin. In addition to gonadal steroids, the corpus luteum of pregnancy secretes a polypeptide hormone called relaxin. Its structure resembles proinsulin (see Fig. 41-3). Plasma levels of relaxin rise early in pregnancy, peak in the first trimester, and then decline somewhat. The production of relaxin by the corpus luteum is stimulated by HCG. Relaxin is also produced by decidual cells. This hormone suppresses myometrial contractions by inhibiting myosin light-chain phosphorylation. It also relaxes pelvic ligaments and increases softening, effacement, and dilation of the cervix. Thus, it may function early to ensure uterine quiescence and to prevent spontaneous abortion, but later it may facilitate passage of the fetus out of the uterus.

Inhibins and related hormones. Maternal plasma inhibin levels exhibit a biphasic rise during pregnancy. Inhibin A reaches an early peak within 7 days of conception. The source of inhibin A at this point is mostly fetal trophoblasts, with some contribution from the corpus luteum in response to stimulation by HCG. A later steady rise in the inhibin A level to a peak at term represents placental production. The inhibin A level falls rapidly after delivery. In contrast, inhibin B levels remain low throughout pregnancy. One maternal role for the increased inhibin A level may be to suppress the mother's FSH secretion and the unneeded ovarian follicle formation.

Both activin A and follistatin levels also increase steadily in maternal plasma. These hormones are derived from placental, decidual, and fetal membrane sources. Activin stimulates HCG and progesterone synthesis by the placenta, whereas follistatin interferes with this effect. The outcome of these interactions may depend on the time at which they occur and on countervailing influences from both mother and fetus.

Other maternal hormonal changes. Pregnancy induces a characteristic series of changes in various maternal endocrine functions. One of the most significant alterations occurs in pancreatic islet β cell function. Insulin secretion, in response to glucose challenge or to meals, increases after the third month of pregnancy. This hypersecretion of insulin reaches its peak during the last trimester; the peak coincides with the peak of the plasma HCS level. Because maternal sensitivity to insulin is greatly diminished during this same period, insulin hypersecretion may be considered largely compensatory. In contrast, basal glucagon levels and responses to stimulation do not change significantly.

Aldosterone secretion increases significantly throughout pregnancy, and it reaches a 6-fold to 8-fold elevation by term. The elevation of aldosterone occurs because both the plasma renin and the renin substrate (angiotensinogen) levels are augmented by the high estrogen levels of pregnancy. Aldosterone hypersecretion may also be stimulated by a reduction in the *effective* circulating maternal blood volume that results from the large placental blood pool. Hyperaldosteronism contributes to the positive sodium balance necessary to maintain a high total maternal plasma volume and to build the extracellular fluid of the fetus. Another mineralocorticoid, deoxycorticosterone (see Chapter 45), is also present in excess in the maternal plasma. It is synthesized in the mother's kidneys exclusively during pregnancy by 21-hydroxylation of the progesterone that originates from the placenta.

The plasma total cortisol level is elevated because of the estrogen-induced increase in cortisol-binding globulin. However, plasma and urinary free cortisol also rise modestly, as do plasma levels of ACTH. The enhanced glucocorticoid activity may contribute to maternal adipose tissue gain and to mammary gland development. This enhanced activity may also be responsible for the plethoric face, thin skin, and susceptibility to bruising of pregnant women. The ultimate cause of maternal hypercortisolism is a large increase in circulating CRH of placental origin. Although the CRH is largely protein bound and nonpulsatile, it stimulates maternal pituitary ACTH secretion and the consequent secretion of cortisol.

The concentration of total plasma thyroid hormones, thyroxine (T_4) and triiodothyronine (T_3), is elevated because of estrogen-induced increases in thyroid-binding globulin. Early in pregnancy, plasma free T_4 and free T_3 concentrations transiently increase above nonpregnancy levels, and they may contribute to the early phase of fetal development. The free T_4 and T_3 levels return toward baseline as pregnancy progresses. Nonetheless, the size of the maternal thyroid gland and its iodine uptake increase throughout pregnancy, as does the basal metabolic rate and the resting pulse rate. These increases may all be caused by the thyrotropic activity of HCG (see above) or by secretion of a placental thyrotropin.

Maternal pituitary growth hormone secretion in response to various stimuli decreases during pregnancy, probably because its anabolic functions are carried out by HCS or by a placental growth hormone variant. Maternal LH and FSH secretion is also suppressed by the high levels of estrogen, progesterone, and inhibin, initially from the corpus luteum, and later from the placenta. In general, the usual circadian rhythms in maternal plasma hormone levels persist. Their transmission to the fetus may help prepare it for extrauterine life.

Calcium absorption from the diet increases during pregnancy, and it offsets the continuing maternal calcium drain created by the growing fetal skeleton. This increase in calcium absorption is mediated by increased maternal levels of 25-OH-vitamin D and 1,25-(OH_2)-vitamin D. The latter active metabolite originates in part from decidual and placental production. As a result, ionized calcium levels are maintained at normal levels, and maternal parathyroid hormone (PTH) secretion is partially suppressed, as manifested by a 50% reduction in maternal PTH levels in the plasma.

Maternal-Fetal Metabolism

During normal pregnancy, the average gain in maternal weight is 11 kg. About half of this weight gain is attributable to changes in maternal tissues, and half to the conceptus. The typical distribution of the excess weight is shown in Fig. 46-36. Approximately 250 to 300 extra kcal/day must be

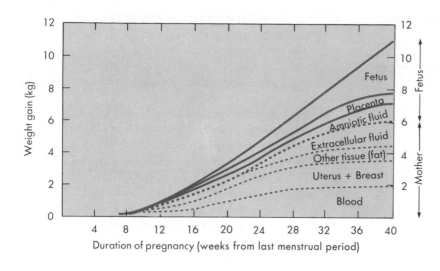

■ **Fig. 46-36** Pattern and components of maternal weight gain during normal pregnancy. (Redrawn from Pitkin RM: In Schneider HA, Anderson CE, Coursin DB, editors: *Nutritional support of medical practice,* New York, 1977, Harper & Row.)

ingested to support this weight gain; 85% ultimately supports fetal metabolism and growth, and 15% is stored in maternal fat. An extra protein intake of 30 g/day ensures adequate supplies for maternal needs and for the accumulation of fetal protoplasm. At birth, the protein content of the fetus has reached 400 to 500 g.

From a metabolic standpoint, pregnancy can be divided into two phases. *During the first half of pregnancy, the mother herself is in an anabolic phase, and the conceptus represents an insignificant nutritional drain. During the second half of pregnancy, and especially the final third, fetal and placental weight increase at an accelerated rate. These demands cause the mother to shift into a metabolic state, which is aptly described as "accelerated starvation."*

The initial anabolic phase is characterized by normal or even increased sensitivity to insulin. Maternal plasma levels of glucose, amino acids, free fatty acids, and glycerol are normal or slightly reduced. Carbohydrate and amino acid loads are readily assimilated. Lipogenesis is increased, and lipolysis is reduced in maternal adipose tissue. Glycogen stores are increased in the liver and muscle, and overall protein synthesis is enhanced. The net effect of these changes is to stimulate growth of the breasts, uterus, and essential musculature in the mother, while preparing her to withstand the metabolic demands of later fetal growth.

During the later catabolic phase of pregnancy, the metabolism of the mother shifts into a mode that effectively accommodates the accelerating needs of the fetus. Insulin sensitivity is replaced by maternal insulin resistance. The assimilation of dietary carbohydrate, protein, and fat by maternal tissues is slowed, which results in elevated postprandial plasma levels of glucose and amino acids. These increases in glucose and amino acids in turn increase the rates of glucose diffusion and of facilitated amino acid transport across the placenta into the fetus. Glucose is the major fuel used by the fetus, and the amino acids are required for fetal protein synthesis. By term, the fetus, is using glucose at a rate of 5 mg/kg/min, compared with the maternal rate of 2.5 mg/kg/min. Hence, the fetus must be supplied with up to 25 g/day of glucose. During fasting intervals, maternal plasma glucose falls more rapidly than in nonpregnant women (see Fig. 40-11), as the fetus continues to siphon this vital energy substrate. Moreover, lipolysis is accelerated in the second half of pregnancy, and maternal plasma free fatty acid, glycerol, and ketoacid levels rise more rapidly than in fasting nonpregnant women (see Fig. 40-11). These changes ensure alternative oxidative fuels for the mother. In addition, ketoacids and, to a lesser extent, free fatty acids are supplied to the fetus, where they may be used instead of some glucose as fuel.

Placental HCS and growth hormone variant are probably the key hormones responsible for insulin resistance and for facilitating lipid mobilization during fasting in the later stage of pregnancy. The rise in the plasma free cortisol level and the large increases in plasma estrogen and progesterone levels may also contribute to these actions.

Along with the other changes in maternal metabolism, plasma cholesterol and triglyceride levels rise throughout pregnancy. The cholesterol is partly used for estrogen and progesterone synthesis. The increased circulating triglycerides are largely the result of an increased hepatic synthesis of VLDL; this synthesis is stimulated by estrogens. Some of the triglycerides are stored in the breasts in preparation for milk production. The triglycerides are shifted away from less specific storage elsewhere by a marked reduction in the levels of adipose tissue lipoprotein lipase.

Parturition

Just as the maintenance of the pregnant state depends on a unique hormonal milieu, its termination probably also depends on specific hormonal changes. However, the exact mechanism by which parturition, or the process of giving birth, is initiated remains unclear. Progesterone, estrogen, cortisol, relaxin, oxytocin, CRH, prostaglandins, and catecholamines all influence the initiation and maintenance of labor and the final uterine evacuation. The most dominant endocrine factor is a decrease in the progesterone effect and an increase in the estrogen effect, commonly on the same targets (Table 46-4). Because species variations exist, it is difficult to extrapolate the results of animal studies directly

■ **Table 46-4** Opposing effects of progesterone and estrogen on factors involved in parturition

	Progesterone	Estrogen
Myometrial quiescence	+	–
Myometrial activation	–	+
Myometrial gap junctions	–	+
Prostaglandins $F_{2\alpha}$ and E production	–	+
Local oxytocin production	NA	+
Oxytocin receptors	–	+
Cervical rigidity	+	–
Matrix metaloproteinase	–	NA
Cervical ripening	–	+

+, Stimulates; –, inhibits; NA, not available.

to humans, even if the studies have been performed in sub-human primates. Figure 46-37 illustrates current concepts of the endocrine regulation of parturition.

Once the conceptus has reached a critical size, distention of the uterus itself and stretching of the muscle fibers increase their contractility. Thus, the inherent contractility of the uterus in itself would probably cause eventual evacuation of the conceptus. Throughout pregnancy, the uterine myometrium exhibits long episodes of low-amplitude contractions, referred to as **contractures.** These are perceived by the mother, beginning at least 1 month before the end of gestation, and they are called **Braxton Hicks** contractions. They are uncoordinated and ineffective. Progesterone helps to maintain this myometrial state of functional quiescence.

The onset of true labor has a circadian rhythm, with a peak between midnight and 5 AM, during which period the sensitivity of the myometrium to stimulation by prostaglandins and oxytocin is heightened and the secretion of maternal oxytocin peaks. Some signal from the fetus probably initiates labor contractions. In sheep, fetal cortisol has been strongly implicated as the signal. Although gestation is prolonged in women when the fetus lacks an intact hypothalamic-pituitary-adrenal unit, the evidence for a surge of fetal cortisol secretion immediately preceding human parturition is weak. However, a late gestational increase in fetal cortisol secretion is important in preparing the fetus for the abrupt transition to extrauterine life (Fig. 46-37). Cortisol stimulates lung maturation, increases stores of liver glycogen, induces intestinal transport systems and important digestive enzymes, such as disaccheridase, and promotes closure of the ductus arteriosus.

Another recent suggestion is that the placenta acts as a clock with an alarm that is set early in gestation. The level of maternal plasma CRH, which comes from the placenta, begins to rise exponentially early in the second trimester, and it reaches a peak during labor. Furthermore, the high maternal levels of a CRH-binding protein fall sharply in the last month of gestation; thus, maternal plasma free CRH levels are very high at the end of gestation. An inverse correlation exists between maternal plasma CRH levels early in gestation and the absolute length of the gestational period. Higher plasma

CRH levels predict a shorter gestation. These observations suggest that the amount of placental CRH production early in pregnancy is at least an indicator of when parturition might begin. Conceivably, CRH also may be a determinant of the time of onset of labor, and it may play an active role in the process.

CRH receptors are present in the uterine muscle, and CRH potentiates the contractile response to prostaglandins and oxytocin. CRH and prostaglandins in the placenta stimulate each other's production. CRH produced by the placenta stimulates the fetal pituitary to secrete ACTH, which in turn increases fetal cortisol and DHEA production. The extra DHEA substrate fuels placental estradiol production (Fig. 46-35), which is also increased by cortisol stimulation. In an unusual positive-feedback effect, the fetal cortisol also amplifies (rather than inhibits, as expected) placental CRH synthesis (see Chapter 43). This phenomenon generates a powerful momentum to increase both factors exponentially.

Even if the precise initiating signal in human parturition is unidentified, current concepts favor a multicomponent process that involves paracrine and endocrine mechanisms. During pregnancy, the opening to the uterus is kept closed by a rigid cervix that prevents expulsion and protects the fetus from an ascending infection. Progesterone maintains rigidity by inhibiting the enzyme matrix metalloproteinase (MMP), which would otherwise lyse the collagen and loosen the tissue. Ripening (softening) of the cervix during labor is produced by estradiol; in addition, relaxin from the placenta opposes the inhibitory effect of progesterone on MMP, and thereby accelerates the dissolution of the cervical matrix. Cervical softening allows the fetus to exit under myometrial propulsion.

The increase in the local concentration of prostaglandins increases myometrial cell Ca^{2+} levels, and it triggers uterine contractions. A drop in the ratio of intrauterine progesterone levels to estrogen levels appears to be largely responsible for augmenting local prostaglandin levels and thereby abolishing uterine quiescence. At term, the increased activity of the enzyme 17β,20α-hydroxysteroid dehydrogenase in the uterine tissue lowers the progesterone/estrogen ratio. This single enzyme reduces the ketone group at position 20 of the steroid nucleus, thereby inactivating progesterone, and generates estradiol from estrone by reducing the ketone at position 17, thereby augmenting the estrogen effect. The fetal amnion and chorion also contribute prostaglandins.

Another major stimulator of myometrial contractions is **oxytocin.** Although the concentration of oxytocin in maternal plasma does not increase consistently just before labor, the frequency of oxytocin pulses does increase. Furthermore, myometrial oxytocin receptor content rises dramatically at term, as does the local synthesis of oxytocin by the decidua and the fetal membranes. Oxytocin may therefore reinforce labor contractions, and it probably maximizes the contractions immediately after delivery, and thereby minimizes maternal blood loss.

Uterine contractions may also be modulated by catecholamines; α-adrenergy is stimulatory and β-adrenergy is

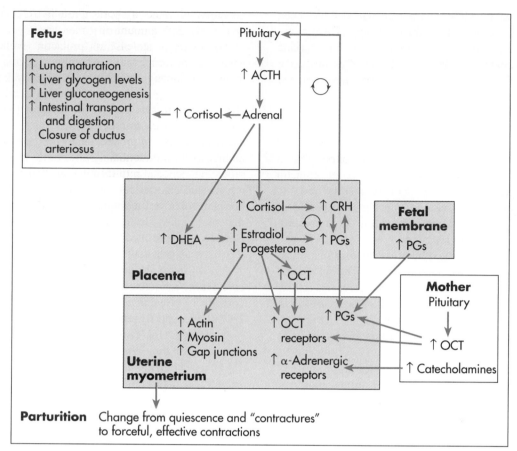

Fetus
- ↑ Lung maturation
- ↑ Liver glycogen levels
- ↑ Liver gluconeogenesis
- ↑ Intestinal transport and digestion
- Closure of ductus arteriosus

Pituitary

↑ ACTH

← ↑ Cortisol ← Adrenal

Placenta

↑ Cortisol → ↑ CRH

↑ DHEA → ↑ Estradiol ↓ Progesterone → ↑ PGs

↑ OCT

Fetal membrane
↑ PGs

Uterine myometrium
- ↑ Actin
- ↑ Myosin
- ↑ Gap junctions

↑ OCT receptors

↑ α-Adrenergic receptors

↑ PGs

Mother
Pituitary

↑ OCT

↑ Catecholamines

Parturition   Change from quiescence and "contractures" to forceful, effective contractions

■ **Fig. 46-37**   Endocrine regulation of parturition. The fetus initiates signals that decrease the ratio of effective progesterone to estrogen in the myometrium. This increases prostaglandin production, which abolishes uterine quiescence and stimulates uterine contractions. Oxytocin produced in the decidua and placenta and a small maternal contribution—combined with markedly increased oxytocin receptors as a result of the higher estrogen/progesterone ratio—may contribute to labor but are not essential. However, oxytocin sustains uterine contractions after expulsion of the fetus in order to minimize maternal loss of blood. Cortisol from the fetal adrenal, stimulated by placental CRH and fetal ACTH, prepares the fetus to adapt to extrauterine life successfully. Placental CRH is greatly augmented by mutual positive feedback effects with cortisol and prostaglandins. CRH is also a myometrial stimulant. In addition, a critical level of CRH may act as a placental alarm that triggers the process.

inhibitory. Both estradiol and prostaglandins increase α-adrenergic receptors. Maternal stress may release more circulating catecholamines, which participate in the final hormonal cascade of parturition.

In addition to uterine contractions, changes that occur in cervical and placental tissue are also important components of labor. Late in pregnancy, increases in the secretion of estradiol by the placenta prepare the myometrium to contract in a forceful and coordinated manner. This goal is accomplished by increasing the concentrations of contractile proteins, myosin and actin, as well as the gap junctions between fibers. These changes are necessary to have coordinated contractions. Oxytocin receptors and prostaglandins are also increased by estradiol. At term, the concentration of inflammatory cytokines, such as interleukin-8, also rises sharply in amniotic fluid. These cytokines are produced by maternal decidua and fetal membranes, probably under hor-

monal paracrine stimulation. The cytokines attract neutrophils, which then release collagenase, which loosens the attachments between the maternal and fetal tissue planes and decreases the cervical resistance to pressure from the fetal head.

Once labor has begun, it proceeds in three clinically recognized stages. In the first stage, which lasts several hours, the uterine contractions, which originate at the fundus and sweep downward, force the head of the fetus against the cervix. Under this pressure, the cervix progressively widens and thins the opening to the vaginal canal. In the second stage, which lasts less than 1 hour, the fetus is forced out of the uterine cavity and through the cervix, and it is delivered from the vagina. In the third stage, which lasts 10 minutes or less, the placenta is separated from the decidual tissue of the uterus, and it is forcefully evacuated. Myometrial contractions during this stage act to constrict the uterine vessels and prevent excessive bleeding. Once the placenta has been removed, all its hormonal products disappear from the maternal plasma, at a rate determined by their characteristic half-lives. In general, by 48 to 72 hours after birth, the steroid and protein hormone concentrations have reached nonpregnancy levels.

LACTATION

Lactation is initiated after delivery by the precipitous drop in estrogen and progesterone levels. Although basal prolactin concentrations gradually decline to normal over the next 4 to 8 weeks, they are acutely elevated during each period of suckling (see Fig. 43-27). This repeated transient hyperprolactinemia helps to sustain milk secretion.

Lactation, which is mediated by prolactin, also suppresses reproductive function in the nursing mother. During the first 7 to 10 days postpartum, plasma FSH and LH levels remain low. FSH then rises to above-normal follicular-phase levels, but LH remains low. The responsiveness of the ovaries to FSH is probably reduced by prolactin, and LH secretion by the pituitary gland is probably inhibited by prolactin. A decrease in the circulating prolactin level, because of cessation of nursing (or by therapeutic administration of a

dopaminergic agonist), plays a role in triggering LH release and in reinitiating the normal menstrual cycle.

The maintenance of high prolactin levels during pregnancy and lactation is facilicated by a decreased sensitivity of the dopaminergic neurons that tonically inhibit prolactin secretion (see Fig. 43-28). In addition to its critical lactogenic effect, prolactin acts through its receptor (increased during pregnancy) in various areas of the brain to stimulate maternal behavior that is beneficial to the neonate. Bonding of mother to child immediately after birth, later sheltering and protective actions, and stimulation of maternal appetite to replace the calories and nutrients donated to the child in breast feeding are all enhanced by prolactin. In contrast, maternal anxiety levels and response to stress are diminished by prolactin.

Maternal provision of nutrients to the newborn begins within 48 hours of delivery. First, a thin fluid, known as **colostrum,** is secreted in very small quantities. This fluid contains lactose and proteins, but little fat. True milk delivery follows shortly afterward (Fig. 46-38). Human breast milk contains 1% protein, largely as casein, lactalbumin, and lactoglobulin. In addition, milk contains 7% lactose and 3.5% fat, which together are equivalent to a concentration of about 70 kcal/100 ml. By 1 week, an average of 550 ml/day

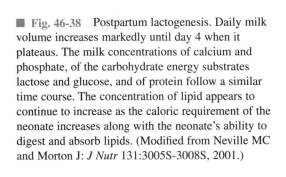

■ Fig. 46-38 Postpartum lactogenesis. Daily milk volume increases markedly until day 4 when it plateaus. The milk concentrations of calcium and phosphate, of the carbohydrate energy substrates lactose and glucose, and of protein follow a similar time course. The concentration of lipid appears to continue to increase as the caloric requirement of the neonate increases along with the neonate's ability to digest and absorb lipids. (Modified from Neville MC and Morton J: *J Nutr* 131:3005S-3008S, 2001.)

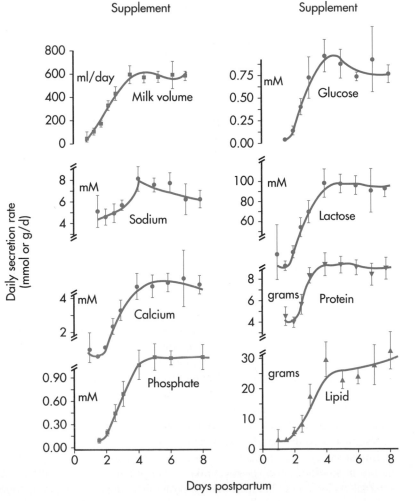

is produced; later, maximal rates of up to 2000 ml/day may be delivered by some mothers. Large quantities of calcium and phosphorus, which are needed by the infant for skeletal growth, are present in milk. During the first 2 to 3 days, high concentrations of lactoferrin are present, as well as immunoglobulin A and oligosaccharides, which help protect the infant from infection. The changes in sodium concentration (Fig. 46-30) reflect closure of tight junctions between ductal cells. This response prevents the paracellular leakage of extracellular fluid and electrolytes into the milk ducts.

Typically, infants nurse for 6 to 12 months. The milk they receive contains a large complement of endocrine-related molecules, which include all pituitary hormones, plus their hypothalamic-releasing and -inhibiting hormones; insulin-like growth factors plus their binding proteins; vitamin D and thyroid and steroid hormones; PTH and PTH-related protein; and prostaglandins. The concentrations of many of these molecules are higher than those in plasma. This disparity indicates local synthesis of these substances in mammary cells, or active transport into the milk. Cortisol, insulin, and, of course, prolactin are essential for maintenance of normal milk production. The functions of other hormones may include (1) supportive effects on breast tissues and milk secretion, (2) assistance in the development and induction of function of the immature gastrointestinal tract of the infant, (3) assistance in development of the immature infant immune system, and (4) endocrine and metabolic effects in the neonate from those substances absorbed by the immature intestinal mucosa. Milk also continues to contain maternal immunoglobulins for several months. These protect the infant against infection while its own immune system matures.

Mammary cells package proteins, lactose, calcium, and phosphate in secretory vesicles and fat in droplets. Prolactin is essential to these processes (Chapter 43). Immunoglobulins are combined with membrane receptors in vesicles when they enter the mammary cells. All of these products are then secreted into the alveoli of the breast ducts. Suckling, and such anticipatory signals as the infant's cry, stimulate oxytocin release via neural sensory pathways and the central **nucleus tractus solitarii** (Fig. 43-36). Oxytocin causes contraction of myoepithelial cells around the alveoli and smooth muscle cells in the duct walls. These contractions "let the milk down" into the areolar area, from which the infant removes it.

Endocrine State of the Fetus

Although fetal pancreatic islets are functional by 14 weeks, insulin and glucagon secretion is relatively low. Neither is critically needed for substrate metabolism, because glucose and amino acids are in plentiful supply from the mother. Fetal pancreatic β cells and α cells respond to their usual stimulators and suppressors in a blunted fashion until birth, when responsiveness rapidly increases. Fetal insulin also contributes to anabolism and to the deposition of adipose tissue.

Fetal **hyperinsulinemia** in the third trimester leads to overweight babies with increases in adipose tissue and lean body mass. This condition occurs in the 4% of pregnancies that are complicated by **gestational diabetes mellitus.** High plasma glucose levels, caused by excessive maternal insulin resistance, are transmitted to the fetus, where they stimulate excessive release of insulin and its anabolic actions. These babies are harder to deliver and may suffer from hypoglycemia shortly after birth.

Fetal growth hormone is not essential for linear growth; although growth hormone levels are high in plasma, growth hormone receptors are deficient in the fetus. Instead, HCS, placental growth hormone variant, and prolactin may subserve the function of growth hormone prenatally. These hormones may be responsible for the ubiquitous presence of IGF-1 and IGF-2 in fetal plasma and tissues. IGF-2 concentration is especially high, and this growth factor may mediate the most important paracrine and autocrine growth effects in fetal life, whereas IGF-1 assumes this role after birth.

Prolactin concentrations are high in fetal plasma and in amniotic fluid. Prolactin may contribute to fetal growth, osmotic regulation, and the production of cortisol and DHEA-S.

The role of fetal thyroid hormone during gestation is not completely defined. A small transfer of maternal T_4 or T_3 to the fetus may be essential for early fetal development. During the last two thirds of gestation, neither maternal nor fetal thyroid hormone may be needed for some developmental processes. At birth, the newborn's own thyroid hormone becomes critical to further central nervous system maturation and somatic growth.

Active transport of calcium across the placenta from mother to fetus is probably stimulated by PTH_{rp} from the fetal parathyroid glands and from the placenta (see Chapter 42); PTH_{rp} keeps fetal plasma calcium levels high. In turn, this slight hypercalcemia inhibits fetal PTH secretion, and it stimulates fetal calcitonin secretion. Calcitonin, combined with $1,25\text{-}(OH)_2$-vitamin D, which is produced in the fetal kidney and in the placenta, promotes fetal bone formation. PTH secretion increases soon after birth, and it assumes its regulatory role in calcium metabolism.

Fetal ACTH is probably not essential for the first 12 to 20 weeks, although later it definitely stimulates production of steroids by the fetal zone of the adrenal cortex. The newborn mounts an immediate stress response, as shown by high levels of cortisol in umbilical cord plasma. If endogenous ACTH and cortisol cannot be secreted at this time, death will ensue unless replacement therapy is provided.

SUMMARY

1. Differences in gonadal function between the genders are derived from the process of sexual differentiation. Genetic material on the Y chromosome determines the development of a testis. Testicular anti-Müllerian hormone suppresses the development of female genital ducts, whereas testosterone and dihydrotestosterone induce masculinization of the genital

ducts and external genitalia. Without this positive input, a female (the neutral) pattern results. Two active X chromosomes are required for oogenesis.

2. Testosterone and estradiol, which is a product of testosterone, are synthesized by common pathways and enzymes in homologous cell lines in the testis and ovary. Both genders exhibit gonadotropin surges in fetal life, quiescence in childhood, activation in puberty, and increases in gonadotropins late in life because of negative feedback resulting from gonadal failure. The monthly cyclic ovulatory burst of LH/FSH is unique to the female.

3. Spermatogenesis proceeds within the seminiferous tubules in a locally conditioned hormonal environment, behind a blood-testis barrier. Sertoli cells, stimulated by FSH, provide growth factors, binding (carrier) proteins for testosterone and for trace metals, inhibin, and other factors to nurture and launch spermatozoa. Sertoli cells also respond to signals from the germ cells.

4. LH stimulates testosterone secretion by Leydig cells. A high local concentration of testosterone is essential to spermatogenesis. This hormone acts indirectly, by affecting Sertoli cells, and possibly by direct access to germ cells.

5. In the ovary, oocytes stimulate formation of a follicle, which is a secluded environment analogous to the seminiferous tubules. Under the influence of FSH, a cohort of immature follicles, with their oocytes suspended in meiosis, begins to develop each month. The surrounding granulosa cells secrete estradiol, which is synthesized from androgen precursors. The precursors are provided by neighboring theca cells under LH stimulation.

6. A single dominant follicle emerges each month. It grows exponentially and secretes sufficient estradiol and inhibin to (1) inhibit cohort follicles, (2) prepare the uterus and fallopian tubes for fertilization, and (3) condition the GnRH-gonadotroph axis to provide an ovulatory LH/FSH surge at the appropriate time.

7. After ovulation takes place, the endocrine cells form a corpus luteum, which secretes progesterone predominantly. The latter acts on the uterus to favor implantation of a zygote.

8. In children during puberty, testosterone in the male and estradiol in the female stimulate linear growth and skeletal maturation as well as enlargement and maturation of the accessory tissues of reproduction.

9. Male and female sexual functioning is stimulated by the autonomic nervous system. An ejaculate of 200 to 400 million sperm requires conditioning (capacitation) in the female genital tract to permit one sperm to fertilize the ovum in the fallopian tube. The zygote is subsequently maintained and protected by secretions from altered uterine cells (decidua) and from placental fetal trophoblastic cells.

10. Implantation of the embryo within the uterus wall requires adhesion, penetration, and invasion. This is also an endocrine and paracrine-regulated process, incorporating signals to and from the endometrium and the embryo.

11. The placenta initially produces human chorionic gonadotropin, which stimulates the corpus luteum; later, the placenta produces its own estrogen and progesterone. In addition, various placental peptides and proteins are synthesized, including human chorionic somatomammotropin, insulin-like growth factors, inhibin, and molecules homologous with those secreted by the hypothalamus and pituitary gland. These hormones affect maternal and possibly fetal metabolism.

12. The mother is in an anabolic state early in pregnancy. This anabolic state facilitates growth of her energy stores and reproductive tissues. The later catabolic phase is marked by insulin resistance, and it facilitates the flow of fuels to the growing fetus.

13. The exact endocrine mechanism of human parturition is unclear, but it includes contributions from an increased estrogen/progesterone ratio within the uterus, from prostaglandins, from oxytocin, and from CRH. A local increase in prostaglandins is the immediate second messenger that causes uterine contractions. A late gestational rise in the fetal cortisol level enhances extrauterine survival.

BIBLIOGRAPHY

Journal articles

Achermann JC et al: Gonadal determination and adrenal development are regulated by the orphan nuclear receptor steroidogenic factor-1, in a dose-dependent manner, *J Clin Endocrinol Metab* 87:1829, 2002.

Adashi EY: The climacteric ovary as a functional gonadotropin-driven androgen-producing gland, *Fertil Steril* 62:20, 1994.

Andersson K-E, Wagner G: Physiology of penile erection, *Physiol Rev* 75:191, 1995.

Blanchard R: Fraternal birth order and the maternal immune hypothesis of male homosexuality, *Horm Behav* 40:105, 2001.

Brann DW et al: Leptin and reproduction, *Steroids* 67:95, 2002.

Bryant-Greenwood GD, Schwabe C: Human relaxins: chemistry and biology, *Endocr Rev* 15:5, 1994.

Brzezinski A: Mechanisms of disease: melatonin in humans, *N Engl J Med* 336:186, 1997.

Burger HG et al: The endocrinology of the menopausal transition: a cross-sectional study of a population-based sample, *J Clin Endocrinol Metab* 80:3537, 1995.

Canning CA, Lovell-Badge R: Sry and sex determination: how lazy can it be? *Trends Genet* 18:111, 2002.

Dean J: Oocyte-specific genes regulate follicle formation, fertility and early mouse development, *J Reprod Immun* 53:171, 2002.

Delemarre-van de Waal HA: Regulation of puberty, *Clin Endocrinol Metab* 16:1, 2002.

Eddy EM: Male germ cell gene expression, *Recent Prog Horm Res* 57:103, 2002.

Fraser LR, Adeoya-Osiguwa SA: Fertilization promoting peptide: a possible regulator of sperm function *in vivo, Vitam Horm* 63:2, 2001.

Grattan DR et al: Prolactin receptors in the brain during pregnancy and lactation: implications for behavior, *Horm Behav* 40:115, 2001.

Groome NP et al: Measurement of dimeric inhibin B throughout the human menstrual cycle, *J Clin Endocrinol Metab* 81:1401, 1996.

Gruber CJ et al: Production and actions of estrogens, *N Engl J Med,* 346:340, 2002.

Habert R et al: Origin, differentiation and regulation of fetal and adult leydig cells, *Mol Cell Endocrinol* 179:47, 2001.

Hawkins JR et al: Mutational analysis of SRY: nonsense and missense mutationsin XY sex reversal, *Hum Genet* 88:471, 1992.

Hayes FJ et al: Differential regulation of gonadotropin secretion by testosterone in the human male: absence of a negative feedback effect of testosterone on follicle-stimulating hormone secretion, *J Clin Endocrinol Metab* 86:53, 2001.

Heckert L, Griswold MD: The expression of the follicle-stimulating hormone receptor in spermatogenesis, *Recent Prog Horm Res* 57:129, 2002.

Hillier SG: Gonadotropic control of ovarian follicular growth and development, *Mol Cell Endocrinol* 179:39, 2001.

Hsueh AJW, Billig H, Tsafriri A: Ovarian follicle atresia: a hormonally controlled apoptotic process, *Endocr Rev* 15:707, 1994.

Hughes IA: Minireview: sex differentiation, *Endocrinology* 142:3281, 2001.

Hull KL, Harvey S: GH as a co-gonadotropin: the relevance of correlative changes in GH secretion and reproductive state, *J Endocrinol* 172:1, 2002.

Illingworth PJ et al: Measurement of circulating inhibin forms during the establishment of pregnancy, *J Clin Endocrinol Metab* 81:1471, 1996.

Jensen TK et al: Inhibin B as a serum marker of spermatogenesis: correlation to differences in sperm concentration and follicle-stimulating hormone levels: a study of 349 Danish men, *J Clin Endocrinol Metab* 82:4059, 1997.

Joseph DR: Structure, function, and regulation of androgen-binding protein/sex hormone-binding globulin, *Vitam Horm* 49:197, 1994.

Josso N et al: Anti-Müllerian hormone and its receptors, *Mol Cell Endocrinol* 179:25, 2001.

Kalra SP: Mandatory neuropeptide-steroid signaling for the preovulatory luteinizing hormone-releasing hormone discharge, *Endocr Rev* 14:507, 1993.

Klein NA et al: Ovarian follicular concentrations of activin, follistatin, inhibin, insulin-like growth factor I (IGF-I), IGF-II, IGF-binding protein-2 (IGFBP-2), IGFBP-3, and vascular endothelial growth factor in spontaneous menstrual cycles of normal women of advanced reproductive age, *J Clin Endocrinol Metab* 85:4520, 2000.

Lessey BA, Arnold JT: Paracrine signaling in the endometrium: integrins and the establishment of uterine receptivity, *J Reprod Immun* 39:105, 1998.

McEwen BS: Genome and hormones: gender differences in physiology invited review: estrogens effects on the brain: multiple sites and molecular mechanisms, *J Appl Physiol* 91:2785, 2001.

McLachlan RI et al: Identification of specific sites of hormonal regulation in spermatogenesis in rats, monkeys, and man, *Recent Prog Horm Res* 57:149, 2002.

McLean M et al: A placental clock controlling the length of human pregnancy, *Nat Med* 1:460, 1995.

Merchant-Larios H, Moreno-Mendoza N: Onset of sex differentiation: dialog between genes and cells, *Arch Med Res* 32:553, 2001.

Neville MC, Morton J: Physiology and endocrine changes underlying human lactogenesis II, *J Nutr* 131:3005S, 2001.

Nilson S et al: Mechanisms of estrogen action, *Physiol Rev* 81:1535, 2001.

Niswender GD et al: Mechanisms controlling the function and life span of the corpus luteum, *Physiol Rev* 80:1, 2000.

Plant TM, Marshall GR: The functional significance of FSH in spermatogenesis and the control of its secretion in male primates, *Endocr Rev* 22:764, 2001.

Reynaud K, Driancourt MA: Oocyte attrition, *Mol Cell Endocrinol* 163:101, 2000.

Riggs BL et al: Sex steroids and the construction and conservation of the adult skeleton, *Endocr Rev* 23:279, 2002.

Roy AK et al: Regulation of androgen action, *Vitam Horm* 55:309, 1999.

Sluijmer AV, Heineman MJ, DeJong FH, Evers JLH: Endocrine activity of the postmenopausal ovary: the effects of pituitary down-regulation and oophorectomy, *J Clin Endocrinol Metab* 80:2163, 1995.

Stern K, McClintock MK: Regulation of ovulation by human pheromones, *Nature* 392:177, 1998.

Stocco DM: StAR protein and the regulation of steroid hormone biosynthesis, *Annu Rev Physiol* 63:193, 2001.

Swaab DF et al: Structural and functional sex differences in the human hypothalamus, *Horm Behav* 40:93, 2001.

Vanderschueren D, Bouillo R: Editorial: Estrogen deficiency in men is a challenge for both the hypothalamus and pituitary, *J Clin Endocrinol Metab* 85:3024, 2000.

Weiss G: Clinical review 118: endocrinology of parturition, *J Clin Endocrinol Metab* 85:4421, 2000.

White MM et al: Estrogen, progesterone, and vascular reactivity: potential cellular mechanisms, *Endocr Rev* 16:739, 1995.

Wilson JD: Androgens, androgen receptors, and male gender role behavior, *Horm Behav* 40:358, 2001.

Wolf U: The serologically detected H-Y antigen revisited, *Cytogenet Cell Genet* 80:232, 1998.

Wolgenmuth DJ et al: Regulation of the mitotic and meiotic cell cycles in the male germ line, *Recent Prog Horm Res* 57:75, 2002.

Wu FCW et al: Ontogeny of pulsatile gonadotropin releasing hormone secretion from midchildhood, through puberty, to adulthood in the human male: a study using deconvolution analysis and an ultrasensitive immunofluorometric assay, *J Clin Endocrinol Metab* 81:1798, 1996.

Books and monographs

Carr BR: The ovary. In Carr BR, Blackwell RE, editors: *Textbook of reproductive medicine,* Norwalk, Conn., 1993, Appleton & Lange.

Carr BR: The normal menstrual cycle: the coordinated events of the hypothalamic-pituitary-ovarian axis and the female reproductive tract. In Carr BR, Blackwell RE, editors: *Textbook of reproductive medicine,* Norwalk, Conn., 1993, Appleton & Lange.

DeKretser DM, Risbridger GP, Kerr JB: Male reproduction: functional morphology. In DeGroot LJ, Jameson LJ, editors: *Endocrinology,* ed 3, Philadelphia, 2001, WB Saunders.

Erickson GF: Folliculogenesis ovulation, and luteogenesis. In DeGroot LJ, Jameson JL, editors: *Endocrinology,* ed 4, Philadelphia, 2001, WB Saunders.

Fisher DA: Endocrinology of fetal development. In Wilson JD et al, editors: *Williams textbook of endocrinology,* Philadelphia, 1998, WB Saunders.

Gooren LJG: Gender identity and sexual behavior. In DeGroot LJ, Jameson JL, editors: *Endocrinology,* ed 4, Philadelphia, 2001, WB Saunders.

Josso N: Anatomy and endocrinology of fetal sex differentiation. In DeGroot LJ, Jameson JL, editors: *Endocrinology,* ed 4, Philadelphia, 2001, WB Saunders.

Junquiera LC, Carneiro J, Kelley RO: The female reproductive system. In *Basic histology,* ed 9, Norwalk, Conn., Appleton and Lange, 1999.

Marshall JC: Hormonal regulation of the menstrual cycle and mechanisms of ovulation. In DeGroot LJ, Jameson JL, editors: *Endocrinology,* ed 4, Philadelphia, 2001, WB Saunders.

Odell WD: Endocrinology of sexual maturation. In DeGroot LJ, Jameson, JL editors: *Endocrinology,* ed 4, Philadelphia, 2001, WB Saunders.

Parker CR Jr: The endocrinology of pregnancy. In Carr BR, Blackwell RE, editors: *Textbook of reproductive medicine,* Norwalk, CT, 1993, Appleton & Lange.

Quigley CA: Genetic basis of sex determination and sexual differentiation. In DeGroot LJ, Jameson JL, editors: *Endocrinology,* ed 4, Philadelphia, 2001, WB Saunders.

Reichlin S: Neuroendocrinology. In Foster D et al, editors: *Williams textbook of endocrinology,* ed 9, Philadelphia, 1998, WB Saunders.

Strauss J III, Coutifaris C: The endometrium and myometrium: regulation and dysfunction. In Yen, SSC, Jaffe RB, editors: *Reproductive endocrinology,* Philadelphia, 1999, WB Saunders.

Turek FW, Van Cauter E: Rhythms in reproduction. In Knobil E, Neil JD, editors: *The physiology of reproduction,* ed 2, New York, 1994, Raven Press.

Veldhuis JD: The hypothalamic-pituitary-testicular axis. In Yen SSC, Jaffe RB, editors: *Reproductive endocrinology,* Philadelphia, 1999, WB Saunders.

Word RA: Parturition. In Carr BR, Blackwell RE, editors: *Textbook of reproductive medicine,* Norwalk, Conn., 1993, Appleton & Lange.

Yamamoto M, Turner TT: Epididymis, sperm maturation, and capacitation. In Lipshultz LI, Howards SS, editors: *Infertility in the male,* St Louis, 1991, Mosby.

Yeh J, Adashi EY: The ovarian life cycle. In Yen SSC, Jaffe RB, editors: *Reproductive endocrinology,* Philadelphia, 1991, WB Saunders.

Yen SSC: The human menstrual cycle: neuroendocrine regulation. In Yen SSC, Jaffe RB, editors: *Reproductive endocrinology,* Philadelphia, 1999, WB Saunders.

Yen SSC: The hypothalamic control of pituitary hormone secretion regulation. In Yen SSC, Jaffe RB, editors: *Reproductive endocrinology,* Philadelphia, 1999, WB Saunders.

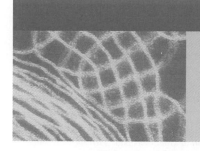

INDEX

A

A band, cardiac muscle electron micrograph of, 306*f*

Abdominal cavity, static lung mechanics and, 464

Abetalipoproteinemia, 618

Absorption, 595-620
  definition of, 539, 595
  filtration and, 376
  intestinal, neural regulation of, 607

Accommodation, action potential and, 39

Accommodation response, autonomic control and, 215

Acetate, hydrolization of acetylcholine to, 46

Acetazolamide, secretion of, by proximal tubule, 650*t*

Acetoacetate, cardiac use of, 421

Acetylcholine
  aldosterone secretion affected by, 906
  automaticity affected by, 290
  autonomic ganglion release of, 211
  calcium conductance and, 280
  as cerebral cortex neurotransmitter, 193
  denervation supersensitivity and, 4
  end plate potential and, 46
  growth hormone secretion affected by, 841
  hydrochloric acid secretion and, 573, 575, 576
  hypothalamus and, 822
  motor neuron release of, 211
  myocardial contractility affected by, 336
  neural control of cardiac function and, 335*f*
  neuromuscular junction as site of release of, 227
  as neurotransmitter, 54
  parasympathetic pathway and, 323
  quantal release of, 46-47
  quantum of, 46
  release of
    gastrointestinal system control and, 547
    salivary gland and, 568, 569
  salivary secretion evoked by, 571*f*
  smooth muscle control and, 253*f*
  smooth muscle regulation and, 258
  in synaptic vesicles, 45
  synthesis of, 46
  vagal nerve release of, 292

Acetylcholine receptor, muscle growth and, 240

Acetylcholine receptor protein, 47-48

Acetylcholinesterase, function of, 45

Achalasia, 551

Achromatopsia, 132

Acid
  dietary production of, 703-704
  excretion of, 705
  renal excretion of, 704-705
  titratable, 704-705

Acid-base balance
  kidney and regulation of, 703-715
  kidney function and, 623
  plasma potassium concentration affected by, 687-688
  potassium excretion affected by, 692

Acid-base disorder, 710-715
  analysis of, 713-715
  mixed, 714
  simple, 712-715
  types of, 712-713

Acidosis
  calcium concentration in plasma and, 794
  calcium homeostasis and, 696
  definition of, 710
  heart function affected by, 338
  hemorrhage and, 440
  hyperchloremic metabolic, 812
  metabolic, 710, 712-713
    plasma potassium concentration affected by, 687-688
    potassium excretion affected by, 692-693, 694*f*
    respiratory acidosis differentiated from, 714
    ventilatory rate affected by, 711
  respiratory, 482, 710, 713

Acinus, lung anatomy and, 447

Acoustic neurinoma, 140

Acromegaly, 840, 844
  G-protein mutation and, 732

Acrosin, fertilization and, 965

Acrosome, formation of, 936

ACTH. *see* Adrenocorticotropic hormone

Actin
  myosin interaction with, 231-232, 380
  smooth muscle content of, 250
  thin, muscle fiber organization and, 224

Action potential
  accommodation and, 39
  axon hillock and, 50
  calcium conductance and, 281*f*
  cardiac, 275
    duration of, 283
    ionic basis of, 275-277
    overshoot of, 279
    phases in, 280*f*
    in slow-response fiber, 286
    tetrodotoxin effect on, 284*f*
  conduction of, 31-43, 39-42
  definition of, 31
  excitability and, 86
  fast response, ionic basis of, 277-283
  in gastrointestinal smooth muscle, 544-545
  generation of, 31-43
  ionic mechanisms of, 34-38
  local response differentiated from, 33
  muscle spindle fibers and, 161
  nerve cell communication and, 26
  neuromuscular transmission and, 45
  neuron, 81
  properties of, 38-39

Action potential—cont'd
  as self-reinforcing signal, 40-41
  sinoatrial node and, 287
  of skeletal muscle, 227, 229*f*
  in smooth muscle, 249, 252
  subthreshold response and, 32-33
  threshold strength and, 33

Active transport
  description of, 644
  secondary, 644

Active zone, synaptic vesicle cycle and, 59

Activin
  intragonadal action of, 926
  luteinizing hormone secretion affected by, 839
  secretion of, during pregnancy, 970
  sexual differentiation and, 924
  testosterone influence on, 940

Acupuncture, pain inhibited with, 112

Adaptation
  rates of, 88
  sensory receptor and, 87-88

Addison's disease, 338, 686, 700, 834, 908

Adefovir, secretion of, by proximal tubule, 650*t*

Adenohypophysis
  description of, 820, 822
  tropic hormones from, 823

Adenoma, thyroid, 867

Adenosine
  blood flow regulation and, 385
  cerebral blood flow affected by, 426
  exercise effect on level of, 434
  mesenteric vascular bed vasodilation by, 427
  reactive hyperemia and, 417
  renal blood flow affected by, 637, 640
  smooth muscle control and, 253*f*
  water secretion stimulated by, 607

Adenosine diphosphate
  platelet aggregation and, 271
  skeletal muscle and, 238
  smooth muscle regulation and, 253-254

Adenosine monophosphate, cyclic. *see* Cyclic adenosine monophosphate

Adenosine triphosphatase
  cellular membrane protein asymmetry and, 5
  f-type, 16
  ion pumping and, 27-28
  ion-transporting, 15, 16
  p-type, 16
  skeletal muscle contraction speed and, 234
  v-type, 16

Adenosine triphosphate
  energy for intense exercise from, 758
  energy generation and, 744
  generation of, 498
  mediated transport and, 15
  muscle energy from, 223
  neural control of cardiac function and, 335*f*
  as neuromodulator, 57
  release of, 910-911
  skeletal muscle and, 237-238
  smooth muscle contraction and, 257